Cancer Surgery

JAMES C. HARVEY, M.D.
Chief, Division of Thoracic Surgery
The Brooklyn Hospital Center
Brooklyn, New York

EDWARD J. BEATTIE, M.D.
Director, Beth Israel Medical Center Cancer Center
New York, New York
Professor of Surgery
Albert Einstein College of Medicine
Bronx, New York

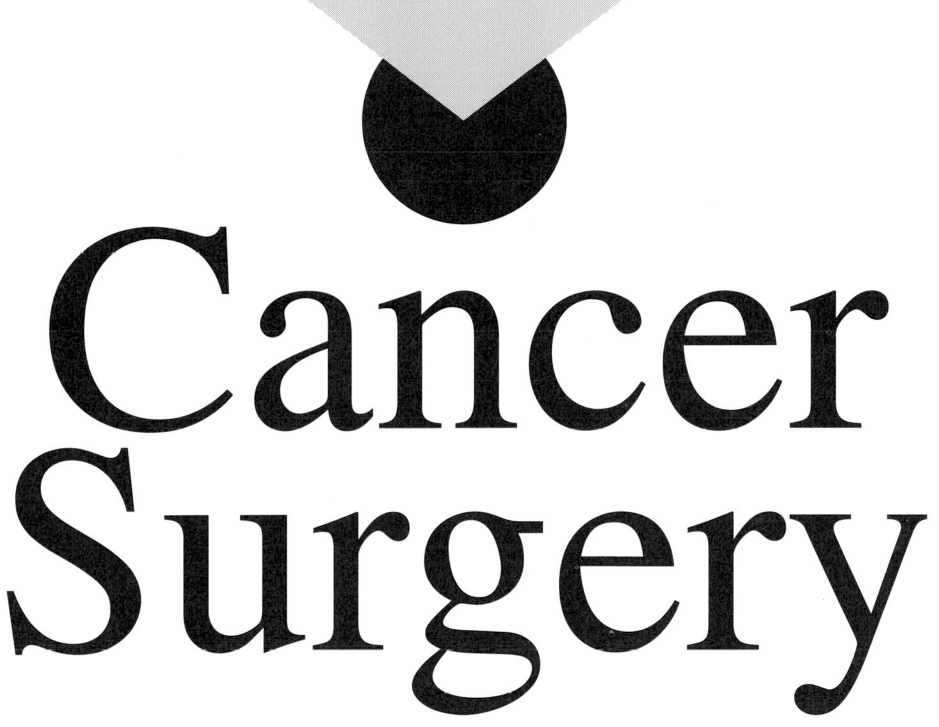

Cancer Surgery

W.B. SAUNDERS COMPANY
A Division of Harcourt Brace & Company
Philadelphia London Toronto Montreal Sydney Tokyo

W.B. SAUNDERS COMPANY
A Division of
Harcourt Brace & Company

The Curtis Center
Independence Square West
Philadelphia, Pennsylvania 19106

Library of Congress Cataloging-in-Publication Data

Cancer surgery/[edited by] James C. Harvey, Edward J. Beattie.—
1st ed.

p. cm.

ISBN 0–7216–5173–9

1. Cancer—Surgery. I. Harvey, James C. II. Beattie, Edward J.,

RD651.C373 1996

616.99′4059–dc20 95–4090

CANCER SURGERY ISBN 0–7216–5173–9

Printed in the United States of America

Last digit is the print number: 9 8 7 6 5 4 3 2 1

To Nicole Beattie, whose patience with us and generosity with her word processing skills helped us immeasurably.

Contributors

EDWARD J. BEATTIE, M.D.

Director, Beth Israel Medical Center Cancer Center, New York, New York; Professor of Surgery, Albert Einstein College of Medicine, Bronx, New York

Tumors of the Esophagus and Gastric Cardia; Lung Cancer: Primary Lung Tumors; Secondary Lung Tumors; Tumors of the Chest Wall and Malignancies of the Pleura: Chest Wall Tumors; Diffuse Malignant Pleural Mesothelioma; Malignant Pleural Effusions

JOHN P. BLANDY, D.M.

Professor of Urology Emeritus, Royal London Hospital, University of London, London, England

Genitourinary Cancer

NORMAN D. BLOOM, M.D.

Clinical Professor of Surgery, New York Medical College, New York, New York; Lecturer in Surgery, Mt. Sinai School of Medicine, New York Medical College, Valhalla, New York, and Mt. Sinai School of Medicine, New York, New York; Chief, Surgical Oncology, Cabrini Medical Center, New York, New York

Tumors of the Chest Wall and Malignancies of the Pleura: Chest Wall Tumors; Soft Tissue Sarcomas: Soft Tissue Sarcomas of the Retroperitoneum; Radical Amputations of the Shoulder and Pelvis and Their Alternatives

MICHAEL A. BREDA, M.D.

Clinical Instructor, Oregon Health Sciences University, Portland, Oregon; Staff Surgeon, Metropolitan Clinic, Portland, Oregon

Hepatobiliary Tumors

RONALD L. BURKES, M.D., F.R.C.P.C.

Associate Professor, University of Toronto Faculty of Medicine, Toronto, Ontario, Canada; Division of Medical Oncology, Mt. Sinai Hospital, Toronto, Ontario, Canada

Tumors of the Mediastinum

MANJEET CHADHA, M.D.

Assistant Professor of Radiation Oncology, Albert Einstein College of Medicine, Bronx, New York; Attending Physician, Radiation Oncologist, Department of Radiation Oncology, Beth Israel Medical Center, New York, New York

Gynecologic Malignancies: Cervical Malignancies

BRUCE J. DAVIDSON, M.D.
Assistant Professor, Department of Otolaryngology–Head and Neck Surgery, Georgetown University Medical Center, Washington, D.C.; Chief of Otolaryngology Section, V.A. Medical Center, Washington, D.C.
Head and Neck Cancer

STEVEN A. DE JONG, M.D.
Associate Professor of Clinical Surgery and Chief, Section of Endocrine Surgery, Loyola University Medical Center, Stritch School of Medicine, Maywood, Illinois; Staff Physician and Surgeon, Hines Veterans Administration Hospital, Hines, Illinois
Cancer of the Pancreas: Neuroendocrine Tumors of the Duodenum and Pancreas

BURTON L. EISENBERG, M.D.
Professor of Surgery, Temple University School of Medicine, Philadelphia, Pennsylvania; Chairman, Surgical Oncology, Fox Chase Cancer Center, Philadelphia, Pennsylvania
Stomach and Small Bowel Cancer: Gastric Cancer; Cancer of the Small Bowel

JOSHUA D. I. ELLENHORN, M.D.
Staff Surgeon, City of Hope National Medical Center, Duarte, California
Head and Neck Cancer

CHRISTOPHER ERDMAN, B.A.
Research Assistant, Department of Surgery, Beth Israel Medical Center, New York, New York
Lung Cancer: Primary Lung Tumors; Secondary Lung Tumors; Tumors of the Chest Wall and Malignancies of the Pleura: Diffuse Malignant Pleural Mesothelioma

RICHARD ESSNER, M.D.
Assistant Director, Surgical Oncology, John Wayne Cancer Institute, Santa Monica, California
Skin Cancers: Melanoma; Basal and Squamous Cancers of the Skin

DANIEL B. FROST, M.D.
Assistant Chief, Division of Surgical Oncology, Department of Surgery, Los Angeles Medical Center, Los Angeles, California; Southern California Permanente Medical Group, Los Angeles, California
Soft Tissue Sarcomas: Soft Tissue Sarcomas of the Extremities

HAROLD FRUCHT, M.D.
Assistant Professor of Medicine, Temple University School of Medicine, Philadelphia, Pennsylvania; Associate Member, Department of Medical Oncology, and Director of Gastroenterology, Fox Chase Cancer Center, Philadelphia, Pennsylvania
Stomach and Small Bowel Cancer: Gastric Cancer

MELVYN GOLDBERG, M.D., F.R.C.S.C.
Professor of Thoracic Surgery, Temple University Medical School, Philadelphia, Pennsylvania; Chief, Thoracic Surgical Oncology, Fox Chase Cancer Center, Philadelphia, Pennsylvania
Tumors of the Mediastinum

MICHAEL GROSS, M.D., F.R.C.S. (C & LOND)
Associate Professor, Department of Surgery, Dalhousie University, Halifax, Nova Scotia, Canada; Staff Surgeon and Trauma Team Surgeon, Division of Orthopaedics, Victoria General Hospital, Halifax, Nova Scotia, Canada
Skeletal Tumors of the Extremities

ALEXANDRE HAGEBOUTROS, M.D.
Fellow, Department of Medical Oncology, Fox Chase Cancer Center, Philadelphia, Pennsylvania
Stomach and Small Bowel Cancer: Gastric Cancer

JAMES C. HARVEY, M.D.
Chief, Division of Thoracic Surgery, The Brooklyn Hospital Center, Brooklyn, New York
Tumors of the Esophagus and Gastric Cardia; Lung Cancer: Primary Lung Tumors; Secondary Lung Tumors; Tumors of the Chest Wall and Malignancies of the Pleura: Chest Wall Tumors; Diffuse Malignant Pleural Mesothelioma; Malignant Pleural Effusions

ALLEN L. HOFFMAN, M.D.
Assistant Director of Liver Transplantation, Cedars–Sinai Medical Center, Los Angeles, California
Hepatobiliary Tumors

JOHN P. HOFFMAN, M.D.
Professor of Surgery, Temple University School of Medicine, Philadelphia, Pennsylvania; Attending Surgeon, Fox Chase Cancer Center, Philadelphia, Pennsylvania
Cancer of the Pancreas; Carcinoma of the Exocrine Pancreas

LAURA HOUGH, R.N.
Nurse Coordinator, Neurosurgery, Department of Neurosurgery, Mt. Sinai School of Medicine, New York, New York
Tumors of the Spine

JAMES E. O. HUGHES, M.D.
Assistant Clinical Professor, Columbia University, New York, New York; Attending Staff, St. Luke's–Roosevelt Hospital Center, New York, New York
Tumors of the Spine

ALLAN J. JACOBS, M.D.
Professor of Obstetrics and Gynecology, Albert Einstein College of Medicine, Bronx, New York; Chairman, Department of Obstetrics and Gynecology, Beth Israel Medical Center, New York, New York
Gynecologic Malignancies: Introduction and Anatomy; Cervical Malignancies; Uterine Cancers; Cancers of the Ovary and Fallopian Tube; Gestational Trophoblastic Neoplasm; Vulvar and Vaginal Malignancies

T. SCOTT JENNINGS, M.D.
Assistant Professor of Obstetrics and Gynecology, Medical University of South Carolina, Charleston, South Carolina; Director, Division of Gynecologic Oncology, Department of Obstetrics and Gynecology, Medical University of South Carolina, Charleston, South Carolina
Gynecologic Malignancies: Cancers of the Ovary and Fallopian Tube

A. ROBERT KAGAN, M.D.
Clinical Professor of Radiation Therapy, UCLA Medical School, Los Angeles, California; Chief, Radiation Oncology, Southern California Permanente Medical Group, Los Angeles, California
Soft Tissue Sarcomas: Soft Tissue Sarcomas of the Extremities

KUSHAGRA KATARIYA, M.D.
Chief Resident, Surgery, Beth Israel Medical Center, New York, New York
Tumors of the Chest Wall and Malignancies of the Pleura: Chest Wall Tumors; Malignant Pleural Effusions

GEORGE KROL, M.D.
Professor, Clinical Radiology, Cornell University Medical School, New York, New York; Chief, Neuroradiology Service and Attending Radiologist, Memorial Sloan-Kettering Cancer Center, New York, New York
Tumors of the Spine; Tumors of the Sacrum

RACHELLE M. LANCIANO, M.D.
Assistant Professor of Radiation Oncology, Medical College of Pennsylvania, Philadelphia, Pennsylvania; Staff Radiation Oncologist, Department of Radiation Oncology, Fox Chase Cancer Center, Philadelphia, Pennsylvania
Stomach and Small Bowel Cancer: Gastric Cancer

KENNETH LEE, M.D.
Chief Resident, Surgery, Beth Israel Medical Center, New York, New York
Lung Cancer: Secondary Lung Tumors

CATHERINE MAHUT, M.D.
General Surgeon, Active Staff, York County Hospital, Newmarket, Ontario, Canada
Cancer of the Colon, Rectum, and Anus: Colorectal Cancer; Cancer of the Anal Canal

LEONARD MAKOWKA, M.D., Ph.D.
Chairman, Department of Surgery, Cedars–Sinai Medical Center, Los Angeles, California
Hepatobiliary Tumors

JOHN E. MEILAHN, M.D.
Assistant Professor of Surgery, Temple University School of Medicine, Philadelphia, Pennsylvania; Attending Surgeon, Temple University Hospital, Philadelphia, Pennsylvania
Cancer of the Pancreas: Periampullary Carcinoma

LESLIE MEMSIC, M.D.
Assistant Director of Surgery, Cedars–Sinai Medical Center, Los Angeles, California
Hepatobiliary Tumors

DONALD L. MORTON, M.D.
Emeritus Professor and Chief of Surgical Oncology, UCLA School of Medicine, Los Angeles, California; Medical Director, Surgeon-in-Chief, John Wayne Cancer Institute, Saint John's Hospital and Health Center, Santa Monica, California
Skin Cancers: Melanoma; Basal and Squamous Cancers of the Skin

R. T. D. OLIVER, M.D.
Sir Maxwell Joseph Professor of Medical Oncology, The Medical College of St. Bartholomew's Hospital and the Royal London Hospital, London, England; Medical Oncology, St. Bartholomew's Hospital, London, England
Genitourinary Cancer

LIDIJA PETROVIC, M.D.
Associate Pathologist, Cedars–Sinai Medical Center, Los Angeles, California
Hepatobiliary Tumors

EDWARD PINA, M.D.
Attending Surgeon, San Jacinito Methodist Hospital, Baytown, Texas
Tumors of the Chest Wall and Malignancies of the Pleura: Malignant Pleural Effusions

JULIANNA PISCH, M.D.
Assistant Professor, Albert Einstein College of Medicine, Bronx, New York; Attending Staff, Radiation Oncology, Beth Israel Medical Center, New York, New York
Tumors of the Esophagus and Gastric Cardia; Lung Cancer: Primary Lung Tumors; Tumors of the Chest Wall and Malignancies of the Pleura: Chest Wall Tumors; Diffuse Malignant Pleural Mesothelioma; Breast Cancer

LUIS G. PODESTA, M.D.
Associate Director, Liver Transplantation Program, Cedars–Sinai Medical Center, Los Angeles, California
Hepatobiliary Tumors

RICHARD A. PRINZ, M.D.
Professor and Chairman, Department of Surgery, Rush-Presbyterian-St. Luke's Medical Center, Chicago, Illinois
Cancer of the Pancreas: Neuroendocrine Tumors of the Duodenum and Pancreas

MARK REINER, M.D.
Assistant Clinical Professor and Section Chief, General and Laparoscopic Surgery, Mount Sinai Medical Center and Bronx VA Medical Center, New York, New York
Tumors of the Sacrum

LEE B. RILEY, M.D., Ph.D.
Clinical Instructor of Surgery, Temple University School of Medicine, Philadelphia, Pennsylvania; Assistant Member, Fox Chase Cancer Center, Philadelphia, Pennsylvania
Stomach and Small Bowel Cancer: Cancer of the Small Bowel

OSCAR RODRIQUEZ, B.S.
Research Assistant, Cedars–Sinai Medical Center, Los Angeles, California
Hepatobiliary Tumors

EVA RUBIN, M.D.
Professor of Diagnostic Radiology, University of Alabama, Birmingham, Alabama; Chief of Mammography Section, University of Alabama, Birmingham, Alabama
Tumors of the Esophagus and Gastric Cardia; Lung Cancer: Primary Lung Tumors; Breast Cancer

RUDY A. SEGNA, M.D.
Assistant Professor of Obstetrics and Gynecology, Eastern Virginia Medical School, Norfolk, Virginia; Chief, Division of Gynecologic Oncology, Department of Obstetrics and Gynecology, Portsmouth General Hospital, Portsmouth, Virginia
Gynecologic Malignancies: Uterine Cancers

JATIN P. SHAH, M.D., F.A.C.S.
Professor of Surgery, Cornell University Medical Center, New York, New York; Chief, Division of Head and Neck Surgery, E.W. Strong Chair in Head and Neck Oncology, Memorial Sloan-Kettering Cancer Center, New York, New York
Head and Neck Cancer

LINDA SHER, M.D.
Associate Director, Liver Transplantation Coordinator, Clinical Trials, Cedars–Sinai Medical Center, Los Angeles, California
Hepatobiliary Tumors

RACHE M. SIMMONS, M.D.
Assistant Professor, The New York Hospital, Cornell University Medical Center, New York, New York; Assistant Director, Strang-Cornell Breast Center, New York, New York
Breast Cancer

ROBERT STENSON, M.D.
Assistant Professor of Obstetrics and Gynecology, Albert Einstein College of Medicine, Bronx, New York; Assistant Attending Staff, Gynecologic Oncologist, Department of Obstetrics and Gynecology, Beth Israel Medical Center, New York, New York
Gynecologic Malignancies: Vulvar and Vaginal Malignancies

ALFRED A. STEINBERGER, M.D.
Assistant Clinical Professor of Neurosurgery, Mt. Sinai Medical Center, New York, New York; Chief of Neurosurgery, Englewood Hospital, Englewood, New Jersey
Tumors of the Sacrum

HARTLEY STERN, M.D., F.R.C.S.(C), F.A.C.S.
Chairman, Department of Surgery, University of Ottawa, Ottawa, Ontario, Canada; Surgeon in Chief, Ottawa Civic Hospital, Ottawa, Ontario, Canada
Cancer of the Colon, Rectum, and Anus: Colorectal Cancer; Cancer of the Anal Canal

NARAYAN SUNDARESAN, M.D.
Clinical Professor of Neurosurgery, Mt. Sinai Medical School, New York, New York; Attending Surgeon, Mt. Sinai Hospital and Lenox Hill Hospital, New York, New York
Tumors of the Spine; Tumors of the Sacrum

BURTON SURICK, M.D.
Instructor of Surgery, Albert Einstein College of Medicine, Bronx, New York; Assistant Attending Staff, Beth Israel Medical Center, New York, New York
Tumors of the Esophagus and Gastric Cardia

CHRISTINE SZARKA, M.D.
Assistant Member, Department of Medical Oncology, Division of Population Science, Fox Chase Cancer Center, Philadelphia, Pennsylvania
Stomach and Small Bowel Cancer: Gastric Cancer

LOUIS M. WEINER, M.D.
Professor of Medicine, Temple University School of Medicine, Philadelphia, Pennsylvania; Chairman, Department of Medical Oncology, Senior Member, Division of Medical Science, Fox Chase Cancer Center, Philadelphia, Pennsylvania
Stomach and Small Bowel Cancer: Gastric Cancer

Preface

This is a surgical oncology text that covers the entire body with the exception of the central nervous system.

Why a textbook of surgical oncology?

The major advance in American medicine began with the development of medical specialization after World War II. In the field of surgery, specialization was chiefly along anatomic lines. Meanwhile, life expectancy in the United States climbed steadily as a result of better food, housing, and sanitation, along with improved medicine, especially for the control of infections.

Today we are becoming a four-generation society with an increasing population over 70 years of age. Cancer is a disease of aging, and now it will develop in approximately one in three persons in the United States. For some time, heart disease and stroke have killed about 750,000 persons annually, with cancer in second place with over more than 500,000 deaths each year. If we can convince our population not to smoke cigarettes and to have blood pressure monitored with effective control of any hypertension, we will approach the state at which cancer will be our prime killer.

Surgery was the first treatment to cure cancer. After the discovery of x-rays and radium a century ago, radiotherapy became the second modality capable of treating cancer for cure. World War II technology and the atom bomb were great boosts to the field of radiotherapy. Both surgery and radiotherapy are aimed at local control with eradication of the primary tumor and control of its regional lymph node spread. A third treatment modality began after World War II and has had rapid expansion: chemotherapy has the advantage of being systemic therapy. Chemotherapy alone has proven its effectiveness in the treatment of leukemia, lymphoma, choriocarcinoma, and germ cell tumors, usually of the testes.

Of recent years, multidisciplinary cancer therapy has had considerable investigation, combining the benefits of surgery, radiotherapy, and chemotherapy. In those instances in which tumors are chemotherapy-sensitive, progress has been made.

Current research at the molecular biologic level has great promise. Gene mapping indicates that genetic causes of cancer will be of great importance, not only for etiology but probably also for early detection and possibly for future therapy.

The role of immunotherapy is still not clear. It should have an important role as the fourth treatment modality, but more information is needed to make it an effective independent therapy.

Since few surgeons are also oncologists, all too frequently medical oncologists and radiation oncologists have made surgical opinions that tumors are "not operable." In the national picture for medicine of the future, it is proposed that nonsurgical primary care physicians play the role of "gatekeepers" to keep patients from specialists. It is in this progressive but reactionary scene that a body of knowledge concerning surgical oncology becomes ever more important for the benefit of the cancer patient. Certain truisms exist:

1. In the United States, 90% of cancers are solid tumors.

2. Early-stage disease has a reasonably high cure rate (70% to 100%) in the five most common killers: lung, breast, colorectal, urologic, and gynecologic cancers.

3. Complete surgical excision is of prime importance in the cure of early-stage tumors, although radiotherapy also is of great importance in accessible tumors such as breast cancer, early laryngeal cancer, and early cervical cancer.

4. Although adjuvant treatment is valuable (radiotherapy-chemotherapy), incomplete surgical excision is much less effective than complete excision.

5. Although cancer treatment requires accurate diagnosis, accurate staging, and aggressive treatment, very frequently the diagnosis is not known until the surgery is being done.

For these reasons, we feel that a surgical text that covers the cancers of the various anatomic regions of the body written by experts in their fields is a valuable source book not only for surgeons who have not made cancer a specialty but also as an up-to-date reference for surgeons who are cancer specialists but who wish to refresh themselves about an area preoperatively. We also hope that this surgical oncology text will prove valuable to our colleagues in medical and radiation oncology. We further hope that promoting the field of surgical oncology will help assure the patient that surgical decisions are made by the appropriate specialists. In this fashion, we hope and believe that the patient stricken with cancer can only be helped.

Our final consideration is that we, as cancer doctors, must aggressively try to cure. Statistics are meaningless in any one patient. And we must not lose sight of our humaneness. When we cannot cure, we still can care. We must relieve pain, and we must support both the patient and his or her family in any way we can.

EDWARD J. BEATTIE, M.D.

JAMES C. HARVEY, M.D.

Acknowledgments

Our thanks to Elena Horohoe, whose management skills allowed us to keep up with voluminous correspondence. Thanks also to Julie Quain, health care researcher, the Boston Consulting Group, New York, New York, and Patricia Gallagher, reference librarian, the New York Academy of Medicine, New York, New York, both of whom were so generous with their time.

Contents

Bruce J. Davidson, M.D.
Joshua D. I. Ellenhorn, M.D.
Jatin P. Shah, M.D.

1

Head and Neck Cancer

SQUAMOUS CELL CARCINOMA OF THE UPPER AERODIGESTIVE TRACT

The upper aerodigestive tract consists of the paranasal sinuses, nasal cavity, nasopharynx, oral cavity, oropharynx, hypopharynx, larynx, and cervical esophagus. Carcinomas of the upper aerodigestive tract mucosa are predominantly of squamous cell origin and in most instances are associated with a long history of tobacco and alcohol use. The fact that most malignant tumors of the upper aerodigestive tract are squamous cell carcinomas means that the diagnostic and treatment modalities used are similar for tumors of different sites. However, each site presents distinct anatomic and pathophysiologic issues relevant to cancer diagnosis and treatment. This section discusses the epidemiology, natural history, pathology, diagnosis, and management of squamous cell carcinoma of the upper aerodigestive tract.

Epidemiology

Incidence

In the United States, squamous cell carcinoma of the upper aerodigestive tract occurs in about 42,000 patients per year, and the number of deaths attributable to this cancer is 11,000 per year.[1] It represents approximately 4% of the more than 1 million cases of cancer diagnosed annually. Approximately half of all squamous cell carcinomas of the upper aerodigestive tract are in the oral cavity. Cancers within the head and neck are predominantly seen in men, and the usual age of onset is 50 to 70 years. Figure 1–1 shows cancer incidence and death estimates by site.

Risk Factors

Genetic-Familial

The strong influence of tobacco and alcohol on the development of cancers of the upper aerodigestive tract obscures underlying genetic predisposition that may exist. However, there is evidence that in a subset of patients, genetic factors may increase cancer susceptibility. Bloom syndrome is an autosomal recessive growth disorder in which individuals have an increased incidence of cancer at a young age, including head and neck carcinomas.[2] Li-Fraumeni syndrome involves mutation, through an autosomal dominant inheritance, of one allele of the p53 tumor suppressor gene. This has been associated with head and neck cancer in some patients with minimal tobacco exposure and may indicate increased susceptibility to environmental carcinogens in these patients.[3]

More subtle forms of susceptibility to tobacco-related cancers may also have a genetic basis. One of these includes heritable variations in carcinogen activation and detoxification pathways, such as those mediated by the P450 and glutathione-*S*-transferase enzyme families.[4] Another form of cancer susceptibility may be demonstrated by the number of chromosomal breaks in peripheral blood lymphocytes cultured in the presence of bleomycin. Head and neck cancer patients appear more sensitive than control smokers to the mutagenic effects of bleomycin.[5] This does not appear to be a tobacco-induced phenomenon and may represent inherent mutagen sensitivity in these individuals.[6]

Dietary

Dietary factors have not been shown to play a direct role in carcinogenesis of the upper aerodigestive tract. However, alcohol is a risk factor in many patients with cancer of the head and neck, and nutritional deficiency is common in alcoholics. Whether this contributes to their risk of cancer development is not clear.

Plummer-Vinson syndrome includes iron deficiency anemia and is associated with squamous carcinomas of the hypopharynx and oral cavity, but there is no evidence that the iron deficiency itself contributes to the development of cancer. While nasopharyngeal cancer appears to have significant genetic and viral associations, the nitrosamine-rich diet in endemic areas of China may contribute to the

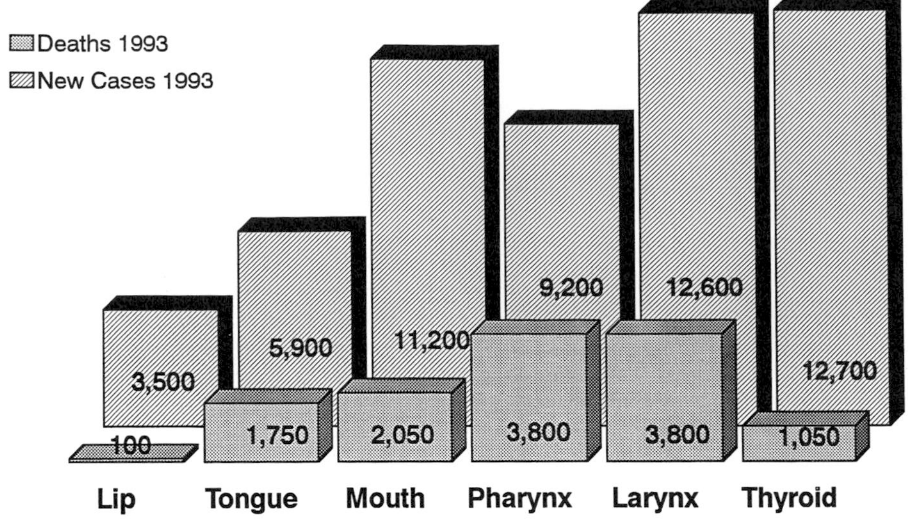

FIGURE 1–1. New cases and deaths from cancers of the upper aerodigestive tract. Thyroid cancer is shown for comparison. (Derived from Boring CC, et al: Cancer statistics, 1993. CA 43:7–26, 1993.)

etiology of this cancer.[7] Although squamous cell carcinomas of the head and neck have not been shown to be attributable to dietary factors, recent endeavors in cancer chemoprevention using vitamin A analogues may indicate nutritional influences on carcinogenesis.

Social

The majority of patients presenting with squamous cell carcinoma of the upper aerodigestive tract report a significant history of tobacco and alcohol consumption. Use of either substance contributes to an increased risk of head and neck squamous cell carcinoma (HNSCC). However, use of both tobacco and alcohol appears to have a synergistic effect, raising the relative risk severalfold compared to that for nonusers (Fig. 1–2).[8]

The oral cavity, pharynx, and esophagus are physically exposed to alcohol, and cancers in these areas more often present with alcohol as a risk factor. In contrast, cancer of the larynx is more often associated with smoking alone. The role of alcohol in carcinogenesis may be to act as a promotor, an irritant, or a solvent to increase the solubility of carcinogens from tobacco. Recently, experimental evidence has suggested that ethanol suppresses the efficiency of DNA repair after exposure to nitrosamine compounds.[9]

In addition to smoking, other forms of tobacco use contribute to the development of HNSCC. These include, in India, the chewing of "pan," a mixture of tobacco, betel (areca) nut, lime, and other substances wrapped in a vegetable leaf. Chronic use of pan is associated with a high incidence of oral carcinoma. In the United States, there has been a recent popularization of chewing tobacco use. This habit has historical roots in the rural South, where it was practiced predominantly by women prior to the social acceptance of cigarette smoking by women. Epidemiologic data from that area of the country has shown a 50-fold increased risk of oral cancer in chronic snuff users.[10] Marijuana smoking has also received attention recently as an etiologic factor in the development of HNSCC, although odds ratios or dose-response relationships have not been reported.[11]

Environmental-Occupational

Occupational factors relevant to carcinoma of the upper aerodigestive tract are best known for their involvement of the nasal cavity and paranasal sinus sites. Risk factors associated with cancers at these sites include nickel refining, woodworking, leather working, and chromium exposure. An increased risk of laryngeal cancer has been associated with occupational exposure to sulfuric acid and asbestos and with textile manufacturing and metal processing.[12]

Viral

Emerging data suggest that viral factors may play a role in the development of carcinoma of the head and neck. Titers against components of the Epstein-Barr virus (EBV) have been described in nasopharyngeal cancer, especially nonkeratinizing and undifferentiated types (World Health Organization [WHO] classes II and III).[13] These titers have been followed serially and appear to correlate with disease status. However, no causal association between EBV and nasopharyngeal cancer has yet been established. It is of interest to note that nasopharyngeal cancer in the United States is more often keratinizing (WHO class I) and is less often associated with elevated EBV titers. In situ hybridization has shown EBV in 68 of 77 undifferentiated nasopharyngeal cancers but in 0 of 8 squamous cell carcinomas from the nasopharynx and in 0 of 15 squamous cell carcinomas from other sites.[14] As with other sites of HNSCC, nasopharyngeal cancer in whites is often associated with tobacco exposure.

An association between human papillomavirus (HPV) infection and HNSCC has been suggested by molecular biologic detection of HPV in 60% to 90% of oral cavity

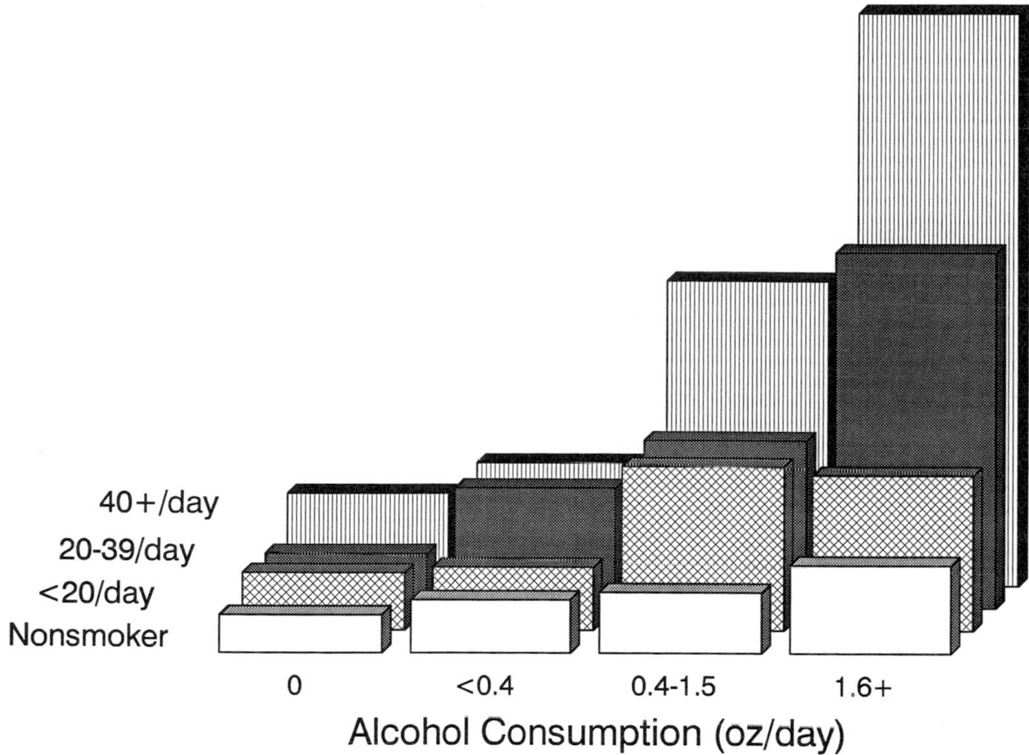

FIGURE 1–2. Increasing risk of cancer of the mouth and pharynx relative to tobacco and alcohol exposure. (Derived from Rothman K, Keller A: The effect of joint exposure to alcohol and tobacco on risk of cancer of the mouth and pharynx. J Chronic Dis 25:711–716, 1972.)

HNSCC.[15, 16] However, establishing an etiologic role for HPV in HNSCC is complicated by the presence of HPV in 40% of normal oral mucosa.[16] Support for an etiologic role has been given by experimental data showing an increased rate of induced transformation by benzo[a]pyrene (a component of tobacco smoke) in oral keratinocytes transfected with HPV.[17] Inverted papilloma is a benign tumor of the nasal cavity that may show a malignant component in 10% of tumors. However, papillomas may have a more direct association with HPV infection than sinonasal cancer, as HPV has been detected in 24% of inverted papillomas but in only 4% of cancers.[18] Recurrent respiratory papillomatosis of the larynx is another benign disease that has revealed malignant transformation in a small number of cases. About half of these cases of malignant transformation have been in patients who received radiation therapy to control recurrent papillomatosis.

Natural History

Approximately one third of patients with HNSCC present with small primary lesions (T1 or T2) and no evidence of regional spread to cervical lymph nodes. In contrast, more than half of patients with HNSCC present with locally advanced disease (T3 or T4) or have cervical lymph node metastases. While traditionally thought to be rare in HNSCC, distant metastases develop in about 20% of patients, as reported in both prospective and autopsy series, but these are seldom discernible at initial diagnosis.[19, 20]

Primary Site

The presentation of early disease is highly dependent on the anatomy of the head and neck. Although vocal cord cancer may present quite early with hoarseness, nearby tumors of the hypopharynx are notorious for late presentation owing to asymptomatic growth. Early tongue tumors may be detected by a fortuitous routine dental examination or may present with a painful ulceration or slurred speech. The singular clinical finding in a patient with early nasopharyngeal cancer may be unilateral otitis media, and any patient presenting with unilateral middle ear effusion requires examination of the nasopharynx.

With locally advanced tumors of the oral cavity, pharynx, or larynx, patients often seek medical attention secondary to severe odynophagia, dysphagia, or aspiration or airway obstruction. Reduced dietary intake due to any of these symptoms may lead to significant weight loss. Airway obstruction may require acute intervention prior to any efforts to obtain pathologic diagnosis and definitively treat the cancer.

Patients with tumors of the nasal cavity and paranasal sinuses are unlikely to present with vocal or swallowing dysfunction. They present with symptoms often mistaken for allergic rhinitis or sinusitis. While recurrent epistaxis, epiphora, diplopia, or cheek swelling is unlikely to be disregarded without a thorough head and neck examination, nasal obstruction also necessitates an investigation. This is particularly true for any unilateral obstruction.

Pain is a common symptom in HNSCC. This pain may be mediated by the trigeminal, glossopharyngeal, or vagus nerve. Tumor necrosis, peritumor inflammation, or local invasion may lead to intense pain in the distribution of the trigeminal nerve. The glossopharyngeal and vagus nerves transmit pain from pharyngeal and laryngeal tumors to the ear. Hypopharyngeal or laryngeal lesions may cause otalgia through Arnold's nerve, the auricular branch of the vagus nerve, while referred pain from oropharyngeal and hypopharyngeal lesions involves Jacobson's nerve, the tympanic plexus of the glossopharyngeal nerve.

The clinical presentation of end-stage primary or locally recurrent HNSCC is also dependent on the anatomy of the head and neck. Symptoms may involve intense pain as previously described. Dysphagia may lead to severe nutritional deficiency. Airway obstruction or recurrent aspiration may cause pulmonary compromise. Invasion of the muscles of mastication may lead to trismus. Invasion may also extend outward to skin and cause a spontaneous orocutaneous fistula.

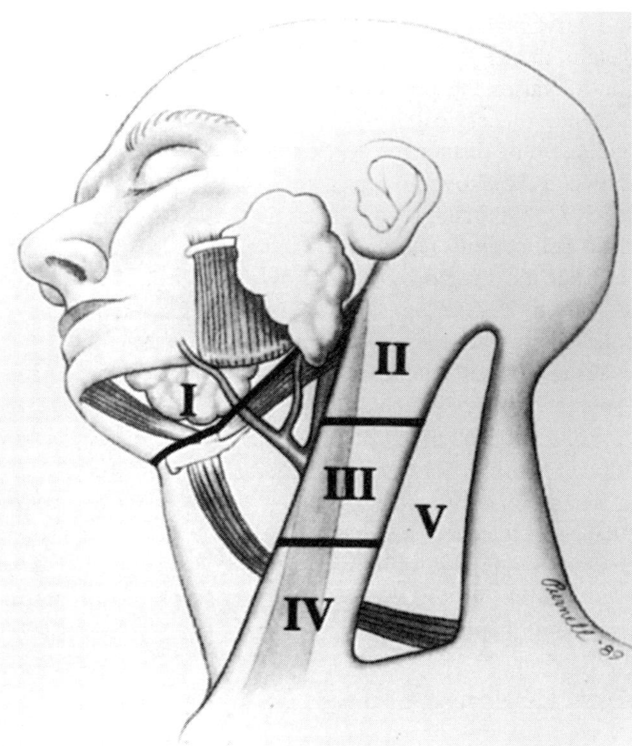

FIGURE 1–3. Diagram of neck showing designated levels for use in describing location of cervical lymphatics.

Cervical Lymphatics

Involvement of cervical lymphatics is common in HNSCC and is the single most important prognostic determinant. Because of this, the diagnosis and treatment of patients with HNSCC require consideration of the status of the cervical lymphatics. Reviews of large numbers of patients have led to an understanding of the patterns of spread to cervical nodes from mucosal sites in the upper aerodigestive tract.[21–23] This knowledge has also guided the search for occult mucosal lesions in patients with metastatic squamous cell carcinoma in a cervical lymph node and no apparent primary lesion.

The cervical lymphatics may be divided into levels I to VII (Fig. 1–3). Level I represents submandibular and submental lymph nodes and includes prevascular facial lymph nodes. Levels II, III, and IV represent upper middle and lower deep jugular lymph nodes. The deep jugular lymph nodes are divided into equal thirds to describe levels II, III, and IV and include jugulodigastric, jugulocarotid, and jugulo-omohyoid groups of lymph nodes. Level V lymph nodes are located in the posterior triangle of the neck and include the spinal accessory chain and transverse cervical chain of lymph nodes. Level VI refers to paratracheal and pretracheal nodes, and level VII refers to nodes of the superior mediastinum.

Primary cancers of the lip or anterior oral cavity predominantly metastasize to level I initially. Lesions of the tongue and posterior oral cavity are more likely to spread to level II.[21] Lesions of the oropharynx, such as the base of the tongue and tonsil, also involve level II initially. Levels II and III are usual sites for metastases from hypopharyngeal and laryngeal primary lesions. Nasopharyngeal carcinoma spreads to levels II and V along the spinal accessory chain. Level V metastases from other sites within the upper aerodigestive tract are rare and usually follow anterior cervical involvement.[24]

The risk of cervical metastases varies between primary sites within the head and neck. The glottic larynx has few lymphatics, and early lesions seldom metastasize. The supraglottic larynx and hypopharynx are associated with cervical metastases in about two thirds of patients at presentation. Oral cavity lesions present with clinical evidence of cervical involvement in one third of patients. However, approximately one third of those with clinically negative necks have occult metastases.[25] A wide variation in the prevalence of cervical metastases is seen between paranasal sinus primary lesions ($\sim 15\%$) and nasopharyngeal primary lesions ($> 90\%$).

Distant Metastases

As stated, distant metastases in HNSCC develop in about 20% of patients. Uncontrolled or recurrent local-regional disease increases the likelihood of distant metastases from 21% to 38%.[19] When analyzed by primary site, the incidence of distant metastasis in nasopharyngeal and hypopharyngeal cancer is about 40% and does not appear to be influenced by local-regional control status. In contrast, oral and laryngeal cancers under local-regional control show distant metastases in only 7% of patients, but loss of control raises the prevalence of metastases to 16%.[19] The presence of cervical metastases in the lower neck is also predictive of distant metastases.[26] A prospective study has shown a 12% overall incidence of distant metastases in HNSCC, but a subgroup of patients with decreased natural killer cell activity had a 50% incidence of distant metastases after local-regional treatment.[27] The majority of metastases from HNSCC are to lung.[20] Less often, metastases to bone, liver, and other sites may be seen.

There is a substantial risk of second primary cancers in patients previously treated for HNSCC. Twenty-five percent of these are lung cancers. This increased risk of second primary cancers in HNSCC patients requires that a lung lesion presenting subsequent to an HNSCC be distinguished between a second primary lesion and metastatic disease. When this distinction cannot be made, the lung lesion should be treated as a primary cancer with aggressive therapy and curative intent.

Local-Regional Anatomy and Pathology

Anatomy

Because tumors of the upper aerodigestive tract are most often of squamous cell histology, it is tempting to consider all HNSCC as one entity. However, as alluded to earlier, tumors of similar histology may behave quite differently in terms of propensity for metastasis. In addition, each primary site affects adjacent anatomic structures in distinct ways. For this reason, a review of upper aerodigestive tract anatomy relevant to tumor behavior is indicated. For more detailed anatomic descriptions, the reader is referred to anatomic texts and surgical atlases.

The upper aerodigestive tract consists of the paranasal sinuses, nasal cavity, nasopharynx, oral cavity, oropharynx, hypopharynx, larynx, and cervical esophagus.

Paranasal Sinuses. The paranasal sinuses consist of four paired sinuses: the frontal, ethmoid, sphenoid, and maxillary. Tumors of the maxillary sinus are most common, followed by tumors of the ethmoid sinus. Extension of maxillary tumors can occur superiorly to the orbit and manifest as lacrimal duct obstruction with epiphora or loss of sensation in the distribution of the infraorbital nerve as well as proptosis or limitation of extraocular movement. Extension from the ethmoid sinus may also involve the orbit or extend superiorly through the roof of the ethmoid (fovea ethmoidalis) into the anterior cranial fossa. Often, sinus tumors cause blockage of normal pathways of mucus secretion. This may lead to opacification of adjacent sinuses in the absence of tumor extension owing to inspissated secretions or mucocele formation.

Nasal Cavity. The nasal cavity extends from the vestibule to the nasopharynx. Each side is defined by the septum medially and three turbinates laterally. The middle meatus is between the inferior and the middle turbinates, and it is through this area that the frontal, maxillary, and anterior ethmoid sinuses drain. As with the paranasal sinuses, tumors of the nasal cavity may be associated with opacification of the paranasal sinuses, indicating tumor extension or simply sinus obstruction. Careful evaluation with computed tomography (CT) or magnetic resonance imaging (MRI) is warranted.

Nasopharynx. The nasopharynx has lateral and posterior walls, and its roof borders the clivus or sphenoid sinus, depending on the aeration of the sphenoid. The eustachian tube orifice is located on the lateral wall. Tumors in this area may cause blockage and produce serous otitis media. Tumors that extend superiorly may enter the sphenoid sinus and from there can gain access to the cranial cavity. Tumors extending laterally may effect cranial nerves IX, X, XI, and XII as they exit the skull base.

Oral Cavity. The oral cavity has several subsites, including the lip, buccal mucosa, anterior tongue, floor of the mouth, alveolar ridge, retromolar trigone, and hard palate. As tumors enlarge, the ability to distinguish the original primary site decreases. Tumors of the floor of the mouth may cause obstruction of Wharton's duct and lead to enlargement of the submandibular gland. Tumor extension in oral cavity lesions may lead to invasion of the mandible. Extensive involvement of the mandible may be detected clinically by sensory deficit in the distribution of the mental nerve. In most cases, mandibular invasion occurs in both dentulous and edentulous patients through a tooth socket or the alveolar process, the path of least resistance.

Oropharynx. The division between the oral cavity and oropharynx is at the circumvellate papillae of the tongue and at the junction of the hard and soft palate. Sites within the oropharynx include the base of the tongue, soft palate, tonsil, and posterior pharyngeal wall. The division between the posterior walls of the nasopharynx, oropharynx, and hypopharynx is somewhat arbitrary, and tumors often extend from one site to another, as there is no anatomic barrier. Tumors of the oropharynx are less likely to invade the mandible than are oral cavity tumors. Tumors of the base of the tongue may involve the deep tongue musculature.

Hypopharynx. The hypopharynx consists of the pyriform sinuses, the posterior pharyngeal wall, and the postcricoid region near the esophageal inlet. The pyriform sinuses lie lateral to the aryepiglottic folds on either side of the larynx. The intimate association of the pyriform sinus with the larynx may lead to similar clinical findings, such as vocal cord paralysis, with tumors from either site. Tumors of the hypopharynx have been shown to cause vocal fold fixation primarily by invasion medially and involvement of the muscles of the intrinsic larynx.[28] Unlike the glottic larynx, however, the pyriform sinus is more likely to metastasize to cervical lymphatics and may also spread to the neck by direct extension laterally.

Larynx. The larynx is divided into supraglottic, glottic, and subglottic regions. The supraglottic larynx has the epiglottis, aryepiglottic folds, and false vocal folds as subsites. The ventricle is a cleft between the false and true vocal cords and marks the separation between the supraglottic and glottic larynx. The glottic larynx includes each true vocal cord and the anterior and posterior commissures. The subglottic larynx begins 10 mm below the margin of the true vocal cords and extends to the lower border of the cricoid cartilage. Vocal cord paralysis may occur secondary to involvement of the recurrent laryngeal nerve or its branches, invasion of the intrinsic muscles of the larynx, or destruction of the cricoarytenoid joint.

Pathology

The majority of cancers of the upper aerodigestive tract are squamous cell carcinomas. These range from well-differentiated to undifferentiated lesions, with distinction in differentiation made by assessing the amount of keratinization. Pharyngeal lesions are more often poorly differentiated. Oral cavity and glottic laryngeal carcinomas tend to be more well differentiated. Verrucous carcinoma is a variant of epidermoid carcinoma that is well differentiated, tends to be exophytic, and has a more favorable prognosis than other HNSCC lesions. Poorly differentiated tumors may be confused with nonepidermoid malignancies such as malignant melanoma and sarcomas and may require immunohistochemical staining for accurate diagnosis.

Preneoplastic lesions may be noted in some patients evaluated for HNSCC. These include the clinical entities of leukoplakia and erythroplakia (literally, white plaque and red plaque, respectively). The pathologic findings in these lesions on biopsy may range from hyperkeratosis to invasive carcinoma. A large study from India found that the relative risk of oral cancer in smokers with homogeneous leukoplakia was 26 times the risk of cancer in smokers without leukoplakia. The relative risk of cancer in leukoplakia with an erythematous base was more than 3246 times greater. Although the risk of oral cancer developing is increased, less than 5% of leukoplakic lesions progress to invasive carcinoma.[29] However, in 30% of those with erythroplasia, carcinoma eventually develops.[30] This difference may simply be a reflection of the higher likelihood of established dysplasia in erythroplastic lesions.

Diagnosis, Screening, Early Detection, and Staging

Diagnosis

In most cases, an adequate examination of the head and neck allows the discovery and characterization of lesions of the upper aerodigestive tract when patients present with symptoms. This examination should be performed using a headlight and mirrors to allow visualization of the pharynx and larynx. Patients having a prominent gag reflex may require evaluation using a flexible fiberoptic endoscope. While lesions of the cervical esophagus or subglottic larynx may not be visible in such a clinical examination, documentation of laryngeal function in tumors arising in these sites is essential.

The discovery of a suspicious mucosal lesion requires biopsy. Biopsy of lesions of the nasal and oral cavities and those in the nasopharynx and oropharynx can often be performed under local or topical anesthesia. Lesions in the hypopharynx and larynx usually require biopsy under general anesthesia. In addition to allowing biopsies, examination under anesthesia provides more accurate assessment of the extent of tumor.

The presentation of a cervical mass in an adult necessitates a thorough examination of the head and neck. Metastatic squamous cell carcinoma may present in the neck with no obvious evidence of a primary lesion. An examination of the upper aerodigestive tract may reveal a primary lesion and allow biopsy without violation of the neck mass. When clinical examination reveals no obvious primary lesion, needle biopsy of the cervical node should be performed. Prior to definitive treatment of the neck, an endoscopic examination of the upper aerodigestive tract with directed biopsies should be performed to rule out an occult primary lesion.

Screening and Early Detection

Unlike some other forms of cancer, HNSCC has no established screening or early detection markers at this time. A thorough clinical examination remains the most sensitive screening device. However, given the relative rarity of HNSCC in developed countries, the use of routine head and neck examinations to screen for cancer is impractical. The incidence of a second primary cancer of the upper aerodigestive tract developing in HNSCC patients is 3% to 4% per year and approaches 25% overall.[31] TNM classification (see below) does not predict the incidence of second primary lesions, so even early-stage lesions require careful follow-up. It is this population, those previously treated for HNSCC, in whom screening by routine head and neck examination is warranted. Likewise, any patients with preneoplastic mucosal lesions warrant routine examination in an effort to detect invasive carcinoma at the earliest possible stage.

Staging

Head and neck cancers are staged using the TNM (tumor-node-metasasis) system put forth by the American Joint Committee on Cancer (AJCC) and the International Union Against Cancer (UICC).[32] In general, stages I and II describe lesions confined to one site in the head and neck without evidence of lymph node metastases. Stages III and IV lesions are locally advanced or involve cervical lymph nodes or both. The T classification breakdown varies with primary site. In the oral cavity and oropharynx, the division between T1, T2, and T3 is 2 cm and 4 cm in greatest dimension. Lesions of the hypopharynx and larynx are T1 if confined to one subsite, T2 when extending to two subsites or associated with impaired vocal cord mobility in glottic carcinoma, and T3 if associated with vocal cord fixation or involvement of the pre-epiglottic space or medial wall of the pyriform sinus. T4 lesions are massive tumors that extend beyond one site or those with bone or muscle invasion.

Classification of nodal metastases is as follows:

NX: Lymph nodes cannot be assessed
N0: No evidence of metastases
N1: Unilateral lymph node less than 3 cm
N2a: Unilateral lymph node 3 to 6 cm
N2b: Multiple ipsilateral nodes
N2c: Contralateral or bilateral nodes
N3: Ipsilateral or contralateral nodes greater than 6 cm

The status of distant disease is designated M0 for no known distant metastases and M1 for confirmed distant disease.

The TNM classification and stage for each new patient should be determined initially by clinical examination. Information from CT, MRI, or examination under anesthesia may be integrated into initial staging. However, it should be realized that new modalities such as MRI may detect subclinical disease and cause lesions to be upstaged in comparison to historical controls. It is best to clarify staging as radiologic or pathologic if this information is used to revise the clinical stage.

Treatment

Several factors affect the choice of treatment of a patient with squamous cell carcinoma of the head and neck. These can be broadly divided into tumor factors, patient factors, and physician factors.

Tumor factors include site, histology, size, depth of invasion, stage of disease, previous treatment, need for reconstructive surgery, and impact on quality of life. Patient factors include general medical condition, patient preference, treatment cost and convenience, and compliance. Physician factors include availability of necessary expertise, comprehensive team requirements, and physician preference.

Each case involves a unique combination of these factors, and thus individualized treatment planning is needed.

Primary Operable Disease—Results and Complications of Treatment

In general, treatment of early (stage I or II) lesions of the head and neck with either radiation or surgery results in equivalent control rates. Decisions regarding which modality should be chosen may depend on the medical condition of the patient, patient compliance, availability of qualified personnel, treatment morbidity, cost, convenience, and so on. Early lesions of the larynx are more likely to be treated with radiotherapy alone at most institutions, with surgery used to salvage recurrent disease if necessary. On the other hand, early lesions of the oral cavity are more suitable for surgical excision. Provided no evidence of nodal metastases exists, these patients may avoid radiotherapy and the associated risks of permanent xerostomia, dental caries, and radionecrosis of the mandible.

Advanced lesions (stage III or IV) require multimodality therapy. In most cases, this involves surgery followed by postoperative radiotherapy. Preoperative radiotherapy has shown no therapeutic advantage and is associated with decreased wound healing and increased risk of surgical complications.[33] Postoperative radiotherapy improves local control and survival, with the 5-year survival rate increased from 31% to 59%.[34] It also improves survival for patients with extracapsular nodal disease and for those with positive surgical margins.[34]

Efforts in laryngeal preservation have led to recent successes using neoadjuvant chemotherapy plus radiotherapy to avoid laryngectomy in the treatment of laryngeal carcinoma.[35, 36] Adjuvant chemotherapy continues to be investigated by randomized trials. Addition of adjuvant chemotherapy is associated with significantly fewer failures in the neck (from 10% to 5%) and fewer distant metastases (from 23% to 15%). However, no survival advantage has been shown for adjuvant treatment.[37]

Management of the Neck

The high prevalence of nodal metastases in HNSCC requires consideration of the treatment of the neck for most primary sites. Management may range from observation to radiotherapy or neck dissection or both. Clinically positive disease in the neck may be treated by surgery or radiotherapy with curative intent if a single node approximately 2 cm or less is noted.[38] Larger nodes or multiple nodes require surgical treatment for the most effective results. This is followed by postoperative radiotherapy for N2 or N3 disease or if the pathology reveals extracapsular spread.

Options in surgical management of the neck have recently been described using a standardized terminology (Table 1–1).[39] Radical neck dissection involves removal of lymph node levels I through V as well as the internal jugular vein (IJV), spinal accessory nerve (cranial nerve [CN] XI), and sternocleidomastoid muscle (SCM). Modified neck dissection also removes all five nodal levels but spares one or more of the IJV, CN XI, or SCM. Components spared should be described specifically in operative records in order to allow clear understanding among health care personnel. Selective neck dissections remove less than five nodal levels and spare the IJV, CN XI, and SCM unless involved by tumor. Common selective neck dissections have been termed supraomohyoid (levels I, II, and III) and anterolateral (levels I to IV) dissections. These operations spare dissection of the posterior triangle, avoiding extensive dissection along CN XI and the resulting shoulder morbidity.

TABLE 1–1
Options in Surgical Management of the Neck

Neck Dissection Type	Lymphatic Levels Included	Nonlymphatic Structures	Clinical Utility
Comprehensive			
Radical	I–V	Includes IJV, CN XI, SCM	N1 and greater All sites
Modified	I–V	Spares IJV and/or CN XI and/or SCM	N1 and N2A All sites (?) Metastatic thyroid cancer
Selective			
Supraomohyoid	I–III	Spares IJV, CN XI, and SCM	N0 and N1 Oral cavity
Posterolateral	II–V	Spares IJV, CN XI, and SCM	N0 Scalp/skin
Lateral (jugular)	II–IV	Spares IJV, CN XI, and SCM	N0 Larynx/pharynx
Anterior (central compartment)	VI	Spares IJV, CN XI, and SCM	N0 Thyroid
Extended Radical	I–V plus others as needed	Includes IJV, CN IX, SCM plus others (CN X, XII, carotid, skin, etc.)	N1 or greater with extension All sites

IJV, Internal jugular vein; CN, cranial nerve; SCM, sternocleidomastoid muscle.

Clinically positive neck disease necessitates radical neck dissection or modified radical neck dissection in most cases. N1 disease has been treated successfully by selective neck dissection, but care must be taken in patient selection. There is a low prevalence of level V metastases in large series of radical neck dissections.[24] Some have suggested that level V may be omitted in neck dissection in all cases.[40] However, this proposal has not been adopted, and most head and neck surgeons prefer radical or modified radical neck dissections in the treatment of clinically positive neck disease.

Elective treatment of N0 neck lesions should be considered when the risk of micrometastases to lymph nodes is greater than 15% to 20%. This may be surgical or radiotherapeutic. However, routine use of elective radiotherapy to N0 neck disease would lead to the loss of salivary and taste function in a high proportion of patients with truly negative neck nodes and would not improve their disease control. For this reason, the use of supraomohyoid neck dissection as a decision-making tool has been adopted for T1N0 and T2N0 oral cavity lesions. Morbidity from selective neck dissection is minimal, and the procedure allows pathologic assessment of nodal histology. If multiple nodal metastases are found or if extracapsular spread is noted, elective radiotherapy is indicated. Spiro et al.[25] have shown a low risk of neck node metastases in superficial carcinomas of the tongue and floor of the mouth. T1 or T2 lesions with tumor thickness less than 2 to 3 mm may be safely observed without treatment.

Control of neck disease has been shown in more than 70% of patients with N2 or N3 disease if surgery is followed by radiotherapy, significantly higher than for single-modality treatment.[41] This same study shows improved neck control for combined treatment versus radiation alone even in N0 or N1 disease (95% vs. 82%). The improvement in survival in advanced neck disease when surgery is followed by radiation has been shown previously.[42]

Unknown Primary Lesion

Approximately 10% of patients with head and neck cancer present with metastases to a cervical lymph node and no obvious primary lesion. A thorough head and neck examination reveals a primary source in a third of these patients. If no mucosal lesion is noted, needle biopsy of the neck mass is indicated. Clinical examination should be augmented by panendoscopy and directed biopsies in order to detect the primary. The nasopharynx, hypopharynx, tonsil, and base of the tongue are sites that require careful inspection and biopsy of any suspicious areas.

If fine-needle aspiration reveals squamous cell carcinoma in the cervical node, and no primary lesion is detected by panendoscopy, radical or modified neck dissection is indicated. Postoperative radiotherapy is indicated if multiple nodes or extracapsular spread is noted or if residual disease remains after resection. Whether to include the mucosa of the potential primary sites within the radiation portals is controversial. Long-term follow-up results in the discovery of a primary lesion in 4% to 16% of patients.[43] The fact that this incidence is similar to the incidence of second primary cancers in HNSCC gives validity to the practice of withholding radiation therapy to mucosal sites if no primary lesion can be identified.[44] Treatment of the second (or late presenting) primary lesion is then dependent on tumor location and previous therapy. Despite this controversy, when patients receive radiotherapy for their neck disease, mucosal sites are included in the radiation portals.

Occasionally, fine-needle aspiration biopsy of the cervical node reveals adenocarcinoma. This may be from a salivary gland primary lesion, but metastasis from distant sites must also be considered. Lymph nodes with metastatic adenocarcinoma are predominantly located in the lower neck,[45] and nodes located in the supraclavicular area are often metastatic from sites below the clavicle. Lung, breast, gastrointestinal, and genitourinary sources must be investigated. These unknown primary adenocarcinomas are aggressive lesions, with frequent metastases to the mediastinum, lung, and bone. The 5-year survival rate of these patients is about 10%.[45] The usual treatment for metastatic adenocarcinoma with unknown primary lesion is chemotherapy and radiation, with surgery included in less than 20% of cases.[45]

In the event that no diagnosis can be made by fine-needle aspiration, an open biopsy is required. The surgeon is wise to be prepared for a formal neck dissection at this time, depending on the frozen section findings. The 5-year survival rate is 86% for unknown primary lesions of squamous cell histology amenable to surgical therapy alone and 63% in those requiring postoperative radiotherapy.[46]

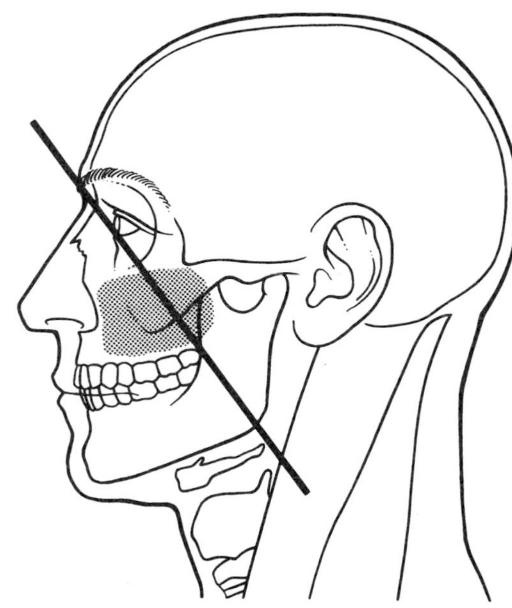

FIGURE 1–4. Lesions inferior to Ohngren's line are more amenable to limited maxillectomy.

Nasal Cavity and Paranasal Sinuses

The surgical options that play a role in the treatment of nasal cavity and paranasal sinus neoplasms range from lateral rhinotomy to extensive craniofacial resections. As with all forms of cancer treatment, the procedure chosen depends on the extent of disease, histology, and other factors.

Medial maxillectomy is indicated for benign neoplasms of the lateral nasal wall, such as inverted papilloma, or for squamous cell cancers localized to this area. The procedure is performed through a lateral rhinotomy via a Weber-Fergusson incision and an ipsilateral upper labial sulcus incision. The resection includes the lateral nasal wall, the inferior turbinate, and variable amounts of ethmoid sinus tissue along with the middle turbinate.

Most maxillary sinus cancers are asymptomatic until they invade surrounding structures. For this reason, many lesions are advanced at presentation. With the use of Ohngren's line, extending from the medial canthus to the angle of the mandible, tumors can be designated as infrastructure or suprastructure lesions (Fig. 1–4). Lesions inferior to Ohngren's line are less likely to have invaded the orbit or skull base and are more amenable to limited resections and offer a favorable prognosis. Cancers confined to the infrastructure can often be resected by a partial maxillectomy. This resection involves removal of a portion of the hard palate and the floor and medial and lateral walls of the maxillary sinus. Tumors extending to the suprastructure are more likely to require removal of the orbital floor. Orbital exenteration is indicated when tumor invades through the periosteal layer lining the orbit.

Tumors extending up to the cranial base require craniofacial resection. This is performed in conjunction with a neurosurgical team, who begin the resection via a frontal craniotomy. This allows assessment of tumor extension superiorly and mobilization of dura and brain from the superior aspect of the tumor. The lower aspect of the resection is performed through a Weber-Fergusson or other facial incision. This combined approach allows en bloc resection of a sinus or nasal cavity tumor with intracranial extension. The skull base is repaired using a galeal-pericranial flap.

Reconstruction of maxillectomy defects requires preoperative evaluation by a maxillary prosthodontist. Preoperative dental impressions allow the creation of a prosthesis to be placed at the completion of the case. The sinus defect may be lined with a skin graft and is packed with gauze as the prosthesis is placed. The final result is a sinus defect left open to the oral cavity, allowing local care of the sinus defect and easy visualization of areas at risk for recurrence. The maxillary prosthodontist also plays an important role in postoperative rehabilitation when resections require orbital exenteration or extensive facial resection. Light, pliable, custom-shaded prostheses provide an acceptable appearance in most cases. More complex reconstructive efforts in craniofacial and maxillectomy resections may require microvascular free flaps of skin, muscle, and bone.

Complications after resection of tumors of the nasal cavity and paranasal sinuses vary with the extent of resection. Medial and partial maxillectomies are tolerated quite well in most patients. Maxillectomy with orbital preservation may lead to postoperative diplopia if a large portion of the orbital floor is removed and the globe is left without support. Craniofacial and extensive extracranial resections may be complicated by cerebrospinal fluid leak. These are managed with bed rest and head elevation initially. Depending on the extent of the defect, spontaneous closure may occur, avoiding the need for surgical repair.

Radiation therapy is used in sinus and nasal carcinomas as postoperative adjunctive treatment. Indications for radiotherapy include positive margins or gross residual disease. In maxillectomy defects in which the orbit is left intact, careful treatment planning is required to avoid radiation injury to the globe and optic nerve. This may entail multiple radiation portals to minimize dosing to these structures.

The overall 5-year cure rate for nasal cavity and sinus cancers is 35% to 40%.[47, 48] Improvement in survival by craniofacial resection for ethmoid and nasal cavity tumors has been reported by numerous authors.[49, 50] The majority of patients in these series are treated by a combination of surgery and radiotherapy. A review of radiotherapy alone for nasal, ethmoid, and sphenoid cancers reports a 52% 5-year survival rate, but 33% of patients had unilateral blindness as a complication of treatment.[51] Cervical lymph node metastases occur in 15% of patients and portend a 10% to 15% 5-year survival rate.

The use of chemotherapy in cancers of the paranasal sinuses remains experimental. While major response rates of more than 80% have been reported in some series, long-term survival has not.[52] The use of cisplatin-based chemotherapy and concomitant radiotherapy has shown a 92% complete response rate in a small group of stage IV tumors of the sinus and nasopharynx. A 58% 3-year survival rate was reported for these patients.[53] These early results are excellent, and further study is merited.

Nasopharynx

Radiation is the treatment of choice for nasopharyngeal cancer. Nasopharyngeal cancer is more radiosensitive than other HNSCC sites. Even massive nodal metastases may respond to radiotherapy alone. The role of surgery in nasopharyngeal carcinoma is limited to localized recurrent disease and to procedures, such as the transpalatal approach,[54] allowing access to the nasopharynx for placement of interstitial implants. Results of treatment of nasopharyngeal cancer depend on the proportion of WHO class I lesions included in the report. Five-year survival rates range from 37% to 62%.[55, 56] A report comparing Asian and white populations in British Columbia shows no difference in histologic distribution or survival between these two groups. However, those with keratinizing squamous cell carcinoma had a 20% 5-year survival rate, while those with the nonkeratinizing type had a 44% survival rate.[57]

Oral Cavity

Early oral cavity cancers can be treated with surgical excision with little compromise in speech or swallowing function. The oral cavity has multiple subsites, and several of these subsites merit distinct surgical approaches.

Small primary lip cancers or areas of severe dysplasia may be treated by lip shave with closure, using an advancement of intraoral mucosa. Invasive cancers of the lip require wedge excision in most cases. Primary closure can be performed if the defect is less than one third the length of the lip. Beyond this length, reconstruction may require use of an Abbé-Estlander or Karapandzic flap. Complications of surgical resection of lip cancers may include loss of oral integrity due to denervation or microstomia after extensive resections. Cure rates for lip lesions approach 95%.

Early buccal lesions may be excised perorally. Reconstruction may involve skin grafting or healing by secondary intention. More advanced lesions may extend to involve the cheek skin, mandible, or oral commissure. Resection of these lesions may require composite resection and may include a full-thickness cheek defect. Reconstruction is likely to require free tissue transfer when such a full-thickness defect exists. Early lesions treated by surgery or radiotherapy have similar cure rates, with 40% to 50% recurrence-free survival.[58, 59] Surgical salvage after radiotherapy is associated with survival in more than 50% but may require full-thickness cheek excision, bone resection, and free tissue transfer, depending on the extent of disease.[60] The 5-year cure rates for buccal cancers range from 50% to 75%.

Surgical options in the treatment of oral carcinoma involving the alveolar ridge range from peroral excision with or without marginal mandibulectomy to composite resection with segmental resection of the involved mandible. These lesions have a higher propensity for nodal metastases than lip or buccal lesions. Therefore, these resections are usually performed in conjunction with some type of neck dissection. Overall cure rates for cancers of the alveolar ridge are approximately 60%.

Small floor of mouth lesions may be resected through the open mouth. Larger lesions may require marginal or segmental mandibulectomy (Figs. 1–5 and 1–6). Thickness of the tumor appears to be a better predictor of nodal disease than surface area of the tumor.[25] Tumors less than 1.5 mm in thickness do not require treatment of the neck. With lesions thicker than 1.5 mm and no clinical evidence of nodal metastases, a selective neck dissection may be performed as a staging procedure in order to determine the need for radiotherapy. Larger lesions require neck dissection for the same reason as well as for surgical access. While control rates are similar for radiotherapeutic and surgical treatment of stage I or II floor of mouth cancer, the complication rates after radiotherapy alone are higher.[61] The 5-year cure rates for floor of mouth lesions are 90% and 70% for stage I and II lesions, respectively. Cure rates for higher-stage lesions are 56% to 75% when surgery and radiotherapy combined-modality treatment is given.[61]

The tongue permits resection of small tumors with primary closure with minimal functional deficit. In most cases, this can be performed easily via the mouth. It is desirable to assess tumor depth at the time of excision in order to determine the risk of cervical metastases. Depth greater than 2 to 3 mm merits a supraomohyoid neck dissection to study levels I, II, and III for evidence of nodal metastases.[25]

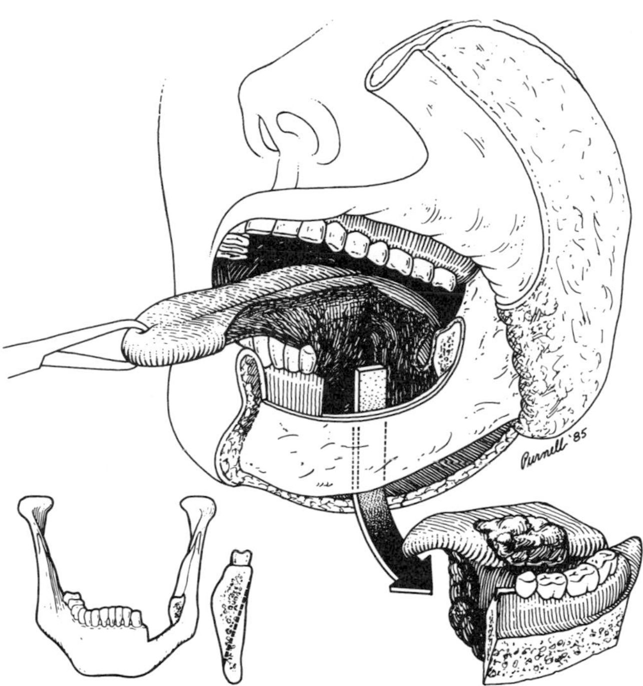

FIGURE 1–5. Diagram of tongue and floor of mouth resection with marginal mandibulectomy. (From Shah JP: Color Atlas of Head and Neck Surgery. Hong Kong: Wolfe Medical Publishing, 1990.)

Decisions regarding the need for postoperative radiotherapy can then be made after assessing the neck pathologically. Other factors that may influence the decision to treat the neck include any evidence of perineural or vascular invasion at the primary site. Each of these factors are reported as indicators of poor survival.[62, 63] T2 and T3 lesions are likely to have nodal metastases in 40% and 70%, respectively. Higher-stage lesions are treated by combined-modality therapy, usually surgery and postoperative radiotherapy. The 5-year overall cure rate is approximately 50%.[64, 65]

Brachytherapy has also been used for cancer of the anterior tongue. While this can provide local control rates in more than 90% of cases, the high doses needed at the primary site by implantation require lower external beam dosing and therefore less radiation to the neck. This has led to failures in the neck in 27%, and the use of brachytherapy has also led to a 13% rate of osteonecrosis.[66] In order to avoid these complications, it is preferable to treat cancer of the anterior tongue with surgical resection, staged neck dissection, and postoperative radiotherapy if indicated.

Hard palate squamous cell carcinomas are rare. While early lesions may be treated by local excision, lesions with bone erosion require surgical approaches similar to those for infrastructure maxillary sinus cancers. These procedures involve a partial palatectomy and require a dental obturator prosthesis.

The use of external beam radiotherapy in the treatment of oral cavity primary lesions is most appropriate as adjunct to surgery for T3 and T4 primary lesions or when gross or microscopic cancer has been left at the site of surgery and re-excision is not possible. As alluded to, external beam radiation and boost to the primary site by implant, reduced-field or intraoral cone provide acceptable control rates in stage I and II cancers of the oral tongue.[67] However, radiotherapy doses of about 70 Gy are required. Radiotherapy to the oral cavity is accompanied by loss of taste and salivary function and raises the risk of osteoradionecrosis of the mandible. The risk of osteoradionecrosis may be increased by preceding or subsequent surgical procedures that devascularize the mandible or by dental extractions, which provide pathways of bacterial invasion. The risk of osteoradionecrosis is close to 20% in some series and argues in favor of surgical treatment for T1 and T2 lesions.[68] Chemotherapy for oral cavity lesions is limited to unresectable and recurrent disease at this time.

Oropharynx

The primary sites of the oropharynx include the soft palate, base of the tongue, tonsil, and pharyngeal wall. The majority of cancers in this region arise in the tonsil. Resection of early lesions at any site within the oropharynx involves more extensive dissection than similarly staged lesions within the oral cavity owing to limited access. Some superficial lesions can be treated by radiotherapy. Advanced lesions are usually treated by surgical resection and postoperative radiotherapy.

The surgical resection used for most base of tongue and tonsillar carcinomas involves a lower-lip–splitting incision.

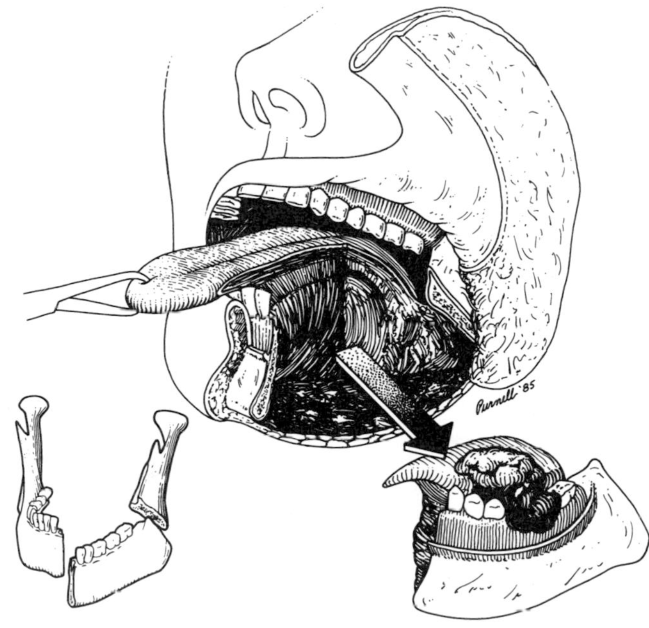

FIGURE 1–6. Diagram of tongue and floor of mouth resection with segmental mandibulectomy. (From Shah JP: Color Atlas of Head and Neck Surgery. Hong Kong: Wolfe Medical Publishing, 1990.)

A paramedian mandibulotomy is then performed, and the mucosal incision is continued along the floor of the mouth to the oropharynx. This allows wide access to the oropharynx without the need to sacrifice a portion of the mandible (Fig. 1–7). Access to tonsillar and lateral tongue base lesions is afforded by this method. In most cases, a neck dissection is done in conjunction with excision of the primary tumor owing to a high incidence of nodal metastases in oropharyngeal cancer. The surgical defect at the site of resection can be repaired by primary closure or may need a myocutaneous pedicled flap or a free flap, depending on the dimensions of the defect.

Radiotherapy is indicated in stage III and IV lesions of the oropharynx following surgical resection or in cases with positive margins. Some T1 and T2 carcinomas can be controlled by radiotherapy alone. When T1 cancer presents with cervical metastases, treatment may involve resection of the primary and neck disease followed by postoperative radiotherapy. However, there is also support for resection of neck disease followed by radiotherapy to control the primary disease.[69] This requires prompt initiation of radiotherapy after neck dissection to avoid progression of disease at the primary site. Careful case selection is advised for such a treatment approach.

Radiotherapy and surgery both give survival rates of 80% to 90% for stage I and II tonsillar cancer.[70] Higher-stage tonsillar cancer requires combined-modality treatment, which offers a 53% 5-year survival rate with surgery and postoperative radiotherapy. The use of primary radiotherapy with surgical salvage gives a similar survival rate.[70] However, surgical resection after full-course radiation is technically more difficult and is associated with an increased risk of complications. Radiotherapy alone is associated with a 29% survival rate.[71]

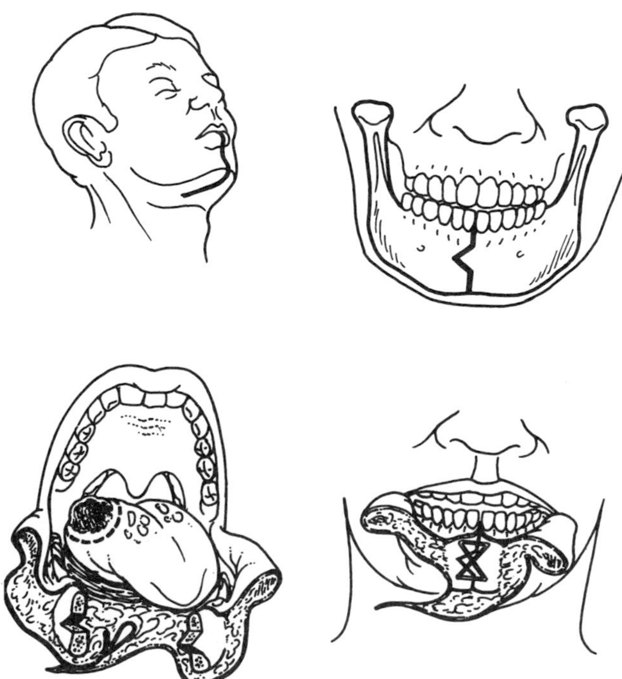

FIGURE 1–7. Diagram showing technique for midline mandibulotomy. Recent modifications include moving most osteotomies to a paramedian position and the increased use of miniplates for repair.

Brachytherapy has an emerging role in the treatment of disease of the base of the tongue. This treatment plan involves external beam radiotherapy to the primary and cervical nodes to a dose of 5000 cGy, followed by neck dissection if the neck was initially positive and implantation of afterloading catheters into the base of the tongue. The boost to the primary site is 2000 to 3000 cGy. Local control and cure rates are reported to be greater than 80%.[72]

Chemotherapy for oropharyngeal cancer has a role in recurrent and unresectable disease and is discussed later. Another role for chemotherapy is in base of tongue disease in which resection would require laryngectomy. This situation arises when a near-total resection of the base of the tongue is required. The loss of the ability to prevent aspiration may necessitate laryngectomy. Induction chemotherapy with cisplatin and 5-fluorouracil is followed by reassessment and radiotherapy if a complete response is noted. This regimen has resulted in a major response in excess of 70% and avoidance of surgery to the tongue. Although no controlled trial has been reported, the 5-year survival rate in this single-arm trial is 42% and compares well with historical controls.[36]

Overall cure rates in patients with oropharyngeal cancer are about 40%. Stage I and II cancers of the oropharynx have a 50% to 60% 5-year survival rate after radiotherapy with surgical salvage.[73, 74] Lesions requiring combined treatment have a 46% 5-year survival rate.[75]

Approach to the Mandible

Cancers of the oral cavity and oropharynx may require attention to the mandible during resection. This may range from mandibulotomy to marginal mandibulectomy to segmental mandibulectomy. Mandibulotomy is useful for obtaining access to the oropharynx for base of tongue or tonsil resections and may occasionally be required in select oral cavity lesions. The mandibulotomy may be placed in the midline, paramedial, or lateral mandible. However, the proximity of the medial incisor roots in most individuals places these teeth in jeopardy if midline mandibulotomy is performed. A major drawback to lateral mandibulotomy is that the bone cut will likely lie in a previous or future radiation portal. For these reasons, the paramedian mandibulotomy is preferred and is usually placed between the lateral incisor and the canine teeth.

Marginal or segmental mandibulectomy is most often considered for gingival, floor of mouth, retromolar trigone, and select buccal and tongue lesions. The decision to perform mandibulectomy is made after clinical assessment of the lesion, with additional information obtained from Panorex films. CT scans are usually not helpful in assessing mandibular invasion.[76] Gross or radiologic involvement of the mandible requires segmental mandibulectomy. In most cases appropriate for marginal mandibulectomy, Panorex films show no erosion of the mandible, and bone resection is performed in order to obtain an adequate margin at the mandibular periosteum. Occasionally, minimal scalloping of the cortex of the mandible may be addressed by marginal mandibulectomy. Closure of the intraoral defect after marginal mandibulectomy may be performed primarily, by placement of a skin graft or by secondary intention.[77]

Reconstruction options for defects left after segmental mandibulectomy have ranged from primary closure without bone reconstruction, to pedicle flap closure of the soft tissue defects with mandibular arch reconstruction using a metal bar or free bone grafts, to microvascular composite graft using fibula or partial thickness of the radius. Primary closure is acceptable in patients who are medically unfit for free flap reconstruction. Nonvascularized mandibular arch reconstruction is not advisable, as free bone tends to resorb over time and metal reconstruction bars extrude as overlying soft tissue retracts with time.

The advantages to microvascular reconstruction include increased tolerance to radiation therapy, presumed resistance to osteoradionecrosis, and improved cosmesis over metal plates or primary closure. Anterior arch defects, in particular, require microvascular free flap reconstruction in order to maximize function and cosmesis. Defects of the body of the mandible also warrant consideration for microvascular reconstruction. Isolated defects of the ramus may require reconstruction in selected circumstances. The technique of fibular free flap reconstruction of the mandible is eloquently discussed by Hidalgo.[78]

Hypopharynx

Hypopharyngeal cancers tend to be asymptomatic until they reach an advanced stage. Fifty percent of lesions present with cervical lymph node metastases. Pyriform sinus lesions may grow laterally into the neck, such that the primary lesion itself is palpable. The advanced stage at presentation seen with hypopharyngeal lesions requires combined-modality treatment.

The surgical options for the treatment of hypopharyngeal lesions are rarely conservative and voice sparing. A few carefully selected lesions may be amenable to either partial pharyngectomy or partial laryngopharyngectomy. The majority of cases require laryngopharyngectomy. This procedure entails a total laryngectomy with a variable pharyngectomy component. Reconstruction of noncircumferential pharyngeal wall defects can be performed with a patch myocutaneous pedicled flap or a thin microvascular free flap such as the radial forearm flap. When there is circumferential involvement of the pharynx, the resection involves removal of the larynx as well as the entire hypopharynx. Reconstruction of the circumferential defect requires use of a jejunal free flap. Extension of the lesion to the cervical esophagus may require total laryngopharyngoesophagectomy and gastric transposition with pharyngogastrostomy. Neck dissection should be performed in conjunction with the resection of hypopharyngeal lesions whether or not disease is clinically palpable. The high incidence of nodal metastases in hypopharyngeal lesions warrants this approach.

Radiotherapy is useful for early lesions of the hypopharynx or for advanced disease as a postoperative adjunctive treatment. Brachytherapy has no established role in hypopharyngeal cancer. Chemotherapy has been used in an attempt at larynx preservation. However, the results of preservation in this subgroup are not as promising as those for lesions of the intrinsic larynx.[79] The cure rate of advanced lesions of the hypopharynx is only 28% at 5 years.

Larynx

Hoarseness is caused by minimal surface alteration of the true vocal cord, and this leads to early discovery of glottic carcinomas in many individuals. This early detection combined with sparse lymphatics and resulting low likelihood of cervical metastases makes early laryngeal cancer amenable to single-modality therapy with excellent results. Surgical options include endoscopic excision with or without carbon dioxide laser for small lesions of the mid–vocal cord. More extensive glottic lesions can be treated using vertical hemilaryngectomy. However, most are treated with external beam radiotherapy, with surgery used for residual or recurrent disease. Cure rates for early glottic cancer are greater than 90% for either treatment modality.[80, 81]

Early lesions of the supraglottic larynx are less likely to cause hoarseness than glottic lesions. For this reason, and because supraglottic cancers are more likely to have cervical metastases, supraglottic tumors are less often detected at an early stage. Surgery for early supraglottic cancers involves supraglottic (horizontal) partial laryngectomy, removing the false vocal folds, epiglottis, and aryepiglottic folds. This surgery preserves a relatively normal voice. However, supraglottic partial laryngectomy should be performed in carefully selected patients, as there are risks of pulmonary compromise owing to aspiration. Chronic aspiration or the need for long-term nutritional support may occur in a small percentage of patients. With these provisos, recurrence-free survival is excellent and has been reported to be greater than 90% in several studies.[82, 83]

External beam radiotherapy is also effective in controlling primary disease in early supraglottic cancer. Control with radiotherapy appears to be slightly less than with surgery, but selection bias may play a role when comparing different studies. Stage I and II supraglottic cancers (i.e., node negative, small lesions) have cure rates greater than 70% with radiotherapy alone.[84] In selected cases, supraglottic laryngectomy may be integrated into a combined treatment modality consisting of partial laryngectomy with or without neck dissection followed by postoperative radiotherapy. This has been associated with a 2-year survival rate and local-regional control in greater than 90% in a group of patients with cancer that varied from stage I to stage IV.[85]

Failure in the neck is associated with a 40% survival rate and argues for considering treatment to the neck in all cases of supraglottic cancer.[84] Early-stage supraglottic cancers treated with radiotherapy should include the cervical lymphatics. When early-stage supraglottic cancers are treated with surgery, decisions about postoperative radiotherapy can be made after surgery if selective neck dissection of levels II, III, and IV is performed to provide pathologic staging of the neck.

Advanced lesions of the larynx may be treated surgically with total laryngectomy. Primary closure of the pharyngeal mucosa is possible unless extensive portions of the pharyngeal mucosa are resected. Ipsilateral thyroid lobectomy should be included in the resection when primary lesions involve the subglottic larynx or pyriform sinus apex. Neck dissection would be indicated in most cases proceeding to laryngectomy. In cases without palpable adenopathy, cervical lymph nodes may be assessed using an anterolateral selective neck dissection (levels II, III, and IV) for staging.

Radiotherapy has a role as postoperative adjunctive treatment in advanced laryngeal cancer. Combined treatment using surgery and radiotherapy is associated with 60% survival rates in patients with stage III and IV laryngeal cancer.[41] While radiotherapy alone has been used in advanced lesions in an effort to avoid laryngectomy,[81] standard care remains surgery followed by postoperative radiotherapy.

Recent trends in the treatment of advanced laryngeal carcinoma have investigated the use of induction chemotherapy followed by radiotherapy to avoid total laryngectomy and allow preservation of laryngeal function. It was in this setting that a multi-institutional randomized Department of Veterans Affairs study was performed that compared larynx preservation and survival between a group treated with induction chemotherapy using cisplatin and 5-fluorouracil followed by radiotherapy in responders and a group treated with surgery and postoperative radiotherapy. Eighty-five percent of patients had a complete or partial response to chemotherapy and therefore went on to receive radiotherapy. At 2-year follow-up, no survival advantage was shown for either group (68% in both groups), and laryngectomy was avoided in 64% of the chemotherapy and radiotherapy group.[35]

Alternative Treatments in Head and Neck Cancer

New dosing schedules in radiotherapy and concomitant radiotherapy and chemotherapy are under investigation in the treatment of HNSCC. Hyperfractioned radiotherapy is associated with greater acute toxicity to normal tissues, but an improvement in 3-year disease-free survival rate, from 30% to 60%, has been shown in stage III and IV cancers.[86] Unfortunately, acute toxicity, such as mucositis, often leads to treatment interruptions. When these interruptions cause delays in the completion of treatment greater than 5 days, local control is compromised.[87] This has prevented widespread adoption of b.i.d. radiotherapy, but protocols utilizing b.i.d. radiotherapy continue to be investigated.

The use of concomitant radiotherapy and cisplatin-based chemotherapy has shown impressive control rates in a series of stage III and IV head and neck cancers. Complete response was 89% for primary tumors and 78% for nodal disease. At 19 months follow-up, 66% had no evidence of disease.[88] In support of this treatment modality, when surgical resection follows concomitant chemotherapy and radiotherapy, more than 80% showed no evidence of tumor. The 5-year survival rate for patients treated using this modality is reported to be 55%.[89] These recent data appear promising, and further investigation is merited.

Recurrent and Incurable Disease—Results and Complications

The treatment of disease that is recurrent depends on the previous treatment given. If a recurrence at the primary site occurring after surgical excision is amenable to complete resection, it is the preferred treatment. This is true whether radiotherapy or chemotherapy or both have been given previously, as long as the initial presentation of disease was resectable. Disease that is initially unresectable that recurs after nonsurgical therapy is unlikely to warrant surgical treatment because it is not possible to define the extent of resection required.

Primary or recurrent cancer of the head and neck may be deemed unresectable owing to involvement of surrounding vital structures. Relative contraindications to surgery include (1) invasion of the skull base, (2) disease involving the common or internal carotid arteries, (3) disease invading the prevertebral fascia. Unresectable recurrent disease in an area that has not previously received radiation may be treated by radiotherapy alone. This is most useful for small-volume disease. Massive recurrent disease or unresectable primary disease is often treated with a combination of chemotherapy and radiation. Current trials are exploring the use of radiotherapy with a concomitant radiosensitizing agent such as cisplatin or mitomycin.

When radiotherapy has previously been given to the area of unresectable disease, this option is no longer available. Chemotherapeutic options include single-agent chemotherapy and combinations of chemotherapeutic agents. The most active agents are methotrexate, cisplatin, 5-fluorouracil, bleomycin, and vinblastine. Response rates for weekly methotrexate infusion range from 8% to 57%.[90] Unfortunately, the duration of response is short (median, 2 to 4 months). Response rates for other single-agent therapies are no better than methotrexate and often involve more serious side effects. Combinations of chemotherapeutic agents have been associated with improved response rates, but duration of response and survival are not improved.[90, 91]

Because of the palliative nature of treatment for unresectable disease, indications for treatment usually revolve around tumor-related symptoms. Also, palliative treatment should not increase patient morbidity if possible, so outpatient treatment of low toxicity is preferred. For this reason, single-agent methotrexate is usually the treatment of choice for symptomatic, unresectable, previously radiated disease. Other agents may be given if disease fails to respond or resistance to methotrexate develops.

Post-treatment Care and Surveillance

Close and long-term follow-up of patients with HNSCC is essential. This is done to detect any evidence of recurrent disease at the earliest possible stage and also because these patients have a significant risk of second primary lesions of the upper aerodigestive tract, esophagus, and lungs owing to the chronic exposure of these areas to alcohol and tobacco. A meta-analysis of more than 40,000 patients with HNSCC shows a prevalence of a second primary lesion in 14.2%. The site of second primary lesions is head and neck in 35%, lung in 25%, and esophagus in 9%. The remaining lesions are at sites outside the upper aerodigestive tract.[92]

The incidence of a second primary lesion is not influenced by whether radiotherapy was used to treat the first primary cancer.[93] However, survival after appearance of a second primary lesion is significantly shorter in patients whose first cancer was treated with radiotherapy.[94] Whether this represents a survival advantage in patients who can still tolerate radiotherapy for the second primary lesion or points to a more aggressive biologic behavior in cancers developing in previously irradiated fields is not clear. Survival following second primary cancers at 2 and 5 years are reported to be 32% and 10%, respectively.[95]

Follow-up surveillance for HNSCC patients is by history, thorough head and neck examinations, and serial chest radiographs. Clinic visits should be scheduled every month for the first year after treatment, every 2 months for the second year, and then quarterly and later semiannually. Chest radiographs should be performed yearly. Examination under anesthesia with endoscopy should be considered if the clinical examination is inadequate to address any symptoms.

Secondary Tumors

Metastases from cancers of the head and neck are most often seen in the lungs. Metastases to bone, liver, and other sites are less common. The treatment of metastatic lesions begins with a careful determination that they are in fact metastases. The high incidence of second primary cancers noted previously should be considered when evaluating lung lesions, since 25% to 40% of second primary cancers after HNSCC arise in the lungs.[92, 96] While the presence of multiple lung lesions is consistent with metastases, a single lung nodule may be primary or metastatic disease. When in doubt, the lung lesion should be treated as a second primary lesion and evaluated for resection. This approach gives the patient the best chance of cure if it truly is a second primary lesion and not metastatic disease. The cure rate after resection of isolated pulmonary nodules in HNSCC patients is about 40%.[97]

Prevention

Prevention for any cancer begins with the control of those factors that increase risk of cancer development. When a disease is caused by genetic factors, little can be done to control exposure. However, with HNSCC, the predominant risk factors are tobacco and alcohol exposure. Limiting exposure to these substances can reduce the risk of HNSCC. Unfortunately, efforts to control these exposures are not particularly successful. Smoking-cessation programs use a number of approaches, including transdermal nicotine, biofeedback, hypnosis, and psychotherapy to attempt to control tobacco addiction. Alcoholics Anonymous remains an effective organization in keeping alcohol addiction under control. Both of these addictions should be actively addressed in any patient with symptoms suspicious for malignancy or with proven HNSCC. Early intervention may reduce the risk of progression to malignancy or development of second primary cancers. Other preventive strategies may arise in the future as more is learned about the risk of HPV infection or dietary factors in the development of HNSCC. At this time, however, our ability to intervene in the pathogenesis of HNSCC depends on effective programs to reduce alcohol and tobacco exposure.

Trials involving vitamin A and vitamin E analogues have shown promise in controlling preneoplastic mucosal disease.[98, 99] In patients previously treated for HNSCC, protocols are under way that attempt to prevent second primary cancers by treating with vitamin A analogues. *Cis*-retinoic acid treatment has been associated with a lower incidence of second primary cancers.[100] However, a high toxicity to *cis*-retinoic acid has prevented its routine use on all HNSCC patients. Current protocols using lower doses of *cis*-retinoic acid are being evaluated in an attempt to maintain efficacy while reducing toxicity.

Future Prospects

Future prospects in the treatment of head and neck cancer can be seen on several fronts. Our ability to perform highly technical surgical procedures is always improving, but progress in this area is approaching a plateau. Likewise, a number of radiotherapy and chemotherapy treatment delivery and dosing options have been investigated, and more will be designed. However, the likelihood that variations in radiotherapy or traditional chemotherapy will cause a substantial improvement in the treatment of HNSCC is small. New treatment modalities will require further understanding of the immunobiology and molecular biology of cancer in general and HNSCC in particular. Through the use of cytokines, antibodies to cancer cell surface molecules, or cancer cell gene transfection, more cancer-specific therapy may be developed. This remains elusive in HNSCC, but substantial improvements in treatment and survival may depend on this technology.

SALIVARY GLAND NEOPLASMS

Malignant tumors of the salivary glands are rare, accounting for about 7% of all tumors of the head and neck, with an incidence of approximately 1 in 100,000 per year.[101] A review of the tumor registry at Memorial Sloan-Kettering Cancer Center yielded 3786 salivary gland neoplasms over a 44-year period.[102] Sixty-five percent were in the parotid gland, 8% in the submandibular gland, and 27% in the minor salivary glands. Only 25% of the parotid tumors were malignant, while nearly 50% of the tumors of the submandibular gland and 81% of the tumors of the minor salivary glands were malignant (Table 1–2).

The etiology of the vast majority of salivary gland cancers remains obscure. Familial clustering of salivary cancers suggests a genetic predisposition to the disease.[103, 104] In addition, the incidence of salivary cancers is increased in patients exposed to ionizing radiation, either for therapeutic reasons[105] or as a result of the atomic bomb explosion at Hiroshima.[106] An increased incidence of salivary gland neoplasms of the nasal cavity and paranasal sinuses appears to be related to wood dust exposure in furniture workers.[107]

Anatomy

The salivary glands consist of a network of both major and minor glands. The major glands are composed of the paired parotid, submandibular, and sublingual glands. The minor salivary glands are small, predominantly mucous glands that are ubiquitous within the submucosa of the upper aerodigestive tract.

The parotid gland is the largest of the salivary glands and weighs approximately 25 g. It is wedged between the mandible and the sternomastoid and overlies both of these structures. The gland lies just inferior to the cartilaginous external auditory canal, the temporomandibular joint, and the zygoma. It is bounded from below by the posterior belly of the digastric muscle, and posteriorly it abuts the sternocleidomastoid muscle. Anteriorly it wraps around the posterior border of the ascending ramus of the mandible, lying over the masseter muscle laterally and over the medial pterygoid muscle on the medial aspect of the mandible. Medially, the gland is adjacent to the parapharyngeal space. The facial nerve, posterior facial vein, and external carotid artery traverse the gland. The parotid duct (of Stensen) arises from the anterior part of the gland and runs over the masseter a fingerbreadth below the zygomatic arch to pierce the buccinator and open through the buccal mucosa opposite the second upper molar tooth.

TABLE 1–2
Distribution of Salivary Neoplasms

	Percent Distribution of All Neoplasms	Percent Malignant
Parotid	65	25
Submandibular gland	8	50
Minor salivary gland	27	81

From Shah JP, Ihde JK: Salivary gland tumors. Curr Probl Surg 27:775–883, 1990. Data from Memorial Sloan-Kettering Cancer Center tumor registry.

The anatomy of the facial nerve is of particular importance to the surgeon operating on the parotid gland. The facial nerve emerges from the stylomastoid foramen and passes laterally around the styloid process. The main trunk of the nerve can be located at the confluence of three structures; the superior aspect of the posterior belly of the digastric muscle, the tip of the mastoid process, and the bony auditory canal. Just beyond this point, the nerve dives into the substance of the parotid gland and bifurcates into its two main divisions. The upper division then further branches into the temporal and zygomatic branches, and the lower division branches into the buccal, mandibular, and cervical branches. Within the substance of the parotid gland, the facial nerve forms a plexus of intermingling connections. There are no actual lobes defined by fascial planes, but the part of the gland located superficial to the facial nerve is designated the superficial lobe (80% of the gland), and the gland deep to the nerve is designated the deep lobe (20% of the gland).

The submandibular gland lies within the submandibular triangle in the neck. It is wedged between the mandible and the mylohyoid and hyoglossus muscles above, and it overlaps the digastric muscle below. Posteriorly it lies adjacent to the parotid gland. Superficial to the gland is the platysma muscle and the marginal mandibular branch of the facial nerve, which courses over the fascia of the gland. The submandibular duct (Wharton's duct) runs forward beneath the mucosa of the floor of the mouth and opens just to the side of the frenulum linguae.

The sublingual gland is the smallest of the paired salivary glands and lies in the immediate submucosal plane of the floor of the mouth just anterior to the submandibular gland. The gland lies just lateral to the lingual nerve and the submandibular duct. It opens by a series of tiny ducts into the floor of the mouth.

Pathology

The same group of neoplasms affects all salivary tissues, but the proportional distribution of each neoplasm differs depending on the gland involved (Table 1–3).[108]

Benign Tumors

Benign Mixed Tumor (Pleomorphic Adenoma). This is the most common tumor arising in the major salivary

TABLE 1–3
Histologic Classification and Incidence of Benign and Malignant Tumors of the Salivary Glands

Benign	Malignant
Pleomorphic adenoma (45.4%)	Mucoepidermoid carcinoma (15.7%)
Warthin's tumor	Low grade
Lymphoepithelial lesion (0.6%)	High grade
Oncocytoma (0.7%)	Adenoid cystic carcinoma (10%)
Monomorphic adenoma (0.2%)	Adenocarcinoma (8%)
Benign cyst (1%)	Acinic cell carcinoma (3%)
	Malignant mixed tumor (5.7%)
	Epidermoid carcinoma (1.9%)
	Other carcinomas (1.3%)

From Spiro RH: Salivary neoplasms: Overview of a 35-year experience with 2,807 patients. Head Neck Surg 8:177–184, 1986. Data from Memorial Sloan-Kettering Cancer Center tumor registry.

glands[109] and accounts for 81% of benign parotid gland tumors.[110] The term pleomorphic adenoma refers to the various histologic components of the tumor, including myxoid, mucoid, chondroid, fibroid, and other elements.

The natural history of the tumor is one of slow growth and relative lack of symptoms. Although the tumor can grow to large proportions, facial nerve dysfunction is rare unless malignant transformation has occurred. Local recurrence is common following inadequate resection,[111] and approximately 2% to 6% of lesions undergo malignant transformation.[112, 113]

Warthin's Tumor (Papillary Cystadenoma Lymphomatosum). This tumor occurs almost exclusively in the parotid gland and accounts for approximately 14% of benign parotid tumors.[114] About 10% of the tumors are bilateral, and about 10% are multifocal. There is an approximate risk of malignant transformation of 0.3%.[115]

Monomorphic Adenoma. Monomorphic adenomas are rare benign tumors involving the parotid gland and minor salivary glands of the upper lip. They represent less than 1% of benign salivary tumors[114] and present as asymptomatic, slow-growing masses. As their name indicates, histologically they have a uniform epithelial pattern.

Oncocytoma. These rare tumors account for less than 1% of all salivary gland tumors. They are slow growing but tend to invade surrounding structures.[116]

Benign Lymphoepithelial Lesions. Originally described as a feature of autoimmune diseases,[117] these lesions are being recognized with increasing frequency in patients with human immunodeficiency virus (HIV). They are thought to represent HIV infection in parotid lymph nodes and are treated with observation alone.[118]

Malignant Tumors

Mucoepidermoid Carcinoma. This tumor represents 44% of the parotid gland cancers, 30% of submandibular gland cancers, and 25% of minor salivary gland cancers.[110] It arises from the salivary duct epithelium and is usually classified according to histologic differentiation as either low, intermediate, or high grade. In general, grade correlates with the degree of aggressiveness. High-grade tumors can invade the facial nerve and cause fixation. On presentation, about half of patients with high-grade tumors have lymph node metastases and about a third of patients have distant metastases.[111, 119]

Malignant Mixed Tumor. This tumor accounts for about 17% of parotid, 19% of submandibular, and 6% of minor salivary gland cancers.[110] The clinical picture is often one of slow growth over many years with a recent history of rapid growth. Many appear to originate in pleomorphic adenomas. Approximately 25% of patients present with involvement of regional lymph nodes.[120] Distant metastases to liver, lung, brain, and bone occur in approximately 30% of cases.

Adenoid Cystic Carcinoma. Adenoid cystic carcinoma makes up about a third of all salivary gland cancers and accounts for about 10% of parotid malignancies.[110] It is characterized by its unpredictable behavior, which is due to local extension beyond apparent gross tumor. It also has a propensity for perineural invasion, adversely affecting local control and survival.[121] Distant metastases occur in almost half of patients.[122] These are predominantly to the lung, where they have a very slow growth rate.

Adenocarcinoma. Adenocarcinomas account for 10% of parotid, 7% of submandibular, and 29% of minor salivary gland malignancies.[110] They commonly affect the minor salivary glands of the nose and paranasal sinuses. The grade of these tumors appears to correlate with outcome.

Squamous Cell Carcinoma. This tumor accounts for less than 10% of all salivary gland malignancies.[110] It must be differentiated from metastases to intra- and periparotid nodes and nodes around the submandibular gland. The tumor is probably derived from duct epithelium. Lymph node metastases occur in about half of patients, and local recurrence is common following resection.[123]

Other Malignant Tumors. Acinic cell carcinoma is a rare tumor mainly affecting the parotid gland. They are generally low grade, and prognosis is good.[124] Undifferentiated carcinomas are fortunately rare but are very aggressive tumors that have a high incidence of lymph node metastases and a very poor prognosis.[125]

Diagnosis and Staging

Physical examination is the most important tool in the diagnosis of salivary malignancies. With regard to the major salivary glands, a hard, fixed mass suggests a malignant process. In addition, facial nerve palsy in the presence of a parotid mass almost always results from a malignancy. Fine-needle aspiration can be helpful in confirming the diagnosis of a malignancy, but a negative finding does not rule out the presence of a cancer.[126] Minor salivary gland cancers are usually diagnosed by biopsy.

CT and MRI scans can be helpful in the diagnosis of both major and minor salivary malignancies. Although they are not necessary for the evaluation of all lesions, they are indispensable in the evaluation of tumors involving the deep lobe of the parotid gland, which are generally not accessible to clinical examination. In addition, CT scanning can be very helpful in the evaluation of minor salivary tumors of the nasal cavity and paranasal sinuses.

Minor salivary gland cancers are staged according to the staging system used for squamous cell cancers depending on each individual site. The staging system for major salivary gland cancers is given in Table 1–4.

Primary Operable Disease

In general, surgical resection is the treatment of choice for salivary gland tumors. Surgical excision should be combined with additional adjuvant radiation therapy for specific indications.

Parotid Gland

The diagnosis of a parotid gland malignancy is usually made at the time of excision of the part of the gland in which the tumor lies. Enucleation of parotid tumors, even when combined with postoperative radiation therapy, is associated with an excessive long-term recurrence rate.[127] In addition, adequate excision of a parotid neoplasm requires the careful identification of the facial nerve and its branches, which are embedded in the gland. For this reason, parotid surgery has been equated with surgery of the facial nerve. Most tumors are located in the superficial lobe of the gland, and excision of that portion of the gland superficial to the plane of the nerve is all that is necessary. Tumors involving the deep lobe of the gland can be approached in a similar fashion. After excision of the superficial lobe and careful identification of the facial nerve, the nerve branches are retracted and the deep lobe containing the tumor is excised. Rare situations necessitate the use of a submandibular approach to the deep lobe of the gland or even the use of a mandibulotomy approach to the parapharyngeal space. With the use of three-dimensional imaging studies, these rare situations can be identified preoperatively.

There has been a trend toward conservatism with respect to the management of the facial nerve in parotid surgery.[128] In general, the nerve can be preserved unless grossly infiltrated by tumor. Occasionally, the nerve is adherent to a malignant tumor, necessitating its careful dissection off the tumor. In such situations, postoperative radiation therapy is warranted. When the main trunk or major branches of the nerve are sacrificed, immediate grafting of the nerve is indicated, provided that tumor-free proximal and distal nerve ends are available. Reconstruction of the nerve is usually accomplished with the use of cable interposition grafts from the cervical plexus or the sural nerve. Successful grafting with the return of most nerve function is accomplished in the majority of patients.[129]

TABLE 1–4
American Joint Committee on Cancer Staging System for Major Salivary Cancer*

Primary Tumor

T0	No evidence of primary tumor
T1	Tumor 2 cm or less in greatest dimension
T2	Tumor more than 2 cm but not more than 4 cm in greatest dimension
T3	Tumor more than 4 cm but not more than 6 cm in greatest dimension
T4	Tumor more than 6 cm in greatest dimension
	Note: All categories are subdivided: (a) no local extension, (b) local extension, defined as clinical evidence of skin, soft tissue, bone, or nerve invasion.

Lymph Nodes

N0	No regional lymph node metastasis
N1	Metastasis in a single ipsilateral lymph node, 3 cm or less in greatest dimension
N2a	Metastasis in a single ipsilateral lymph node more than 3 cm but not more than 6 cm in greatest dimension
N2b	Metastasis in multiple ipsilateral lymph nodes, none more than 6 cm in greatest dimension
N2c	Metastasis in bilateral or contralateral lymph nodes, none more than 6 cm in greatest dimension

Distant Metastasis

M0	No distant metastasis
M1	Distant metastasis

Stage Grouping

Stage I	T1a	N0	M0
	T2a	N0	M0
Stage II	T1b	N0	M0
	T2b	N0	M0
	T3a	N0	M0
Stage III	T3b	N0	M0
	T4a	N0	M0
	Any T (except T4b)	N1	M0
Stage IV	T4b	Any N	M0
	Any T	N2, N3	M0
	Any T	Any N	M1

*1988 revision.

Submandibular Glands

Adequate therapy for tumors of the submandibular gland usually requires en bloc resection of the contents of the submandibular triangle.[130] Mandibular resection should be considered for those patients with adherent tumors. Large or extensively infiltrating tumors often require resection of adjacent nerves and muscle, including the lingual and hypoglossal nerves and the digastric and mylohyoid muscles, in addition to the adjacent floor of the mouth.

Minor Salivary Glands

Surgical management of salivary gland neoplasms varies depending on the site involved. In general, resection should be similar to that required for the management of squamous cancers of the same site.

Cervical Lymph Nodes

With the exception of high-grade mucoepidermoid carcinoma and primary squamous cell carcinoma, the incidence of cervical lymph node metastases in patients with malig-

TABLE 1–5
Cervical Lymph Node Involvement in Salivary Gland Carcinoma

Time of Appearance	Parotid (%) (N = 623)	Submandibular (%) (N = 129)	Minor (%) (N = 526)
Initially	20	33	13
Subsequently	5	4	9
Total	25	37	22

Derived from Shah JP, Ihde JK: Salivary gland tumors. Curr Probl Surg 27:775–883, 1990.

nant salivary neoplasms is relatively low (Table 1–5).[110] Therefore, a selective approach to the management of cervical lymph nodes is justified. For patients with clinically positive cervical lymph nodes, neck dissection is mandatory. In addition, patients with high-stage or high-grade tumors are candidates for elective node dissections. In the absence of gross or histologic lymph node involvement, the dissection can be modified to excise selectively only those lymph node levels at highest risk for metastatic involvement (levels I, II, and III).

Adjunctive and Alternative Therapy

Radiation Therapy

The indications for the use of adjuvant radiation therapy in the management of salivary gland neoplasms are not absolute. Proposed indications include those situations in which a potentially high rate of recurrence can be diminished with the use of radiotherapy and include the following: positive margins, advanced tumor stage, high-grade histology, deep lobe involvement, positive neck nodes, and tumor spillage at the time of surgery.[131–134] Radiotherapy using fast neutrons for advanced salivary gland malignancy shows early promising results with improved local control, meriting further investigation.[135]

Chemotherapy

Chemotherapy has a minimal role in the treatment of primary salivary gland malignancy and is utilized as palliative treatment in the management of recurrent or metastatic tumors. A number of agents, including doxorubicin-5, fluorouracil, methotrexate, cyclophosphamide, and cisplatin, have demonstrated responses when used either alone or in combination.[136] Complete responses are unfortunately rare, and response durations are relatively short.

Results

A number of factors are important determinants of outcome, including the following: tumor stage, grade, site, and histologic subtype.

Stage

Stage is the most important prognostic factor in all salivary neoplasms.[114, 137] The overall 10-year survival rate for stage I tumors is approximately 90%; for stage II, 65%; and for stage III, 22% (Fig. 1–8).[114]

Grade

Grade clearly has an impact on survival regardless of specific histologic diagnosis (see Fig. 1–8).[114] The 10-year survival rate of patients with low-grade tumors approaches

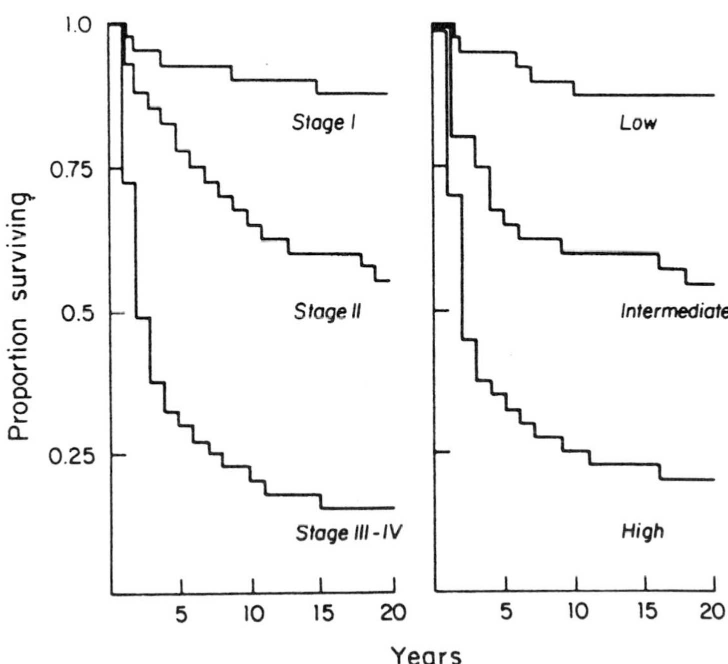

FIGURE 1–8. Survival from salivary cancer by tumor stage and grade. (From Spiro RH: Salivary neoplasms: Overview of a 35-year experience with 2,807 patients. Head Neck Surg 8:177–184, 1986.)

90%, while that of patients with high-grade tumors is only about 25%.

Site

Site of origin of salivary neoplasms clearly has an impact on survival. In general, submandibular gland tumors are considered to be more aggressive than parotid tumors. In addition, minor salivary tumors located in places that are less accessible to clinical examination (i.e., sinuses and larynx) carry a worse prognosis (Fig. 1–9).[114]

Histology

Survival is significantly influenced by the histology of the tumor.[137] It is better in those patients with acinic or low-grade mucoepidermoid carcinoma than in those with adenocarcinoma, malignant mixed tumor, high-grade mucoepidermoid carcinoma, squamous carcinoma, or adenoid cystic carcinoma (Fig. 1–10).

THYROID CANCER

Thyroid cancer affects about 13,000 people a year in the United States; just less than 10% die as a result of the disease.[138] The true incidence of subclinical thyroid cancer is probably much higher. Studies of patients dying of other causes demonstrate occult thyroid cancer in up to 13% of routine autopsies.[139]

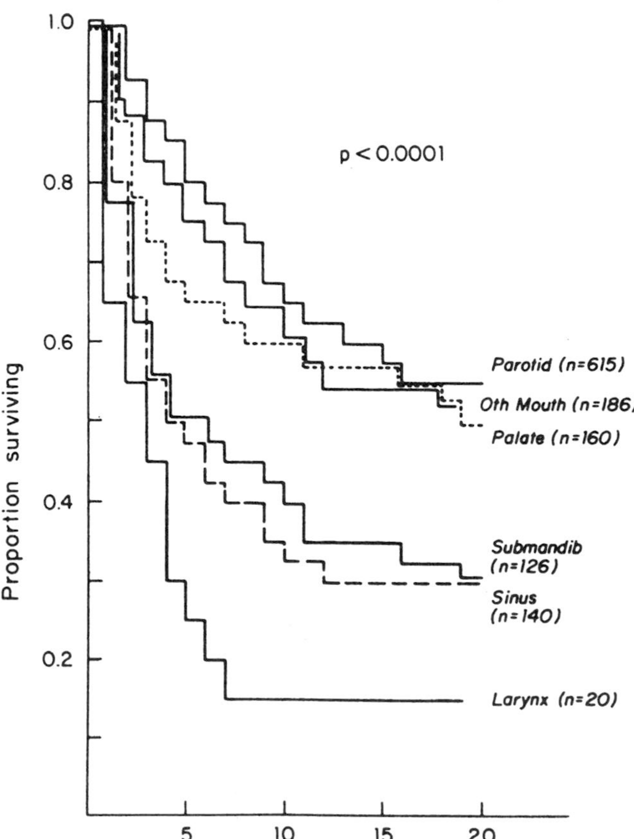

FIGURE 1–9. Survival from salivary cancer by primary site. (From Spiro RH: Salivary neoplasms: Overview of a 35-year experience with 2,807 patients. Head Neck Surg 8:177–184, 1986.)

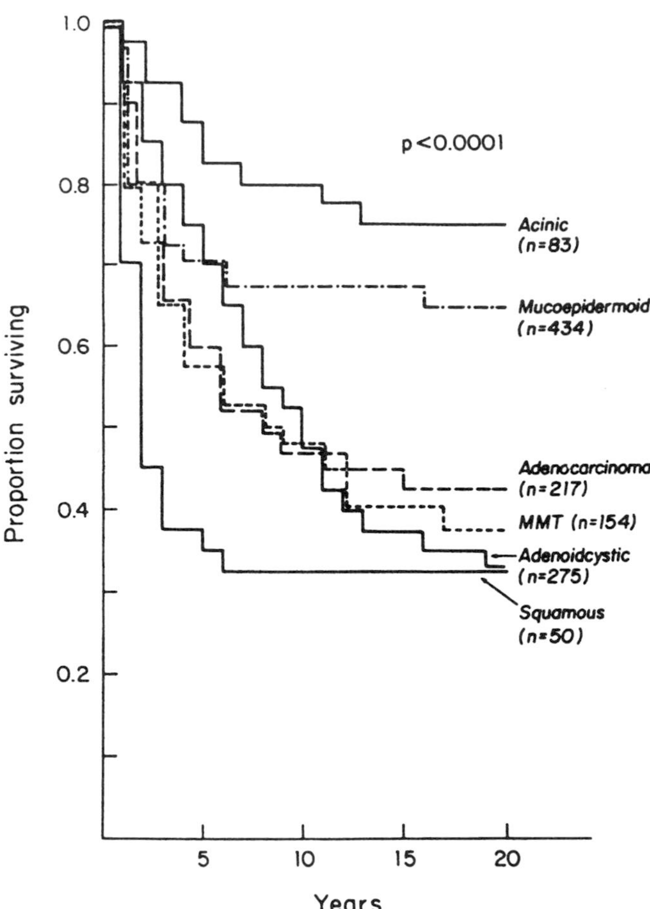

FIGURE 1–10. Survival from salivary cancer by tumor histology. MMT, Malignant mixed tumor. (From Spiro RH: Salivary neoplasms: Overview of a 35-year experience with 2,807 patients. Head Neck Surg 8:177–184, 1986.)

Epidemiology

There is a clear relationship between exposure to ionizing radiation and the later development of thyroid cancer.[140] The risk of thyroid cancer developing is related to the dose of radiation and increases with as little as 6.5 cGy to as much as 1200 cGy.[141] With doses higher than 2000 cGy, the incidence of thyroid cancer declines because the epithelium of the thyroid gland becomes defunct. An increased incidence of thyroid cancer has been demonstrated both in survivors of nuclear fallout[142–145] and in patients with a history of low-dose therapeutic radiation to the head and neck.[146, 147] The occurrence of thyroid cancer often follows exposure to radiation by 20 to 35 years.[146] Fortunately, the incidence of radiation-induced thyroid cancer appears to be decreasing owing to the more judicious use of radiation therapy.[148]

There is considerable controversy in the medical literature as to whether a relationship between benign thyroid disease and thyroid malignancy exists. If such an association does exist, it is of only marginal clinical significance.[149] The thyroid malignancy that is most affected by genetic factors is medullary carcinoma of the thyroid (MCT). Approximately 20% of patients have multiple endocrine neoplasia (MEN) type 2A or type 2B.[150] In addition, up to 15% of patients belong to familial non-MEN kindreds.[151] Two familial syndromes can include other differentiated thyroid cancers. These are Gardner's syndrome (polyposis)[152] and Cowden's disease (multiple hamartoma syndrome).[153] Evidence of a genetic relationship for most differentiated thyroid tumors is weak. A hormonal relationship with thyroid cancer is suggested by the female predominance of the disease.[138]

Anatomy of the Thyroid and Parathyroid Glands

The thyroid gland is composed of the isthmus, the lateral lobes, and an inconstant pyramidal lobe. The isthmus overlies the second to the fourth tracheal rings, the lateral lobes extend from the side of the thyroid cartilage down to the sixth tracheal ring, and the pyramidal lobe projects up from the isthmus. Anteriorly, the gland is enclosed by the pretracheal fascia, which lies just deep to the strap muscles anteriorly and the sternocleidomastoid muscle anterolaterally. The larynx and the trachea are deep to the gland, with the pharynx and esophagus behind them. The carotid sheath sits just lateral to the gland on either side.

The two nerves that are important in thyroid surgery are the recurrent laryngeal nerve and the external branch of the superior laryngeal nerve. The recurrent laryngeal nerve courses up from the mediastinum within the tracheoesophageal groove, and the external branch of the superior laryngeal nerve lies deep to the upper pole of the thyroid and passes in an oblique manner to the cricothyroid muscle.

Two arteries supply the thyroid gland, and three veins drain the gland. The superior thyroid artery arises from the external carotid and passes to the upper pole, often in close proximity to the external branch of the superior laryngeal nerve. The inferior thyroid artery comes from the thyrocervical trunk and passes behind the carotid sheath to the posterior aspect of the gland. The thyroidea ima is an inconstant artery arising from the arch of the aorta or the innominate artery and coursing up to the inferior aspect of the isthmus of the gland. The venous drainage of the gland is less constant in both number and position. In general, the superior thyroid vein drains the upper pole of the gland into the internal jugular vein, the middle thyroid vein drains from the lateral side of the gland into the internal jugular vein, and the inferior thyroid vein drains the lower pole into the innominate vein.

Most people have four parathyroid glands, but the number of glands can range from two to six. Normally the glands lie in close proximity to the thyroid gland, but about 10% are aberrant; these are invariably the inferior glands. The superior glands usually lie at the middle of the posterior border of the lobe of the thyroid above the level at which the inferior thyroid artery crosses the recurrent laryngeal nerve. The inferior parathyroids are most often situated below the inferior artery near the lower pole of the thyroid gland. The next most common site is within 1 cm of the lower pole of the thyroid gland. Aberrant inferior parathyroids may descend along the inferior thyroid veins in front of the trachea and may even track into the superior mediastinum along with thymic tissue. Aberrant superior glands may lie posteriorly, close to the esophagus or even in the posterior mediastinum. Rarely, the glands can be buried within the thyroid tissue.

Pathology

The various thyroid histologies and their frequencies, as reported by the Head and Neck Service at Memorial Sloan-Kettering Cancer Center, are listed in Table 1–6.[154]

The most common variant of thyroid cancer is papillary adenocarcinoma, which constituted 54% of cases. Follicular carcinoma is the next most common thyroid malignancy. Together, these two histologies along with the less common Hürthle cell carcinoma are commonly referred to as "differentiated" thyroid cancers. Other less common histologies include medullary carcinoma, anaplastic or undifferentiated carcinoma, sarcoma, and lymphoma.

Papillary Carcinoma

Papillary carcinoma accounts for the majority of malignant tumors of the thyroid gland. It affects women more commonly than men,[155] with the highest incidence occurring in the third through sixth decades. Most papillary carcinomas contain varying amounts of follicular tissue; however, when the predominant histology is papillary, it is considered to be papillary. Papillary carcinomas demonstrate multifocal intraglandular involvement in 38% to 87% of cases.[154, 156, 157] However, the clinical significance of this finding is unclear.[158, 159] Papillary carcinoma also has a tendency to metastasize to regional lymph nodes.[160–162] Less

TABLE 1–6
Distribution of Thyroid Cancer Pathology, Head and Neck Service, Memorial Sloan-Kettering Cancer Center, 1930 to 1980

Histology	Patients	
	No.	*%*
Papillary carcinoma	731	66.0
Follicular carcinoma (plus Hürthle cell)	200	18.1
Medullary carcinoma	66	6.0
Anaplastic carcinoma	97	8.8
Unclassified	13	1.2
Total	1107	100.0

commonly, papillary carcinoma can become locally invasive.

Follicular Carcinoma

Follicular carcinoma makes up about 13% of all primary thyroid cancers.[154] As with papillary carcinoma, women are more commonly affected than men.[155] It is biologically more aggressive than papillary carcinoma, and, although it is less likely to metastasize to regional lymph nodes, it spreads more frequently to distant sites than papillary carcinoma.[163] The pathologic distinction between follicular adenoma and follicular carcinoma can be difficult. Rather than relying on cellular features, one makes the distinction on the basis of capsular invasion at the interface of the tumor and the thyroid gland.[164]

Hürthle Cell Carcinoma

Hürthle cell neoplasms make up about 6% of all primary thyroid cancers.[154] Hürthle cells are considered to be a variant of follicular cells. The clinical behavior of Hürthle cell carcinoma is similar to that of follicular carcinoma except for a greater tendency for lymph node metastases. As with follicular neoplasms, the histologic diagnosis of Hürthle cell carcinoma is made on the basis of capsular invasion or metastases.

Medullary Carcinoma of the Thyroid

MCT accounts for about 10% of thyroid cancers.[154] The tumor develops from the parafollicular or C cells of the thyroid[165] and produces the humoral agent calcitonin, which distinguishes this tumor from other thyroid malignancies. The serum calcitonin level is an exquisitely sensitive marker for the presence of the disease. Elevations are found in the presence of C-cell hyperplasia, which is the precursor lesion of MCT.[166] Elevations are also found in the presence of locally unresected or metastatic disease.[167] Calcitonin secretion from malignant or hyperplastic cells can be stimulated by a number of agents, including pentagastrin,[168] calcium,[169] or a combination of both.[170] Provocative screening with a calcitonin stimulation test is useful in the relatives of patients with familial forms of MCT.

MCT tends to spread by local invasion of surrounding structures, by metastases to regional lymph nodes, and by hematogenous metastases to distant sites. In addition, patients with familial forms of the disease almost always have bilobar involvement of the gland. The standard therapy for MCT is surgery and includes thyroidectomy along with a dissection of the lymph nodes within the central compartment of the neck.[171] In the presence of familial disease or clinical bilobar involvement, total thyroidectomy is preferred. Hemithyroidectomy is appropriate in patients with sporadic disease and unilateral involvement.

Anaplastic Carcinoma

Anaplastic carcinoma is the most lethal form of thyroid cancer. Fortunately, it accounts for less than 10% of thyroid malignancies. However, many of these patients present with locally advanced disease, lymph node metastases, and distant metastatic disease. Patients often have an antecedent history of differentiated thyroid cancer.[172] With surgery alone, the disease is almost invariably fatal. Recent reports of combined radiation therapy, chemotherapy, and surgery for anaplastic carcinoma have yielded improved results, but the durable complete response rate remains less than 20%.[173]

Thyroid Lymphoma

Lymphomas make up less than 2% of all thyroid malignancies,[174] and they are almost always non-Hodgkin's lymphomas of intermediate grade. The primary role of surgery in this disease is to establish a tissue diagnosis. In selected cases of tumor isolated to the thyroid gland, total thyroidectomy can be considered therapeutic.[175] Disease beyond the confines of the gland is treated with either radiation therapy or combined-modality therapy, depending on the extent of the tumor.

Diagnosis

Most thyroid cancers present as thyroid nodules. Thyroid nodules are present in about 6% of the adult population and are even more common in people who have undergone prior radiation treatment to the neck.[176] However, only about 10% to 20% of thyroid nodules are malignant. The clinical circumstances and examination are important in the evaluation of thyroid nodules. Nodules are three times more likely to be malignant in males than in females. Nodules in children under age 20 are more likely to be malignant, as are nodules in patients with a history of radiation exposure.[176] A change in the size of a nodule, hoarseness, dysphagia, and dyspnea are more likely to be associated with malignancy. On physical examination, the presence of lymphadenopathy along with a palpable thyroid mass suggests malignancy. Other findings predictive of malignancy include a history of rapid growth, vocal cord paralysis, Horner's syndrome, fixation to surrounding structures, firmness on palpation, and tracheal invasion.

Fine-needle aspiration of thyroid nodules has become a mainstay in the diagnosis of thyroid masses. Adequate specimens can be obtained in 90% of patients using a 22-gauge needle.[177] With the availability of a competent cytopathologist, the diagnostic accuracy of fine-needle aspiration can be as high as 95%.[178] There are limitations to the technique, especially when dealing with follicular and Hürthle cell lesions, for which demonstration of capsular invasion may be required to diagnose malignancy.

Ultrasonography is of limited value in the routine evaluation of thyroid nodules. It can be helpful in monitoring the involution of a multinodular gland during medical therapy, in evaluating nodules during pregnancy, and for repeatedly examining a patient with a history of radiation therapy to the thyroid.

Radioisotope scanning of the thyroid gland is also of limited value in the evaluation of a thyroid mass in a euthyroid patient.[178] While malignant masses tend to be cold (nonfunctioning), only 10% to 20% of cold nodules are malignant. Hot (functioning) nodules suggest benign disease, but malignant disease cannot be ruled out.[179] Similarly, subjecting patients with suspicious nodules to a trial of thyroid-stimulating hormone (TSH) suppression can yield misleading results and delay appropriate surgical therapy.

Staging

The staging system for thyroid cancer is given in Table 1–7. All anaplastic cancers are designated stage IV. The stage designations for papillary and follicular cancers differ from the designations for MCT; however, both take into account tumor size and extent, lymph node involvement, and distant metastases.

TABLE 1–7
American Joint Committee on Cancer Staging System for Thyroid Cancer*

Primary Tumor

All categories may be subdivided: (a) solitary, (b) multifocal—measure the largest for classification

TX	Primary tumor cannot be assessed
T0	No evidence of primary tumor
T1	Tumor 1 cm or less in greatest dimension limited to the thyroid
T2	Tumor more than 1 cm but not more than 4 cm
T3	Tumor more than 4 cm in greatest dimension limited to the thyroid
T4	Tumor of any size extending beyond the thyroid capsule

Lymph Node

Regional nodes are the cervical and upper mediastinal lymph nodes

NX	Regional lymph nodes cannot be assessed
N0	No regional lymph node metastasis
N1	Regional lymph node metastasis
N1a	Metastasis in ipsilateral cervical lymph nodes
N1b	Metastasis in bilateral, midline, or contralateral cervical or mediastinal lymph nodes

Distant Metastasis

MX	Presence of distant metastasis cannot be assessed
M0	No distant metastasis
M1	Distant metastasis

Stage Grouping

Separate stage groupings are recommended for papillary and follicular, medullary, and undifferentiated

Papillary or Follicular

Under 45 years of age	
Stage I	Any T, Any N, M0
Stage II	Any T, Any N, M1
45 years of age and over	
Stage I	T1, N0, M0
Stage II	T2, N0, M0
	T3, N0, M0
Stage III	T4, N0, M0
	Any T, N1, M0
Stage IV	Any T, Any N, M1

Medullary

Stage I	T1	N0	M0
Stage II	T2	N0	M0
	T3	N0	M0
	T4	N0	M0
Stage III	Any T	N1	M0
Stage IV	Any T	Any N	M1

Undifferentiated

All cases are stage IV	
Stage IV	Any T Any N Any M

*1988 revision.

Differentiated Thyroid Cancer—Primary Operable Disease

The optimum treatment for differentiated thyroid cancer is resection. However, the extent of thyroid gland resection in a patient with a solitary thyroid nodule in one lobe is a matter of debate in the literature. Advocates of total thyroidectomy for the treatment of differentiated thyroid cancer point to the relatively low morbidity of this procedure in experienced hands and the incidence of contralateral lobe recurrence following lobectomy alone.[180, 181] The use of postoperative radioactive iodine (RAI) scanning and treatment is also facilitated by total thyroidectomy.[182]

In fact, the risks of total thyroidectomy can be significant.[183] Total thyroidectomy places both recurrent and superior laryngeal nerves at risk, and all of the parathyroid glands are placed at risk.[157] In addition, the issue of residual or recurrent disease in the contralateral remaining lobe has been addressed in a number of large series.[157, 181, 184] Although unilateral lobectomy is associated with a small but increased incidence of local recurrence,[157, 181] survival is not affected by lobectomy versus total thyroidectomy. Total thyroidectomy for the purpose of facilitating the routine use of RAI ablative therapy following resection is unjustified.[185] There are no well-controlled studies to support the routine use of RAI following surgery.[154]

The recent review of a 50-year experience at Memorial Sloan-Kettering Cancer Center elucidates the significant prognostic factors in differentiated thyroid cancer.[158] By multivariate analysis, factors predictive of poor outcome included older age, follicular histology, large tumor size, extrathyroidal extension, and distant metastases. An additional poor prognostic factor by univariate analysis was male sex. The effect of clinical factors on survival is demonstrated in Figure 1–11. These findings correlated with similar findings from both the Lahey Clinic and the Mayo Clinic.[181, 186]

On the basis of predicted prognosis, patients can be separated into high- and low-risk groups (Table 1–8) and treatment can be individualized. The typical high-risk patient is a man over age 45 with a high-grade lesion, extrathyroidal extension, and/or distant metastases. A low-risk individual is a woman under age 45 with an intracapsular, low-grade tumor without distant metastases. The extent of thyroidectomy should depend on the gross extent of tumor at the time of surgery and the likelihood of needing RAI

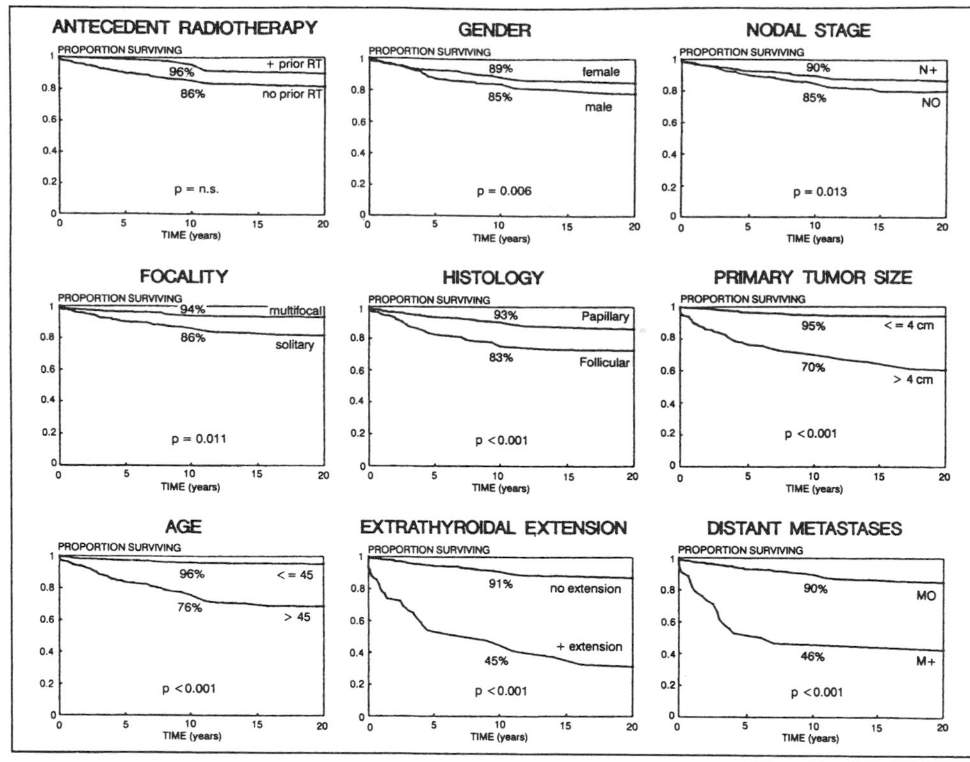

FIGURE 1–11. Survival from differentiated thyroid carcinoma by clinical and pathologic variables. (From Shah JP, et al: Prognostic factors in differentiated carcinoma of the thyroid gland. Am J Surg 164:658–661, 1992.)

treatment. Indications for total thyroidectomy include documented distant metastases, multifocal gross tumor nodules involving both lobes, and the presence of a large primary tumor with extrathyroidal extension. RAI treatment should be reserved for patients who have tumor left behind at the time of surgery, distant metastases, and a history of massive regional lymph node metastases in the central compartment of the neck and mediastinum.

Management of regional lymph nodes in differentiated thyroid cancer should be conservative. Although the significance of cervical lymphadenopathy has been raised by some investigators,[187, 188] the presence of tumor in regional lymph nodes does not appear to affect survival.[158, 181, 186] However, if left untreated, neck metastases can become bulky and symptomatic. For this reason, patients should be examined preoperatively and again intraoperatively for the presence of cervical metastases. If cervical metastases are found, the patient should undergo a modified neck dissection, preferably preserving the sternocleidomastoid muscle, the accessory nerve, and the internal jugular vein. In spite of the presence of micrometastases in as many as 50% of the patients with clinically negative neck disease, elective neck dissection does not improve prognosis and is not recommended.[154]

TABLE 1–8
Risk Groups for Differentiated Thyroid Cancer

High-Risk Patients	Low-Risk Patients
Age over 45	Age under 45
Male gender	Female gender
Extrathyroid extension	Intracapsular tumor
High-grade lesion	Low-grade histology
Distant metastases	No distant metastases

Post-treatment Care and Surveillance

Lifelong thyroid hormone therapy has been recommended in order to suppress TSH secretion. The reasoning behind this therapy comes from the theory that TSH not only stimulates normal thyroid cells but can also stimulate thyroid tumor cells. Although it has been disputed,[189] an overall and disease-free survival advantage to patients who undergo TSH suppression therapy is suggested by retrospective data.[190, 191]

Patients who have undergone successful treatment of thyroid cancer should be followed with periodic history and physical examination in order to detect recurrent or metastatic disease. In patients who undergo thyroid lobectomy, careful attention should be paid to the contralateral gland because of the increased risk for local recurrence. A periodic chest radiograph is indicated to look for pulmonary metastases. In addition, a rising serum thyroglobulin level can be a helpful indicator in the early diagnosis of metastases.

PARATHYROID CANCER

Cancer of the parathyroid gland accounts for only 0.5% to 4% of cases of primary hyperparathyroidism.[192] Patients usually present with severe hypercalcemia, with an average serum calcium concentration of 15 mg/dl. About a third of patients have a palpably enlarged parathyroid mass at presentation.[193]

Parathyroid carcinoma has a tendency to invade surrounding structures. The thyroid gland is most commonly involved, followed by the recurrent nerve, strap muscles, esophagus, and trachea. Cervical and mediastinal lymph nodes are involved in about 17% of patients, and distant metastases to the lung, bone, and liver affect about a quarter of patients at some point in the couse of their disease.[193]

A preoperative diagnosis of parathyroid carcinoma is usually not possible in a patient with hyperparathyroidism, but the diagnosis is suggested by the findings of severe hypercalcemia, a palpable mass, and vocal cord paralysis. At the time of exploration, a carcinoma often presents as a "sticky" mass adherent to surrounding structures, often with a thick, dense, fibrotic, whitish capsule.[194]

If the diagnosis of parathyroid cancer is made at the time of operation, an en bloc resection should be performed. This may require thyroid lobectomy, resection of strap muscles, and resection of the recurrent nerve. Although elective neck dissection has been recommended,[195] most surgeons reserve radical neck dissection for patients with grossly involved nodes.[193]

The 5-year survival rate following resection of parathyroid malignancy is 50% to 60%.[195, 196] Local and distant metastases usually manifest as recurrent hypercalcemia, which can be severe and symptomatic. Localization of metastatic disease can be assisted by the use of a thallium-201 chloride scan in addition to standard radiographic techniques. Recurrent and metastatic disease should be aggressively resected to palliate symptomatic hypercalcemia because other forms of therapy are generally ineffective.[197]

References

1. Boring CC, Squire TS, Tong T: Cancer statistics, 1993. CA 43:7–26, 1993.
2. Berkower AS, Biller HF: Head and neck cancer associated with Bloom's syndrome. Laryngoscope 98:746–748, 1988.
3. Li FP, Correa P, Fraumeni JF: Testing for germ line p53 mutations in cancer families. Cancer Epidemiol Biomarkers Prev 1:91–94, 1991.
4. Davidson BJ, Hsu TC, Schantz SP: The genetics of tobacco-induced malignancy. Arch Otolaryngol Head Neck Surg 119:1198–1205, 1993.
5. Hsu TC, Spitz MR, Schantz SP: Mutagen sensitivity: A biological marker of cancer susceptibility. Cancer Epidemiol Biomarkers Prev 1:83–89, 1991.
6. Bondy ML, Spitz MR, Halabi S, et al: Association between family history of cancer and mutagen sensitivity in upper aerodigestive tract cancer patients. Cancer Epidemiol Biomarkers Prev 2:103–106, 1991.
7. The Biology of Nasopharyngeal Carcinoma. Geneva: International Union Against Cancer, 1982.
8. Rothman K, Keller A: The effect of joint exposure to alcohol and tobacco on risk of cancer of the mouth and pharynx. J Chronic Dis 25:711–716, 1972.
9. Mufti S, Salvagnini M, Lieber C, Garro A: Chronic ethanol consumption inhibits repair of dimethylnitrosamine-induced DNA alkylation. Biochem Biophys Res Comm 152:423–431, 1988.
10. Winn D, Blot W, Shy C: Snuff dipping and oral cancer among women in the southern United States. N Engl J Med 304:745–749, 1981.
11. Donald P: Marijuana smoking: Possible cause of head and neck carcinoma in young patients. Otolaryngol Head Neck Surg 94:517–521, 1986.
12. Cann C, Fried M, Rothman K: Epidemiology of squamous cell cancer of the head and neck. Otolaryngol Clin North Am 18:367–388, 1985.
13. Pearson G, Weiland L, Neel H: Applications of Epstein-Barr virus (EBV) serology to the diagnosis of North American nasopharyngeal carcinoma. Cancer 51:260–268, 1983.
14. Niedobitek G, Hansmann M, Herbst H, et al: Epstein-Barr virus and carcinomas: Undifferentiated carcinomas but not squamous cell carcinomas of the nasopharynx are regularly associated with the virus. J Pathol 165:17–24, 1991.
15. Watts SL, Brewer EE, Fry TL: Human papillomavirus DNA types in squamous cell carcinomas of the head and neck. Oral Surg Oral Med Oral Pathol 71:701–707, 1991.
16. Woods KV, Shilltoe EJ, Spitz MR, Schantz SP, Adler-Storthz K: Analysis of human papillomavirus DNA in oral squamous cell carcinomas. J Oral Pathol 22:101–108, 1993.
17. Li S, Kim MS, Cherrick HM, Doniger J, Park N: Sequential combined tumorigenic effect of HPV-16 and chemical carcinogens. Carcinogenesis 13:1981–1987, 1993.
18. Kashima HK, Kessis T, Hruban RH, Wu TC, Zinreich SJ, Shah KV: Human papillomavirus in sinonasal papillomas and squamous cell carcinoma. Laryngoscope 102:973–976, 1992.
19. Leibel SA, Scott CB, Mohiuddin M, et al: The effect of local-regional control on distant metastatic dissemination in carcinoma of the head and neck: Results of an analysis from the RTOG head and neck database. Int J Radiat Oncol Biol Phys 21:549–556, 1991.
20. Zbaren P, Lehmann W: Frequency and sites of distant metastases in head and neck squamous cell carcinoma. Arch Otolaryngol Head Neck Surg 113:762–764, 1987.
21. Shah JP, Candela FC, Poddar AK: The patterns of cervical lymph node metastases from squamous carcinoma of the oral cavity. Cancer 66:109–113, 1990.
22. Candela FC, Shah J, Jaques DP, Shah JP: Patterns of cervical node metastases from squamous carcinoma of the larynx. Arch Otolaryngol Head Neck Surg 116:432–435, 1990.
23. Medina JE, Byers RM: Supraomohyoid neck dissection: Rationale, indications and surgical technique. Head Neck 11:111–122, 1989.
24. Davidson BJ, Kulkarny V, Delacure MD, Shah JP: Posterior triangle metastases of squamous cell carcinoma of the upper aerodigestive tract. Am J Surg 166:395–398, 1993.
25. Spiro RH, Huvos AG, Wong GY: Predictive value of tumor thickness in squamous carcinoma confined to the tongue and floor of mouth. Am J Surg 152:420–423, 1986.
26. Ellis ER, Mendenhall WM, Rao PV, Parsons JT, Spangler AE, Million RR: Does node location affect the incidence of distant metastases in head and neck squamous cell carcinoma? Int J Radiat Oncol Biol Phys 17:293–297, 1989.
27. Schantz SP, Goepfert H: Multimodality therapy and distant metastases. Arch Otolaryngol Head Neck Surg 113:1207–1213, 1987.
28. Tani M, Amatsu M: Discrepancies between clinical and histopathologic diagnoses in T3 pyriform sinus cancer. Laryngoscope 97:93–96, 1987.
29. Pindborg JJ: Studies in oral leukoplakia. J Am Dent Assoc 76:767–770, 1968.
30. Silverman S, Rozen RD: Observations on the clinical characteristics and natural history of oral leukoplakia. J Am Dent Assoc 76:772–776, 1968.
31. Cooper JS, Pajak TF, Rubin P, et al: Second malignancies in patients who have head and neck cancer: Incidence, effect on survival and implications based on the RTOG experience. Int J Radiat Oncol Biol Phys 17:449–456, 1989.
32. American Joint Committee on Cancer: Manual for Staging of Cancer. Philadelphia, JB Lippincott, 1993, pp 27–62.
33. Mantravadi RVP, Skolnik EM, Applebaum EL: Complications of postoperative radiation therapy in head and neck cancers. Arch Otolaryngol 107:690–693, 1981.

34. Huang DT, Johnson CR, Schmidt-Ullrich R, Grimes M: Post-operative radiotherapy in head and neck carcinoma with extracapsular lymph node extension and/or positive resection margins: A comparative study. Int J Radiat Oncol Biol Phys 23:737–742, 1992.
35. Department of Veterans Affairs Laryngeal Cancer Study Group: Induction chemotherapy plus radiation compared with surgery plus radiation in patients with advanced laryngeal cancer. N Engl J Med 324:1685–1690, 1991.
36. Pfister DG, Strong EW, Harrison L: Larynx preservation with combined chemotherapy and radiation therapy in advanced but resectable head and neck cancer. J Clin Oncol 9:850–859, 1991.
37. Laramore GE, Scott CB, Al-Sarraf M, et al: Adjuvant chemotherapy for resectable squamous cell carcinoma of the head and neck: Report on intergroup study 0034. Int J Radiat Oncol Biol Phys 23:705–713, 1992.
38. Million RM: Management of Head and Neck Cancer: A Multidisciplinary Approach. Philadelphia: JB Lippincott, 1984.
39. Robbins KT, Medina JG, Wolfe GT: Standardizing neck dissection terminology. Arch Otolaryngol Head Neck Surg 117:601–605, 1991.
40. Schuller DE, Platz CE, Krause CJ: Spinal accessory lymph nodes: A prospective study of metastatic involvement. Laryngoscope 88:439–449, 1978.
41. Spaulding CA, Hahn SS, Constable WC: The effectiveness of treatment of lymph nodes in cancers of the pyriform sinus and supraglottis. Int J Radiat Oncol Biol Phys 13:963–968, 1987.
42. Vikram B, Strong EW, Shah JP, Spiro R: Failure in the neck following multimodality treatment for advanced head and neck cancer. Head Neck 6:724–729, 1984.
43. Coster JR, Foote RL, Olsen KD, Jack SM, Schaid DJ, Desanto LW: Cervical nodal metastases of squamous cell carcinoma of unknown origin: Indications for withholding radiation therapy. Int J Radiat Oncol Biol Phys 23:743–749, 1992.
44. Freeman D, Mendenhall WM, Parsons JT, Million RR: Unknown primary squamous cell carcinoma of the head and neck: Is mucosal irradiation necessary? Int J Radiat Oncol Biol Phys 23:889–890, 1992.
45. Lee NK, Byers RM, Abbruzzese JL, Wolf P: Metastatic adenocarcinoma to the neck from an unknown primary source. Am J Surg 162:306–309, 1991.
46. Wang RC, Goepfert H, Barber AE, Wolf P: Unknown primary squamous cell carcinoma metastatic to the neck. Arch Otolaryngol Head Neck Surg 116:1388–1393, 1990.
47. Spiro JD, Soo KC, Spiro RH: Squamous cell carcinoma of the nasal cavity and paranasal sinuses. Am J Surg 158:328–332, 1989.
48. Lavertu P, Roberts JK, Kraus DH, et al: Squamous cell carcinoma of the paranasal sinuses: The Cleveland clinic experience 1977–1986. Laryngoscope 99:1130–1136, 1989.
49. Shah JP, Kraus DH, Arbit E, Galicich JH, Strong EW: Craniofacial resection for tumors involving the anterior skull base. Otolaryngol Head Neck Surg 106:387–393, 1992.
50. Ketcham AS, Van Buren JM: Tumors of the paranasal sinuses: A therapeutic challenge. Am J Surg 150:406–413, 1985.
51. Parsons JT, Mendenhall WM, Mancuso AA, Cassisi NJ, Million RR: Malignant tumors of the nasal cavity and ethmoid and sphenoid sinuses. Int J Radiat Oncol Biol Phys 14:11–22, 1988.
52. LoRusso P, Tapazoglou E, Kish JA, et al: Chemotherapy for paranasal sinus carcinoma: A 10-year experience at Wayne State University. Cancer 62:1–5, 1988.
53. Choi KN, Rotman M, Aziz H, Potters L, Stark R, Rosenthal JC: Locally advanced paranasal sinus and nasopharynx tumors with hyperfractionated radiation and concomitant infusion of cisplatin. Cancer 67:2748–2752, 1991.
54. Harrison LB, Sessions RB, Fass DE, Armstrong JG, Hunt M, Spiro RH: Nasopharyngeal brachytherapy with access via a transpalatal flap. Am J Surg 164:173–175, 1992.
55. Perz CA: Carcinoma of the nasopharynx. In Brady LW, Perez CA (eds): Principles and Practice of Radiation Oncology. Philadelphia: JB Lippincott, 1992, pp 617–644.
56. En-Pee Z, Pei-Gun L, Kuang-Long C: Radiation therapy of nasopharyngeal carcinoma: Prognostic factors based on a 10-year follow-up of 1,302 patients. Int J Radiat Oncol Biol Phys 16:301–305, 1989.
57. Flores AD, Dickson RI, Riding K, Coy P: Cancer of the nasopharynx in British Columbia. Am J Clin Oncol 9:281–291, 1986.
58. Bloom ND, Spiro R: Carcinoma of the cheek mucosa: A retrospective analysis. Am J Surg 149:556–559, 1980.
59. Nair MK, Sankaranarayanan R, Padmanabhan TK: Evaluation of radiotherapy in cancer of the buccal mucosa. Cancer 61:1326–1331, 1988.
60. Cherian T, Sebastian P, Ahamed MI, et al: Evaluation of salvage surgery in heavily irradiated cancer of the buccal mucosa. Cancer 68:295–299, 1991.
61. Rodgers LW, Stringer SP, Mendenhall WM, Parsons JT, Cassisi NJ, Million RR: Management of squamous cell carcinoma of the floor of mouth. Head Neck 15:16–19, 1993.
62. Soo KC, Carter RL, O'Brien CJ, Barr L, Bliss JM, Shaw HJ: Prognostic implications of perineural spread in squamous carcinomas of the head and neck. Laryngoscope 96:1145–1148, 1986.
63. Close LG, Brown PM, Vuitch MF, Reisch J, Schaefer SD: Microvascular invasion and survival in cancer of the oral cavity and oropharynx. Arch Otolaryngol Head Neck Surg 115:1304–1309, 1989.
64. Hanha IWF, Moui RF, Nicholson R: Survival results for cancer of the tongue, Westminster Hospital, 1947–1976. Br J Radiol 58:781–782, 1985.
65. Franceschi D, Gupta R, Spiro RH, Shah JP: Improved survival in the treatment of squamous carcinoma of the oral tongue. Am J Surg 166:360–365, 1993.
66. Wendt CD, Peters LJ, Delclos L, et al: Primary radiotherapy in the treatment of stage I and II oral tongue cancers: Importance of the proportion of therapy delivered with interstitial therapy. Int J Radiat Oncol Biol Phys 18:1287–1292, 1990.
67. Wang CC: Radiotherapeutic management and results of T1N0, T2N0 carcinoma of the oral tongue: Evaluation of boost techniques. Int J Radiat Oncol Biol Phys 17:287–291, 1989.
68. Morton ME: Osteoradionecrosis: A study of the incidence in the north west of England. Br J Oral Maxillofac Surg 24:323–331, 1986.
69. Byers RM, Clayman GL, Guillamondequi OM, Peters LJ, Goepfert H: Resection of advanced cervical metastases prior to definitive radiotherapy for primary squamous carcinomas of the upper aerodigestive tract. Head Neck 14:133–138. 1992.
70. Wong CS, Ang KK, Fletcher GH, et al: Definitive radiotherapy for squamous cell carcinoma of the tonsillar fossa. Int J Radiat Oncol Biol Phys 16:657–662, 1989.
71. Kajanti MJ, Mantyla MJ: Carcinoma of the nasopharynx. Acta Oncol 29:611–614, 1990.
72. Harrison LB, Zelefsky MJ, Sessions RB, et al: Base-of-tongue cancer treated with external beam irradiation plus brachytherapy: Oncologic and functional outcome. Radiology 184:267–270, 1992.
73. Johansen LV, Overgaard J, Avergaard M, Birkler N, Fisker A: Squamous cell carcinoma of the oropharynx: An analysis of 213 consecutive patients scheduled for primary radiotherapy. Laryngoscope 100:985–990, 1990.
74. Bataini JP, Bernier J, Jaulerry C, Brunin F, Pontvert D: Impact of cervical disease and its definitive radiotherapeutic management on survival: Experience in 2013 patients with squamous cell carcinomas of the oropharynx and pharyngolarynx. Laryngoscope 100:716–723, 1990.
75. Gehanno P, Depondt J, Guedon C, Kebali C, Koka V: Primary and salvage surgery for cancer of the tonsillar region: A retrospective study of 120 patients. Head Neck 15:185–189, 1993.
76. Shaha AR: Preoperative evaluation of the mandible in patients with carcinoma of the floor of mouth. Head Neck 13:398–402, 1991.
77. Shaha AR: Marginal mandibulectomy for cancer of the floor of the mouth. J Surg Oncol 49:116–119, 1992.
78. Hidalgo D: Aesthetic mandibular reconstruction. Plast Reconstr Surg 88:574–585, 1991.
79. Kraus DH, Pfister DG, Harrison LB, et al: Larynx preservation with combined chemotherapy and radiation therapy in advanced hypopharynx cancer. Otolaryngol Head Neck Surg 111:31–37, 1994.
80. Rucci L, Gallo O, Fini-Storchi O: Glottic cancer involving anterior commissure: Surgery vs radiotherapy. Head Neck 13:403–410, 1991.
81. Mendenhall WM, Parsons JT, Stringer SP, Cassissi NJ, Million RR: The role of radiation therapy in laryngeal cancer. CA 40:150–165, 1990.
82. Lee NK, Goepfert H, Wendt CD: Supraglottic laryngectomy for intermediate-stage cancer: UT MD Anderson Cancer Center experiance with combined therapy. Laryngoscope 100:831–836, 1990.
83. Desanto LW: Early supraglottic cancer. Ann Otol Rhinol Laryngol 99:593–597, 1990.
84. Levendag P, Sessions RB, Vikram B, et al: The problem of neck

relapse in early stage supraglottic larynx cancer. Cancer 63:345–348, 1989.
85. Spaulding CA, Constable WC, Levine PA, Cantrell RW: Partial laryngectomy and radiotherapy for supraglottic cancer: A conservative approach. Ann Otol Rhinol Laryngol 98:125–129, 1989.
86. Johnson CR, Schmidt-Ullrich RK, Wazer DE: Concomitant boost technique using accelerated superfractionated radiation therapy for advanced squamous cell carcinoma of the head and neck. Cancer 69:2749–2754, 1992.
87. Cox JD, Pajak TF, Marcial VA, et al: Interruptions adversely affect local control and survival with hyperfractionated radiation therapy of carcinomas of the upper respiratory and digestive tracts. Cancer 69:2744–2748, 1992.
88. Fontanesi J, Beckford NS, Lester EP, et al: Concomitant cisplatin and hyperfractionated external beam irradiation for advanced malignancy of the head and neck. Am J Surg 162:393–396, 1991.
89. Slotman GJ, Doolittle CH, Glicksman AS: Preoperative combined chemotherapy and radiation therapy plus radical surgery in advanced head and neck cancer. Cancer 69:2736–2743, 1992.
90. Jacobs C, Meyers F, Hendrickson C: A randomized phase III study of cisplatin with or without methotrexate for recurrent squamous cell carcinoma of the head and neck. Cancer 52:1563–1569, 1983.
91. Vogl SE, Schoenfeld DA, Kaplan BH: A randomized prospective comparison of methotrexate with a combination of methotrexate, bleomycin and cisplatin in head and neck cancer. Cancer 56:432–442, 1985.
92. Haughey BH, Arfken CL, Gates GA, Harvey J: Meta-analysis of second malignant tumors in head and neck cancer: The case for an endoscopic screening protocol. Ann Otol Rhinol Laryngol 101:105–112, 1992.
93. Parker RG, Enstrom JE: Second primary cancers of the head and neck following treatment of initial primary head and neck cancers. Int J Radiat Oncol Biol Phys 14:561–564, 1988.
94. Robinson E, Neugut AI, Murray T, Rennert G: A comparison of the clinical characteristics of first and second primary head and neck cancers. Cancer 68:189–192, 1991.
95. Fijuth J, Mazeron J, Le Phechoux C, et al: Second head and neck cancers following radiation therapy of T1 and T2 cancers of the oral cavity and oropharynx. Int J Radiat Oncol Biol Phys 24:59–64, 1992.
96. Licciardello JT, Spitz MR, Hong WK: Multiple primary cancer in patients with cancer of the head and neck: Second cancer of the head and neck, esophagus and lung. Int J Radiat Oncol Biol Phys 17:467–476, 1989.
97. Sercarz J, Holmes EC, Ellison D, Calcaterra TC: Isolated pulmonary nodules in head and neck cancer patients. Ann Otol Rhinol Laryngol 98:113–118, 1989.
98. Benner S, Winn R, Lippman S, Poland J, Hansen K, Luna M: Regression of oral leukoplakia with alpha-tocopherol: A community clinical oncology program chemoprevention study. J Natl Cancer Inst 85:44–47, 1993.
99. Lippman S, Batsakis J, Toth B, et al: Comparison of low-dose isotretinoin with beta carotene to prevent oral carcinogenesis. N Engl J Med 328:15–20, 1993.
100. Hong WK, Lippman SM, Itrim LM: Prevention of second primary tumors with isotretinoin in squamous-cell carcinoma of the head and neck. N Engl J Med 323:795–801, 1990.
101. Million RR, Cassisi NJ, Clark JR: Cancer of the head and neck. In DeVita VT, Hellman S, Rosenberg SA (eds): Cancer: Principles and Practice of Oncology. Philadelphia: JB Lippincott, 1989, pp 488–590.
102. Shah JP, Ihde JK: Salivary gland tumors. Curr Probl Surg 27:775–883, 1990.
103. Hollander L, Cunningham MP: Management of cancer of the parotid gland. Surg Clin North Am 53:113–119, 1973.
104. Merrick Y, Albeck H, Nielsen NH, Hansen HS: Familial clustering of salivary gland cancer in Greenland. Cancer 57:2097, 1986.
105. Maxon HR, Saenger EL, Buncher CR, et al: Radiation-associated carcinoma of the salivary glands. A controlled study. Ann Otol Rhinol Laryngol 90:107–108, 1981.
106. Takeichi N, Hirose F, Yamamoto H: Salivary gland tumors in atomic bomb survivors, Hiroshima, Japan. I. epidemiologic observations. Cancer 38:2462–2468, 1976.
107. Hadfield EH, Macbeth RG: Adenocarcinoma of ethmoids in furniture workers. Ann Otol Rhinol Laryngol 80:699–703, 1971.
108. Wells SA, Baylin SB, Leight GS, Dale JK, Dilley WG, Farndon JR: The importance of early diagnosis in patients with hereditary medullary thyroid carcinoma. Ann Surg 195:595–599, 1982.
109. Foote FB, Frazell EL: Tumors of the major salivary glands. Cancer 6:1065–1069, 1953.
110. Layfield LJ, Glasgow BJ: Diagnosis of salivary gland tumors by fine-needle aspiration cytology: A review of clinical utility and pitfalls. Diagn Cytopathol 1991 7:267–272, 1993.
111. Pownell PH, Brown OE, Pransky SM, Manning SC: Congenital abnormalities of the submandibular duct. Int J Pediatr Otorhinolaryngol 24:161–169, 1992.
112. Spiro RH, Huvos AG, Strong EW: Adenocarcinoma of salivary origin. Clinicopathologic study of 204 patients. Am J Surg 144:423–431, 1982.
113. LiVolsi VA, Perzin KH: Malignant mixed tumors arising in salivary glands. I. Carcinomas arising in benign mixed tumors: A clinicopathologic study. Cancer 39:2209–2230, 1977.
114. Granick MS, Erickson ER, Hanna DC: Accuracy of frozen-section diagnosis in salivary gland lesions. Head Neck Surg 7:465–467, 1985.
115. Batsakis JG: Tumors of the Head and Neck, Clinical and Pathological Considerations. Baltimore: Williams & Wilkins, 1979.
116. Brandwein MS, Huvos AG: Oncocytic tumors of major salivary glands. A study of 68 cases with follow-up of 44 patients. Am J Surg Pathol 15:514–528, 1991.
117. Godwin J: Benign lymphoepithelial lesion of the parotid gland. Cancer 5:1089–1103, 1952.
118. Bruner J, Cleary K, Smith F, Batsakis J: Immunocytochemical identification of HIV antigen in parotid lymphoid lesions. J Laryngol Otol 103:1063–1066, 1989.
119. Evans HL: Mucoepidermoid carcinoma of salivary glands: A study of 69 cases with special attention to histologic grading. Am J Clin Pathol 81:696–701, 1984.
120. Carlson GW, Schusterman MA, Guillamondegui OM: Total reconstruction of the hypopharynx and cervical esophagus: A 20-year experience. Ann Plast Surg 29:408–412, 1992.
121. Vrielinck LJ, Ostyn F, van Damme B, van den Bogaert W, Fossion E: The significance of perineural spread in adenoid cystic carcinoma of the major and minor salivary glands. Int J Oral Maxillofac Surg 17:190–193, 1988.
122. Nascimento AG, Amaral AL, Prado LA, Kligerman J, Silveira TR: Adenoid cystic carcinoma of salivary glands. A study of 61 cases with clinicopathologic correlation. Cancer 57:312–319, 1986.
123. Wysocki GP, Wright BA: Intraneural and perineural epithelial structures. Head Neck Surg 4:69–71, 1981.
124. Spiro RH, Huvos AG, Strong EW: Acinic cell carcinoma of salivary origin. Cancer 41:924–935, 1978.
125. Bullerdiek J, Takla G, Bartnitzke S, Brandt G, Chilla R, Haubrich J: Relationship of cytogenetic subtypes of salivary gland pleomorphic adenomas with patient age and histologic type. Cancer 64:876–880, 1989.
126. O'Dwyer P, Farrar WB, James AG, Finkelmeier W, McCabe DP: Needle aspiration biopsy of major salivary gland tumors. Its value. Cancer 57:554–557, 1986.
127. Dawson AK, Orr JA: Long-term results of local excision and radiotherapy in pleomorphic adenoma of the parotid. Int J Radiat Oncol Biol Phys 11:451–455, 1985.
128. Spiro RH, Spiro JD: Cancer of the salivary glands. In Sven J, Myers E (eds): Cancer of the Head and Neck, 2nd ed. New York: Churchill Livingstone, 1989, pp 645–668.
129. Adams G: Malignant tumors of the paranasal sinuses and nasal cavity. In McQuarrie DG (ed): Head and Neck Cancer Clinical Decisions and Management Principles Chicago: Year Book Medical Publishers, 1986, pp 311–334.
130. Weber RS, Byers RM, Petit B, Wolf P, Ang K, Luna M: Submandibular gland tumors. Adverse histologic factors and therapeutic implications. Arch Otolaryngol Head Neck Surg 116:1055–1060, 1990.
131. Armstrong JG, Harrison LB, Spiro RH, Fass DE, Strong EW, Fuks ZY: Malignant tumors of major salivary gland origin. A matched-pair analysis of the role of combined surgery and postoperative radiotherapy. Arch Otolaryngol Head Neck Surg 116:290–293, 1990.
132. Harrison LB, Armstrong JG, Spiro RH, Fass DE, Strong EW: Postoperative radiation therapy for major salivary gland malignancies. J Surg Oncol 45:52–55, 1990.

133. Fu KK, Leibel SA, Levine ML, Friedlander LM, Boles R, Phillips TL: Carcinoma of the major and minor salivary glands: Analysis of treatment results and sites and causes of failures. Cancer 40:2882–2890, 1977.
134. Awan AM, Vokes EE, Weichselbaum RR: Recent advances in radiation therapy for head and neck cancer. Hematol Oncol Clin North Am 5:635–654, 1991.
135. Buchholz TA, Laramore GE, Griffin BR, Koh WJ, Griffin TW: The role of fast neutron radiation therapy in the management of advanced salivary gland malignant neoplasms. Cancer 69:2779–2788, 1992.
136. Dimery IW, Legha SS, Shirinian M, Hong WK: Fluorouracil, doxorubicin, cyclophosphamide, and cisplatin combination chemotherapy in advanced or recurrent salivary gland carcinoma. J Clin Oncol 8:1056–1062, 1990.
137. Spiro RH, Armstrong J, Harrison L, Geller NL, Lin SY, Strong EW: Carcinoma of major salivary glands. Recent trends. Arch Otolaryngol Head Neck Surg 115:316–321, 1989.
138. Boring CC, Squires TS, Tong T: Cancer statistics, 1993. CA 43:7–26, 1993.
139. Nishiyama R, Ludwig G, Thompson N: The prevalence of small papillary thyroid carcinoma in 100 consecutive necropsies in an American population. In DeGroot L (ed): Radiation Associated Thyroid Cancer. Orlando: Grune & Stratton, 1977, pp 123–136.
140. Duffy BJ, Fitzgerald BJ: Cancer of the thyroid in children: A report of 28 children. J Clin Endocrinol Metab 10:1296–1299, 1950.
141. Norton JA, Doppman JL, Jensen RT: Cancer of the endocrine system. In DeVita VT, Hellman S, Rosenberg SA (eds): Cancer: Principles and Practice of Oncology. Philadelphia: JB Lippincott, 1989, pp 1269–1344.
142. Takeichi N, Ezaki H, Dohi K: A review of forty-five years study of Hiroshima and Nagasaki atomic bomb survivors. Thyroid cancer: Reports up to date and a review. J Radiat Res 32 (Suppl):180–188, 1991.
143. Ezaki H, Takeichi N, Yoshimoto Y: Thyroid cancer: Epidemiological study of thyroid cancer in A-bomb survivors from extended life span study cohort in Hiroshima. J Radiat Res 32 (Suppl):193–200, 1991.
144. Rallison ML, Dobyns BM, Keating FR Jr, Rall JE, Tyler FH: Thyroid nodularity in children. JAMA 233:1069–1072, 1975.
145. Conard RA, Dobyns BM, Sutow WW: Thyroid neoplasia as late effect of exposure to radioactive iodine in fallout. JAMA 214:316–324, 1970.
146. Schneider AB, Shore-Freedman E, Ryo UY, Bekerman C, Favus M, Pinsky S: Radiation-induced tumors of the head and neck following childhood irradiation. Prospective studies. Medicine (Baltimore) 64:1–15, 1985.
147. Hancock SL, Cox RS, McDougall IR: Thyroid diseases after treatment of Hodgkin's disease. N Engl J Med 325:599–605, 1991.
148. Mehta NT, Goetowski PG, Kinsella TJ: Radiation induced thyroid neoplasms 1920 to 1987: A vanishing problem? J Radiat Oncol Biol Phys 16:1471–1475, 1989.
149. Schneider AB: Carcinoma of follicular epithelium: Pathogenesis. In Braverman LE, Utiger RD (eds): Werner and Ingbar's: A Fundamental and Clinical Text. The Thyroid, 6th ed. Philadelphia: JB Lippincott, 1991, pp 1121–1129.
150. Saad MF, Ordonez NG, Rashid RK, et al: Medullary carcinoma of the thyroid. A study of the clinical features and prognostic factors in 161 patients. Medicine (Baltimore) 63:319–342, 1984.
151. Ponder BAJ: Familial medullary thyroid cancer—screening the family of the apparently sporadic case. Br J Cancer 53:436–437, 1986.
152. Delamarre J, Capron JP, Armand A, Dupas JL, Deschepper B, Davion T: Thyroid carcinoma in two sisters with familial polyposis of the colon. Case reports and review of the literature. J Clin Gastroenterol 10:659–662, 1988.
153. Thyresson HN, Doyle JA: Cowden's disease (multiple hamartoma syndrome). Mayo Clin Proc 56:179–184, 1981.
154. Shah JP: Differentiated thyroid cancer. In Bloom HJG, Hanham IWF, Shaw HJ (eds): Head and Neck Oncology. New York: Raven Press, 1986, pp 207–214.
155. Rossi RL, Cady B: Differentiated thyroid cancer. In Cady B, Rossi RL (eds): Surgery of the Thyroid and Parathyroid Glands, 3rd ed. Philadelphia: WB Saunders, 1991, pp 139–151.
156. Tollefsen HR, Shah JP, Huvos AG: Follicular carcinoma of the thyroid. Am J Surg 126:523–528, 1973.
157. Tollefsen HR, Shah JP, Huvos AG: Papillary carcinoma of the thyroid. Recurrence in the thyroid gland after initial surgical treatment. Am J Surg 124:468–472, 1972.
158. Shah JP, Loree TR, Dharker D, Strong EW, Begg C, Vlamis V: Prognostic factors in differentiated carcinoma of the thyroid gland. Am J Surg 164:658–661, 1992.
159. Crile G Jr, Antunez AR, Esselstyn CB Jr, Hawk WA, Skillern PG: The advantages of subtotal thyroidectomy and suppression of TSH in the primary treatment of papillary carcinoma of the thyroid. Cancer 55:2691–2697, 1985.
160. Noguchi S, Noguchi A, Murakami N: Papillary carcinoma of the thyroid. II. Value of prophylactic lymph node excision. Cancer 26:1061–1064, 1970.
161. Noguchi S, Noguchi A, Murakami N: Papillary carcinoma of the thyroid. I. Developing pattern of metastasis. Cancer 26:1053–1060, 1970.
162. Attie JN, Khafif RA, Steckler RM: Elective neck dissection in papillary carcinoma of the thyroid. Am J Surg 122:464–471, 1971.
163. Ruegemer JJ, Hay ID, Bergstralh EJ, Ryan JJ, Offord KP, Gorman CA: Distant metastases in differentiated thyroid carcinoma: A multivariate analysis of prognostic variables. J Clin Endocrinol Metab 67:501–508, 1988.
164. Kahn NF, Perzin KH: Follicular carcinoma of the thyroid: An evaluation of the histologic criteria used for diagnosis. Pathol Ann 18 (Part 1):221–253, 1983.
165. Van Heerden JA, Grant CS, Gharib H, Hay ID, Ilstrup DM: Long-term course of patients with persistent hypercalcitoninemia after apparent curative primary surgery for medullary thyroid carcinoma. Ann Surg 212:395–400, 1990.
166. Telander RL, Zimmerman D, Sizemore GW, VanHeeden JA, Grant CS: Medullary carcinoma in children: Results of early detection and surgery. Arch Surg 124:841–843, 1989.
167. Tisell LE, Hansson G, Jansson S: Surgical treatment of medullary carcinoma of the thyroid. Horm Metab Res Suppl 21:29–31, 1989.
168. Cooper CW, Schwesinger WH, Mahgoub AM, Ontjes DA: Thyrocalcitonin: Stimulation of secretion by pentagastrin. Science 172:1238–1240, 1971.
169. Block MA, Jackson CE, Tashjian AH Jr: Medullary thyroid carcinoma detected by serum calcitonin assay. Arch Surg 104:579–586, 1972.
170. Samaan NA, Schultz PN, Hickey RC: Medullary thyroid carcinoma: Prognosis of familial versus sporadic disease and the role of radiotherapy. J Clin Endocrinol Metab 67:801–805, 1988.
171. Duh QY, Sancho JJ, Greenspan FS, et al: Medullary thyroid carcinoma. The need for early diagnosis and total thyroidectomy. Arch Surg 124:1206–1210, 1989.
172. Sisson JC: Medical treatment of benign and malignant thyroid tumors. Endocrinol Metab Clin North Am 18:359–387, 1989.
173. Tennvall J, Tallroth E, el Hassan A, et al: Anaplastic thyroid carcinoma. Doxorubicin, hyperfractionated radiotherapy and surgery. Acta Oncol 29:1025–1028, 1990.
174. Rossi RL, Cady B: Undifferentiated carcinoma and lymphoma of thyroid gland. In Cady B, Rossi RL (eds): Surgery of the Thyroid and Parathyroid Glands, 3rd ed. Philadelphia: WB Saunders, 1991, pp 179–188.
175. Rosen IB, Sutcliffe SB, Gospodarowicz MK, Chua T, Simpson WJ: The role of surgery in the management of thyroid lymphoma. Surgery 104:1095–1099, 1988.
176. Rojeski MT, Gharib H: Nodular thyroid disease: Evaluation and management. N Engl J Med 313:428–434, 1985.
177. Hall TL, Layfield LJ, Philippe A, Rosenthal DL: Sources of diagnostic error in fine needle aspiration of the thyroid. Cancer 63:718–725, 1989.
178. Ashcraft MW, Van Herle AJ: Management of thyroid nodules. II. Scanning techniques, thyroid suppressive therapy, and fine needle aspiration. Head Neck Surg 3:297–322, 1981.
179. Katz AD, Zager WJ: The malignant "cold" nodule of the thyroid. Am J Surg 132:459–462, 1976.
180. Clark OH: Total thyroidectomy: The treatment of choice for patients with differentiated thyroid cancer. Ann Surg 196:361–370, 1982.
181. Hay ID, Grant CS, Taylor WF, McConahey WM: Ipsilateral lobectomy versus bilateral lobar resection in papillary thyroid carcinoma: A retrospective analysis of surgical outcome using a novel prognostic scoring system. Surgery 102:1088–1095, 1987.
182. Beierwaltes WH, Rabbani R, Dmuchowski C, Lloyd RV, Eyre P,

Mallette S: An analysis of "ablation of thyroid remnants" with I-131 in 511 patients from 1947–1984: Experience at University of Michigan. J Nucl Med 25:1287–1293, 1984.
183. Harness JK, Fung L, Thompson NW, Burney RE, McLeod MK: Total thyroidectomy: Complications and technique. World J Surg 10:781–786, 1986.
184. Hoie J, Stenwug AE, Brennhovd IO: Surgery in papillary thyroid carcinoma: A review of 730 patients. J Surg Oncol 37:147–151, 1988.
185. Snyder J, Gorman C, Scanlon P: Thyroid remnant ablation: Questionable pursuit of an ill-defined goal. J Nucl Med 24:659–665, 1983.
186. Cady B, Rossi R: An expanded view of risk-group definition in differentiated thyroid carcinoma. Surgery 104:947–953, 1988.
187. Coburn MC, Wanebo HJ: Prognostic factors and management considerations in patients with cervical metastases of thyroid cancer. Am J Surg 164:671–676, 1992.
188. Sellers M, Beenken S, Blankenship A, et al: Prognostic significance of cervical lymph node metastases in differentiated thyroid cancer. Am J Surg 164:578–581, 1992.
189. Cady B, Cohn K, Rossi RL, et al: The effect of thyroid hormone administration upon survival in patients with differentiated thyroid carcinoma. Surgery 94:978–983, 1983.
190. Mazzaferri EL, Young RL, Oertel JE, Kemmerer WT, Page CP: Papillary thyroid carcinoma: The impact of therapy in 576 patients. Medicine (Baltimore) 56:171–196, 1977.
191. Staunton MD, Greening WP: Treatment of thyroid cancer in 293 patients. Br J Surg 63:253–258, 1976.
192. Shortell CK, Andrus CH, Phillips CE Jr, Schwartz SI: Carcinoma of the parathyroid gland: A 30-year experience. Surgery 110:704–708, 1991.
193. Obara T, Fujimoto Y: Diagnosis and treatment of patients with parathyroid carcinoma: An update and review. World J Surg 15:738–744, 1991.
194. Kaplan EL, Yashiro T, Salti G: Primary hyperparathyroidism in the 1990's: Choice of surgical procedures for this disease. Ann Surg 215:300–317, 1992.
195. Holmes EC, Morton DL, Ketcham AS: Parathyroid carcinoma: A collective review. Ann Surg 169:631–640, 1969.
196. Wang CA, Gaz RD: Natural history of parathyroid carcinoma. Diagnosis, treatment, and results. Am J Surg 149:522–527, 1985.
197. Sandelin K, Thompson NW, Bondeson L: Metastatic parathyroid carcinoma: Dilemmas in management. Surgery 110:978–986, 1991.
198. Spiro RH: Salivary neoplasms: Overview of a 35-year experience with 2,807 patients. Head Neck Surg 8:177–184, 1986.
199. Shah JP: Color Atlas of Head and Neck Surgery. Hong Kong: Wolfe Medical Publishing, 1990.

2

James C. Harvey, M.D. • Julianna Pisch, M.D.
Burton Surick, M.D. • Eva Rubin, M.D.
Edward J. Beattie, M.D.

Tumors of the Esophagus and Gastric Cardia

Cancer of the esophagus accounts for only 1% of the annual new cancers in the United States, but few tumors are more lethal. In 1995 the death rate was predicted to be 90% of the incidence rate, with 10,900 deaths and 12,100 new cases.[1] The rate of increase in incidence of adenocarcinoma of the esophagus and of the probably related adenocarcinoma of the proximal stomach is among the highest of all tumors.[2]

Surgical treatment options, and nonsurgical options, at this time are similar for tumors of the esophagus and tumors of the gastric cardia. Furthermore, the epidemiology of adenocarcinoma of the gastric cardia is more similar to that of adenocarcinoma of the esophagus than to distal stomach cancers.

RISK FACTORS

Sex

In areas of the world where squamous cell carcinoma of the esophagus (SCCE) is of relatively low incidence, men have higher incidence rates than women (1.7 times as many men as women in the United States), but the difference tends to disappear in endemic areas such as the Transkei in South Africa and the Caspian littoral of Iran.[3, 4] For adenocarcinoma of the esophagus (ACE), the risk among white men in the United States is increasing steeply, with a male to female ratio of 3:7.[2]

Racial

Urban African Americans have a higher risk of SCCE, about triple that of Americans of European ancestry (14.0 vs. 4.2 in 100,000), and an epidemic of squamous cell carcinoma has been noted among South African blacks, especially in the Transkei.[1–4] However, socioeconomic factors may be of greater significance than racial propensity, since Bantu peoples of other parts of Africa have an incidence rate lower than that of American whites.[5]

For ACE, white race is a risk factor: a study at a large health maintenance organization (HMO) found that 97% of ACE cases occurred among whites, compared with only 84% of cases of squamous cell carcinoma of the distal esophagus.[6]

Genetic-Familial

It has been difficult to separate genetic and familial risks from environmental influences except for keratosis palmaris et plantaris (tylosis), an autosomal dominant trait.[1]

Dietary

Endemic areas, such as the Caspian littoral of Iran and certain mountainous, rural regions of China, have been characterized as arid lands with poor soil quality whose inhabitants have monotonous, monocereal diets of wheat or maize. Diets in these areas are typically deficient in calories, protein, fats, trace minerals, and vitamins. Studies in the Transkei of South Africa have demonstrated that high-risk areas are found in association with soil having low agricultural potential, high alkalinity, trace metal deficiency, and high boron levels. These characteristics are similar to those of soils found in the historically endemic areas of China and Iran. Certain areas of the Transkei where soils are derived from dolerite and are rich in many minerals, including iron, magnesium, calcium, and phosphates have produced few cancers. It has also been noted in Africa that diets based on maize are associated with high risk for SCCE, whereas more traditional diets of sorghum, cassava, millet, and peanuts are associated with low risk.[3, 5, 7]

Among specific food deficiencies associated with SCCE

are milk, meat, fresh fruit and vegetables, vitamins (riboflavin, vitamin A, vitamin C), and minerals (zinc, iron, molybdenum).[2–4]

In the United States, deficiencies in vitamins A and C have not been implicated in SCCE. In the case of vitamin A from animal sources, at least one study determined that increased intake has a dose-related increased risk.[2] Total fat intake has also been found to have a dose-related association with SCCE in this country. Body mass index has been found to be inversely related to SCCE even when controlled for the weight-loss effects of dysphagia (by using self-reported weights 5 years prior to diagnosis of SCCE).

For ACE, total fat intake and vitamin A from animal sources have been found to have a dose-related risk, but vitamin A from plant sources did not. Vitamin C intake did not seem to influence the risk. High fiber intake is protective. Differences in body mass index have not been found to influence the risk of ACE.[2]

Social

Tobacco

Cigarette smoking is strongly implicated as a risk factor for SCCE in almost all studies. The risk increases with the number of cigarettes smoked per day and the duration of exposure. The risk diminishes when the habit is abandoned. Pipe and cigar smoking seemed not to have as strong a role.[3]

For ACE, the association with cigarette smoking has been controversial. Kabat and colleagues[2] believe that the failure to detect an association has been due to failure to compare ACE patients with appropriate controls. A problem that the authors noted in some studies was that "controls" had smoking-associated diseases. In their own study, Kabat and coworkers found an elevated and dose-related risk for smokers, both current and former and both men and women.[2] However, compared with the risk of SCCE, the association was weak. Again, pipe and cigar smoking were not implicated.

Alcohol

In most studies, alcohol intake has been associated with SCCE with a dose-related relationship. Drinkers of more than 4 oz of whiskey per day have a greater than 10-fold risk compared with nondrinkers.[3, 4]

For ACE, Kabat et al.[2] found a twofold risk among men who drink compared with women but no dose-related response; no relationship could be verified among women, but the sample size was small in this predominantly male disease. Compared with the risk of SCCE, the association of ethanol intake with ACE is, at best, weak, with some studies failing altogether to verify a relationship.[2]

Other Social Habits

Snuff, betel quid, and thermal irritation associated with drinking "burning-hot" tea or coffee have all been associated with SCCE, but these exposures are not as important as tobacco in endemic areas.[3, 4]

Environmental-Occupational

Exposure to irradiation, asbestos, heavy metals, solvents, and dyes has been associated with tumors of the esophagus. Plant pathogens invading kernels of weakened plants growing in the poor soil of endemic areas, *Alternaria alternata* on Iranian wheat and *Fusarium moniliforme* on corn in China and the Transkei, have been shown to enhance tumor growth in the nitrosamine model at levels lower than those occurring in the human diet in endemic areas.[5, 7, 8]

Barrett's Esophagus

Columnar epithelium is a known risk factor for development of ACE. The condition is believed by most investigators to be related to gastroesophageal reflux, but not all have been able to verify the association. Certainly, the condition has been described in patients without symptoms of reflux. Successful treatment of reflux does not reverse the metaplasia, nor does it reduce the risk of subsequent carcinoma. Once columnar metaplasia develops, the incidence rate of subsequent cancer is in the range of 1 per 52–441 patient-years.

Studies involving multiple endoscopic biopsies have demonstrated a very high risk of subsequent invasive adenocarcinoma among subjects with severe dysplasia. High-grade dysplasia is verified in 83% to 100% of resected adenocarcinomas whenever it is specifically sought by examining pathologists. Some authorities have recommended esophagectomy for patients with severe dysplasia for these reasons.[9, 10]

Esophageal Dysmotility

Achalasia is a risk factor for carcinoma of the esophagus, mostly in the middle third. Tumors are estimated to develop in about 20% of patients, with peak incidence 17 years after diagnosis.[11] Cricopharyngeal[12] and epiphrenic[13] diverticula have rarely been reported to harbor mural squamous cell carcinomas.

Corrosive Strictures

Squamous carcinomas arise in less than 5% of chronic strictures, usually following a prolonged latent period of 20 to 40 years.[14]

Previous Tumors of the Aerodigestive Tract

Second primary tumors arise elsewhere in the aerodigestive tract at a rate of 3% to 4% per year following successful treatment of a reference tumor.[15, 16]

LIFE HISTORY OF CANCER OF THE ESOPHAGUS

In the United States, dysphagia for solids and progressing to liquids is the most frequent presenting complaint. The patient may sense a level of obstruction, but the true level is not reliably predicted by history alone.[17]

Tumor in proximity to the airway may compress or invade, resulting in symptoms of stridor, cough, or choking. At times, the symptoms are thought to indicate "aspiration" pneumonia. Fistulization into airways (Fig. 2–1) complicates about 10% of tumors in proximity to the airway (i.e., unresected tumors of the cervical and upper thoracic esophagus).[18] Fistulization from more distal esophagus directly into the lung may also occur, as may fistulization into the aorta (Fig. 2–2), presenting as lethal massive hematemesis.

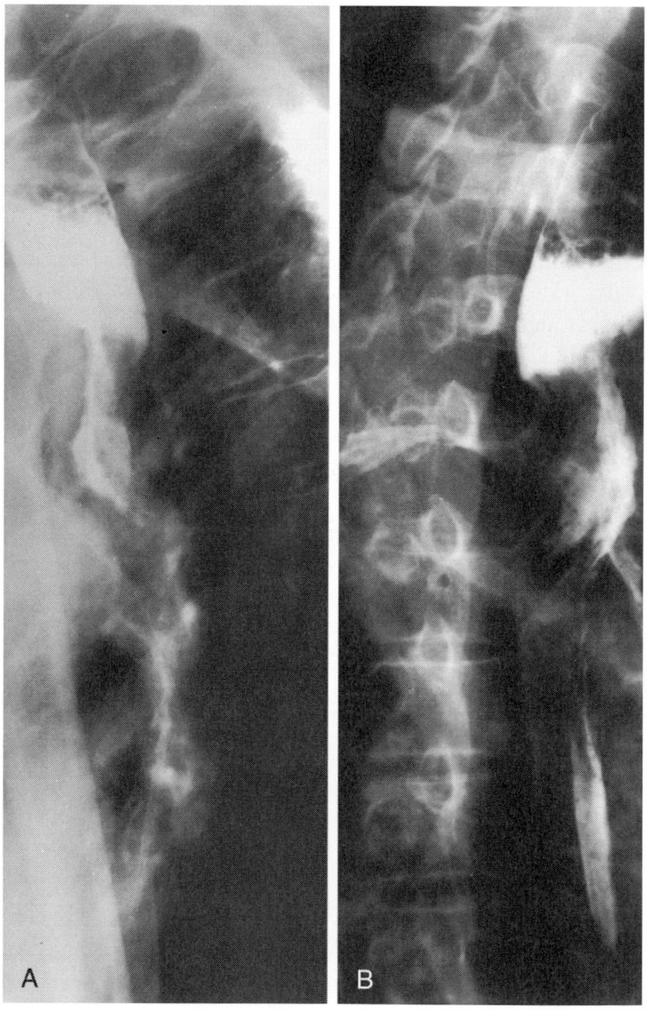

Only 40% of patients have symptoms of distant metastases, including nerve paralysis, at presentation. However, disseminated disease is present in the majority of patients at the time of diagnosis, even among those believed resectable for cure.[19] This is verified by autopsy observations and also by life-history studies demonstrating that most patients die of distant disease even when local control has been achieved by radiotherapy or surgery.[20] Anorexia and weight loss preceding dysphagia suggest distant metastases.

Patients who cannot or do not receive specific antitumor treatment in some form, either chemotherapy, radiotherapy, or surgery, almost all die within a year owing to malnutrition or pulmonary complications related to aspiration.

A B

FIGURE 2–1. *A,* Esophagram of a 66-year-old man with dysphagia and recurrent left lower lobe pneumonia. Luminal narrowing and mucosal irregularities are seen in the midesophagus with overhanging edges at the superior margin, indicating tumor extending over a length of at least 5 cm. The esophagus is dilated proximal to the tumor, and only a trickle of barium has passed distally. *B,* The same patient showing a fistulous communication from area of tumor to proximal left main stem bronchus.

LOCAL-REGIONAL ANATOMY

The esophagus is a tubular structure originating in the neck as a continuation of the pharynx. Proximal anatomic landmarks for the esophagus are the caudal portion of the cricoid cartilage, the lower border of the cricopharyngeal muscle, and the sixth cervical vertebra. It continues through the thoracic inlet into the posterior mediastinum in proximity to the membranous trachea to the point of airway bifurcation at the fifth thoracic vertebra, where the trachea deviates slightly to the right so that the esophagus lies posterior to the left main bronchus at this level. Caudally it lies posterior to the pericardium before it descends through the esophageal hiatus to the abdominal cavity, joining the stomach at the cardia opposite the eleventh thoracic vertebra. The length of the esophagus varies with the individual's proportions, but the average distance from the incisor teeth to the cardia is 40 cm (Fig. 2–3).

The esophagus is usually considered in four segments: the cervical, upper thoracic, midthoracic, and lower esophagus. The cervical segment is from the cricopharyngeal muscle to the suprasternal notch. The upper thoracic portion is from the thoracic inlet to the bifurcation of the trachea, approximately 24 cm from the incisors. The midthoracic segment is the proximal half of the esophagus distal to the tracheal bifurcation, approximately 32 cm from the incisors. The lower thoracic part is the lower half of the esophagus distal to the bifurcation of the trachea, including the abdominal portion.

The esophagus lacks a serosal layer; only loose adventitia separates the organ from surrounding structures. The muscle wall of the esophagus comprises an outer longitudinal muscle layer and an inner circular muscle layer (Fig. 2–4). The upper portion of muscle is striated, the lower esophageal muscle is smooth muscle, and between are mixed muscle layers. Deep to the muscle layers are submucosa, muscularis mucosa, and mucosa. Stratified squamous epithelium lines the esophagus from the pharynx to just proximal to the cardia, where an abrupt transition into columnar epithelium normally takes place.

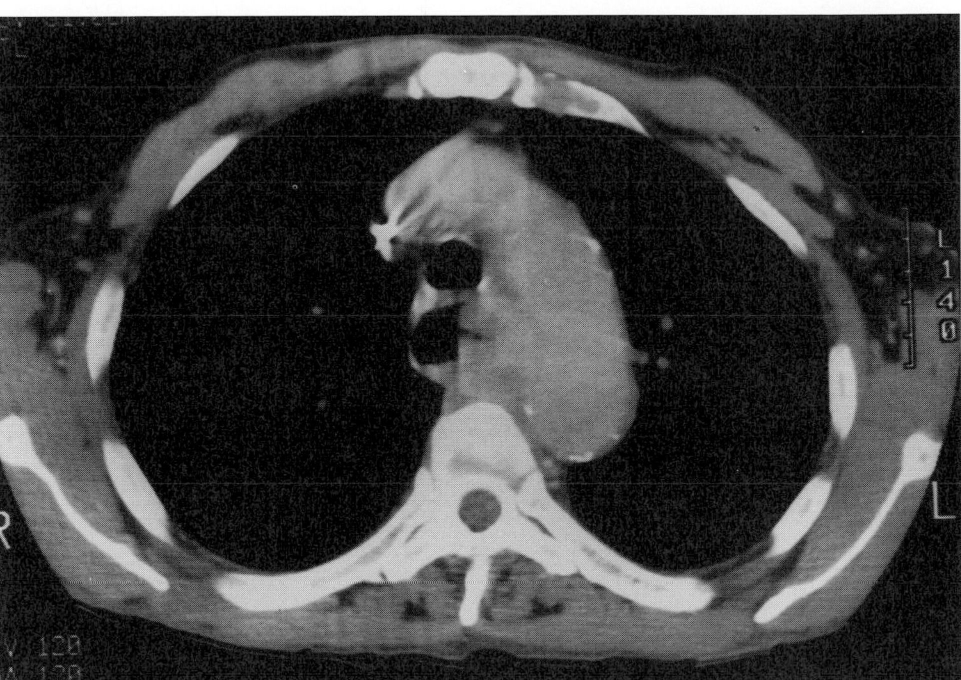

FIGURE 2–2. Computed tomogram showing bulky inhomogeneous tumor mass encroaching on esophageal lumen from the left side. The interface between the esophagus and the aorta is obliterated.

The blood supply to the esophagus originates from the inferior thyroid arteries in the neck; from the bronchial arteries, aorta, and right intercostal arteries in the chest; and from the inferior phrenic arteries and branches of the left gastric and short gastric arteries in the abdomen.

The lymphatic channels drain longitudinally in the submucosa for variable distances before penetrating muscle layers into regional lymph nodes or continuing to course along adventitial longitudinal lymphatics. Ultimately, drainage may include nodes in the neck, mediastinum, left gastric, perigastric, cardiac, and lesser curvature areas of the stomach.

PATHOLOGY

Grossly, esophageal tumors may be fungating, ulcerative, or infiltrating. The predominant cell type had been squamous cell carcinoma, mostly in the midesophagus[21, 22]; however, in recent years there has been a tendency toward a predominance of adenocarcinomas of the distal esophagus—the incidence rate quadrupling over 35 years in the tumor registry of one large HMO.[6] Only 4 of 557 esophageal tumors reviewed for the 35 years up to 1988 at the Southern California Permanente Medical Group were other than squamous cell carcinomas or adenocarcinomas (Table 2–1).

Tumors of either of the predominant cell types spread via lymphatics, coursing longitudinally in the submucosa, often considerable distances before penetrating muscle layers. Cells may either be deposited in local lymph nodes or course through adventitial longitudinal lymphatics before depositing in more distant nodes. This longitudinal course explains why submucosal involvement may be found as far as 10 cm from the primary mucosal tumor in about 5% of cases, and also why involved nodes may be quite distant from the primary site, with uninvolved nodes between them and the primary tumor. Bloodborne metastases are frequently found in adrenals, bone, brain, liver, lung, and peritoneum.[20]

SCREENING AND DIAGNOSIS

In the United States, carcinoma of the esophagus is sufficiently rare that screening and early detection programs for squamous cell carcinoma are not economically feasible. Early detection is of demonstrated value in endemic areas, where excellent cure rates have been demonstrated.[23] Tumor cells may be discovered in cytology samples collected by means of withdrawing swallowed sponges, balloons, or brushes.

Some have recommended frequent (several times per year) endoscopic biopsies of patients with Barrett's esophagus (Fig. 2–5) because, as dysplasia progresses to high grade, occult invasive carcinomas are frequent.[9, 10] We have reported invasive carcinoma discovered in a biopsy speci-

TABLE 2–1
Distribution of 557 Tumors of the Esophagus

	SCC	AC	Others
Cervical and proximal thorax	95	3	0
Middle thorax	227	10	0
Distal thorax and abdominal	124	94	4

SCC, Squamous cell carcinoma; AC, adenocarcinoma.

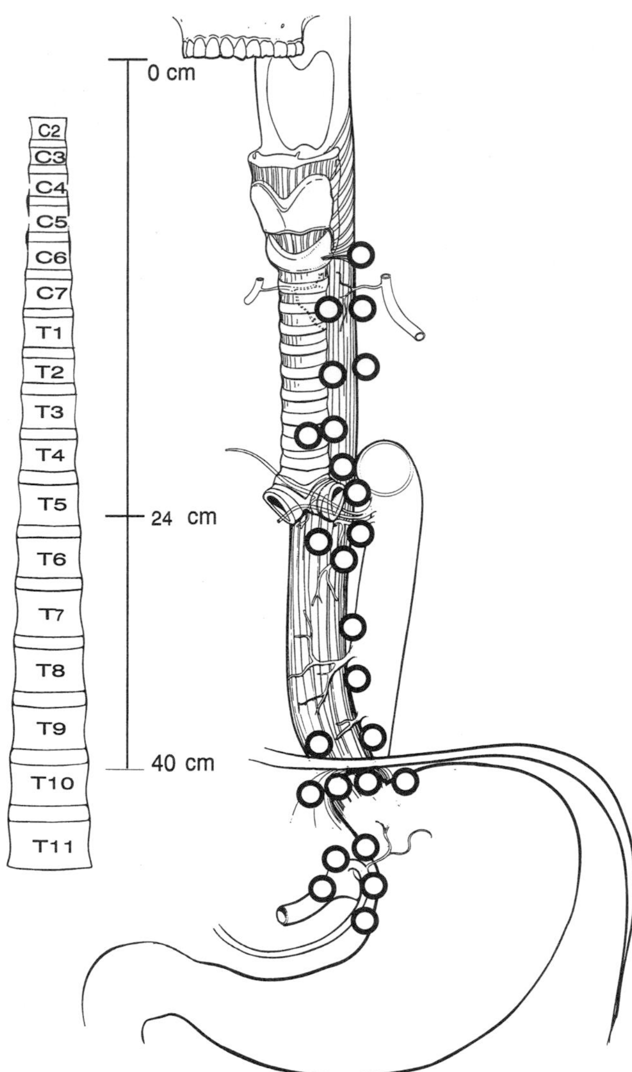

FIGURE 2–3. Outline of anatomic relationships of the esophagus. The length is about 3 cm from the incisor teeth to the esophagogastric junction. The spinal column is drawn as a reference point for these relationships.

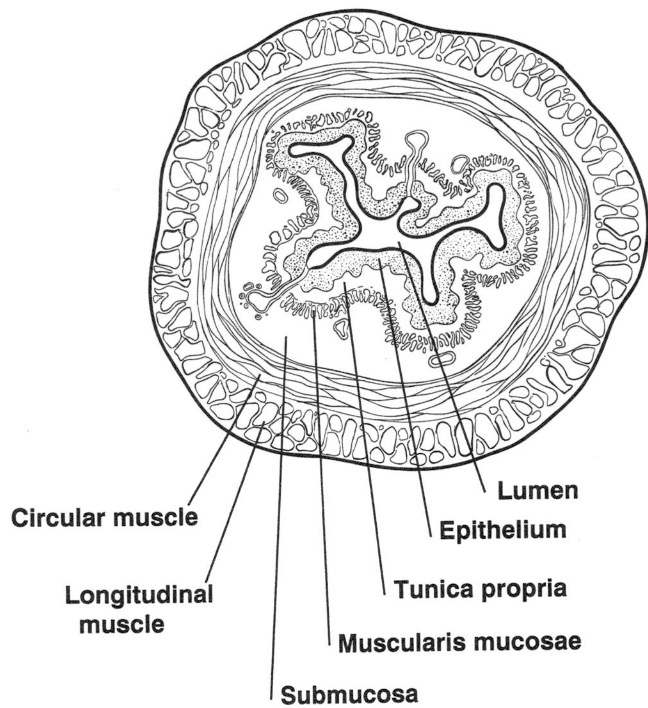

FIGURE 2–4. Cross section of the esophagus demonstrating the two muscular layers and absence of the cirrhosal layer.

men of a "superficial erosion" seen at surveillance endoscopy in a patient with Barrett's esophagus.[24] The cost efficiency of this approach is controversial, but we tentatively endorse it as the only means to increase the early detection rate for adenocarcinoma.

Most patients with esophageal carcinoma present with progressive dysphagia, often associated with weight loss. Pain is reported by approximately 30% of patients. Cough or hoarseness is unusual except when the tumor is close to the airway, in which case the incidence of these symptoms may approach 20%. The history frequently reveals risk factors, such as smoking and alcohol abuse.

Barium swallow generally confirms mucosal abnormalities (see Fig. 2–1). Esophagoscopy is required to obtain tissue for diagnosis and to search for other mucosal defects (Figs. 2–6 and 2–7). Bronchoscopy is routinely used to assess airway invasion by cervical and upper thoracic tumors.[17] Computed tomography (CT) is useful in assessing tumor dimensions; encroachment or invasion into neighboring structures; adenopathy; and spread to lungs, liver, and adrenals.[25] When clinical suspicions dictate, special studies such as bone scans, brain scans, and CT scans (or magnetic resonance imaging [MRI] scans) of the brain

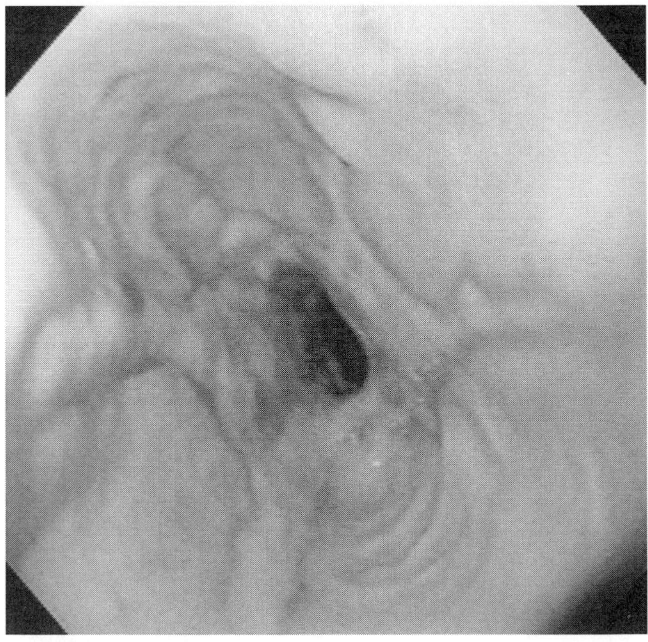

FIGURE 2–5. Endoscopic view of a transition from stratified squamous esophageal mucosa onto columnar-lined Barrett's esophagus just proximal to the esophagogastric junction.

are helpful, but their use is not routine.[26, 27] Esophageal ultrasonography (EUS) is useful in estimating tumor dimensions and transmural spread. Some studies have found EUS more accurate than CT in assessing depth of tumor invasion, especially in early tumors.[28, 29]

STAGING

Staging systems represent attempts to correlate the extent of disease with its prognosis. Surgical scholars have been able to demonstrate the value of systems similar to that of Dukes used for colorectal carcinoma in that wall penetration and accurate assessment of nodal spread are the most important prognostic indicators of local-regional disease.[30] It is not surprising that esophageal tumors should have prognostic indicators similar to those of other gastrointestinal tract tumors, but staging systems requiring study of the surgical specimen preclude easy comparison of surgical results with patients treated nonsurgically or treated by other means prior to surgery. Despite limitations of clinical staging, surgeons must begin to report results based on clinical staging as well as pathologic staging in order to compare their results with those in which resection either is not employed or is used following neoadjuvant therapy. EUS, 82% accurate in assessing depth of invasion and 73% accurate in determining node involvement,[31] will more frequently be used in estimating clinical stage of disease.

We recommend the use of the system proposed by the American Joint Commission on Cancer (AJCC) in cooperation with the Union Internationale Contre le Cancer (UICC).[32] In this system, the esophagus is divided into four anatomic regions: cervical, upper thoracic, midthoracic, and lower thoracic, which includes the abdominal portion. The system applies to squamous cell carcinomas and to adenocarcinomas because treatment options and outcomes are similar and no purpose is served in separating these two most common cell types. Other cell types are rare and are considered separately.

A TNM system is used (Table 2–2). T designations describe the depth of invasion of the primary tumor, ranging from in situ (Tis) and progressing to invasion of adjacent structures (T4). In this system, the length of tumor or whether it is circumferential plays no part, acknowledging that these factors are not as important as depth of invasion extending through the four layers of the esophagus—mucosa, submucosa, muscularis, and adventi-

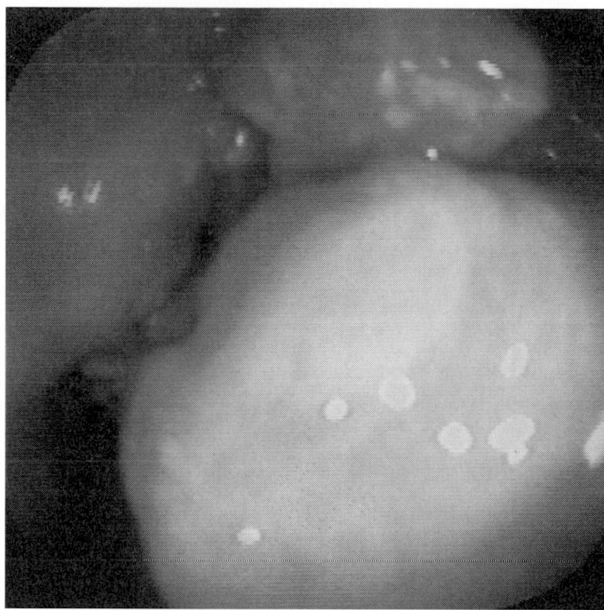

FIGURE 2–7. Endoscopic view of an advanced squamous cell carcinoma of the esophagus with near-total occlusion of the lumen.

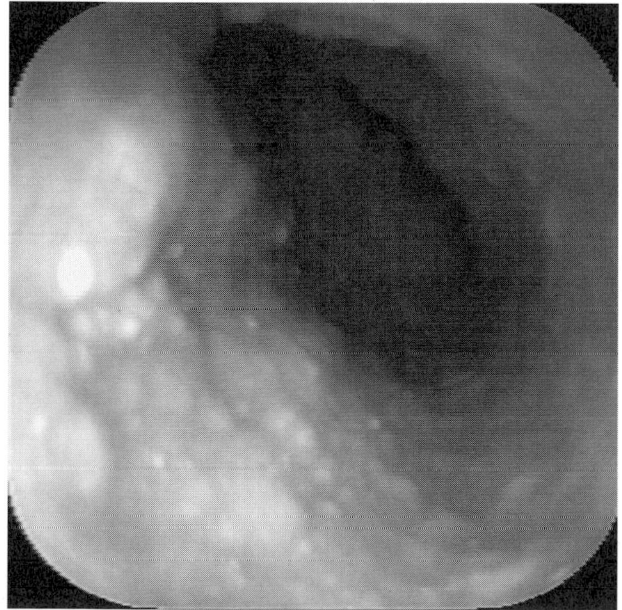

FIGURE 2–6. Endoscopic view of an early squamous cell carcinoma of the midthoracic esophagus.

TABLE 2–2
Definition of TNM System

Primary Tumor (T)	
TX	Primary tumor cannot be assessed
T0	No evidence of primary tumor
Tis	Carcinoma in situ
T1	Tumor invades lamina propria or submucosa
T2	Tumor invades muscularis propria
T3	Tumor invades adventitia
T4	Tumor invades adjacent structures
Regional Lymph Nodes (N)	
NX	Regional lymph nodes cannot be assessed
N0	No regional lymph node metastasis
N1	Regional lymph node metastasis
Distant Metastasis (M)	
MX	Presence of distant metastasis
M0	No distant metastasis
M1	Distant metastasis

tia. N designates regional lymph node involvement, with lymph node distributions designated as regional in relationship to the four anatomic regions of the esophagus or as metastatic if outside these regional lymphatic drainage boundaries (Table 2–3). M designates metastatic sites. TNM stage groupings are represented (Table 2–4).

For purposes of clinical staging, routine radiographic examination (CT, MRI, ultrasonography) and biopsy of accessible nodes may be used. When comparing results of surgery with those of radiation therapy, it is important to remember that a bias in favor of surgery may be introduced when pathologic staging results in "upstaging." In radiation therapy series, bias is introduced by the assumption that patients are incurable and by withholding curable attempts from all but early tumors in fit patients.[33]

SURGICAL TREATMENT

Resection

Standard operations for esophageal cancer attempt wide excision of the organ and its lymphatic drainage with 10-cm margins whenever possible.

We perform a midline abdominal incision for mobilization of the stomach. The left gastric artery is divided close to its origin so that lymph nodes along the lesser curvature are taken with the specimen. Care is taken to preserve the gastroepiploic arcade and right gastric artery. A pyloromyotomy or pyloroplasty is routine. After the Kocher maneuver, the fundus of the stomach reaches the neck without tension. A chest incision is performed through the fifth intercostal space, and the esophagus is mobilized proximal to the divided azygos vein or to the neck, if required, in order to achieve the preferred 10-cm margins.

The stomach is delivered through the manually dilated hiatus into the thorax. The specimen is excised using a surgical stapler along the lesser curvature. The specimen generally involves esophagus, periesophageal tissue, portions of fundus, cardia, and lesser curvature of the stomach en bloc with regional nodes. Resection of a generous portion of the lesser curvature and part of the fundus creates a stomach "tube" for esophageal replacement, a less bulky structure with fewer emptying problems than intact stomach used for the same purpose.

Staple lines are reinforced with sutures, and the anastomosis is generally accomplished with a circular anastomotic stapling device high in the thorax (Fig. 2–8). If a neck incision is required, our anastomosis is performed in two layers of interrupted braided absorbable suture (Fig. 2–9).

A nasogastric tube is passed into the stomach at completion of the anastomosis (and sutured to the nose to prevent

TABLE 2–3
Specific Regional Lymph Nodes

Cervical esophagus
Scalene
Internal jugular
Upper cervical
Periesophageal
Supraclavicular
Cervical, NOS
Intrathoracic esophagus—upper, middle, and lower
Internal jugular
Tracheobronchial
Perigastric (excluding celiac)
Carinal
Hilar (pulmonary roots)
Periesophageal
Left gastric
Cardiac
Nodes of lesser curvature of stomach
Mediastinal, NOS

NOS, Not otherwise specified.

TABLE 2–4
Stage Grouping

Stage 0	Tis	N0	M0
Stage I	T1	N0	M0
Stage IIA	T2	N0	M0
	T3	N0	M0
Stage IIB	T1	N1	M0
	T2	N1	M0
Stage III	T3	N1	M0
	T4	Any N	M0
Stage IV	Any T	Any N	M1

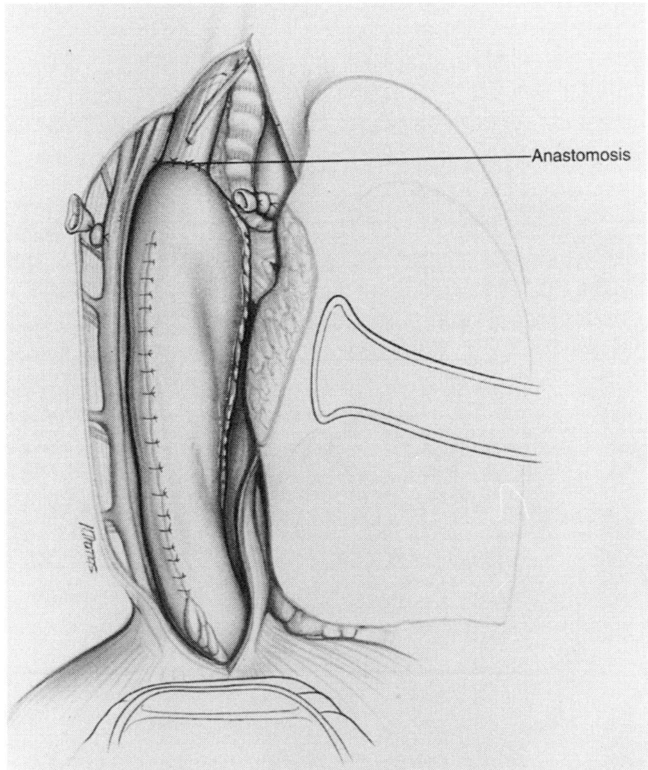

FIGURE 2–8. Stomach tube with esophagogastric anastomosis proximal to the divided azygos vein. The stapled suture lines are reinforced with interrupted sutures.

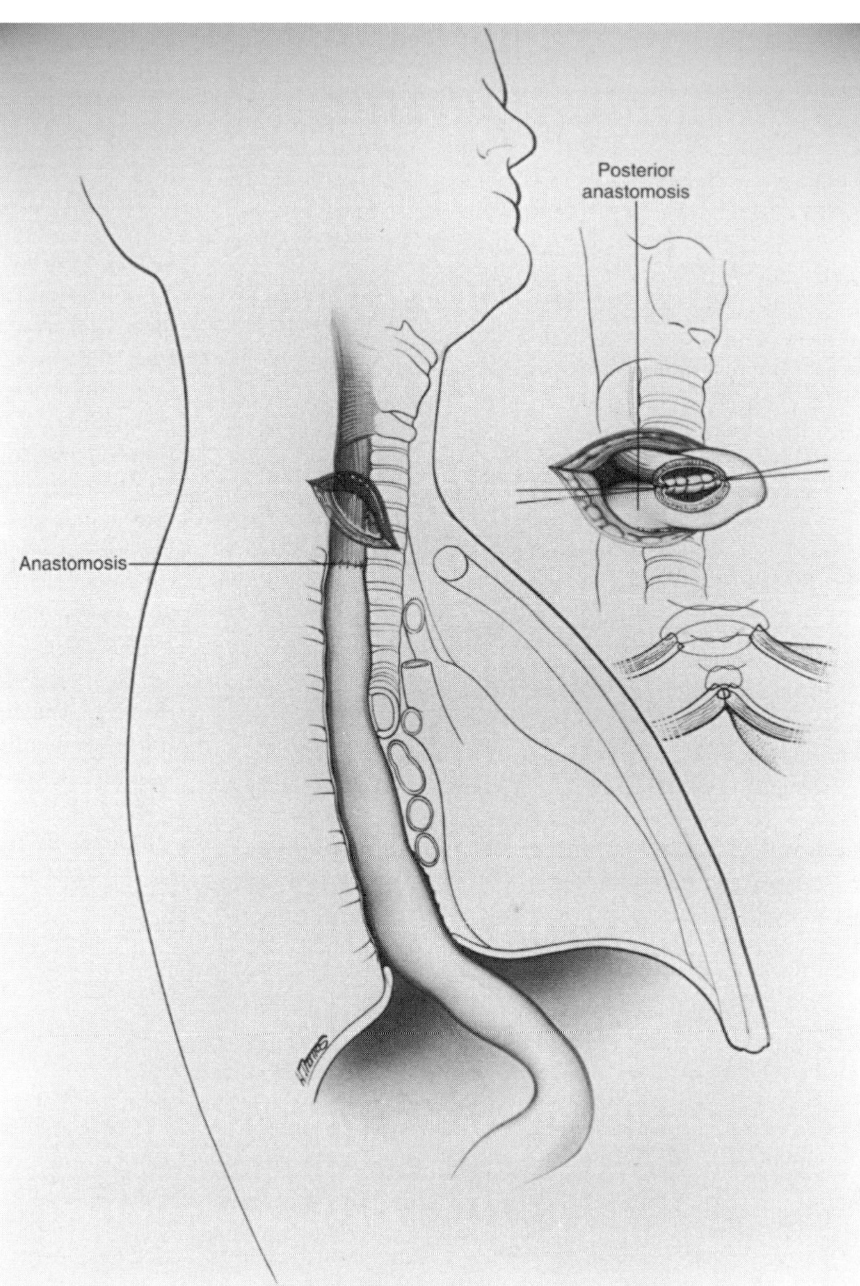

FIGURE 2–9. Stomach tube in the posterior mediastinum after a two-layered anastomosis performed in the neck.

dislodgment prior to transporting the patient from the operating room). Anterior and posterior chest tubes are positioned in the right thorax, and a feeding jejunostomy is performed prior to abdominal closure. We insert a left chest tube after repositioning the patient to supine, because drainage from the operative field to the dependent side is inevitable and must be presumed contaminated. Tube feedings are begun early in uncomplicated cases, and clear liquids are initiated on the eighth postoperative day if constrast studies confirm no leak and good gastric emptying (Fig. 2–10).[17]

Less extensive esophageal resections performed through the left chest have been advocated for tumors of the distal esophagus and cardia. An objection to this approach is that submucosal tumor extension is occasionally quite proximal to the required margins estimated at endoscopy and it is more difficult to extend the operation proximally in the left chest compared with the right because of aortic arch vessels. Nonetheless, admirable results have been obtained when this approach has been selected by some experts, and we sometimes use it for tumors of the cardia and intra-abdominal esophagus.[34]

Transhiatal, blunt esophagectomy involves the standard abdominal mobilization of the stomach along with a neck incision to mobilize the esophagus. With neck and abdominal tension applied to the esophagus, it is bluntly dissected

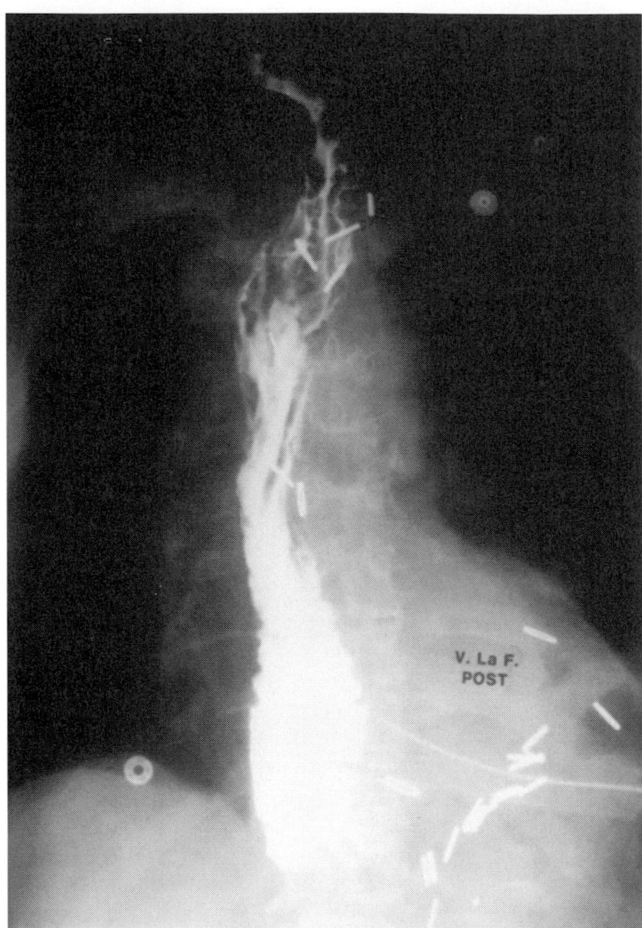

FIGURE 2–10. A barium swallow performed on the eighth postoperative day demonstrating no anastomotic leak and emptying of the stomach tube.

from mediastinal structures. Hemoclips are applied through the hiatus to the small segmental vessels at the aorta, which are then divided. The esophagus is gently dissected from the airway through the neck incision. When it is freed, the organ is divided at the neck. The esophagus is then withdrawn through the hiatus into the abdomen. The specimen is as described for the "standard" operation: esophagus, periesophageal tissue, and node-bearing area of the lesser curvature of the stomach. The fundus is then sutured to a rubber drain, which is passed from the neck. By gently pushing the stomach while pulling the drain, the fundus is delivered into the neck (Fig. 2–11), where a two-layer anastomosis is performed. Cardiac rhythm disturbances or hypotension are frequent while the surgeon's hand displaces the heart, but the operation can generally continue, allowing a recovery period to follow intervals of dissection. If palpation reveals a tumor too adherent for safe dissection, a standard resection is performed.

Akiyama et al.[35] have recommended a more radical operation in which special care is taken to dissect nodes from the posterior mediastinum, including tracheobronchial, paraesophageal, para-aortic, and pulmonary hilar nodes, along with an extensive abdominal node dissection. They found that even when tumor is located in the upper thoracic esophagus, abdominal node metastases are found in more than 30% of cases, and that with distal esophageal tumors, positive nodes are found in the superior mediastinum in about 10%. They recommend that thoracic and abdominal esophagectomy along with extensive thoracic and abdominal lymphadenectomy be performed.[35]

Skinner and colleagues[30] recommend a radical en bloc dissection that, in addition to providing 10-cm margins from the primary tumor, excises all resectable tissue in the posterior mediastinum, including both pleural surfaces, pericardium, thoracic duct, mediastinal nodes, and azygos vein. The abdominal portion of the specimen includes a 10-cm margin on the gastric side, spleen, a cuff of esophageal hiatus, and regional nodal tissue. Patients with "unfavorable pathology," defined as those having both transmural tumor and more than four positive nodes, are excluded and receive a lesser operation.[30]

DeMeester et al.[36] extend the en bloc operation of Skinner and coworkers to include the proximal 75% of the stomach. The specimen involves a tissue block of thoracic and abdominal esophagus, proximal stomach, and all potentially involved nodes. The operation is restricted to tumors of the middle and distal esophagus. Patients with "unfavorable pathology" as defined by Skinner et al. are not offered this operation. Colon interposition (Fig. 2–12) is used to re-establish intestinal continuity.[36]

Postoperative Care

Esophageal resection may involve entry into the neck, thorax, and abdomen, a relatively large area of trauma. Large volumes of fluids are sometimes required for the first 48 hours, and it is usually necessary to transfuse the patient. Many of the patients undergoing esophagectomy are elderly and have impaired cardiovascular-respiratory systems. They must often be monitored with central venous pressure lines or Swan-Ganz catheters. Flow sheets monitoring trends and daily weights are kept.

Jejunostomy is the preferred route of postoperative fluid, electrolyte, and calorie administration, eliminating the need for prolonged parenteral nutrition. The nasogastric tube can be placed on free drainage, since the main concern is that the stomach does not become distended.

It is important that the patient be encouraged to cough well. Chest physiotherapy is necessary. Blind nasotracheal aspiration is avoided because of risk of injury to the esophagogastric anastomosis. In cases of insufficient cough, respiratory secretions are aspirated by means of a catheter inserted into the airway with the assistence of a laryngoscope.

Cervical drainage should be minimal. Saliva in the cervical drains indicates an anastomotic leak. On the seventh day, a Gastrografin swallow is performed in the upright position to ascertain that the fluid goes through the stomach

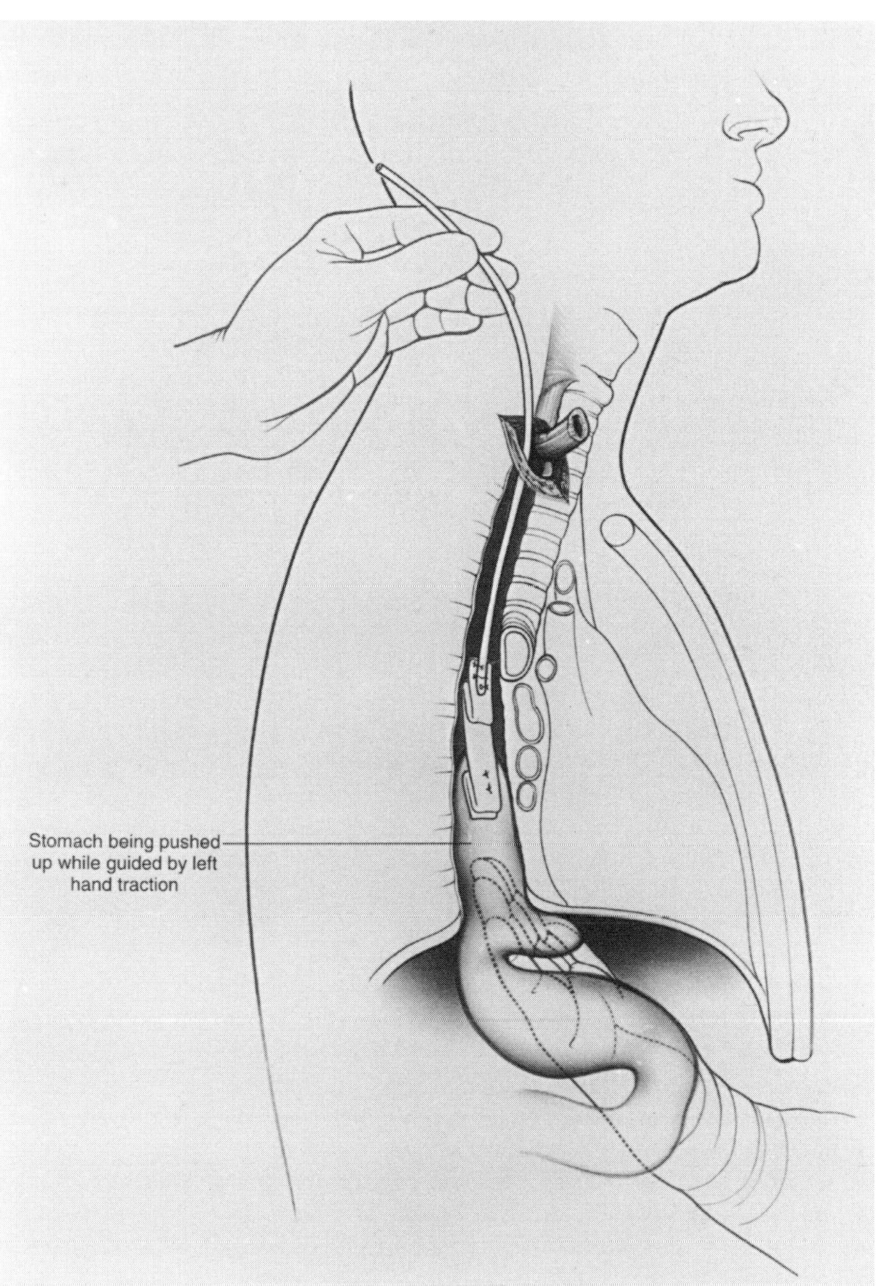
Stomach being pushed
up while guided by left
hand traction

FIGURE 2–11. Stomach tube being delivered into the neck by pushing through the hiatus and gently pulling the fundus.

and into the duodenum without delay or leak. The nasogastric tube is then removed. Oral intake begins with sips of clear liquids. Daily radiographs ascertain that the stomach is not distended. If the patient tolerates sips of fluids the first day, 4 oz of clear liquids are given per hour on day 2, followed by full liquids on the third day and then by a mechanical soft diet in five small meals per day. The patient is ready for discharge about 12 days postoperatively.

Throughout life, the patient must sleep with his head elevated to avoid aspiration, since there is free regurgitation. Frequent small meals are better tolerated than normal-sized ones three times per day.

Results of Resection

A 35-year review of patients in the tumor registry of the Southern California Permanente Medical Group showed an operative mortality rate of 9% and 12.7% for resections of tumors of the distal and middle esophagus, respectively, when surgery was the initial treatment. In this cohort, there was no difference in mortality for "curative" compared with palliative resections. In cases of "complete" resection, median survival was 381 days, 2-year survival was 28%, and 5-year survival was 20%. Stage of disease in retrospective studies is difficult to determine, but most were stage IIB or III.[6, 21, 22, 37]

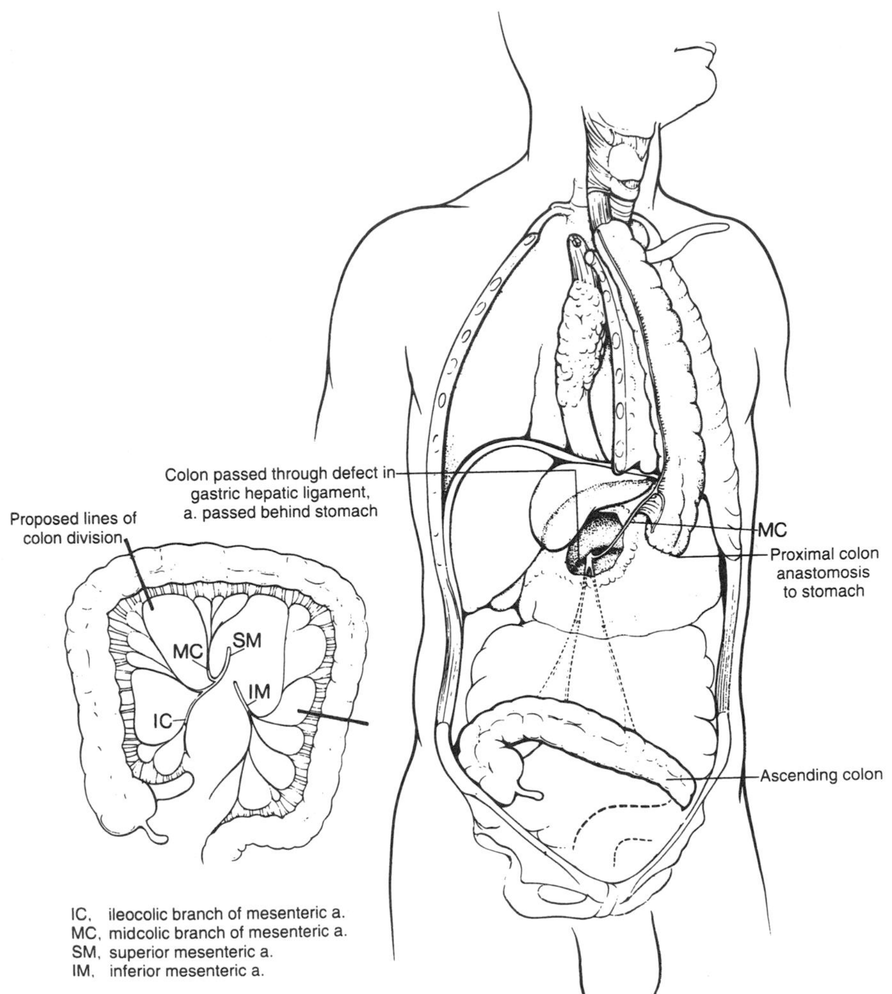

FIGURE 2–12. Depiction of a colon interposition using middle colon. Right and left colon may also be selected. A midesophageal tumor is in place in this drawing as it would be for a colon bypass.

An extensive review by Müller and colleagues[38] included all publications on surgical treatment of esophageal carcinoma appearing in a Western European language during the interval 1980 to 1988. After exclusion of editorials, reviews, case reports, papers dealing primarily with head and neck tumors, papers dealing primarily with adenocarcinomas of the cardia, and republications of the same material, the population reviewed comprised 76,911 patients described in 130 papers.

Müller and coworkers found that operability (the fitness of the patient to tolerate the procedure) and resectability (whether the removal of the tumor is technically feasible and reasonable) depend on policy or philosophy rather than on measurable differences in extent of disease. Aggressive surgeons, who believe in the value of palliative or incomplete resections, report resectability in the neighborhood of 90%,[34] but most surgeons forgo resection in cases of extensive local invasion, involvement of major abdominal organs, or distant metastases.

Mortality rates were similar for series reporting squamous cell carcinomas and those mixing squamous cell carcinomas and adenocarcinomas. No differences in mortality were related to the tumor level. The mean mortality rate for "curative" resections was lower than that for palliative resections, 11% ± 7% versus 19% ± 8%. Transthoracic resections, either right or left, had similar mortality rates when the anastomoses were performed in the chest (median, 13% vs. 14%), but cervical anastomosis reduced the mortality rate to a median of 10%. A lower mortality rate (median, 8%) was found with transhiatal esophagectomy, but Müller et al. remind us that since this operation has only recently been introduced to many centers, better mortality rates may be associated with recent improvements in postoperative care rather than with a truly less morbid operation. The lowest operative mortality rates, by any approach, were published by surgeons with greater personal experience. A "learning curve" is demonstrated by the fact that improved results are demonstrated by surgeons publishing over long intervals (e.g., Ellis with 20% mortality in 1960 and 2% in 1985).

Japanese studies report considerably lower mortality rates (6%) than those from other countries, but it has been observed that Japanese studies have addressed earlier disease with more superficial tumors and fewer positive nodes.[39, 40] American series involve tumors that more often have deeper penetration into (or through) the esophageal wall and positive lymph nodes, so "better" results reflect biologic variation rather than surgical triumph.

There are no convincing survival data to prove the superiority of any operative option. Survival rates are similar with approaches from the chest or with transhiatal resections. Improved survival attributed to extensive lymph node dissections is more likely the result of a lower proportion of advanced disease among patients undergoing extensive resections. Abe and coworkers[41] found that extensive en bloc resections, such as described by Akiyama et al.,[35] failed to result in 5-year survival if more than one node was positive; they found that when the number of nodes per patient and the number of positive nodes per patient were compared in their study and in that of Akiyama and colleagues, these numbers were similar. Abe et al. report a 50.9% 5-year survival rate if fewer than two nodes are positive, but a 0% 5-year survival rate if two or more nodes are positive. Radical en bloc resections have a very limited role if so few patients benefit.

The results of DeMeester et al.[36] for radical en bloc resection have been reported for 14 patients, with one perioperative death and only one patient available for 5-year follow-up. Actuarial survival was 66% at 2 years, but only five patients were evaluable beyond that time. This survival for the 14 highly selected patients of DeMeester and colleagues' cohort[36] is not significantly different from the 50% 2-year survival reported by Orringer[42] for 15 stage I and stage II patients treated by transhiatal esophagectomy. It has been noted that a statistical analysis of the results of DeMeester and others showing improved survival of patients undergoing radical en bloc resection compared with their other patients does demonstrate an improvement that is unlikely to be due to chance, but the data do not prove that the better outcome is due to the more radical operation rather than to patient selection factors.[43]

Palliative Resections

We recommend palliative resection in low-risk patients because survival is as good as with other means of treatment (~ 15% 1-year survival) and relief of aspiration and dysphagia are superior. In addition, resection and reconstruction prevent fistulization, abscess formation, and bleeding.[44] Other treatment options, such as laser therapy, palliative radiation, chemotherapy, and attempts to maintain a patent lumen with a combination of laser therapy, dilations, and endoprostheses, are preferable for those incurable patients with poor performance status.

Complications of Resection

The review by Müller et al.[38] revealed an average complication rate of 36%, but, since the reviewed authors seemed to focus only on serious problems or on those associated with technique, this figure probably represents an underestimate. The most frequent serious or lethal problems are anastomotic leaks, pneumonia, respiratory failure, and myocardial infarction.[45]

Pneumonia and atelectasis are less frequent among transhiatal esophagectomy patients than among thoracotomy patients, and respiratory failure is halved (13% vs. 27%) when thoracotomy is avoided.[38] Fan and colleagues[46] found that age greater than 65; arterial Po_2 less than 10 kPa (normal range, 11 to 14.4 kPa); serum albumin less than 39 g/L (normal range, 35 to 50 g/L); peak expiratory flow rate less than 65% predicted; and a procedure requiring three surgical wounds were incremental risk factors for postoperative pulmonary morbidity. Myocardial infarction has been reported in 2% to 5% of recent series. Atrial fibrillation and premature ventricular contractions are common minor complications but are occasionally major management problems.[38, 46] We administer prophylactic digitalis to reduce the incidence of postoperative supraventricular arrhythmias.

Anastomotic leaks complicate 10% of esophageal reconstructions, whether the anastomosis is performed in the neck or in the chest. Fatal complications, however, are less frequent in the neck. Leak incidence rates are similar with one- or two-layer hand-sutured anastomoses and stapled anastomoses but are lower with absorbable than nonabsorbable sutures (7% vs. 11%).[38] Fan et al.[47] reported that 62% of esophageal fistulas heal with conservative measures (total parenteral nutrition and adequate drainage) within 4 weeks in the absence of extensive sepsis, intestinal discontinuity, distal obstruction, or epithelialization of the fistulous tract. However, incomplete resections or low preoperative albumin levels were associated with low spontaneous closure. Surgical repair is recommended in cases of persisting drainage for 4 weeks. Early repair must be considered in cases of low albumin or residual disease. One third of the patients whose fistulas failed to heal within 4 weeks died of sepsis.[47]

Hoarseness, usually temporary, complicates up to 10% of esophageal resections.[48] Chylothorax is an infrequent complication of esophagectomy but is accompanied by a high mortality rate (up to 50% in some series).[49] If brief conservative management (drainage and total parenteral nutrition) fails, better outcomes result from thoracic duct ligation. Reoperation should be performed on the previously operated side so that leaking vessels may be identified and individually ligated, because thoracic duct ligation alone has not been uniformly successful.[50] The problem has also been successfully treated with insertion of a pleuroperitoneal shunt by Little et al.,[51] who reported complete resolution in two patients treated.

Bypass

Retrosternal bypass, using either stomach or colon, has been employed for palliation of advanced esophageal tumors. The procedure is conceptually attractive, especially for tracheoesophageal fistulas (TEFs), but results have been disappointing because of high mortality and brief survival.[52] We found that an occasional patient with an airway fistula benefits if disease is confined to the thorax and he has not yet had any other treatment. We have found the procedure futile in patients whose TEFs present as part of an extensive disease process, in those already in a debilitated state after previous treatment failure, or in those in whom pulmonary sepsis is already established.[18] We recommend only comfort measures for these patients.

Burt and colleagues[53] found superior survival (median, 77 days) for TEF patients bypassed compared with all other modes of treatment, but these were very select patients (28 of 207), and there was a 25% 30-day mortality rate.

Gastrostomy and Jejunostomy

Gastrostomy and jejunostomy, taken alone, fail to palliate esophageal cancer patients because they do not protect them from aspiration, nor do they restore the consolation of normal swallowing. Palliative attempts must be directed toward dysphagia rather than toward nutrition alone.[44] Cervical esophagostomy diverts oral secretions from the respiratory tract but, obviously, is no substitute for the comforts of swallowing. A feeding enterostomy of some sort, with or without diversion, may have a role while nonsurgical treatment is in progress.

In Burt and colleagues' review of TEF,[53] the 14% of patients treated with exclusion had a median survival of only 29 days, not significantly different from those patients treated with supportive measures only (the majority of patients).

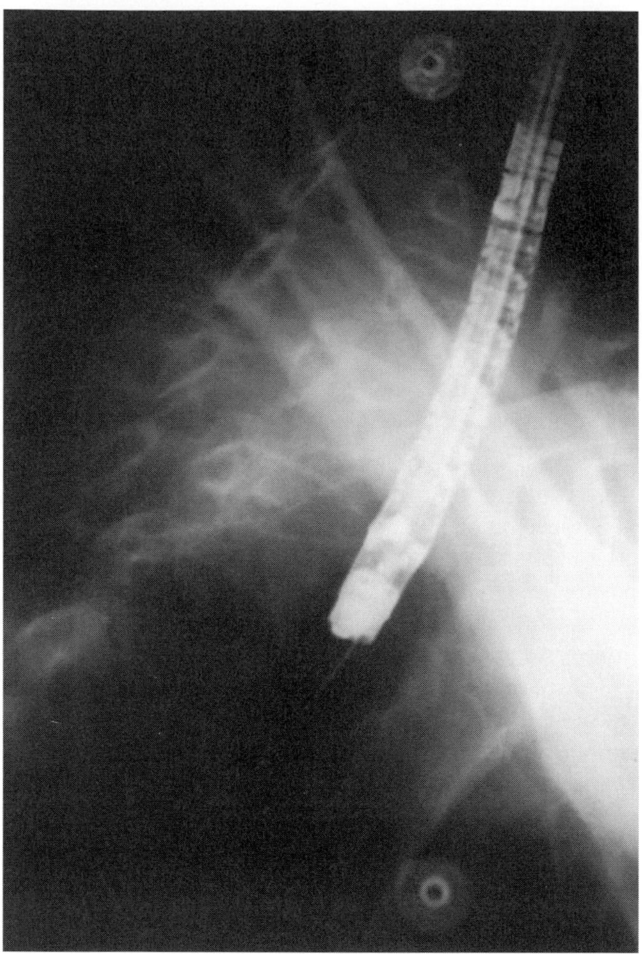

FIGURE 2–13. An endoscope at the level of the narrowed esophagus and a guide wire to the tip being positioned thoracoscopically below the narrowing.

Endoscopic Palliative Procedures

Dilatation

A variety of outpatient endoscopic treatments are useful in relieving dysphagia. These involve repeated dilatation, alone or accompanied by other modalities. The duration of benefit of dilatation alone is brief.[54] It does provide symptomatic relief during the interval of staging and treatment planning. Subsequent dilatations are required at decreasing time intervals unless treatment in addition to dilatation is employed. Repeated dilatations become increasingly difficult and painful.

Endoscopic techniques have almost entirely replaced "blind" insertion of mercury-filled dilators in many medical centers. A guide wire is passed through the stricture and fluoroscopically positioned in the stomach. Serial dilatations with graduated dilators may progress over the guide wire under fluoroscopic visualization (Figs. 2–13 and 2–14). Another method is a balloon system, which exerts a radial force to dilate the narrowed lumen.[55]

In conjunction with other modalities, such as laser therapy,[56, 57] stents,[58] bicap tumor probe,[59] and intraluminal brachytherapy,[60, 61] relief of dysphagia may be significantly prolonged.

Our preference is to accompany dilatation with high dose rate intraluminal radiation. Duration of palliation equivalent to that provided by external beam radiation (4.5 months of a life expectancy of 5.8 months) has been accomplished in less than 30 minutes' total treatment time. The cost efficiency and efficacy compare favorably with other combinations and may be delivered to a population too frail for repeated endoscopy or return trips to the radiation therapy suites.[60, 61]

Perforation is the most serious complication of dilatation. Small perforations, recognized early when the procedure is performed for benign disease, are frequently treated conservatively. This is less often a successful option in the case of stricture due to carcinoma in which obstructive tumor is distal to the defect. In the case of perforation during diagnostic endoscopy of a patient who is an operative candidate, an urgent resection is preferred treatment. An esophageal exclusion, with mediastinal and thoracic drainage, is sometimes required in nonoperative candidates,[62] but this is suboptimal palliation. In theory, it is preferable to complete the dilatation and pass a stent, whenever possible, but results are generally poor.[53]

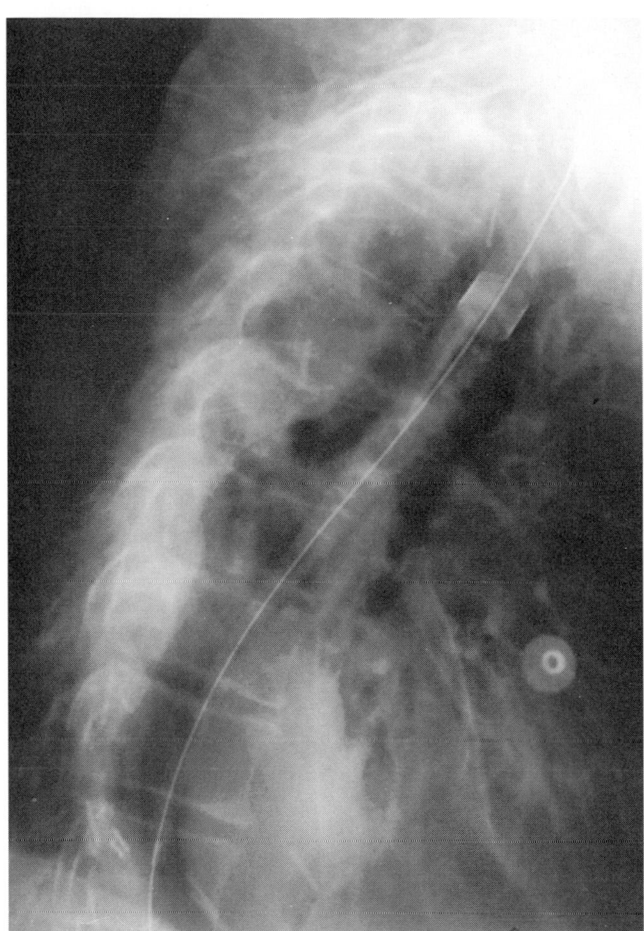

FIGURE 2–14. Dilators being passed through the strictured area to the previously positioned guide wire.

Laser Treatments

Endoscopic Nd:YAG laser treatment for esophageal tumors was first reported by Fleischer and Kessler.[56] The Nd:YAG laser is a monochromatic light source that is able to be easily focused and delivered. Light energy is converted to heat energy at the tissue focal point, where, depending on the temperature that is created, the effect on the cell varies from cell death and edema at low levels to tissue vaporization at higher temperatures. The tumor is dilated so that the endoscope can be passed beyond its distal extent and treated in a retrograde fashion until an adequate lumen is created. The procedure is repeated in 48 to 72 hours to ensure that an adequate lumen has been created.

A functional success in 70% to 85% of patients is possible, with benefit lasting up to 3 months. The procedure can be repeated when symptoms recur.[56, 63]

Bipolar Electrocoagulation

Bipolar electrocoagulation can be used to locally reduce the tumor. The main problem with the bicap tumor probe is that it treats in a circumferential manner and therefore can lead to stricture formation if normal esophageal mucosa is treated.[59]

Endoprostheses

The palliative treatment of esophageal obstruction via the insertion of an esophageal prosthesis dates to the nineteenth century. Since then, there have been an assortment of prosthesis shapes, sizes, and designs. The goal for effective palliation with an esophageal prosthesis is to maintain a patent lumen and to relieve dysphagia. The limiting factor to using a prosthesis is the anatomic location of the lesions. Tumors located within 2 cm of either the cricopharyngeal muscle or the esophagogastric junction are difficult to palliate with this method. The prosthesis must be placed so that it extends at least 2 cm beyond both the proximal and the distal margins (Fig. 2–15). Major complications of prostheses are migration and erosion of the tubes. Malignant overgrowth may also occur, resulting in recurrent dysphagia. Respiratory compromise may be caused by compression of the airway (Fig. 2–16).[55]

In a comparison of the palliation derived from endo-

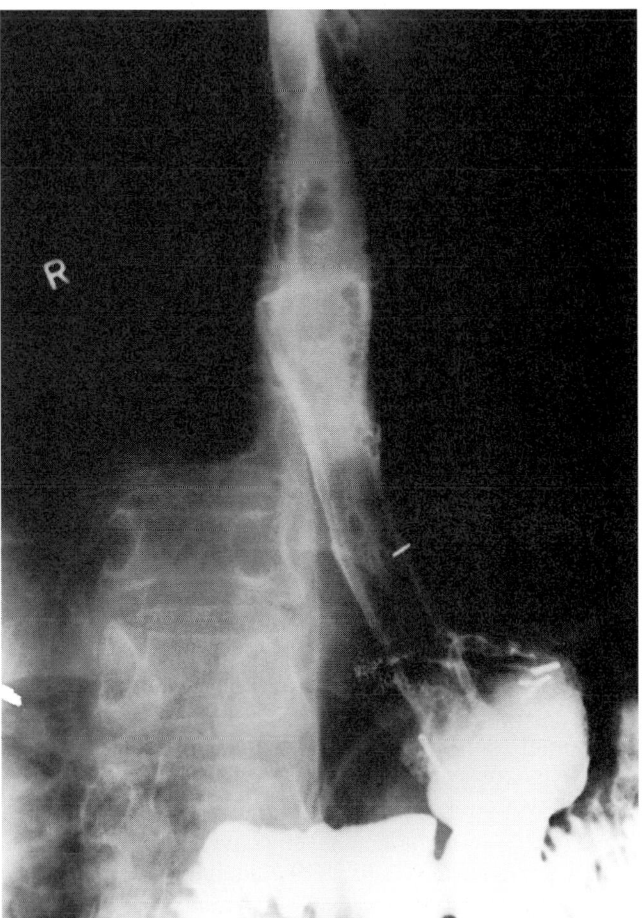

FIGURE 2–15. A barium swallow showing contrast passing through a tube prosthesis into the stomach. The prosthesis was placed for recurrence after a limited esophagogastrectomy performed for tumor.

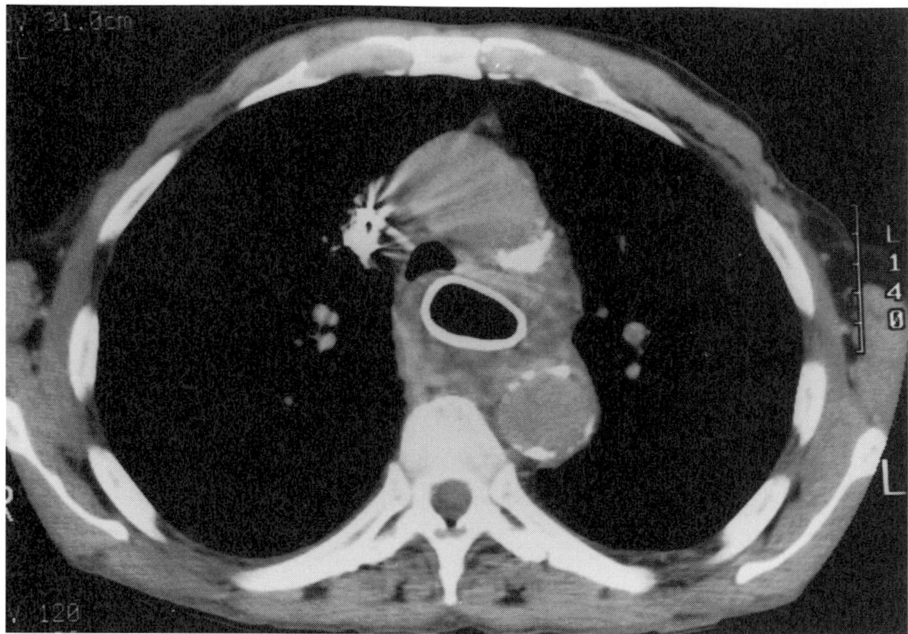

FIGURE 2–16. Computed tomogram showing area just above the carina. An esophageal Atkinson stent is in place surrounded by tumor, which encroaches on posterior trachea and extends into azygoesophageal recess and left hilum.

scopic stent placement versus laser palliation for malignant obstruction, both modalities offered immediate improvement. The mean survival was similar for both groups, with 6.1 months in the laser group and 5.1 months in the prosthesis group. Those patients who were treated with laser palliation required more procedures (an average of 1.4 procedures for the stent group versus 4.6 procedures for the laser group) and spent more time in the hospital (averaging 9 days for the stent group versus 14 days for the laser group), but prosthesis insertion was associated with more complications. The incidence of perforation was 13% in the stent group as compared to 2% in the laser group. Neither group had any procedure-related mortalities. In this study, patients treated with laser had better overall relief of the symptoms of dysphagia and were better able to tolerate solid food when compared to the group with the prosthesis insertion.[64]

RADIOTHERAPY

External Beam Radiation

External beam doses of 6000 to 7000 cGy in fractions of 180 to 200 cGy/day, 5 days a week, are required to control gross tumor, but lesser doses suffice for subclinical disease. The treatment field must include generous margins because of the propensity for wide drainage within the muscular walls of the esophagus. Treatment fields include nodal areas from the supraclavicular to the celiac (Figs. 2–17 and 2–18). Shielding of the spinal cord is essential because its radiation tolerance is in the neighborhood of only 4500 cGy.[65]

Complications

Short-term complications of radiotherapy frequently include esophagitis, pneumonitis, pericarditis, skin changes, hair loss, transient myelosuppression, gastrointestinal complaints (including nausea, vomiting, anorexia, and weight

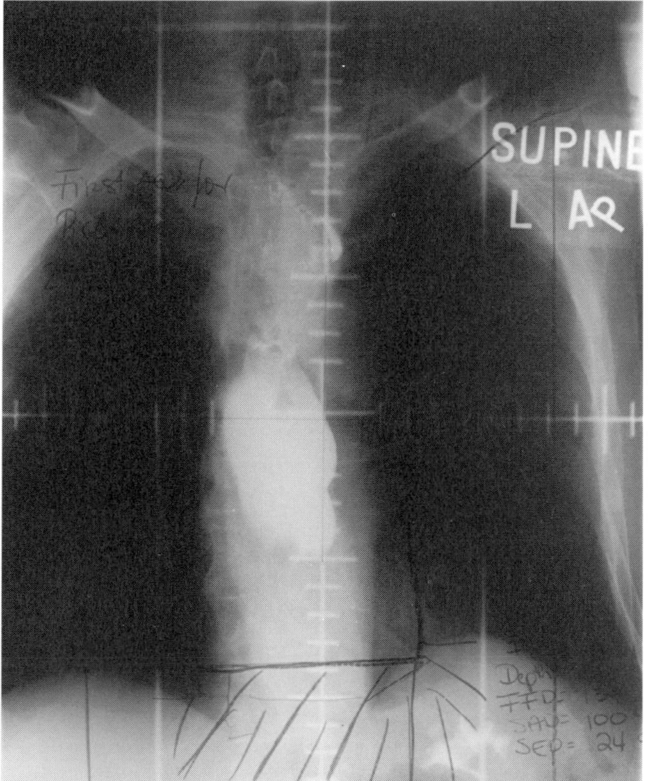

FIGURE 2–17. Anteroposterior fields for treatment of esophagus cancer. Barium is in the esophagus to help outline treatment area.

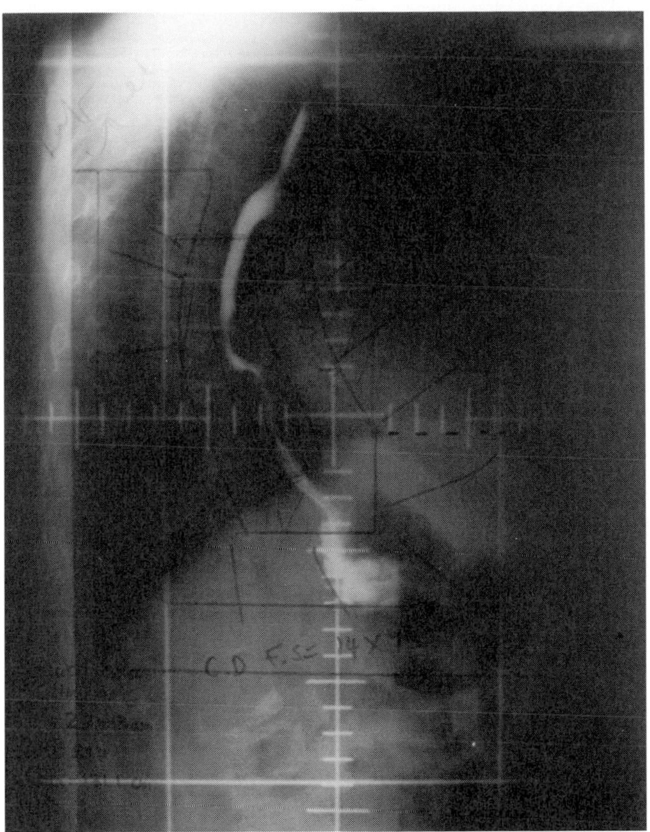

FIGURE 2–18. Cone down lateral fields include the tumor with a 5-cm margin.

loss), and fatigue. Perforation with fistulization or hemorrhage is often listed as a complication but should be considered a complication of disease progression rather than of treatment, since radiation only hastens the inevitable by killing tumor cells already invading airway or aorta.[33]

Longer-term complications include stricture, pulmonary fibrosis, pericardial constriction, myocarditis, bone necrosis, and transverse myelitis. Transient dysphagia is common, but fibrous strictures require approximately 3 months to develop. Occasionally, strictures refractory to dilatation necessitate resection for palliation; nondilatable postradiation strictures frequently represent tumor recurrence.[66, 67]

Survival

In retrospective studies reported from the tumor registry of a large HMO, primary radiotherapy yielded survival rates similar to those with surgery: 20% 5-year survival among those treated for cure, but less than 20% 1-year survival among patients treated for palliation.[6, 21, 22] However, only palliative treatment was provided to 80% of patients. Selection criteria excluding so many radiotherapy patients from curative attempts are difficult to determine in a retrospective study, but an assumption of futility on the part of some treating therapists prevents planning curative treatment.

A high attrition rate was reported in a large collective review in which it was found that most patients failed to complete a full course of curative irradiation.[33] If only the most fit and motivated patients with early disease are given curative treatment, the true potential for cure will not be tested or fairly compared with surgery. Nonetheless, several studies demonstrate cure rates that are similar for external beam radiotherapy and resection.[33, 68] Duration of survival with palliative radiation is as long as that with palliative resection, but relief of dysphagia is improved and prolonged with resection.

Intraluminal Brachytherapy

Many patients referred for radiation therapy have advanced disease with such poor performance status that a full treatment course cannot be expected. In these cases, we have found it useful to perform a short course of intensive intraluminal radiation delivered via a nasogastric tube inserted following dilatation of the tumor (Fig. 2–19). A low dose rate cesium 137 source may be used to deliver 160 to 170 cGy/hour, for a total dose of 2000 cGy delivered in three sessions over 1 week.[60] Alternatively, a high dose rate iridium 192 source may be used to provide 200 cGy/minute, for a total dose of 1250 cGy in one session.[61] Either dose rate provided significant improvement in dysphagia to the extent that most patients retained or regained their ability to swallow solid foods until death from distant disease.

This expeditious, efficient, and uncomplicated mode of delivery is especially useful for the very sick patient who

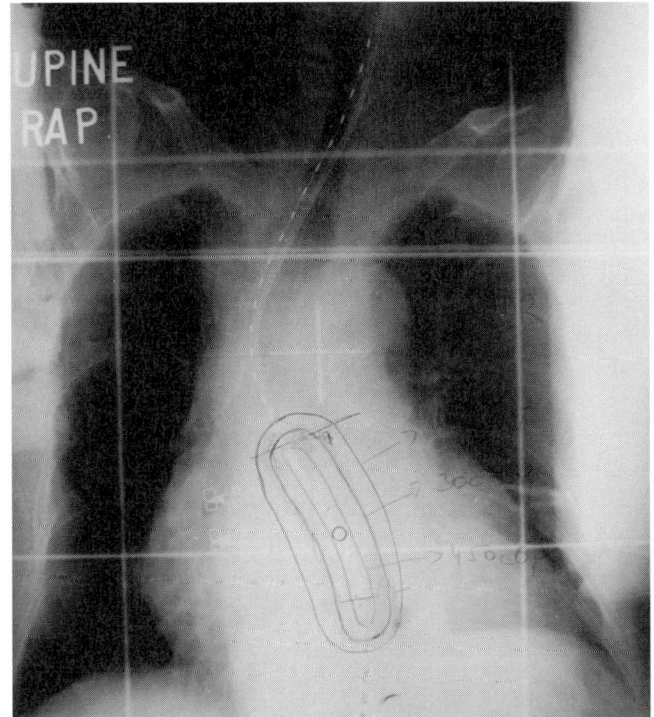

FIGURE 2–19. Endoluminal high dose rate planning photographs with isodose lines superimposed over the tumor.

would otherwise have only intubation and hospice care as options, usually patients with a predicted survival of less than 6 months. We also advise consideration of intraluminal radiotherapy for postoperative use in cases of microscopic positive margins.

Combined External Beam and Intraluminal Radiation

High dose rate iridium 192 radiation has been combined with external beam radiation for treatment of localized disease in curative doses and also for palliative treatment.[69, 70]

Pakisch and colleagues[70] achieved prolonged satisfactory palliation, defined as intake of at least semisolid food, in 96% of patients with tumors of the esophagus and gastric cardia that they described as nonresectable. Stage I and II patients achieved a 66% 1-year survival rate (mean survival, 19 months); stage III and IV patients had a mean survival of 6.9 months.[70]

Hashikawa and colleagues[69] reported their experience with 66 "limited disease" thoracoesophageal tumors treated with a combination of 6000 cGy external beam radiation over 6 weeks followed by 1200 cGy high dose rate intraluminal radiation. Two- and 5-year survival rates were 37% and 18% respectively. Two-year local control rate was 64%. The same regimen employed for 82 patients with extensive disease resulted in a 2-year survival rate of 7%, but still a local control rate of 45%. Serious complications among these 148 patients included ulceration (28%), stricture (10%), and fistula (4%), with 10 patients requiring surgery for treatment of these complications.[69]

Hareyama and coworkers[71] reported results treating squamous cell carcinomas with 5500 to 6000 cGy external beam radiation over 5.5 to 6 weeks followed by 1500 to 2000 cGy intraluminal radiation delivered in two or three fractions. Local control was achieved in 32% of 161 patients with an actuarial 5-year survival rate of 43% for stage I, 21% for stage II, and 0% for stages III and IV tumors. They reported five benign, radiation-induced ulcers among their long-term survivors, leading them to conclude that the treatment schedule was close to maximal tolerance of the esophagus.[71]

Any advantages of this combination over external irradiation alone remain to be clarified. Certainly, local control is very good but at the expense of a high incidence of local complications, some of which necessitated surgery for their treatment.

Preoperative Radiotherapy

Preoperative radiotherapy has been delivered by a variety of methods with the expectation that it would decrease tumor bulk and improve resectability, reduce metastases induced by operative manipulation, and destroy residual tumor left following resection. However, prospective randomized trials have been unable to verify an impact on operability, resectability, or survival. Furthermore, complete response rates have been less than 10%.[72] Diehl[73] reviewed 10 historically controlled series and 3 prospective randomized studies and concluded that no clear value for preoperative radiation has been established.

Postoperative Radiotherapy

In the past, postoperative radiotherapy has been given in the hope of destroying residual tumor in the operative field. The delivery of tumoricidal dose is limited by the sensitivity to radiation of the replacement organ, usually stomach. A prospective randomized controlled study has revealed that postoperative radiotherapy reduces the local recurrence rate among patients receiving palliative resections compared with nonradiated controls (P = .04) and decreases the incidence of tracheobronchial obstruction among patients with residual disease in the mediastinum (P = .03). There was no observed reduction in extrathoracic or anastomotic recurrence.

Complications occurred in the intrathoracic stomach in 37% of irradiated patients and in only 6% of controls (P = .0001), with a 21% death rate, as a result of bleeding, among patients in whom complications developed. Overall median survival was reduced from 15.2 months in the control group to 8.7 months in the irradiated group (P = .02) because of the lethality of bleeding in the irradiated stomach and because of the earlier onset of distant metastases among the irradiated palliative resection group (5.1 months) as compared to the nonirradiated controls (8.5 months, P = .05). The authors concluded that postoperative radiotherapy should be limited to patients with residual disease in the mediastinum, in which case the incidence of obstruction of the tracheobronchial tree is significantly reduced.[74]

CHEMOTHERAPY

Because it is known that the majority of patients with cancer of the esophagus already have disseminated disease at the time of diagnosis, there has been much interest in discovering combinations of drugs effective against this tumor.[19] Pioneering efforts carried out by investigators at Memorial Sloan-Kettering Cancer Center initially used combinations of drugs with demonstrated effects against head and neck tumors (cisplatin and bleomycin). When these drugs were used prior to surgery in patients with local-regional disease, half of the patients experienced subjective improvement in swallowing, even though only 14% had objective partial responses. Similar objective response rates were documented among patients with extensive disease. The later addition of the *Vinca* alkaloid vindesine improved survival in a subsequent cohort of patients with local-regional disease treated prior to surgery and improved the partial response rate among patients with extensive disease.[75] When Kelsen et al.[76] performed a randomized prospective trial comparing cisplatin-bleomycin-vindesine chemotherapy with preoperative external beam radiotherapy at 5500 cGy, similar objective responses were found in both cohorts. They concluded that chemotherapy was as good as radiotherapy for local control of squamous cell carcinoma.[76]

Other drugs have been effective in combination with cisplatin: mitoguazone, originally substituted for bleomycin in an attempt to avoid the pulmonary toxicity of bleomycin; methotrexate with folinic acid rescue; 5-fluorouracil (5-FU); and mitomycin C. In the hands of experienced medical oncologists, a variety of combinations, doses, and schedules have produced objective responses, including complete response rates greater than 20% documented by study of surgical specimens. Others have verified the observation of Kelsen et al.[76] that even modest objective responses may result in significant relief of dysphagia among patients with extensive disease. Several combinations have been found useful, either alone or in combination with other palliative efforts (dilatation, endoprostheses), in relieving dysphagia in patients too ill to withstand standard radiation or surgery.[77–79]

Cisplatin plays a key role in modern protocols for chemotherapy of carcinoma of the esophagus. There are now several reports of cisplatin-based chemotherapy combinations resulting in response rates of greater than 50% for squamous cell carcinomas and also for adenocarcinomas. Muggia[78] described several areas that may become clinically important in expanding the use of cisplatin. Sodium thiosulfate has been shown to permit intensive high doses of cisplatin with diminished nephrotoxicity, neurotoxicity, and anemia. Circadian dosing strategies may improve efficacy, as has been reported for evening doses in treating gynecologic cancers. Prediction of response may be feasible from studies of the ability of tissues to retain platinum-DNA adducts prior to drug administration. Since enhanced repair of platinum-DNA adducts has been implicated in tumor resistance, there may be a role for pretreatment study to predict resistance and also a clinical application of drugs that inhibit DNA repair to enhance cytotoxicity.[78] Hyperthermia accelerates the cellular uptake of cisplatin and its binding with DNA even among resistant cells.[80]

COMBINATION THERAPY

Preoperative Chemotherapy

Preoperative chemotherapy is an in vivo test of efficacy of the selected combination against a *particular* tumor, and, in the case of response, the resectability rate should be improved. Furthermore, in theory, chemotherapy administered prior to surgery is more effective against microscopic disease and in minimizing selection of resistant clones.[81, 82] These considerations, along with the fact that most esophageal cancers have already metastasized by the time they are diagnosed,[20] promoted an interest in neoadjuvant, or preoperative, chemotherapy.[19]

Kelsen et al.[76] performed a prospective trial for squamous cell carcinoma comparing preoperative radiotherapy with preoperative chemotherapy consisting of two courses of cisplatin, vindesine, and bleomycin. Radiation was delivered at 4500 cGy to the primary tumor with 5-cm proximal and distal margins and to regional nodes, followed by a boost to 5500 cGy to the primary tumor with a 2-cm margin. Patients in the chemotherapy limb of the study received cisplatin, 120 mg/m^2 on days 1 and 29; vindesine, 3 mg/m^2 on days 1, 8, 15, 22, 29, 38, and 43; and bleomycin, 10 U/m^2 intravenous bolus followed by a 4-day continuous infusion at 10 U/m^2/day beginning on day 3 and ending on day 7 and beginning on day 31 and ending on day 36. No deaths were attributed to induction therapy.

Surgery was performed during the eighth week following initiation of therapy. Patients who had complete resection of T1–2, N0, M0 tumors were considered to have curative resections and received no further treatment. Resections were considered palliative if margins were microscopically positive, lymph nodes were positive, or tumor had penetrated into periesophageal tissue. These patients received postoperative radiotherapy if initially on the chemotherapy limb and vice versa. Most (75%) of the chemotherapy patients were operable, and 58% were resectable, with an operative mortality rate of 11%. The median survival of patients with resectable tumors was 16 months, but that of responders was 26.6 months.

Kelsen et al.[76] concluded that the results with preoperative radiotherapy and with chemotherapy were similar but that the impact on survival, even with all three modes (because of the crossover design of the study) was poor and not better than results with surgery alone. They mentioned that the phenomenon of "responders" doing better than "nonresponders" may not be a causal relationship. They concluded that more effective chemotherapy combinations remain to be discovered and that surgery remains standard care outside of carefully designed clinical trials.[76]

Ajani et al.[83] at the M.D. Anderson Cancer Center evaluated prolonged perioperative courses of etoposide, 5-FU, and cisplatin (EFP) for adenocarcinoma of the esophagus or gastroesophageal junction. They planned a total of six courses, two preoperatively and four postoperatively, and a median of five courses were actually administered, with a 77% major response rate. There was modest toxicity associated with the protocol, but no deaths were attributable to complications of chemotherapy. This study showed complete resection to be associated with improved survival and demonstrated that up to six courses of cisplatin-based chemotherapy could be provided, but they could not conclude that EFP imparted survival benefit in this pilot study.[83]

More recent studies have confirmed that neoadjuvant protocols based on cisplatin and 5-FU are well tolerated, with no increased operative mortality associated. A complete clinical response of 20% to 40% is not uncommon; however, when microscopic disease is sought, active tumor may still be found in up to 90% of resected specimens.[84, 85] Actuarial survivals, when compared with historical controls, (1) may be prolonged, (2) may[85] or may not[84] be correlated with complete clinical response, and (3) are improved among those completely resected. When evaluating results such as these, it is important to keep in mind that actuarial survivals tend to overestimate the eventual observed survival.[43] Also, improved survival compared with historical controls may result from selection factors or other improvements in treatment rather than the chemotherapy. We agree with Ginsberg's comments urging participation in prospective randomized trials required to answer questions regarding the utility of neoadjuvant therapy.[86]

Chemoradiotherapy Without Surgery

Laboratory data have demonstrated the ability of 5-FU, cisplatin, and other agents to potentiate tissue radiation sensitivity, leading Leichman and Berry[77] to conclude that all future trials involving radiotherapy should also include chemotherapy. They have reported results of trials demonstrating improved survival of patients treated with chemoradiation compared with radiation alone and with chemoradiation followed by surgery compared with radiation followed by surgery.[77]

Investigations are in progress to attempt to improve the therapeutic ratio of chemoradiation, especially to decrease the toxicity sometimes observed with simultaneous chemoradiation. When radiation is administered following the planned dose of chemotherapy, the reduction in toxicity is thought to be accompanied by a reduced intensity of treatment. Looney and Hopkins[87] have demonstrated that a strategy of alternating intensive doses of chemotherapy with radiation allows delivery of both treatments at initiation of induction therapy. They believe that alternating dosing reduces toxicity while minimizing buildup of resistance of tumor cells to either technique and, of course, provides early chemotherapy for this "sandwich" technique in locally advanced tumors of the hypopharynx and proximal esophagus.

Coia et al.[88] reported results of 5-FU and mitomycin C chemotherapy combined with external beam radiation. Fifty-seven patients with stage I or II disease were treated with 6000 cGy in 6 to 7 weeks, along with 5-FU (1000 mg/m^2/24 hours) as a continuous intravenous infusion for 96 hours beginning on days 2 and 29 and mitomycin C (10 mg/m^2) as a bolus on day 2. Median survival was 18 months, with actuarial 3- and 5-year survivals of 29% and 18%, respectively. An element of local failure appeared in 48%, with a 72% distant failure rate noted. Thirty-three stage III–IV patients received palliative treatment, the same chemotherapy with 5000 cGy, with 9- and 7-month survivals, respectively.[88]

Uncontrolled studies, such as the previously mentioned one, have led some radiation therapists to speculate on dispensing with surgery in the treatment of esophageal cancer.[89] This opinion represents a backward step in the present multidisciplinary era as long as local failure is expected to be recognized in about 50% of nonsurgically treated patients (and to be truly present in considerably more than those in whom it is recognized).[85] Furthermore, several randomized trials have failed to reveal a benefit of chemoradiation over radiation alone. Negative trials include those of the Eastern Cooperative Oncology Group,[90] the Radiation Therapy Oncology Group,[91] and the Second Scandinavian Trial in Esophageal Cancer.[92]

Hyperthermia has been applied concomitantly with bleomycin and irradiation because exposure to hyperthermia results in a substantial decrease in growth of esophageal tumor cells in a time- and temperature-dependent manner in laboratory studies.[93] A precipitous decrease in growth was observed at 42.5°C in human esophageal cancer cell lines, and the effect was enhanced by the addition of bleomycin and radiation compared with treatment with only one or two of these modalities. Optimal fractionations remain to be determined, but early results for early-stage tumors show that tumor can be eradicated with minimal morbidity and potential for long-term survival.[94] In a review of the subject, Maehara et al.[95] concluded that "immediate improvement of subjective complaints and decrease or elimination of the cancer lesion are so distinct that this treatment, by means of an endotract antenna, shows promise as a modality for esophageal lesions."

Preoperative Chemoradiotherapy

Orringer et al.[96] reported results of a prospective multidisciplinary protocol involving an intensive in-hospital chemoradiation protocol followed by transhiatal esophagectomy. External beam radiotherapy was administered at 150 cGy twice daily for 5 days per week to a dose of 4500 cGy simultaneously with cisplatin (20 mg/m^2/day) by continuous infusion on days 1 through 5 and days 17 through 21; vinblastine (1 mg/m^2/day) by intravenous bolus on days 1 through 4 and days 17 through 20; and 5-FU (300 mg/m^2/day) by continuous infusion for the entire 21 days. Transhiatal esophagectomy was scheduled after a 3-week rest. Two patients died of sepsis due to bone marrow suppression. The overall operability was 95%, with complete resection thought accomplished in all but 1 of 39 patients operated on. There was a single operative death (2%).[96] Pathologically negative (complete response) patients had a median survival of 70 months and a 60% 5-year survival rate. Median survival was 29 months, with a 34% 5-year survival rate. Importantly, 32% of patients with residual tumor in their esophagectomy specimens were long-term survivals, suggesting a benefit to esophagectomy in multidisciplinary protocols.[97] The authors conclude that their intensive multidisciplinary management resulted in an approximate doubling of survival compared with results

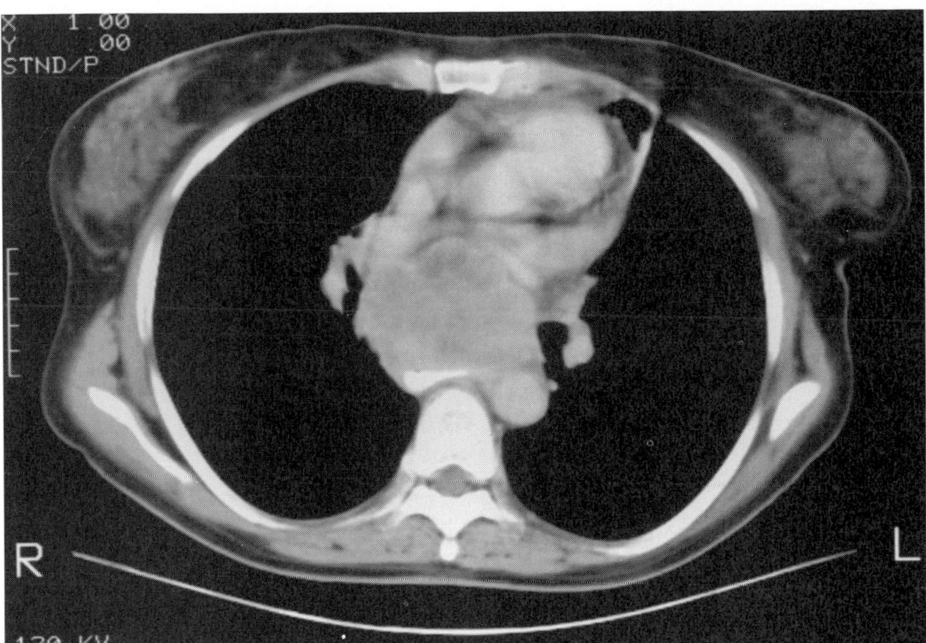

FIGURE 2–20. A large posterior mediastinal mass seen encroaching on contrast-filled esophageal lumen. Distinct borders around this mass separate it from aorta and other structures. At surgery, it was found to be a metastatic tumor from a small primary lung mass.

reported with surgery alone. A randomized trial comparing this preoperative regimen with surgery alone is in progress at the University of Michigan.

We[98] and others[99] have found that preoperative chemoradiotherapy, delivered in less intensive protocols than that employed by Orringer and colleagues,[96] did not yield significant improvement in survival compared with surgery (historical controls). Treatments have been well tolerated, though, with no increase in surgical complications attributed to neoadjuvant therapy.

A prospective randomized trial comparing neoadjuvant hyperthermochemoradiation with chemoradiation in squamous cell carcinomas found an improved complete response rate with hyperthermia (26% vs. 8%).[100] Western investigators have not yet reported large-scale experiences with this combination.

POST-TREATMENT SURVEILLANCE

Because recurrence is expected following treatment of esophageal tumors, it is the norm for patients to require the skills of a multidisciplinary team. Patients benefit from contact with physicians and surgeons who anticipate the failure of their own modalities of treatment and quickly investigate the slightest dysphagia (or change in baseline post-treatment dysphagia) so that prompt alternative treatments are initiated to maintain the ability to swallow—the principal goal of treatment.

In the case of prolonged survival, second primary cancers of the aerodigestive tract are expected at the rate of 3% to 4% per year, so routine chest radiographs and examinations of the head and neck are advised.[15, 16]

SECONDARY TUMORS

The incidence of secondary esophageal involvement by a variety of primary neoplasms has been reported to be as high as 3.2%.[101] Clinical and imaging characteristics simulate benign mural lesions because of great bulk in the presence of intact mucosa.[102]

We have had experience with an 8-cm mural mass secondary tumor (Fig. 2–20) from a 1-cm pulmonary mass, which we were able to enucleate through a long esophageal myotomy, leaving mucosa intact. Dysphagia was totally relieved up until the time of the patient's death from widespread metastases several months later.[103]

PREVENTION

The incidence rate of squamous cell cancer of the esophagus would be reduced by avoidance of tobacco, especially cigarettes; moderation in use of alcohol; and consumption of fresh fruits and vegetables.[104]

The long-term effects of school-based education programs remain to be evaluated, but measurable changes in attitudes regarding cigarette and alcohol use have been reported internationally. This is true as early as the sixth grade of school.[105] Massive antismoking campaigns[106] and no-smoking rules on the job are also effective,[107] as are labor intensive personal antismoking education programs by physicians, nurses, and friends.[108] Smoking-cessation programs have not reliably resulted in long-term success except among the highly motivated.[109] We therefore favor those educational programs that initially focus on developing motivation.

Aspirin and other nonsteroidal anti-inflammatory drugs

have been demonstrated to inhibit prostaglandin synthesis and tumor growth in experimental systems. A prospective study found death rates for cancers of the esophagus, stomach, colon, and rectum to be 40% lower in a population using 16 or more aspirins per month for at least a year compared with those who used no aspirin. There was a trend of decreasing risk with more frequent aspirin use, strongest among those who had used aspirin more than 10 years.[110]

High-dose 13-*cis*-retinoic acid has attracted interest in preventing tumors of the lung and esophagus because of its established chemopreventive activity in suppressing oral premalignancy and second primary head and neck cancers. These studies are still in their early stage and so are not yet of established value. Furthermore, the toxicity of high-dose treatment makes the drug not ideal for widespread use.[111, 112]

In a case-control study, vitamin supplements were found protective against oral and esophageal tumors.[113] Vitamin C was protective among current smokers as was vitamin B. Vitamin E, an antioxidant, was also found protective. Vitamin E has been found to reduce ethanol-mediated carcinogenesis in *N*-nitrosomethylbenzylamine (NMBza)–induced tumors among laboratory animals.[114, 115]

Several Chinese teas have the ability to inhibit the occurrence of esophageal tumors in laboratory models. Among the effects noted have been blockage of the formation of NMBza and also inhibition of the carcinogenic activity of preformed NMBza and its precursors.[116, 117]

FUTURE PROSPECTS

Reducing the death rate of esophageal tumors depends on improved methods of prevention, early detection, and treatment of systemic disease. Preventive lifestyle modifications are already known. The problem is discovering cost-efficient means of motivating people to avoid or abandon risky habits. Behavioral scientists are attempting to meet this challenge.

Early detection is unlikely to be funded for a low-incidence disease (squamous cell carcinoma of the esophagus) thought related to "bad habits" if it is not recommended for a high-incidence disease (lung cancer) caused primarily by one of the same habits. At this time, it remains the official position of the American Cancer Society that screening is not cost efficient in the early detection of lung cancer, even among high-risk smokers.

Surgery or radiation therapy with or without chemotherapy most often provides satisfactory local control, but most patients still die of their disease with present-day chemotherapy. Realistically speaking, achieving superior local control should remain our primary objective while we test newer toxic combinations in our quest for the elusive cure.

References

1. Wingo PA, Tong T, Bolden S: Cancer Statistics 1995 CA 45:8–30, 1995.
2. Kabat GC, Ng SKC, Wynder EL: Tobacco, alcohol intake, and diet in relation to adenocarcinoma of the esophagus and gastric cardia. Cancer Causes Control 4:123–132, 1993.
3. Day NE, Munoz N: Esophagus. In Schottenfeld D, Fraumeni JF (eds): Cancer Epidemiology and Prevention. Philadelphia: WB Saunders, 1982, pp 596–623.
4. Blot WJ: Epidemiology of esophageal cancer. In Roth JA, Ruckdeschel JC, Weisenburger TH (eds): Thoracic Oncology. Philadelphia: WB Saunders, 1989, pp 295–304.
5. VanRensburg SJ: Oesophageal cancer. Risk factors common to endemic regions. S Afr Med J 70(Suppl):9–11, 1987.
6. Harvey JC, Kagan AR, Ahn C, et al: Adenocarcinoma of the esophagus: A survival study. J Surg Oncol 45:29–32, 1990.
7. VanRensburg SJ: Epidemiologic and dietary evidence for a specific nutritional predisposition to esophageal cancer. J Natl Cancer Inst 67:243–251, 1981.
8. Warwick GP: Some aspects of the epidemiology and etiology of oesophageal cancer with particular emphasis on the Transkei, South Africa. Cancer Res 17:81–86, 1973.
9. Pera M, Trastek VF, Pairolero PC: Barrett's disease: Pathophysiology of metaplasia and adenocarcinoma. Ann Thorac Surg 56:1191–1197, 1993.
10. Reid BJ, Weinstein WM: Barrett's esophagus and adenocarcinoma. Annu Rev Med 38:477–492, 1987.
11. MacFarlane SD: Carcinoma of the esophagus. In Hill L, Kozarek R, McCallum R, Mercer CD (eds): The Esophagus: Medical and Surgical Management. Philadelphia: WB Saunders, 1988, pp 237–256.
12. Belsey R: Functional disease of the esophagus. J Thorac Cardiovasc Surg 52:164–188, 1966.
13. McGregor DH, Mills G, Bardet RA: Intramural squamous cell carcinoma of the esophagus. Am J Gastroenterol 80:325–329, 1985.
14. Hopkins JRA, Postlethwait RW: Caustic burns and carcinoma of the esophagus. Ann Surg 194:146–148, 1992.
15. Vikram B, Strong EW, Shah JP, Spiro R: Second malignant neoplasms in patients successfully treated with multimodality treatment for advanced head and neck cancer. Head Neck Surg 6:734–737, 1984.
16. Tepperman BS, Fitzpatrick PJ: Second respiratory and upper digestive tract cancers after oral cancer. Lancet 2:547–549, 1981.
17. Harvey JC, Pisch J, Beattie EJ: Esophagus. In Beattie EJ, Bloom ND, Harvey JC (eds): Thoracic Surgical Oncology. New York: Churchill Livingstone, 1992, pp 185–236.
18. Hause DW, Kagan AR, Fleischman E, Harvey JC: Tracheoesophageal fistula complicating carcinoma of the esophagus. Am Surg 58:441–442, 1992.
19. Kelsen D: Neoadjuvant therapy of esophageal cancer. Can J Surg 32:410–414, 1989.
20. Anderson LL, Lad TE: Autopsy findings in squamous cell carcinoma of the esophagus. Cancer 50:1587–1590, 1982.
21. Harvey JC, Kagan AR, Frankl H, et al: Squamous carcinoma of the distal esophagus: A survival study. J Surg Oncol 46:97–99, 1991.
22. Harvey JC, Davidson W, Frankl H, et al: Squamous carcinoma of the mid-esophagus: A survival study. Am Surg 57:615–617, 1992.
23. Shao LF, Gao ZG, Yang NP, et al: Results of surgical treatment in 6123 cases of carcinoma of the esophagus and gastric cardia. J Surg Oncol 42:170–174, 1989.
24. Harvey JC, Kagan AR, Hause D, et al: Adenocarcinoma arising in Barrett's esophagus. J Surg Oncol 45:162–163, 1990.
25. Sharma OP, Subnani S: Role of computerized tomography imaging in staging oesophageal carcinoma. Semin Surg Oncol 5:355–358, 1989.
26. Germanov AB, Spivack PB, Lukjanchenko AB, Mazneva NL: Preoperative diagnosis of esophageal cancer spread. Semin Surg Oncol 8:50–54, 1992.
27. Dachman AH, Levine MS: Radiology of the esophagus. Gastroenterol Clin North Am 20:635–658, 1991.
28. Lightdale CJ, Botet JF: Esophageal carcinoma: Preoperative staging and evaluation of anastomotic recurrence. Gastrointest Endosc 36(Suppl 2):s11–s16, 1990.
29. Snady H: Endoscopic ultrasonography: An effective tool for diagnosing gastrointestinal tumors. Oncology 6:63–81, 1992.

30. Skinner DB, Ferguson MK, Soriano A, et al: Selection of operation for esophageal cancer based on staging. Ann Surg 204:391–401, 1986.
31. Rice TW, Boyce GA, Spivak MV, et al: Esophageal ultrasound assessment of preoperative chemotherapy. Ann Thorac Surg 53:972–977, 1992.
32. Beahrs OH, Henson DE, Hutter RVP, Kennedy BJ (American Joint Committee on Cancer) (eds): Manual for Staging of Cancer, 4th ed. Philadelphia: JB Lippincott, 1992, pp 57–59.
33. Earlam R, Cunha-Melo JR: Oesophageal squamous cell carcinoma. II. A critical review of radiotherapy. Br J Surg 67:457–461, 1980.
34. Ellis FH: Treatment of carcinoma of the esophagus or cardia. Mayo Clin Proc 64:945–955, 1989.
35. Akiyama H, Tsurumaru M, Kamamara T, Ono Y: Principles of surgical treatment for carcinoma of the esophagus. Ann Surg 194:438–446, 1981.
36. DeMeester TR, Zaninotto G, Johansson K-E: Selective therapeutic approach to cancers of the lower esophagus and cardia. J Thorac Cardiovasc Surg 95:42–54, 1988.
37. Peddada AJ, Harvey JC, Anderson PJ, et al: High dose rate (HDR) intraluminal radiation in a combined modality treatment plan for carcinoma of the esophagus. J Surg Oncol 52:160–163, 1993.
38. Müller JM, Erasmi H, Stelzner M, et al: Surgical therapy of esophageal carcinoma. Br J Surg 77:845–857, 1990.
39. Orringer MB: Ten year survival after esophagectomy for carcinoma: Surgical triumph or biologic variation? Chest 96:970–971, 1989.
40. Iizuka T, Isono K, Kakegawa T, Watanabe H: Parameters linked to 10-year survival in Japan of selected esophageal carcinoma. Chest 96:1005–1011, 1989.
41. Abe S, Tachibana M, Shiraishi M, Nakamura T: Lymph node metastases in resectable esophageal cancer. J Thorac Cardiovasc Surg 100:287–291, 1990.
42. Orringer MB: Transhiatal esophagectomy without thoracotomy for carcinoma of the thoracic esophagus. Ann Surg 200:282–288, 1984.
43. Kirklin JW, Blackstone EH: The DeMeester paper on carcinoma of the esophagus. J Thorac Cardiovasc Surg 100:456–458, 1990.
44. Belsey R, Hiebert CA: An exclusive right thoracic approach for cancer of the middle third of the esophagus. Ann Thorac Surg 18:1–15, 1974.
45. King RM, Pairolaro PL, Trastek VF, et al: Ivor Lewis esophagogastrectomy for carcinoma of the esophagus: Early and late functional results. Ann Thorac Surg 44:119–122, 1987.
46. Fan ST, Lau WY, Yip WC, et al: Prediction of postoperative pulmonary complications in oesophagogastric cancer surgery. Br J Surg 74:408–410, 1987.
47. Fan ST, Lau WY, Yip WC, et al: Healing of esophageal fistulas after surgical treatment for carcinoma of the esophagus and upper part of the stomach. Surg Gynecol Obstet 166:307–310, 1988.
48. Hankins JR, Miller JE, Attar S, McLaughlin JS: Transhiatal esophagectomy for carcinoma of the esophagus: Experience with 26 patients. Ann Thorac Surg 44:123–127, 1987.
49. Robinson CLN: The management of chylothorax. Ann Thorac Surg 39:90–95, 1985.
50. Ferguson MK, Little AG, Skinner DB: Current concepts in the management of chylothorax. Ann Thorac Surg 40:542–545, 1985.
51. Little AG, Kadowaki MH, Ferguson MK, et al: Pleuro peritoneal shunting. Ann Surg 208:443–450, 1988.
52. Orringer MB: Substernal bypass of excluded thoracic esophagus—results of an ill-advised operation. Surgery 96:467–470, 1984.
53. Burt M, Diehl W, Martini N, et al: Malignant esophagorespiratory fistula: Management options and survival. Ann Thorac Surg 52:1222–1229, 1991.
54. Tytgat GN, den Hartog Jager FCA: To dilate or intubate. Gastrointest Endosc 29:58–68, 1983.
55. Parker CH, Peura DA: Palliative treatment of esophageal carcinoma using esophageal dilation and prosthesis. Gastroenterol Clin North Am 20:717–729, 1991.
56. Fleischer D, Kessler F: Endoscopic Nd:YAG laser therapy for carcinoma of the esophagus: A new palliative approach. Am J Surg 143:280–283, 1982.
57. Reilly HF, Fleischer DE: Palliative treatment of esophageal carcinoma using laser and tumor probe therapy. Gastroenterol Clin North Am 20:731–742, 1991.
58. Loizou LA, Grigg D, Atkinson M, et al: A prospective comparison of laser therapy and intubation for malignant dysphagia. Gastroenterology 100:1303–1310, 1991.
59. Johnston JH, Fleischer D, Petrini J, et al: Palliative bipolar electrocoagulation therapy of obtructing esophageal cancer. Gastrointest Endosc 33:349–353, 1987.
60. Fleischman EH, Kagan AR, Bellotti JE, et al: Effective palliation for inoperable esophageal cancer with intensive intracavitary radiation. J Surg Oncol 44:234–237, 1990.
61. Harvey JC, Fleischman EH, Bellotti JE, Kagan AR: Intracavitary radiation in the treatment of advanced esophageal carcinoma: A comparison of high dose rate versus low dose rate brachytherapy. J Surg Oncol 52:101–104, 1993.
62. Michel L, Grillo HC, Malt R: Esophageal perforation. Ann Thorac Surg 33:203–210, 1982.
63. Pietrafitta JJ, Dwyer RM: New laser technique for treatment of malignant esophageal obstruction. J Surg Oncol 35:157–162, 1987.
64. Loizou LA, Rampton D, Atkinson M, et al: A prospective assessment of life after endoscopic intubation and laser therapy for malignant dysphagia. Cancer 70:386–391, 1992.
65. Fisher S, Brady L: Esophagus. In Perez CA, Brady LW (eds): Principles and Procedure of Radiation Oncology. Philadelphia: JB Lippincott, 1992, pp 853–870.
66. Beatty J, Rider W: Carcinoma of the esophagus: Pretreatment assessment, correlation of radiation treatment parameters with survival and identification and management of radiation treatment failure. Cancer 43:2254–2259, 1975.
67. O'Rourke I, Tiver K, Bull C, et al: Swallowing performance after radiation therapy for carcinoma of the esophagus. Cancer 61:2022–2026, 1988.
68. Earlam R, Johnson L: 101 oesophageal cancers: A surgeon uses radiotherapy. Ann R Coll Surg Engl 72:32–40, 1990.
69. Hashikawa Y, Kurisu K, Taniguchi M, et al: High dose rate intraluminal brachytherapy for esophageal cancer: 10 years experience in Hyogo College of Medicine. Radiother Oncol 21:107–114, 1991.
70. Pakisch B, Kohek P, Poier E, et al: Iridium-192 high dose rate brachytherapy combined with external beam irradiation in nonresectable oesophageal cancer. Clin Oncol 5:154–158, 1993.
71. Hareyama M, Nishio M, Kagami Y, et al: Intracavitary brachytherapy combined with external beam irradiation for squamous cell carcinoma of the esophagus. Int J Radiat Oncol Biol Phys 24:235–240, 1992.
72. Gignoux M, Roussel A, Paillot B, Gillet M: The value of preoperative radiotherapy in esophageal cancer: Results of a study of the EORTC. World J Surg 11:426–432, 1987.
73. Diehl LF: Radiation and chemotherapy in the treatment of esophageal cancer. Gastroenterol Clin North Am 4:765–774, 1991.
74. Fok M, Sham JS, Choy SW, et al: Postoperative radiotherapy for carcinoma of the esophagus: A prospective randomized controlled study. Surgery 113:138–147, 1993.
75. Kelsen DP, Bains M, Hilaris B, et al: Combined modality therapy of esophageal cancer. Semin Oncol 11:169–177, 1984.
76. Kelsen DP, Minsky B, Smith M, et al: Preoperative therapy for esophageal cancer: A randomized comparison for chemotherapy versus radiation therapy. J Clin Oncol 8:1352–1361, 1990.
77. Leichman L, Berry BT: Experience with cisplatin in treatment regimens for esophageal cancer. Semin Oncol 18(Suppl 3):64–72, 1991.
78. Muggia F: Cisplatin update. Semin Oncol 18(Suppl 3):1–4, 1991.
79. Coia LR: The use of mitomycin in esophageal cancer. Oncology 50(Suppl1):53–60, 1993.
80. Miyahara T, Ueda K, Akaboshi M, et al: Hyperthermic enhancement of cytotoxicity and increased uptake of *cis*-diamminedichloroplatinum (II) in cultured human esophageal cancer cells. Jpn J Cancer Res 84:336–340, 1993.
81. Goldie J, Coldam A: The genetic origin of drug resistance in neoplasms: Implications for systemic therapy. Cancer Res 44:3643–3646, 1984.
82. Fisher B, Gunduz N, Soffer EA. Influence of the interval between primary tumor removal and chemotherapy on kinetics and growth of metastases. Cancer Res 43:1488–1492, 1983.
83. Ajani JA, Roth JF, Ryan B, et al: Evaluation of pre- and postoperative chemotherapy for resectable adenocarcinoma of the esophagus or gastroesophageal junction. J Clin Oncol 8:1231–1238, 1990.
84. Hoff SJ, Stewart JR, Sawyers JL, et al: Preliminary results with neoadjuvant therapy and resection for esophageal carcinoma. Ann Thorac Surg 56:282–287, 1993.

85. Carey RW, Hilgenberg AD, Wilkins EW, et al: Long-term follow-up of neoadjuvant chemotherapy with 5-FU and cisplatin with surgical resection and possible postoperative radiotherapy and/or chemotherapy in squamous cell carcinoma of the esophagus. Cancer Invest 11:99–105, 1993.
86. Ginsberg RJ: Discussion. Ann Thorac Surg 56:286, 1993.
87. Looney WB, Hopkins HA: Rationale for different chemotherapeutic and radiation therapy strategies in cancer management. Cancer 67:1471–1483, 1991.
88. Coia LR, Engstrom PF, Paul AR, et al: Long term results of infusional 5-FU, mitomycin-C, and radiation as primary management of esophageal carcinoma. Int J Radiat Oncol Biol Phys 20:29–36, 1991.
89. Coia LR: Esophageal cancer: Is esophagectomy necessary? Oncology 3:110–111, 1989.
90. Earle JD, Gelber RD, Moertel CG, et al: A controlled evaluation of combined radiation and bleomycin therapy for squamous cell carcinoma of the esophagus. Int J Radiat Oncol Biol Phys 6:457–461, 1980.
91. Herskovic A, Martz K, Al-Sarraf M, et al: Intergroup esophageal study: Comparison of radiotherapy to radio-chemotherapy combination: A phase III trial. Proc Am Soc Clin Oncol 10:135, 1991 (abstract).
92. Hatlevoll R, Hagen S, Hansen HS, et al: Bleomycin/cis-platin as neoadjuvant chemotherapy before radical radiotherapy in localized, inoperable carcinoma of the esophagus. A prospective randomized multicenter study: The second Scandinavian trial in esophageal cancer. Radiother Oncol 24:114–116, 1992.
93. Matsuoka H, Sugimachi K, Mori M, et al: Effects of hyperthermochemoradiotherapy on KSE-1 cells, a newly established human squamous cell line derived from esophageal carcinoma. Eur Surg Res 21:49–59, 1989.
94. Matsuoka H, Tsutsui S, Morita M, et al: Hyperthermochemoradiotherapy as definitive treatment for patients with early esophageal cancer. Am J Clin Oncol 15:509–514, 1992.
95. Maehara Y, Kuwano H, Kitamura K, et al: Hyperthermochemoradiotherapy for esophageal cancer. Am J Clin Oncol 15:509–514, 1992.
96. Orringer MB, Forastiere AA, Perez-Tamayo C, et al: Chemotherapy and radiation therapy for transhiatal esophagectomy for esophageal carcinoma. Ann Thorac Surg 49:348–354, 1990.
97. Forastiere AA, Orringer MB, Perez-Tamayo C, et al: Preoperative chemoradiation followed by transhiatal esophagectomy for carcinoma of the esophagus: Final report. J Clin Oncol 11:1118–1123, 1993.
98. Peddada AV, Harvey JC, Anderson PJ, et al: High dose rate intraluminal radiation in a combined modality treatment plan for carcinoma of the esophagus. J Surg Oncol 52:160–163, 1993.
99. Terz JJ, Leong LA, Lipsett JA, Wagman LD: Preoperative chemotherapy and radiotherapy for cancer of the esophagus. Surgery 114:71–75, 1993.
100. Sugimachi K, Kitamura K, Baba K, et al: Hyperthermia combined with chemotherapy and irradiation for patients with carcinoma of the esophagus—a prospective randomized trial. Int J Hyperthermia 8:289–295, 1992.
101. Toreson WE: Secondary carcinoma of the esophagus as a cause of dysphagia. Arch Pathol 38:82–84, 1944.
102. Orringer MB, Skinner DB: Unusual presentation of primary and secondary esophageal malignancies. Ann Thorac Surg 11:305–314, 1971.
103. Bakshandeh N, Beattie EJ, Harvey JC: Enucleation of a secondary esophageal mural tumor. J Surg Oncol 50:204–205, 1992.
104. Jaskiewicz K: Oesophageal carcinoma: Cytopathology and nutritional aspects in aetiology. Anticancer Res 9:1847–1852, 1989.
105. Kreutter KJ, Gewirtz H, Davenny JE, Love C: Drug and alcohol prevention project for sixth graders: First-year findings. Adolescence 26:287–293, 1991.
106. Tilgren P, Haglund BJ, Gilljam H, Holm LE: A tobacco quit and win model in the Stockholm cancer prevention programme. Eur J Cancer Prev 1:361–366, 1992.
107. Brenner H, Mielck A: Smoking prohibition in the workplace and smoking cessation in the Federal Republic of Germany. Prev Med 21:252–261, 1992.
108. Schwartz JL: Methods of smoking cessation. Med Clin North Am 76:451–476, 1992.
109. Oei TP, Hallam J: Behavioral strategies used by long-term successful self-quitters. Int J Addict 26:993–1002, 1991.
110. Thun MJ, Namboodiri MM, Calle EE, et al: Aspirin use and the risk of fatal cancer. Cancer Res 53:1322–1327, 1993.
111. Gerawal HS, Sampliner RE, Fennerty MB: Chemoprevention studies in Barrett's esophagus: A model premalignant lesion for esophageal adenocarcinoma. Monogr Natl Cancer Inst 13:51–54, 1992.
112. Lippman SM, Hong WK: 13-*cis*-Retinoic acid and cancer chemoprevention. Monogr Natl Cancer Inst 13:111–115, 1992.
113. Barone J, Taioli E, Hebert JR, Wynder EL: Vitamin supplement use and risk for oral and esophageal cancer. Nutr Cancer 18:31–41, 1992.
114. Odeleye OE, Eskelson CD, Mufti SI, Watson RR: Vitamin E inhibits the carcinogenicity of *N*-nitrosomethylbenzylamine. Ann NY Acad Sci 669:368–370, 1992.
115. Odeleye OE, Eskelson CD, Mufti SI, Watson RR: Vitamin E inhibition of lipid peroxidation and ethanol-mediated promotion of esophageal tumorigenesis. Nutr Cancer 17:223–234, 1992.
116. Zhu JQ, Xiao Y, Liu ZQ, et al: The effects of Chinese tea on the methylation of DNA by the esophageal carcinogen *N*-nitrosomethylbenzylamine. Biomed Environ Sci 4:225–231, 1991.
117. Han C, Xu Y: Chinese tea inhibits the occurrence of oesophogeal tumours induced by *n*-nitrosomethylbenzylamine and blocks its formation in rats. IARC Sci Publ 105:541–545, 1991.

3

Stomach and Small Bowel Cancer

Gastric Cancer

Burton L. Eisenberg, M.D. • Christine Szarka, M.D.
Harold Frucht, M.D. • Rachelle M. Lanciano, M.D.
Alexandre Hageboutros, M.D.
Louis M. Weiner, M.D.

Gastric adenocarcinoma continues to present a challenge to the cancer surgeon worldwide despite compelling evidence of an absolute decrease in incidence in the United States and in many other countries. The true incidence of the disease has declined in the United States by more than 40% in the last 30 years. However, gastric carcinoma remains the eighth most common cause of cancer-related mortality, with approximately 15,000 deaths in the United States each year.[1] Worldwide frequency has likewise diminished, albeit less dramatically. Yet gastric carcinoma remains the leading cause of cancer mortality in Japan, in some of Latin America, and in Northern Europe.

Cure rates for gastric adenocarcinoma reported in the Western literature have changed little in the past three decades. Generally, the 5-year survival rate following surgery remains in the range of 15%.[2, 3] Since early gastric cancer cure rates can exceed 90%, these poor survival statistics are thought to be the result of the advanced stage of disease at the time of initial diagnosis. In a 1989 American College of Surgeons study, 66% of patients with stomach cancer had locally advanced or metastatic disease (stage III or IV) at presentation.[4] The onset of specific symptoms is often associated with bulky or ulcerative cancer within the stomach. In many cases, these symptoms are initially managed with medications for benign gastric conditions, delaying the diagnosis of cancer. Advanced disease precludes resection with curative intent in a large proportion of patients. Only 30% of patients with gastric cancer are candidates for attempted curative resections (complete gross tumor removal). Single institutional experiences report operability rates of 85%, with approximately 66% of these patients actually having a gastric resection.[5, 6] A 1983 10-year review of Western literature supports an overall resection rate (curative and palliative) of approximately 50%.[7]

Patients with gastric cancer who undergo attempted curative resection in the United States have 5-year survival rates ranging from 20% to 57%, varying by stage of disease.[7–9] In contrast, a compilation of reports from Japan suggests improved curative resection rates and subsequent 5-year survival statistics (Table 3–1).[10] The apparent enhancement in survival reported in the Japanese literature may be accounted for by a notable increase in the incidence of early gastric cancer, in addition to a more accurate and standardized nodal staging system combined with a more aggressive surgical resection. As demonstrated in Table 3–1, the noted comparative survival advantages seem to be limited to node-positive patients.

In addition to prognostic implications associated with advanced disease at presentation, there has been a proportional shift in the location of gastric adenocarcinoma to the proximal stomach. Recent reports suggest that more than

TABLE 3–1
Five-Year Survival Rates (%) After Gastrectomy in Japan and the United States

Stage		Japan	United States
N0	T1	80	90
	T2	60	58
	T3	30	50
	T4	5	20
N1		53	20
N2		26	10
N3		10	—
N4		3	—

From Smith JW, Brennan MF: Surgical treatment of gastric cancer. Surg Clin North Am 72:381–399, 1992.

one third of stomach cancers are located in the upper fundus or gastric cardia.[11, 12] This may in part be accounted for by a relative increase that has accompanied a diminishing number of patients with distal gastric cancers. This proximal location complicates the surgical management and adversely affects survival.[13] Equally important with reference to surgical cure rates is the trend toward an increasing incidence of undifferentiated gastric cancers, including an increase in the signet-ring variety of adenocarcinoma. In addition, approximately 15% of patients present with diffuse submucosal cancer spread and the scirrhous changes of linitis plastica.

The surgical treatment of stomach cancer is complicated, then, by the locally advanced nature of the disease at presentation, its natural history of early lymphatic permeation through the upper retroperitoneum, and tumor cell penetration through the gastric wall.

This chapter reviews the present data relevant to the surgical management of gastric cancer. Emphasis is placed on the management of adenocarcinoma, since this cell type is found in more than 90% of the patients with gastric cancer.

EPIDEMIOLOGIC CONSIDERATIONS

Incidence

Approximately, 24,000 new cases of gastric carcinoma are diagnosed yearly in the United States. The incidence and mortality of gastric cancer increase with age. Very few cases are reported prior to age 30, with a sharp increase after age 50. In the United States, the disease is more common in men than in women (1.6:1.0). Other countries have reported male to female ratios as high as 2.5:1.0.[14]

While gastric cancer remains a significant health problem, the death rate from this disease has decreased from 16 in 100,000 in 1960 to 6 in 100,000 in 1988, representing a 62% and 67% decrease in mortality among men and women, respectively.[1] This decline in mortality has been attributed to a decreased incidence of gastric cancer that is not fully understood. While the epidemiology of this disease varies throughout the world, most countries have observed a similar decline, including Korea, Costa Rica, Russia, Japan, China, and Chile, which have the highest mortality rates from gastric cancer.[14] It is uncertain whether this phenomenon is related to mass screening efforts or the same unidentified factors responsible for the decline in incidence and mortality in other countries.

Genetics

Certain families have demonstrated multiple occurrences of gastric cancer, suggesting an inherited susceptibility. While a specific genetic linkage has not been identified, studies involving blood typing and migration effect support a familial relationship.

In 1953, Aird et al.[15] observed that patients with gastric cancer frequently had blood group A. Subsequent studies supported this finding.[16] However, the relative risk ratio for gastric cancer in persons with blood group A compared with those with blood group O is only 1.2. Therefore, the overall risk is only minimally increased.

The intercountry variation associated with gastric cancer has provided epidemiologists the opportunity to study the effect of migration. Populations emigrating from high-risk to low-risk areas experience a significant decrease in disease occurrence over one generation. Although this suggests involvement of an environmental factor, these first-generation immigrants continue to be at higher risk than natives of the low-risk area.[17] This persistent elevated risk suggests genetic predisposition to be important in subsequent disease occurrence.

Further studies clarifying genetic linkage need to be conducted, since specific genetic factors have not been identified and generally the environmental exposure in families with multiple occurrences of gastric cancer is similar.

Predisposing Conditions

Chronic Atrophic Gastritis and Intestinal Metaplasia

Chronic atrophic gastritis and intestinal metaplasia, prevalent in individuals with gastric cancer, are often considered predisposing or precancerous lesions. Animal models have shown that atrophic gastritis and intestinal metaplasia often precede overt cancer, suggesting a continuum of disease.[18] Clinical studies attempting to characterize the natural history of precancerous gastric lesions have also suggested a sequential relationship.[19, 20] However, chronic atrophic gastritis and intestinal metaplasia are being found with increasing frequency in older normal individuals. Although there appears to be a continuum between these disorders and gastric cancer, they are too prevalent to be sensitive indicators of cancer. Studies are under way to clarify this matter.

Helicobacter pylori Infections

The identification of *Helicobacter pylori* in chronic inflammatory conditions of the stomach has stimulated interest in its potential role in carcinogenesis. *H. pylori* is not easily eliminated by the host's normal defense system and probably persists for life in most patients. It is speculated that *H. pylori* is related to the superficial gastritis that progresses to chronic atrophic gastritis, a presumed precursor of gastric cancer.[21, 22]

A high prevalence of infection has been found in areas at high risk for gastric cancer in the United States and other parts of the world. Individuals with intestinal metaplasia, chronic atrophic gastritis, and gastric cancer are commonly infected with *H. pylori*.[23, 24] The prevalence of this infectious agent in individuals with chronic atrophic gastritis ranges from 40% to 90%.[25] The relative risk for gastric cancer is increased 3.6 to 6 times in individuals infected with *H. pylori*. Still, many *H. pylori*–positive individuals do not go on to have gastric cancer.[26] *H. pylori* commonly affects 50% of North Americans over age 50, and in some developing countries it affects almost all adults.[27] Clearly, other critical factors must be operative in the pathogenesis of gastric cancer.

An association between *H. pylori* and gastric cancer could be important in the prevention of this disease. Serologic tests for the detection of *H. pylori* have been developed and are used worldwide. The enzyme-linked immunosorbent assay has proved to be sensitive and specific for the detection of active disease.[28] Following detection, triple-therapy treatment with bismuth subcitrate, tetracycline, and metronidazole has shown excellent eradication of *H. pylori*.[29] Eradicating this infectious agent with antibiotics in individuals at high risk for gastric cancer might be a way to decrease the incidence and subsequent mortality of gastric cancer.

Gastric Polyps and Ulcers

The relationship between gastric polyps and ulcers with gastric cancer has been studied extensively. It is generally agreed that gastric polyps rarely progress to malignant lesions. True adenomatous polyps are quite rare and have a malignant potential. However, unlike in colon cancer, the sequence of cancer progression in gastric adenomatous polyps is not well documented. Chronic benign gastric ulcers, even though they share many features with gastric cancer, such as intestinal metaplasia and a high incidence of gastritis, do not appear to be precursors of gastric carcinoma.[30]

Partial Gastrectomy

Several studies have shown an increased incidence of gastric cancer in individuals who underwent resection for benign gastric disease. The typical lag time for such a cancer developing is 15 to 40 years. The reason for this association is not clear but may be due to the elevated gastric pH that results following such surgery. This may allow for the overgrowth of nitrite-producing bacteria in the gastric remnant and the subsequent development of intestinal metaplasia.[31, 32]

Pernicious Anemia

Autopsy studies years ago revealed an increased incidence of gastric cancer in patients with pernicious anemia. Clinical studies have confirmed the relationship with an incidence of 5% to 10%. It is estimated that gastric cancer is 20 times more common in patients with pernicious anemia than in age-matched controls.[33]

Diet

Diet has been implicated as a possible etiologic factor in gastric cancer. Despite inherent difficulties in dietary investigation (such as reliance on an individual's dietary recall and retrospective analysis over long periods of time), numerous investigators from several countries have formed general conclusions with regard to gastric cancer.[34, 35]

Dose-response relationships have been observed with foods high in sodium, such as pickled vegetables, salted fish, salted meat, and smoked foods, in multiple logistic regression analysis.[36] Items containing nitrates and nitrites may contribute to the development of gastric cancer. Nitrates are thought to be precursors of mutagens that target epithelial cells.[37, 38] Nitrates are common constituents of our diet found in vegetables, cured meat, and even drinking water. While nitrites are ingested, they are mainly derived from the conversion of nitrates. An increase in nitrite-forming bacteria has been seen in the upper gastrointestinal tract of individuals predisposed to gastric cancer, including those with achlorhydria, atrophic gastritis, pernicious anemia, and previous gastrectomy.[39, 40]

Gastric cancer is inversely associated with consumption of fresh vegetables, citrus fruits, vitamin C, and whole milk.[34, 35] Vitamin C and citrus fruits high in vitamin C inhibit nitrosation (the conversion of nitrates to nitrosamines and nitroamides). It is thought that refrigeration has contributed to the decline of gastric cancer through a decreased reliance on nitrates as a food preservative and the ability of cold temperatures to inhibit the conversion of nitrates to nitrites.[34]

Social Habits

In the past, no relationship between alcohol and tobacco use and gastric cancer was thought to exist. Several subsequent studies have confirmed no direct link with alcohol consumption.[34, 36] However, many studies have shown cigarette smoking associated with an increased risk for gastric cancer.[34–36] A relative risk of 2.0 is seen in individuals who smoke regularly.[34]

Occupation

A number of occupations have been associated with increased gastric cancer rates. These include coal mining, timber processing, rubber production, and those requiring manual labor. It is unknown whether these occupations are causally linked with the disease or merely reflect the often low socioeconomic status of the employees. In the United States and in Western Europe, gastric cancer occurs twice as frequently in lower as compared to higher socioeconomic groups.[34] Asbestos exposure has been related to gastric cancer in some studies but not all.[41, 42]

NATURAL HISTORY AND RECURRENCE PATTERN

Intraperitoneal failure represents the majority of treatment failures following gastric resection. Beginning with Wangensteen and coworkers' second-look operations for gastric cancer,[43] databases have been developed specifically to address the issue of disease-related failure patterns. In 1982, Gunderson and Sosin[44] reviewed Wangensteen and colleagues' data for the purpose of developing radiation portals that would encompass disease recurrence sites. In this review, 29% of patients had limited local-regional failure as the only site of disease recurrence and in another 53% failure was within the peritoneal cavity as a whole (defined as a combination of peritoneal implants and local-regional tumor recurrence). In only 6% of patients was the development of distant metastases the sole site of failure. Other series have supported these findings by analysis of autopsy data following attempted curative gastric resection (Table 3–2).[45, 46] It is of importance to note that even in lymph node–positive patients, 75% of the treatment failures are confined to the peritoneal cavity, suggesting that distant metastatic spread in patients with gastric cancer is generally seen only in end-stage disease and is not an early finding in recurrence patterns. This information is relevant to developing treatment schemes for primary therapy of gastric cancer.

The pattern of lymphatic failure is quite well documented in gastric carcinoma and is independent of the extent of lymphadenectomy or type of gastrectomy in the University of Minnesota series.[47] In patients with positive regional nodes at the time of definitive gastric resection, recurrence is overwhelmingly within the lymphatic pathways of the upper abdomen; in only 10% is the development of liver spread a component of the recurrence.[44] Whether extended lymphadenectomies of the R2 or R3 variety will ultimately change these patterns of recurrence, as suggested in the Japanese literature, remains unproven by prospective analysis. One would surmise, however, that tumor emboli or intraperitoneal viable tumor cells noted in patients with numerous positive nodes or gross serosal penetration will ultimately lead to recurrent disease after extensive surgical clearing without effective adjuvant therapy. The anatomic limitations for complete lymphatic clearing within the upper abdomen present a substantial obstacle to prevention of lymphatic-associated recurrence. With increasing nodal involvement, the removal of one tier of nodes beyond those harboring metastatic disease, as advocated by proponents of extensive lymphadenectomy, becomes less feasible.

Anastomotic recurrence in gastric cancer is related to extent of primary disease and the status of the surgical margins. A minimum proximal tumor-free margin of 2 cm is required for localized cancer. This should be extended to 5 cm or greater for large bulky tumors, T3 tumors, or those displaying diffuse characteristics. The distal margin of resection should be through the duodenal bulb unless the distal cancer is within 2 cm of the pyloric channel. If this is the case, the surgical margin should be between the first and the second portion of the duodenum. A 30% incidence rate of cases in which tumor extends into the duodenum and past the pyloric ring has been documented when gross cancer is within 2 cm of the distal margin. The mode of duodenal extension is generally via serosal spread or subserosal lymphatics, in contrast to esophageal spread, which more often involves the submucosal lymphatics.

Although the esophageal margin is more commonly microscopically positive, the presence of microscopic disease at either margin significantly worsens the prognosis in any patient other than those who have a planned palliative resection. In one study, there were no 5-year survivors noted in patients with both stage II (T3, N0) and stage III

TABLE 3–2
Patterns of Local-Regional Failure, Reoperation, and Autopsy Series

Failure Area	University of Minnesota Reoperation Series (No. of Patients)	McNeer et al. Autopsy Series (No. of Patients)	Thomson and Robins Autopsy Series (No. of Patients)
Gastric bed	55.2% (58/105)	52.2% (48/92)	67.9% (19/28)
Anastomosis or stumps	26.7% (28/105)	59.8% (55/92)	53.6% (15/28)
Abdominal or stab wounds	4.7% (5/105)	—	—
Lymph nodes	42.9% (45/105)	52.2% (48.92)	—

From Kern K: Natural history of surgically treated gastric cancer. In Sugarbaker P (ed): Management of Gastric Cancer. Boston: Kluwer Academic Publishers, 1991, pp 1–16.

disease when a microscopic surgical margin was positive.[48] The substantial effect of positive margins on disease-free survival supports the routine use of intraoperative frozen section analysis of surgical margins. One must caution, however, that with obvious bulky serosal disease and extensive submucosal tumor spread, the presence of positive duodenal or esophageal margins, or both, is indicative of incurability. Rather than risk extended or repeated resections in an attempt to obtain negative margins, a microscopically positive margin can be acceptable in a palliative procedure.

LOCAL-REGIONAL ANATOMY

The stomach begins at the gastroesophageal junction and ends at the pylorus (Fig. 3–1). It is therefore likely that direct spread of gastric cancer can involve both the esophagus and the duodenum. The stomach can be divided into segments consisting of the cardia, fundus, body, and pylorus. The cardia usually begins 3 cm below the esophageal hiatus. The fundus, which is the dome-shaped portion, lies to the left and about 3 to 5 cm cephalad to the cardia. The largest portion of the stomach is the body, which contains the antrum. The pylorus can be identified by the pyloric vein of Mayo, crossing the stomach at the junction of the pylorus and the duodenum. The medial border of the stomach is known as the lesser curvature and provides attachment for the lesser omentum. The lateral border of the stomach is the greater curvature and attaches the greater omentum.

The blood supply to the stomach is derived from the celiac axis through the left gastric artery; the gastroduodenal and right gastric arteries from the hepatic artery; the right gastroepiploic artery from the gastroduodenal artery; the left gastroepiploic and short gastric arteries from the splenic artery. The venous drainage parallels the arterial supply.

The stomach is quite rich in lymphatics. These all interconnect, but there are three main trunks: the left gastric chain, the splenic chain, and the hepatic chain. Thus, lymphatic involvement from gastric cancer can extend to the hilum of the spleen, up to the portal vein, across the pancreas, and along the inferior portion of the duodenum. This complex lymphatic drainage makes the prediction of lymphatic flow from a gastric cancer site more difficult than predicting usual patterns for locations of direct lymphatic involvement from colorectal cancer. The initial lymphatic spread from a distal gastric cancer follows the distribution of the hepatic and left gastric chains rather than proximal flow to the splenic chain or toward the esophagus. This is the rationale for a subtotal gastrectomy without a necessary routine splenectomy for distal gastric cancer. As gastric cancer lymphatic spread becomes more extensive, the third and fourth nodal echelons can be involved even to the point of diffuse retrograde spread into the peritoneal lymphatics.

The anatomic position of the stomach in the upper abdomen places it in close proximity to the spleen, tail of the pancreas, transverse colon and mesocolon, and left lateral segment of the liver. All of these structures can be involved in contiguous spread of transmural gastric cancer.

PATHOLOGY

The most widely used histopathologic classification of gastric carcinoma is that described by Lauren.[49] It is useful as both an epidemiologic and a prognostic indicator. This system emphasizes two main types of gastric cancer with presumably two different etiologies: intestinal type and diffuse type. These account for 90% of all gastric adenocarcinomas, with the remaining 10% designated as mixed, demonstrating features of both. Within these broad categories, tumors can be graded as well differentiated, poorly differentiated, or undifferentiated.

The cells of the intestinal type of gastric cancer are reminiscent of normal columnar intestinal cells exhibiting striated borders. The intestinal type is associated with atrophic gastritis and metaplasia and tends to be "epidemic" in worldwide distribution. Thus, its occurrence is increased in those geographic areas where the incidence of gastric cancer is high. It is thought to be closely associated with diet-induced mucosal dysplastic changes. Generally, the growth pattern is by outward expansion and is manifested by intraluminal fungating masses, bulky disease, and ulceration. This type is noted more often in men and in patients over age 60 and predominates in high-risk areas.[50] The worldwide decrease in stomach cancer is due to a decrease in the incidence of the intestinal variety.[51] This type of gastric cancer usually metastasizes to the liver as circumscribed lesions, unlike the diffuse variety, which has a greater tendency for peritoneal spread owing to early transmural penetration.

Diffuse gastric cancer infiltrates the stomach wall early without forming large masses. It is "endemic" in worldwide distribution, with equal occurrence in countries that have both a high and a low incidence of gastric cancer. Diffuse gastric cancer tends to be found more often in women, young patients, and populations at low risk for gastric cancer. It is generally thought to be less associated with dietary factors than the intestinal type. The diffuse variety is composed of dispersed neoplastic cells lacking adhesive characteristics and without organized glandular patterns. This variety can produce mucin with a signet-ring cell appearance, and in an extensive diffuse pattern produce the characteristic linitis plastica. Prognostically in one series, the diffuse type was more often associated with advanced disease.[52]

Gross morphology of advanced gastric cancer (tumors extending into or beyond the muscularis propria) can be classified into a scheme originally devised by Bormann (Fig. 3–2).[53] This classification includes four distinct gross categories:

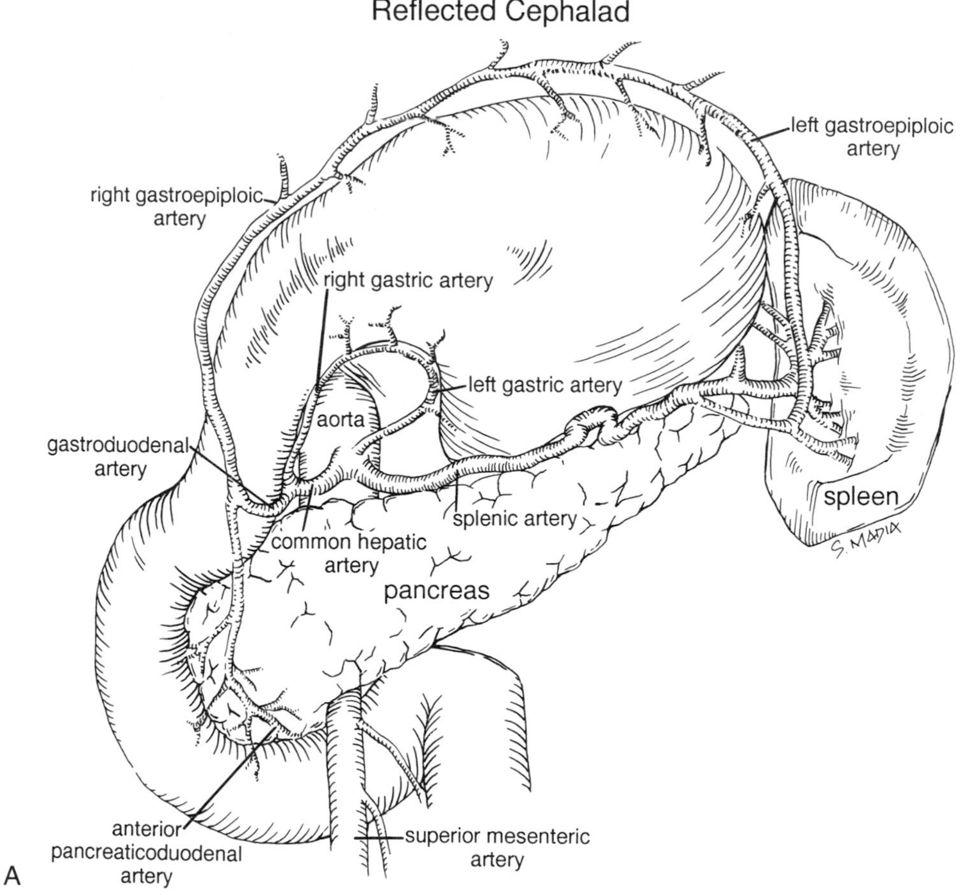

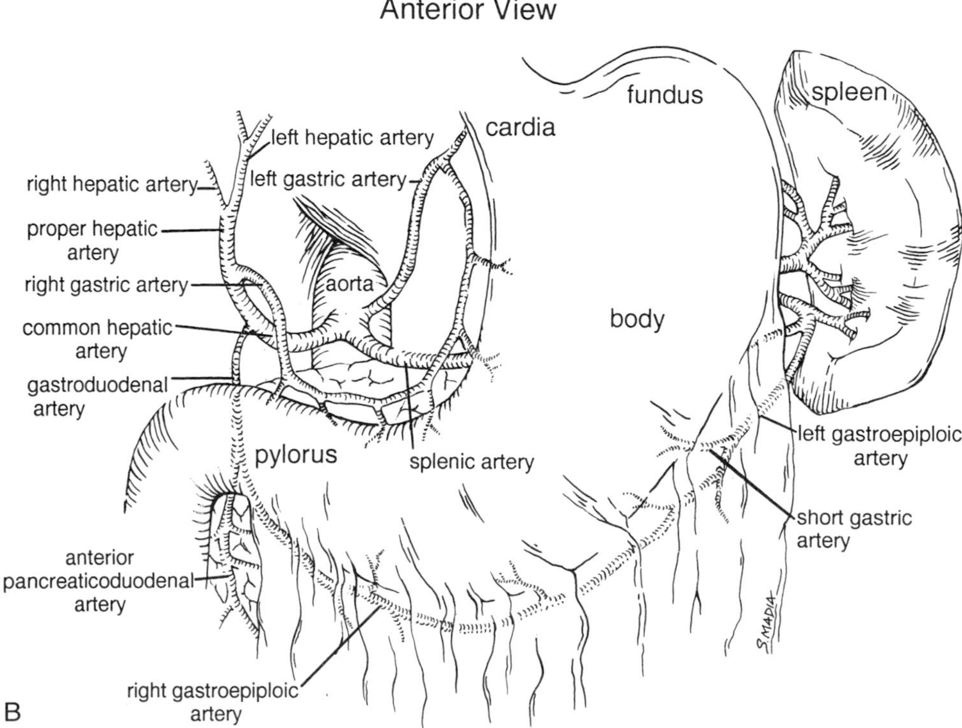

FIGURE 3–1. Anatomic relationships of the stomach. *A,* View reflected cephalad. *B,* Anterior view.

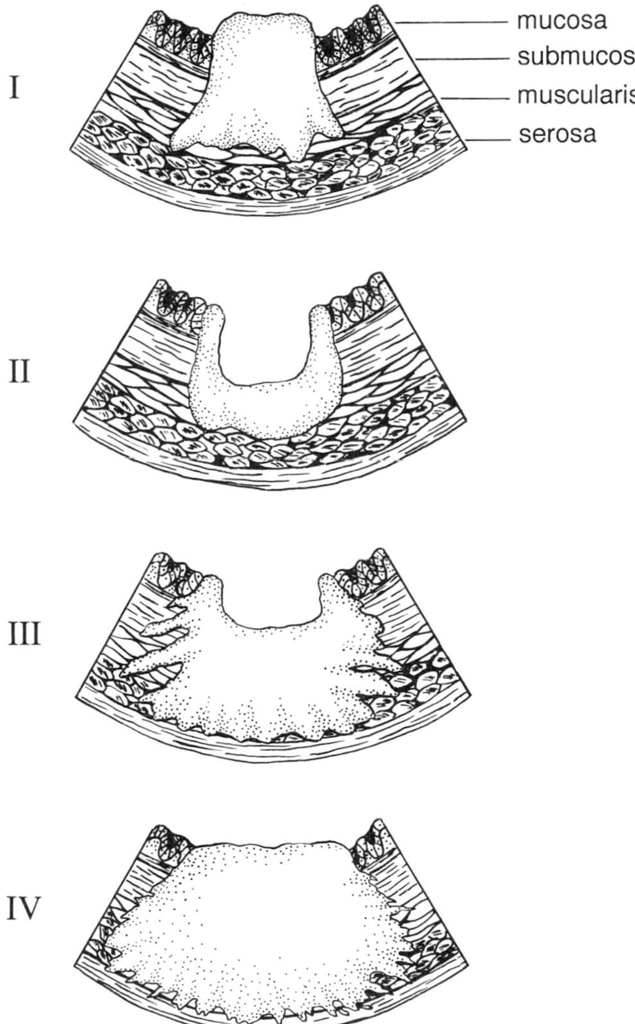

FIGURE 3–2. Bormann's morphologic classification of advanced gastric cancer.

- Type I—polypoid
- Type II—ulcerating with sharply defined margins
- Type III—combined ulcerating and infiltrating without clear-cut margins
- Type IV—diffusely infiltrating

Type I tumors are unusual and represent approximately 7% of the subtypes. Type II tumors account for 25% and are grossly difficult to distinguish from a benign ulcer. Type III is the commonest subtype, accounting for approximately 36%. Type IV accounts for 26% and correspondingly is associated with the worst prognosis. This morphologic classification has relevance to surgical results, since types III and IV are rarely, if ever, amenable to curative surgical resection and have a combined 5-year overall survival rate in the range of 5% to 10%.

A similar morphologic classification has been developed by Marakami[54] to describe the endoscopic appearance of a early gastric cancer, as noted in Figure 3–3. It is possible that the protruding and the depressed or ulcerative type of early gastric cancer may have a more favorable prognosis (95% 5-year survival rate) than the elevated type II (85% 5-year survival rate).[55, 56] However, there is no evidence that prognosis can be based on this gross morphologic classification of early gastric cancer. Regardless of the morphology, early gastric cancer can be multifocal in origin up to 50% of the time.[57]

Molecular Aspects

DNA analysis by flow cytometry is being used with increasing frequency for predicting prognosis in various solid tumors. Ploidy has not been evaluated extensively in gastric cancer, but in several studies there has been a correlation established between aneuploid predominance and poor prognosis, particularly in proximal gastric adenocarcinoma.[58]

The presence of oncogene mutation has been studied in small patient series from the United States and Japan. Although *ras* oncogene mutation may be an important event in colorectal cancer, it does not appear to be present in most gastric cancers. However, mutant p53 and Her-2/neu protein overexpression probably occurs in 10% to 40% of stomach cancer and may signify a poorer outcome.[59, 60] Obviously, molecular markers for prognostication either before or after therapy will be valuable in designing treatment schemes. Additional data collection and evaluation are necessary before the pathologic description of gastric cancer can include these aspects of tumor biology.

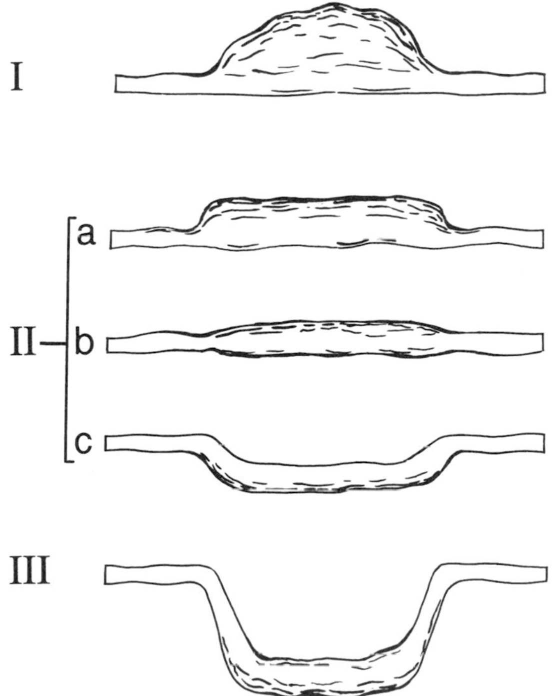

FIGURE 3–3. Morphologic and endoscopic classification of early gastric cancer. I, Protruded or polypoid type; II, superficial type; IIa, elevated; IIb, flat; IIc, depressed; III, excavated type.

Studies of gastrointestinal cancer receptor biology has broadened the understanding of necessary growth regulation of local cancer extension and metastatic potential. Interesting observations concerning the presence of high-affinity gastrin receptors in certain gastric adenocarcinomas may eventually contribute to novel methods of therapy.[61] In addition, the presence of an autocrine growth regulator (epidermal growth factor receptor) may be important in the progression of certain gastric cancer. Approximately one third of gastric cancers exhibit a higher rate of epidermal growth factor receptor than adjacent normal gastric epithelium.[62]

DIAGNOSIS

Clinical Presentation

The initial symptoms of gastric cancer are usually vague and nonspecific; often there is a lag time between the onset of symptoms and the confirmation of a diagnosis.[63, 64] As a result, the disease is commonly advanced or metastatic at the time of diagnosis.

Seventy to 80% of patients present with weight loss, making this the most common presenting symptom. This is often associated with anorexia and a specific distaste for beef products. Nonspecific pain is present in about 70% of patients with gastric cancer. The localization of pain can be epigastric, substernal, or spinal; it can mimic peptic ulcer disease and respond transiently to antisecretory medications. Cancers involving the antral and pyloric regions of the stomach can present with manifestations of gastric outlet obstruction. The pain produced, in this instance, is exacerbated by food intake and results in nausea relieved by vomiting, which produces limitations on food intake and further weight loss. Constipation frequently results from the restricted food intake. The blood loss of gastric cancer is usually in the form of occult blood in the stool. Uncommonly, hematemesis and melena can occur. When they do, associated disseminated intravascular coagulation should be suspected.[65] As a result of chronic blood loss, anemia can develop, leading to fatigue and weakness, exacerbation of cardiac dysfunction, and a decreased performance status. Carcinomas of the cardia or gastroesophageal junction can produce progressive dysphagia, further exacerbating weight loss and constipation.

Physical Examination

The physical examination of a patient with gastric carcinoma can be normal. Usually, it is remarkable for signs of systemic debilitation. Signs of anemia can result from chronic blood loss. Weight loss is generally present as a result of anorexia and dysphagia. Additional physical signs of gastric carcinoma relate to the pattern of spread: direct extension, nodal metastases, hematogenous metastases, and intraperitoneal dissemination.

Direct extension of tumor can result in a palpable abdominal mass. If gastric outlet obstruction is present, abdominal distention and gastric peristalsis can be visualized, and a succession splash may be evident.

When lymphatic spread involves distant nodal groups, the patient may present with a left supraclavicular node (Virchow's node) via the thoracic duct. In approximately 5% of patients with advanced gastric carcinoma, left axillary nodes can be palpated.

Hematogenous spread of gastric carcinoma is usually to the liver, although, rarely, pulmonary and bone metastases are also noted. Extra-abdominal metastases are unlikely in the absence of advanced intra-abdominal spread. Gastric carcinoma involving the liver can result in jaundice, ascites, hepatomegaly, or palpable liver metastasis.

Peritoneal spread can manifest as ascites or a palpable mass on rectal examination (Blumer's shelf). Peritoneal spread to the ovaries (Krukenberg's tumor) can present as a mass on pelvic examination. When peritoneal spread involves the umbilical area, at times nodules can be palpated, which are called Sister Mary Joseph nodes.

Laboratory Studies

Routine laboratory studies are commonly normal in gastric cancer. With advanced symptomatic disease, however, laboratory abnormalities often confirm clinical signs and symptoms. A microcytic anemia secondary to chronic gastrointestinal blood loss, or a macrocytic anemia secondary to pre-existing pernicious anemia, can be found. With metastatic disease to the liver, abnormal liver function tests can be detected.

Once a diagnosis of gastric carcinoma is determined, nutritional parameters such as albumin and transferrin should be assessed and followed as a determination of adequate nutritional repletion. Carcinoembryonic antigen (CEA) can be obtained and, if elevated, can serve as an indicator of response to therapy.

Radiologic Studies

Single-contrast barium study of the upper gastrointestinal tract is commonly the first diagnostic study ordered to evaluate symptoms referable to the upper gastrointestinal tract.[66] In most instances, the study detects more than 80% of gastric cancers, although this method frequently misses early gastric cancer.[67] Significant findings include a mass lesion in the gastric lumen, an obstructing lesion of the antrum or cardia, an ulcerated mass resembling a benign ulcer, enlarged gastric folds, or a nondistensible stomach. A more accurate test for detecting early gastric carcinoma is the double-contrast barium study with external compression.[68] The obvious disadvantage of the barium study is the lack of biopsy capability, with resulting lack of histologic confirmation of malignancy. In addition, at least 10% of gastric cancers can be missed by barium study.

When the barium study reveals an ulcer within 1 cm of

the pyloric channel, the likelihood is high that it is a benign lesion, and it is reasonable to treat this medically with follow-up radiographic study or endoscopy. An upper endoscopy and biopsy should be performed on any patient when the ulcer is not located in proximity to the pylorus. A routine course of medical therapy with only a follow-up radiologic study is inappropriate in these instances. A small percentage of malignant ulcers can heal with medical antisecretory treatment, and these might be missed without initial endoscopy and biopsy.[69]

The most useful role for the barium study in gastric cancer is as a complementary examination to endoscopy. This serves two useful purposes. In cases of infiltrative gastric cancer, such as the linitis plastica variety, nondistensibility of the stomach is common. This should serve as an indicator to the endoscopist that multiple biopsies of the same area should be performed to get deeper samples to increase the yield of malignant tissue. The barium study is also very useful localizing test to help direct the endoscopist to the abnormal area that needs careful examination and biopsy.

Endoscopic Evaluation

Upper gastrointestinal endoscopy enables the direct visualization, photographic documentation, and biopsy of gastric lesions. Although a visual diagnosis is accurate in 90% of patients with gastric cancer, biopsies and cytologies must be done for histologic confirmation. In exophytic lesions, Winawer et al.[70] showed that a tissue diagnosis can be established by biopsy or cytology in 92% of patients. In gastric cancer of the infiltrative type, diagnosis was made by biopsy and cytology in only 50% of patients. Subsequent studies have shown that increasing the number of biopsy samples taken, as well as performing brush cytology of a lesion, can increase the yield of a positive histologic diagnosis.

In a study by Graham et al.,[71] patients with esophageal and gastric cancers were evaluated by endoscopy. This study showed that a single biopsy resulted in a tissue diagnosis in 70% of patients with gastric carcinoma. When four biopsy samples were taken, the diagnosis was made in 95% of patients; when seven samples were taken, the diagnosis was made in 98% of patients with gastric cancer. When biopsy and cytology samples were obtained, the diagnosis was possible in all patients with gastric carcinoma.

When a gastric lesion is detected endoscopically, a minimum of six biopsy samples and a brush cytology sample for exophytic lesions should be obtained. When a lesion is infiltrative, multiple biopsy samples in the same area should be obtained in an attempt to sample tissue from a level deeper than the mucosa. This technique is commonly referred to as the well technique. When available, photographic documentation by videoendoscopy should be done, as this will enable determination of efficacy of various presurgical neoadjuvant chemotherapeutic regimens by comparing pre- and post-treatment films.

Several benign lesions are associated with gastric cancer. Most notable are those lesions in patients with a history of pernicious anemia. At present, there is no evidence that the yield of routine screening endoscopy for cancer detection in asymptomatic patients with pernicious anemia, atrophic gastritis, or prior gastric resection is cost effective. However, elderly patients with new onset of persistent dyspeptic symptoms should be initially evaluated by endoscopy, especially if they are known to have a history of atrophic gastric mucosal changes. Endoscopic evaluation is still the most accurate method available for the diagnosis of early stomach cancer in symptomatic patients.

Preoperative Staging

Once the diagnosis of gastric carcinoma has been established, the extent of disease and therefore its resectability should be evaluated. Computed tomography (CT) or magnetic resonance imaging (MRI) scans should be obtained, specifically for evaluation of hepatic metastases. With good distention of the stomach, CT scans can assess the extent of gastric wall thickening but cannot definitively determine depth of cancer penetration through the layers of the gastric wall. CT scans may demonstrate extension into contiguous organs such as pancreas, transverse colon, or spleen. In addition, extension into the perigastric fat may be visualized by stranding beyond the gastric wall. Ascites suggesting incurable disease can usually be visualized by CT scan. Regional lymph node spread can be predicted when nodes are greater than 2 cm (Fig. 3–4).

CT evaluation, however, has been reported to both understage and overstage disease. In one series, 61% of patients were understaged by CT criteria.[72] In addition, in

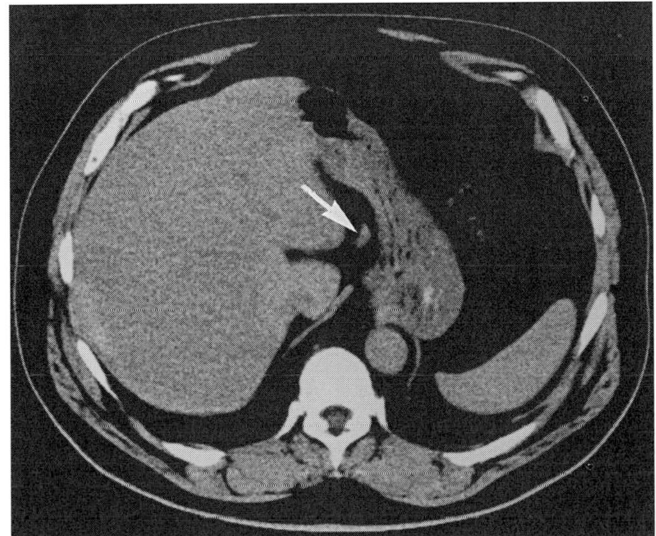

FIGURE 3–4. Computed tomogram of upper abdomen of patient with gastric adenocarcinoma. Arrow indicates a perigastric (N1) lymph node enlargement.

another report the sensitivity for evaluating regional lymph nodes by CT scan was 67%, with a specificity of only 61%.[73] Importantly in this series, CT failed to predict carcinomatosis in 6 of 20 patients. It is clear that in many cases, CT disease assessment should serve only as a supplement to laparotomy in assessing resectability.

Endoscopic intraluminal ultrasound is a newly developed technique that is showing great promise in preoperative staging of gastric carcinoma. The accuracy of endoscopic ultrasound in determining the depth of penetration through the gastric wall is upward of 80%, and the accuracy of determining lymph node involvement is approximately 65%.[74] With a great number of clinical trials under way, the accuracy of this technique should increase rapidly. Endoscopic ultrasound should be considered a complementary diagnostic test in conjunction with CT scanning or MRI.

Recently, video-assisted laparoscopy has been shown to supplement preoperative staging prior to definitive laparotomy. Laparoscopy can provide a sensitive evaluation for visualization of the entire peritoneal cavity to assess peritoneal seeding, organ involvement outside the stomach, and lymph node involvement and can provide access to peritoneal washings for cytologic evaluation. Future preoperative staging protocols may include the routine use of video-assisted laparoscopy, especially in designing neoadjuvant protocols for the treatment of gastric carcinoma.

Special Studies

Abnormalities of serum markers and gastric acid have been noted in patients with gastric cancer. Detection of these abnormalities is not useful in establishing the diagnosis of gastric carcinoma because a causal relationship has not been established and the sensitivities of the tests are low. Some may be useful in post-treatment surveillance.

Studies of gastric acid secretion often reveal achlorhydria or hypochlorhydria, indicating the presence of chronic atrophic gastritis or pernicious anemia.[75] Associated elevation of serum gastrin levels due to the hypochlorhydria or achlorhydria is common.

Serum tumor markers such as CEA, cancer antigen (CA) 19-9, and alpha-fetoprotein (AFP) are commonly elevated in patients with gastric carcinoma. However, they are also elevated in benign conditions and are therefore not specific in the diagnosis of gastric cancer.[76] As many as 50% of patients with gastric cancer have an elevation of one or a combination of these tumor markers. In these patients, the tumor markers can be followed for recurrence if they have normalized during the course of surgical or medical therapy. Their usefulness in this regard for improving patient survival has not been substantiated.

In addition, other markers have been evaluated in patients with gastric cancer. Serum pepsinogen I is low in patients with gastric cancer.[77] Fetal sulfoglycoprotein antigen has been detected in the gastric secretions of up to 96% of patients with gastric cancer but has also been detected in up to 15% of patients with benign gastric disease.[78]

Surgical Staging and Survival

The TNM staging system for gastric adenocarcinoma is the result of an international agreement made in 1985 and modified in 1987.[79] The basis for the present staging system was developed from concepts first introduced in "The General Rules for the Gastric Cancer Study in Surgery and Pathology" presented by the Japanese in 1962 and subsequently published in English in 1981.[80] These general concepts resulted from several prior retrospective analyses examining large gastric cancer patient series in which three important prognostic indicators were identified. The three variables that corresponded to the most significant prognostic indicators correlating with survival consisted of the depth of invasion of the primary tumor into the gastric wall (T), the lymph node status (N), and the presence of metastatic disease (M). Thus, these three indicators are the basis for the present staging system (Tables 3–3 and 3–4).

It should be emphasized that a uniform staging system is absolutely critical in establishing a database for clinical trials evaluating either the surgical management or the adjuvant treatment of gastric cancer. The noted discrepancies between published series analyzing data from the Western literature and similar series from Japan are certainly the result of a lack of uniformity of staging methodology, particularly with reference to lymph node involvement. Any meaningful survival comparison of gastric cancer patient populations extrapolated from the U.S. and Japanese experiences and then correlated to disease stage is quite difficult because of the potential for understaging in Western patient series. This is particularly relevant to the presence or absence of lymph node metastases. Many Western series do not report or systematically assess the involvement of regional nodes other than perigastric lymph nodes. The inaccuracies of clinical and pathologic staging

TABLE 3–3
International Staging of Gastric Cancer

T—Primary Tumor

T_1	Tumor limited to the mucosa or mucosa and submucosa
T_2	Tumor involves the muscularis propria or subserosa
T_3	Tumor penetrates the serosa
T_4	Tumor involves contiguous structures

N—Regional Lymph Nodes

N_0	No metastases to regional lymph nodes
N_1	Involvement of perigastric lymph nodes within 3.0 cm of the primary tumor
N_2	Involvement of regional lymph nodes more than 3.0 cm from the primary tumor, including those located along the left gastric, common hepatic, splenic, and celiac arteries *Note:* Involvement of other intra-abdominal lymph nodes is regarded as distant metastases.

From Cushieri A: Tumors of the stomach. In Moosa AR, et al (eds): Comprehensive Textbook of Oncology, vol 1, 2nd ed. Baltimore: Williams & Wilkins, 1991, p 877.

TABLE 3–4
Gastric Cancer Staging

Stage Groupings				Cumulative Average Survival (%)*
Stage	*pT*	*pN*	*M*	
Ia	pT_1	pN_0	M_0	88
Ib	pT_1	pN_1	M_0	80
	pT_2	pN_0	M_0	
II	pT_1	pN_2	M_0	55
	pT_2	pN_1	M_0	
	pT_3	pN_0	M_0	
IIIa	pT_2	pN_2	M_0	30
	pT_3	pN_1	M_0	
	pT_4	pN_0	M_0	
IIIb	pT_3	pN_2	M_0	9
	pT_4	pN_1	M_0	
	pT_4	pN_2	M_0	
IV	Any	Any	M_1	0

From Cushieri A: Tumors of the stomach. In Moosa AR, et al (eds): Comprehensive Textbook of Oncology, vol 1, 2nd ed. Baltimore: Williams & Wilkins, 1991, p 877.
p, Pathologic staging.
*80% of patients are stage III or IV at the time of initial diagnosis.

by inspection, and of in situ assessment of regional node involvement at the time of the operative procedure, are documented.[81] The average number of 30 lymph nodes examined in the Japanese series is not obtainable in most Western series. Lymph node size is a predictor of tumor involvement, but up to 18% of reported positive lymph nodes are less than 5 mm in diameter.[10]

There are several important features of the present American Joint Committee on Cancer (AJCC) TNM staging system. First, this system excludes tumor size, grade, location, and degree of serosal involvement. N3 and N4 lymph nodes are classified as M (metastatic disease). Stage I is divided into Ia (absence of nodal involvement) and Ib (involvement of N1 nodes within 3 cm of the primary tumor); stage III is divided into IIIa (T2-N2, T3-N1, T4-N0) and IIIb (T3-N2 and any T4 with node involvement). A T2 tumor may penetrate the muscularis propria and extend into the gastrocolic or gastrohepatic ligaments or into the greater or lesser omentum but is not considered a T3 lesion unless there is perforation of the covering visceral peritoneum.

There are important differences between the AJCC TNM staging system and the clinical staging system suggested by the Japanese Research Society for Gastric Cancer (JRSGC) in a review of the Japanese literature (Table 3–5).[82, 83] These differences reinforce the complexity of the JRSGC system, which also includes the location of the primary tumor, designated C (fundus and cardia), M (corpus), and A (antrum), or combinations (e.g., AM). The location of the primary tumor is quite significant in the JRSGC clinical system, since it determines the extent of the planned gastric resection as well as the designated level of a particular regional lymph node group.

The JRSGC system quantitates the degree of gastric wall involvement and incorporates this information into the staging system. The serosal involvement is designated ss (subserosa), s (serosa suspected), se (serosa definite), and si (gross contiguous invasion). Survival statistics are known to vary considerably with the degree and pattern of serosal involvement, ranging from a 43% 5-year survival rate for s to 23% for si.[84] In addition, one would expect positive correlation between the extent of serosal involvement and the potential for peritoneal seeding. Indeed, Itsuka et al.[85] reported that with serosal invasion greater than 15 cm^2, free cancer cells were detected in nearly all peritoneal lavage specimens, which predicted a particularly bad prognosis.

In the JRSCG staging system, regional lymph nodes are divided into four groups designated N1 through N4. Within these nodal groupings are 16 possible anatomic locations and the N1-N4 designations, and incidence of metastatic involvement for any particular nodal group varies with the site of the primary tumor (Tables 3–6 and 3–7). As indicated in Table 3–6, the N1 nodes are in closest proximity to the tumor, the N2 nodes follow the distribution of the celiac axis, and the N3 nodes are farther away from the stomach and located in the portahepatic, retropancreatic region and base of the mesentery. The N4 nodes are located at the base of the middle colic artery and in the para-aortic areas. This complex node designation is in contradistinction to the TNM classification of N1 and N2 nodal designation, which loosely resembles the N1 and N2 designation of the JRSCG system. The Japanese additionally categorize the type of surgical procedure performed based on the extent of lymph node echelon removed. Therefore, an R0 resection implies incomplete removal of the N1 nodes; an R1 resec-

TABLE 3–5
Comparison Between AJCC TNM and JRSGC Classification for Stomach Cancer

TNM Classification	JRSGC Classification
Primary Tumor	*Primary Tumor*
Tis	m
T1	sm
T2	pm, ss
T3	se, s
T4	sei, si
Nodal Involvement	*Nodal Involvement*
N0	n(−)
N1	n1
N2	n2
M	n3
M	n4

Adapted from Fujimoto S, et al: New trends in therapy for gastric malignancy. In Sugarbaker P (ed): Management of Gastric Cancer. Boston: Kluwer Academic Publishers, 1991.
AJCC, American Joint Committee on Cancer; JRSGC, Japanese Research Society for Gastric Cancer; m, mucosa, including muscularis mucosa; sm, submucosa; pm, muscularis propria; ss, subserosa; s, serosa; se, cancer cells existing on the serosal surface and exposed to the peritoneal cavity; si, cancer cells invading the adjacent tissue; sei, the coexistence of se and si.

TABLE 3–6
Anatomic Groupings of Lymph Nodes* According to Site of Primary Tumor

Group	Location of Tumor			
	Entire Stomach	*Lower Third*	*Middle Third*	*Upper Third*
Group 1 (N^1 or perigastric nodes)	1–6	3–6	1, 3–6	1–4
Group 2 (N^2)	7–11	1, 7–9	2, 7–11	5–11
Group 3 (N^3)	12–14	2, 10–14	12–14	12–14

From Behrns KE, et al: Extended lymph node dissection for gastric cancer. Surg Clin North Am 72:433, 1992.

1, Right cardial; 2, left cardial; 3, along the lesser curvature; 4, along the greater curvature; 5, suprapyloric; 6, infrapyloric; 7, along the left gastric artery; 8, along the common heptic artery; 9, around the celiac artery; 10, at the splenic hilus; 11, along the splenic artery; 12, in the hepatoduodenal ligament; 13, at the posterior aspect of the pancreas; 14, at the root of the mesentery.

tion complete N1 group lymph node removal; an R2 resection complete removal of both N1 and N2 nodal groups; and an R3 resection complete removal of nodes designated N1, N2, and N3.

In general, nodal labeling and clearance reported for Western gastric cancer patient series are neither as comprehensive nor as selective as the Japanese series describing N1 or N2 nodal location and surgical removal. Most Western reports of nodal spread constitute N1 involvement, since rarely will a complete N2 nodal removal be accomplished and subsequently analyzed. This hampers survival comparisons between U.S. and Japanese clinical series. Twenty to 25% of patients who have macroscopic involvement of the N1 nodes will additionally have microscopic N2 nodal involvement. This means that some patients included in disease stage I and II (T1, N1; T2, N1) in U.S. series are pathologically understaged and actually have more advanced disease (stage II [T1, N2] and stage III [T2, N2]). Therefore, some of the patients reported in U.S. series (see Table 3–1) designated as having N1 nodal involvement with an associated combined 20% 5-year survival rate may in fact have understaged pathologic N2 nodal metastasis. This subset of understaged N2 patients would then compare more favorably with the reported 26% 5-year survival rate in the collective Japanese series for patients with N2 nodal disease spread. Similarly, the exclusion of patients who actually have N2 involvement from the N1 node-positive group should improve the 5-year survival rate of the collective U.S. series for patients with N1 nodal disease.

TABLE 3–7
Location of Lymph Node Metastasis of Advanced Gastric Cancer (%)* Based on Primary Site Within the Stomach

Lymph Node Group	Total	Location of Tumor		
		Upper Third	*Middle Third*	*Lower Third*
Right cardiac	19.9	33.2	20.6	10.9
Left cardiac	7.2	18.0	5.4	2.2
Lesser curvature	44.5	39.7	48.4	43.5
Greater curvature	32.7	17.6	37.5	37.4
Suprapyloric	7.7	2.4	7.1	11.6
Infrapyloric	30.5	8.4	25.5	49.1
Left gastric artery	27.6	24.8	29.7	27.2
Common hepatic artery	21.2	12.3	18.8	29.2
Celiac axis	17.0	16.4	16.5	17.9
Splenic hilum	6.4	13.9	7.2	1.0
Splenic artery	8.6	13.2	8.1	6.3
Hepatoduodenal ligament	5.2	2.4	3.6	8.6
Retropancreatic	1.7	0.7	0.9	3.1
Mesenteric root	2.0	1.7	1.5	2.8
Middle colic	1.1	1.7	0.5	1.2
Para-aortic	5.3	5.8	5.3	5.1
Total cases	1754	416	666	672

From Noguchi Y, et al: Radical surgery for gastric cancer: A review of the Japanese experience. Cancer 64:2053–2062, 1989.

*Results from the National Cancer Institute of Japan for 1754 evaluable cases with extensive lymph node dissection.

Survival data for gastric adenocarcinoma correlates with disease stage and in general follows predictable attrition rates based on extent of tumor penetration into the stomach wall and the presence of positive regional lymph nodes (see Table 3–4). In a collective Japanese review, Maruyama et al.[114] compared overall survival by stage based on the present TNM classification where all patients had N2 nodes removed. Overall reported survival rates were as follows: stage I (96%), stage II (70%), stage III (36%), and stage IV (12%).[86] Most prior reports from Western literature sources do not analyze results by subset of the TNM staging system. Reports generally include either overall survival for the entire group of patients being evaluated or survival statistics that are separately based on either lymph node disease or serosal involvement. However, several recent survival reports from the Western literature can be extrapolated into the present TNM system. These compare more favorably to the large series reported by Maruyama (Table 3–8).[13, 87, 88] It must be noted, however, that survival statistics from these series are based on the fact that the majority of patients had R2 node dissections (removal of N2 lymph nodes) and thus were subject to more comprehensive pathologic staging.

Early Gastric Cancer

The reported improved survival statistics on gastric cancer from Japan may in part be due to the increasingly

TABLE 3–8
Comparison of Survival Based on TNM Classification

Series	No. of Patients	5-Year Overall Survival Rate (%) by Stage					
		I	*II*	*III*	*IIIa*	*IIIb*	*IV*
Maruyama et al.[114]	10,812	89	70	36	50	24	12
Gall and Hermanek[13]	1,636		70	30			
Lawrence and Shiu[87]	60	85	36				
Rohde et al.[88]	994	62	35		32	18	13

common finding of early gastric cancer. This fact alone could account for a 27% improvement in overall survival of gastric carcinoma compared to U.S. series, in which early gastric cancer remains a small percentage of the total group.[89] The definition of early gastric cancer is a T1 primary lesion regardless of lymph node status. Thus, early gastric cancer can be classified as stage Ia, Ib, or II. The presence of positive lymph nodes is generally not reported to be a significant prognostic factor in early gastric cancer. However, it is important to note that positive lymph nodes are unusual, occurring in only 10% of cases, and thus have not been accounted for in most survival statistics for early gastric cancer. These cancers are generally found in the prepyloric and antral regions of the stomach. Mass screening programs in Japan over the last 30 years have increased the incidence of early gastric cancer to nearly 50%, and, correspondingly, gastric cancer survival has significantly increased during this time period. This explains why Japan is the only country where the mortality from gastric cancer is declining more rapidly than the incidence. Patients in Japan with this entity tend to be 5 to 10 years younger at diagnosis than those with advanced gastric cancer, perhaps reflecting the effectiveness of screening programs in place. It is not clear that all gastric cancers follow an established pattern of early gastric cancer slowly progressing to advanced gastric cancer.

The symptoms of early gastric cancer generally mimic those of acid peptic disease.[90] The duration of symptoms is generally longer in patients with early gastric cancer than reported for patients with advanced gastric cancer. This is perhaps indicative of a slower natural history of disease progression in patients with early gastric cancer. Gastroscopy with multiple directed and random biopsies is a highly sensitive and specific test for the diagnosis of this entity.[91]

Multicentricity is an important aspect of early gastric cancer and may be present in up to half of patients.[92] Subtotal gastrectomy as a primary treatment is associated with a low recurrence rate and excellent survival even with multicentricity.[87] The extent of surgical resection for these lesions is somewhat controversial. Curability rates are high and do not seem to vary by extent of gastric resection (provided negative margins are obtained) or by extent of lymphadenectomy. In a summary of the North American experience in early gastric cancer reporting a 5-year survival rate of 85%, 87% of patients had less than total gastrectomy and only 7% had radical regional lymphadenectomy.[93]

The variables favoring long-term survival include small tumor size (<1.5 cm) and lack of submucosal invasion.[93] There is evidence that extension into the submucosa can be a factor denoting a more aggressive lesion. The recurrence rate for lesions extending into the submucosa has been reported to be 8.4%, compared with 2.2% for mucosal lesions. Since lymph node involvement is so infrequent, the impact of extending the node dissection may not be realized when evaluating retrospective data. In addition, several reports indicate a higher incidence of nodal involvement in patients with submucosal disease. Therefore, the standard operative procedure should include at least resection of the appropriate N1 nodes (R1 resection) and consideration of removal of the appropriate N2 nodes (R2 resection) if the lesion appears larger than 1.5 cm or if there is clinical evidence of perigastric nodal involvement. Infirm patients with small mucosal polypoid lesions may be managed by endoscopic ablative techniques.[94]

PRIMARY OPERABLE DISEASE

Surgical Options

Since the only effective method of curing gastric cancer is surgery, the therapeutic management of this disease revolves around two important issues. These relate to the extent of gastric resection and the extent of regional lymphadenectomy. These issues are addressed separately.

Perioperative Considerations

Since the majority of patients diagnosed with stomach cancer are elderly, any underlying significant medical problem, including nutritional repletion, should be addressed and optimized prior to surgery. Patients should undergo bowel cleansing prior to surgery because of the possibility of transverse colon or mesocolon involvement. Preoperative antibiotics are indicated because of potential colonization of bacteria in the obstructed or achlorhydric stomach.

Patient positioning on the operative table is important, especially in proximal gastric cancers, for which a thoracoabdominal approach might be necessary for proximal tumor clearance. If body habitus permits, extension into the right chest can be accomplished with an angled elevation of the patient's right upper abdomen and chest to obviate the need for a full lateral thoracotomy.

A feeding jejunostomy tube should be placed during surgery in all patients with a planned gastric resection, particularly after total gastrectomy. Closed suction drains are not used routinely except when a pancreatic resection is performed. Unless the patient has a particularly wide costal angle, we prefer a midline approach with a mechanical retractor to elevate the ribs and the left hepatic lobe.

Gastric Resection

Total radical or extended total radical gastrectomy was the procedure of choice in all instances of gastric cancer in the 1950s and 1960s.[95] However, there is no substantial evidence to insist on its routine use. To the contrary, there are existing data to suggest that its routine use is not warranted.[96–98] Additionally, in many reports, mortality following total or extended total gastrectomy exceeds that following subtotal gastrectomy. Mortality rates of 11% to 23% have been reported for total gastrectomy, in comparison to 3% to 10% for subtotal gastrectomy.[13, 96–99] One must also take into account the nutritional consequences of routine total gastrectomy. In comparison to subtotal gastrectomy, total gastrectomy is associated with more profound weight loss and fat depletion, regardless of the method of reconstruction of the esophageal anastomosis (gastric reservoir or not, duodenal transit preservation or not).[100, 101]

Within the general principles of en bloc resection for cancer surgery, it is reasonable to expect a similar outcome from subtotal gastrectomy and total gastrectomy. However, total gastrectomy is necessary when the gastric cancer occupies a portion of the stomach such that adequate margins cannot be obtained without resection of the entire stomach. Tumors of the gastric cardia are often considered for routine total gastrectomy, since the associated problems of an esophageal anastomosis cannot be circumvented owing to the necessity of the proximal resection margin. In this instance, a proximal subtotal gastrectomy may be disadvantageous because of subsequent problems due to alkaline reflux esophagitis. The preference may be for a better functional anastomosis employing an esophagojejunal Roux-en-Y reconstruction.

The performance of extended total gastrectomy in all instances of resectable gastric cancer, consisting of routine en bloc resection of the pancreatic tail and spleen, has not improved survival. Although routine use of extended gastric resection for stomach cancer has been associated with better disease control in a few select series, this appears to benefit only a small subset of patients with early-stage disease, and the attendant morbidity does not justify its routine use.[102] Importantly, reports have suggested a negative prognostic role for routine splenectomy. This is true even for proximal cancers, with which there is normally a higher probability of splenic hilar nodal involvement (see Table 3–7).[103, 104] Extended gastrectomy, consisting of en bloc splenectomy and pancreatectomy along with gastrectomy, is necessary when the patient presents with a bulky gastric tumor extending posteriorly into the pancreatic tail or laterally into the splenic hilum. In these instances, 5-year survival rates of 10% to 20% have been reported in select patients. An occasional patient may present with direct macroscopic invasion of the colon, mesocolon, or left lobe of the liver without evidence of widespread peritoneal disease. En bloc resection in these instances can result in 5-year survival rates of 5% to 10%. In the clinical situation in which there is only microscopic disease extension or "tumor" adhesions, 5-year survival rates in the 30% range have been reported when the gastric resection includes contiguous structures. One must add, however, that this applies to a select group of patients in whom other prognostic factors (e.g., the absence of peritoneal disease) are favorable.

It is largely believed that radical lymph node dissection can be accomplished to a similar degree regardless of whether the patient undergoes a total or a subtotal gastrectomy. The N2 nodes around the celiac axis, common hepatic artery, and left gastric artery can all be removed without performing a total gastrectomy (see Fig. 3–7). Similarly, the right and left paracardial nodes, which are routinely removed with a total gastrectomy, can likewise be resected with a high subtotal gastrectomy. These nodes are considered N1 nodes for cancers of the middle and upper stomach (see Table 3–6). Their removal can be accomplished with a complete resection of the lesser curvature of the stomach and a limited dissection along the left gastroesophageal junction (see Fig. 3–6). In one report, the number of nodes removed from the paracardial nodal group was similar regardless of whether a total or a subtotal gastrectomy was performed.[97]

Lymphadenectomy

The rich lymphatic drainage of the stomach has been appreciated for a number of years and was illustrated quite well by Sunderland et al.[105] in relation to gastric cancer spread. At that time, radical lymph node dissection, as described by McNeer and colleagues,[106] was reported as part of the standard surgical procedure for the management of gastric cancer. However, in 1969, Gilbertsen[107] noted an excessive morbidity and mortality associated with the standard application of radical lymph node dissection, and its routine use in the United States was curtailed.

Currently, the concept of radical lymphadenectomy included in the gastric resection is advocated and practiced as a routine procedure for gastric cancer in Japan and in some European centers. This routine application of radical lymphadenectomy for all cases of operable gastric cancer has been proposed as an important factor in the seemingly dramatic difference in improved survival from gastric cancer noted in the overall Japanese experience. These differences can also be attributed to the increase in the numbers of early gastric cancer in the Japanese series when compared to Western reports. It has been suggested that improved survival reported by Japanese surgeons may be a manifestation of carefully applied and uniform staging techniques compared with Western survival statistics, which are often based on patients who are actually surgically understaged. In addition, low postoperative morbidity and mortality (2% and 1%, respectively) in the Japanese patients have improved the Japanese long-term postoperative survival statistics when comparison is made to similar operations performed in Western series. All of these factors play a role in examining the notable differences.

There are no prospective randomized trials from Japan to prove that more radical lymph node clearing is the underlying important factor in their reported enhanced survival from gastric cancer. In all instances, despite large numbers of patients in reviews from the Japanese literature, comparison of improved survival is invariably made to their historical controls. Selective review of these large operative series reveals that there has been a profound decrease in the percentage of patients with either positive nodes or transmural cancers over the last 30 years. In a series reported by Soga and coworkers,[108] the decline in the percentage of patients with positive regional lymph nodes dropped from 62% in the 1960s to 38% in the early 1980s. A similar decline in the percentage of transmural cancers, from 50% to 30%, was also observed in this time period.[108] It is difficult to ascribe the apparent improvement in gastric cancer outcome to the increased radicality of nodal extirpation without considering the effect of the changing patterns of the disease. This question cannot be answered in a retrospective review.

A multi-institutional European prospective randomized trial is under way to compare the R1 versus the R2 node dissection. Dent et al.[109] published the only randomized trial to date and did not demonstrate a significant difference in survival outcome between the R1 and R2 node dissection. It is important to note that in this series, out of a total population of 608 gastric cancer patients, only 43 actually qualified for a curative resection and were randomized to either a R1 or R2 lymph node dissection. This exemplifies the difficulty in accrual of patients who can undergo curative surgery. It has been estimated that in order to detect a survival difference of 15% between the two operative procedures, approximately 1100 patients with gastric cancer will have to be entered into a randomized trial, considering that the proportion of curative resections will remain at 30% of the total group.

One argument against extended lymphadenectomy for gastric cancer is the reported increase in postoperative morbidity and mortality associated with the R2 and R3 node dissections. However, two recent studies suggest that there are no apparent differences in complications or mortality associated with the performance of an R1 versus an R2 lymph node dissection after an initial "learning curve."[110, 111]

The surgical principles involved in performing radical lymphadenectomy for gastric cancer are soundly based on an en bloc resection technique, which includes a wide resection of the primary tumor, the intervening lymphatics, and the regional lymph nodes. Patients who are likely to benefit from such an approach are those whose disease can be encompassed by this extension of primary tumor resection. This represents a rather small proportion of patients who initially present with the diagnosis of gastric cancer.

The standards for what constitutes a curative resection for gastric cancer in Japan are well described by the JRSGC. A resection in Japan is considered to be performed with curative intent when the patient's gastric cancer fulfills the following criteria: cancer confined to the gastric wall (ss) or only suspected serosal involvement (s); no peritoneal metastases or only minimal involvement of adjacent peritoneum above the transverse colon, including the omentum; no evidence of nodal involvement extending into the N3 or N4 nodal group; and no evidence of distant metastatic disease. This description limits the applicability of the R2 resection to a fairly select group of patients. A report from the Japanese literature included 1906 gastric cancer patients, and only 367 (19%) underwent a potentially curative resection.[112]

A review of the Japanese series in Table 3–9 indicates that the real impact of radical lymph node dissection over a 24-year period is found in those patients presenting with pathologically confirmed N0 or N1 disease.[10] Shiu et al.[96] noted that radical lymphadenectomy in patients with N0 or N1 nodal disease appeared to be of benefit when the group of nodes removed was one echelon higher than the group of nodes found to be pathologically involved. Thus, a standard R2 nodal resection should benefit only patients with clinical N0 disease (some of whom may actually have microscopic N1 disease) and patients with N1 disease. It is also possible that select patients with minimal or microscopic involvement of N2 nodes may benefit from an R2 dissection, particularly those whose tumors do not penetrate the gastric wall. Analysis of the literature concerning the incidence of positive lymph nodes indicates that N2 nodes will be positive in T2 gastric cancers with an incidence of 20%; in T3 primary gastric cancers, N2 nodes will be positive more than 40% of the time.[86]

The logical assumption would be that a routine R3 nodal resection would be beneficial for all patients with N2 disease. However, this has not been the case. A complete removal of the N3 nodes represents an extensive addition to the surgical procedure, and patients with grossly evident N2 node involvement most likely have microscopic or macroscopic disease beyond the N2 nodal group. Because of the extent of lymphatic involvement, the disease in these patients will not be completely encompassed by an R3 dissection. Large databases on advanced but resectable gastric cancer have been used to evaluate the extent and location of lymph node metastases based on the anatomic

TABLE 3–9
Results of Radical Surgery in Gastric Carcinoma (5-Year Survival Rate [%] According to Lymph Node Metastasis [Microscopic])*

Period	N0	N1	N2	N3	N4
1946–50	68	44	22	10	0
1951–55	69	48	21	9	0
1956–60	77	47	27	5	8
1961–65	83	62	30	16	6
1966–70	85	60	25	11	0
Total	80	53	26	10	3
Cases	1016	863	967	240	59

From Noguchi Y, et al: Radical surgery for gastric cancer: A review of the Japanese experience. Cancer 64:2053–2062, 1989.

*Results from the Cancer Institute Hospital for solitary curative cases, 1946 to 1970. N2 disease with radical surgery had a 26% survival rate. The only apparent improvement in survival is seen in the N0 and N1 groups, despite (presumably) more aggressive lymph node dissection in more recent years. Much of the improvement in the N0 group will be from early gastric cancer. (Data modified from the Japanese Research Society for Gastric Cancer).

location of the primary tumor site (see Table 3–7). It is apparent from these studies that the N3 lymph nodes are rarely involved in resectable gastric cancer, which suggests that their removal will not present a considerable survival advantage. Data from the literature imply that there is no survival advantage in N3 node removal (R3 dissection) when compared to complete removal of N2 nodes (R2 dissection).[112] A 1988 report evaluated the value of complete N3 lymph node dissection versus incomplete N3 lymph node dissection (just grossly involved nodes removed) for patients with clinically evident N3 nodal disease and indicated no difference in 5-year survival between the two groups.[113] In the Japanese literature over the last 30 years, the 5-year survival rate remains at 10% and essentially unchanged in those patients with N3 nodal involvement despite increasingly radical nodal clearing surgery for gastric cancer.[114] Therefore, routine clearance of the N3 nodes cannot be recommended, since involvement of these nodes indicates disease beyond surgical cure.

Node involvement at the splenic hilum and splenic artery (sites 10 and 11 in Table 3–6) poses a particularly difficult problem for the surgeon. Although not common in distal gastric cancer, splenic hilar nodal involvement is more common in proximal tumors. Obviously, splenectomy provides the only means of adequately assessing the involvement of these nodes. Involved nodes along the splenic artery frequently necessitate distal pancreatectomy for complete clearance. These nodes, however, are infrequently positive unless there is obvious clinical involvement of nodes in the celiac axis and primary transmural tumor spread. The 5-year survival rate of patients with splenic nodal involvement varies from 2.7% to 40%, depending on the presence or absence of other nodal disease. However, it is distinctly uncommon for patients to have isolated involvement of splenic arterial or hilar nodes (only 2.1% in one series), and thus most patients with this pattern will have extensive N2 nodal disease.[115] Since the number of positive lymph nodes has been related directly to curability, the value of routine lymph node dissection of the splenic hilum and along the splenic artery by extended radical gastrectomy is small.[116] The morbidity of routinely extending the surgical resection for gastric cancer to include the spleen and tail of the pancreas for the purpose of removal of nodal groups 10 and 11 outweighs the benefit. Extending the gastrectomy to include the spleen and tail of the pancreas is justified in patients with clinically evident direct extension of tumor into these organs.

Clinical trials are required to verify the efficacy of extended lymphatic resection for gastric cancer. However, until more effective adjuvant chemotherapy or radiation therapy protocols are designed, the R2 nodal resection may offer the only method of long-term disease control in patients with potentially curable gastric carcinoma.

Method of Lymphadenectomy

The R2 node dissection can be accomplished with either subtotal or total gastrectomy (see Table 3–6 for N1 or N2 designation based on the anatomic location of the primary tumor). Initially, the greater omentum is completely detached from the transverse colon together with the anterior leaf of the transverse mesocolon. The dissection continues until the pancreatic body is visualized at the base of the mesocolon. The omentum and anterior sheet of the mesocolon are taken en bloc with the stomach, since this area can harbor microscopic disease extension. This will also ensure the removal of lymph nodes in level 4 (Fig. 3–5). The dissection plane is continued to the right, and the hepatic flexure is separated from the duodenum and head of the pancreas (this can be accomplished with clamps and sharp dissection techniques). At this point, the origins of the right gastroepiploic artery (from the gastroduodenal artery) and gastroepiploic vein (from the superior mesenteric vein) are visualized. These vessels are ligated as close to their origins as possible. This will encompass the lymph nodes in level 6 (see Fig. 3–5). The uncinate process of the pancreas is in close proximity to this area.

Next, attention is turned to the lesser omentum, which is divided near the liver, and the right gastric artery is located and divided at its origin. The lymph nodes in level 5 are removed in this area as the common hepatic artery and the head of the pancreas are visualized (Fig. 3–6).

The duodenum is then divided at the duodenal bulb with a linear stapling device. It is not necessary to invert the staple line with suture. The stomach is then retracted upward for better exposure. The head of the pancreas is clearly seen, and the pylorus and resected portion of duodenum are easily cleared off this area. Nodes covering the common hepatic artery are then dissected, and these are designated level 8 (Fig. 3–7). Care is taken to either clip or tie small vessels extending over the hepatic artery in this area, since bleeding can obscure node clearing. As the common hepatic artery is skeletonized, the left gastric artery and coronary vein come into view. The left gastric artery is taken at its origin for nodes in level 7 (see Fig. 3–7). The coronary vein is likewise individually ligated. When there is a large amount of fatty tissue surrounding these vessels, it is easier to ligate them from a retrogastric approach, utilizing the mobilized stomach to provide countertraction. The nodes in level 9 are then dissected from the anterior border of the celiac axis (see Fig. 3–7).

The splenic artery is cleaned for about 7 to 8 cm from the celiac axis to the proximity of the posterior gastric artery for nodes in level 11 (Fig. 3–8). Continued dissection beyond this point may involve intrapancreatic dissection and potential injury to the pancreas. Further dissection of nodes in level 11 and nodes in level 10 requires distal pancreatectomy and splenectomy.

The stomach can then be transected with a linear stapler at a location providing a safe proximal margin around the tumor. The nodes at level 3 can be removed en bloc during resection of a portion of, or all of, the lesser curvature of the stomach, depending on the location of the primary tumor (see Fig. 3–5). Care must be taken to ligate the left

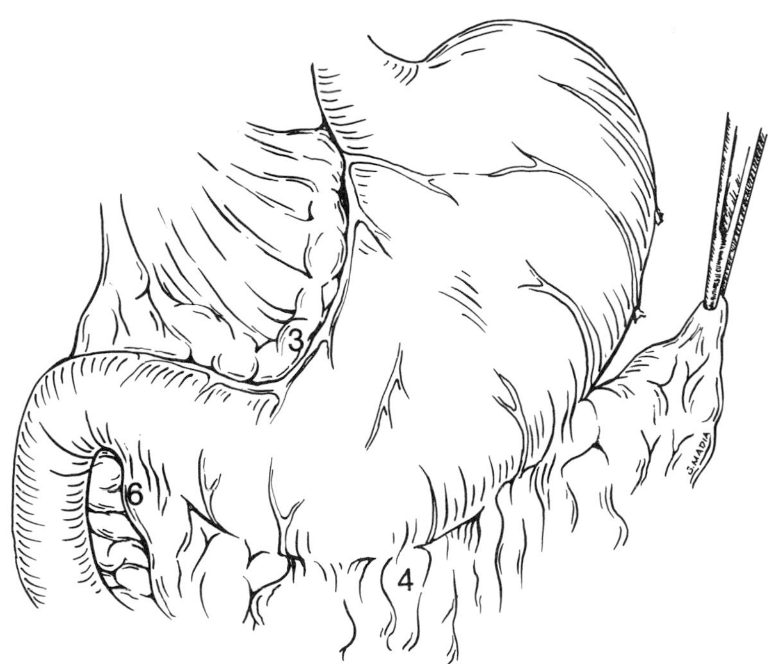

FIGURE 3–5. Resection of regional nodes, levels 3, 6, and 4. 3, Lesser curvature nodes; 6, infrapyloric nodes; 4, greater curvature nodes.

gastric arterial branches located within the lesser curvature fat pad prior to selection of a suitable area for transecting the stomach. The level 1 nodes at the highest point of the lesser curvature, where the esophagus meets the stomach, can be removed with either a total or a subtotal gastrectomy (see Fig. 3–6). With a subtotal gastrectomy, the majority of the lesser curvature is removed to ensure dissection of these nodes. When a total gastrectomy is performed with splenic preservation, the dissection skirts the lower pole of the spleen, ligating the short gastric vessels with division of the suspensory ligament and the lienorenal fold and continuing cephalad toward the esophageal hiatus. The left paracardial nodes in level 2 can be removed in this process (see Fig. 3–6).

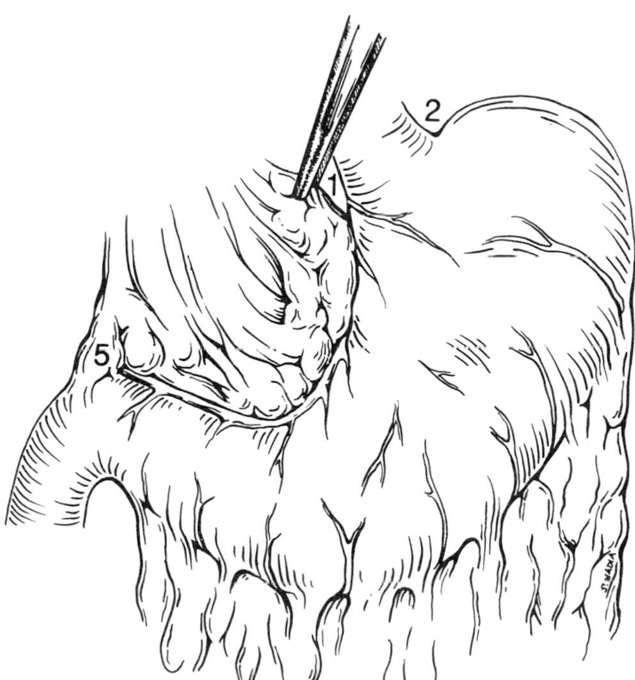

FIGURE 3–6. Resection of regional nodes, levels 1, 2, and 5. 1, Right cardial nodes; 2, left cardial nodes; 5, suprapyloric nodes.

NONSURGICAL OPTIONS

Adjuvant Radiation Therapy

There are few data available to support the efficacy of adjuvant external beam radiation therapy alone in preventing recurrence following surgery for the primary treatment of gastric cancer. The most comprehensive study to date representing a randomized trial of postoperative radiation was carried out by the British Stomach Cancer Group.[117] This three-arm study comparing surgery alone with either postoperative radiation therapy or chemotherapy indicated no significant benefit to either adjuvant treatment.

Data derived from intraoperative radiation trials, although limited, have provided better evidence for recurrence and survival benefit. This is particularly true in a randomized trial from Kyoto University in Japan, where Abe and Takahashi[118] have shown 5-year survival benefit using intraoperative radiation for stage II, III, and IV disease compared to surgery alone. A small nonrandomized trial from Spain by Calvo et al.[119] utilized a treatment scheme of surgery plus intraoperative radiation followed by external beam radiation for patients with stage II, III, and IV gastric cancer as well as recurrent gastric cancer. On the basis of historical data, patients with either cancer

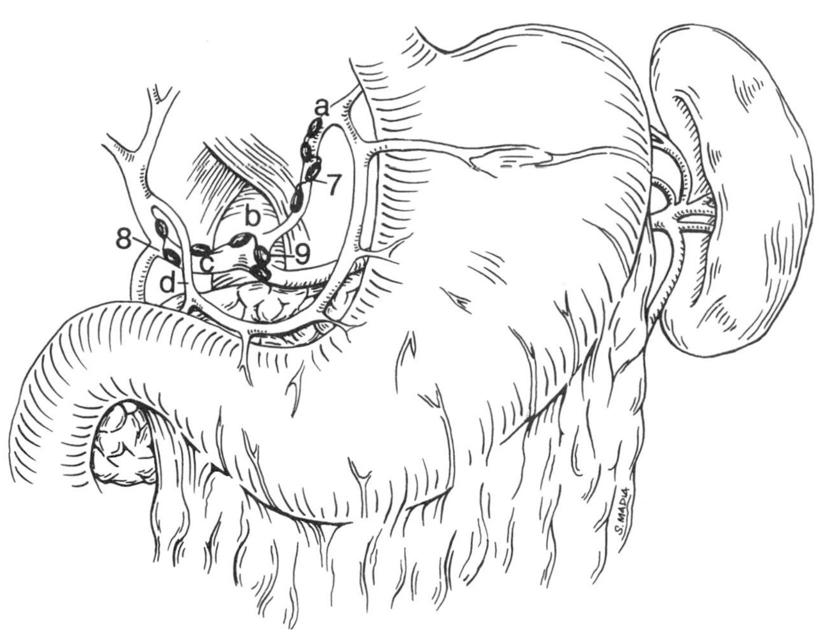

FIGURE 3–7. Resection of regional nodes, levels 7, 8, and 9. 7, Left gastric artery nodes; 8, common hepatic artery nodes; 9, celiac artery nodes; a, left gastric artery; b, aorta; c, common hepatic artery; d, right gastric artery.

penetrating into the stomach muscular wall or with positive regional nodes appeared to benefit from this scheme of radiation compared to surgery alone. Subsequent studies by the Radiation Therapy Oncology Group (RTOG) have further indicated the feasibility of this approach.[120] In the only prospective randomized trial of intraoperative radiation in the United States, completed at the National Cancer Institute (NCI), patients were randomized to either intraoperative radiation alone or external radiation alone.[121] There was no difference in survival comparison between the two groups; however, there was improved local-regional control in the intraoperative radiation group.

These data suggest that any further clinical application of radiation therapy and particularly intraoperative radiation following surgery for gastric cancer should be used only in the context of a defined clinical study. Currently, there is no definitive role for adjuvant radiation in gastric cancer outside of this rationale. Both RTOG and intergroup studies utilizing either external beam or intraoperative radiation for high-risk patients with gastric cancer are under way. Results of these trials may clarify the future role for radiation as a combined modality in resectable gastric cancer.

Combined Radiation Therapy and Chemotherapy

Few randomized trials have investigated the effect of combined adjuvant chemotherapy and radiation therapy for resectable gastric cancer. Most of the data come from series of patient trials in which disease was either unresectable

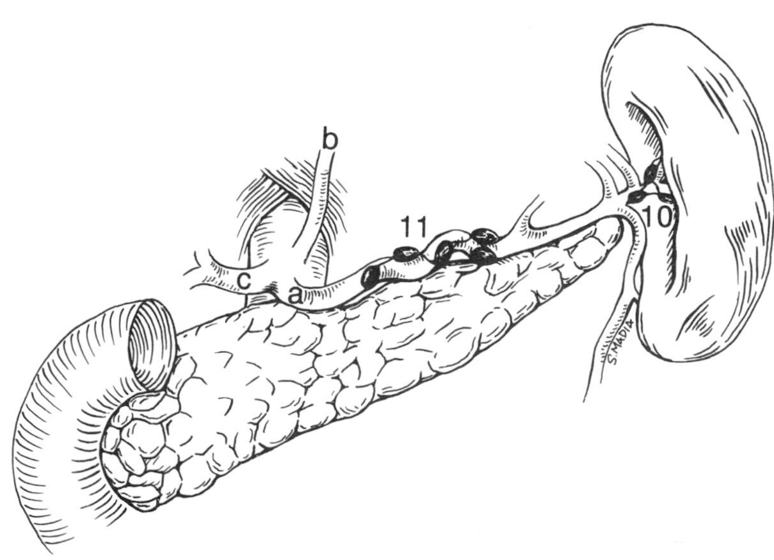

FIGURE 3–8. Resection of regional nodes, levels 10 and 11. 10, Splenic hilum nodes; 11, splenic artery nodes; a, splenic artery; b, left gastric artery; c, common hepatic artery.

or residual following surgical exploration and attempted resection.

The Gastrointestinal Tumor Study Group (GITSG) combined chemotherapy and radiation versus chemotherapy alone, and, although the initial toxicity of the combined treatment was higher, the 4-year follow-up favors a survival advantage for the combined-modality arm, particularly in those patients with minimal residual disease after resection.[122] A similar GITSG study indicated an advantage for surgery followed by combined chemotherapy and radiation versus surgery alone.[123] However, this study was difficult to analyze because of small numbers and the fact that a large portion of the patients randomized to the treatment arm refused adjuvant therapy. Therefore, there are no data to support the routine use of combined-modality therapy after gastric resection.

Adjuvant Chemotherapy

Single-agent adjuvant chemotherapy does not provide survival benefit over surgery alone. Trials employing combination chemotherapy have been investigated. The only positive randomized trial to date was reported by the GITSG. This study randomized between a control arm of surgery alone versus 5-fluorouracil (5-FU) and methyl-CCNU (chloroethyl-cyclohexyl-nitrosourea) for 18 months postoperatively. There was a statistically significant benefit for the chemotherapy group (43% vs. 27% for 5-year survival).[124] These results were not confirmed by two subsequent similar trials.

There have been a number of other trials conducted to evaluate the efficacy of combined chemotherapy in the adjuvant setting. These included newer regimens with improved activity for metastatic disease, such as FAM (5-FU, doxorubicin [Adriamycin], mitomycin C). To date, none has given a positive result.[125]

Chemotherapy prior to surgery for gastric cancer (neoadjuvant) is under investigation. Two neoadjuvant regimens, ELP (etoposide, 5-FU, cisplatin) and EAP (etoposide, Adriamycin, cisplatin [Platinol]) have shown efficacy in nonrandomized studies, particularly in tumor size reduction and increased resectability. Some complete responses have been noted.[126, 127] A small clinical trial in Germany indicated that preoperative chemotherapy did increase resectability in patients initially believed to be locally unresectable.[127] Methods of combined treatment that can "downstage" gastric cancer prior to surgery might provide an important benefit to the surgical management of gastric cancer and should be the subject of future clinical trials.

PALLIATIVE PROCEDURES FOR INCURABLE DISEASE

Patients presenting with locally advanced or metastatic gastric cancer are those too infirm to undergo a surgical procedure (inoperable), those who are relatively asymptomatic and can be managed nonoperatively, and those that are symptomatic and operable. Bleeding or obstruction can often be palliated with an Nd:YAG laser with repeated treatments in patients with life expectancy of a few months or less. However, the majority of patients with obstructive symptoms or bleeding can be effectively palliated by resection. Many series support the value of gastric resection in symptomatic patients over gastric bypass for relief of obstructive symptoms and quality of life.[128, 129]

It is difficult to comment on the issue of duration of survival following a resection versus a bypass procedure, since selection bias and lack of randomization hamper any meaningful analysis in this regard. It is stressed that resection in the face of diffuse disease manifested as peritoneal dissemination, massive ascites, multiple or extensive liver metastases (>25% liver volume), or widespread gross nodal involvement has not been shown to be beneficial.[130] Although it was previously believed that postoperative morbidity and mortality were increased in patients undergoing palliative versus curative gastric resections, more recent data suggest that there are no substantial differences in postoperative complications between these two groups of patients.[131]

In an extension of a palliative resection, total gastrectomy may be considered for relief of symptoms in patients with advanced gastric cancer in the proximal stomach or when the tumor occupies a large portion of cardia and gastric fundus. In this situation, microscopically positive margins are acceptable. Butler et al.[131] reported an operative mortality rate of 4% with a 48% postoperative morbidity rate in 27 patients undergoing total gastrectomy for palliation. The median survival in this group was 15 months. In a similar series of palliative surgery, Bozzetti and colleagues[132] reported an operative mortality rate of 14% following total gastrectomy, with a 10% mortality rate following either subtotal resection or gastric bypass. Patient selection criteria are very important determinants for the success of a palliative total gastrectomy. With this in mind, when the bulk of the disease is resectable in a symptomatic patient, a gastric resection (either subtotal or total) should be considered.

POSTOPERATIVE SURVEILLANCE

Normally, follow-up of patients after potentially curative gastric resection should take place every 3 months during the first 18 months to 2 years. Patients are then seen every 6 months until 5 years, after which they undergo yearly follow-up. Several modalities are useful for surveillance for recurrent disease. The tumor markers CEA, CA 19-9, or AFP can be used if they were elevated preoperatively and normalized after tumor resection. These are easy to obtain and would be indicative of recurrence if they began to rise in the postoperative follow-up period.

Imaging modalities such as upper gastrointestinal barium

studies are often of poor quality because of the altered postoperative anatomy, with frequent underfilling of the gastric pouch or inflammation of the anastomotic surgical site. Extraluminal recurrence can be detected by CT scanning; however, peritoneal involvement can easily be missed by this modality. Endoscopy with biopsy is effective in detecting recurrence in the gastric pouch. The appropriate frequency of surveillance endoscopy is controversial, although we recommend yearly screening for the first 5 years.

Once recurrent disease is proven, the majority of patients are not cured following reoperation. Exceptions may be seen in those cases of multicentric early gastric cancer and in patients with recurrence confined to the gastric remnant or anastomosis. In many cases, however, palliative surgery can improve quality of life.

FUTURE DIRECTIONS

Adenocarcinoma of the stomach continues to have an overall poor prognosis. Although earlier detection improves survival, mass screening of asymptomatic patients in the United States is not cost effective with present technology.

To date, the use of chemotherapy or radiation therapy has not improved outcome, and patients with advanced gastric cancer should be routinely considered for standard surgical therapy alone unless they are entered into a clinical trial. Present clinical studies from the NCI and the RTOG are attempting to evaluate the role of cytoreduction with preoperative combination chemotherapy followed by a standardized surgical procedure, which includes a careful R2 node dissection for accurate pathologic staging. The RTOG trial includes intraoperative radiation therapy to consolidate local control. Response rates to this neoadjuvant chemotherapy approach have been initially favorable, with most patients demonstrating at least a partial response, indicated by improvement of symptoms. It is, however, difficult to quantitate response by available imaging and endoscopic techniques, and those patients who do not display disease progression must be explored and carefully staged to evaluate pathologic response criteria. The hematologic toxicity of these regimens, especially in elderly and debilitated patients, is considerable and contributes to dose modification in many patients. These problems can be overcome with better regimens providing enhanced response rates that can be given over a short time period prior to surgery.

In addition, the realization of the importance of local control in decreasing the recurrence of gastric cancer has prompted studies employing a combination of surgery and radiation therapy schemes to improve local control rates. Modulated 5-FU combined with postoperative radiation therapy is currently being evaluated in a phase III intergroup trial. Analysis of this trial will be important in standardizing future treatment with adjuvant therapy. It is possible that increasing insight into the molecular aspects of gastric adenocarcinoma will provide therapeutic regimens that are not now available and will ultimately enhance the surgical management of this difficult disease.

Gastric Lymphoma

Gastric lymphoma accounts for the most frequent type of extranodal non-Hodgkin's lymphoma. It represents approximately 5% of gastric malignancies. The general presentation of a patient with gastric lymphoma is a man (2:1 frequency over women) over 50 years of age with weight loss, upper abdominal pain, early satiety, and, rarely, gastrointestinal bleeding or perforation. Diagnosis is generally made by endoscopic biopsy and brush cytology, with a diagnostic yield of 50% to 90%.[133] The pattern of spread of primary gastric lymphoma is not dissimilar to adenocarcinoma (i.e., local extension into adjacent organs and regional lymph node metastases tend to precede distant metastases).

The origin of gastric lymphoma is unclear, but most are derived from mucosa-associated lymphoid tissue (MALT).[134] There is clear evidence that high-grade lymphomas of gastric origin can arise from a blastic transformation of MALT lymphomas.[135] The majority of gastric lymphomas are classified morphologically as diffuse histiocytic or mixed lymphomas in the Rappaport classification or as diffuse large cell or mixed small and large cell lymphomas in the working formulation. Once the diagnosis of gastric lymphoma is established, staging is accomplished by CT scan, bone marrow biopsy, and chest radiograph. Poor prognostic features include tumor size greater than 10 cm, three or more extranodal disease sites, and the presence of regional or distant nodal involvement.

The staging of gastric lymphoma is based on the Ann Arbor system used for staging Hodgkin's lymphoma (Table 3–10). This system of staging is not adequate to document the prognostic differences between the stage II patient with two limited nodal sites on one side of the diaphragm and the stage II patient presenting with a 10-cm bulky gastric mass. For this reason, an additional staging system proposed by the NCI includes poor prognostic features related to B symptoms and bulk of disease in gastric lymphoma (Table 3–11).

Surgery is considered the main treatment for gastric lymphoma. Resection provides for accurate staging, removes bulk disease, and alleviates symptoms. Surgical therapy consists of gastric resection either by subtotal or by total gastrectomy to remove all gross disease. Lymphadenectomy should be limited to grossly positive regional lymph nodes. Rosen and coworkers[136] noted that splenic involvement in their series of 84 patients was limited to disease by direct extension, with no patient displaying metastatic involvement of the spleen. This suggests that routine splenectomy or liver biopsy is unnecessary in the absence of gross abnormality in these organs. Resectability

TABLE 3–10
Ann Arbor Staging Classification for Hodgkin's Disease

Stage	Characteristics
I	Involvement of a single lymph node region (I) or a single extralymphatic organ or site (IE)
II	Involvement of two or more lymph node regions on the same side of the diaphragm (II) or localized involvement of an extralymphatic organ or site (IIE)
III	Involvement of lymph node regions on both sides of the diaphragm (III) or localized involvement of an extralymphatic organ or site (IIIE) or spleen (IIIS) or both (IIISE)
IV	Diffuse or disseminated involvment of one or more extralymphatic organs with or without associated lymph node involvement.
	The organ(s) involved should be identified by a symbol: A, asymptomatic; B, fever, sweats, weight loss >10% of body weight.

From Longo DL, et al: Lymphocytic lymphomas. In DeVita VT, Hellman S, Rosenberg SA (eds): Cancer, Principles and Practice of Oncology, 4th ed. Philadelphia: JB Lippincott, 1993, pp 1859–1927.

rates in gastric lymphoma vary from 66% to 88%, depending on initial clinical stage of disease and the indications for surgery.[137] Resectability rates are obviously better in those series reporting the majority of operable patients having stage IE or IIE disease. The 5-year survival rate following complete surgical resection of gastric lymphoma varies from 50% to 80%, depending on initial disease stage.[138] It must be noted that the variables in most surgical series, including stage of disease and use of postoperative treatment modalities, are not usually analyzed independently when reporting postoperative survival results. Therefore, although patients treated initially by surgery appear to do comparatively better than those patients treated with nonoperative management, it has not been established whether selection factors such as earlier tumor stage or less extensive tumor in the same stage are as important to patient outcome as the resection itself.

Radiation therapy plays an important role in this disease as well, and although there is evidence that radiation alone may provide the same benefit as surgical resection, most series support radiation as only an adjunct to surgery when positive surgical margins are noted or when there is gross disease left behind at the time of resection.[139, 140] Although combination chemotherapy is routinely applied in advanced-stage (stages III and IV) gastric lymphoma, its use in stage I or II disease is more controversial. Because of the high frequency of relapse following surgical management alone, trials have been designed to evaluate the role of adjunctive chemotherapy following surgery. One such trial did demonstrate that the combination of surgery and chemotherapy was beneficial in operable patients with gastric lymphoma.[141] Also, studies have suggested that for stage IE and IIE gastric lymphoma, CHOP-BLEO (cyclophosphamide, hydroxydaunomycin, vincristine [Oncovin], prednisone, bleomycin) chemotherapy and radiation are efficacious without surgical resection. In one such study, combined chemotherapy and radiation therapy resulted in a 5-year survival rate of 73% and, importantly, 92% of the patients did not require gastric resection.[142]

Because of the lack of prospective trials and the obvious selection bias associated with the results obtained in surgically treated patients, an answer as to the definitive role of surgery in patients with gastric lymphoma is undetermined. It is likely, however, that patients with bulky or symptomatic disease will ultimately respond better to attempted complete surgical resection. Microscopically positive margins or diffuse residual disease should be managed by chemotherapy alone or in combination with radiation therapy to enhance local control. Surgical resection in the patient with locally extensive disease provides superior palliation and prevents treatment-related gastric bleeding or perforation. Total gastrectomy in this setting is unnecessary unless the actual bulk of gross disease throughout the stomach necessitates its use. It is possible that patients with locally aggressive but early-stage nonbulky gastric lymphoma may be adequately managed nonsurgically with combined chemotherapy and radiation therapy with anticipated survivals similar to those in surgical series.

TABLE 3–11
National Cancer Institute Modified Staging for Intermediate- and High-Grade Lymphomas

Stage	Characteristics
I	Localized nodal or extranodal disease (Ann Arbor stage I or IE)
II	Two or more nodal sites of disease or a localized extranodal site plus draining nodes with none of the following: performance status ≤70, B symptoms, any mass >10 cm in diameter (particularly gastrointestinal), serum lactate dehydrogenase >500, three or more extranodal sites of disease
III	Stage II plus any poor prognostic features

From Longo DL, et al: Lymphocytic lymphomas. In DeVita VT, Hellman S, Rosenberg SA (eds): Cancer, Principles & Practice of Oncology, 4th ed. Philadelphia: JB Lippincott, 1993, pp 1859–1927.

Gastric Sarcomas

The stomach is the most common site of smooth muscle tumors of the gastrointestinal tract, accounting for 50%. Most are benign leiomyomas. Leiomyosarcomas of the stomach are generally larger and more necrotic or hemorrhagic. The distinction between the two entities relates to the aggressiveness seen on histologic analysis. Leiomyosarcomas tend to be larger and have mitotic counts exceeding 10 per high-power field. Those with mitotic rates of greater than 50 per high-power field have an increased incidence of liver and lung metastases.

These gastric muscle tumors often form well-circumscribed nodules that may be multilobulated and are in the submucosa or the submucosa and intramuscular layer of the stomach. They are generally surrounded by a pseudocapsule and may ulcerate and bleed. Larger tumors are associated with symptoms of obstruction, pain, or acute hemorrhage. Ulcerative leiomyosarcoma can also be the cause of chronic blood loss and iron deficiency anemia.

The preferred treatment is wedge resection if the lesion is small. Larger tumors are treated by partial gastrectomy with a 2-cm margin. Enucleation is not advocated, even if the lesion is expected to be benign, since there is a high rate of recurrence associated with this method.[143]

References

1. Wingo PA, Tong T, Bolden S: Cancer statistics 1995. CA 45:8–30, 1995.
2. Boddie AW, McBride CM, Balch CM: Gastric cancer. Am J Surg 157:595–606, 1989.
3. Kern KA: Gastric cancer: A neoplastic enigma. J Surg Oncol Suppl 1:34–39, 1989.
4. Wanebo HJ: Gastric cancer: Patient care evaluation survey. Audio-Digest Surg 36:1–4, 1989.
5. Cady B, Rossi R, Silverman ML, et al: Gastric adenocarcinoma: A disease in transition. Arch Surg 124:303–308, 1989.
6. McGuire WL, Sugarbaker PH (eds): Cancer Treatment and Research: Management of Gastric Cancer. Boston: Kluwer Academic Publishers, 1991.
7. Diehl JT, Hermann RE, Cooperman AM, et al: Gastric carcinoma: A ten year review. Ann Surg 198:9–12, 1983.
8. Shiu MH, Moore E, Sanders M, et al: Influence of the extent of resection on survival after curative treatment of gastric carcinoma. Arch Surg 122:1347–1351, 1987.
9. Breaux JR, Bringaze W, Chappuis C, et al: Adenocarcinoma of the stomach: A review of 35 years and 1710 cases. World J Surg 14:580–586, 1990.
10. Noguchi Y, Imada T, Matsumoto A, et al: Radical surgery for gastric cancer: A review of the Japanese experience. Cancer 64:2053–2062, 1989.
11. Correa P: Clinical implications of recent developments in gastric cancer pathology and epidemiology. Semin Oncol 1:2–10, 1985.
12. Meyers W, Damiano RJ, Postlethwait RW, et al: Adenocarcinoma of the stomach: Changing patterns over the last four decades. Ann Surg 205:1–8, 1987.
13. Gall FP, Hermanek P: New aspects in the surgical treatment of gastric carcinoma—a comparative study of 1636 patients operated on between 1969 and 1982. Eur J Surg Oncol 11:219–225, 1985.
14. American Cancer Society: Cancer Facts and Figures. Selected Cancer Sites. New York: ACS, 1992, pp 3–5.
15. Aird I, Bentall HH, Roberts JAF: A relationship between cancer of the stomach and the ABO blood groups. Br Med J 1:799–801, 1953.
16. Nomura A, Glober G, Terasaki P, Stemmermann GG: HLA antigens in stomach cancer. Int J Cancer 25:195–196, 1980.
17. Gregorio DI, Flannery JT, Hansen H: Stomach cancer patterns in European immigrants to Connecticut, United States. Cancer Causes Control 3:215–221, 1992.
18. Saito T, Sasaki O, Matsukuchi T, Iwamatsu M, Inokucki K: Experimental gastric cancer: Pathogenesis and clinicohistopathologic correlation. In Herfath C, Schlag P (eds): Gastric Cancer. New York: Springer-Verlag, 1979, p 22.
19. Correa P, Haenszel W, Cuello C, et al: Gastric precancerous process in a high-risk population: Cohort follow-up. Cancer Res 50:4737–4740, 1990.
20. Correa P, Haenszel W, Cuello C, et al: Gastric precancerous process in a high-risk population: Cross-sectional studies. Cancer Res 50:4731–4736, 1990.
21. Blaser MJ: *Helicobacter pylori* and the pathogenesis of gastroduodenal inflammation. J Infect Dis 161:626–633, 1990.
22. Villako K, Siurala M: The behavior of gastritis and related conditions in different population samples. Ann Clin Res 13:114–118, 1981.
23. Talley NJ, Zinsmeister AR, Weaver A, et al: Gastric adenocarcinoma and *Helicobacter pylori* infection. J Natl Cancer Inst 83:1734–1738, 1991.
24. Parsonnet J, Friedman GD, Vandersteen DP, et al: *Helicobacter pylori* infection and the risk of gastric carcinoma. N Engl J Med 325:1127–1136, 1991.
25. Karnes WE Jr, Samloff IM, Siurala M, et al: Positive serum antibody and negative tissue staining for *Helicobacter pylori* in subjects with atrophic body gastritis. Gastroenterology 101:167–174, 1991.
26. Young GP, Demediuk BH: The genetics, epidemiology and early detection of gastrointestinal cancers. Curr Opin Oncol 4:728–735, 1992.
27. Parsonnet J: The epidemiology of *C. pylori.* In: Blaser MJ (ed): *Campylobacter pylori* in Gastritis and Peptic Ulcer Disease. New York: Igaku-Shoin, 1989, pp 51–60.
28. Morris A, Ali MR, Brown P, et al: *Campylobacter pylori* infection in biopsy specimens of gastric antrum: Laboratory diagnosis and estimation of sampling error. J Clin Pathol 42:727–732, 1989.
29. George LL, Borody TJ, Andrews P, et al: Cure of duodenal ulcer after eradication of *Helicobacter pylori.* Med J Aust 153:145–149, 1990.
30. Lee S, Iida M, Yao T, et al: Risk of gastric cancer in patients with non-surgically treated peptic ulcer. Scand J Gastroenterol 25:1223–1226, 1990.
31. LaVecchia C, Negri E, D'Avanzo B, et al: Partial gastrectomy and subsequent gastric cancer risk. J Epidemiol Community Health 46:12–14, 1992.
32. Lacaine F, Houry S, Huguier M: Stomach cancer after partial gastrectomy for benign ulcer disease. A critical analysis of epidemiological reports. Hepatogastroenterology 39:4–8, 1992.
33. Brinton LA, Gridley G, Hrubec Z, et al: Cancer risk following pernicious anemia. Br J Cancer 59:810–813, 1989.
34. Kneller RW, McLaughlin JK, Bjelke E, et al: A cohort study of stomach cancer in American population. Cancer 68:672–678, 1991.
35. Boeing H: Epidemiological research in stomach cancer: Progress over the last ten years. J Cancer Res Clin Oncol 117:133–143, 1991.
36. Hiroshima Y, Sasabat T: A case control study of single and multiple stomach cancers in Saitama Prefecture, Japan. Jpn J Cancer Res 83:937–943, 1992.
37. Pocock SJ: Nitrates and gastric cancer. Human Toxicol 4:471–474, 1985.
38. Chen VW, Abu-Ely Azeed RR, Zavala DE, et al: Risk factors of gastric precancerous lesions in a high risk Columbian population. Nutr Cancer 13:67–72, 1990.
39. Ruddell WSJ, Bone ES, Hill MJ, Walters CL: Pathogenesis of gastric cancer in pernicious anemia. Lancet 1:521–523, 1978.
40. Schlag P, Ulrich H, Merkle P, et al: Are nitrate and *N*-nitroso compounds in gastric juice risk factors for carcinoma in the operated stomach? Lancet 1:727–729, 1980.
41. Selikoff I: Cancer risk of asbestos exposure. In Hiatt HH, Watson JD, Winsten JA (eds): Origins of Human Cancer, Book C. New York: Cold Spring Harbor Laboratory, 1977, pp 1765–1784.
42. de Klerk NH, Armstrong BK, Musk AW, Hobbs MS: Cancer mortality in relation to measures of occupational exposure to crocidolite at Witlenoom Gorge in Western Australia. Br J Ind Med 46:529–536, 1989.
43. Wangensteen O, Lewis F, Archilger S, et al: An interim report upon the "second look" procedure for cancer of the stomach, colon, and rectum and for limited intraperitoneal carcinomatosis. Surg Gynecol Obstet 99:257–267, 1954.
44. Gunderson L, Sosin H: Areas of failure in a re-operation series (second or symptomatic look). Clinicopathologic correlation and implications for adjuvant therapy. Int J Radiat Oncol Biol Phys 8:1–11, 1982.
45. McNeer G, Vandenberg H, Donn F: A critical evaluation of subtotal gastrectomy for the cure of cancer of the stomach. Ann Surg 134:2–7, 1951.
46. Thomson F, Robbins R: Local recurrence following subtotal resection for gastric carcinoma. Surg Gynecol Obstet 95:341–344, 1952.
47. Kern K: Natural history of surgically treated gastric cancer. In Sugarbaker P (ed): Management of Gastric Cancer. Boston: Kluwer Academic Publishers, 1991, pp 1–16.
48. British Stomach Cancer Group: Resection line disease in stomach cancer. Br Med J 289:601–603, 1985.
49. Lauren P: The two histological main types of gastric carcinoma: Diffuse and so-called intestinal type carcinoma. Acta Pathol Microbiol Scand 64:31–49, 1965.

50. Munoz N, Correa P, Cuello C, et al: Histologic types of gastric carcinoma in high- and low-risk areas. Int J Cancer 3:809–818, 1968.
51. Sipponen P, Jarvi O, Kekki M, Siurala M: Decreased incidences of intestinal and diffuse types of gastric carcinoma in Finland during a 20 year period. Scand J Gastroenterol 22:865–871, 1987.
52. Hagustvedt T, Viste A, Eide G, et al: Is Lauren's histopathological classification of importance in patients with stomach cancer? A national experience. Eur J Surg Oncol 18:124–130, 1992.
53. Bormann R: Geschwuelste des Magens and Duodenums. In Henke F, Lunarsch D (eds): Handbuch der Spezieller Pathologischen Anatomie und Histologie, vol 4. Berlin: Julius Springer, 1926.
54. Marakami T: Pathomorphological diagnosis: Definition and gross classification of early gastric cancer. In Gann Monograph on Cancer Research. Tokyo: Tokyo University Press, 1971, pp 53–55.
55. Green PHR, O'Toole KM, Slonim D, et al: Increasing incidence and excellent survival of patients with early gastric cancer: Experience in an United States Medical Center. Am J Med 85:658–661, 1988.
56. Kodama V, Inokuchi K, Soejima K, et al: Growth patterns and prognosis in early gastric carcinoma. Cancer 51:320–326, 1981.
57. Brandt D, Muramatsu Y, Ushio K, et al: Synchronous early gastric cancer. Radiology 173:649–652, 1989.
58. Nanus DM, Kelsen DP, Niedzwiecki D, et al: Flow cytometry as a predictive indicator in patients with operable gastric cancer. J Clin Oncol 7:1105–1112, 1989.
59. Tamura G, Kihana T, Namura K, et al: Detection of frequent P53 gene mutations in primary gastric cancer by call sorting and polymerase chain reaction single strand conformation polymorphism analysis. Cancer Res 51:3056–3058, 1991.
60. Yonemura Y, Ninomiya I, Yamaguchi A, et al: Evaluation of immunoreactivity for *erb*-B2 protein as a marker for poor short term prognosis in gastric cancer. Cancer Res 51:1034–1038, 1991.
61. Weinstock J, Baldwin GS: Binding of gastrin 17 to human gastric carcinoma cell lines. Cancer Res 48:932–937, 1988.
62. Yasui W, Sumiyoshi H, Hata J: Expression of epidermal growth factor receptor in human gastric and colonic carcinoma. Cancer Res 48:137–141, 1988.
63. Oleorchyk AS: Gastric carcinoma: A critical review of 243 cases. Am J Gastroenterol 70:25–45, 1978.
64. Cassell P, Robinson JO: Cancer of the stomach: A review of 854 patients. Br J Surg 63:603–607, 1976.
65. Fung WB, Barr A: Fulminant disseminated intravascular coagulation in advanced gastric carcinoma. Am J Gastroenterol 171:210–212, 1979.
66. Cooley RN: The diagnostic accuracy of upper gastrointestinal radiologic studies. Am J Med Sci 242:628–650, 1961.
67. Mitty WF, Rousselot LM, Grace WJ: Carcinoma of the stomach. Am J Dig Dis 5:249–258, 1960.
68. Laufer I: A simple method for routine double contrast study of the upper gastrointestinal tract. Radiology 117:513–518, 1975.
69. Veterans Administration Cooperative Study of Gastric Ulcer. Gastroenterology 61:567–654, 1971.
70. Winawer SJ, Sherlock P, Hajdu SI: The role of upper gastrointestinal endoscopy in patients with cancer. Cancer 37:440–448, 1976.
71. Graham DY, Schwartz JT, Cain D, Gyorkey F: Prospective evaluation of biopsy number in the diagnosis of esophageal and gastric carcinoma. Gastroenterology 82:228–231, 1982.
72. Cook AO, Levine BA, Sirinek KR: Evaluation of gastric adenocarcinoma: Abdominal computed tomography does not replace celiotomy. Arch Surg 121:603–606, 1986.
73. Sussman SK, Halvorsen RA, Illescas FF, et al: Gastric adenocarcinoma: CT versus surgical staging. Radiology 167:335–340, 1988.
74. Botet JF, Lightdale CJ, Zauber AG, et al: Preoperative staging of gastric cancer: Comparison of endoscopic US and dynamic CT. Radiology 181:426–432, 1991.
75. Everson TC: Carcinoma of the stomach. In Everson TC, Cole WH (eds): Cancer of the Digestive Tract, Clinical Management. New York: Appleton-Century-Crofts, 1969, pp 11–73.
76. Heymer B, Quentmeier A: Biological markers for staging of gastric cancer. In Herfarth C Schlag P (eds): Gastric Cancer. New York: Springer Verlag, 1979, pp 157–162.
77. Nomura AMY, Stemmermann GN, Samloff IM: Serum pepsinogen I as a predictor of stomach cancer. Ann Intern Med 93:537–540, 1980.
78. Hakkinen I, Viikari S: Occurrence of fetal sulphoglycoprotein antigen in the gastric juice of patients with gastric diseases. Ann Surg 165:277–284, 1969.
79. Kennedy BJ: The unified international gastric cancer staging classification system. Scand J Gastroenterol 22(Suppl 133):11–13, 1987.
80. Japanese Research Society for Gastric Cancer: The general rules for the gastric cancer study in surgery and pathology. I. Clinical classification. Jpn J Surg 11:127, 1981.
81. Imada T, Noguchi Y, Abe M, et al: Lymph node metastasis in gastric cancer. Eur Surg Res 19(Suppl 1):90, 1987 (abstract).
82. Mishima Y, Hirayama R: The role of lymph node surgery in gastric cancer. World J Surg 11:406–411, 1987.
83. Fujimoto S, Kasanuki J, Yoshida S, Okui K: New trends in therapy for gastric malignancy. In Sugarbaker P (ed): Management of Gastric Cancer. Boston: Kluwer Academic Publishers, 1991, pp 307–324.
84. Kaibara N, Itsuka Y, Kimura A, et al: Relationship between area of serosal invasion and prognosis in patients with gastric carcinoma. Cancer 60:136–139, 1987.
85. Itsuka Y, Kaneshima S, Tanida O, et al: Intraperitoneal free cancer cells and their viability in gastric cancer. Cancer 44:1476–1480, 1979.
86. Jessup J, Posner M, Huberman M, et al: Efficacy of multimodality therapy in gastric adenocarcinoma. Semin Surg Oncol 9:19–26, 1993.
87. Lawrence M, Shiu M: Early gastric cancer: Twenty-eight year experience. Ann Surg 213:327–334, 1991.
88. Rohde H, Bauer P, Stutzer H, et al: Proximal compared with distal adenocarcinoma of the stomach: Differences and consequences. German Gastric Cancer TNM Study Group. Br J Surg 78:1242–1248, 1991.
89. Brennan M: Editorial: Radical surgery for gastric cancer—a review of the Japanese experience. Cancer 64:2063, 1989.
90. Bringaze W, Chappuis C, Cohn I, et al: Early gastric cancer: 21 year experience. Ann Surg 204:103–107, 1986.
91. Longo W, Zucker K, Edon M, et al: Detection of early gastric cancer in an aggressive endoscopy unit. Am Surg 55:100–104, 1989.
92. Friesen G, Dockerty M, Remine W: Superficial carcinoma of the stomach. Surgery 51:300–312, 1962.
93. Farley D, Donohue J: Early gastric cancer. Surg Clin North Am 72:401–421, 1992.
94. Haruma K, Sumii K, Inoue K, et al: Endoscopic therapy in patients with inoperable early gastric cancer. Am J Gastroenterol 85:522–526, 1990.
95. McNeer G, Bowden L, Booker R: Elective total gastrectomy for cancer of the stomach. Ann Surg 192:30–37, 1974.
96. Shiu M, Moore E, Saunders M, et al: Influence of the extent of resection on survival after curative treatment of gastric carcinoma. A retrospective multivariate analysis. Arch Surg 122:1347–1351, 1987.
97. Bozzetti F: Total versus subtotal gastrectomy in cancer of the distal stomach: Facts and fantasy. Eur J Surg Oncol 18:572–579, 1992.
98. Salo J, Saario I, Kivilaakso E, et al: Near total gastrectomy for gastric cancer. Am J Surg 155:486–489, 1988.
99. Papachristou D, Fortner J: Choice of operative procedure for adenocarcinoma of the gastric antrum: A study based on TNM classification. J Surg Oncol 21:241–244, 1982.
100. Bozzetti F, Ravera E, Dossena G, et al: Comparing the nutritional status after total or subtotal gastrectomy. Nutrition 6:371–375, 1990.
101. Gouzi J, Huguier M, Fagniez P, et al: Total versus subtotal gastrectomy for adenocarcinoma of the gastric antrum: A French prospective controlled study. Ann Surg 209:162–166, 1989.
102. Papachristou D, Fortner J: Adenocarcinoma of the gastric cardia: The choice of gastrectomy. Ann Surg 192:58–64, 1979.
103. Shiu M, Papachristou D, Kosloff C, et al: Selection of operative procedure for adenocarcinoma of the midstomach. Twenty years experience with implications for future treatment strategy. Ann Surg 192:730–737, 1980.
104. Shiu M, Perrotti M, Brennan M: Adenocarcinoma of the stomach. A multivariate analysis of clinical pathologic and treatment factors. Hepatogastroenterology 36:7–12, 1989.
105. Sunderland D, McNeer G, Ortega L, et al: The lymphatic spread of gastric cancer. Cancer 6:987–996, 1953.
106. McNeer G, Sunderland D, McInnes G, et al: A more thorough operation for gastric cancer: Anatomic bias and description of technique. Cancer 4:957–967, 1951.
107. Gilbertsen V: Results of treatment of stomach cancer: An appraisal of efforts for more extensive surgery and a report of 1983 cases. Cancer 23:1305–1308, 1969.

108. Soga J, Ohyama S, Mujashita K, et al: A statistical evaluation of advancement in gastric cancer surgery with special reference to the significance of lymphadenectomy for cure. World J Surg 12:398–405, 1988.
109. Dent D, Madden M, Price S: Randomized comparison of R1 and R2 gastrectomy for gastric carcinoma. Br J Surg 75:110–112, 1988.
110. Bonenkamp J, Van de Vedde C, Sasako M, et al: R2 compared with R1 resection for gastric cancer: Morbidity and mortality in a prospective randomized trial. Eur J Surg 158:413–418, 1992.
111. Smith J, Shiu M, Kelsey L, et al: Morbidity of radical lymphadenectomy in the curative resection of gastric carcinoma. Arch Surg 126:1469–1473, 1991.
112. Kaibara N, Sumi K, Yonekawa M, et al: Does extensive dissection of lymph nodes improve the results of surgical treatment of gastric cancer? Am J Surg 159:218–221, 1990.
113. Korenaga D, Tsujitani S, Haraguchi M, et al: Longterm survival in Japanese patients with far advanced carcinoma of the stomach. World J Surg 12:236–240, 1988.
114. Maruyama K, Kokabayashi K, Kinoshita T: Progress in gastric cancer surgery in Japan and its limits of radicality. World J Surg 11:418–425, 1987.
115. Ohashi I, Takagi K, Ohta H, et al: Pancreaticosplenectomy for advanced gastric carcinoma: With special reference to lymph node metastases. Jpn J Gastroenterol Surg 12:993–999, 1979.
116. Makino M, Moriwaki S, Yoneskawa M, et al: Prognostic significance of the number of metastatic lymph nodes in patients with gastric cancer. J Surg Oncol 47:12–16, 1991.
117. Allum WH, Hallissey MT, Ward LC, Hockey MS: A controlled, prospective, randomised trial of adjuvant chemotherapy or radiotherapy in resectable gastric cancer: Interim report. Br J Cancer 60:739–744, 1989.
118. Abe M, Takahashi M: Japanese gastric trials in intraoperative radiation therapy. Int J Radiat Oncol Biol Phys 15:1431–1433, 1988.
119. Calvo FA, Santos M, Alberro JA, et al: Intraoperative and external radiotherapy in resectable gastric cancer: Updated report of a phase II trial. Int J Radiat Oncol Biol Phys 24:729–736, 1992.
120. Radiation Therapy Oncology Group: Progress Report, 1/89–4/91, vol 1. July 1991.
121. Sindelar WF, Kinsella TJ, Tepper JE, et al: Randomized trial of intraoperative radiotherapy in carcinoma of the stomach. Am J Surg 165:178–187, 1993.
122. Tepper JE: Combined radiotherapy and chemotherapy in the treatment of gastrointestinal malignancies. Semin Oncol 19:96–101, 1992.
123. Moertel C, Childs D, O'Fallon J: Combined 5-FU and radiation therapy as a surgical adjuvant for poor prognosis gastric carcinoma. J Clin Oncol 2:1249–1254, 1984.
124. The Gastrointestinal Tumor Study Group: Controlled trial of adjuvant chemotherapy following curative resection for gastric cancer. Cancer 49:1116–1122, 1982.
125. Macdonald JS, Gagliano R, Fleming T, et al: A phase III trial of FAM (5-fluorouracil, Adriamycin, mitomycin-C) chemotherapy vs control as adjuvant treatment for resected gastric cancer: A Southwest Oncology Group Trial—SWOG 7804. Proc Am Soc Clin Oncol 11:168, 1992 (abstract).
126. Ajani JA, Ota DM, Jackson DE: Current strategies in the management of locoregional and metastatic gastric carcinoma. Cancer 67:260–265, 1991.
127. Wilke H, Preusser P, Fink U, et al: Preoperative chemotherapy in locally advanced and non-resectable gastric cancer. A phase II study with etoposide/Adriamycin plus cisplatin. J Clin Oncol 7:1318–1326, 1989.
128. Hallissey M, Allum W, Roginski C, et al: Palliative surgery for gastric cancer. Cancer 62:440–444, 1988.
129. Haugstvedt T, Viste A, Eide G, et al: The survival benefit of resection in patients with advanced stomach cancer: The Norwegian multicenter experience. World J Surg 13:617–622, 1989.
130. Viste A, Haugstvedt T, Eide G, et al: Postoperative complications and mortality after surgery for gastric cancer. Ann Surg 207:7–13, 1988.
131. Butler J, Dubrow T, Trezama T, et al: Total gastrectomy in the treatment of advanced gastric cancer. Am J Surg 158:602–605, 1989.
132. Bozzetti F, Bonfanti G, Audisio R: Prognosis of patients after palliative surgical procedures for carcinoma of the stomach. Surg Gynecol Obstet 164:151–154, 1987.
133. Spinelli P, Gullo C, Pizzetti P: Endoscopic diagnosis of gastric lymphomas. Endoscopy 12:211–214, 1980.
134. Isaacson PG, Spencer J: Malignant lymphoma of mucosa-associated lymphoid tissue. Histopathology 11:445–462, 1987.
135. Chan JKC, Ng CS, Isaacson PG: Relationship between high-grade lymphoma and low-grade B-cell mucosa-associated lymphoid tissue lymphoma (MALToma) of the stomach. Am J Pathol 136:1153–1164, 1990.
136. Rosen C, VanHeerden J, Martin J, et al: Is our aggressive approach to the patient with gastric lymphoma warranted? Ann Surg 205:634–640, 1987.
137. Frazee R, Roberts J: Gastric lymphoma treatment. Medical versus surgical. Surg Clin North Am 72:423–431, 1992.
138. Donohue J, Habermann T: The management of gastric lymphoma. Surg Oncol Clin North Am 2:213–232, 1993.
139. Hermann R, Panahon A, Barros M: Gastrointestinal involvement in non-Hodgkin's lymphoma. Cancer 46:215–222, 1980.
140. Shimm D, Dosoretz D, Anderson T, et al: Primary gastric lymphoma: An analysis with emphasis on prognostic factors and radiation therapy. Cancer 52:2044–2048, 1983.
141. Sheridan W, Medley G, Brodie G: Non-Hodgkin's lymphoma of the stomach: A prospective pilot study of surgery plus chemotherapy in early and advanced disease. J Clin Oncol 3:495–500, 1985.
142. Maor M, Velasquez W, Fuller L, et al: Stomach conservation in Stages IE and IIE gastric non-Hodgkin's lymphoma. J Clin Oncol 8:266–271, 1990.
143. Cushieri A: Tumors of the stomach. In Moosa AR, Schimpff C, Robson M (eds): Comprehensive Textbook of Oncology. Baltimore: Williams & Wilkins, 1991, p 877.

Cancer of the Small Bowel

Lee B. Riley, M.D., Ph.D.
Burton L. Eisenberg, M.D.

Both benign and malignant tumors intrinsic to the small intestine are quite rare. Together they account for less than 6% of all the tumors found in the gastrointestinal tract. Malignant tumors of the small intestine, constituting approximately two thirds of all small bowel tumors, represent only 1% to 3% of all gastrointestinal cancers.[1–5] It is anticipated that, in 1995, 4600 new malignant small bowel tumors would be diagnosed in the United States.[5a] Adenocarcinomas, malignant carcinoids, lymphomas, and sarcomas are the most common small intestinal cancers, with adenocarcinomas accounting for nearly 50% of these.

The rarity of primary small intestinal cancers has prevented a detailed understanding of both the clinical aspects and the etiologic mechanisms of cancer found within the small bowel. Malignant lesions of the duodenum are detailed elsewhere in this text. Therefore, this chapter summarily focuses on malignant lesions of the jejunum and ileum.

LOCAL-REGIONAL ANATOMY AND PATHOLOGY

Anatomy

The small intestine is divided into three segments: the duodenum, the jejunum, and the ileum. The duodenum, the section with the largest diameter, begins at the pylorus and ends at the ligament of Treitz. For descriptive purposes, it is divided into superior, descending, horizontal, and ascending regions.

The jejunum and ileum make up the remainder of the small intestine and together average 22 feet in length. Several features distinguish the jejunum from the ileum. The plicae circulares are large in the proximal bowel, resulting in a thicker wall. Distally, the small bowel diameter diminishes, the mesentery contains less fat, and the number of lymphatics and lymph nodes increase. The blood supply to the small bowel originates from the superior mesenteric artery, which branches to give the inferior pancreaticoduodenal, jejunal, and ileal arteries. The jejunal and ileal arteries, 10 to 16 in number, enter the mesentery and unite distally, forming the arterial arcades. The arterial arcades increase in number in the ileum because of shorter vasa recta (Fig. 3–9).[6] The venous drainage of the small intestine originates from tributaries that correspond to the arterial arcades and unite to form the superior mesenteric vein. The superior mesenteric vein joins the splenic vein to form the portal vein.

PATHOLOGY

Embryologically, the small bowel is derived from the distal foregut and the midgut and comprises all three germ layers. The mucosal elements arise from the endoderm, and the muscular, vascular, lymphatic, and connective tissues arise from the mesoderm. The ectoderm is responsible for the neural elements and the enterochromaffin cells, from which carcinoid tumors are thought to arise.[7]

Because the small intestine is composed of all three germ layers, virtually every histologic type of neoplasm has been reported. Benign tumors make up about 30% to 40% of all small bowel tumors, with adenomatous polyps, leiomyomas, and lipomas constituting the majority of these.[5] Malignant lesions make up the remaining 60% to 70% and tend to be found distally, with their location dependent on their histology (Table 3–12).

TABLE 3–12
Location of Small Bowel Malignancies

Location	Adenocarcinoma	Carcinoid	Lymphoma	Totals
Duodenum				
Coit, 1992[20*]	559 (45%)	55 (7%)	26 (6%)	640 (26%)
Reiner, 1976[20a]	418 (40%)	54 (7%)	43 (10%)	515 (23%)
Total	977 (42%)	109 (7%)	69 (8%)	1155 (24%)
Jejunum				
Coit	413 (33%)	73 (9%)	147 (36%)	633 (25%)
Reiner	399 (38%)	75 (10%)	160 (36%)	634 (28%)
Total	812 (35%)	148 (9%)	307 (36%)	1267 (27%)
Ileum				
Coit	276 (22%)	709 (85%)	235 (58%)	1220 (49%)
Reiner	234 (22%)	622 (83%)	236 (54%)	1092 (49%)
Total	510 (22%)	1331 (84%)	471 (56%)	2312 (49%)
Total				
Coit	1248 (50%)	837 (34%)	408 (16%)	2493
Reiner	1051 (47%)	751 (34%)	439 (20%)	2241
Total	2299 (49%)	1588 (34%)	847 (18%)	4734

*This series additionally reported sarcomas; however, for comparison to Reiner's data, they have been deleted.

Histology

Adenocarcinomas of the proximal small intestine generally present with a papillary configuration. In contrast, more distal adenocarcinomas present with napkin-ring deformities. About 20% of small bowel adenocarcinomas have either polypoid or fungating appearances. Microscopically, the majority of adenocarcinomas of the small intestine are moderately well differentiated tumors with mucin and carcinoembryonic antigen reactivity.[8] Endocrine cells, identified by their reactivity with a number of peptide hormones, are frequently seen in small bowel adenocarcinomas.[9] Small cell carcinomas, adenosquamous carcinomas, adenosquamous carcinomas, and anaplastic carcinomas of the small bowel have also been described.

Carcinoid tumors arise from the argentaffin cells described by Kulchitsky in the base of the crypts of Lieberkühn. Microscopically, they are composed of solid masses of cells with small nuclei and fine nucleoli. The cytoplasm contains pleomorphic secretory granules. Immunohistochemically, they react with both epithelial and neuroendocrine markers (i.e., keratin and neuron-specific enolase, respectively). Other histologic variants of carcinoid tumors include trabecular, glandular, undifferentiated, and mixed.[10]

Two major forms of primary small intestinal lymphoma (PSIL) occur. Western lymphoma is microscopically characterized by highly pleomorphic large cells with immunoblastic features. The majority of these tumors are derived from the B-cell lineage.[11] The second form of PSIL is immunoproliferative small intestinal disease (IPSID), and the majority are large B-cell lymphomas. These tumors are frequently associated with abnormal heavy chains from immunoglobulin A (IgA) (see later). Occasionally, these tumors are associated with an intense eosinophilic infiltrate, which complicates the diagnosis.[12]

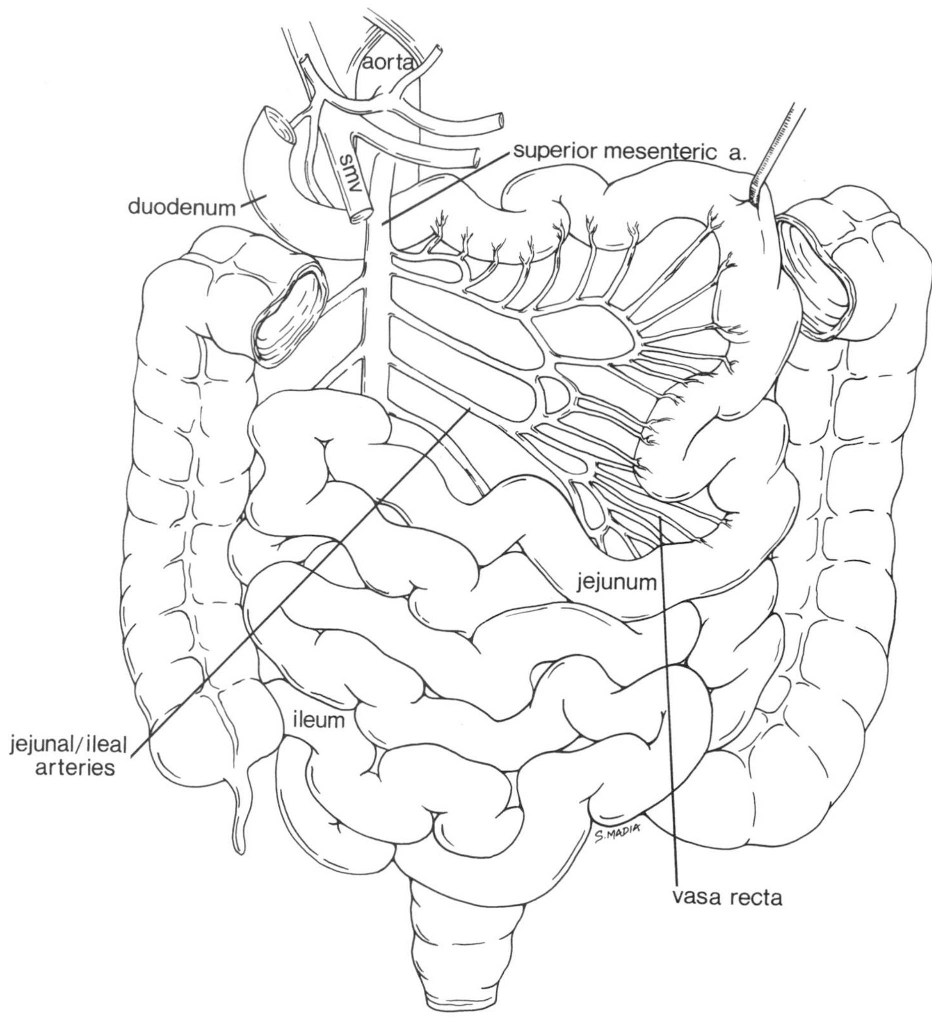

FIGURE 3–9. Anatomy of the small intestine.

Leiomyosarcomas represent the most common sarcoma of the small intestine. These cancers are spindle shaped and react with vimentin and actin (desmin is rarely present). Distinguishing between benign and malignant lesions is very difficult, and therapeutic decisions should not be based on frozen section diagnoses.

EPIDEMIOLOGY

Incidence

When all histologies are combined, there is a slight preponderance of small bowel cancers in males, but there is no consistent trend in racial or socioeconomic subgroups.[6, 13] The majority of cancers arise in the fourth, fifth, and sixth decades of life.[1] Table 3–12 compares two large studies separated by two decades and indicates that adenocarcinomas occur more commonly in the proximal small bowel, whereas carcinoids and lymphomas generally occur in the distal small bowel.[20, 20a] However, sarcomas are evenly distributed throughout the small bowel. The relative location of these tumors does not appear to have undergone substantial change in the 20 years between these two collected series. Adenocarcinomas of the small bowel are more common in western countries, and their regional prevalence rates within geographic areas correlate with those of carcinoma of the colon but not of the stomach.[20, 20a] Further, a recent analysis of the Japan-Hawaii Cancer Study suggests that after migration small bowel neoplasms develop in Japanese men at a rate similar to the increased incidence rate seen in colon cancer.[13, 15]

Primary small intestinal lymphoma represents 17% of all small bowel malignancy and is the second-most frequent site of extranodal lymphoma (preceded only by gastric lymphoma). Two broad categories of small bowel lymphoma exist. Western lymphoma, which is the most common variety, occurs predominantly in men during their sixth decade.[16] Mediterranean lymphoma, which is the most common lymphoma seen in Middle Eastern countries, occurs with equal sex distribution and generally presents before the age of 30. There appears to be an association between intestinal lymphoma and ethnic origin from the Middle East. There is also a strong association in patients with an antecedent history of chronic celiac disease and chronic immunodeficiency diseases.[17, 18] In the pediatric population, lymphomas are reported to be the most common malignant tumor of the small bowel.

Carcinoid tumors are the second-most common malignant tumor of the small bowel. Eighty-five percent of small bowel carcinoids are located within the ileum. Carcinoid tumors of the small intestine are most commonly reported during the sixth and seventh decades of life, in contrast to carcinoids of the appendix (the most common primary gastrointestinal anatomic site), for which the peak incidence is approximately two decades earlier. Carcinoid tumors are equally distributed among the sexes and are occasionally reported to be familial.[19]

Sarcomas account for 11% of small bowel cancers and have been reported in all ages. Most tumors present after age 50, and they affect men and women equally.[20]

Etiologic Factors

The small intestine makes up approximately 75% of the length of the gastrointestinal tract and therefore more than 90% of the surface area. Additionally, the crypt cells within the small intestinal mucosa replicate rapidly and can replace the entire mucosal surface of the small bowel in less than 7 days. Despite these notable facts, the small intestine is the site of less than 2% of all gastrointestinal malignancies. Although there has been considerable interest in this phenomenon, little is known about the etiology of small bowel malignancies. Several hypotheses have been advanced, but none is known to be consistent with all the data.

The influence of local-regional parameters, which include the liquidity and rapid transit of the small bowel contents, the low bacterial population in the small intestine, and the alkaline pH, may all be potentially protective against tumorigenesis.[13, 14] Celik et al.[21] using an animal model for human colon cancer, cast serious doubt on suppressive influences of these local-regional effects. Surgical transposition of the left colon to the proximal jejunum, followed by treatment with dimethylhydrazine (a chemical carcinogen that induces colon and small bowel tumors in a distribution similar to that observed in humans), still induced adenocarcinomas in the transposed colon but did not induce tumors in the segments of jejunum similarly transposed to the left colon.[21] These experiments suggest that factors inherent in the small intestine mucosa or mucosal cells but not found in the colon (i.e., different detoxifying enzyme systems) may contribute to the phenomenon.[23]

Patient populations that are chronically immunosuppressed have an increased incidence of small bowel neoplasms; consequently, immunologic mechanisms have been invoked to explain the lack of adenocarcinomas in the distal small intestine. Support for this comes from the increased number of T cells as well as IgA producing B-cell lymphocyte populations in the distal small bowel, which may perhaps be in sufficient numbers to reject early tumors or neutralize oncogenic viruses.[14] In animal models, transplanted allogeneic tumors survive better in the stomach, which lacks a substantial lymphocyte pool relative to the small intestine.[13, 14, 22, 23] These arguments do not, however, account for the equal distribution of sarcomas in the gastrointestinal tract, nor the focality of carcinoids located within the ileum.

Lipkin and Quastler[23a] proposed that carcinomas cannot establish a dominant cell mass because the relatively few but rapidly proliferating progenitor cells found in the small bowel mucosa extrude these developing cell populations into the lumen. It is also possible that malignant cells, which actually have a slower proliferation rate, would not be competitive with the rapidly dividing adjacent normal mucosa. This hypothesis, however, is not consistent with the high frequency of adenomas (0.3%) that have been identified in autopsy series.[24]

Genetic Factors

Because of the rarity of small bowel neoplasms, the genetics of these tumors is poorly understood. Because there are numerous reports of small bowel carcinomas arising from adenomas, it would be logical to implicate a similar mechanism as reported in the Vogelstein colon carcinoma model.[25] The fact that small bowel cancers are associated with histologically different metachronous tumors suggests that individuals who present with small bowel tumors may have a diffuse genetic susceptibility to all these neoplasias. As far as a familial incidence is concerned, Lynch et al.[31] reported nine cases of small bowel neoplasms in kindreds with the Lynch II syndrome, and there are other isolated reports within the literature. While the APC (familial adenomatous polyposis coli), DCC (deleted in colorectal cancer), MCC (mutated in colorectal cancer), and p53 genes play a substantial role in the etiology of colon carcinomas, their involvement in the genesis of small bowel cancers has not been established.

Other Risk Factors

The majority of patients with small bowel neoplasms have no known risk factors; nevertheless, several conditions place patients at greater risk, including other neoplasms, inherited polyposis syndromes, chronic small intestinal inflammatory disease from any etiology, and immunosupression.[25–27]

Twenty-five percent of patients with small bowel tumors are noted to have additional gastrointestinal as well as other unrelated cancer sites.[20] The prevalence of colon cancer in various countries is linearly related to that of small bowel cancer. In contrast, no relationship exists between the incidence of small intestinal cancers and that of gastric or esophageal cancer.[14] The inheritable polyposis syndromes, including familial polyposis, Peutz-Jeghers syndrome, and Gardner's syndrome, have all been implicated as risk factors for the development of small bowel adenocarcinomas.[28, 29] In patients with Peutz-Jeghers syndrome, the developing adenocarcinomas are usually at distinct sites from the classic hamartomas seen in these patients.[30] In patients with familial polyposis or Gardner's syndrome, the lesions tend to be periampullary cancers rather than true small bowel cancers.[32] As mentioned, Lynch et al.[31] described nine small bowel cancers in patients belonging to pedigrees of the Lynch II syndrome. Overall, the number of these cases is small, but the consistent theme remains that patients with familial gastrointestinal syndromes tend to have an increased incidence of small bowel carcinoma.

Patients with inflammatory conditions of the small bowel, including Crohn's disease and celiac sprue, are also at increased risk of small bowel tumors. The majority of these tumors are lymphomas, but adenocarcinomas have been reported.[32] The disease state typically precedes the development of tumors by several years. The increased risk of a small bowel cancer developing in patients with either of these diseases is estimated to be between 80 and 100 times that in the normal population.[33]

Patients who are chronically immunosuppressed, either from inherited immunodeficiency syndromes (e.g., Wiskott-Aldrich syndrome), immunosuppressive therapy (e.g., cyclosporine), or acquired immunodeficiency syndrome (AIDS), tend to develop extranodal lymphoma. A significant percentage of these lymphomas are reported to involve the small intestine.[34–36]

Additionally, diet appears to be an added risk factor. Populations known to consume larger quantities of fat in their staple diet also have an increased incidence of small bowel carcinomas.[37]

DIAGNOSIS

Several radiologic techniques are particularly applicable to the small bowel. Radiologic examination of the small intestine is possible by upper gastrointestinal barium study with small bowel follow-through, as well as the increasingly sensitive technique of enteroclysis. This technique involves the installation of barium directly into the small bowel by oral intubation techniques or instillation of barium into distal small bowel through the colon. The quantity of dye is increased compared with that which is swallowed and eventually passed through the stomach, and therefore smaller lesions are easily detected. In addition, when a patient presents with a palpable abdominal mass, a computed tomography (CT) scan with contrast can be helpful in delineating a primary small bowel tumor in relation to contiguous structure involvement.

Endoscopically, two techniques are gaining increased use. The first of these is push enteroscopy. This involves the use of a long endoscope, which is orally intubated and advanced through the stomach into the small bowel. Although these endoscopes are not long enough to examine the entire small bowel, they can be used to obtain biopsy samples for histologic diagnosis. If a lesion is more distal in the small bowel, this may be detected by sonde enteroscopy. This technique involves the use of a long, narrow endoscope, which is nasally intubated and allowed to advance to the distal small bowel by physiologic peristalsis. After several hours, the sonde is radiologically proven to be in the terminal small bowel and is then withdrawn while the endoscopist visualizes the mucosa of the small bowel. Although the sonde endoscope can be advanced slightly by insufflation of a balloon on the terminal tip, several centimeters of small bowel at a time can conceivably be missed because of sliding of the small bowel off the tip of the endoscope. These small-diameter endoscopes currently cannot be used to obtain biopsy samples or to perform therapeutic techniques.

STAGING

Although there are approximately 4600 new cases of small bowel cancer a year, most single institutional clinical series are limited to a small number of patients. Only a few of these series have attempted to stage patients with small bowel cancer in a reproducible fashion.[2, 38] Collected series such as those presented in Table 3–12, which report on a large number of patients, are limited in their ability to assess prognosis, since there is no standardized staging system currently available for small bowel cancers. A few clinical series have reported their results using the Astler-Coller modification of the Dukes staging system for colon cancer. The significant prognostic variables for small bowel cancer are similar to those for colon cancer, and the risk factors are also similar. Therefore, it is quite reasonable to adapt the TNM staging system used for colon carcinoma in reporting small bowel adenocarcinomas (Fig. 3–10). A method for reporting tumor location should also be incorporated into this small bowel staging system.

The classic staging of lymphomas uses the Ann Arbor staging system; however, Blackledge et al.[39] established a specific staging system adapted to small bowel lymphomas (Table 3–13). This system incorporates tumor perforation as a prognostic variable (see later).

Staging systems in the literature for carcinoid tumors of

TABLE 3–13
Blackledge Staging System for Small Bowel Lymphomas

Stage	Description
I	Tumor confined to the gastrointestinal tract
II	Tumor with local mesenteric nodal involvement
III	Tumor with perforation
IV	Tumor with distant (para-aortic and beyond) nodal involvement
V	Tumor with visceral or bone marrow involvement

Data from Blackledge G, et al: A study of gastrointestinal lymphoma. Clin Oncol 5:209–219, 1979.

Definition of TNM

T	X	Primary tumor cannot be assessed
	0	No evidence of primary tumor
	is	Carcinoma in situ
	1	Tumor invades submucosa
	2	Tumor invades muscularis propria
	3	Tumor invades through the muscularis propria into the subserosa
	4	Tumor perforates the visceral peritoneum, or directly invades other organs or structures
N	X	Regional lymph nodes cannot be assessed
	0	No regional lymph node metastasis
	1	Lymph node metastasis within the vasa recta
	2	Lymph node metastasis between the vasa recta and superior mesenteric artery
	3	Metastasis in nodes along the superior mesenteric artery
M	X	Presence of distant metastasis cannot be assessed
	0	No distant metastasis
	1	Distant metastasis

Stage Grouping

Stage	T	N	M
0	Tis	N0	M0
I	T1	N0	M0
	T2	N0	M0
II	T3	N0	M0
	T4	N0	M0
III	Any T	N1	M0
	Any T	N2	M0
IV	Any T	N3	M0
	Any T	Any N	M1

Histopathologic Grade

Gx	Grade cannot be assessed
G1	Well differentiated
G2	Moderately well differentiated
G3	Poorly differentiated
G4	Undifferentiated

FIGURE 3–10. Proposed staging system for adenocarcinomas of the small intestine. The N staging has been modified to accommodate anatomic differences between the small and large intestine. Additionally, physicians are encouraged to report the number of involved lymph nodes.

the small bowel have varied. In 1990, Moesta and Schlag[40] prospectively compared tumor size versus local tissue invasion to predict outcome. The depth of tumor penetration predicted lymph node involvement and was superior to tumor size as a predictor of regional and distant metastasis. Survival data were not presented; nevertheless, on the basis of this analysis, they proposed a pathologic staging system for carcinoid tumors (Table 3–14).[40]

In 1992, a staging system for gastrointestinal leiomyosarcomas was proposed.[41] Univariate and multivariate analyses of 139 patients with gastrointestinal leiomyosarcomas demonstrated the importance of several prognostic variables. A staging system based on this analysis is shown in Figure 3–11.

TREATMENT—SURGICAL AND NONSURGICAL OPTIONS

Adenocarcinoma

Adenocarcinoma is the most common cancer found in the small bowel, representing approximately 50% of all

TNM Classification

T1	<5 cm
T2	>5 cm
T3	Contiguous organ involvement or peritoneal implants
T4	Tumor rupture
G1	Low grade
G2	High grade
M0	No metastases
M1	Metastases present

Staging

Stage	TNM	5-Year Survival
I	T1, G1, M0	75%
II	T2, G1, M0	52%
III	T1-2, G2, M0 T3, any G, M0	28%
IVA	M1 or residual disease after surgery	12%
IVB	T4	7%

FIGURE 3–11. TNM classification and staging system proposed by Ng et al.[41]

malignant tumors of that site (see Table 3–12). Forty percent of small bowel adenocarcinomas are located in the duodenum, and they occur with decreasing frequency from the duodenum to the ileum. The presentation and treatment of duodenal adenocarcinomas differ from those of jejunoileal tumors and are presented elsewhere in this text.

When combined, jejunoileal adenocarcinomas compose the majority of small bowel adenocarcinomas. Most adenocarcinomas of the small intestine are symptomatic (ranging from days to years), while 95% of benign small bowel tumors are asymptomatic.[42] Adenocarcinomas usually present with the acute signs and symptoms of intestinal obstruction (nausea, vomiting, pain) or the chronic signs and symptoms of occult gastrointestinal bleeding (melena, weakness).[43, 44] Weight loss is a relatively frequent finding, a palpable mass is found in about one fourth of patients, and perforation occurs in less than 10%.[44] If the lesion is in the duodenum, it can usually be identified and pathologically diagnosed preoperatively. More distal adenocarcinomas can be diagnosed with enteroclysis studies in up to 90% of cases.[44a]

The majority of jejunoileal adenocarcinomas are resectable at exploration; however, about 35% to 50% have nodal involvement and 10% to 20% have distant metastases.[2, 38, 45] Small bowel adenocarcinomas should be resected with an adequate proximal and distal margin (a definitive margin has not been established, although some authors recommended a 10-cm margin) as well as sufficient mesentery to remove the draining lymph node basin.[42] The wide mesenteric resection should include all mesentery supplying the affected bowel down to the superior mesenteric vessels. Curative treatment for tumors of the terminal ileum includes a right hemicolectomy. Palliative procedures include partial resection or bypass procedures, or both, depending on the individual circumstances. Twenty percent of patients with small bowel tumors have additional tumors, and most of these are in the colon. Consequently, a thorough exploration for synchronous lesions should be performed at laparotomy.

Table 3–15 shows the reported 5-year survival rates for small bowel adenocarcinomas. The weighted mean of these studies gives an overall survival rate of 19%. Unfortunately, this dismal rate is consistent with older studies as well. The most important prognostic indicator is lymph node status. The 5-year survival rate for patients with negative nodes ranges from 55% to 70%, which decreases to 12% to 13% when nodal metastases are present.[38, 46] Histologic grade has also been shown to be a significant prognostic indicator. The 5-year survival rate with well-differentiated lesions is 75%, compared to 25% for less-differentiated lesions.[38, 40, 46, 49] The depth of bowel wall penetration has been proposed as a significant prognostic

TABLE 3–14
Staging System for Carcinoid Tumors

Stage	Description
I	Primary tumor confined to the submucosa
II	Primary tumor confined to the muscularis propria
III	Primary tumor confined to the serosa
IV	Primary tumor involving adjacent structures

Data from Moesta KT, Schlag P: Proposal for a new carcinoid tumour staging system based on tumour tissue infiltration and primary metastasis: A prospective multicentre carcinoid tumour evaluation study. Eur J Surg Oncol 16:280–288, 1990.

TABLE 3–15
Survival Rates for Adenocarcinoma

Investigator(s)	Year	No. of Patients	5-Year Survival
Martin[1]	1986	87	21
Cicarelli et al.[2]	1987	17	12
Brophy and Cahow[84]	1989	18	36
Lioe and Biggart[85]	1990	25	16
Kusumoto et al.[86]	1992	19	10
Serour et al.[87]	1992	14	18

indicator.[38, 43, 46] The prognostic utility of DNA ploidy, oncogenes, or tumor suppressor genes remains to be addressed.

Experience with either chemotherapy or radiotherapy is quite limited. One partial response to a 5-fluorouracil 5-FU–based regimen has been reported; however, there were 13 nonresponders noted in this clinical trial.[47]

Carcinoid Tumors

Carcinoid tumors develop from the enterochromaffin cells, which are of neuroectodermal origin and biochemically utilize the amine precursor and decarboxylation (APUD) system. Historically, carcinoid tumors were classified as either benign or malignant; however, all carcinoid tumors should be regarded as having metastastic potential and treated as such. Carcinoid tumors represent the second-most common malignancy of the small bowel. They occur most frequently in the sixth decade of life and affect men twice as often as women. In a collected series of 3718 abdominal carcinoid tumors, Wilson et al.[48] found the appendix to be the most common site (45%), followed by the small bowel (33%), rectum (16%), and other sites (6%). Eighty-five percent of small bowel carcinoids occur in the ileum (see Table 3–12). Twenty-five percent of patients with carcinoid tumors present with multiple sites, while, as with all small bowel tumors, the risk of second malignancies (both synchronous and metachronous) is also high (see earlier).[49]

The clinical presentation of these tumors depends on whether systemic endocrine effects are manifested. Patients without classic "carcinoid syndrome" often present with signs of obstruction or vague abdominal pain. This pain may relate to the extensive desmoplastic reaction that can accompany many of these lesions.[50] This fibrotic reaction, thought to be secondary to secreted byproducts from the tumor itself, may cause shortening of the bowel mesentery, leading to a partial obstruction or a potential vascular compromise.[51] Approximately 15% of patients with small bowel carcinoids present with the typical carcinoid syndrome (more than one half of patients with malignant carcinoid eventually have the carcinoid syndrome).[52] The patient presents with carcinoid syndrome usually only after significant hepatic involvement by the tumor and with subsequent findings of elevated levels of urinary 5-hydroxyindoleacetic acid (5-HIAA). Hepatomegaly is appreciated in 70% of patients with the carcinoid syndrome. The more common symptoms of this syndrome include cutaneous flushing (75%), diarrhea (70%), endocardial lesions (50%), venous telangiectasis (50%), edema (52%), and bronchospasm (20%). Occasionally, pellagra, peptic ulcers, arthralgia, and retroperitoneal fibrosis can develop.[53] Normally, only a small fraction of dietary-ingested tryptophan is used for the biosynthesis of serotonin; however, in patients with the carcinoid syndrome, the majority of tryptophan is directed toward serotonin synthesis. Consequently, the syndrome can be precipitated by ingesting foods rich in serotonin precursors (e.g., cheese, chocolate).[54, 55]

The diagnosis of small bowel carcinoids is seldom made preoperatively unless the carcinoid syndrome is present. Small bowel studies with barium are generally less diagnostically rewarding than in patients with adenocarcinoma because of the submucosal location of the carcinoid tumors and their limited intraluminal size.[55] CT scans may reveal extensive lymphatic or hepatic disease but are not useful for identifying the primary lesions. Angiography may show the fibroplastic mesenteric arterial changes or a "tumor blush" at the primary site.[55] Scintigraphy using a radiolabeled somatostatin analogue may be a useful technique in the near future. In an initial report, Dorr and colleagues[56] were able to detect 83% of the primary carcinoids and 90% of the metastatic lesions.

Several prognostic variables for patients with gastrointestinal carcinoid tumors have been established. Agranovich et al.[57] staged patients using a modified Astler-Coller system and found a significant correlation between stage and survival.[57] Other prognostic variables included the presence of residual disease after resection, histologic differentiation, and urinary levels of 5-HIAA. In addition to these variables, other studies have shown increasing age and the occurrence of a second malignancy to be independent predictors of a poor prognosis.[58]

At exploration, grossly these lesions appear as firm, tan, submucosal nodules. Localized tumors should be resected in a fashion similar to that done for adenocarcinoma. This includes a wide resection of the involved bowel and its associated mesentery. Lesions of the terminal ileum are removed with a right hemicolectomy. A careful search of synchronous lesions should be undertaken. Primary lesions should be resected even in the face of hepatic disease. Debulking patients with unresectable disease significantly extends their survival.

Soreide and coworkers[59] retrospectively evaluated 75 patients with abdominal carcinoid tumors. The median survival of patients who underwent intra-abdominal tumor debulking (139 months) was significantly longer than that of those who did not (69 months).[59] Patients with recurrent disease fair better if reresected. Because of the difficult problems associated with the carcinoid syndrome, hepatic metastases should also be addressed. In Soreide and colleagues' series, patients with hepatic metastases who were treated with either resection of their metastases, hepatic artery ligation, or artery embolization survived significantly longer than those who were not treated (median survival, 216 months for treated metastases versus 48 months for untreated metastases).[59]

In general, if only a few superficial hepatic metastases are present, they should be excised. If there is diffuse liver involvement, hepatic artery ligation in conjunction with cholecystectomy (to avoid ischemic cholecystitis) should be considered. Alternative treatments for diffuse hepatic metastases include arterial embolization, although this frequently requires repeated embolization procedures and the response tends to be of short duration owing to the rich collateral blood supply within the liver.[60]

A multitude of agents have been used in the palliative management of the symptoms associated with the carcinoid syndrome. Cyproheptadine is useful for improving diarrhea but has little effect on the cutaneous flushing. The long-acting somatostatin analogue SMS-201 has had impressive results in palliation of the symptoms of the syndrome, and measurable partial tumor regressions have been noted as well.[61] Currently, no evidence shows that somatostatin or its analogue should be used in asymptomatic patients.

Single chemotherapy agents, including dacarbazine, doxorubicin, streptozocin, and 5-FU, have been tried but with only marginal response rates (17% to 26%). The most effective chemotherapy combination employs streptozocin and 5-FU, with a response rate of 33%. In either modality, the response rates are not durable. Radiotherapy for palliation of painful bone metastases has been reported; otherwise, there is little role for radiotherapy in this disease.[62]

In sharp contrast to adenocarcinomas, carcinoid tumors of the small bowel are slow-growing neoplasms and may take an indolent course. The median survival is 15 years for patients with resectable nodal disease. The overall 5-year survival rate for carcinoid tumors of the small bowel is 54%: 75% in tumors without regional or distant metastases, 59% in tumors with regional metastases, and 9% in tumors with distant metastases.[63]

Lymphomas

The gastrointestinal tract is the most common site of extranodal lymphoma. The stomach is the most common gastrointestinal site, followed by decreasing frequency in the small bowel and finally the colon. Primary small intestinal lymphoma (PSIL) is distinct from extranodal lymphoma with gastrointestinal involvement and must meet strict criteria, including

1. No involvement of peripheral or mediastinal lymph nodes.
2. A normal peripheral blood smear.
3. No evidence of hepatic or splenic involvement.[64, 65]

There are two main forms of PSIL, each with its own clinical presentation. Western PSIL is characterized by discrete single or multiple nodules in the small bowel; has a bimodal age distribution, occurring in children under 10 and in adults in the fifth and sixth decades; and has a male to female ratio of 2:1. The majority of Western PSIL cases are diffuse, histiocytic, non-Hodgkin's lymphomas and occur in the ileum; 25% are well-differentiated lymphocytic lymphomas. Using the Kiel classification scheme, which is based on phenotypic makers, Domizio et al.[11] found that 66% of small bowel lymphomas were of B-cell origin and 34% were of T-cell origin. High-grade lymphomas predominated in both the T-cell and the B-cell groups.

The second form of PSIL, immunoproliferative small intestinal disease (IPSID), includes a number of conditions, including Mediterranean lymphoma, primary upper small intestinal lymphoma, and alpha-chain disease. The majority of cases of IPSID occur in Middle Eastern countries and typically affect adults in their second or third decade with a history of poor hygiene and a high incidence of enteric and parasitic infections. IPSID has an equal sex distribution, and there is no documented racial susceptibility. In contrast to Western PSIL, IPSID usually affects long segments of the second, third, and fourth portions of the duodenum and upper jejunum.[66] In the early stage, IPSID is a prelymphomatous B-cell proliferative disorder containing 90% mature plasma cells. Macroscopically, the mucosa appears thickened and granular. In the more advanced stage, the cells become dysplastic in appearance and invade the muscularis mucosa. Tumor nodules develop and can invade adjacent organs. Individual patients may show distinct lesions at various stages of development.[66] Alpha-chain disease is a subgroup of patients with IPSID that expresses a mutant form of the alpha heavy chain of IgA.

Burkitt's lymphoma can also originate within the small intestine.[67] This disease usually affects children and young adolescents. Because of its rapid growth rate, intestinal obstruction is a frequent complication.

The most common presenting symptom in patients with Western PSIL is abdominal pain (75% to 100%), while the most common physical finding is an abdominal mass (16%).[66] In contrast to patients with Western lymphoma, those with IPSID present with a high incidence of diarrhea (70% to 100%), anorexia and weight loss (87% to 100%), and malabsorption (60% to 78%).[66] Enteroclysis studies detect small bowel abnormalities in 90% of patients with intestinal lymphoma.[64] These lesions typically show luminal narrowing, mucosal ulceration, and minimal proximal dilatation.[68, 69] Displacement of adjacent small bowel loops is seen in approximately 50% of patients. Endoscopy is of little utility in Western PSIL but is frequently useful in IPSID, in which biopsy of the proximal lesions can be performed.[70]

Because of the vague nature of the chronic symptoms and the urgency of the acute symptoms, Western PSIL is frequently diagnosed at the time of exploratory celiotomy. If PSIL is encountered intraoperatively, the involved bowel should be resected along with its mesentery. Previously, extensive resections have been performed, however, in more recent years more conservative resections have been recommended.[71, 72] Palliative resections to relieve immediate symptoms are indicated in the presence of extensive disease. Patients with bulky disease are generally treated postoperatively with chemotherapy or radiotherapy. At the time of laparotomy, specimens from the liver and the mesenteric and para-aortic lymph nodes should be obtained for biopsy. With aggressive chemotherapy, most current series report 5-year survival rates of greater than 50%.[20] IPSID is frequently diagnosed prior to surgical intervention by either peroral jejunal biopsy or the presence of alpha heavy chains in the serum or jejunal aspirate.

Remissions have been achieved in patients with early-stage IPSID treated with tetracycline-based antibiotics.[73] However, the combination of tetracycline, prednisone, and cyclophosphamide appears to provide more durable remissions. Patients with gross tumor nodules can be successfully treated with chemotherapy and enjoy complete remissions, which may last for months to years. Eventually the disease recurs and follows a progressive course, intermittently interrupted with periods of clinical improvement. The role of surgery in this setting is palliation. The prognosis is poor, with 5-year survival rates around 20%.[71]

Patients with Burkitt's lymphoma frequently present with massive tumors that should be completely resected if possible. Unresectable disease should be optimally debulked (>90%), as this has been shown to be of significant benefit as well.[74] Systemic chemotherapy with cyclophosphamide as a single agent or in combination with other agents remains the mainstay of treatment for patients with Burkitt's lymphoma. Prior to the recognition of tumor lysis syndrome, 10% of patients with Burkitt's lymphoma died during chemotherapy induction.[75] This syndrome occurs almost exclusively in patients with large bulky tumors and further exemplifies the need for tumor debulking.

Sarcomas

Sarcomas of the small bowel are uncommon, composing 11% to 13% of small bowel cancers. Leiomyosarcomas constitute the majority of sarcomas originating within the small bowel, although sarcomas of adipose, connective, neural, and vascular origin have been reported. Leiomyosarcomas can occur at any age, but 75% occur in the fifth and sixth decades of life with a male to female ratio of 2:1. In Wilson and coworkers' series of 432 leiomyosarcomas of the small bowel,[76] 9% occurred in the duodenum, 37% in the jejunum, and 53% in the ileum, or approximately the same number of leiomyosarcomas per unit length of small bowel. In general, the clinical presentation of small bowel sarcomas is similar to other small bowel cancers except that 75% of small bowel leiomyosarcomas grow to greater than 5 cm prior to detection, and consequently most patients have a clinically palpable mass at presentation. Typically, these lesions grow exenterically and cause obstruction from extrinsic compression of the small intestine. Additionally, 75% of patients with leiomyosarcomas present with hemorrhage, 25% with sufficient blood loss to cause hematochezia.[77]

The treatment of sarcomas of the small intestine is surgical extirpation. The various histologic types of sarcomas should be treated similarly because a definitive distinction between benign and malignant lesions often cannot be reliably obtained with frozen sections. Curative resection involves the removal of the primary tumor with a wide margin of normal bowel. Although sarcomas do not typically metastasize via lymphatic pathways, regional nodal metastases have been reported in 10% to 15% of small bowel leiomyosarcomas. Because of the attendant morbidity with local recurrence, a wide resection of the mesentery, if it can be accomplished safely, should be considered. Palliative resections should be performed if possible, otherwise an intestinal bypass is appropriate in symptomatic patients.

The 5-year survival rate of patients with small bowel sarcomas is approximately 50%. Significant prognostic variables include tumor size, resectability, grade, presence of perforation, and extension to other organs (Table 3–16) (see Fig. 3–11).[41, 78–80] Survival based on the TNM system proposed by Ng et al.[41] is shown in Figure 3–11. There is currently no proven benefit of adjuvant chemotherapy or radiotherapy for sarcomas of the small bowel. Several chemotherapeutic regimens (mostly in combination with doxorubicin) have reported response rates of 35% to 65% in patients with unresectable or metastatic disease, and these regimens should be considered in symptomatic patients.

Metastatic Disease

Metastases to the small bowel are a frequent though rarely isolated event.[81] Small bowel metastases can be classified as originating from either abdominal or extra-abdominal sites. Melanoma is the most common primary tumor causing small bowel metastasis. Sixty percent of patients dying of melanoma have gastrointestinal involvement.[82] Other extra-abdominal cancers that metastasize to the small intestine include cervix, lung, esophagus, breast, head and neck, thyroid, and skin.[5, 83] Intra-abdominal metastases can occur from virtually any intra-abdominal organ. The clinical presentation of metastases to the small bowel is similar to other small bowel tumors and includes obstruction, bleeding, and perforation.

A mean survival for patients with small bowel metastatic cancer was approximately 6 months in one study, with all patients dying within 19 months of treatment.[81] However, palliation is an important goal and should be considered in patients with focal areas of high-grade obstruction or bleeding. Multiple areas of obstruction, however, are more problematic and should be subject to palliative surgery only rarely.

TABLE 3–16
Prognostic Variables for Small Bowel Sarcomas

	Favorable Category	Unfavorable Category
Size	<5 cm (71%)*	>5 cm (27%)
Grade	Low (62%)	High (12%)
Resection	Complete (50%)	Palliative (25%)

*Numbers in parentheses represent 5-year survival rates.[78]

CONCLUSIONS

The rarity of occurrence of small bowel cancer prevents a better understanding of the basic science and clinical questions concerning these tumors. Thus, the question posed by Lowenfels more than 20 years ago—why are small bowel tumors so rare?—remains unanswered today.[14] Compared with cancers of the large intestine, little is known regarding the role of oncogenes and tumor suppressor genes in small bowel cancer. Furthermore, the rarity of these tumors has resulted in the publication of series containing only a small number of patients. For collected series to provide meaningful data regarding the natural history of these tumors, there needs to be a consensus concerning the staging and reporting of small bowel cancers, and the TNM system proposed herein seems a reasonable first approach. It is unlikely that routine screening for small bowel cancers using new markers or better diagnostic techniques will improve earlier detection in the next decade; consequently, if improvements are to be made in survival, therapeutic modalities must be enhanced.

References

1. Martin RG: Malignant tumors of the small intestine. Surg Clin North Am 66:779–785, 1986.
2. Cicarelli O, Welch JP, Kent G: Primary malignant tumors of the small bowel: The Harford Hospital experience. Am J Surg 153:350–354, 1987.
3. Johnson AM, Harman PK, Hanks JB: Primary small bowel malignancies. Am Surg 51:31–36, 1985.
4. Barclay THC, Schapira DV: Malignant tumors of the small intestine. Cancer 51:878–881, 1983.
5. Herbsman H, Wetstein L, Rosen Y, et al: Tumors of the small intestine. Curr Probl Surg 17:123–128, 1980.

5a. Wingo PA, Tong T, Bolden S: Cancer statistics 1995, CA 45:8–30, 1995.

6. Healey JE, Hodge J: Surgical Anatomy. Philadelphia: BC Decker, 1990.
7. Langman J: Medical Embryology. Baltimore: Williams & Wilkins, 1981.
8. Blackman E, Nash S: Diagnosis of duodenal and ampullary epithelial neoplasms by endoscopic biopsy. A clinicopathologic and immunohistochemical study. Hum Pathol 16:901–910, 1985.
9. Iwafuchi M, Watanabe H, Ishihara N, et al: Neoplastic endocrine cells in carcinomas of the small intestine. Histochemical and immunohistochemical studies of 24 tumors. Hum Pathol 18:185–194, 1987.
10. Johnson L, Lavin P, Moertel CG, et al: Carcinoids. The association of histologic growth pattern and survival. Cancer 51:882–889, 1983.
11. Domizio P, Owen RA, Shepherd NA, et al: Primary lymphoma of the small intestine. A clinicopathological study of 119 cases. Am J Surg Pathol 17:429–442, 1993.
12. Sheperd NA, Blackshaw AJ, Hall PA, et al: Malignant lymphoma with eosinophilia of the gastrointestinal tract. Histopathology 11:115–130, 1987.
13. Lightdale CJ, Loepfell TC, Sherlock P: Small intestinal cancer. In Schottenfeld D, Fraumeni J (eds): Cancer Epidemiology and Prevention. Philadelphia: WB Saunders 1982, pp 692–702.
14. Lowenfels AB: Why are small bowel tumors so rare? Lancet 1:24–26, 1973.
15. Stemmermann GN, Goodman MT, Nomura MY: Adenocarcinoma of the proximal small intestine, a marker for familial and multicentric cancer? Cancer 70:2766–2771, 1992.
16. McGovern VT: Lymphomas of the gastrointestinal tract. In Yardley JH, Morson BC, Abell MR (eds): The Gastrointestinal Tract. Baltimore: Williams & Wilkins, 1977, pp 184–205.
17. Harris OD, Cooke WT, Thompson H, et al: Malignancy in adult coeliac disease and idiopathic steatorrhoea. Am J Med 42:899–912, 1967.
18. Dutz W, Asvadi S, Sadri S, et al: Intestinal lymphoma and sprue: A systematic approach. Gut 12:804–810, 1971.
19. Moertel CG, Dockerty MG: Familial occurrence of metastasizing carcinoid tumors. Ann Intern Med 78:389–390, 1973.
20. Coit DG: Cancer of the small intestine. In DeVita VT, Hellman S, Rosenberg SA (eds): Cancer Principles and Practice of Oncology. Philadelphia: JB Lippincott, 1993, pp 915–928.

20a. Reiner MA: Primary malignant neoplasms of the small bowel. Mt Sinai J Med 43:274–280, 1976.

21. Celik C, Mittelman A, Paolini NS, et al: Effects of 1,2-symmetrical dimethylhydrazine on jejunocolic transposition in Sprague-Dawley rats. Can Res 41:2908–2911, 1981.
22. Calman KC: Why are small bowel tumors rare? An experimental model. Gut 15:552–554, 1974.
23. Wattenberg LW: Studies of polycyclic hydrocarbon hydroxylases of the intestine possibly related to cancer effect of diet on benzpyrene hydroxylase activity. Cancer 28:99–102, 1971.

23a. Lipkin M, Quastler H: Cell retention and incidence of carcinoma in several portions of the gastrointestinal tract. Nature 194:1198–1199, 1962.

24. Spiro HM: Small intestinal tumors. In Spiro HM (ed): Clinical Gastroenterology. Toronto: McMillan, 1970, pp 140–164.
25. Jagelman DG, DeCosse JJ, Bussey HJ: Upper gastrointestinal cancer in familial adenomatous polyposis. Lancet 1:1149–1151, 1988.
26. Reid JD: Intestinal carcinoma in the Peutz-Jeghers syndrome. JAMA 229:883–886, 1974.
27. Savoca PE, Ballantyne GH, Cahow CE: Gastrointestinal malignancies in Crohn's disease. A 20-year experience. Dis Colon Rectum 33:7–11, 1990.
28. Perzin KH, Bridge MF: A clinicopathologic review of 51 cases and a study of their relationship to carcinoma. Cancer 48:799–808, 1981.
29. Ross JE, Mara JE: Small bowel polyps and carcinoma in multiple intestinal polyposis. Arch Surg 108:736–742, 1974.
30. Spigelman AD, Murday V, Phillips RK: Cancer and the Peutz-Jeghers syndrome. Gut 30:1588–1590, 1990.
31. Lynch HT, Smyrk TC, Lynch PM: et al: Adenocarcinoma of the small bowel in Lynch syndrome II. Cancer 64:2178–2183, 1989.
32. Swinson CM, Slavin G, Coles EC, Booth CC: Coeliac disease and malignancy. Lancet 1:111–115, 1983.
33. Fresko D, Lazarus SS, Doltan J, Reingold M: Early presentation of carcinoma of the small bowel in Crohn's disease ("Crohn's carcinoma"): Case reports and review of the literature. Gastroenterology 82:783–789, 1988.
34. Ioachim HI: Neoplasms associated with immune deficiencies. Pathol Ann 22:177–222, 1987.
35. Penn I, First MR: Development and incidence of cancer following cyclosporine therapy. Transplant Proc 18(Suppl 1):210–213, 1986.
36. Ziegler JL, Beckstead JA, Volberding PA, et al: Hodgkin's disease lymphoma in 90 homosexual men—relationship to generalized lymphadenopathy and the acquired immunodeficiency syndrome. N Engl Med 311:565–570, 1984.
37. Lowenfels AB, Sonni A: Distribution of small bowel tumors. Cancer Lett 3:83–86, 1977.
38. Quriel K, Adams J: Adenocarcinoma of the small intestine. Am J Surg 147:66–71, 1984.
39. Blackledge G, Bush H, Dodge OG, Crowther D: A study of gastrointestinal lymphoma. Clin Oncol 5:209–219, 1979.
40. Moesta KT, Schlag P: Proposal for a new carcinoid tumour staging system based on tumour tissue infiltration and primary metastasis; a prospective multicentre carcinoid tumour evaluation study. West German Surgical Oncologists' Group. Eur J Surg Oncol 16:280–288, 1990.
41. Ng EH, Pollock RE, Munsell MF, et al: Prognostic factors influencing survival in gastrointestinal leiomyosarcomas. Implications for surgical management and staging. Ann Surg 215:68–77, 1992.
42. Nelson R: Adenocarcinoma of the small intestine. In Nelson RL, Nyhus LM (eds): Surgery of the Small Intestine. Norwalk: Appleton & Lange, 1987, pp 223–230.
43. Adler SN, Lyon DT, Sullivan PD: Adenocarcinoma of the small bowel—clinical features, similarity to regional enteritis and analysis of 338 documented cases. Am J Gastroenterol 77:326–330, 1982.
44. Desa L, Bridger F, Grace PA, et al: Primary jejunoileal tumors: A review of 45 cases. World J Surg 15:81–87, 1991.

44a. Ekberg O, Ekholm S: Radiography in primary tumors of the small bowel. Acta Radiol 21:79–84, 1980.
45. Zollinger RM, Sternfeld W, Schreiber H: Primary neoplasms of the small intestine. Am J Surg 151:654–658, 1986.
46. Bridge MF, Perzin KH: Primary adenocarcinoma of the jejunum and ileum: A clinicopathologic study. Cancer 36:1876–1887, 1975.
47. Jigyasu D, Bediklan AY, Stroehlein JR: Chemotherapy for primary adenocarcinoma of the small bowel. Cancer 53:23–25, 1984.
48. Wilson H, Cheek RC, Sherman R, Storer EH: Carcinoid tumors. Curr Probl Surg 7:1–23, 1970.
49. Alexander JW, Altemeier WA: Association of primary neoplasms of the small intestine with other neoplastic growths. Ann Surg 167:958–964, 1968.
50. Sjoblom SM: Clinical presentation and prognosis of gastrointestinal carcinoid tumors. Scand J Gastroenterol 23:779–787, 1988.
51. Makridis C, Oberg K, Juhlin C, et al: Surgical treatment of mid-gut carcinoid tumors. World J Surg 14:377–385, 1990.
52. Moertel CG, Sauer WG, Dockerty MB, Baggenstoss AH: Life history of the carcinoid tumor of the small intestine. Cancer 14:901–912, 1961.
53. Kaplan EL: The carcinoid syndrome. In Friesen SR (ed): Surgical Endocrinology: Clinical Syndromes. Philadelphia: JB Lippincott, 1978.
54. Vinick AI, McLeod MK, Fig M, et al: Clinical features, diagnosis and localization of carcinoid tumors and their management. Gastrointest Clin North Am 18:865–896, 1989.
55. Udekwu A, Kaplan EL: Carcinoid tumors of the small intestine and their carcinoid syndromes. In Nelson RL, Nyhus LM (eds): Surgery of the Small Intestine. Norwalk: Appleton & Lange, 1987, pp 231–242.
56. Dorr U, Rath U, Schurmann G, et al: Somatostatin receptor scintigraphy. A new imaging procedure for the specific demonstration of carcinoids of the small intestine. ROFO 158:67–73, 1993.
57. Agranovich AL, Anderson GH, Manji M, et al: Carcinoid tumour of the gastrointestinal tract: Prognostic factors and disease outcome. J Surg Oncol 47:45–52, 1991.
58. Greenberg RS, Baumgarten DA, Clark WS, et al: Prognostic factors for gastrointestinal and bronchopulmonary carcinoid tumors. Cancer 60:2476–2483, 1987.
59. Soreide O, Berstad T, Bakka A, et al: Surgical treatment as a principle in patients with advanced abdominal carcinoid tumors. Surgery 111:48–54, 1992.
60. Malton PN: The carcinoid syndrome. JAMA 260:1602–1605, 1988.
61. Kvols LK: The carcinoid syndrome: A treatable malignant disease. Oncology 2:33–39, 1988.
62. Gaitan-Gaitan A, Rider WD, Bush RS: Carcinoid tumor-cure by irradiation. Int J Radiat Oncol Biol Physics 1:9–13, 1975.
63. Godwin JD: Carcinoid tumors, an analysis of 2837 cases. Cancer 36:560–569, 1975.
64. Cooper BT, Read AE: Small intestinal lymphoma. World J Surg 9:930–937, 1985.
65. Dawson IM, Cornes JS, Morson MC: Primary malignant lymphoid tumors of the intestinal tract. Report of 37 cases with a study of factors influencing prognosis. Br J Surg 40:80–88, 1961.
66. Al-Mondhiry H: Primary lymphomas of the small intestine: East-West contrast. Am J Hematol 22:89–105, 1986.
67. Rachmilewitz D, Okon E: Primary small intestinal lymphoma. In Berk JE (ed): Gastroenterology. Philadelphia: WB Saunders, 1985, pp 1867–1873.
68. Gourtsoyiannis NC, Nolan DJ: Lymphoma of the small intestine: Radiological appearances. Clin Radiol 39:639–645, 1988.
69. Iida M, Suekane H, Tada S, et al: Double-contrast radiographic features in primary small intestinal lymphoma of the 'western' type: Correlation with pathological findings. Clin Radiol 44:322–326, 1991.
70. Barakat MH: Endoscopic features of primary small bowel lymphoma: A proposed endoscopic classification. Gut 23:36–41, 1982.
71. Al-Bahrani AR, Al-Mondhiry H, Bakin F, Al-Saleem T: Clinical and pathologic subtypes of primary intestinal lymphoma. Experience with 132 patients over a 14 year period. Cancer 52:1666–1670, 1983.
72. Weingrad DN, DeCosse JJ, Sherlock P, et al: Primary gastrointestinal lymphoma: A 30 year review. Cancer 49:1258–1262, 1982.
73. Rambaud JC: Small intestinal lymphomas and alpha-chain disease. Clin Gastroenterol 12:743–750, 1983.
74. Magrath IT, Lwanga S, Carswell W, Harrison N: Surgical reduction of tumor bulk in the management of abdominal Burkitt's lymphoma. Br Med J 12:308–312, 1977.
75. Cohen LF, Balow JE, Magrath IT, et al: Acute tumor lysis syndrome. Am J Med 68:486–491, 1980.
76. Wilson JM, Melvin DB, Gray GF, Thorbyarnarson B: Primary malignancies of the small bowel. Ann Surg 179:175–181, 1974.
77. Akwari OE, Dozois RR, Weiland LH, Beahrs OH: Leiomyosarcoma of the small and large bowel. Cancer 42:1375–1384, 1978.
78. Shiu MH, Farr GH, Egeli RA, et al: Myosarcomas of the small and large intestine: A clinicopathologic study. J Surg Oncol 24:67–73, 1983.
79. Chiotasso PJ, Faxio VW: Prognostic factors of 28 leiomyosarcomas of the small intestine. Surg Gynecol Obstet 155:197–202, 1982.
80. Kimura H, Yonemura Y, Kadoya N, et al: Prognostic factors in primary gastrointestinal leiomyosarcoma: A retrospective study. World J Surg 15:771–777, 1991.
81. de Castro CA, Dockerty MB, Mayo CW: Metastatic tumors of the small intestines. Surg Gynecol Obstet 105:159–165, 1987.
82. Ihde JK, Coit DG: Melanoma metastatic to the stomach, small bowel and colon. Am J Surg 162:208–211, 1991.
83. Phillips DL, Benner KG, Keeff EB, Traweek ST: Isolated metastasis to small bowel from anaplastic thyroid carcinoma: With a review of extra-abdominal malignancies that spread to the bowel. J Clin Gastroenterol 9:563–567, 1987.
84. Brophy C, Cahow DE: Primary small bowel malignant tumors. Am Surg 55:408–412, 1989.
85. Lioe T, Biggart JD: Primary adenocarcinoma of the jejunum and ileum: Clinicopathological review of 25 cases. J Clin Pathol 43:533–536, 1990.
86. Kusumoto H, Takahashi I, Yoshida M, et al: Primary malignant tumors of the small intestine: Analysis of 40 Japanese patients. J Surg Oncol 50:139–143, 1992.
87. Serour F, Dona G, Birkenfeld S, et al: Primary neoplasms of the small bowel. J Surg Oncol 49:29–34, 1992.

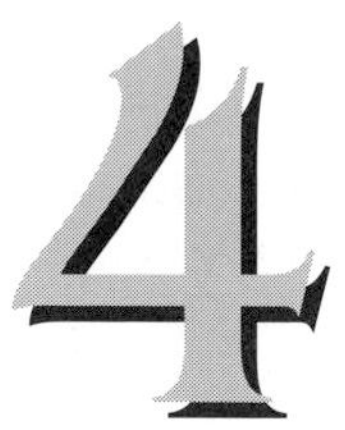

Michael A. Breda, M.D. • Allen L. Hoffman, M.D.
Linda Sher, M.D. • Luis G. Podesta, M.D.
Oscar Rodriquez, B.S. • Lidija Petrovic, M.D.
Leslie Memsic, M.D. • Leonard Makowka, M.D., Ph.D.

Hepatobiliary Tumors

HEPATOCELLULAR CARCINOMA

Epidemiology

Hepatocellular carcinoma may be the most common fatal malignancy in the world, causing an estimated 1,250,000 deaths each year. Even more striking is the tremendous geographic variation in incidence. In North America and Western Europe, hepatocellular carcinoma is relatively rare, with an incidence of less than 5 in 100,000. Approximately 2500 cases of hepatocellular carcinoma occur in the United States annually, or less than 2% of all cancers, making it the twenty-second commonest form of cancer. In marked contrast, this malignancy is rampant in several regions of the world, notably sub-Saharan Africa and Southeast Asia, where it represents up to 50% of all cancers. As can be seen in Table 4–1, Mozambique and Taiwan have an incidence of more than 100 in 100,000 population annually, and among men in Taipei the incidence is an astounding 1158 in 100,000.

TABLE 4–1
Geographic Incidence of Hepatocellular Carcinoma

Country	Incidence/100,000/Year	
	Men	*Women*
United Kingdom	1.1	0.4
Canada	1.3	0.5
USA		
White	2.4	0.6
Black	8	1.8
Japan	12	2.9
China		
Shanghai	32	9.1
South Africa		
Black	28	
White	1.2	
Zimbabwe	65	25
Mozambique	113	31
Taiwan		
Taipei	1158	

Male predominance is universal and is more pronounced in regions of high incidence. In reports from Africa and Asia, the male to female ratio varies between 4:1 and 8:1; in low-incidence areas, it is closer to 2:1. As will be discussed, this variation reflects the underlying risk factor distribution for the disease.

Racial and ethnic discrepancies have also been noted, most particularly in South Africa. There, the incidence among blacks is 28.4 in 100,000, in contrast to 1.2 in 100,000 among whites—similar to that in the United States and Europe. Blacks in the United States have a nearly fourfold higher risk for hepatocellular carcinoma than whites (8.8 vs. 2.4 in 100,000). Asians living in the United States have an incidence intermediate between that in their native countries and that in the United States, suggesting that the discrepancies in incidence are more related to environmental factors than to genetic predisposition to the disease.

The age distribution also demonstrates marked geographic variability (Table 4–2). In Africa, the tumor predominantly affects people in their thirties and forties, as opposed to in regions of low incidence, where patients tend to be in their sixties and seventies. In Asia, the incidence of hepatocellular carcinoma peaks between 40 and 60 years, intermediate between that in Africa and North America.

The fibrolamellar variant of hepatocellular carcinoma behaves differently. There is no sex predilection and, even in regions of low prevalence such as the United States, it affects a much younger population, usually between 20 and 40 years of age. Unlike other forms of hepatocellular

TABLE 4–2
Age Distribution of Hepatocellular Carcinoma

Location	Common Age Range (Yr)
Africa	30–50
Asia	40–60
North America	60–80

carcinoma, this cancer is not associated with cirrhosis or hepatitis B.

Etiology

Worldwide, hepatitis B infection is the leading cause of hepatocellular carcinoma. The unrelated hepatitis C virus is increasingly recognized as a separate cause of this malignancy. In regions of low prevalence, such as the United States, hepatitis B infection is relatively rare, and the chronic process of liver injury and regeneration (i.e., cirrhosis) becomes etiologically more important. A variety of other environmental and dietary carcinogens have been identified (Table 4–3).

Hepatitis B

The hepatitis B virus is endemic in those parts of the world where the incidence of hepatocellular carcinoma is highest. It is estimated that 300 million people are chronically infected with this virus. Hepatitis B can be transmitted vertically via breast milk, an important factor in the high incidence of hepatocellular carcinoma in endemic areas. Most individuals with hepatocellular carcinoma in these areas have evidence of prior hepatitis B infection, and 66% to 95% of these patients are hepatitis B surface antigen (HBsAG)–positive, in contrast to 8% to 15% of the general population.[1, 2] A prospective study by Beasley et al.[3] in Taiwan of 22,707 men showed that the incidence of primary hepatocellular carcinoma among carriers of HBsAg was 1158 in 100,000, versus 5 in 100,000 noninfected men, giving a relative risk of 223. In the United States and Western Europe, the carrier rate of hepatitis B among patients with hepatocellular carcinoma is much lower, between 10% and 26%.[4, 5]

Integrated hepatitis B DNA can be identified in the chromosomes of hepatomas developing in chronic carriers of hepatitis B, suggesting a possible genetic mechanism for malignant transformation. In mice, integration and expression of the hepatitis B virus x-protein result in the induction of hepatocellular carcinoma in 90% of animals.[6] It is hoped that widespread vaccination against hepatitis B will eventually reduce the occurrence of hepatocellular carcinoma.

TABLE 4–3
Causes of Hepatocellular Carcinoma

Hepatitis B
Hepatitis C
Alcoholic cirrhosis
Aflatoxin
Medications (anabolic steroids, estrogens?)
Congenital
Tyrosinemia
Hemochromatosis
$Alpha_1$-antitrypsin deficiency

Hepatitis C

As testing for hepatitis C became possible, the virus was noted to have a close association with hepatocellular carcinoma, with prevalence rates among patients with this tumor of 50% to 75%.[7] Cirrhosis develops in up to one third of patients with hepatitis C. In certain countries, such as Japan, hepatitis C shares a closer association with hepatocellular carcinoma than does hepatitis B.

The induction of malignancy is attributed to chronic hepatocyte injury, inflammation, regeneration, and fibrosis, leading to cirrhosis, which alone may be a premalignant condition. In one study, 45% of HBsAg-negative Western patients with cirrhosis were positive for antibodies to hepatitis C.[8] Hepatitis C may act as a cofactor with hepatitis B in the induction of malignancy.

Alcoholic Cirrhosis

In Western countries, hepatocellular carcinoma commonly develops in association with alcoholic cirrhosis. Autopsy studies show that as many as 55% of former alcoholics have foci of hepatocellular carcinoma, and the lifetime risk for development of clinically evident disease approaches 15%. Eighty percent to 90% of Western patients with hepatocellular carcinoma have underlying cirrhosis.

The pathogenesis of the induction of malignancy in this setting is thought to be due to the chronic cycle of injury and repair, much as in the case of chronic viral hepatitis. The combination of alcoholic cirrhosis and hepatitis B infection leads to a higher incidence of hepatocellular carcinoma than does either process individually.

Aflatoxin

Aflatoxin B_1 is a product of the ubiquitous fungus *Aspergillus flavus*, a frequent contaminant of a variety of stored foodstuffs, including grains and ground nuts. It has long been known that in areas where aspergillus contamination is common, the incidence of hepatocellular carcinoma is likewise high.[9] Livers of patients with hepatocellular carcinoma in endemic areas have high levels of aflatoxin, as compared to those of controls from these same regions.

In the laboratory, aflatoxin is the most potent hepatic carcinogen known. Although the mechanism by which aflatoxin causes hepatocellular carcinoma is unclear, recent work suggests that exposure to this agent causes a unique mutation in codon 249 of the tumor suppressor gene p53.[10]

Medications

Medications are not a major cause of hepatocellular carcinoma. There appears to be a weak association between chronic usage of anabolic steroids or estrogens and the development of hepatocellular carcinoma.

Congenital

Several inherited conditions are associated with an increased risk of hepatocellular carcinoma. Hepatocellular carcinoma eventually develops in all patients with tyrosinemia, and this disease is an indication for transplantation. Hemochromatosis and alpha$_1$-antitrypsin insufficiency with resulting cirrhosis are associated with a 200-fold increased risk of malignancy.

Pathology

Macroscopic Appearance

The gross appearance of hepatocellular carcinoma varies depending on the condition of the underlying hepatic parenchyma (Table 4–4). In a noncirrhotic liver, the tumor commonly presents as a single large mass in the right lobe, which may contain regions of necrosis and hemorrhage. This presentation has been described as the *massive* type of hepatocellular carcinoma. The cut surface appears multilobular. Satellite tumors are frequently clustered around the larger primary lesion. Most resectable tumors are of this type.

In a cirrhotic liver, hepatocellular carcinoma is usually multifocal, with lesions of various sizes scattered throughout the liver. A section through apparently uninvolved liver often reveals unsuspected minute tumor nodules. This morphology has been termed the *nodular* type of hepatocellular carcinoma. It is not uncommon for the malignancy nearly to replace the residual liver prior to manifesting clinically.

A third type, the *diffuse* form, is rare. This form infiltrates widely and may not be distinguishable grossly or radiologically from surrounding cirrhosis. These tumors are not resectable.

Through mass screening efforts, the Japanese and Chinese have uncovered a population of patients with small, isolated hepatocellular carcinomas, 3 to 5 cm in diameter, which have been called *minute* carcinomas. Whether these represent earlier stages of one of the above three morphologies or a separate, fourth type is unclear. These tumors have a thick, fibrous capsule and are generally well differentiated and slow growing. They have a high resectability rate and a more favorable prognosis than the above three morphologies.

Of special importance is the *fibrolamellar* carcinoma, a type of hepatocellular carcinoma that is distinct in several ways. The tumor has a slight predilection for the left lobe. The characteristic features are fibrous septa apparent on cross section grossly as well as on cross-sectional imaging studies.

TABLE 4–4
Morphologic Classification of Hepatocellular Carcinoma

Massive	Minute
Nodular	Fibrolamellar
Diffuse	

TABLE 4–5
Distribution of Metastases in Hepatocellular Carcinoma

Lymph nodes	Adrenal
Lung	Brain
Bone	

Hepatocellular carcinomas derive their blood supply primarily from the hepatic artery, an observation of great therapeutic importance. Neovascularity from surrounding structures such as the diaphragm, stomach, colon, omentum, and anterior abdominal wall can develop.

Vascular invasion is common. Obstruction of the portal vein can lead to portal hypertension, resulting in ascites or varices. Invasion and obstruction of the inferior vena cava may lead to lower extremity edema or renal vein thrombosis. Blockage of the hepatic veins can result in the Budd-Chiari syndrome. Invasion of the major bile ducts by tumor is rare but can account for hemobilia.

Hepatocellular carcinoma is primarily locally invasive until the late stages of the disease, when metastatic spread to lymph nodes, lung, bone, adrenal, and brain, in order of decreasing frequency, is seen (Table 4–5).

Histology

One of the striking features of hepatocellular carcinoma is the dramatic dichotomy between the tumor's aggressive biologic nature and its often innocuous histology. Well-differentiated hepatocellular carcinoma cells closely resemble normal hepatocytes. The tumor often grows in a trabecular pattern, distinguished from normal liver by the presence of more than two to three cell layers between endothelial-lined sinusoids (Fig. 4–1). The compact type of histology is characterized by cellular aggregates without recognizable sinusoids. The cells are smaller and more atypical, with increased nuclear pleomorphism and reduced cellular cytoplasm. The presence of bile either intracellularly or between cells is pathognomonic for hepatocellular carcinoma.

The acinar or pseudoglandular histology consists of malignant cells forming glandlike structures surrounding central spaces, which may contain bile (Fig. 4–2). Portions of a hepatocellular carcinoma may consist of clear cells containing large amounts of glycogen.

The most malignant histology consists of highly atypical, bizarre cells with tremendous nuclear pleomorphism. Mitoses are common. Polynuclear giant cells may be present (Fig. 4–3).

Although the above schema is useful in describing individual tumors, it must be recognized that the histologic appearance of a tumor can vary tremendously from one zone to another.

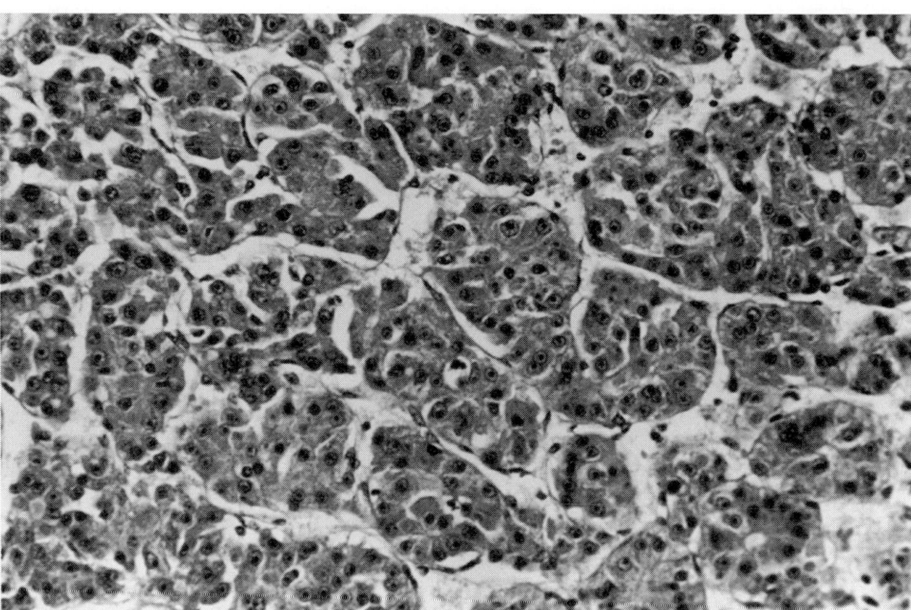

FIGURE 4–1. Hepatocellular carcinoma, well-differentiated, trabecular variant (hematoxylin-eosin, ×400).

The fibrolamellar variant histologically consists of large, uniform eosinophilic polygonal cells separated by intersecting bands of fibrous stroma. Nuclei are vesicular with a single nucleus. Mitoses are rare.

Presentation

Hepatocellular carcinoma remains one of the most lethal solid cancers precisely because, in its early and most treatable stages, symptoms are few or absent. In the cirrhotic patient, the development of hepatocellular carcinoma may manifest as a worsening of the patient's pre-existing signs and symptoms of liver failure (Table 4–6). Frequent complaints are weakness, fatigue, anorexia, and weight loss. Abdominal pain centered over the tumor is seen in the majority of patients. Radiation to the shoulder suggests involvement of the diaphragm. Recurring or continuous fever, occasionally quite dramatic, in the cirrhotic patient should raise concern. Jaundice is a rare and grave sign, often implying near-complete replacement of the liver with tumor. Particularly in areas of high incidence, such as South Africa, young patients may initially present with exsanguinating intra-abdominal hemorrhage caused by rupture of the tumor. This presentation, although rare, is also recognized in the United States and other areas of low incidence.

Early hepatocellular carcinomas are associated with few if any abnormal physical findings. In contrast, advanced

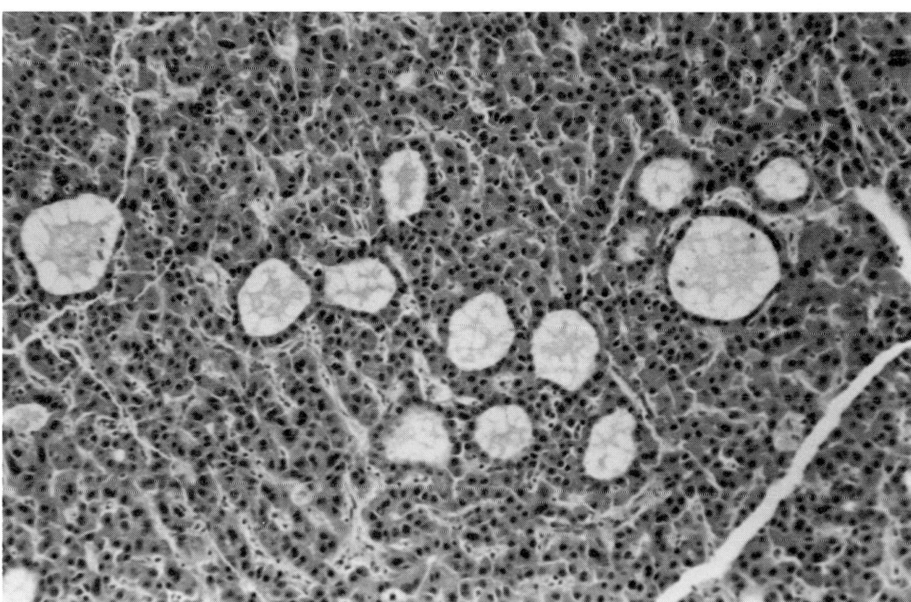

FIGURE 4–2. Hepatocellular carcinoma, well-differentiated, acinar (pseudoglandular) variant (hematoxylin-eosin, ×100).

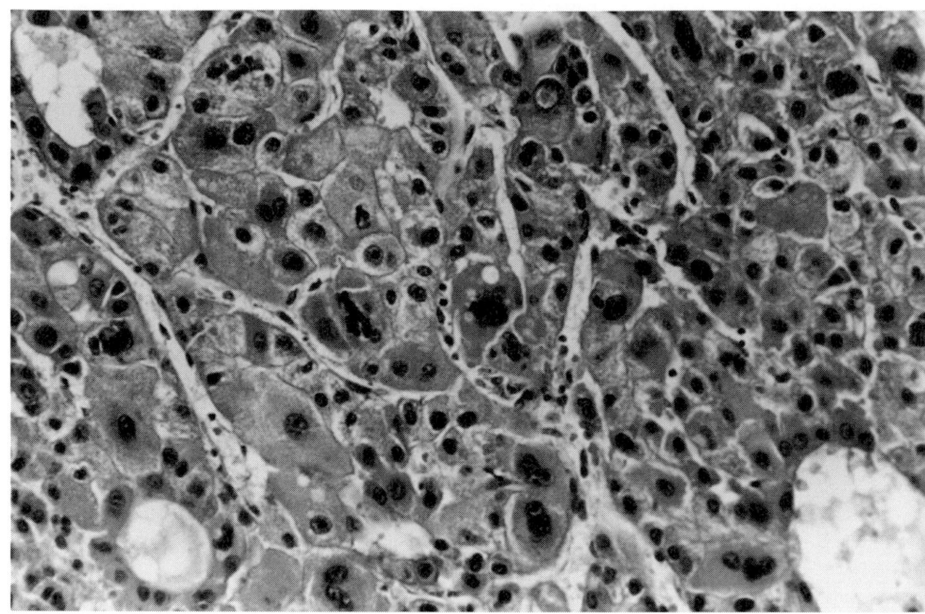

FIGURE 4–3. Hepatocellular carcinoma, giant cell variant (hematoxylin-eosin, ×400).

tumors can easily be recognized by the presence of hard, irregular, nontender hepatomegaly, commonly massive in degree. The tumor can often be recognized by simple visual inspection of the abdomen. A hepatic bruit is a nonspecific supportive finding. Associated signs such as splenomegaly and ascites are seen in the minority of patients. Lymphadenopathy is vanishingly rare.

Paraneoplastic syndromes are seen in 4% to 5% of patients and can lead to the early diagnosis of this malignancy if recognized. The most common syndromes are hypoglycemia, hypercholesterolemia, and erythrocytosis, although a wide spectrum of other paraneoplastic syndromes associated with hepatocellular carcinoma have been described.[11]

Screening

Screening of high-risk patients may have an important role in identifying subclinical and potentially curable cases of hepatocellular carcinoma, particularly in those regions of the world, such as Japan and China, where the tumor is often not associated with advanced liver disease.[12] Tsukuma and colleagues[13] recently reported the results of a large screening program in Osaka. A total of 917 patients with either compensated cirrhosis or chronic hepatitis were followed. Among patients with cirrhosis, the cumulative risk for development of hepatocellular carcinoma was 12.5% at 3 years. The risk among patients with hepatitis was 3.8% at 3 years. Particular risk factors for the development of hepatocellular carcinoma identified from this study were elevated alpha-fetoprotein (AFP) levels at entry and positive serum markers for hepatitis B and C. Clinical outcome for those patients identified with hepatocellular carcinoma was not reported in this paper.

TABLE 4–6
Signs and Symptoms of Hepatocellular Carcinoma

Increasing liver failure	Weight loss
Ascites, coagulopathy, encephalopathy	Fever
	Jaundice
Abdominal pain	Intra-abdominal hemorrhage
Weakness	Mass, hepatomegaly
Fatigue	Hepatic bruit
Anorexia	Paraneoplastic symptoms

The role for screening in Western countries is less clear. In a large prospective Italian trial, 447 patients with well-compensated cirrhosis (62% due to viral hepatitis) were followed from 1985 to 1990 with serial AFP levels and ultrasonography. Thirty hepatocellular carcinomas were found on admission and 29 during follow-up. Seventeen potentially resectable tumors were identified, but only four of the tumors detected on follow-up were thought to be resectable. Twelve patients underwent surgery, with a 1-year survival rate of 67% and a 60% recurrence rate at 1 year. From this study, the yearly incidence rate of hepatocellular carcinoma in Western cirrhotic patients can be estimated to be 3%.[14]

Although unproven in Western countries, it is generally recommended that patients with known risk factors for hepatocellular carcinoma undergo, at a minimum, biannual measurements of their AFP levels and annual computed tomography (CT) or ultrasound examinations of their liver. The estimated cost of such a screening program is $35,000 per year per patient diagnosed with hepatocellular carcinoma.

Evaluation

Laboratory Studies

All patients being evaluated for any hepatobiliary tumor should undergo baseline prothrombin time and liver func-

TABLE 4–7
Routine Liver Function Tests

Prothrombin time	Alanine aminotransferase
Bilirubin: total, direct, indirect	Alkaline phosphatase
Aspartate aminotransferase	Gamma glutamyltransferase

tion tests to measure synthetic function, presence of ongoing hepatocyte injury, and canalicular enzymes and bilirubin to determine signs of biliary obstruction (Table 4–7).

Baseline tumor markers routinely obtained include AFP, carcinoembryonic antigen (CEA), and carbohydrate antigen CA 19-9. Measurement of AFP level is the most valuable test. This protein is produced by fetal liver hepatocytes and dedifferentiated liver cells. Seventy-five percent to 95% of patients with hepatocellular carcinoma have elevated AFP levels. The upper limit of normal by the radioimmunoassay is approximately 30 to 40 ng/ml. Levels above 400 ng/ml are highly suggestive of hepatocellular carcinoma. False-positive tests are noted in testicular carcinoma, embryonal carcinoma, and teratocarcinoma, and, rarely, hepatic metastases and benign hepatic disease such as cirrhosis and in regenerating liver. AFP levels should be measured preoperatively and then followed in the postoperative period. If the resection is complete, AFP levels should return to normal within 6 weeks. Any elevation during follow-up should immediately prompt an investigation for recurrence.

A variety of other substances have been detected in association with hepatocellular carcinoma, most notably des-gamma-carboxyprothrombin.[15] Experience with these assays is still limited, but they may become clinically important in the future.

Imaging Studies

Patients being referred to the hepatobiliary surgeon have almost invariably had an abdominal ultrasound or CT scan, or both. These studies are often complementary in visualizing tumors. Although the CT scan gives clear anatomic definition, it is occasionally inadequate in visualizing the hepatic vasculature. Occasionally tumors are isodense and not well visualized by CT. Magnetic resonance angiography (MRA) and CT portography are the most effective and sensitive studies to assess resectability. The use of magnetic resonance imaging (MRI) and MRA avoids the use of intravenous contrast, provides adequate resolution, and also provides multiplanar images of the tumor. Standard celiac arteriography is being used less frequently than in the past but still has a role in situations in which preoperative arterial embolization is desired. The occasional arterial anomaly not detected on preoperative MRA can easily be identified at the time of resection. MRI is also reliable in differentiating hepatocellular carcinoma from such benign lesions as hemangiomas and simple and complex cysts. With the availability of MRI, we believe that liver-spleen imaging with technetium Tc 99m, sulfur colloid has little additional utility.

Before a treatment strategy is embarked on, an aggressive metastatic evaluation is indicated. A CT examination of the lungs as well as a bone scan helps exclude metastatic disease. In the very rare circumstance of the patient with neurologic signs, imaging by CT or MRI of the brain is necessary.

Biopsy Studies

Preoperative percutaneous core needle biopsy is useful in establishing the diagnosis unless a large, noncystic hepatic mass is demonstrated concurrent with an extremely elevated AFP level. Simultaneous biopsy of the uninvolved liver is recommended to exclude underlying cirrhosis. Although very uncommon, seeding of the skin has been reported following percutaneous biopsy.[16]

Laparoscopy and laparoscopically guided liver biopsy can be useful preoperative tools in assessing both the tumor and, often more importantly, the status of the uninvolved liver. Peritoneal spread is easily visualized. Laparoscopy is not helpful in assessing the porta hepatis and retroperitoneum, especially in the presence of portal hypertension.

Intraoperative Imaging Studies

When preoperative imaging of the liver has been inconclusive, or when there is particular concern that tumors exist outside of the planned resection, intraoperative ultrasound can be used. Laparoscopic ultrasound probes are being developed. Early reports suggest that intraoperative ultrasound may be as sensitive as MRI or CT portography in detecting occult hepatic metastases. Carbon dioxide contrast infusion can further enhance intraoperative imaging by ultrasound.[17]

Staging

No universally accepted staging system has been developed for hepatocellular carcinoma. The most commonly used scheme is that developed by Okuda et al.[18] using pooled data from three prominent Japanese centers (Table 4–8). This staging system reflects the tumor size and three variables (ascites, albumin, bilirubin) associated with the underlying liver function and degree of cirrhosis. No attempt is made to classify patients by presence or absence of metastases or to subclassify the extent of malignancy

TABLE 4–8
Okuda Classification of Hepatocellular Carcinoma

	Tumor Size		Ascites		Albumin		Bilirubin	
	>50%	*<50%*			*<3 g/dl*	*>3 g/dl*	*>3 mg/dl*	*<3 mg/dl*
Stage	+	−	+	−	+	−	+	−
I								
II				1 or 2 +				
III				3 or 4 +				

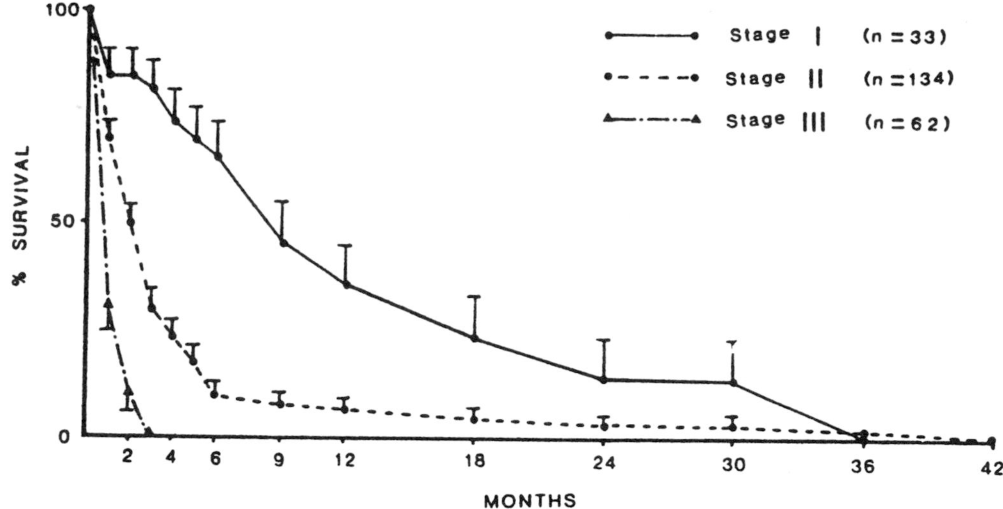

FIGURE 4–4. Survival of 229 patients with hepatocellular carcinoma who received no specific therapy. Median survival for stage I was 8.3 months, stage II 2.0 months, stage III 0.7 months. (From Okuda K, et al: Natural history of hepatocellular carcinoma and prognosis in relation to treatment study of 850 patients. Cancer 56:918–928, 1985.)

other than to delineate those patients whose tumor replaced less than or more than 50% of the liver volume. Although simplistic, this staging system effectively predicts survival irrespective of treatment, as seen in Figure 4–4.

An alternative staging system is the TNM pathologic classification (Table 4–9).

Treatment

Hepatocellular carcinoma remains one of the most highly lethal forms of cancer and, in the majority of cases, is incurable. The essence of the problem is, in a word, multicentricity. As previously described, most cases of hepatocellular carcinoma, particularly in the Western world, arise in a cirrhotic liver. The continuous cycle of injury and repair leading to cirrhosis also predisposes the entire parenchyma to malignant changes. Thus, it is not unexpected that attempts to cure this disease with resectional or local ablative procedures have a high failure rate. Acknowledging the common multicentricity of this tumor, several groups have explored total hepatectomy and orthotopic liver transplantation in the treatment of hepatic malignancies.

TABLE 4–9
pTNM Classification of Hepatocellular Carcinoma

Stage I	T1	N0	M0
Stage II	T2	N0	M0
Stage III	T1	N1	M0
	T2	N1	M0
	T3	N0, N1	M0
Stage IVA	T4	Any N	M0
Stage IVB	Any T	Any N	M1

T1: Solitary, ≤2 cm, without vascular invasion
T2: Solitary, ≤2 cm, with vascular invasion
Multiple, one lobe, ≤2 cm, without vascular invasion
Solitary, >2 cm, without vascular invasion
T3: Solitary, >2 cm, with vascular invasion
Multiple, one lobe >2 cm, with or without vascular invasion
T4: Multiple, > one lobe
Invasion of major branch of portal or hepatic veins
N1: Regional
M1: Distant metastases

In this section, the results of therapy, including surgical resection, transplantation, nonsurgical ablative procedures, chemotherapy, chemoembolization, and radiation, are reviewed.

Surgical Resection

Surgical resections are made possible in large part by the normal liver's remarkable regenerative capacity. In animal models, resection of up to two thirds of the liver volume is followed within 24 hours by a burst of DNA synthesis, and within 48 hours the liver mass is doubled. It can be expected that by 7 to 10 days the liver mass will be fully reconstituted. The biochemistry orchestrating this fascinating transformation of a quiescent organ into a rapidly growing one, and then equally amazingly stopping the explosive growth once the animal's requisite liver mass has been regenerated, has been the subject of extensive scientific inquiry, but it is beyond the scope of this chapter.

Considerations

Age

The issue of whether resection is warranted in the aged has been studied. In a comparative study by Nagasue et al.[19] 32 patients 70 or more years old underwent hepatic resection for hepatocellular carcinoma, with a 1-month operative mortality rate of 12.5% and a 5-year survival rate of 17.6%, including hospital mortalities. Although comparison with a concurrent group of patients younger than 50 years undergoing resection demonstrated higher long-term survival in the younger patients (48.6% at 5

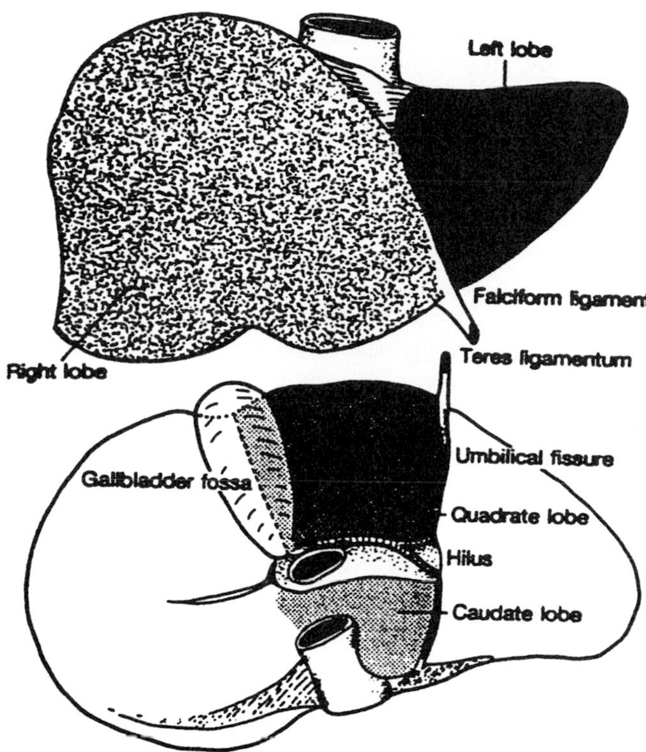

FIGURE 4–5. Morphologic anatomy of the liver. (From Bismuth H, et al: World J Surg 6:10, 1982.)

years, excluding hospital deaths), the acceptable results in the older patients support continued attempts at curative resection irrespective of age per se.

Cirrhosis

Cirrhosis has been considered a contraindication to hepatic resection owing to the increased risk of hepatic insufficiency and bleeding. However, with refinement of operative technique and careful patient selection, anatomic resections, including formal right or left hepatectomies, can be performed safely in patients with well-compensated cirrhosis.[20] Particular care must be taken to exclude multifocal malignancies, which, as discussed earlier, are very common in this setting. Nonetheless, the morbidity and mortality of hepatic resection significantly increase in patients with cirrhosis. For example, in a series of 119 patients undergoing resections for hepatocellular carcinoma at Keio University, 67% had cirrhosis. Overall operative and hospital mortality rates were 9.2% and 5.9%, respectively; however, 17 of the 18 deaths were among the subgroup with cirrhosis.[21]

Principal Resections

Surgical resection remains the only proven, potentially curative treatment for hepatocellular carcinoma. Unfortunately, only 10% to 20% of patients typically referred to the surgeon prove to be resectable, this low rate usually being due to multicentric disease, metastases, or involvement of major vascular structures.[22, 23] In the patient with advanced liver disease, manifested by jaundice, ascites, coagulopathy, or signs of portal hypertension, resection is usually not feasible.

Five principal liver resections are performed, determined for the most part by involvement of the key vascular structures. If no major vessels are involved and the tumor is located peripherally, a simple *nonanatomic* wedge resection can be done. This usually entails temporary local hepatic compression by a noncrushing clamp, excision of the lesion with a 1- to 2-cm margin, and local hemostasis. The remaining resections are termed *anatomic*, since they are based on the vascular anatomy of the liver as defined by Couinaud (Figs. 4–5 to 4–7).

The most common of the anatomic resections, the right hepatectomy, is performed by ligating the right branches of the hepatic artery, portal vein, and bile duct. The liver is fully mobilized by division of the right triangular and coronary ligaments and dissection of the liver off the diaphragm, exposing the entire vena cava. The right, and occasionally the middle, hepatic veins are then divided near their ostia with the vena cava. On completion of these steps, a clear vascular demarcation between right and left lobes is apparent. A temporary Pringle maneuver can be performed using a bulldog clamp. The hepatic parenchyma

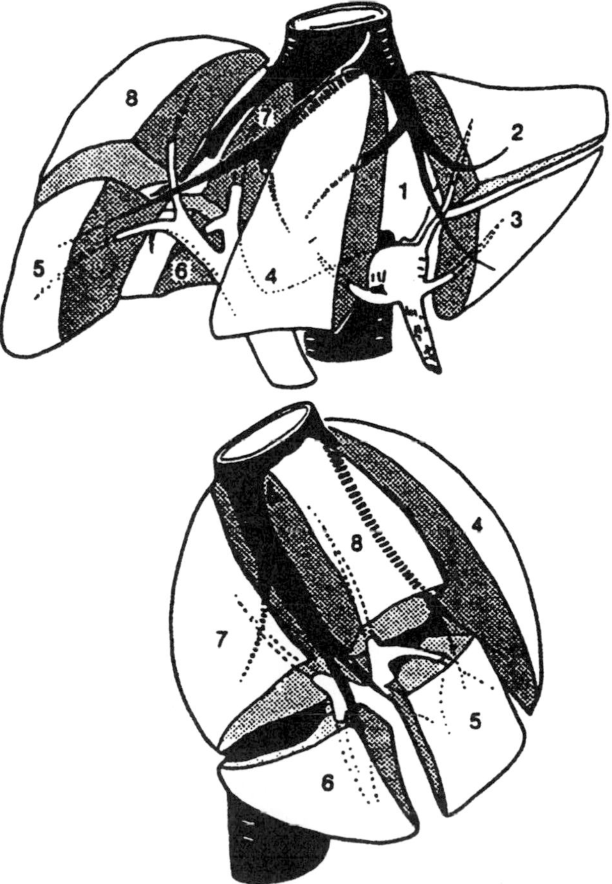

FIGURE 4–6. Functional anatomy of the liver (according to Couinaud). (From Bismuth H, et al: World J Surg 6:10, 1982.)

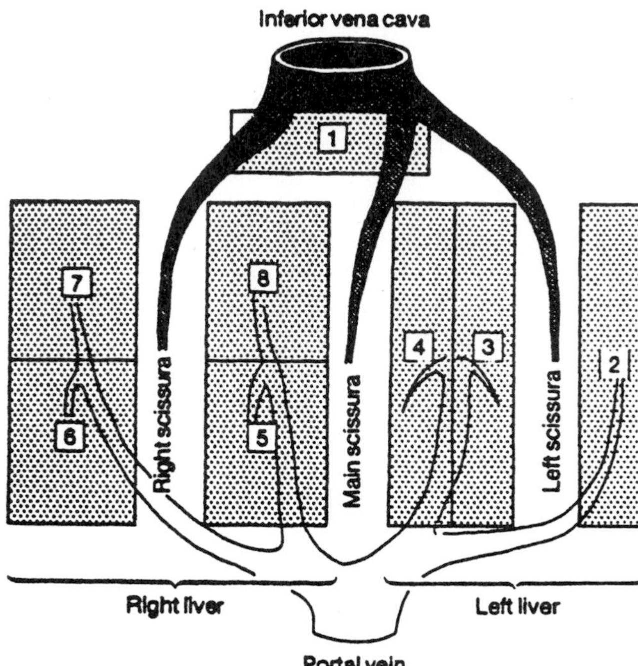

FIGURE 4–7. Simplified schematic diagram of functional anatomy (according to Couinaud). (From Bismuth H, et al: World J Surg 6:10, 1982.)

can best be divided using the simple technique of taking small bites of tissue with a tonsil clamp and ligating with 2-0 silk. We have found this technique to be superior to more cumbersome methods, such as use of the ultrasonic dissector. The plane of division, Cantlie's line, is usually readily apparent, running between the gallbladder bed and the vena cava. Topical hemostatic agents, including fibrin glue, are applied, and compression is maintained for 20 minutes after removal of the Pringle clamp. With the use of this technique, most major parenchymal divisions can be accomplished within 30 minutes and are associated with minimal blood loss (Figs. 4–8 to 4–15).

The left hepatectomy is in principle the mirror image of the right hepatectomy (Figs. 4–16 and 4–17). Mobilization of the left lobe is technically easier, and of course this resection preserves approximately 60% of the hepatic parenchyma, as compared to 40% for the right hepatectomy. The left lateral segmentectomy involves vascular division of the vessels to segments II and III of the liver, followed by resection lateral to the falciform ligament.

Not infrequently, tumors are found that cross Cantlie's line, the anatomic (vascular) division between right and left lobes. In this situation, resection requires either a left or a right trisegmentectomy, or extended hepatectomy in the European nomenclature (Fig. 4–18). Right trisegmentectomies are performed more often than left. The remarkable ability of the liver to regenerate its preresection functional volume within months of operation makes this a perfectly feasible option in the absence of underlying liver disease. The right trisegmentectomy requires resection of the entire right lobe and medial segment of the left lobe. Essentially, all structures to the right of the falciform ligament are resected. The procedure is similar to that for the right hepatectomy except that the gallbladder need not be separately resected and a meticulous division of the "feedback" vessels to segment IV, carefully preserving the remaining vessels and ducts to the left lateral segments, must be performed. This operation removes nearly 80% of the liver parenchyma. Typical results of trisegmentectomy for hepatocellular carcinoma are given by al-Hadeedi et al.[24] from Hong Kong, who reported an operative mortality rate of 12%, a median survival of 9.7 months, and 1-year, 2-year, and 3-year survival rates of 46%, 33%, and 22%, respectively.

Text continued on page 101

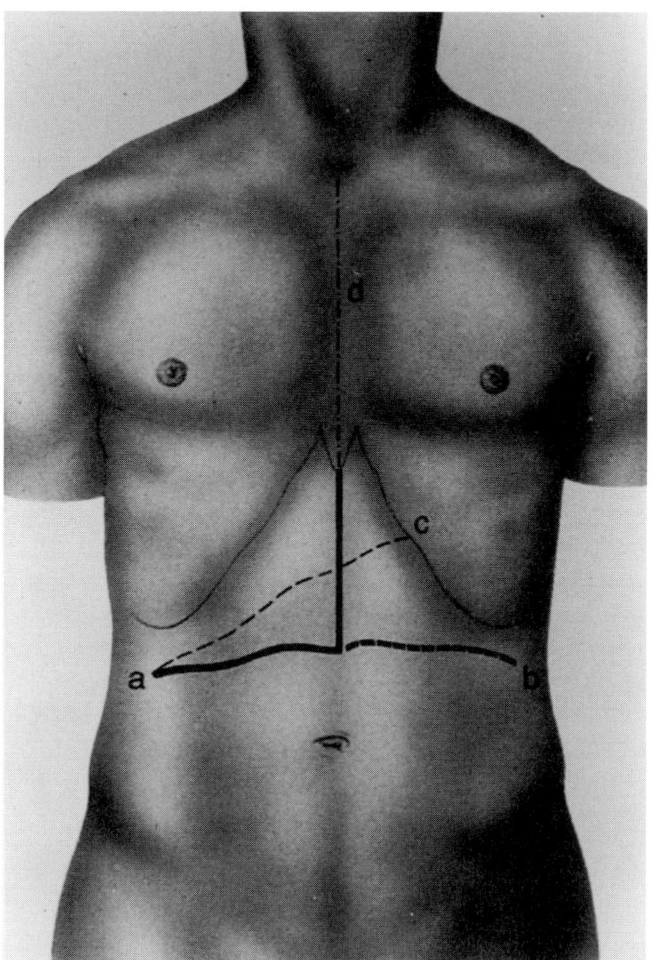

FIGURE 4–8. Standard incisions for hepatic resections. Right-sided resections are best approached via a right transverse incision (a) with a midline extension to the xiphoid. Extension of the transverse incision to the left (b) is performed when necessary. Left-sided resections are approached similarly but usually require at least partial incision of the left rectus muscle (c). Thoracoabdominal incisions are almost never needed. Median sternotomy (d) is very rarely required. (From Kremer B, Henne-Bruns D: Surgical techniques. In Lygidakis NJ, Tytgat GNJ [eds]: Hepatobiliary and Pancreatic Malignancies. Stuggart: Georg Thieme Verlag, 1989, pp 195–218.)

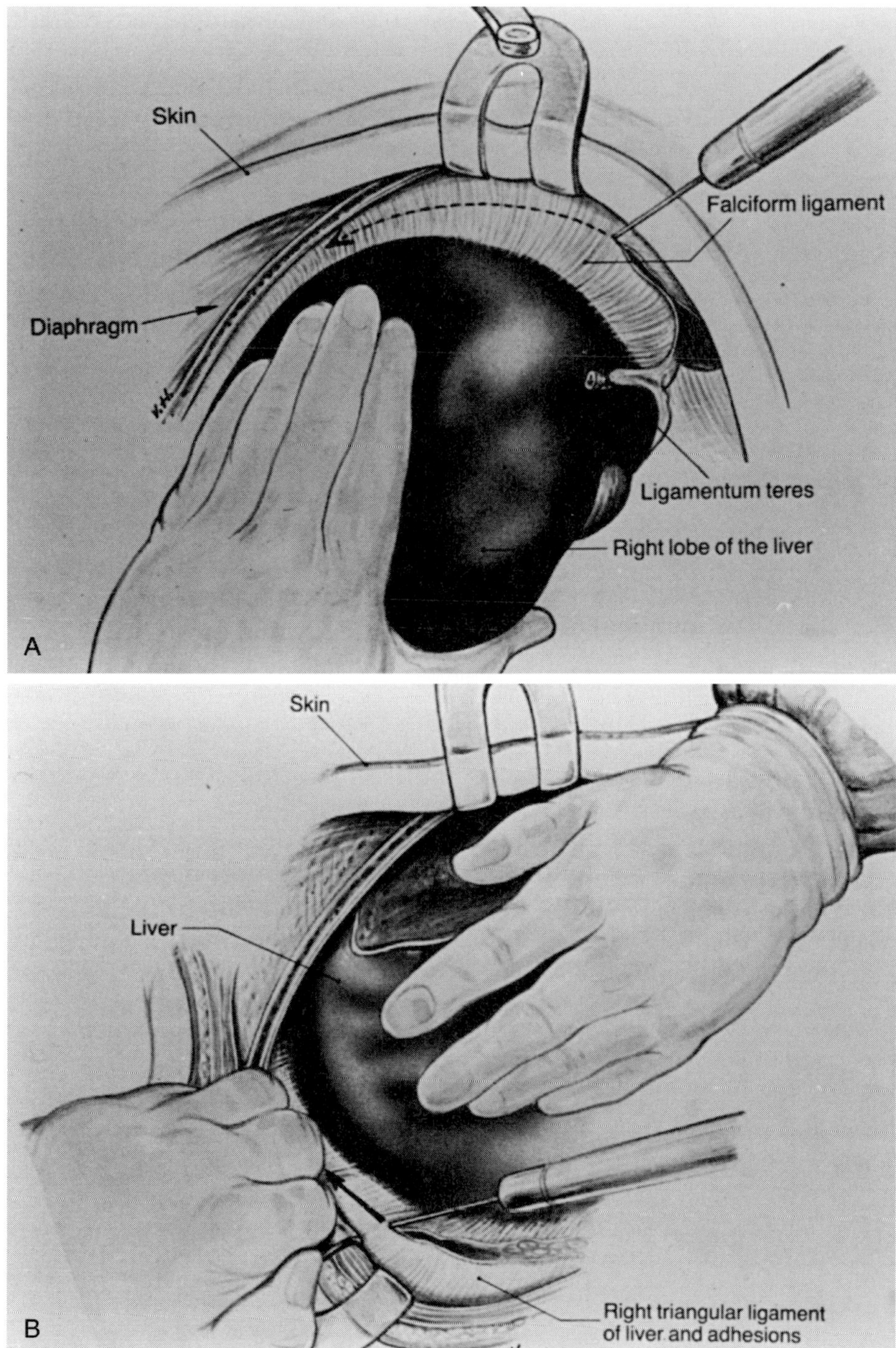

FIGURE 4–9. *A*, Mobilization of the liver. After ligation of the ligamentum teres, the falciform ligament is divided. *B*, The right triangular and coronary ligaments are divided. (From Kremer B, Henne-Bruns D: Surgical techniques. In Lygidakis NJ, Tytgat GNJ [eds]: Hepatobiliary and Pancreatic Malignancies. Stuggart: Georg Thieme Verlag, 1989, pp 195–218.)

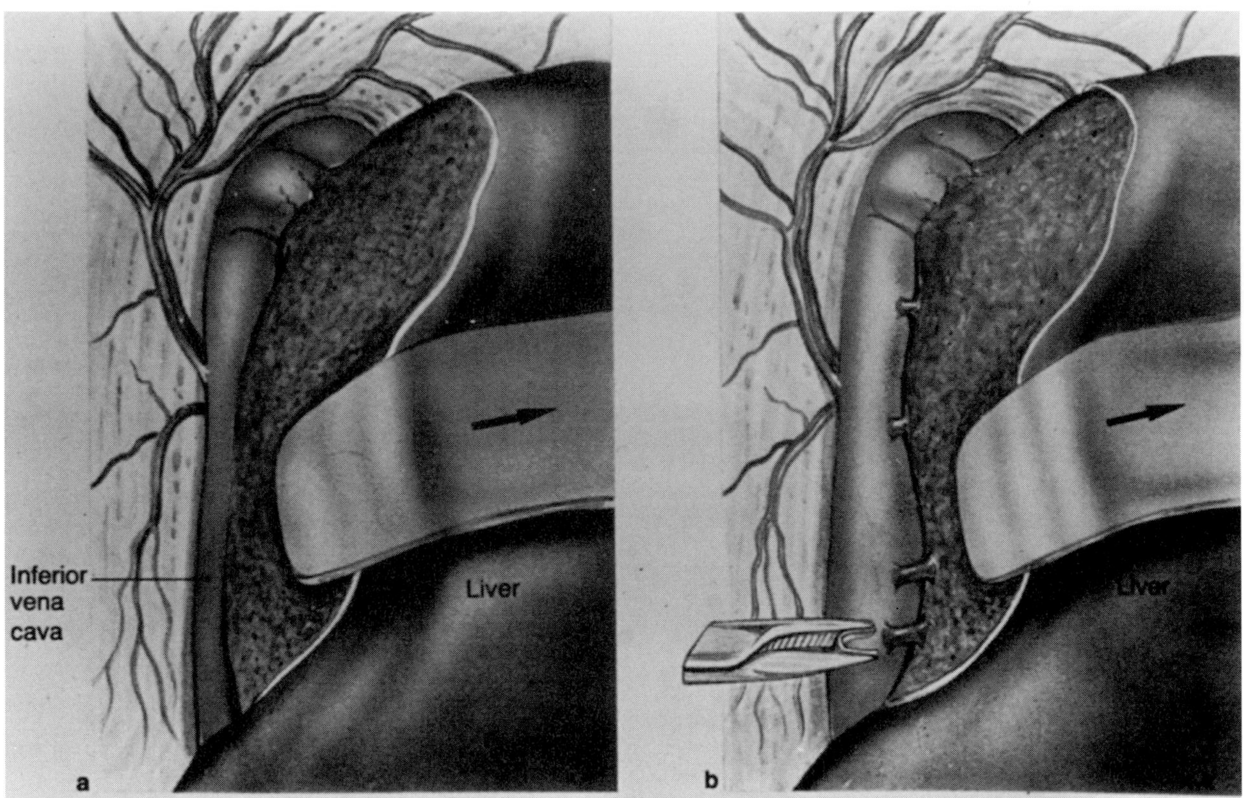

FIGURE 4–10. *A*, Medial traction on the right lobe allows exposure to the infrahepatic vena cava. *B*, Multiple hepatic veins draining segment IV are divided to mobilize the liver off of the cava, exposing the right hepatic vein. (From Kremer B, Henne-Bruns D: Surgical techniques. In Lygidakis NJ, Tytgat GNJ [eds]: Hepatobiliary and Pancreatic Malignancies. Stuggart: Georg Thieme Verlag, 1989, pp 195–218.)

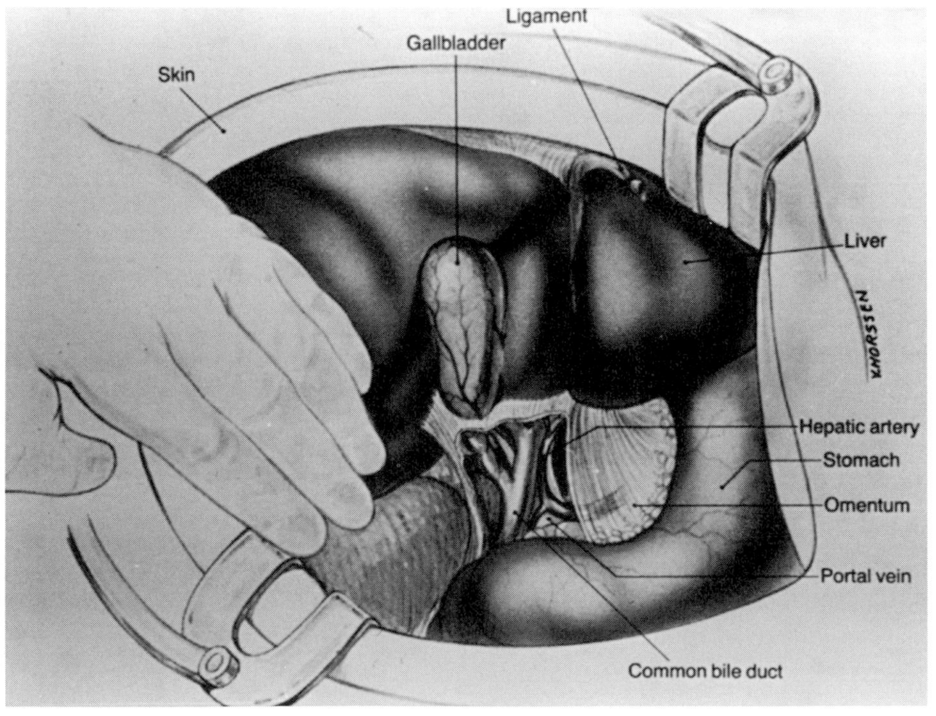

FIGURE 4–11. Operative exposure to the porta hepatis. The bifurcations of the hepatic artery, portal vein, and hepatic duct must be clearly identified. (From Kremer B, Henne-Bruns D: Surgical techniques. In Lygidakis NJ, Tytgat GNJ [eds]: Hepatobiliary and Pancreatic Malignancies. Stuggart: Georg Thieme Verlag, 1989, pp 195–218.)

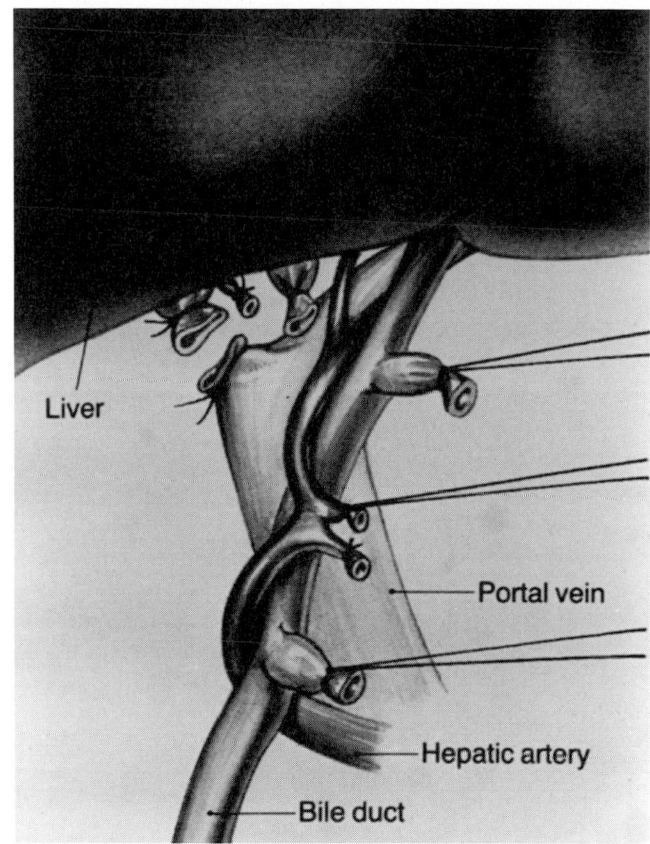

FIGURE 4–12. Schematic appearance of the porta hepatis following division of the right branches of the hepatic artery, portal vein, and hepatic duct. (From Kremer B, Henne-Bruns D: Surgical techniques. In Lygidakis NJ, Tytgat GNJ [eds]: Hepatobiliary and Pancreatic Malignancies. Stuggart: Georg Thieme Verlag, 1989, pp 195–218.)

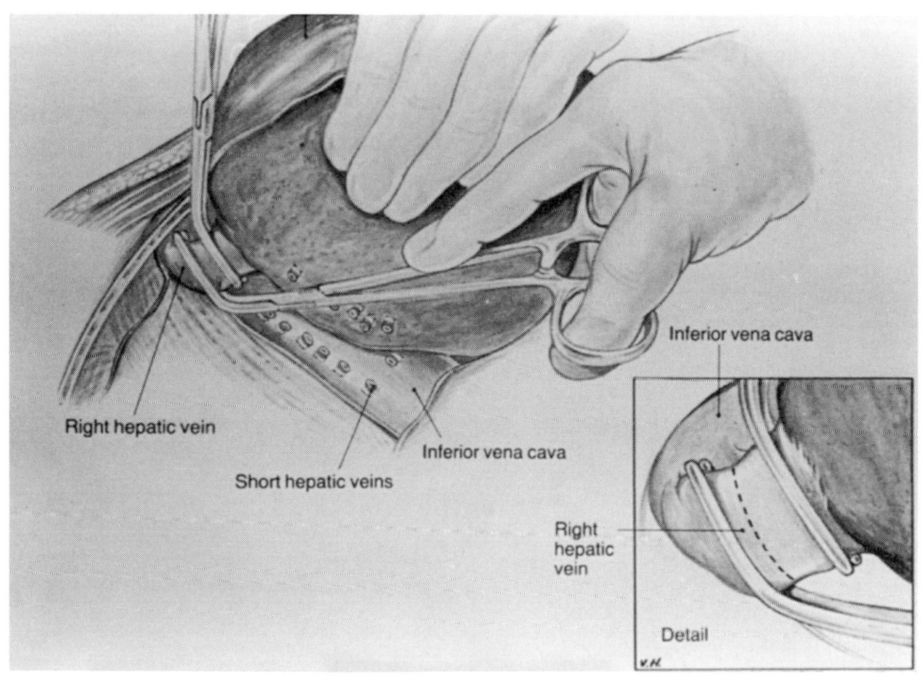

FIGURE 4–13. Division of the right hepatic vein between vascular clamps. The middle hepatic vein can be similarly divided if necessary. (From Kremer B, Henne-Bruns D: Surgical techniques. In Lygidakis NJ, Tytgat GNJ [eds]: Hepatobiliary and Pancreatic Malignancies. Stuggart: Georg Thieme Verlag, 1989, pp 195–218.)

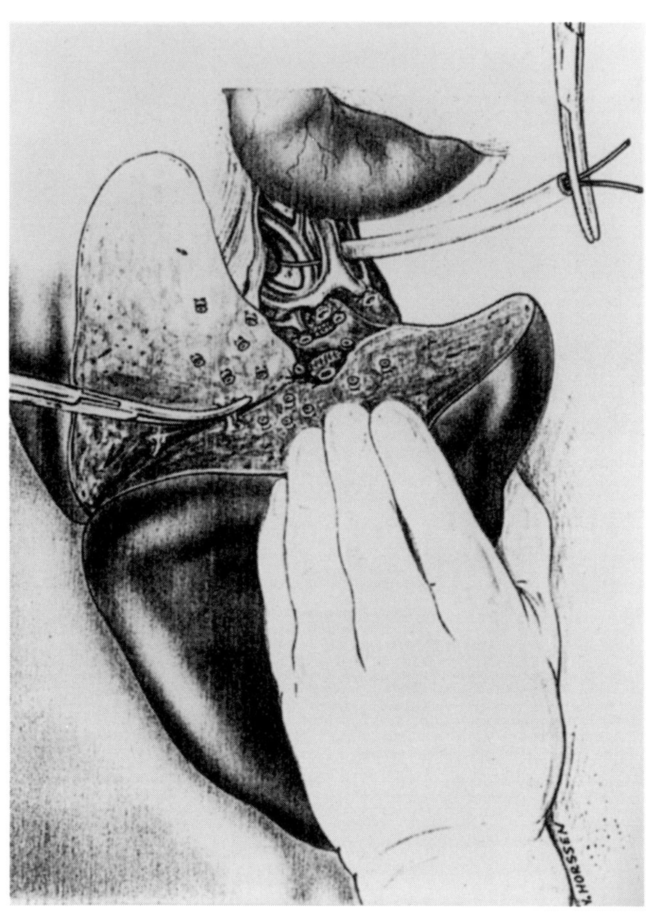

FIGURE 4–14. Division of the hepatic parenchyma. Control of vascular inflow with a Pringle maneuver reduces blood loss. (From Kremer B, Henne-Bruns D: Surgical techniques. In Lygidakis NJ, Tytgat GNJ [eds]: Hepatobiliary and Pancreatic Malignancies. Stuggart: Georg Thieme Verlag, 1989, pp 195–218.)

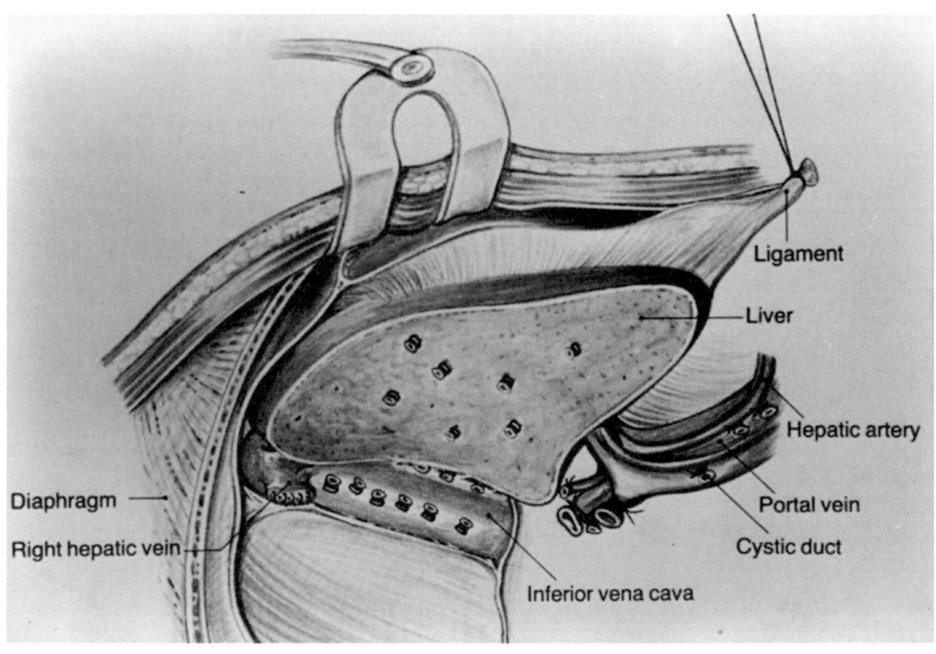

FIGURE 4–15. Completed right hepatectomy. Note that the right hepatic vein orifice has been sutured. (From Kremer B, Henne-Bruns D: Surgical techniques. In Lygidakis NJ, Tytgat GNJ [eds]: Hepatobiliary and Pancreatic Malignancies. Stuggart: Georg Thieme Verlag, 1989, pp 195–218.)

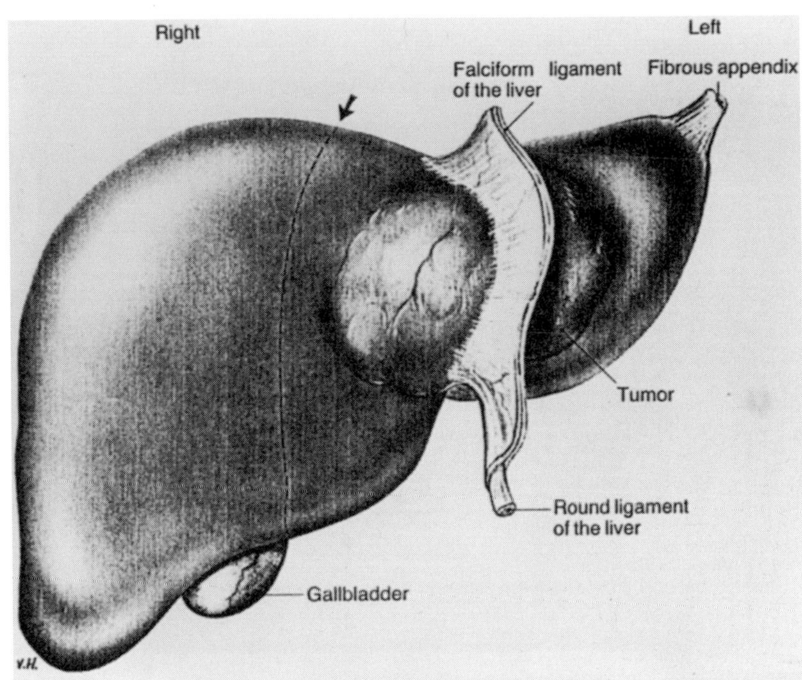

FIGURE 4–16. Plane of division for left hepatectomy. (From Kremer B, Henne-Bruns D: Surgical techniques. In Lygidakis NJ, Tytgat GNJ [eds]: Hepatobiliary and Pancreatic Malignancies. Stuggart: Georg Thieme Verlag, 1989, pp 195–218.)

Formerly, major hepatic resections were associated with massive transfusion requirements. However, over the last 10 to 15 years with the advent of liver transplantation, the vascular anatomy of the liver has become much better understood, allowing for more controlled surgical techniques and subsequently less bleeding. Jamieson and coworkers[25] reported on a series of 75 hepatic resections, including 21 right or left hepatectomies, with a median blood replacement of 0 units; 63% of patients did not receive blood products. In the setting of major hemorrhage, intraoperative autotransfusion is a viable alternative. Although there is a theoretic risk of hematogenous tumor dissemination, a recent retrospective review of 39 patients receiving autologous transfusion during the course of hepatic resections showed no increased risk of metastasis over that predicted for similarly staged patients.[26] Nevertheless, the need for autotransfusion should be rare.

Our approach to difficult resections, particularly if the tumor is encroaching on the vena cava, is to perform total vascular exclusion (Fig. 4–19). This is accomplished by occlusion of the hepatic artery and portal vein at the porta hepatis (Pringle maneuver) and crossclamping of the infra-

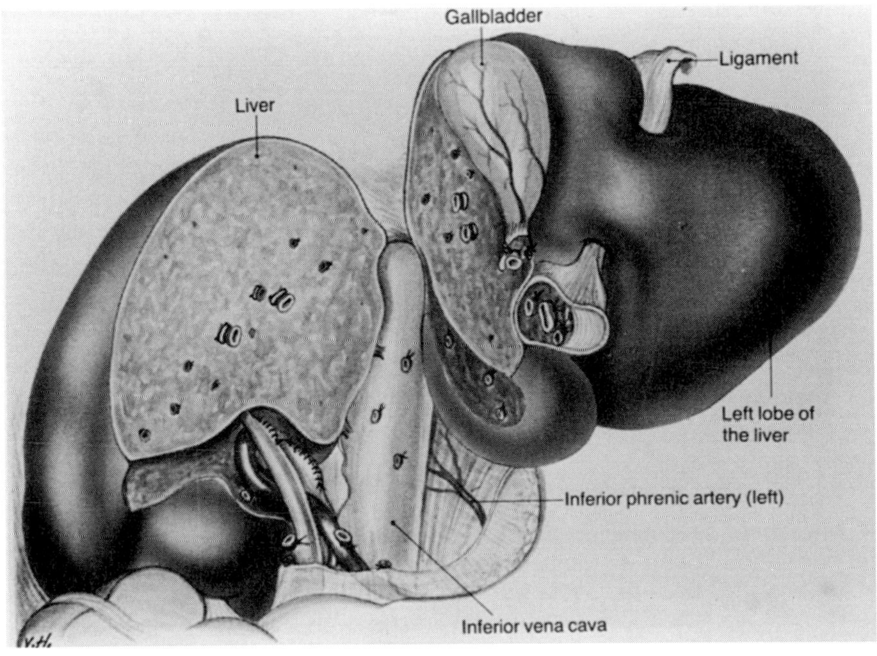

FIGURE 4–17. Completed left hepatectomy. Note division of the left branches of the hepatic artery, portal vein, and hepatic duct. Generally, the gallbladder is removed prior to parenchymal division to facilitate exposure of the porta hepatis. (From Kremer B, Henne-Bruns D: Surgical techniques. In Lygidakis NJ, Tytgat GNJ [eds]: Hepatobiliary and Pancreatic Malignancies. Stuggart: Georg Thieme Verlag, 1989, pp 195–218.)

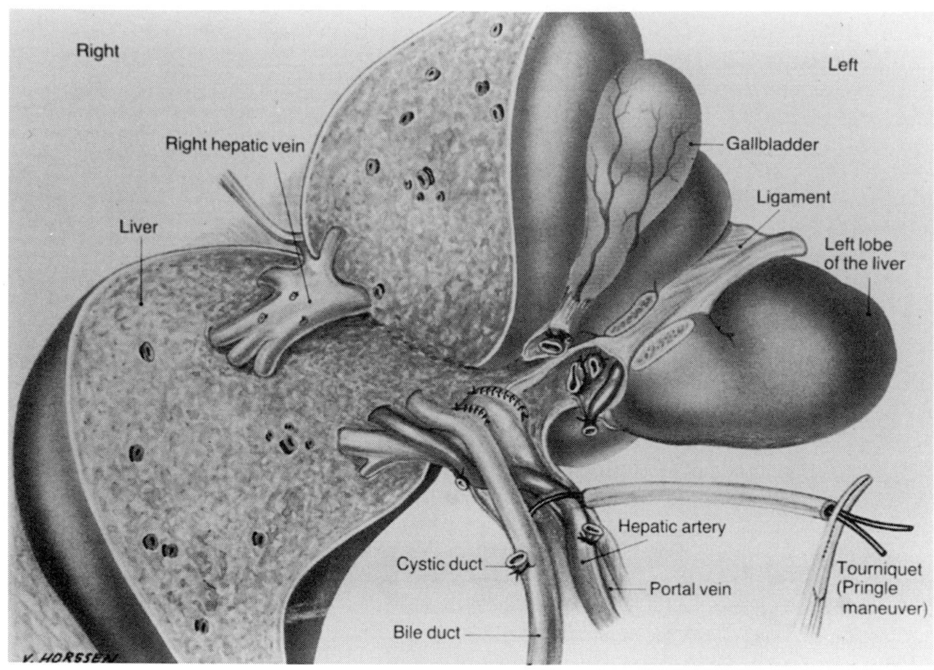

FIGURE 4–18. Left trisegmentectomy (extended left hepatectomy). (From Kremer B, Henne-Bruns D: Surgical techniques. In Lygidakis NJ, Tytgat GNJ [eds]: Hepatobiliary and Pancreatic Malignancies. Stuggart: Georg Thieme Verlag, 1989, pp 195–218.)

and suprahepatic inferior vena cava. Adequate exposure for these maneuvers can be obtained with the standard bilateral subcostal incision with midline extension, including xyphoidectomy; thoracoabdominal incisions are rarely indicated. The large majority of patients tolerate occlusion of the vena cava with minimal hemodynamic compromise. The liver can tolerate 60 minutes of normothermic ischemia. In a series of 53 hepatic resections using portal triad clamping alone (28 cases) or in conjunction with vena caval clamping (25 cases), patients were examined on the basis of the period of normothermic hepatic ischemia. The overall mortality rate was 5.7%, and it was 0% in the 15 patients subjected to more than 1 hour of ischemia. There was no difference in liver function tests or postrecovery liver histology between those patients made ischemic for less than 30 minutes, 30 minutes to 1 hour, or more than 1 hour.[27]

Should the patient not tolerate caval crossclamping, venovenous bypass using a centrifugal force pump can be employed (Fig. 4–20). This is usually instituted by insertion of a perfusion cannula into the inferior vena cava via an open saphenous vein cutdown, plus or minus insertion of a portal vein cannula, with outflow from the pump into the superior vena cava via the axillary vein. Among 521 patients undergoing liver resection by Yamaoka and colleagues[28] at Kyoto University, vascular exclusion and double venovenous bypass were used in 20 patients, 8 of whom were cirrhotic. All patients tolerated vascular exclusion well, except one patient with cirrhosis, who underwent 70 minutes of hepatic ischemia and who died of liver failure.[28]

Recurrence Following Resection

Despite "curative" hepatic resections, most patients with hepatocellular carcinoma have recurrences. Belghiti et al.[29] studied 47 cirrhotic patients after resection of solitary tumors with free margins of greater than 1 cm. Synchronous lesions were carefully excluded with CT following intra-arterial injection of Lipiodol and by intraoperative ultrasound. Survival was 35% at 3 years and 17% at 5 years. Recurrence was 81% at 3 years and 100% at 5 years.

In general, the Japanese find a lower risk of recurrence, probably representing the somewhat different forms of the disease seen in Asia. Typical statistics are from Ikeda et al.[30] They report 1-, 2-, and 3-year recurrence rates of 37.0%, 57.1%, and 71.6%, respectively.

Management of these patients is controversial. Options include reresection if anatomically feasible, intratumoral ethanol injection, chemoembolization, or no treatment. In a large Japanese series from Osaka, 100 patients were followed after resection. There was a 9% operative mortality rate. Forty percent of the remaining 91 patients had recurrences. Re-exploration was carried out in 22 of these patients: 16 underwent reresection, and 6 underwent operative ethanol injections and intra-arterial chemotherapy. Of the 22 patients, 15 were alive at the time of the report, a considerably better outcome than that for the patients with recurrence who were managed nonoperatively.[31]

Nagasue and colleagues[32] followed 161 patients after resection of primary hepatocellular carcinomas. There were 18 operative deaths, and 69 patients had recurrences. Two thirds of the recurrences occurred within 1.5 years. Sex, presence of hepatitis B, type of tumor, tumor encapsulation, extent of resection, and postoperative chemotherapy did not influence the rate of recurrence. Cirrhosis was associated with a higher rate of recurrence. Twenty selected patients achieved a 26.8% 5-year survival rate following reresection.

Park and coworkers[33] analyzed the efficacy of percutaneous arterial chemoembolization in 87 patients with recur-

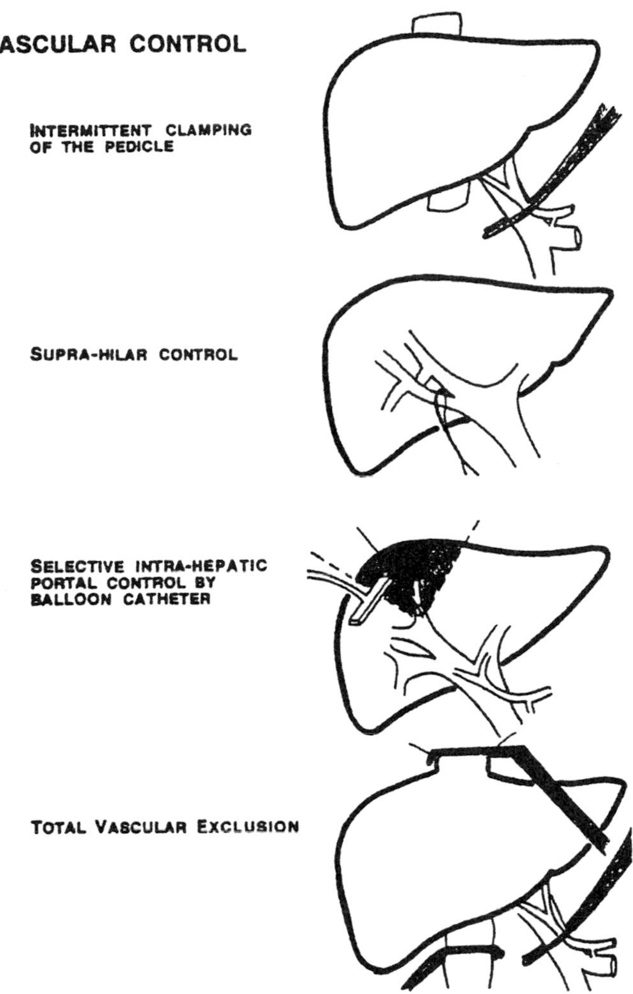

FIGURE 4–19. Techniques of vascular control or exclusion. (From Bismuth H, et al: World J Surg 6:10, 1982.)

rent hepatocellular carcinoma. They achieved 1- and 2-year survival rates of 74.7% and 55.0%, respectively, despite the often multinodular pattern of recurrence.

There have been no careful prospective, randomized trials comparing these different treatment approaches; therefore, although some results seem promising, there is a large element of selection bias, and conclusions must remain tentative.

Complications Following Resection

Complications following liver resections are still frequent in most series, ranging from 11% among noncirrhotic patients in the series by Nagasue et al.[34] to 74% as reported by Fortner and colleagues[35] in 1981. The most common complications are wound infections, bile leaks, bleeding, subphrenic abscesses, liver failure, renal failure, pleural effusions, and pneumothorax.

Series dating prior to 1970 documented operative mortality rates for hepatic resection of between 25% and 45%. Despite the tremendous improvement in operative safety in the current era, there is still a widely held impression, particularly among nonsurgeons, that liver resections are particularly hazardous ventures.

Transplantation

Interest in total hepatectomy and orthotopic liver transplantation for advanced hepatocellular carcinoma is understandable given the frequent multifocality and high recurrence rate for this malignancy, especially in light of the improving safety of liver transplantation. Iwatsuki and colleagues[36] in 1991 reported a comparison between 76 patients with hepatocellular carcinoma undergoing resection and 105 patients subjected to transplantation. The 1- and 5-year survival rates were 71.1% and 32.9%, respectively; for the resection group, compared to 65.7% and 35.6%, respectively, for the transplant group. Long-term survivors tended to have early-stage tumors or the fibrolamellar variant of hepatocellular carcinoma. For small (<3 cm) tumors

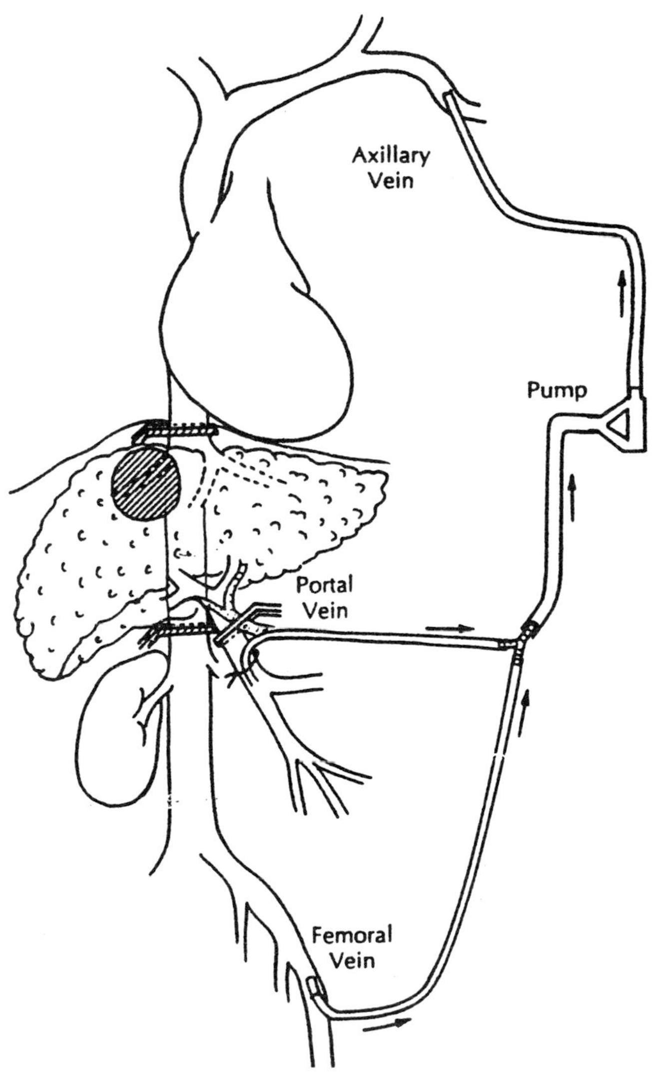

FIGURE 4–20. Venovenous bypass. Caval and portal venous blood is returned to the axillary vein via a centrifugal pump. (From Yamaoka Y, et al: Total vascular exclusion for hepatic resection in cirrhotic patients. Application of venovenous bypass. Arch Surg 127:276–280, 1992.)

in cirrhotic livers, the survival rate at 3 years following resection was only 18%, as compared to 55% following transplantation. Risk factors for recurrence included tumors greater than 5 cm, multiple or noncircumscribed lesions, or vascular invasion. Patients with positive lymph nodes do not survive more than 1 year, whereas patients with node-negative tumors have been reported to have a 2-year actuarial survival of 36%.[37]

In a careful analysis of their extensive experience with transplantation for hepatocellular carcinoma, Ringe and coworkers[38] found an overall median survival of 8.9 months following transplantation. Median survival for patients with stage II (pT2, pN0, pM0) was 120 months, but it was only 11.9 months for stage III (pT1-3, pN0-1, pM0) and less for patients with more advanced lesions. All patients with stage IVB disease (M1) died within 2 months, and all patients with positive lymph nodes died within 1 year. Cirrhosis was associated with a 34.5% operative (30-day) mortality rate, but overall survival was the same between cirrhotic and noncirrhotic patients. Preoperative AFP levels did not influence outcome in this series.

In the University of California, Los Angeles, experience, 28 patients were transplanted for malignancy of the 413 patients transplanted during that period. Sixteen patients had hepatocellular carcinoma, 12 of whom had associated cirrhosis. Seven patients received either chemotherapy or chemoembolization, but all of these patients died. Four patients died in the first 3 months, and 8 others had recurrences. Three patients were surviving at the time of the report.[39]

O'Grady and coworkers[40] reported the experience at King's College Hospital, Cambridge, with transplantation for malignancy between 1968 and 1987. Ninety-three patients underwent transplantation, 50 of whom had primary hepatocellular carcinoma. Nineteen patients in this subgroup had cirrhosis, and seven were found to have the fibrolamellar variant. Among patients with cirrhotic livers, 6 had solitary tumors ranging in size from 2.7 to 6 cm, and 13 had multifocal lesions up to 10 cm in size. Nineteen of the 31 patients with noncirrhotic livers had solitary lesions 8 to 21 cm in size, and 12 had multiple masses. Routine metastatic screening included CT scans of the abdomen and thorax, radioisotope bone scanning, and, in five patients, limited exploratory laparotomy.

In O'Grady and colleagues' study, the survival rate at 3 months was 68.5% for cirrhotic patients and 77.4% for noncirrhotic patients, with deaths being due to hemorrhage (42%), graft failure (25%), sepsis (25%), and rejection (8%). The 1- and 2-year survival rates were 42.5% and 37.3%, respectively, for cirrhotic patients and 48.5% and 38.3%, respectively, for noncirrhotic patients. Twelve patients survived more than 1 year, but only two patients were surviving 5 years after transplantation. One patient was alive 11.8 years following transplantation.

Tumor recurrence occurred in 64.9% of patients surviving beyond 3 months. Recurrence was diagnosed by rising AFP levels or on the basis of radiologic tests. Recurrence was equally common in the liver or lung (57.9%), followed by adrenal (42.1%), bone (26.3%), abdominal cavity (21.1%), and skin (15.8%). Fibrolamellar tumors recurred in three of the seven patients at 6, 9, and 18 months; one patient died of sepsis related to hepatitis-induced cirrhosis; and three patients were alive and free of detectable tumor at 3 months, 1.8 years, and 4.5 years. O'Grady et al. found a significant difference in median interval between transplantation and recurrence when comparing well-differentiated tumors (2 years) and moderate or poorly differentiated tumors (33 weeks). No difference in recurrence intervals was noted between patients with cirrhotic and noncirrhotic livers. Interestingly, patients in the more contemporary era treated with cyclosporine-based immunosuppression appeared to fare better, with a median interval to recurrence of 12 months (range, 4 weeks to 1.2 years).

Somewhat more optimistic results have been reported by Haug et al.[41] from the Boston Center for Liver Transplantation. Of 383 transplant recipients, 24 underwent transplant for treatment of unresectable hepatocellular carcinoma. Actuarial survival was 71%, 56%, and 42% at 1, 2, and 3 years, respectively. Recurrence was noted in 5 of the 20 patients who survived more than 3 months.

Penn[42] published results of liver transplantation for malignancies reported to the Cincinnati Transplant Tumor Registry from centers around the world. A total of 637 patients were studied, 429 of which had hepatocellular carcinomas. Patients ranged in age from 5 months to 71 years, the average being 42 years. Approximately half of the patients had coexisting cirrhosis, chronic hepatitis, or other chronic liver disease. Among the patients with a preoperative diagnosis of hepatocellular carcinoma, there was a 39% recurrence rate at the time of the report, associated with a 91% mortality rate. Life-table analysis showed a 30% 2-year survival rate and, at 5 years, an 18% survival rate. Thirty-one patients had hepatomas discovered only incidentally on examination of the explanted liver, and of these only four had recurrences. Actuarial 5-year survival was 57%, although only three patients from the group had been followed for this length of time. Patients with fibrolamellar hepatomas fared approximately the same, with a 39% recurrence rate. Three patients were alive at 5 years, and the estimated 5-year survival rate was 55% with or without recurrent tumor.

Surgical resection is the preferred approach for hepatocellular carcinoma whenever possible. Given the survival and recurrence data outlined here, transplantation for advanced, unresectable hepatocellular carcinoma presents an ethical dilemma. There are no other potentially curative options for these patients and, clearly, approximately 20% of such patients would achieve long-term cure following transplantation. However, donor organs are an increasingly precious resource, and approximately 25% of patients die while awaiting transplantation. Patients with benign liver disease would be expected to have much higher survival rates following transplantation than patients with cancer. We conclude that, at present, indications for transplantation in the setting of hepatocellular carcinoma should be limited to patients with end-stage liver discase and concurrent early-stage (single lesions < 5 cm) primary malignancies and perhaps to patients with fibrolamellar carcinomas confined to the liver.

Nonsurgical Ablative Procedures

Ethanol Injection

Absolute ethanol, when injected into or around a hepatic tumor, causes local tissue necrosis. As such, it has been used for both curative and palliative purposes in the treatment of hepatocellular carcinoma. The procedure is usually performed under ultrasound guidance.

Shiina and colleagues[43] from the University of Tokyo reported on a series of 146 patients receiving 1048 ethanol injections; 98 patients were treated with curative intent. Two to 8 ml of absolute ethanol was injected per treatment session, performed two to three times per week. Total volume of ethanol was calculated by the formula $V = (4/3)\pi(r + 0.5)^3$ where V is the volume of ethanol in milliliters and r is the radius of the tumor. Histologic evaluation in 21 patients showed 100% tumor necrosis in 15 patients and 90% necrosis in 5 patients. Survival rates among the 98 patients treated for cure were 85% at 1 year, 70% at 2 years, 62% at 3 years, and 52% at 4 and 5 years. Recurrences were common (60% at 5 years) but almost invariably occurred in untreated portions of the liver. These results were confirmed by Tanaka et al.[44] who found that percutaneous ethanol injection significantly increased tumor necrosis, as compared to transcatheter arterial embolization alone, and led to improved medium-term prognosis (1- and 3-year survival rates, 100% and 85% respectively). The Barcelona group[45] has cautioned that tumors larger than 3 cm do not respond as favorably to alcohol injection therapy.

Percutaneous ethanol injection does carry some morbidity. Neoplastic seeding has been described,[46] and the procedure can result in liver abscess.[47]

Cryoablation

In a technique conceptually similar to ethanol injection, the Yale group[48] has utilized liquid nitrogen–cooled probes intraoperatively to freeze a variety of liver tumors in 32 patients, including 3 with hepatocellular carcinoma. Although outcome was generally poor in this heterogeneous group of patients, the authors note that only three patients suffered recurrence at the treatment site.

There do not seem to be any advantages to this technique over ethanol injection, and the instrumentation required is far more complex and expensive.

Transcatheter Embolization

Capitalizing on the fact that large hepatocellular carcinomas derive much of their blood supply from the hepatic artery, investigators have proposed transcatheter arterial embolization as a means to treat these tumors. A single comparative (but not randomized) study of this form of therapy versus resection has been published. Kanematsu and colleagues[49] reported results in 135 patients with early-stage hepatocellular carcinoma treated between 1983 and 1987. Sixty-seven patients underwent hepatic resection, while 68 had transcatheter arterial embolization as their principal therapy. Twenty of the embolization-treated patients were thought, by radiologic and functional criteria, to be potentially resectable. The 1-, 3-, and 5-year survival rates for the surgically treated patients were 89.1%, 74.6%, and 54.6%, respectively. For the 20 potentially resectable patients treated with embolization, corresponding survival rates were 90.0%, 50.0%, and 17.5%, suggesting that surgical resection remains preferable therapy for resectable lesions.

An important indication for tumor embolization is in the patient who presents with shock and a ruptured, bleeding hepatocellular carcinoma. Almost all such patients are men with cirrhosis. Emergency surgery for either resection or ligation of the hepatic artery is associated with a prohibitive mortality rate. The recommended initial approach toward such patients is emergency transcatheter embolization.[50]

Chemotherapy

Standard chemotherapy has been disappointing. The most active single agent, doxorubicin, has yielded measurable responses in only 11% to 17% of patients, and median survival with therapy has been less than 4 months in all trials reported to date. For example, in a randomized trial of 106 unresectable patients given doxorubicin (60 to 75 mg/m^2) versus no therapy, there was only a 3.3% partial response rate. Fatal cardiotoxicity or sepsis occurred in 25% of the treated patients. Median survival in the treated group was 10.6 weeks versus 7.5 weeks in the untreated group.[51]

Other antibiotic chemotherapeutic agents, such as mitomycin C and actinomycin D, have no proven efficacy. Numerous trials have been conducted in search of more active chemotherapeutic agents. None of the alkylating agents, including cyclophosphamide, alanine mustard, and chlorethyl-cyclohexyl-nitrosourea (CCNU), have been shown to be superior to placebo. Similarly, the various antimetabolites, including methotrexate, 6-mercaptopurine, cytosine arabinoside, and 5-fluorouracil (5-FU), are ineffective. Vinblastine and cisplatin have no proven value, but etoposide, another of the plant alkaloids, has shown minimal efficacy in one trial but no advantage in others.

Combination chemotherapy has resulted only in increased toxicity without any increase in response. No series of combination chemotherapy has achieved mean survivals of greater than 5 months, with most series reporting survivals of 2 to 3 months. Hormonal therapy with the antiestrogen tamoxifen has been unsuccessful, as have trials with the biologic response modifiers interferon (IFN)-α, IFN-β, and IFN-γ.

Intra-arterial Chemotherapy

Hepatocellular carcinomas derive their vascular supply from the hepatic artery, and thus intra-arterial chemotherapy should maximize tumor dose while minimizing systemic toxicity. However, no prospective trials have shown that this treatment is any more effective than standard chemotherapy. Extensive experience with intra-arterial chemotherapy for colon metastases to the liver failed to demonstrate a survival advantage, although some reduction in tumor size, at the expense of significant toxicity, was seen.

Several small, uncontrolled trials of intra-arterial chemotherapy for hepatocellular carcinoma have suggested some potential benefit. Nonami et al.[52] reported on the use of postresection combination intra-arterial chemotherapy with doxorubicin, mitomycin C, and 5-FU in 23 patients with high-risk tumors (margin <1 cm, intrahepatic metastasis, tumor embolus, lack of capsule formation). Four patients were excluded from further analysis, leaving 19 patients in the treatment group. A nonrandomized comparison group consisted of 113 surviving postoperative patients (of an original 193 patients undergoing hepatectomy) with similar risk factors for recurrence who did not receive chemotherapy. Limited follow-up at 1 year showed that 18 of the 19 treated patients remained alive. Survival in the comparison group was 85% at 1 year. A lasting benefit from chemotherapy remains to be proved.[52]

Complications of intra-arterial therapy, including infection, thrombosis of the hepatic artery, bleeding, and gastric or duodenal ulceration, have been reported.

Chemoembolization

The term chemoembolization describes a variety of techniques used to embolize the arterial supply to a tumor and simultaneously infuse chemotherapeutic agents. In theory, the combination of embolization and chemotherapy should increase the local concentration and time of exposure of the drug to the malignancy. Many different approaches have been tried. The arterial supply can be interrupted permanently with Gelfoam particles or stainless steel coils or temporarily with starch microspheres. The chemotherapeutic agent can be bound to the embolic material or administered intra-arterially in conjunction with the embolic material. Agents used have included doxorubicin, mitomycin C, and maleic acid conjugated to a lymphographic agent, and iodized oil combined with a variety of agents.

Several enthusiastic reports have shown tumor responses to this form of therapy, but all suffer from significant selection bias.[53–56] At present, there are no prospective, randomized trials to assess the value of this form of therapy. Nagasue and coworkers[57] reported a retrospective analysis of their large series of patients treated for hepatocellular carcinoma. Of 138 patients with resectable tumors, 31 had undergone preoperative chemoembolization. Clinical features of the two groups were similar. Chemoembolization had no impact on long-term survival or rate of recurrence, although chemoembolization was associated with a significantly accelerated time of recurrence (7.4 months vs. 16.0 months). Chemoembolization was associated with increased operative difficulty due to adhesions and neovascularity, hepatic or gallbladder infarctions, and postinfarction abscess formation.

Chemoembolization may have a role in downsizing large, otherwise unresectable lesions. Yu and colleagues[58] from Shanghai Medical University used a combination of cisplatin, mitomycin C, 5-FU, and ethiodized oil (Lipiodol) or absorbable gelatin sponge in 30 patients with large tumors, ranging in size from 5.6 to 12.0 cm. Chemoembolization was delivered was delivered every 4 to 6 weeks for one to five sessions, followed by a 1- to 4-month waiting period. Tumors shrank an average of 31.6%. Five patients had complete histologic necrosis of their resected tumors, but the other 25 still had variable amounts of viable cancer despite chemoembolization. These authors reported survival rates of 89%, 77%, and 77% at 1, 2, and 3 years, respectively.

Kuroda et al.[59] reported similar results but, again, found viable tumor cells in 9 of 14 small hepatocellular carcinomas resected following pretreatment with chemoembolization. Importantly, they found that chemoembolization was completely ineffective in treating nonencapsulated intrahepatic metastases, an indication for which chemoembolization has been advocated.[60] The reason appears to be that small tumors can derive their blood supply from the portal venous system and are thus not rendered ischemic by embolization of the regional arteries.

Radiation

External

The liver tolerates external beam radiation poorly, with exposures above 3000 to 4000 cGy causing lethal radiation hepatitis and necrosis. Lesser doses of radiation have not been shown to improve survival. Combining external beam radiation with chemotherapeutic agents has not consistently improved outcomes.

Internal and Radiopharmaceutical

Order and colleagues[61] at Johns Hopkins have pioneered the use of isotopically labeled antibodies to selectively irradiate hepatocellular carcinomas. Using a combination of external beam radiation, systemic doxorubicin plus 5-FU, and antiferritin antibodies labeled with iodine 131, this group achieved clinical responses in 30 of 66 patients. Median survival was between 5 and 7 months.

Sitzmann and Abrams[62] reported on the use of combination chemotherapy and external beam radiation as well as ^{131}I-antiferritin to downsize unresectable tumors in 10 patients, allowing resection. The 5-year survival rate in this poor-risk group was 48%, similar to the 45% 5-year survival rate in a group of 21 resectable patients treated primarily with resection. Yttrium 90 may replace iodine 131 as a more powerful beta-emitting isotope in this form of therapy.

Prognosis

The natural history of hepatocellular carcinoma is simply not known. There are no historical series with accurate staging that document the prognosis of untreated patients with resectable tumors. It is clear that patients presenting with obvious advanced disease and liver failure have a dismal prognosis, with survival measured in terms of weeks. However, the natural history of the typical patient referred to a surgeon for consideration of resection is unclear. This essential deficiency in our knowledge makes meaningful analysis of post-treatment results difficult, if not impossible. Unfortunately, given the increasing number of potentially efficacious therapies, a true randomized trial using a nontreated control arm may never be done.

Prognosis following surgical resection depends on several variables, including age, gender, tumor stage, presence or absence of cirrhosis, presence or absence of hepatitis, hepatic reserve, presence or absence of portal hypertension, the patient's baseline performance status, and perhaps use of adjuvant therapy. A comprehensive analysis of these variables has been reported by Iwatsuki and coworkers.[63] All surgical series are inherently distorted by selection bias, not only on the part of the surgeons but also by local referral patterns.

The large multi-institutional Japanese review by Okuda et al.[18] provides the best available data of survival as a function of disease stage and treatment. Among 850 patients with hepatocellular carcinoma, overall median survival was 4.1 months. Patients with stage I disease had a median survival of 11.5 months, stage II 3.0 months, and stage III 0.9 months. Survival for untreated patients is clearly influenced by stage, as shown in Fig. 4–4. A comparison of surgical versus nonsurgical treatment for patients with stage I or II disease shows significantly prolonged survival in the resected patients, although it must be stressed that this was a purely retrospective analysis, and it can be assumed that operative candidates represented a selected group with better prognostic factors (Fig. 4–21). It can be seen in Figure 4–22 that for patients with stage I disease none of the nonsurgical treatments (arterial embolization, arterial chemotherapy, systemic chemotherapy) had much impact compared to no treatment, and that, in fact, systemic chemotherapy had a negative effect on survival as compared to no treatment. The causes of death were, in order of frequency, hepatic failure, gastrointestinal hemorrhage, intra-abdominal hemorrhage, and cancer cachexia.

Representative survival statistics following resection are reported by the Japanese group of Nagasue et al.[64] Among 229 patients with primary hepatocellular carcinoma treated by radical hepatic resection over 11 years, the 30-day operative mortality rate was 7.0%, and 5- and 10-year survival rates were 26.4% and 19.4%, respectively. Tsuzuki et al.[21] reported a 5-year actuarial survival of 39%, after excluding the 15.1% of patients who died in the hospital following resection. Arii and coworkers[65] had 1-, 3-, and 5-year cancer-free survival rates after partial hepatectomy of 54.8%, 32.5%, and 25.6%, respectively. In one of the largest American series, Savage and Malt[66] from Massachusetts General Hospital reported a 25% 5-year survival rate following resection in 42 patients with hepatocellular carcinoma. Patients with normal AFP levels had a 37% 5-year survival rate, in contradistinction to patients with elevated AFP levels, none of whom survived 3 years. Patients with positive resection margins or spread to regional lymph nodes had an 8% 5-year survival rate.

Recurrence of hepatocellular carcinoma following resection to clear margins is common, if not universal. Recurrence statistics were discussed earlier. The large majority of recurrences occur in the residual liver (93%), with bone and lung metastases representing only 5% and 2%, respec-

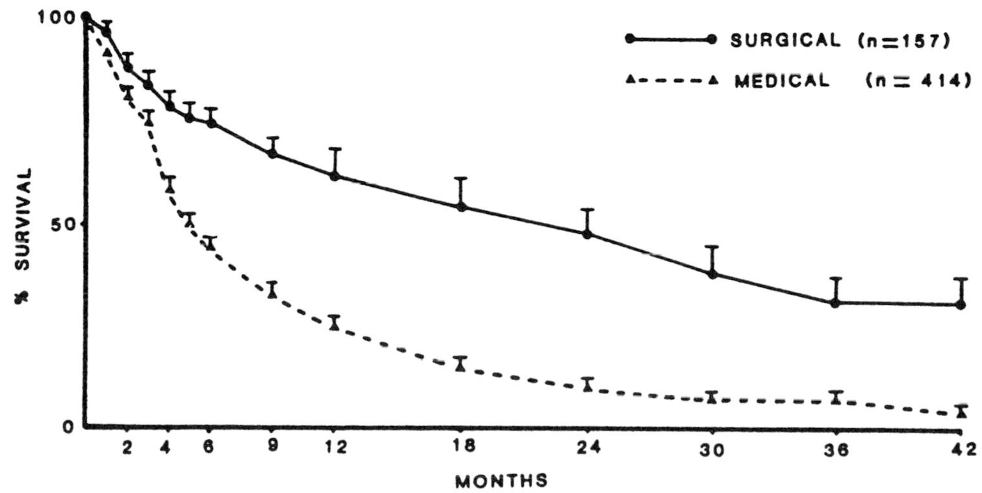

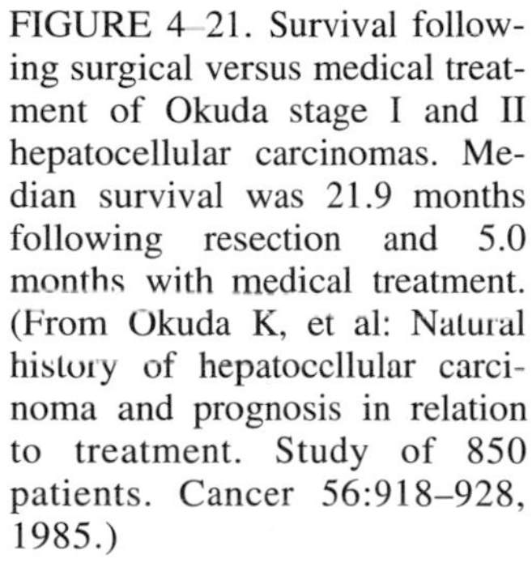
FIGURE 4–21. Survival following surgical versus medical treatment of Okuda stage I and II hepatocellular carcinomas. Median survival was 21.9 months following resection and 5.0 months with medical treatment. (From Okuda K, et al: Natural history of hepatocellular carcinoma and prognosis in relation to treatment. Study of 850 patients. Cancer 56:918–928, 1985.)

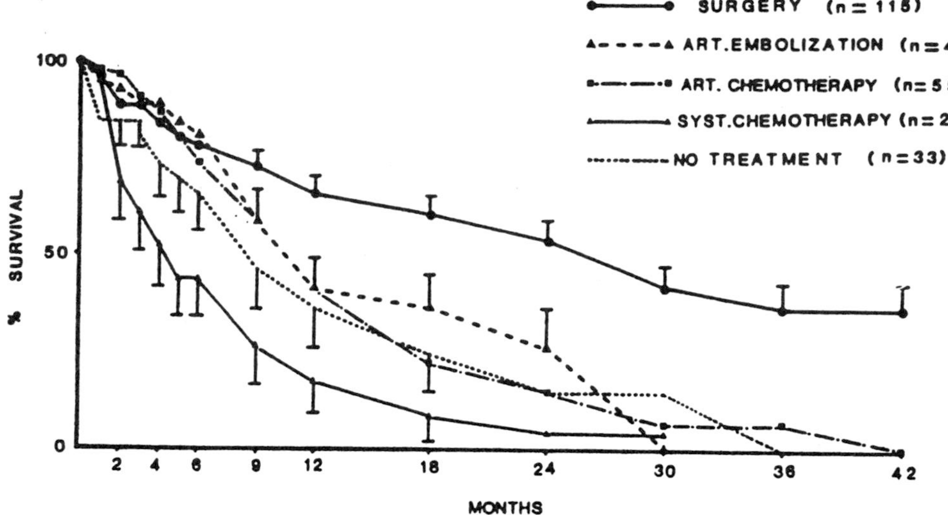

FIGURE 4–22. Comparison of surgery versus other therapies or no treatment for Okuda stage I hepatocellular carcinoma. Median survivals were 25.6 months following surgery, 10.4 months following arterial embolization, 10.3 months following arterial chemotherapy, 4.3 months with systemic chemotherapy, and 8.3 months with no treatment. (From Okuda K, et al: Natural history of hepatocellular carcinoma and prognosis in relation to treatment. Study of 850 patients. Cancer 56:918–928, 1985.)

tively. Most recurrences occur within the first year (56%), with a decreasing rate of recurrence thereafter.[67]

Whether or not patients with the fibrolamellar variant of hepatocellular carcinoma have a better prognosis following resection or transplantation remains unclear. In a retrospective, nonrandomized review of 20 patients with fibrolamellar carcinoma, 14 of whom underwent resection and 6 of whom had total hepatectomies and orthotopic transplantation, the overall survival rate was 36.6% at 5 years, with a median survival rate of 44.5 months following resection versus 28.5 months following transplantation.[68] It is the general consensus that the fibrolamellar form of hepatocellular carcinoma grows more slowly and is more often resectable.

Prognosis of patients with hepatocellular carcinoma and cirrhosis is, in most series, worse than in patients with otherwise normal livers. In a Japanese study by Sasaki et al.,[69] 142 cirrhotic patients were compared with 48 noncirrhotic patients. Five-, 7-, and 9-year survival rates were 44%, 32%, and 26%, respectively, in patients with cirrhosis versus 68%, 57%, and 57% respectively, in patients without cirrhosis. The major cause of death in both groups was cancer recurrence. The smaller American series of Savage and Malt cited above did not find a correlation between cirrhosis and prognosis, which may represent different tumor biology in the Western forms of the disease. In highly selected cirrhotic patients with isolated, peripheral lesions, good results can be achieved, as attested to by the report of Paquet and colleagues[70] from Germany, who performed 23 limited resections. One- and 5-year survival rates were 77% and 49%, respectively.

The presence of concurrent diseases can influence the outcome following hepatic resection. Diabetes mellitus is associated with higher operative morbidity, particularly hepatic decompensation and abdominal sepsis, but mortality in properly managed patients is unaffected.[71] Insulin is known to be important in hepatic regeneration, perhaps accounting for this association.

Nuclear DNA content has proven to be a useful prognostic indication for a variety of malignancies. However, a careful analysis of this variable in 46 patients operated on at the Mayo Clinic showed a diploid pattern in 33%, tetraploid or polyploid in 30%, and aneuploid in 37%. There was no correlation between nuclear ploidy, pathologic findings, or survival.[72] Others have confirmed these findings.[73]

Hepatocellular carcinoma in childhood has a particularly grave prognosis, representing the often far-advanced stage at which these children present. In the largest series found by us, 71 Taiwanese children from 3 to 17 years of age were described.[74] Most presented with abdominal pain and mass, often associated with anorexia, fever, and internal bleeding. Resectability was only 9.8%. The 1-year survival rate was 10%, and only two children are known to have survived 5 years.

HEPATOBLASTOMA

Epidemiology

Hepatoblastoma is a highly malignant neoplasm of the liver, occurring most commonly in infants and young children.[75] Hepatoblastoma constitutes only 0.6% of childhood malignancies but is the most common primary malignant liver tumor of children. The median age at diagnosis is 1 year, and most cases arise in children under 3 years of age. Unusual cases of hepatoblastoma occurring in adults have been reported.[76, 77] There is a 2.3:1 male to female predominance.[78]

The etiology is unknown, although numerous associations have been reported. There is a clear link between the familial adenomatous polyposis syndrome and hepatoblastoma.[79–81] Several trisomy syndromes, including trisomy 2, trisomy 18, and trisomy 20, are associated with hepatoblastoma.[82–84] There may be an increased incidence among siblings and twins.[85] Hemihypertrophy and renal and adrenal gland anomalies are associated. Several toxic exposures, including fetal alcohol syndrome and maternal exposure to metal fumes, petroleum products, paints, and selenium, are reported to increase the risk of hepatoblastoma.[86]

Pathology

Hepatoblastoma commonly presents as a large, solitary tumor in the right lobe of the liver, measuring 10 to 12 cm in diameter. The tumors are faintly lobulated and in about half of cases are encompassed in a fibrous capsule. Hemorrhage and necrosis are characteristic. There may be variable amounts of bile staining.

Microscopically the tumor consists of various combinations of epithelial and mesenchymal cells. The tumor has been subtyped into anaplastic, embryonal, fetal, mixed, and teratoid histotypes.[87] Embryonal and fetal histologies are most common. The embryonal histology is characterized by sheets of immature, small, dark-stained cells with little cytoplasm and prominent neucleoli arranged in a trabecular pattern. Squamous and ductal elements may be present. The fetal pattern consists of more mature–appearing cells containing an increased amount of cytoplasm relative to the embryonal type. Sinusoids and canaliculi may be present. A variable amount of mesenchymal tissue consisting of spindle, osteoid, chondroid, or muscle cells may be seen. The highly malignant anaplastic subtype consists of actively dividing cells with scant cytoplasm. This tumor is highly invasive.

Presentation

Most children present for evaluation of an abdominal mass. Associated symptoms include anorexia, weight loss, fever, weakness, and pain. Precocious puberty in boys due to ectopic production of human chorionic gonadotropin has been reported.[88]

Physical examination demonstrates a large, nontender hepatic mass. Anemia and thrombocytopenia are common. AFP level is frequently elevated but is not specific for hepatoblastoma.

Treatment

Without treatment, hepatoblastoma is rapidly fatal. The best treatment currently available is complete surgical resection. Outcome appears to be better for the fetal subtype. However, despite adequate resection, at least 50% of children have recurrent or metastatic disease within 6 months. Because of the high recurrence rate, chemotherapy is usually recommended as adjuvant therapy, and also as neoadjuvant therapy for patients with bulky tumors in an effort to downstage them and improve their chance for resection.

A large variety of chemotherapeutic regimens have been tested. Using a regimen of cisplatin, vincristine, and 5-FU, the Pediatric Oncology Group reported a 90% 5-year disease-free survival rate for 21 patients with stage I or II disease, a 67% 5-year disease-free survival rate for 31 patients with stage III disease, but only 1 survivor out of 8 children treated for metastatic disease.[89] Thirty-seven patients with unresectable tumors were treated; following therapy, 26 underwent successful resection. Follow-up has shown equivalent disease-free survival between these patients treated with neoadjuvant therapy and a group of patients with resectable tumors treated postoperatively.[90]

The Childrens Cancer Study Group reported satisfactory results with a protocol of continuous-infusion doxorubicin and cisplatin. Among 26 patients with unresectable hepatoblastoma, 25 responded to treatment. A total of 22 patients underwent subsequent surgery: 9 had no evidence of residual malignancy at exploration, 7 had complete resections, and 6 were not completely resectable despite chemotherapy.[91]

Another option for patients failing standard chemotherapy is chemoembolization. The Japanese have reported success with intrahepatic arterial injection of cisplatin-phosphatidylcholine-Lipiodol in the control of an unresectable hepatoblastoma.[92]

The Pittsburgh group and others have reported excellent preliminary survival results among a small group of children who have undergone total hepatectomy and orthotopic liver transplantation for otherwise unresectable tumors.[93, 94]

ANGIOSARCOMA

Although the most common mesenchymal malignancy of the liver, angiosarcoma is one of the rarest of cancers, with only 25 cases per year diagnosed in the United States. The tumor originates from the endothelial cells lining the hepatic sinusoids. The tumor occurs in elderly people and is more common in men by a ratio of 3:1.

A number of specific carcinogens are associated with angiosarcoma, even though in 70% of patients no risk factors can be identified. Thorium dioxide (Thorotrast) is an alpha-emitting radioisotope that was used between 1930 and 1953 as a contrast agent. It is taken up by Kupffer cells, thus exposing the liver to chronic low-level radiation. The latency for malignant degeneration appears to be more than 20 years. Industrial vinyl chloride exposure increases the risk of developing angiosarcoma 400-fold. Other potential carcinogens include arsenic, anabolic steroids, radium, and inorganic copper.

The tumor is usually multicentric and involves both lobes. Usually the tumor consists of blood-filled cysts along with solid tumor nodules. Histologically, the malignancy may have areas of sinusoidal infiltration, solid growth into macroscopic tumor nodules, and/or cavernomatous differentiation (Fig. 4–23). Vascular invasion is the rule. The tumor stains positive with antibodies to factor VIII and vimentin. This tumor can be difficult to differentiate from

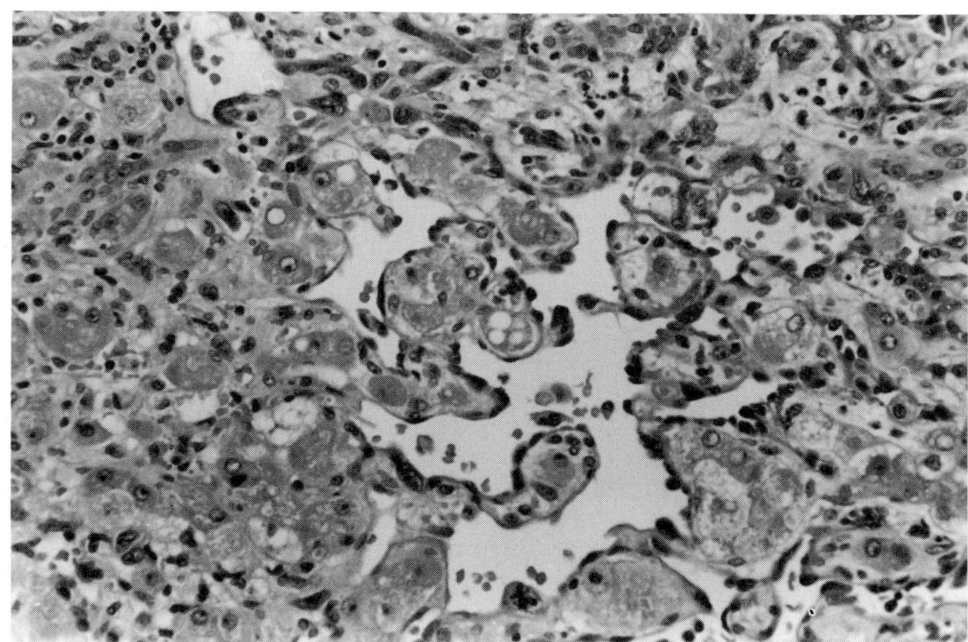

FIGURE 4–23. Hemangiosarcoma, diffuse variant (hematoxylin-eosin, ×400).

epithelioid hemangioendothelioma, but clinically the distinction is important, as the latter responds quite well to liver transplantation, in some cases even in the presence of metastatic disease.

Patients with angiosarcoma present late with symptoms of hepatic failure. The possibility of resection is exceedingly low, as the tumor grows diffusely throughout the liver. Prognosis is dismal, with mean survival less than 6 months. Chemotherapy and radiation are generally ineffective.

PRIMARY CARCINOID TUMOR

A carcinoid is a low-grade malignancy originating from enterochromaffin cells. These cells are part of the neuroendocrine system and are characterized by neurosecretory granules and the metabolic pathway for amine precursor uptake and decarboxylation (APUD). Most carcinoids originate in the appendix, ileum, and rectum, but a small number arise in the liver, gallbladder, and bile ducts.[95]

Like gastrointestinal carcinoids metastatic to the liver, primary hepatic carcinoids may result in the carcinoid syndrome, with flushing, diarrhea, asthma, and right-sided valvular disease.

The indications for resection are

1. Primary hepatic carcinoid tumor not involving extrahepatic vascular or biliary structures, the inferior vena cava, or all four lobes.
2. Debulking of metastatic disease causing the carcinoid syndrome that is refractory to medical management with octreotide or chemotherapy.

Owing to the slow growth of this tumor, patients can have many years of palliation following hepatic debulking of carcinoid tumors.

Hepatic artery embolization and chemoembolization can also be effective in controlling the symptoms related to carcinoid syndrome.[96, 97] Chemotherapy with streptozocin and 5-FU can achieve partial responses in 30% of patients treated.

COLONIC METASTASES

Patients with unresected hepatic metastases from colonic carcinomas seldom survive 5 years, with median survival rates of 3 to 24 months in various series.[98] Surgical resection is associated with a 5-year survival rate ranging from 20% to 50%, depending on selection factors.[99] The multi-institutional study reported by Hughes et al.[100] showed a 33% overall survival rate and a 25% disease-free survival rate at 5 years following resection. Even the presence of positive hilar lymph nodes is not necessarily incompatible with long-term survival.[101]

Despite the significantly improved survival following hepatic resection, recurrence following resection is common, occurring in up to 80% of patients.[102] In 25% and 40% of individuals, recurrence is limited to the liver, and as such is potentially resectable. Several series have proven that reresection in highly selected patients can be performed safely and lead to long-term survival in about 40% of patients.[103, 104] In selected patients, even tertiary reresection or metastasectomy outside of the liver is warranted and can result in significant prolongation of good quality life.

Relative contraindications to liver resection of colonic metastases include synchronous metastases outside of the liver, more than four separate liver tumors, or medical contraindications to hepatic resection. Size of the tumor is

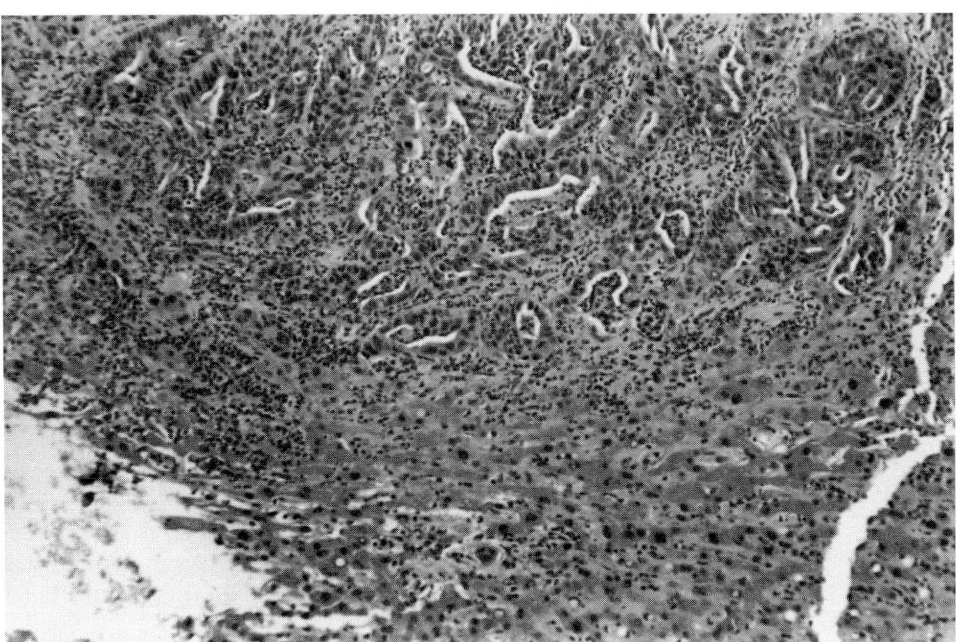

FIGURE 4–24. Metastatic adenocarcinoma, moderately differentiated (hematoxylin-eosin, ×100).

not, in and of itself, a contraindication to resection. Original Dukes stage does not appear to affect subsequent survival.

Factors affecting survival have been analyzed by Savage and Malt.[66] In their series, 104 patients underwent resection of metastases from colorectal primary tumors; the 5-year survival rate was 18%. Resection margins proved to be important. Patients with margins less than or equal to 5 mm had a 9% 5-year survival rate, while those with margins greater than 5 mm had a 27% 5-year survival rate. No patients with tumor outside of the resection margin or with positive lymph nodes survived 5 years. No patients with poorly differentiated primary tumors survived 3 years, as opposed to a 20% 5-year survival rate for patients with well-differentiated or moderately differentiated cancer (Fig. 4–24).

GALLBLADDER CARCINOMA

Epidemiology

Gallbladder carcinoma is the fifth most common gastrointestinal malignancy and is the most common cancer of the biliary tract. In the United States, 2.5 in 100,000 residents are diagnosed with this aggressive malignancy, and autopsy series suggest that the incidence is much higher. Approximately 6500 deaths from gallbladder carcinoma occur in the United States each year.

Gallbladder carcinoma is primarily a disease of older women. The average age at detection is 72 years, with nearly two thirds of patients being over age 70. Women outnumber men by 2.7:1. Nevertheless, gallbladder carcinoma can occur as early as the third decade of life.

There is wide geographic variation in the incidence of gallbladder carcinoma. In Chile, it is the most frequent cause of cancer-related death, and similar high rates of incidence are reported in other South American countries and in Native Americans.[105] Hispanic Americans and Japanese have an intermediate incidence, while the disease is less common among whites.

Risk factors for gallbladder carcinoma are not well defined. Gallstones are found concurrently in 75% to 90% of patients, while approximately 1% of gallbladders resected for symptomatic cholelithiasis harbor an occult carcinoma. Populations with a high frequency of cholelithiasis have an increased incidence of gallbladder cancer. Gallstones larger than 2.5 cm increase the risk of malignancy. It is hypothesized that chronic irritation from gallstones induces mucosal dysplasia, which may progress to carcinoma in situ and eventually to invasive carcinoma. Since the risk of gallbladder carcinoma is only 1% in the general population with cholelithiasis, asymptomatic cholelithiasis is not an indication for cholecystectomy. However, it is interesting to note that there have been several documented cases of gallbladder carcinoma developing in patients treated with gallbladder-preserving therapies for cholelithiasis.[106]

There is a nearly 20% risk of malignancy in association with the calcified or "porcelain" gallbladder, making this rare finding an absolute indication for cholecystectomy.

Whether benign adenomas are premalignant remains unclear. Adenomas larger than 1.5 cm have been noted to contain foci of malignancy, lending support to the hypothesis regarding progression of adenoma to carcinoma. Tumors larger than 2 cm, particularly in elderly women, should be resected. Smaller tumors or tumors in young patients can be followed with serial ultrasound examinations. Adenomyomatosis may have some malignant potential but does not warrant cholecystectomy in and of itself.

Pathology

A variety of malignant tumors can originate in the gallbladder. Data from the SEER (Surveillance, Epidemiology, and End Results) program of the National Cancer Institute demonstrate that 75.8% of tumors are adenocarcinomas, followed by papadenocarcinomas (5.8%) and mucinous (4.8%), adenosquamous (3.6%), squamous (1.7%), and oat cell (0.5%) carcinomas. Approximately 8% of the tumors were not classified.[107] Adenocarcinomas may be further characterized as mucinous, signet-ring cell, clear cell, and intestinal type. Primary carcinoid tumors, lymphoma, Kaposi's sarcoma, melanoma, and undifferentiated malignancies must also be included in the histologic classification of gallbladder malignancies.[108]

Different staging definitions have been used, complicating the interpretation of the literature on this tumor. The TNM system is shown in Table 4–10. Grossly, gallbladder carcinoma can be difficult to recognize, presenting only as local or diffuse thickening of the gallbladder wall. Occasionally, a discrete nodule or polyp is present, which can easily be identified after the gallbladder is opened in the operating room.

Gallbladder carcinoma is locally invasive, with frequent spread into the adjacent liver and regional lymph nodes. Celiac and periaortic nodes are frequently involved in more advanced disease. Vascular and intraductal spread is common.

Presentation

Twenty percent to 30% of gallbladder carcinomas are discovered incidentally at the time of routine cholecystectomy or postoperatively by the pathologist. Only 25% of patients have disease confined to the gallbladder at the time of diagnosis, while 70% already have invasion of adjacent organs or, less commonly, distant metastases (stage III to IV) at the time of presentation. Symptoms mimic those of cholelithiasis. Seventy percent of patients complain of right upper quadrant pain, often accompanied by nausea, vomiting, anorexia, and weight loss. Jaundice is an ominous finding, associated with unresectable disease in approximately 80% of patients. Patients with advanced disease may also present with a palpable abdominal mass, ascites from carcinomatosis, or anemia due to chronic hemobilia.

TABLE 4–10
TNM Staging of Gallbladder Carcinoma

Stage		Definition	
I		T1	Tumor limited to mucosa and muscularis
		N0	No lymph node metastases
		M0	No metastases
II		T2	Tumor invading subserosa
		N0	
		M0	
III		T3	Tumor into liver (<2 cm) or one adjacent organ
	or	N1	Lymph node involvement
		M0	
IV		T4	Tumor >2 cm into liver or invading two or more adjacent organs
		N0 or N1	
	or	M1	Distant metastases

Evaluation

Laboratory findings are nonspecific. Elevated serum bilirubin and alkaline phosphatase suggest biliary tract obstruction. Tumor markers such as CEA and CA 19-9 are occasionally elevated, raising the suspicion of malignancy.

Evaluation of a patient with signs or symptoms referable to the biliary system should begin with an ultrasound examination. Although small polypoid tumors of the gallbladder are readily visualized with this modality, the frequent presence of gallstones obscures the presence of a concurrent tumor in most cases. Ultrasound is very useful in identifying bile duct dilatation as well as hepatic metastases larger than 2 cm, when present. A HIDA (hepatoiminodiacetic acid) scan that reveals nonvisualization of the gallbladder may be due to acute cholecystitis or, rarely, tumor obstructing the cystic duct. Obstruction of the common bile duct due to advanced gallbladder carcinoma can be visualized with endoscopic retrograde cholangiopancreatography (ERCP) or percutaneous transhepatic cholangiography (PTC), although often the etiology of the bile duct obstruction remains unclear. CT or MRI can document the extent of advanced disease and identify hepatic as well as extrahepatic metastases.

Treatment

Surgery

The only potentially curative therapy remains surgical extirpation. Unfortunately, most patients found to have gallbladder carcinoma have unresectable disease. In these cases, the extent of disease should be documented and the diagnosis verified with frozen section biopsy.

Recommendations for treatment of gallbladder carcinoma are difficult to substantiate owing to the poor prognosis regardless of therapy and the lack of any randomized surgical trials. What is clear is that more than 90% of all patients who have survived more than 5 years with gallbladder carcinoma (any stage) had no therapy beyond cholecystectomy.

Subclinical carcinoma discovered only on histologic examination is adequately treated with cholecystectomy alone, but this point remains controversial. Some have suggested that reoperation with local hepatic resection and radical regional lymphadenectomy be performed in such cases.[109, 110] However, a more recent Japanese series failed to find residual carcinoma in any of the operative specimens following reoperation for subclinical gallbladder carcinoma, drawing into question the utility of reoperation.[111]

Therapy for tumors more extensive than stage I is also

controversial. Most patients with stage II or III disease undergo extended cholecystectomy, which consists of a 2-cm or greater wedge resection of the gallbladder bed plus complete dissection of the porta hepatis with resection of the cystic, periportal, and peripancreatic lymph nodes. Dissection can be extended to include celiac and periaortic nodes. Several Japanese groups have advocated even more radical resections, including resections of the extrahepatic bile ducts with or without pancreaticoduodenectomy and/or right trisegmentectomy for locally invasive tumors.

Using such an aggressive approach, Matsumoto and colleagues[112] reported on a series of 48 patients with carcinoma of the gallbladder, 28 of whom had potentially curative resections based on clear pathologic margins, including 9 of 27 patients with stage IV disease. Surgical morbidity was 14.5% and mortality 4%. It is clear from this study that the patients with potentially curative resections had better average survival lengths (32 months) than those with noncurative resections (10 months) and that patients with early-stage tumors did better than those with advanced disease. Several patients with extended cholecystectomy in conjunction with duct resection, pancreaticoduodenectomy, or liver resection were alive on follow-up to 65 months. Using a similar approach, Nakamura and coworkers[113] reported 54% 1-year survival, 23% 2-year survival, and 15% 5-year survival rates for patients with TNM stage IV disease. Although encouraging, data such as these do not allow one to infer that such radical surgery is superior to cholecystectomy alone without a randomized prospective trial.

Endoscopic and Percutaneous Stents

The dramatic advances in both endoscopic and radiologically guided percutaneous stent placement that have taken place in the last decade have made operative bypass in cases of unresectable carcinoma largely unnecessary. For patients with distal common bile duct obstruction, an endoscopically placed stent can provide excellent palliation for the life of the patient. More proximal obstructions can be better palliated with a percutaneously placed stent, providing both internal and, if necessary, external drainage. It is rare for such patients to live long enough to require stent replacement because of sludge deposition.

Radiation Therapy

Gallbladder carcinoma is not considered radiosensitive. External beam radiation may offer some palliative benefit. Intraoperative irradiation in conjunction with maximal surgical resection has been reported to increase the 3-year survival rate to 10% for patients with stage IV disease.[114]

Chemotherapy

No chemotherapeutic protocol has shown significant efficacy in controlling gallbladder carcinoma. 5-FU alone or in combination with radiotherapy or other chemotherapeutic agents has been used; however, few patients show any response, and survival does not appear to be increased.

Prognosis

Despite advances in surgical care, gallbladder carcinoma remains one of the most rapidly lethal malignancies. In pooled data of 5703 patients with gallbladder carcinoma, the overall 5-year survival rate was 2.5%.[115] Among 3038 patients followed in the SEER program from 1977 to 1986, survival rates at 2 years were 45% for tumors confined to the gallbladder, 15% if regional lymph nodes were involved, 4% if local extension to adjacent organs had occurred, and 2% for patients with metastases. Yamaguchi and Tsuneyoshi[111] reported a 100% 5-year survival rate for stage I tumors in their series, but these results have not been replicated in Western countries. The reason for this discrepancy is not known. Finally, despite the grim prognosis for patients with advanced gallbladder carcinoma, the occasional patient survives long term after attempted curative resection, justifying a continued hopeful approach to the patient who presents with this dreaded disease.

CHOLANGIOCARCINOMA

Epidemiology

Cholangiocarcinoma represents only about 5% to 7% of primary hepatobiliary malignancies. Approximately 4500 cases are reported annually in the United States. As with gallbladder carcinoma, this is a disease primarily of elderly patients, with a peak incidence in the eighth decade. Unlike gallbladder carcinoma, there is a male predominance of approximately 2:1.

Chronic infection with the liver fluke *Clonorchis sinensis*, as well as the parasites *Opisthorchis felineus* and *O. viverrini*, is associated with cholangiocarcinoma. This may explain the increased incidence of cholangiocarcinoma in Southeast Asia, where such infestations are more common.[116]

There is a well-recognized risk of cholangiocarcinoma developing in patients with choledochal cysts and in those with Caroli's disease. The lifetime risk of malignancy increases to 14% in adults with unresected choledochal cysts.[117]

Cholangiocarcinoma develops in approximately 10%–30% of patients with long-standing sclerosing cholangitis. The development of cholangiocarcinoma in the patient with sclerosing cholangitis is often associated with a rapid deterioration in clinical status. In a prospective study of 70 patients with sclerosing cholangitis followed an average of 30 months, 12 patients died, and of these 5 were found on autopsy to have cholangiocarcinoma.[118] Generally, malignancy develops in the setting of advanced disease, and the prognosis is especially poor in this setting, with a median survival of 5 months. There may be an increased incidence of cholangiocarcinoma in patients with ulcerative colitis, independent of the known association of ulcerative colitis and sclerosing cholangitis.

Various benign biliary tumors, including papillomas and adenomas, are considered to have malignant potential. The familial adenomatous polyposis syndromes, including Gardner's disease, are associated with an increased risk of ampullary cholangiocarcinomas.[119]

Pathology

Cholangiocarcinomas typically present as small, fibrous, irregular masses. Grossly, there are three primary morphologies: diffuse, nodular, and papillary. The diffuse form usually affects the intrahepatic ducts and proximal extrahepatic ducts. The cancer spreads throughout the biliary tree, causing multiple focal narrowings, which can closely mimic the appearance of sclerosing cholangitis. The nodular form, as the name implies, is caused by a nodular growth of the proximal bile ducts with resulting local stenosis. The most common form of this disease is due to a carcinoma at the bifurcation of the left and right bile ducts, the so-called Klatskin tumor. Finally, the papillary tumor grows intraluminally in the distal bile duct in the vicinity of the ampulla.

Histologically, cholangiocarcinoma is an adenocarcinoma with ductular differentiation. Ducts may contain mucus but not bile. Extensive fibrosis surrounding individual tumor acini is typical. Cytologically, the tumor can be recognized by prominent nucleoli and cellular polymorphism. Rarely, primary malignant bile duct obstruction can be due to squamous carcinoma, rhabdomyosarcoma, melanoma, lymphoma, carcinoid tumors, and other rare forms.

Presentation

The clinical presentation of patients with cholangiocarcinoma depends, in large part, on the location of the tumor. Patients with intrahepatic malignancies usually present very late into their illness. Symptoms may be due to cholangitis superimposed on bile duct obstruction. Patients may note the subtle onset of anorexia, weight loss, and malaise. Pain, usually mild, is seen in half of patients. Jaundice is rare, but patients may note acholic stools or bilirubinuria. Patients with tumors of the bifurcation and distal bile duct present at an earlier stage, usually with jaundice and pruritus. Hepatomegaly is not infrequent with complete bile duct obstruction. Cirrhosis and liver failure can develop rapidly if the obstruction is not treated.

On examination, the prominent sign of malignant bile duct obstruction is jaundice. Cholangiocarcinomas are rarely palpable. If the obstruction is distal to the cystic duct, a distended, nontender gallbladder may be palpable. Hepatomegaly is often found. Heme-positive stools in the jaundiced patient suggest a biliary malignancy, usually in the periampullary region.

Evaluation

Characteristically, a patient harboring a cholangiocarcinoma will have an elevation of alkaline phosphatase and, to a lesser degree, direct bilirubin. Transaminases are usually only mildly elevated. CA 19-9 levels are elevated in many patients with gastrointestinal, pancreatic, as well as hepatobiliary carcinomas. This assay has a reported sensitivity of 33% to 89% and specificity of 89% to 97%.

A right upper quadrant ultrasound is an excellent test to document bile duct dilatation, evaluate for gallstones, and, on occasion, identify an obstructing tumor. Liver metastases and ascites can usually be detected when present. Thin-section dynamic CT scanning is useful in assessing resectability as well as giving complementary information regarding hepatic and nodal metastases. In a study evaluating 380 patients with malignant bile duct obstruction, CT was found to have an 89% positive predictive value for determining unresectability and an 80% positive predictive value for determining resectability.[120] In cases in which particular concern exists regarding vascular involvement by the tumor, MRA provides adequate imaging without subjecting the patient to the potential complications associated with standard angiography.

Cholangiography can define the nature and extent of the tumor. ERCP is preferred for distal lesions, as it provides better information regarding the duodenum, pancreatic duct, and distal bile duct. Endoscopic bushings may allow cytologic confirmation of the malignancy. Decompressive stents can be inserted to alleviate the bile duct obstruction temporarily. The major limitation of ERCP is the occasional difficulty in visualizing the proximal extent of disease, particularly in cases of high-grade or total duct obstruction. When the patient has documented bile duct obstruction and intrahepatic bile duct dilatation, PTC is preferable, as it will clearly demonstrate the site or sites of proximal obstruction. As with ERCP, PTC can easily be combined with placement of a palliative decompressive stent, allowing either external or, if the lesion is traversable, combined internal and external drainage. Despite the technical facility with which decompressive stents can now be placed, it has been demonstrated in several studies that routine preoperative biliary drainage increases cost and the risk of sepsis while not lessening morbidity or mortality of the subsequent operation. Selected patients with signs of cholangitis or hepatic dysfunction may still benefit from a short period of preoperative drainage.[121, 122] Cameron and coworkers[123] find placement of percutaneous stents useful in the intraoperative identification of the right and left hepatic ducts and in stenting the biliary anastomosis.

Treatment

Surgery

Improvement in nonoperative palliative drainage procedures has dramatically altered the indication for surgery in this disease. Only patients who appear to be resectable on the basis of an extensive preoperative evaluation should be considered for surgery. Criteria for unresectability include invasion or encasement of the portal vein or hepatic artery, the presence of diffuse or bilobar intrahepatic disease, metastatic disease including liver metastases, lymph node involvement or peritoneal seeding, or local hepatic invasion felt to be too extensive for en bloc resection. Of these exclusion criteria, local vessel involvement is the most frequent cause for tumors to be unresectable. Cholangiocarcinoma tends to remain localized, and metastases are seen in less than 25% of patients. Nevertheless, only one in four patients evaluated is potentially resectable.

The patient's general medical condition should be optimized. Patients with a prolonged period of biliary obstruction may be nutritionally depleted and may benefit from a preoperative period of either enteral or parenteral alimentation. Vitamin K should be administered routinely. Control of cholangitis with preoperative drainage and antibiotics is indicated in selected cases.

Resection

Intrahepatic cholangiocarcinomas are treated in much the same way as discussed for hepatocellular carcinomas. Initial abdominal exploration should exclude any evidence of metastases. Meticulous dissection of the hilar plate is performed to identify and isolate the right and left bile ducts, portal veins, and hepatic arteries in anticipation of anatomic lobectomy. This dissection is facilitated by cholecystectomy. Any suspicious portal nodes should be submitted for frozen section examination. Regional spread of intrahepatic cholangiocarcinoma carries with it a grim prognosis and would ordinarily be considered a contraindication to resection.

Tumors involving the bifurcation—Klatskin tumors—pose a unique and challenging problem. To determine resectability, one approach is to initially dissect between the portal vein and the common hepatic duct. If the tumor invades or encompasses the portal vein, it is considered unresectable. Some groups have reported success with more radical resections involving portal vein or hepatic artery resection with graft interposition[124, 125]; however, in our opinion, such heroic efforts are rarely justified given the poor prognosis of cholangiocarcinoma even with "curative" resection, as will be discussed.

Once the tumor has been determined to be resectable, the distal common bile duct is divided and the surgical margin submitted for frozen section. This is an important step, as cholangiocarcinoma tends to have extensive submucosal spread along the bile ducts, often far in excess of what is noted grossly by the surgeon. If a tumor-free distal margin cannot be obtained, consideration should be given to pancreaticoduodenal resection (Whipple procedure) in continuity with radical excision of the bile duct. The proximal margins are divided at or above the secondary biliary bifurcations. Proximal margins should likewise be submitted for frozen section. In the situation of either gross or microscopic extension of the malignancy into one or the other hepatic lobes, the surgeon should be prepared to perform in-continuity hepatic resection.

Following resection of the tumor, reconstruction is performed with a Roux-en-Y limb of jejunum anastomosed to the proximal ducts. Unless the ducts are markedly dilated, we use internal or external stents fixed to the level of the anastomosis with an absorbable suture. Drains are placed dependently. Antibiotics are continued for 48 hours, unless preoperative cholangitis was present, in which case a full course of antibiotics is warranted. Cholangiography is performed on postoperative day 7 prior to removing the drains. Patients are usually discharged home soon thereafter. External stents are removed 3 months following surgery.

Transplantation

Because of the low resectability rates and very high local recurrence rates of standard surgical approaches, several centers have attempted total hepatectomy followed by orthotopic liver transplantation in the care of patients with proximal bile duct malignancies. The Transplant Tumor Registry documents the outcome of 109 patients transplanted for cholangiocarcinoma. Recurrence was the leading cause of death. Actuarial 2-year survival (seven patients) was 30%, and 17% survived 5 years. Ringe and colleagues[126] from Hanover transplanted 10 patients with cholangiocarcinoma. Two patients died in the perioperative period. All of the other patients died, most within 6 months of surgery. The experience of the Boston group was better, with five of nine patients alive on follow-up up to 80 months.[127] The Cambridge group reported on 26 patients with cholangiocarcinoma undergoing transplantation. The 3-month survival rate was 53.8%, but most deaths were due to sepsis. All but one patient surviving the perioperative period died of recurrent disease, with death occurring at a median of 34 weeks for patients with central cholangiocarcinomas and 1.1 years for peripheral tumors. One remarkable patient with a 13-cm tumor remained alive at over 6 years follow-up.[128]

Cholangiocarcinoma remains a controversial indication for transplantation, especially given the poor results to date and the critical shortage of donor organs.

Bypass

The number of open surgical biliary bypasses has dramatically declined in recent years owing to the advances in radiologic imaging and percutaneous or endoscopic stenting of the biliary system. Occasionally, patients with diffuse intrahepatic disease present with multiple intrahepatic strictures. If drainage of the dominant stricture or strictures is not effective and tissue diagnosis of cholangiocarcinoma is confirmed, efforts should be directed at comfort measures.

Unresectable intrahepatic cholangiocarcinomas do not require drainage unless tumor has obstructed both right and left systems or the patient has cholangitis or pain.

Unresectable Klatskin tumors can be surgically drained by creation of an anastomosis between the duct of segment III in the umbilical fissure of the left lobe and a limb of bowel. This anastomosis is particularly successful when the tumor has not blocked communication between right and left lobes. The Longmire procedure, consisting of partial resection of the left lateral segments with anastomosis of the exposed biliary radicals and a loop of intestine, is very rarely performed owing to the availability of more easily accomplished percutaneous stenting procedures.

Endoscopic and Percutaneous Stents

Palliative stenting can be performed endoscopically or percutaneously under fluoroscopic guidance. All palliative stenting devices have relative advantages as well as significant drawbacks, and often the choice between various approaches depends on the local expertise available at any one institution.

Endoscopic Stents

Endoscopic stents are placed at the time of ERCP, often concurrent with the initial diagnostic procedure. Their insertion generally requires performance of a sphincterotomy, which carries with it a 3% to 10% risk of major hemorrhage, perforation, pancreatitis, or cholangitis. Overall mortality is reported to be less than 2%.[129, 130]

The procedure is best suited for low biliary tumors. Proximal lesions or bilateral lesions may not be amenable to endoscopic placement. Often the insertion procedure is staged to allow for initial decompression, followed by ductal biopsy or brushings and placement of a larger endoprosthesis.

The primary advantage to internally placed endoscopic stents is patient comfort, as no external drains are required. Endoscopically placed nasobiliary stents are satisfactory only in the short term. In patients expected to live beyond several months, one can expect that biliary sludge will obstruct the stents every few months, occasionally complicated by episodes of cholangitis. Many physicians recommend regular endoscopic stent exchanges every 3 to 4 months to obviate this expected complication.

Percutaneous Stents

Radiologically guided percutaneous stenting allows specific drainage of that portion of the liver obstructed by the tumor. The initial success rate is between 75% and 100%, in contrast to the approximately 50% success rate expected with endoscopic techniques.

This technique is preferred for high or bilateral lesions. Percutaneous stents offer more therapeutic options than endoprostheses, as drainage can be external to a bag in cases of complete obstruction or can be combined internal-external drainage when the catheter can be passed beyond the tumor. Occasionally, a well-functioning stent can be completely internalized and buried under the skin, allowing a degree of comfort comparable to endoprostheses.

Percutaneous access allows one to flush the catheter on a daily basis in cases of extensive associated biliary sludge and sediment. Catheter exchange is a straightforward outpatient procedure requiring only local anesthetic. Complications associated with percutaneous stent placement occur in 40% to 69% of patients. The most frequent complication is cholangitis, which occurs in 20% to 40% of patients. Other complications include bile leaks, hemorrhage, pleural effusion or pneumothorax, hepatic abscess, and tumor dissemination.[131–134] Procedure-related mortality is 2% to 9%.

Chemotherapy

As with most other malignancies of the liver, no truly effective chemotherapy exists to date. Partial responses have been seen in several clinical trials using a variety of agents, including 5-FU, doxorubicin (Adriamycin), or mitomycin C (FAM), alone or in combination. Responses tend to be short-lived, and no documentation of clear survival benefit has been reported.[135]

Radiation

Cholangiocarcinoma is a locally invasive malignancy with a relatively low incidence of distant metastasis. As such, radiation therapy either as an adjuvant to surgery or as a primary treatment for unresectable disease should hold significant promise. Unfortunately, the malignancy is poorly responsive to radiotherapy, and high doses (5000 to 6000 cGy) of external beam radiation are required to see any response.

Alternatively, radiation can be administered internally by placement of percutaneous or endoscopic stents loaded with iridium 192 or cobalt 60 to achieve much higher local doses of up to 60,000 cGy.

To date, no large controlled trials have been done to assess the efficacy of any form of radiotherapy, although anecdotal reports of prolonged survival do exist. Veeze-Kuijpers et al.[136] reported on a series of 31 patients with unresectable bile duct cancer and 11 patients with residual tumor following surgical resection. A combination of external beam and ^{192}Ir-wire internal radiotherapy was used. Median survival was 10 months. Complications are rare but include fibrosis and strictures of the liver, biliary tract, and duodenum. Right renal failure has been reported.

Prognosis

Cholangiocarcinoma has a very poor prognosis. Although a rare patient can be cured following complete resection, statistics suggest that no current form of therapy has a significant impact on overall survival rates. Untreated, the median survival of patients with proximal cholangiocarcinoma is on the order of 2 to 3 months. The 5-year survival rate is less than 10%, even after "curative" resections, and in many series approaches 0%.

Using an aggressive surgical approach to 136 patients

with hilar cholangiocarcinoma, Bismuth and colleagues[137] explored 122 patients and was able to resect the cancer in 23. Hepatic resection was required in 13 patients, and 9 of the original 136 patients had microscopically clear surgical margins. Of the 23 patients undergoing resection, survival at 1, 2, and 3 years was 87%, 63%, and 25%, respectively, with a median survival of 24 months.

Similar results are reported by Hadjis and associates[138] from London: Of 131 patients evaluated, 27 underwent radical surgical extirpation, including liver resection in 16. Hospital mortality was 7.4%. Median survival among the successfully resected patients was 25 months, and four patients remained alive at the time of the report.

Nimura and coworkers[139] reported on a series of 29 patients who underwent combined portal vein and hepatic resection for proximal biliary (16 bile duct, 13 gallbladder) malignancies. They achieved 1-, 3-, and 5-year survival rates of 48%, 29%, and 6%, respectively, with an operative mortality rate of 17%.

Palliative bypasses are associated with median survivals of approximately 5 months.[140]

References

1. Song E, Dusheiko GM, Bowyer S, Kew MC: Hepatitis B viral replication in Southern African Blacks with HBsAg-positive hepatocellular carcinoma. Hepatology 3:817, 1983.
2. Chung WK, Sun HS, Park DH, et al: Primary hepatocellular carcinoma and hepatitis B virus infection in Korea. J Med Virol 11:99–104, 1983.
3. Beasley RP, Hwang LY, Lin CC, Chien CS: Hepatocellular carcinoma and hepatitis B virus: A prospective study of 22,707 men in Taiwan. Lancet 2:1129–1133, 1981.
4. Hadziyannis SJ: Hepatocellular carcinoma and type B hepatitis. Clin Gastroenterol 9:117–134, 1980.
5. Yarrish RL, Werner BG, Blumberg BS: Association of hepatitis B virus infection with hepatocellular carcinoma in American patients. Int J Cancer 26:711–715, 1980.
6. Kim C-M, Koike K, Saito I, et al: HBx gene of hepatitis B virus induces liver cancer in transgenic mice. Nature 351:317–320, 1991.
7. Takeda S, Nagafuchi Y, Tashiro H, et al: Antihepatitis C virus status in hepatocellular carcinoma and the influence on clinicopathological findings and operative results. Br J Surg 79:1195–1198, 1992.
8. Colombo M, deFranchis R, Del Ninno E, et al: Hepatocellular carcinoma in Italian patients with cirrhosis. N Engl J Med 325:675–680, 1991.
9. Alpert ME, Hutt MSR, Wogen GN, et al: The association between aflatoxin content of food and hepatoma frequency in Uganda. Cancer 28:253–260, 1971.
10. Hsu IC, Metcalf RA, Sun T, et al: Mutational hotspot in the p53 gene in human hepatocellular carcinomas. Nature 350:427–428, 1991.
11. LaBrecque DR: Neoplasia of the liver. In Kaplowitz N (ed): Liver and Biliary Diseases. Baltimore: Williams & Wilkins, 1992, pp 347–388.
12. McMahon BJ, London T: Workshop on screening for hepatocellular carcinoma. J Natl Cancer Inst 83:916–919, 1991.
13. Tsukuma H, Hiyama T, Tanaka S, et al: Risk factors for hepatocellular carcinoma among patients with chronic liver disease. N Engl J Med 328:1797–1801, 1993.
14. Colombo M, de Franchis R, Del Ninno E, et al: Hepatocellular carcinoma in Italian patients with cirrhosis. N Engl J Med 325:675–680, 1991.
15. Okuda K, Okuda H: Primary liver cell carcinoma. In McIntyre N, Benhamou J, Bircher J, Rizzetto M, Rodes J (eds): Oxford Textbook of Clinical Hepatology. Oxford: Oxford University Press, 1991, p 1033.
16. Russi EG, Pergolizzi S, Mesiti M, et al: Unusual relapse of hepatocellular carcinoma. Cancer 70:1483–1487, 1992.
17. Takada T, Yasuda H, Uchiyama K, et al: Contrast-enhanced intraoperative ultrasonography of small hepatocellular carcinomas. Surgery 107:528–532, 1990.
18. Okuda K, Ohtsuki T, Obata H, et al: Natural history of hepatocellular carcinoma and prognosis in relation to treatment. Study of 850 patients. Cancer 56:918–928, 1985.
19. Nagasue N, Chang YC, Takemoto Y, et al: Liver resection in the aged (seventy years or older) with hepatocellular carcinoma. Surgery 113:148–154, 1993.
20. MacIntosh EL, Minuk GY: Hepatic resection in patients with cirrhosis and hepatocellular carcinoma. Surg Gynecol Obstet 174:245–254, 1992.
21. Tsuzuki T, Sugioka A, Ueda M, et al: Hepatic resection for hepatocellular carcinoma. Surgery 107:511–520, 1990.
22. Bismuth H, Houssin D, Ornowski J, Meriggi F: Liver resections in cirrhotic patients: A Western experience. World J Surg 110:311, 1986.
23. Okamoto E, Tanaka N, Yamanaka N, Toyosaka A: Results of surgical treatments of primary hepatocellular carcinoma: Some aspects to improve long-term survival. World J Surg 8:360–366, 1984.
24. al-Hadeedi S, Choi TK, Wong J: Extended hepatectomy for hepatocellular carcinoma. Br J Surg 77:1247–1250, 1990.
25. Jamieson GG, Corbel L, Campion JP, Launois B: Major liver resection without a blood transfusion: Is it a realistic objective? Surgery 112:32–36, 1992.
26. Zulim RA, Rocco M, Goodnight JE, et al: Intraoperative autotransfusion in hepatic resection for malignancy. Is it safe? Arch Surg 128:206–211, 1993.
27. Huguet C, Gavelli A, Chieco PA, et al: Liver ischemia for hepatic resection: Where is the limit? Surgery 111:251–259, 1992.
28. Yamaoka Y, Ozawa K, Kumada K, et al: Total vascular exclusion for hepatic resection in cirrhotic patients. Application of venovenous bypass. Arch Surg 127:276–280, 1992.
29. Belghiti J, Panis Y, Farges O, et al: Intrahepatic recurrence after resection of hepatocellular carcinoma complicating cirrhosis. Ann Surg 214:114–117, 1991.
30. Ikeda K, Saitoh S, Tsubota A, et al: Risk factors for tumor recurrence and prognosis after curative resection of hepatocellular carcinoma. Cancer 71:19–25, 1993.
31. Matsuda Y, Ito T, Oguchi Y, et al: Rationale of surgical management for recurrent hepatocellular carcinoma. Ann Surg 217:28–34, 1993.
32. Nagasue N, Yukaya H, Chang YC, et al: Assessment of pattern and treatment of intrahepatic recurrence after resection of hepatocellular carcinoma. Surg Gynecol Obstet 171:217–222, 1990.
33. Park JH, Han JK, Chung JW, et al: Postoperative recurrence of hepatocellular carcinoma: Results of transcatheter arterial chemoembolization. Cardiovasc Intervent Radiol 16:21–24, 1993.
34. Nagasue N, Kohno H, Chang YC, et al: Liver resection for hepatocellular carcinoma. Results of 229 consecutive patients during 11 years. Ann Surg 217:375–384, 1993.
35. Fortner JG, Maclean BA, Kim DK, et al: The seventies evolution in liver surgery for cancer. Cancer 47:2162–2166, 1981.
36. Iwatsuki S, Starzl TE, Sheahan DG, et al: Hepatic resection versus transplantation for hepatocellular carcinoma. Ann Surg 214:221–228, 1991.
37. Ismail T, Angrisani L, Gunson BK, et al: Primary hepatic malignancy: The role of liver transplantation. Br J Surg 77:983–987, 1990.
38. Ringe B, Wittekind C, Bechstein WO, et al: The role of liver transplantation in hepatobiliary malignancy. Ann Surg 209:88–98, 1989.
39. Olthoff KM, Millis JM, Rosove MH, et al: Is liver transplantation justified for the treatment of hepatic malignancies? Arch Surg 125:1261–1268, 1990.
40. O'Grady JG, Polson RJ, Rolles K, et al: Liver transplantation for malignant disease. Results in 93 consecutive patients. Ann Surg 207:373–379, 1988.
41. Haug CE, Jenkins RL, Rohrer RJ, et al: Liver transplantation for primary hepatic cancer. Transplantation 53:376–382, 1992.
42. Penn I: Hepatic transplantation for primary and metastatic cancers of the liver. Surgery 110:726–735, 1991.
43. Shiina S, Tagawa K, Niwa Y, et al: Percutaneous ethanol injection therapy for hepatocellular carcinoma: Results on 146 patients. Am J Roentgenol 160:1023–1028, 1993.

44. Tanaka K, Nakamura S, Numata K, et al: Hepatocellular carcinoma: Treatment with percutaneous ethanol injection and transcatheter arterial embolization. Radiology 185:457–460, 1992.
45. Vilana R, Bruix J, Bru C, et al: Tumor size determines the efficacy of percutaneous ethanol injection for the treatment of small hepatocellular carcinoma. Hepatology 16:353–357, 1992.
46. Cedrone A, Rapaccini GL, Pompili M, et al: Neoplastic seeding complicating percutaneous ethanol injection for treatment of hepatocellular carcinoma. Radiology 183:787–798, 1992.
47. Isobe H, Fukai T, Iwamoto H, et al: Liver abscess complicating intratumoral ethanol injection therapy for HCC. Ann J Gastroenterol 85:1646–1648, 1990.
48. Ravikumar TS, Kane R, Cady B, et al: A 5-year study of cryosurgery in the treatment of liver tumors. Arch Surg 126:1520–1523, 1991.
49. Kanematsu T, Matsumata T, Shirabe K, et al: A comparative study of hepatic resection and transcatheter arterial embolization for the treatment of primary hepatocellular carcinoma. Cancer 71:2181–2186, 1993.
50. Dewar GA, Griffin SM, Ku KW, et al: Management of bleeding liver tumours in Hong Kong. Br J Surg 78:463–466, 1991.
51. Lai EC, Wu PC, Chan GCB, et al: Doxorubicin versus no antitumor therapy in inoperable hepatocellular carcinoma: A prospective randomized trial. Cancer 62:479–483, 1988.
52. Nonami T, Isshiki K, Katoh H, et al: The potential role of postoperative hepatic artery chemotherapy in patients with high-risk hepatomas. Ann Surg 213:222–226, 1991.
53. Kirk S, Blumgart R, Craig B, et al: Irresectable hepatoma treated by intrahepatic iodized oil doxorubicin hydrochloride: Initial results. Surgery 109:694–697, 1991.
54. Takayasu K, Shima Y, Muramatsu Y, et al: Hepatocellular carcinoma: Treatment with intraarterial iodized oil with and without chemotherapeutic agents. Radiology 163:345–351, 1987.
55. Kanematsu T, Furuta T, Takenaka K, et al: A 5-year experience of lipiodolization: Selective regional chemotherapy for 200 patients with hepatocellular carcinoma. Hepatology 10:98–102, 1989.
56. Ohishi H, Yoshimura H, Uchida H, et al: Transcatheter arterial embolization using iodized oil (lipiodol) mixed with an anticancer drug for the treatment of hepatocellular carcinoma. Cancer Chemother Pharmacol 23(Suppl):33–36, 1989.
57. Nagasue N, Galizia G, Kohno H, et al: Adverse effects of preoperative hepatic artery chemoembolization for resectable hepatocellular carcinoma: A retrospective comparison of 138 liver resections. Surgery 106:81–86, 1989.
58. Yu YQ, Xu DB, Zhou XD, et al: Experience with liver resection after hepatic arterial chemoembolization for hepatocellular carcinoma. Cancer 71:62–65, 1993.
59. Kuroda C, Sakurai M, Monden M, et al: Limitation of transcatheter arterial chemoembolization using iodized oil for small hepatocellular carcinoma. A study in resected cases. Cancer 67:81–86, 1991.
60. Park JH, Han JK, Chung JW, et al: Postoperative recurrence of hepatocellular carcinoma: Results of transcatheter arterial chemoembolization. Cardiovasc Intervent Radiol 16:21–24, 1993.
61. Order SE, Stillwagon GB, Klein JL, et al: Iodine 131 antiferritin, a new treatment modality in hepatoma: A Radiation Therapy Oncology Group Study. J Clin Oncol 3:1573–1582, 1985.
62. Sitzmann JV, Abrams R: Improved survival for hepatocellular cancer with combination surgery and multimodality treatment. Ann Surg 217:149–154, 1993.
63. Iwatsuki S, Starzl TE, Sheahan DG, et al: Hepatic resection versus transplantation for hepatocellular carcinoma. Ann Surg 214:221–229, 1991.
64. Nagasue N, Kohno H, Chang YC, et al: Liver resection for hepatocellular carcinoma. Results of 229 consecutive patients during 11 years. Ann Surg 217:375–384, 1993.
65. Arii S, Tanaka J, Yamazoe Y, et al: Predictive factors for intrahepatic recurrence of hepatocellular carcinoma after partial hepatectomy. Cancer 69:913–919, 1992.
66. Savage AP, Malt RA: Survival after hepatic resection for malignant tumours. Br J Surg 79:1095–1101, 1992.
67. Nagao T, Inoue S, Yoshimi F, et al: Postoperative recurrence of hepatocellular carcinoma. Ann Surg 211:28–33, 1990.
68. Ringe B, Wittekind C, Weimann A, Pichlmayr R: Results of hepatic resection and transplantation for fibrolamellar carcinoma. Surg Gynecol Obstet 175:299–305, 1992.
69. Sasaki Y, Imaoka S, Masutani S, et al: Influence of coexisting cirrhosis on long-term prognosis after surgery in patients with hepatocellular carcinoma. Surgery 112:515–521, 1992.
70. Paquet KJ, Koussouris P, Mercado MA, et al: Limited hepatic resection for selected cirrhotic patients with hepatocellular or cholangiocellular carcinoma: A prospective study. Br J Surg 78:459–462, 1991.
71. Yanaga K, Matsumata T, Hayashi H, et al: Effect of diabetes mellitus on hepatic resection. Arch Surg 128:445–448, 1993.
72. McEntee GP, Batts KA, Katzmann JA, et al: Relationship of nuclear DNA content to clinical and pathologic findings in patients with primary hepatic malignancy. Surgery 111:376–379, 1992.
73. Chen MF, Hwang TL, Tsao KC, et al: Flow cytometric DNA analysis of hepatocellular carcinoma: Preliminary report. Surgery 109: 455–458, 1991.
74. Ni YH, Chang MH, Hsu HY, et al: Hepatocellular carcinoma in childhood. Clinical manifestations and prognosis. Cancer 68:1737–1741, 1991.
75. Brown BF, Drehner DM, Saldivar VA: Hepatoblastoma: A rare pediatric neoplasm. Milit Med 158:51–55, 1993.
76. Altmann HW: Epithelial and mixed hepatoblastoma in the adult. Histological observations and general considerations. Pathol Res Pract 188:16–26, 1992.
77. Sugino K, Dohi K, Masuyama T, et al: A case of hepatoblastoma occurring in an adult. Jpn J Surg 19:489–493, 1989.
78. Hartley AL, Birch JM, Kelsey AM, et al: Epidemiological and familial aspects of hepatoblastoma. Med Pediatr Oncol 18:103–109, 1990.
79. Hughes LJ, Michels VV: Risk of hepatoblastoma in familial adenomatous polyposis. Am J Med Genet 43:1023–1025, 1992.
80. Bernstein IT, Bulow S, Mauritzen K: Hepatoblastoma in two cousins in a family with adenomatous polyposis. Report of two cases. Dis Colon Rectum 35:373–374, 1992.
81. Lesher AR, Castronuovo JJ Jr, Filippone AL Jr: Hepatoblastoma in a patient with familial polyposis coli. Surgery 105:668–670, 1989.
82. Bardi G, Johansson B, Pandis N, et al: Trisomy 2 as the sole chromosomal abnormality in a hepatoblastoma. Genes Chromosomes Cancer 4:78–80, 1992.
83. Tanaka K, Uemoto S, Asonuma K, et al: Hepatoblastoma in a 2-year-old girl with trisomy 18. Eur J Pediatr Surg 2:298–300, 1992.
84. Mascarello JT, Jones MC, Kadota RP, Krous HF: Hepatoblastoma characterized by trisomy 20 and double minutes. Cancer Genet Cytogenet 47:243–247, 1990.
85. Riikonen P, Touminen L, Seppa A, Perkkio M: Simultaneous hepatoblastoma in identical male twins. Cancer 66:2429–2431, 1990.
86. Buckley JD, Sather H, Ruccione K, et al: A case-control study of risk factors for hepatoblastoma. A report from the Childrens Cancer Study Group. Cancer 64:1169–1176, 1989.
87. Pollice L, Zito FA, Troia M: Hepatoblastoma: A clinico-pathologic review. Pathologica 84:25–32, 1992.
88. Watanabe I, Yomagochi M, Kasai M: Histologic characteristics of gonadotropin producing hepatoblastoma: A survey of seven cases from Japan. J Pediatr Surg 22:406, 1987.
89. Douglass EC, Reynolds M, Finegold M, et al: Cisplatin, vincristine, and fluorouracil therapy for hepatoblastoma: A Pediatric Oncology Group Study. J Clin Oncol 11:96–99, 1993.
90. Reynolds M, Douglass EC, Finegold M, et al: Chemotherapy can convert unresectable hepatoblastoma. J Pediatr Surg 27:1080–1083, 1992.
91. Ortega JA, Krailo MD, Haas JE, et al: Effective treatment of unresectable or metastatic hepatoblastoma with cisplatin and continuous infusion doxorubicin chemotherapy: A report from the Childrens Cancer Study Group. J Clin Oncol 9:2167–2176, 1991.
92. Sue K, Ikeda K, Nakagawara A, et al: Intrahepatic arterial injections of cisplatin-phosphatidylcholine-Lipiodol suspension in two unresectable hepatoblastoma cases. Med Pediatr Oncol 17:496–500, 1989.
93. Tagge EP, Tagge DU, Reyes J, et al: Resection, including transplantation, for hepatoblastoma and hepatocellular carcinoma: Impact on survival. J Pediatr Surg 27:292–296, 1992.
94. Koneru B, Flye MW, Busuttil RW, et al: Liver transplantation for hepatoblastoma. The American experience. Ann Surg 213:118–121, 1991.
95. Andreola S, Lombardi L, Audisio RA, et al: A clinicopathologic

study of primary hepatic carcinoid tumors. Cancer 65:1211–1218, 1990.
96. Ruszniewski P, Rougier P, Roche A, et al: Hepatic arterial chemoembolization in patients with liver metastases of endocrine tumors. A prospective phase II study in 24 patients. Cancer 71:2624–2630, 1993.
97. Hajarizadeh H, Ivancev K, Mueller CR, et al: Effective palliative treatment of metastatic carcinoid tumors with intra-arterial chemotherapy/chemoembolization combined with octreotide acetate. Am J Surg 163:479–483, 1992.
98. Bengmark S, Hafstrom L: The natural history of primary and secondary malignant tumors of the liver. I. The prognosis for patients with hepatic metastases from colonic and rectal carcinoma by laparotomy. Cancer 23:198–202, 1969.
99. Ekberg H, Tranberg K-G, Andersson R, et al: Determinants of survival in liver resection for colorectal secondaries. Br J Surg 73:727–731, 1986.
100. Hughes KS, Simon R, Songhorabodi S, et al: Resection of the liver for colorectal carcinoma metastases: A multi-institutional study of patterns of recurrence. Surgery 100:278–284, 1986.
101. Nakamura S, Yokoi Y, Suzuki S, et al: Results of extensive surgery for liver metastases in colorectal carcinoma. Br J Surg 79:35–38, 1992.
102. Hughes KS, Simon R, Songhorabodi S, et al: Resection of the liver for colorectal carcinoma metastases: A multi-institutional trial of the indications for resection. Surgery 103:278–288, 1988.
103. Stone MD, Cady B, Jenkins RL, et al: Surgical therapy for recurrent liver metastases from colorectal cancer. Arch Surg 125:718–722, 1990.
104. Griffith KD, Sugarbaker PH, Chang AE: Repeat hepatic resections for colorectal metastases. Surgery 107:101–104, 1990.
105. de Aretxabala X, Roa I, Burgos L, et al: Gallbladder cancer in Chile. A report on 54 potentially resectable tumors. Cancer 69:60–65, 1992.
106. So CB, Gibney RG, Scudamore CH: Carcinoma of the gallbladder: A risk associated with gallbladder-preserving treatments for cholelithiasis. Radiology 174:127–130, 1990.
107. Henson DE, Albores-Saavedra J, Corle D: Carcinoma of the gallbladder. Histologic types, stage of disease, grade, and survival rates. Cancer 70:1493–1497, 1992.
108. Albores-Saavedra J, Henson DE, Sobin LH: The WHO histological classification of tumors of the gallbladder and extrahepatic bile ducts. A commentary on the second edition. Cancer 70:410–414, 1992.
109. Bergdahl L: Gallbladder carcinoma first diagnosed at microscopic examination of gallbladders removed for presumed benign disease. Ann Surg 191:19–22, 1980.
110. de Aretxabala X, Roa I, Araya JC, et al: Operative findings in patients with early forms of gallbladder cancer. Br J Surg 77:291–293, 1990.
111. Yamaguchi K, Tsuneyoshi M: Subclinical gallbladder carcinoma. Am J Surg 163:382–386, 1992.
112. Matsumoto Y, Fujii H, Aoyama H, et al: Surgical treatment of primary carcinoma of the gallbladder based on the histologic analysis of 48 surgical specimens. Am J Surg 163:239–245, 1992.
113. Nakamura S, Sakaguchi S, Suzuki S, Muro H: Aggressive surgery for carcinoma of the gallbladder. Surgery 106:467–473, 1989.
114. Todoroki T, Iwasaki Y, Orii K, et al: Resection combined with intraoperative radiation therapy (IORT) for stage IV (TNM) gallbladder carcinoma. World J Surg 15:357–366, 1991.
115. Foster J: Carcinoma of the gallbladder. In Way LW, Pellegrini CA (eds): Surgery of the Gallbladder and Bile Ducts. Philadelphia: WB Saunders, 1987, pp 471–485.
116. Srivatanakul P, Parkin DM, Jiang YZ, et al: The role of infection by *Opisthorchis viverrini*, hepatitis B virus, and aflatoxin exposure in the etiology of liver cancer in Thailand. A correlation study. Cancer 68:2411–2417, 1991.
117. Yamaguchi M: Congenital choledochal cyst. Analysis of 1,433 patients in the Japanese literature. Am J Surg 140:653–657, 1980.
118. Rosen CB, Nagorney DM, Wiesner RH, et al: Cholangiocarcinoma complicating primary sclerosing cholangitis. Ann Surg 213:21–25, 1991.
119. Spigelman AD, Farmer KC, James M, et al: Tumours of the liver, bile ducts, pancreas and duodenum in a single patient with familial adenomatous polyposis. Br J Surg 78:979–980, 1991.
120. Gulliver DJ, Baker ME, Cheng CA, et al: Malignant biliary obstruction: Efficacy of thin-section dynamic CT in determining resectability. AJR 159:503–507, 1992.
121. Pitt HA, Gomes AS, Lois JF, et al: Does preoperative biliary drainage reduce operative risk or increase hospital cost? Ann Surg 201:545–552, 1985.
122. McPherson GAD, Benjamin IS, Hodgson HJF, et al: Preoperative percutaneous transhepatic biliary drainage: The results of a controlled trial. Br J Surg 71:371–375, 1984.
123. Cameron JL, Gayler BW, Zuidema GD: The use of silastic transhepatic stents in benign and malignant biliary strictures. Ann Surg 188:552, 1978.
124. Blumgart LH: Cancer of the bile duct. In Blumgart LH (ed): Surgery of the Liver and Biliary Tract. London: WB Saunders, 1982, pp 208–235.
125. Lygidakis HJ, Van der Heyde MN: Surgical approaches for unresectable primary carcinoma of the hepatic hilus. Surg Gynecol Obstet 166:107–114, 1988.
126. Ringe B, Wittekind C, Bechstein WO, et al: The role of liver transplantation in hepatobiliary malignancy. A retrospective analysis of 95 patients with particular regard to tumor stage and recurrence. Ann Surg 209:88–98, 1989.
127. Haug CE, Jenkins RL, Rohrer RJ, et al: Liver transplantation for primary hepatic cancer. Transplantation 53:376–382, 1992.
128. O'Grady JG, Polson RJ, Rolles K, et al: Liver transplantation for malignant disease. Results in 93 consecutive patients. Ann Surg 207:373–379, 1988.
129. Walta DC, Fausel CS, Brant B: Endoscopic biliary stents and obstructive jaundice. Am J Surg 153:444–447, 1987.
130. Marks WM, Freeny PC, Ball TJ, et al: Endoscopic retrograde biliary drainage. Radiology 152:357–360, 1984.
131. Passariello R, Pavone P, Rossi P, et al: Percutaneous biliary drainage in neoplastic jaundice: Statistical data from a computerized multicenter investigation. Acta Radiol 26:681–688, 1985.
132. Yee ACN, Ho C-S: Complications of percutaneous biliary drainage: Benign vs malignant diseases. AJR 148:1207–1209, 1987.
133. Carrasco CH, Zornoza J, Bechthel WJ: Malignant biliary obstruction: Complications of percutaneous biliary drainage. Radiology 152:343–346, 1984.
134. Joseph PK, Bizer LS, Sprayregen SS, et al: Percutaneous transhepatic biliary drainage: Results and complications in 81 patients. JAMA 255:2763–2767, 1986.
135. Wanebo HJ, Falkson G, Order SE: Cancer of the hepatobiliary system. In DeVita VT Jr, Hellman S, Rosenberg SA (eds): Cancer. Principles & Practice of Oncology. Philadelphia: JB Lippincott, 1989, pp 867–868.
136. Veeze-Kuijpers B, Meerwaldt JH, Lameris JS, et al: The role of radiotherapy in the treatment of bile duct carcinoma. Int J Radiat Oncol Biol Phys 18:63–67, 1990.
137. Bismuth H, Nakache R, Diamond T: Management strategies in resection for hilar cholangiocarcinoma. Ann Surg 215:31–38, 1992.
138. Hadjis NS, Blenkharn JI, Alexander N, et al: Outcome of radical surgery in hilar cholangiocarcinoma. Surgery 107:597–604, 1990.
139. Nimura Y, Hayakawa N, Kamiya J, et al: Combined portal vein and liver resection for carcinoma of the biliary tract. Br J Surg 78:727–731, 1991.
140. Lammer J, Neumayer K: Biliary drainage endoprostheses: Experience with 201 placements. Radiology 159:625–629, 1986.

5

Cancer of the Pancreas

Carcinoma of the Exocrine Pancreas

John P. Hoffman, M.D.

This section includes data regarding only exocrine cancers of the pancreas. Since adenocarcinomas account for 98% to 99% of exocrine tumors, the discussion refers to these unless any of the rarer malignancies are specified.[1]

EPIDEMIOLOGY

Incidence

The incidence of pancreatic adenocarcinoma in the United States doubled between 1930 and 1970 and has plateaued at roughly 28,000 new cases annually since then.[2] Worldwide incidence figures show a similar increase, although the rise in Japan has been sevenfold since 1950.[3–6] These statements are tempered by the fact that 40% to 60% of the patients reported do not have histologic confirmation of the diagnosis.[6] Both metastases from other sites and primary periampullary cancers from bile duct, ampulla, and duodenum could be falsely inflating the incidence rates. However, modern diagnostic methods should identify a carcinoma of the pancreas better than those of the 1920s, so the increase is very likely real.[7]

Deaths in the United States from pancreatic cancer have been approximately 25,000 annually, exceeded only by those from lung, breast, large bowel, and prostate cancers. Although the American Cancer Society predicts a nearly equal incidence according to gender, in most countries the incidence is higher for men than women by a ratio of nearly 2:1.[4] The majority of cancers occur in individuals over 60 years of age.

The incidence is highest in the industrialized countries (6 to 10 in 100,000).[2, 5] Maoris in New Zealand and African Americans in Alameda County, California, have the highest reported incidence (12 to 16 in 100,000).[2, 4] African Americans in the United States appear to have a higher incidence than whites, regardless of gender, except in Connecticut, where the rates for both are 8 in 100,000.[4]

Risk Factors

Genetic-Familial

The influence of genetic, environmental, and socioeconomic factors is still unclear but does not appear to be marked. Seven families have been reported from 1973 to 1987 with more than one family member with pancreatic cancer.[5] Since the cases are so rare, and most of the patients have other risk factors, it is generally accepted that genetic influences are weak or nonexistent.

Dietary

Diets high in meat, fat, simple sugars, and total calories have been variably and weakly related to the development of pancreatic cancer.[3–6, 8–10] Some studies have shown a decreased risk for those who ingest raw vegetables (especially carrots) and fruits.[11–13] There appears to be an increase in pancreatic cancer development in immigrants to the United States or Australia, but rates then decrease in subsequent generations. This may indicate that any change in the diet is more influential than any specific dietary elements.[5] Since cholecystokinin and secretin have been shown to potentiate the development of experimental pancreatic cancers, it has been postulated that diets rich in fats and proteins may be carcinogenic by increasing these hormonal mediators.[14] However, most studies have shown no association between remotely previous cholecystectomy (which increases cholecystokinin levels) and pancreatic cancer incidence.[15–17] Furthermore, it is difficult to relate simple sugar intake (a proven risk factor) with cholecystokinin release.[8]

Coffee has been the most controversial risk factor. MacMahon et al.[18] first noted a strong association in a study that was later criticized because it had a control group composed of inpatients on a gastroenterology ward (many of whom may have been counseled to avoid coffee). Many subsequent studies have examined this issue and found minimal to no correlation between coffee drinking (either with or without caffeine) and cancer of the pancreas.[19] Tea is even less of a risk factor.[19]

Social: Drugs and Alcohol

Cigarette smoking is the strongest known risk factor for the future development of pancreatic cancer.[4–6, 9–11, 19] Most studies have shown the risk to be two to three times that for nonsmokers. There is a clearly increased risk with increased intake, and ex-smokers have a decreased risk compared with current smokers.[20] Pipe and cigar smoking have been shown to be associated with increased risk by only one of several studies.[21]

Only a few studies have implicated alcoholic beverages as risk factors.[6, 22, 23] Since so many investigations have shown no relationship, it is unlikely that alcohol is a strong risk factor for pancreatic cancer development.

Environmental-Occupational

Urban and developed environments give rise to more cancers of the pancreas. Past medical conditions that may have an influence on future pancreatic cancer are cholecystectomy, gastrectomy, pernicious anemia, diabetes mellitus, and pancreatitis.[13, 17, 24, 25] Since pancreatitis and diabetes often accompany and may be caused by pancreatic cancer, it would seem unlikely that they are predisposing conditions.[26] Accordingly, diabetes has been noted to be a risk factor that decreases in power the longer the time of onset from the onset of pancreatic cancer. When only those patients with diabetes that preceded the onset of pancreatic cancer by more than 1 year were examined, the risk for men was no longer greater than normal.[27, 28] However, female diabetics still had a standardized mortality ratio of 1.82 for pancreatic cancer.[27] A more recent but smaller study has not confirmed this observation.[29]

Pancreatic cancer incidence has not increased in survivors of the atomic bomb or in nuclear plant workers. A fivefold increase in cancer of the pancreas was noted in workers exposed to benzidine and betanaphthylamine.[30] A similarly increased risk was noted in Japanese chemical workers.[6] DDT exposure was recently shown by a case-control study to be associated with risk four to seven times that for the nonexposed, depending on the duration of exposure.[31] Meter instrument repair and assembly workers, electricians, and textile workers were noted to have a risk two to four times that of normal.[6] Other workers shown to have an increased risk are commercial press workers, chemists, coke and gas plant workers, and those involved in dry cleaning, oil refining, jewelry making, petrochemicals, and paper manufacturing.[4–6, 10] No chemical or class of chemicals has been found to be common to these various exposures.

NATURAL HISTORY

The natural history of stage I tumors is the least described. Obertop and colleagues[32] reported five patients who had resectable cancers but whose medical conditions obviated resection. They all expired from their tumors within 1 year. Fourteen stage I patients without resection were noted in the Vermont tumor registry from 1954 to 1972.[33] Median survival was 9 months, and the longest survival was 13 months. Sener and coworkers[34] noted the median survival to be 6.8 months for 181 patients with clinical stage I cancer and without resection. Some of these patients had radiotherapy and chemotherapy. Pollard et al.[35] noted 32 stage I patients with bypass only and no further therapy. Median survival was 2.2 months, and the 1-year survival rate was 11%.

Table 5–1 lists median survival rates for patients with locally unresectable tumors with and without nodal positivity who had no therapy, and Table 5–2 lists those for patients with distant metastases. Those with locally advanced cancer judged by their surgeons to be candidates for bypass procedures had the longest median survivals (6 to 6.5 months), while those with distant metastases or regional tumor so advanced as to preclude bypass lived only 1 to 2 months.

Forrest and Longmire[40] and Nakase and colleagues[41] reported survival figures for large groups receiving bypass procedures. However, they did not report the stage of the patients and whether chemotherapy or radiotherapy was given. Mean survival reported by Carter and Comis[39] was 5.7 months and for Forrest and Longmire's group was 6.8 months (range, 0 to 24 months), while Nakase et al. reported that 1000 of 1006 patients with cancer of the head of the pancreas having palliative bypasses lived less than 12 months (average, 4.6 months). The 240 cases with cancers of the pancreatic body and tail had a mean survival of 3.1 months, and none lived more than 1 year.[41]

In 1950, Mikal and Campbell[42] reported a series of 100 consecutive autopsies of patients who died from pancreatic cancer. It is unlikely that any of these patients had any sort of antemortem treatment. Eighteen were found to have

TABLE 5–1
Natural History of Patients with Locally Advanced Pancreatic Cancer

Authors	No. of Patients	Median Survival (Mo)	Range (Mo)	Comment
Mallinson et al.[36]	11	3		Local disease only
Hermreck et al.[37]	36	2.5	0–12	Locally advanced, negative nodes, biopsy only
	22	6.5	0–48	Locally advanced, negative nodes, bypass only
	51	1	0–4	Locally advanced, positive nodes, biopsy only
	16	6	0–48	Locally advanced, positive nodes, bypass only
Moertel and Reitemeier[38]	67	8.8		Locally advanced only
Pollard et al.[35]	17	2.5		Locally advanced, laparotomy only
Pollard et al.[35]	66	3.2		Locally advanced, bypass only

cancer limited to the primary area ("considered as curable"). Gross pancreatitis with fat necrosis was noted in 23, and microscopic evidence of pancreatitis was noted in 49%. Large cysts (up to 12 cm) were seen in 5%.

LOCAL-REGIONAL ANATOMY

Figure 5–1 shows the relations of the regional lymph nodes and major blood vessels to the pancreas. The American Joint Committee on Cancer (AJCC) and Japanese nodal classifications differ in that there is no distinction between N1 and N2 nodes in the AJCC classification.[43, 44] If a positive node is found in the middle colic or hepatic duct area, the patient is classified as having a positive N2 node in Japan and as having a distant metastasis in the United States. Other nodes considered N2 by the Japanese rules are the para-aortic, inferior and superior body, and celiac nodes.[44] These, with the exception of contralateral aortic nodes, are classified as regional nodes in the AJCC system.

Note that as the superior mesenteric vein (SMV) and its continuation into the portal vein course toward the liver, the superior mesenteric artery (SMA) continues straight upward to its origin at the aorta (Fig. 5–2). The retropancreatic dissection should follow the SMA to its origin, with retraction of the portal vein.

DIAGNOSIS

Issues of greatest import in the diagnosis of pancreatic cancer are those of accuracy, determination of resectability, and early diagnosis. The latter is addressed in the next section, but it is important to realize how tiny a fraction of cases are currently diagnosed at a stage that allows for possible curative therapy. A recent 3-year survey of the tumor registry of Manitoba noted only 2 of 214 patients with stage I (AJCC) cancers.[45] A retrospective review of 213 consecutive patients with pancreatic cancer diagnosed by dynamic computed tomography (CT) scan at a large U.S. teaching hospital between 1982 and 1992 revealed only three patients with tumors less than 3 cm that had not spread to surrounding tissues or nodes.[46]

The reason for the tardiness of diagnosis is in large part because the cancers are silent until most have reached an advanced stage. Still, two studies, from Norway and the United States, noted patient delay from the time of symptoms to the first physician visit to average 2 to 4 months.[47, 48] The time from first physician visit to diagnosis averaged 1.5 to 2.5 months but was 5.4 months in a group of patients with unresectable cancers.[48]

The family physician, internist, and gastroenterologist should be aware that weight loss, late adult-onset diabetes mellitus or hyperglycemia, unexplained pancreatitis, or epigastric or back pain can be early symptoms of pancreatic cancer.[47–49] Painless jaundice occurs as the first symptom in only 10% to 30% of patients, and 10% of those with jaundice have fluctuations in bilirubin level.[47–49]

Once the diagnosis is suspected, the algorithm of tests to be used depends both on the goals (is resectability analysis or presurgical drainage in the jaundiced patient desired?) and on the individual institutional expertise in

TABLE 5–2
Natural History of Patients with Distant Metastatic Pancreatic Cancer

Authors	No. of Patients	Median Survival (Mo)	Range (Mo)	Comment
Mallinson et al.[36]	19	2.2	1–19	No treatment control group; 11 local only, 8 liver and local
Mallinson et al.[36]	8	1.75		Hepatic metastases
Hermreck et al.[37]	98	1.6	0–12	Distant metastases, biopsy only
Hermreck et al.[37]	77	3	0–36	Distant metastases, bypass only
Moertel and Reitemeier[38]	50	2.5		Liver metastases
Moertel and Reitemeier[38]	27	4.2		Nonhepatic abdominal metastases
Pollard et al.[35]	131	1.2		Laparotomy only
Pollard et al.[35]	154	2.2		Bypass only

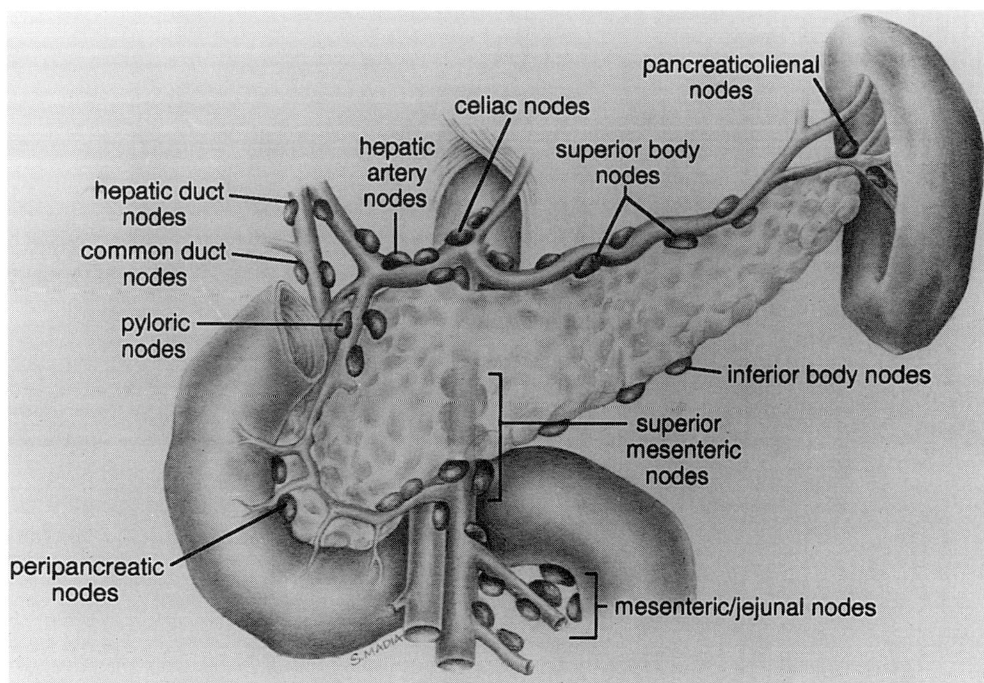

FIGURE 5–1. Anterior view of the pancreas, surrounding blood vessels, and regional lymph nodes.

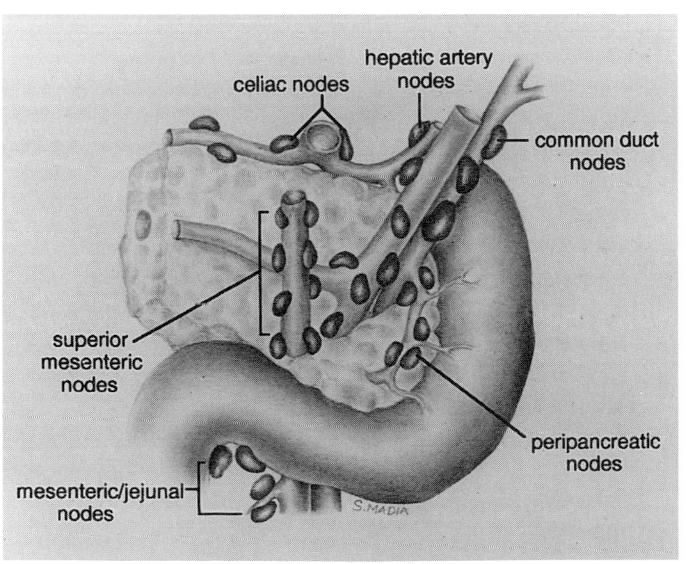

FIGURE 5–2. Posterior view of the head of the pancreas and its regional lymph nodes.

the tests that are operator-dependent (CT scan, ultrasound, endoscopic retrograde cholangiopancreatography [ERCP], and radiologic stent placement). Unfortunately, the sensitivity of all tests decreases as the pancreatic cancer is smaller and more potentially curable.[47, 49]

DIAGNOSTIC AND THERAPEUTIC ALGORITHMS

At least four major philosophies govern the formation of a diagnostic and therapeutic algorithm:

1. *Operation reserved for resectable cases, transcoelomic needle biopsies dangerous:* optimal diagnosis and resectability determinations without biopsy.
2. *Operation for all cases:* high suspicion after initial tests, surgery does the rest.
3. *Operation not advised under any circumstances:* (optimal) diagnosis with biopsy, no surgery.
4. *Preoperative chemoradiotherapy for all localized cases:* optimal diagnosis and resectability determinations, biopsy required.

These are opinions that are held without comparative trials, in terms of either cost effectiveness or patient quality or quantity of life analyses. Each is based on an assumption that remains questionable, yet proponents of each method are convinced of the superiority of their chosen algorithm.

The standard algorithm is ultrasound or CT of the upper abdomen for the patient presenting with jaundice or epigastric or back pain, followed by ERCP if a mass in the pancreas or dilated bile ducts is noted.[47, 49–52] Endoscopic ultrasound may eventually have an important place early in the scheme, since it is very sensitive to smaller lesions in the pancreas.[53]

If the diagnosis is highly suspected or secure at this point, most would recommend further tests to determine resectability.[46, 47, 49–52, 54–66] Splanchnic arteriography, laparoscopy, CT portography, and dynamic CT scan each have their proponents. They all have the ability to detect either liver or peritoneal metastases or local vascular involvement by the tumor that would proscribe resection.

Others would prefer operative intervention at this point, feeling that biopsy and resectability determination are costly, potentially dangerous, and best performed at the operating table.[48, 67–69] This position is supported by two studies that look at whether the average pancreatic cancer is discovered at an earlier stage now than in the era preceding the availability of ultrasound, CT scanning, and ERCP. A decrease in the number of diagnostic laparotomies was seen, but no decrease in tumor size or diagnostic delay or increase in resectability or survival was noted.[70, 71] However, one of the groups advocating this algorithm also showed that 4 of 36 (11%) patients having a pancreatoduodenectomy based only on the surgeon's suspicion of cancer (no biopsy done) actually had benign disease.[68] This is similar to the 12% error (false-positive) rate in intraoperative diagnoses noted in a review of 11 published series.[72] More cogent arguments against this approach are the lack of information about central hepatic metastases and about tumor encroachment on vessels at the mesentery of the pancreas.

Many nonsurgeons prefer a tissue diagnosis before considering surgery, and some surgeons use tissue diagnosis to obviate an operation.[69, 73] Either ERCP-obtained fluid or biopsy or fine-needle aspiration biopsy with CT, ultrasonic, or fluoroscopic guidance may be used, but the yield is higher with the latter procedures.[73, 74] There is controversy regarding the possibility of implanting cancer cells into the needle track by the percutaneous techniques.[75–78] Most reports describe implants in patients with metastatic cancer and in those who underwent biopsies by needles thicker than the recommended 22 gauge, although there is one case of needle track spread in which 10 passes were taken over 2 days with a 22-gauge needle.[76] While cutaneous implants are decidedly rare (Smith[78] estimates 1 in 20,000), it may be that cells are spread intraperitoneally. Warshaw[79] implicates this technique as causing both unresectability and decreased survival in those patients undergoing such biopsies. However, his biopsy patients may have had larger, more advanced tumors, since a very small percentage were able to have a resection. There are certainly no well-controlled trials to give us an idea of the magnitude of risk, if any, involved with thin-needle aspiration biopsies.

Those who prefer adjuvant radiotherapy and chemotherapy delivered before surgical extirpation must obtain a tissue diagnosis by either of the above methods, by brushings taken from externally placed biliary stents, or by aspiration of pancreatic juice by ERCP.[80, 81]

We have followed this routine for 28 consecutive patients. Three patients had unsuccessful biopsies, requiring surgery: one had islet cell cancer, one experienced pancreatitis after a rapid core biopsy and elected to proceed with surgery, and one underwent two different fine-needle aspiration attempts without success and later underwent open transduodenal core needle biopsy, which showed adenocarcinoma. Thus, the technique was 89% accurate in our hands, with no episodes of pancreatitis associated with the 22-gauge needle. Fifteen (60%) patients underwent a successful biopsy on the first attempt, but eight required 2 separate days of biopsy and two required 3 separate days early in the series. We have found that having a cytologist with a scanning microscope in the CT or fluoroscopy suite helps to obviate multiple visits for the patient.

Twelve of the 25 patients who underwent fine-needle aspiration biopsies had pancreatic resections, compared with only 1 of 12 of Warshaw's patients.[79] Two of the eight patients with recurrence had liver metastases only, one had mesenteric node metastases only, and the other five had peritoneal metastases as a component of their recurrence pattern. Of the 13 patients who had no resection, only 1 had a peritoneal component of the disease persistence (10 had liver metastases and 2 had local progression). Four of

11 patients who underwent either open or ERCP biopsies had recurrences, but only 1 had a peritoneal component. This pattern is not significantly different from that seen with transcoelomic aspirations but is trending in that direction. We will follow these patterns with great interest.

In summary, the diagnostic algorithm used by any individual is now largely dependent on his or her beliefs in five areas of contention and how strongly they are held:

1. Palliative pancreatectomy.
2. Transcoelomic aspiration biopsy.
3. All diagnostic and resectability tests.
4. Pancreatic cancer curability by resection.
5. Preoperative chemoradiation.

Thus, transcoelomic biopsies are done by nihilists and those convinced of the value of, or of studying, preoperative adjuvant therapy, and they are eschewed by those convinced of their danger or irrelevance. Tests to improve resectability (arteriography, CT portography, and possibly laparoscopy) and to minimize operative danger (arteriography) are ordered by those who believe that nonoperative biliary bypass is preferable to surgical bypass in the jaundiced patient with distant metastases and by those who are convinced that an accessory right hepatic artery or a median arcuate ligament syndrome with total arterial flow to the liver via the pancreaticoduodenal arteries poses a significant risk to the patient if not recognized by the surgeon performing resection. Finally, a large fraction of family physicians, internists, and gastroenterologists are convinced that even the smallest pancreatic cancer is a death sentence, requiring minimal diagnostic and therapeutic intervention.

DIFFERENTIAL DIAGNOSIS

Pancreatitis, periampullary cancers, rarer types of pancreatic cancer, pancreatic lymphoma, and penetrating duodenal ulcer are part of the differential diagnosis in a patient with a mass in the pancreas.[82–86] They are almost all more benign, with the exception of the extremely rare microadenocarcinoma.[87] All but pancreatitis, lymphoma, and ulcer necessitate resection if localized, so the identification of these three processes preoperatively or intraoperatively is most important. It is also important to sample every pancreatic malignancy for biopsy at celiotomy if no prior biopsy has been done, precisely to identify those few cases of lymphoma that are potentially curable.

The differentiation between cancer and pancreatitis is often difficult, since pancreatitis is often associated with cancer and can look and feel like cancer. A good history reveals previous alcoholic intake or gallstones. Pancreatic cancer tends to produce a higher bilirubin level that continues to rise.[83] ERCP with biopsy or pancreatic juice cytology is the most discriminating test except for operative exploration and biopsy.[84] However, a small fraction of patients remain either with small cancers surrounded by pancreatitis or with very localized pancreatitis in whom distinction is impossible until after resection. Multiple attempts at transduodenal core needle biopsies are recommended in such instances, but so is resection if the suspicion of cancer remains in a good operative candidate.[40, 48, 88, 89]

DETERMINATION OF RESECTABILITY

Before one discusses tests that determine resectability, one must address the wide range of criteria for resectability advised by various groups and authors (Table 5–3). There is near consensus that size alone should not prohibit resection, although several studies have shown increasing size to be associated with unresectability and incurability.[44, 101–105] It also seems fair to say that most surgeons would avoid resection if a large number of regional nodes were proven to contain metastases, and virtually all would stop at hepatic or superior mesenteric arterial encasement or direct invasion. Some would consider focal lateral portal or SMV abutment or tethering grounds for lateral vein wall resection and closure, but most surgeons in the United States would eschew resection of any tumor that even abuts these veins.

Some of the objections to resecting mesenteric vein segments stem from discomfort on technical grounds, but all of the criteria against resection of tumors associated with positive nodes and most against resection of tumors abutting, surrounding, or invading large vessels reflect a belief that virtually all of these patients will soon have distant or locally recurrent cancer. As more data emerge regarding the mortal effect of positive margins, these should further discourage attempts to remove tumors even within 1 to 2 cm of the planned vena caval and superior mesenteric venous and arterial borders of resection unless adjuvant therapy can be shown to alter the natural history of resections with cancer cells close to any margin.[80, 106]

It is clear that "resectability" as it is used in the surgical literature for this malignancy is a misnomer. It does not connote the technical ability of a surgeon to remove a particular cancer but, rather, whatever resection and adjuvant therapy contemplated by the surgeon offer a safe passage out of the hospital and a reasonable chance of long-term survival benefits. Unfortunately, each of these clinical situations (large tumors, regionally positive nodes, and various types of large vessel or margin involvement) has not been extensively investigated, so the responsible surgeon must face difficult decisions when confronting them, especially in this age of preoperative, chemotherapy-enhanced adjuvant radiation therapy, one of the major effects of which is an improvement in local control.[80] However, postoperative chemoradiotherapy did not produce a statistically significant improvement in survival or local control in those patients with positive margins at pancreato-

TABLE 5–3
Variations in Operative Criteria for Resectability

Author(s)	Year	Tumor	Nodes	Vessel Relations	Other
Cattell and Pyrtek[90]	1949	No local invasion; any size	No positive nodes	No SMV, SMA involvement	
Porter[91]	1958	No size criteria	None positive below transverse mesocolon	No SMA, SMV invasion or encasement after 1958	Only metastases outside the limits of the proposed resection
Longmire[92]	1966	No size criteria	No celiac, SMV; middle colic accepted	5 portal vein segments resected, 3 recurred 3–11 mo (basis for unresectability)	
Brooks and Culebras[93]	1976	No size criteria	No positive nodes		
Forrest and Longmire[40]	1979	No size criteria	Not mentioned	Not mentioned	Not age >70; tumor immovable
Herter et al.[94]	1982	Allow grossly adequate clearance	No biliary, hepatic, suprapancreatic	Portal vein freedom	"Any cancer that because of its size requires a total pancreatectomy should not be resected"
Moossa[49]	1982	No size criteria	Not mentioned	Not mentioned	Distant metastases, age >70, life expectancy <3 yr when surgeon inexperienced in this field
Piorkowski et al.[95]	1982	No size criteria	No positive nodes	No portal vein involvement	
Malt[96]	1983	No size criteria	Only a few juxtapancreatic	Not into wall of SMA, SMV, portal vein	Not age>70
Kellum et al.[88]	1983	<3 cm	Positive	No portal vein invasion	
Trede[97]	1985	No size criteria	Not mentioned	No SMA, hepatic artery invasion	"Policy to remove every technically operable tumor even if the risks are considerable"
Pellegrini et al.[98]	1989	No size criteria	Not mentioned	Not mentioned	"If . . . no overt evidence of extrapancreatic tumor and if it seemed possible to remove the entire lesion"
Warshaw et al.[61]	1990	No size criteria	Not mentioned	No encasement or occlusion of celiac or SMA and major branches, splenic, portal, and SMV	
Gall et al.[99]	1991	No size criteria	No distant nodes	No large vessel invasion	Massive retroperitoneal invasion, invasion of mesenteric root or hepatoduodenal ligament
Ishikawa et al.[44, 100]	1992	Tumor >4 cm	No distant nodes	No bilateral narrowing or occlusion of portal vein, SMV	No invasion of root of transverse mesocolon or mesojejunum
Hoffman et al.[80]	1993	No size criteria	No N2 nodes	No portal vein, SMV occlusion, SMA, hepatic artery invasion or encasement	

SMV, Superior mesenteric vein; SMA, superior mesenteric artery.

duodenectomy treated at Massachusetts General Hospital.[106]

Large Vessel Proximity or Invasion

It is possible but not proven that a patient with tumor or pancreatitis (it is often difficult or impossible to distinguish them) at the right lateral wall of the SMV has a better outlook with a resection and pre- or postoperative chemoradiotherapy than in the past with surgery alone. This needs further investigation because the number of such patients reported in the past is small. For instance, Longmire[92] and Aston and Longmire[107] reported five patients with lateral SMV or portal vein resection along with the observation that three died from 3 to 11 months after resection of liver metastases. The fates of the other two were not reported, yet it is suggested that resection is not indicated in this situation. There is also no reported comparable series of patients with only this clinical picture treated with bypass alone.

We have resected tumors from five patients after they had preoperative chemoradiation with angiographic bilateral impingement on the SMV (Fig. 5–3). Three died with pleural, diffuse, and peritoneal recurrence at 8, 9, and 29 months, respectively, while one is alive with lung metastases at 37 months and another is alive without recurrence at 20 months after tissue diagnosis. Another with a carcinoma originating in the body and medial tail of the pancreas with both splenic arterial and venous occlusion has survived 5 years after tissue diagnosis (57 months after resection). Those with bilateral portal vein and SMV impingement are declared by Ishikawa et al.[100] as unable to be helped even by super-radical resection, since none of their seven cases survived 18 months after total pancreatectomy with portal vein resection and extensive lymphadenectomy. Fifteen patients with this type of narrowing and distant metastases lived just as long without resection. They did not study splenic vessel occlusion.

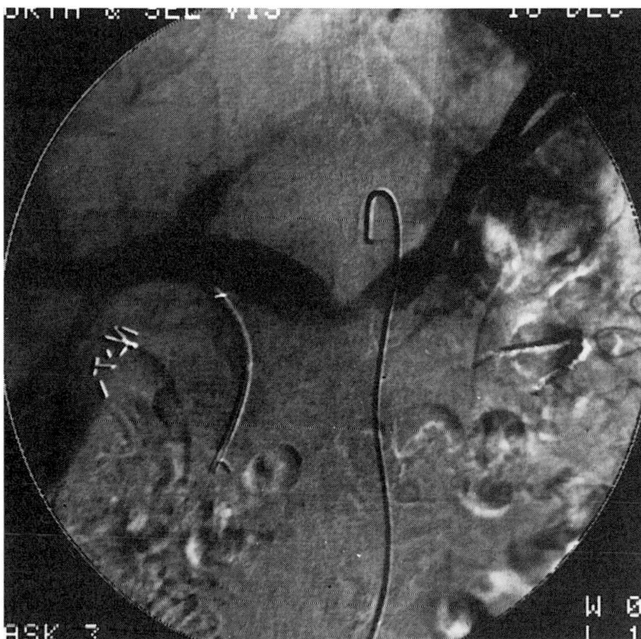

FIGURE 5–3. Late portal views after celiac artery injection of radiopaque dye. Note superior and inferior impingement of the portal vein at its junction with the splenic vein (at right).

The categories of portal vein/SMV involvement reported by Ishikawa et al.[100] were as follows:

I: normal
II: smooth shift without narrowing
III: unilateral narrowing
IV: bilateral narrowing
V: bilateral narrowing and the presence of collateral veins

Seven of 17 patients with type I to III narrowing lived more than 3 years after pancreatoduodenectomy with portal vein and SMV replacement and extensive lymphadenectomy. None of four patients with arterial (SMA 3, hepatic 1) resection and replacement survived that long. In fact, there are no long-term survivors reported who had resection of hepatic or mesenteric arteries that proved to be involved with cancer. Thus, there is less evidence for resectability of tumors surrounding or invading these two arteries than with any other local-regional indicator.

Regional Lymph Node Involvement

Data regarding regional node invasion and resectability should be complete by now but are not. There is no question that nodal involvement negatively influences prognosis more than any feature other than grossly positive margins or large artery invasion in patients having pancreatic resections. However, the site and number of involved nodes have not been examined closely enough to allow us to know the implication of a single involved node in a given position or the critical number of involved nodes to render a patient incurable after resection.

A recent report from Memorial Sloan-Kettering Cancer Center noted only 1 5-year survivor of 69 patients having resections for node-positive cancers.[103] Median survival was 13 months. The report does not mention the size, number, or location of involved nodes. Similarly, a series from Germany reports no survivors beyond 32 months of 35 node-positive patients with tumor resection.[105] Median survival was only 6.8 months. Another series from Germany noted 4 of 12 patients surviving 5 years with just one positive node, but none of 54 with multiple positive nodes survived that long (their median survival was 6.1 months).[99] Others also have reported occasional long-term survivors. Mannell and colleagues[108] noted 10 of 23 3-year survivors with positive lymph nodes, and four other groups[109–112] noted 6 patients surviving more than 5 years after resection.

Ishikawa and coworkers[44] are the only ones reporting a series of resections who have categorized nodal involvement to some extent. They noted one of eight patients with positive N2 nodes and three of seven patients with positive N1 nodes surviving 3 years after extended resection (see section on local-regional anatomy for definitions). They claimed that the reason for the increased survivorship was an extended lymphadenectomy. There were no node-positive patients surviving 3 years of 22 patients who had standard pancreatoduodenectomy. Extended lymphadenectomy produced more long-term survivals (4 of 15) in node-positive patients than in those with tumors greater than 4 cm in diameter who also had direct retroperitoneal invasion, in whom no 3-year survival was obtained.

Since only one patient with an N2 node is reported as a long survivor, the presence of involved N2 nodes should contraindicate resection unless a procedure such as Ishikawa et al.[44] recommend is contemplated. Unfortunately, they have not reported survival according to the N2 nodal positions. It is doubtful that patients with positive nodes at the hepatic duct bifurcation, the celiac origin, and the contralateral para-aortic positions could be salvaged by even radical surgery combined with adjuvant irradiation. Those with nodes in the mesocolon or ipsilateral aortocaval areas close to the primary cancer may benefit from a wide resection and adjuvant radiotherapy. Positive N1 nodes may allow an occasional long survival after resection and therefore should not constitute an impediment to resection for the patient and surgeon ready for the procedure.

We noted 3 of 23 (13%) patients with pancreatoduodenectomy after chemoradiotherapy who had positive nodes found in the specimens: one with three positive N1 nodes is alive without recurrence 9 months after tissue diagnosis; one with positive N1(4) N2(1) nodes died of peritoneal recurrence at 11 months; and one with one positive N1 node is living with liver metastases at 20 months. We are quite certain that the preoperative therapy is downstaging the nodes, since the median tumor size in our series is 4 cm and two thirds of the patients had some angiographic SMV and portal vein involvement. All other series of resections treated without preoperative radiotherapy have more than 40% of patients with positive nodes.[103, 105, 106, 109, 113] In that there are so few node-positive patients in preoperative radiotherapy trials, the significance of an initially (or at resection) positive node is even less well understood than in studies involving surgery only or surgery plus postoperative adjuvant chemoradiation.

Clearly, when one treatment method is able to produce long-term survivors in categories of patients unable to be helped with past methods, criteria for resectability for that particular method require amendment. At the same time, data generated from these new methods should be as precise as possible regarding the tumor and its margins, nodes, and large vascular relationships in order for these criteria to be rationally formulated and understood.

Preoperative and Intraoperative Determination of Resectability

Preoperative determination of resectability is best accomplished by those methods most accurately identifying distant metastases, invasion of hepatic and superior mesenteric arteries, and the proximal (with respect to blood flow) SMV. There is not much question regarding the supremacy of celiac and SMA arteriography to detect local vessel invasion, although Freeny and coworkers[46] argue that dynamic CT scanning is more sensitive, as 12 of 60 patients were not seen on angiogram to have vascular involvement (tumor-vessel contiguity or encasement of the SMA or SMV) noted by dynamic CT.[46] Fuhrman et al.[63] believe dynamic CT scanning with thin cuts at the level of the SMA origin is preferable to arteriography for this purpose. Even if others agreed, it would still be sensible to obtain both studies in order to fully understand the patient's vascular anatomy.[54–56] Metastases are most frequently in the liver, peritoneum, and lung. CT portography and intraoperative ultrasound are the most sensitive tests for liver secondary tumors.[65] Warshaw and colleagues[61] found that laparoscopy with peritoneal washings discovered many more liver and peritoneal metastases than did dynamic CT scanning. Chest CT scan should be done to detect pulmonary metastases, although the majority are seen on a chest radiograph.

The surgeon should examine the peritoneal surfaces, liver, and N2 nodal areas carefully. Any large or firm N2 nodes should be sent for frozen section examination. The small bowel mesentery and the SMV as it crosses the duodenum should be carefully palpated for nodes or tumor extension (even if the surgeon is prepared for SMV resection, proximal involvement of the vein prohibits reanastomosis). Finally, the SMA can best be approached for palpation from its left side just above the left renal vein (Fig. 5–4). We have not found any tumors unresectable where angiography demonstrated uninvolved SMA and hepatic

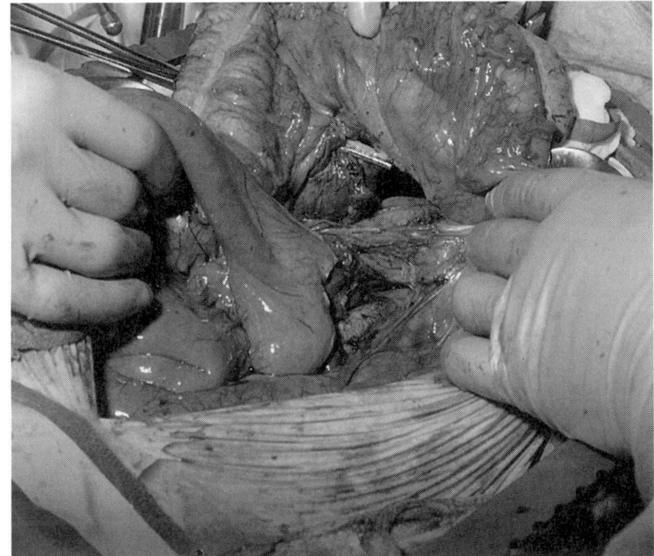

FIGURE 5–4. View from the patient's left side of the dissection behind the superior mesenteric vessels and anterior to the aorta. The superior mesenteric artery is the structure directly anterior to the aorta. Note the lymphatics preserved on its left side in order to preserve lymphatic flow from the small bowel.

arteries, although many tumor masses with surrounding pancreatitis have been in very close approximation to the vein. In 15 resections where SMV and portal vein studies showed Ishikawa grade II to IV narrowing, we have not noted a single positive vascular margin. Thus, we currently consider any SMV and portal vein venogram without occlusion as grounds for resection. The reader should be advised that this is probably unwise for those patients not having had preoperative chemoradiotherapy, particularly if postoperative radiotherapy is not planned.

We have used intraoperative hepatic ultrasound to detect occult hepatic metastases but have not found any lesions by this method that CT portography or surgical exploration failed to identify. However, two patients had false-positive CT portograms, produced by areas of cholangitis with microabscess formation from long-term, ERCP-placed biliary stents (Fig. 5–5).

SCREENING AND EARLY DETECTION

The only efficacy test of early detection of pancreatic cancer was performed by Moossa and Levin[114] at the University of Chicago between 1974 and 1980. A total of 238 patients were enrolled in their study by fulfilling entry criteria that were revised to more restrictive criteria in 1978. The early criteria were any of the following: obstructive jaundice, weight loss greater than 10% of normal body weight, epigastric or lumbar pain, suspected pancreatic mass; or any two of the following: vague, unexplained dyspepsia, weight loss less than 10% of normal body weight, sudden onset of diabetes mellitus without a family history, unexplained thrombophlebitis, unexplained steatorrhea. Of the first 186 patients enrolled by these early criteria, 104 (56%) were found after testing and laparotomy to have a cancer, and 73 (39%) had a pancreatic cancer.

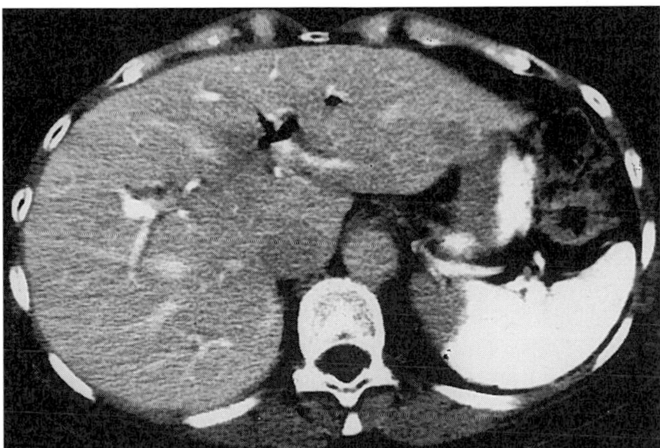

FIGURE 5–5. CT portogram of the liver that was read as showing a metastasis to the left lateral segment of the liver. This was later shown to be an area of microabscess formation with surrounding fibrosis.

The later criteria (jaundice, unexplained back or upper abdominal pain less than 1 year in duration, weight loss greater than 10% of normal body weight, unexplained pancreatitis in a patient over 50 years old, and adult-onset diabetes mellitus in a patient over 50 years old) elicited 52 patients, 45 of whom after testing underwent surgery. Thirty-one cancers (29 pancreatic cancers [56%]) were discovered. Thirty-nine of the 102 pancreatic cancers from both cohorts (38%) were resected. Nearly one third of these were "early" (size < 2 cm, no capsular invasion, no nodal or distant metastases).

Considering that this kind of tumor constitutes only 2% to 5% of most groups of patients with resection, the Chicago experience was highly successful.[115, 116] It is surprising that more attention has not been paid to the effort. Perhaps a quirk of fate that brought death to 12 of these patients from other causes has dampened what should have been enthusiasm. It is also unclear why Moossa and Levin[114] reported five 5-year survivors and a later publication from the same institution noted only 3 such survivors from 1946 to 1983.[112]

The only rational, cost-effective way to screen people at high risk in the community (smokers, those with positive criteria for the Moossa and Levin study) must be to await a sensitive, inexpensive serum marker for pancreatic cancer that could then be used in concert with ultrasound.[117] CA 19-9, the most sensitive marker, is reserved for confirmation of other tests in the diagnosis of pancreatic cancer and for following patients after resection.[118–121] CA 19-9 is elevated in only 60% of those with cancers less than 2 cm and in only 78% of those with cancers greater than 2 cm but less than 4 cm.[122] Moreover, a large number of false-positive readings occur in patients with general medical complaints.[123]

STAGING

Distribution

Carcinomas of the head of the pancreas outnumber those in the body and tail by 4 or 5:1.[3, 34, 39, 104, 124–127] Stage distribution in all series is at least 50% for those presenting with metastatic disease. Of the remaining 40% to 50% of patients at least one half present with locally advanced cancer. A few of these may be resectable, but most have concurrent or eventual distant metastases. Thus, only 20% to 25% of patients have tumors lending themselves to standard resection; half of these (10% of all) have node-negative cancers. One tenth (1% to 2% of all) have cancers less than 2 cm in diameter; one third of these (<1% of all) have these small cancers without capsular or nodal invasion.[39, 115, 116]

Staging Systems

A provisional system was used to study the best staging correlation to survival in the United States in the past decade.[35] This system has persisted with only minor changes over the past 12 years.[43] The design was to capture the surgically treatable patients in stage I, those with locally present but unresectable tumors in stage II, those with regional node involvement in stage III, and those with distant metastatic involvement in stage IV. Unfortunately, the surgeon's judgment about resectability, discussed earlier as being highly variable, was inherent in the system. Thus, the T3 category was defined only as "incompatible with surgical resection."[39] This was refined to become the present AJCC system, whereby a T3 tumor is any "which extends directly to any of the following: stomach, spleen, colon, or adjacent large vessels."[43] The only other substantive changes were to subdivide the T1 category as to tumor size (greatest dimension ≤2 cm [T1a or T1b]) and to specifically limit the T1 category to exclude tumors extending beyond the pancreatic capsule. Histology, location of the tumor, resection margins, and DNA characteristics, all shown to strongly influence survivorship in resectable lesions, are not included.[44, 106, 113, 128–131]

Although the current AJCC system has been refined, the issue of extension to blood vessels is unclear and will hinder future data collection. Actual wall invasion or occlusion is now coded the same as tumor and vessel proximity as noted by either a surgeon at operation or a radiologist examining a CT scan. There are clear differences among these clinical situations, yet the staging system will not detect them as currently written.[100, 106] This is particularly relevant to those patients declared "unresectable" and then treated by nonoperative techniques. Until these distinctions can be made, most claims of improved therapy for this group of patients (either surgical or nonsurgical) must be viewed with skepticism.

No distinction is made between N1 and N2 nodes in the North American or European systems (see the section on local-regional anatomy for a further discussion of these differences).

PRIMARY OPERABLE DISEASE—RESULTS AND COMPLICATIONS OF TREATMENT

Surgical Options

Once the diagnosis is highly suspicious or made, the surgeon decides what further testing he or she will order to help with the future decision of resectability (see the section on resectability). The individual surgeon's experience, capability, and criteria for resectability should all be reviewed prior to embarking on an exploratory celiotomy for this type of cancer.

Treatment options differ for each of several clinical scenarios: cancer in the superolateral head, medial head, or uncinate process abutting or invading the SMV; a large or small tumor in the head or pancreatic tail or body. Adjuvant therapy options are discussed later. Surgical options include pylorus-preserving pancreatectomy, standard Whipple pancreatoduodenectomy, and total pancreatectomy, with or without adjacent organ or vessel resection and replacement. These procedures have never been compared in a prospective, randomized trial.

Extent of Lymphadenectomy

All of the surgical options just mentioned involve the question of the extent of lymphadenectomy and where to divide the pancreas in a Whipple procedure. The latter issue is addressed in the next section. Only the nonrandomized study of Ishikawa et al.[44] attempted to answer this question. They claimed that a lymphadenectomy encompassing all of the lymphatic tissue between the supraceliac aorta and the origin of the inferior mesenteric artery, and from the left of the aorta to the hepatic duct bifurcation, resulted in improved survivorship. The "control" group had a more standard lymphadenectomy, which was still probably more extensive than most surgeons in the United States would perform, since the celiac axis and hepatic artery were skeletonized. There was a decrease in local recurrence favoring extended lymphadenectomy in those with T2 tumors and those with retroperitoneal capsular invasion, and there was a difference in survival favoring the extended procedure. Other than in the descriptions for extended procedures, there are no descriptions of lymphadenectomy extent in reported cohorts of those treated by standard or total pancreatectomy.

Studies of the spread of pancreatic cancer have shown the majority of involved nodes to be those along the pancreaticoduodenal vessels, followed by the nodes in the central vascular mesentery at the SMV and SMA in the superior body inferior to the bifurcation of the celiac axis, and next to and anterior to the aorta at the level of the left renal vein.[93, 131–135] In order to optimize local control, it would seem prudent to include these areas with pancreatic resection.

Partial or Total Pancreatoduodenectomy?

A tumor at the superolateral head of the pancreas obviates the decision for pylorus-preserving pancreatectomy but leaves that regarding partial versus total pancreatoduodenectomy (TP). There have been claims for a superior lymphadenectomy with TP, but of course there are nodes to the left of the aorta along the superior and inferior borders of the pancreas and splenic hilus that are removed by TP but not by Whipple-type pancreatoduodenectomy. These are seldom, if ever (splenic hilus), involved with metastases from cancers in the head of the pancreas.[131–135] Any N1 or N2 nodes are just as removable with Whipple pancreatoduodenectomy as with TP, with the possible exception of nodes to the far left of the inferior and superior body groups.

Two other reasons for selecting TP are the putative increase in safety and curability provided by the lack of a pancreatojejunostomy and the complete resection of lesions that are multicentric.[136–140] No one has demonstrated decreased mortality and morbidity with TP, although a scientific trial, making the type of operation the only changing variable with otherwise equal patient, tumor, and surgeon variables, has never been done.

Multicentricity has been reported in 17% to 37% of TP specimens removed for pancreatic cancer.[136–139, 141] However, many of the cases reported were actually direct spread of cancer from the head into the body or tail. This would probably be discovered at frozen section examination of the divided pancreas during the Whipple procedure. The percentage of truly discontinuous lesions in resectable cases is still in doubt but is probably not as high as the 20% figure first published by Brooks et al.[136, 141–144] More sophisticated histologic staining techniques show that the vast majority of pancreatic head lesions extending into the tail do so in continuity.[135, 136, 142–144] Frozen section analysis of the divided pancreas is obviously indicated in order to obtain clear margins in these 5% to 10% of cases.[40] We have performed frozen section analysis of both pancreatic and hepatic duct margins in 18 consecutive Whipple procedures. There was one false-negative reading and no false-positive results. The clinical significance of residual microfoci of tumor in the pancreatic tail was questioned by Kloppel and colleagues,[142] who found that recurrence after Whipple pancreatoduodenectomy did not originate from the pancreatic remnant. Our one patient with a positive pancreatic margin had a liver metastasis 12 months after resection. There was no evidence of recurrence in the pancreatic remnant.

In favor of the Whipple procedure are the preservation of the pancreatic tail and spleen. Moossa et al.[140] have argued that pancreas preservation to avoid diabetes mellitus is irrational, since at least a third of patients with pancreatic cancer already have the ailment. However, death from insulin coma or hyperglycemia is unusual in these patients presenting with diabetes, and it frequently improves after tumor excision. Several of the major TP series report at least one or two deaths from insulin shock.[94, 137, 139, 145, 146] Pancreatojejunostomy leak, with subsequent morbidity and mortality, is avoided by TP. However, modern series have noted a decreasing incidence of morbidity and mortality from these leaks.[110, 146–149] It may be that the advent of somatostatin analogues for reduction in flow of the pancreatic juice has further reduced the virulence of this complication.[150, 151] While definitions of chemical leak differ, such that comparisons are dangerous, we have had only 2 of 13 patients with duct-mucosa pancreatojejunostomies with a chemical leak, defined as drain amylase greater than serum amylase. Of five patients with intussuscepting anastomoses, there was one clinical and one chemical leak. The clinical leak required percutaneous drainage, then resolved without reoperation. Others have also noted a decrease in pancreatic fistulas after preoperative radiotherapy.[152]

Splenic preservation may have more than theoretic benefit. A study from Norway did not detect differences in the mortality or morbidity of the Whipple procedure and TP but did show a significant increase in mortality for those with splenectomy.[153] The groups were not randomized. However, because of the danger of postsplenectomy sepsis, one should try to preserve the splenic vein and spleen if performing TP to avoid pancreatojejunostomy and microscopic tumor in the tail.

Cancer At the Portal Vein: Is Any Resection Justified? What Type of Resection?

A cancer abutting or invading the SMV or portal vein demands that a decision be made between resection and no resection, between partial, total, and extended pancreatoduodenectomy, and between methods of vein resection and reconstruction.

As discussed in the sections concerning resectability and staging, there is a great difference between (1) pancreatitis at a portal vein wall, (2) cancer at the wall, (3) cancer directly invading the wall focally, and (4) cancer invading and occluding the vein. The first three situations are unlikely to be distinguishable by the operating surgeon until the procedure is nearly complete, or perhaps until microscopic analysis is performed. Many surgeons will declare all of the above circumstances unfit for resection (see Table 5–3). Tepper and coworkers[154] noted that one third (35 of 114) of those patients deemed unresectable at the time of surgery were thought so because of local disease extent only. Since it is known that most of these tumors can be technically resected, it must be that the operating surgeons thought that future distant disease and local recurrence were inevitable. However, a potentially curable, small tumor in the head that produces periportal pancreatitis may give rise to this intraoperative scenario. One must also remember the autopsy findings of Mikal and Campbell[42] showing that a substantial number of patients were found (18%) who had died with local disease only.

If it is known from preoperative tests that the tumor mass approaches the SMV or portal vein without occluding them, it would seem prudent for the surgeon unprepared for partial or complete vein excision to refer the patient to one who is. The surgeon is much more likely to encounter a patient with this clinical situation than one with a T1a lesion. A surgical excision with clean margins can be accomplished in any but the fourth scenario (vein occlusion), particularly when preoperative adjuvant chemoradiotherapy has been used.[80, 155]

The decision to proceed with resection is usually made preoperatively. Unless distant cancer or extension completely surrounding the SMA or hepatic artery (true encasement) is noted at operation, the surgeon familiar with the anatomy will proceed with the resection based on arteriographic and CT scan findings. The operative findings will influence the decision by the ease or difficulty of separating the pancreas from the SMV. If there is no direct vein wall invasion, there will be two glistening surfaces (pancreatic capsule and vein) that are separable. Invasion is likely and vein excision demanded when there is no dissectable plane between the two structures. If the venogram showed only unilateral venous impingement by the tumor, it is very likely that a lateral SMV wall excision (with the vein partially occluded by a curved vascular clamp) and either direct or vein patch venorrhaphy will suffice. If the venogram shows bilateral impingement, the surgeon should be prepared for possible segmental SMV resection. If the vein is occluded, segmental vein excision is the only possible chance for complete tumor excision.

Free proximal and distal sections of the vein must be available to control and reapproximate. If lateral vein–tumor approximation is present, the decision is either to separate the two, to excise the lateral vein wall, or to segmentally resect the vein. Unfortunately, available data are not helpful to the surgeon making the decision.

The first recorded SMV resection with pancreatectomy was in 1951.[156] The patient died with diffuse liver and peritoneal metastases, but no tumor was present at the venovenostomy. Fortner published a series of operations, including segmental portal vein and SMV resection, extended lymphadenectomy, and occasional arterial resection, in 1973 and named the procedure regional pancreatectomy.[145, 157–159] Others have reported results from similar operations, but none has reported a 5-year survivor with portal vein invasion.[99, 145, 157–165] Manabe et al.[161, 162] resected 42 tumors with "portal vein involvement" (the depth and extent were not specified); no patient lived beyond 1.5 years from the time of surgery. Ishikawa and colleagues[100] reported 7 of 19 patients living after 3 years (5 alive without recurrence from 3 to 4.5 years), all of whom had histologic portal vein and SMV invasion but confined to less than a semicircle of the lateral wall and less than 2 cm in length. They compared these to 18 patients with angiographic portal vein and SMV bilateral impingement with greater than 1.2 cm of narrowing. None of these patients lived beyond 1.5 years. However, they do not say what adjuvant therapy was used with the extended procedures.[100] Nagakawa et al.[165] reported "5-year survivors" in the group with portal vein adventitial or medial invasion, while both patients with invasion completely through the portal vein wall died within 2 years. Their lymphadenectomy extends to both kidneys and to an area below the aortic bifurcation. They note that diarrhea commonly accompanies the resection and so recommend skeletonization of only the right half of the SMA in stage I and II cases, but they report no data supporting the efficacy of this maneuver.

Perioperative mortality rates for these extended procedures vary from 8% (Fortner's later series) to 32% (his earlier series), and morbidity is greater than with standard TP or Whipple pancreatoduodenectomy.[145, 157–159] It is clear that many of the tumors removed could not be removed by any lesser operation. It may be that patients with extremely advanced local lesions are better palliated by massive excision than by other, nonoperative means. However, no trial has been performed. With a median survival of 6 months and a less than 20% chance to survive 1 year, it is unlikely that nonoperative alternatives would be substantially worse in terms of both quality and quantity of life. Until comparative data are available, one must question the use of any excisional procedure alone for patients with frank SMV and portal vein invasion or occlusion. As noted in the section on resectability, we have two patients with SMV bilateral impingement living beyond 28 months and another without recurrence at 20 months following treatment with preoperative radiotherapy and resection (only one of the three required vein resection). The vein margins and pancreatic margins at the vein were all negative in these cases, undoubtedly owing to the preoperative radiotherapy. There are no data available to assess whether postoperative radiotherapy could similarly sterilize venous margins after subtotal surgical excisions. Patients with unilateral SMV impingement (Ishikawa stages II and III) probably have a better prognosis, although only Ishikawa et al.[100] and our group[80] have published relevant survival data. Since Ishikawa and coworkers have published results of preoperative radiotherapy elsewhere and did not specify whether the patients reported with vascular classifications had adjuvant therapy,[166] the outlook for such patients with resection alone must remain unclear. We have treated six patients with Ishikawa stage II and III lesions with resection after preoperative chemoradiotherapy. Lateral SMV resection was necessary for one. Lymphadenectomy extended to the anterior aortic and vena caval walls and to the right lateral wall and origin of the SMA. All pancreatic margins at the vein and the one vein wall resected contained no cancer. One patient (stage III) is alive without recurrence at 34 months; two (stage III and II) are alive with distant metastases at 19 and 20 months, respectively; two (stage II and III) died with liver metastases at 7 and 11 months, respectively; and one died postoperatively of sepsis.

Focal involvement of the hepatic or superior mesenteric arteries is also resected by proponents of extended pancreatectomy, although no long-term survivors are reported. It is likely that such arterial involvement and diffuse SMV and portal vein invasion or occlusion are signs of cancer extending beyond the area of excision. Patients with splenic artery and vein involvement or occlusion are staged as T2 (tumor extension beyond the capsule), as if the vessel involvement were insignificant.[39, 43] Reports of treatment for distal pancreatic cancer do not mention patients with vascular involvement.[40, 167–169] We have performed distal pancreatectomy to the right of the SMV after preoperative radiotherapy on two patients with tumors of the tail and body of the pancreas that occluded both splenic artery and vein: one died with distant recurrence at 14 months, and the other is alive without recurrence 60 months after treatment. The latter patient required lateral portal venorrhaphy at the splenic vein entrance for clearance.

Pylorus-Preserving Pancreatectomy?

The rare small tumor in the head of the pancreas may be resected by pylorus-preserving or standard, pylorus-sacrificing pancreatoduodenectomy, although proponents of both total and extended pancreatectomy have expressed opinions that these operations will produce more cures for patients with small lesions. While faster liquid gastric emptying, more normal gastrin and secretin secretion, and a lesser incidence of postgastrectomy syndromes have been shown for pylorus-preserving pancreatectomy, there is concern with its efficacy in removing pancreatic cancers.[170–174]

Sharp and colleagues[173] reported two cases with intramural spread of pancreatic cancer into the duodenum and antrum and another case of recurrent tumor within the pylorus after a pylorus-preserving resection. The largest comparative trial (there have been no randomized trials) revealed an inferior survival rate for patients with stage III pancreatic cancers treated by pylorus-preserving versus pylorus-excision pancreatectomy.[174] Lymphadenectomy was not standardized, and the decision for the type of operation was according to the preference of the surgeon, so there may have been hidden biases. However, since the benefits of the procedure are not marked, and it is the smallest lesion that may be the only one potentially cured by surgery alone, pylorus-preserving pancreatoduodenectomy should probably not be used in the treatment of pancreatic cancer beyond a prospective trial.

How Should the Pancreatic Tail or Body Lesion Be Approached?

Cancer at the pancreatic tail prompts decisions about what neighboring organs to resect and how far to proceed medially. The same decisions exist with cancers involving the pancreatic neck and body, although the decision to continue to TP is more strongly considered in such cases. Since most cases of cancer in the pancreatic body and tail are discovered at stage III or IV, it is reasonable to consider preoperative radiotherapy in order to improve local control.[40, 94, 167–169] If the aorta or the origins of the celiac axis or SMA are involved, tumor excision should not be attempted. Since the disease-free survival of those patients with adjacent organ or nodal extension has been so poor, preoperative or postoperative adjuvant radiotherapy with chemopotentiation is recommended.

Nonsurgical Options

Since the report by Haslam et al.[175] in 1973, there has been much work by radiotherapists in attempting to control localized, "irresectable" pancreatic cancer.[176–188] There are three fundamental problems with the effort:

1. A mass or a cancer in the periampullary area may not have arisen in the pancreas.[46, 189]
2. Opinions about resectability vary widely.
3. There is no staging system to allow comparison of results to other therapies.

Thus, every radiotherapy series should elicit doubt about the nature and extent of the primary tumor.

Nevertheless, work over the past two decades has shown that chemotherapy and radiotherapy potentiate the effects of each other on pancreatic cancer and that either interstitial implantation of radioactive seeds or intraoperative radiotherapy increases local control (defined as no radiologically detectable growth in the irradiated tumor volume) as compared to external radiotherapy alone.[175, 176, 179–181, 183, 185] Komaki and coworkers[190] developed a protocol in which patients with locally advanced lesions received radiotherapy and 5-fluorouracil (5-FU) along with prophylactic hepatic radiotherapy, since so many patients with pancreatic cancer die of and with hepatic metastases. Liver metastases developed in only 2 of the original 18 patients.[190] However, a confirmatory study of the same method did not show the same good results: documented liver metastases developed in only 32% of the patients, but only 10% survived at 1 year.[191]

Curiously, no series has a better 30-month survival rate than the 21% reported by Haslam et al.[175] in 1973, in which patients received 6000 cGy to the tumor (three cycles of 2000 cGy with 2-week breaks between) with bolus 5-FU both during and indefinitely after the radiotherapy. One patient "with biopsy proof of adenocarcinoma" was surviving without recurrence 72 months after diagnosis. While these results are superb (30-month survival rates in resection series range from 15% to 50%, depending on the initial tumor stage), it is likely that the long-term survivors either had duodenal or ampullary cancer (both much more responsive to radiotherapy) or had much less tumor volume than those in other cohorts of "irresectable" patients. To avoid making erroneous conclusions about future treatment strategies, it would be desirable to develop a staging system that specifically addresses this group of patients. Whittington et al.[181] and Mohiuddin and colleagues[185] used a system similar to the AJCC system in staging their patients, but it is difficult to understand. Stage II patients have no involved lymph nodes (how do we know?) and are unresectable (what are the criteria?). Stage III patients may be resectable but must have positive lymph nodes (which nodes? why was no resection done?). A system that staged the degree of central vascular encroachment, the amount of tumor volume, and the number and location of involved nodes would obviously be preferable, just as it would for the cases with resection.

Questions remaining to be answered involve the place of several brachytherapy and chemopotentiating modalities in the treatment of the patient with locally advanced cancer. No trials of radiosensitizers such as misonidazole or SR-2508 versus or combined with 5-FU, mitomycin C, or platinum derivatives have been done, either with external beam, interstitial, or intraoperative radiotherapy.

Combination Therapy: Pre- and Postoperative Radiotherapy

The phenomena of antitumor activity with radiotherapy and chemotherapy-enhanced radiotherapy in the locally advanced patient and poor results with surgery alone for the patient with "resectable" tumors brought to many authors the question of whether results could be improved by combination therapy.[125, 154, 192–195]

The Only Prospective, Randomized Trial

The now defunct Gastrointestinal Tumor Study Group (GITSG) began a randomized trial of excisional surgery plus postoperative radiotherapy and 5-FU versus surgery in 1974.[195–198] Patients in the treatment group received two courses of 2000 cGy to the entire pancreas through anterior and posterior portals, separated by a 2-week treatment break. Bolus 5-FU was given on the first 3 days of each radiotherapy cycle and weekly thereafter for a total of 2 years or until recurrence was noted. Accrual to the trial was slow (6 patients per year), but nonetheless the number of patients in each group (20 and 21, respectively) were adequate to show a statistically significant difference in median survival favoring the combined-therapy cohort (20 vs. 11 months, $P = .035$). The findings were substantiated by a second cohort of 30 patients treated in exactly the same fashion except that three- and four-field techniques were used for the radiotherapy.[196]

Ten-year follow-up showed that the only 10-year survivors were in the treatment group (19% vs. 0%).[198] Unfortunately, the sizes of the tumors were not all measured (only 14 of 21 of the control group and 18 of 20 of the first treatment group). However, pathologically clear resection margins (not otherwise specified) were a requirement for entry to the protocol. Local recurrence was found in 7 of 21 of the control arm but in 21 of 41 of those treated with postoperative therapy. However, only four patients had autopsies, so these findings must be viewed with some doubt. The fact remains that treatment did not markedly decrease local recurrence rates and may have had no effect on them.

This raises the question of local recurrence after pancreatectomy. Even at autopsy, it is necessary to define what one means by local. Theoretically, it should be recurrence within the margins of the original operation, but these margins are pushed inward by surrounding tissue as soon as the procedure is completed. Recurrence in the distal mesenteric (SMA, SMV) tree would be in nodes not dissected by the operation but that would be "local-regional" relative to the tumor bed. Definitions of local recurrence have varied from being any recurrence in the retroperitoneum, to a recurrence in the tumor bed or para-aortic lymphatics, to no definition.[106, 154, 184, 185, 199] The only recurrences strictly local are those at the pancreatic and biliary anastomoses and those anterior to the aorta and inferior vena cava just above and below the left renal vein. There is no standard staging system for recurrences. Until there is, it will be difficult to compare various treatment programs that address the problem of local control. Future authors are encouraged to define clearly their criteria for labeling a recurrence "local," and readers are advised to examine closely those criteria in any paper.

Other methods of adjuvant therapy combined with surgery have included intraoperative radiotherapy at the time of resection and varied forms of chemotherapy with preoperative or postoperative radiotherapy.[80, 125, 200–209]

Adjuvant Intraoperative Radiotherapy

Hiraoka[200] reported 16 patients with extended pancreatectomy and intraoperative radiotherapy (IORT) and compared their survival and recurrence patterns with those of patients he had treated with standard pancreatectomy with and without IORT and extended resection without IORT. Tumor stages were similar in all groups. The only patients surviving more than 3 years were those with extended resection and IORT. He claims a 40% 5-year survival rate for those 12 patients with clear margins of resection, but only 1 patient in that group has actually survived more than 5 years. Three others are alive free of recurrence from 3 to 4 years. Only one patient had an autopsy, and microscopic cancer was found in the left para-aortic position just above the left renal vein (within the radiotherapy field). As expected, those with extended resections all had watery diarrhea postoperatively and required total parenteral nutrition for 4 to 16 months postoperatively.

A less extended resection has been combined with preoperative radiotherapy and continuous 5-FU and IORT by Evans et al.[155, 201] End results from this trial will be available in 2 to 3 years.

Neither group has used postoperative chemotherapy.

Postoperative Radiotherapy With or Without Chemotherapy

All studies of postoperative treatment other than the GITSG trial mentioned above have compared either sequential historical cohorts or patients within the same time frame either given or not given chemotherapy and/or radiotherapy. As one might expect, the latter reports have shown no advantage to the therapy, while the former types have (with contemporary cohorts, it is usually the patient with the more advanced, aggressive cancer who is given the added therapy).

Thus, Appelqvist et al.[125] and Whittington and colleagues[202] reported an increased survival in those patients with postoperative radiotherapy and chemotherapy, but Cameron and coworkers[203] and Geer and Brennan[103] were able to demonstrate no positive effect of the adjuvant treatment in larger cohorts. Whittington et al. reported the most impressive results, with a 3-year actuarial survival rate of 59% in 17 patients with clear margins of resection. At least 11 of these patients had positive nodes. Median tumor volume was 78 cm^3. Patients received 4500 to 4860 cGy in 180-cGy fractions with two 96-hour infusions of 5-FU (1000 mg/m^2/day) and a single bolus of mitomycin C (10 mg/m^2) on the first day of treatment.

Not for purposes of comparison but, rather, for a degree of perspective, the 2- and 3-year actuarial survival results from the most highly selected cohorts treated with no or occasional adjuvant therapy vary from 20% to 30% for 2- and 3-year survival for all patients with resection (those with positive lymph nodes included).[88, 103, 109, 203] Figures for those with negative nodes are 30% to 65% for both 2- and 3-year survival.[88, 103, 109, 203] Almost all of the patients with such high survival results had tumors less than 3 cm in diameter. Results from series with more liberal selection criteria were considerably worse, with median survival ranging from 12 to 18 months.[112, 182]

Preoperative Radiotherapy With or Without Chemotherapy

The concept of presurgical radiotherapy for patients with pancreatic cancer was published as early as 1975 by Tepper and colleagues.[154] The theoretic advantages are the following:

1. Increased vulnerability of the cancer cells to radiotherapy because of no vascular interruption by surgery.
2. Sterilization of cells at the boundaries of resection before manipulation.
3. Increased patient tolerance (thus an increased likelihood that more of a dose will be delivered).
4. An ability to reduce the amount of radiotherapy-injured bowel both by treating small bowel that is not tethered into the radiotherapy field by postoperative adhesions and by resecting much of what was in the field during the radiotherapy.
5. Patients destined to have extrapancreatic metastases would have another 3 months in which to display them (improved selection).
6. Fewer pancreatojejunostomy leaks.

Pilepich and Miller[192] and Kopelson[193] first reported treatment by preoperative radiotherapy without chemotherapy in the early 1980s. The therapy resulted in at least two 5-year survivors from at least 17 patients so treated between 1972 and 1981. No chemotherapy was given in addition to the 4000 to 5000 cGy delivered by a two-field technique in 200-cGy fractions. Patients must have been considered resectable by the Tufts surgeons to have been offered this therapy, although many of them had been previously explored elsewhere and judged to have unresectable tumors. Three fourths of the patients had cancers greater than 5 cm in diameter. Of the 17 reported, 6 never came to second surgery because of progressive local or distant cancer, or both; 5 were found unresectable (1 locally, 4 because of distant peritoneal metastases) at second surgery; and 6 had Whipple resections.

Since these reports, several groups have added chemotherapy to preoperative radiotherapy in an attempt to improve the results.[80, 155, 201, 204, 205] The only series reporting even preliminary end results is ours, in which resectability based on CT scan, arteriography, and intraoperative ultrasonography was 58%.[80, 204] Median size of the tumors was 4 cm^2, and 15 of the 21 patients with arteriograms had at least some portal vein involvement, indicating that these were largely locally advanced lesions. Only 3 of 23 patients with resection had a positive margin (1 with cancer cells at a divided pancreatic tail, 1 one high-power field [HPF] away at the same location, and 1 one HPF away from the distal SMV margin). Only 2 of 12 patients having a recurrence had a local recurrence as a component of the failure, and none had local recurrence alone. Median follow-up from the time of diagnosis for the 13 patients still alive after resection is 19 months (5 to 61 months), and 10 remain free of recurrence from 5 to 61 months (median, 18 months). The 2- and 3-year actuarial survival rate is 60% for those with resections in the Fox Chase pilot protocol.[204] Other experiences began later than ours, and thus survival outcomes are not available.[155, 205]

One can observe resectability, margins of resection, local recurrence, and survival for patients treated with preoperative therapy, but it is impossible to assure oneself that the tumors being treated are similar to those with surgical (postresectional) staging. Even if Ishikawa venographic staging were reported for patients with surgery alone or postoperative adjuvant therapy for comparative purposes, the nodal status and original extent of spread in the preoperative therapy group would be unknown. Thus, for any true comparison to be made of these two sequencing programs, a randomized trial would be necessary in order to make the groups equal. Before such a trial can exist, data from both preoperative and postoperative adjuvant therapy trials must continue to mature to a point at which the results can be better analyzed, and consensus must be developed regarding the type and delivery method of chemotherapy.

RECURRENT AND UNRESECTABLE DISEASE—RESULTS AND COMPLICATIONS

Surgical Options

Although patients with inoperable pancreatic cancer and palliative bypass seldom live more than 1 year, it is important to understand that most patients with cancers of the pancreatic head and body eventually have biliary obstruction and at least 20% have obstruction of the duodenum.[41, 206, 207] Those with cancers of the body or tail may have sinistral portal hypertension and subsequent gastric variceal bleeding from splenic vein thrombosis by the tumor. None of these situations dictates a prophylactic operation in an asymptomatic patient. However, when the surgeon has entered the abdomen for a resection and finds an inoperable tumor, biliary and duodenal bypass for those with tumors of the pancreatic head and splenectomy for those with left-sided portal hypertension should be considered.

Much has been written about the relative merits of cholecystojejunostomy and choledochojejunostomy.[206, 207] Most experienced authors favor bypasses at the bile duct as being more durable conduits, but none has proven this bias. Certainly, if one entertains bypass by the gallbladder, one must be sure that the cystic duct enters the common bile duct well above the malignancy. Duodenal bypass is more controversial, since only 20% to 30% of patients experience duodenal obstruction and gastrojejunostomy is often inadequate palliation, as food often continues to enter and distend the obstructed duodenum. Lucas et al.[208] recommended antrectomy with gastrojejunostomy as a procedure able to provide better palliation for these patients. The intraoperative decision should be governed primarily by the clinical situation. If the tumor is impinging on the duodenum, gastrojejunostomy with or without antrectomy should probably be performed in any patient with a life expectancy of greater than 1 month. The stomach should probably be sewn to the jejunum beyond the Roux jejunojejunostomy for best emptying results.[208] If the tumor extends to the hepatic duct bifurcation, the options are prosthetic bypass and cholangiojejunostomy at the segment III hepatic duct.

Nonsurgical Options

Transhepatic and endoscopically placed biliary stents are available for those patients presenting with stage IV cancer or with tumor recurrence resulting in obstructive jaundice. Wire mesh stents can be internalized through transhepatic stents. These can last for several months after placement. The relative value of endoscopic and radiologic stents will continue to be debated by their proponents, but it is clear that individual skills vary widely for each method of stenting and that it is far easier to replace a clogged transhepatic stent than one placed endoscopically. Trials comparing surgical and radiologic or endoscopic bypass have shown contradictory results, probably indicating selection bias and variance in technical skill.[209–212] Recurrent jaundice and cholangitis are least in those patients having surgical bypass.[209–211] Since any of the prosthetic stents is liable to occlusion after 4 to 5 months, it is prudent to select one that can be easily changed. For the patient with obstructive jaundice about to embark on a preoperative radiotherapy program, a percutaneous stent is far preferable to an endoscopically placed stent, since there is often more debris in the ducts of these patients, requiring multiple stent changes.

For those with gastric outlet or bowel obstruction, an endoscopically placed gastrostomy tube is often the only palliation. This is often impossible because of an inability to approximate the gastric remnant to the anterior abdominal wall. Celiac plexus blocks can be useful for pain control in those with para-aortic recurrences. For a more detailed discussion of these issues, see the following subchapter on periampullary carcinoma.

Systemic chemotherapy offers the only palliation that can affect pancreatic cancer in all of its locations. Unfortunately, response rates are no better than 7% to 15% with currently available therapy. However, 50% of patients have stable disease for a period of time (median, 3 months), and 20% have stable disease from 6 to 25 months.[213] This is clearly superior to the natural history of pancreatic cancer.

POST-TREATMENT CARE AND SURVEILLANCE

Post-treatment care consists primarily of dietary instruction and insulin management for those with total pancreatectomy. Patients usually require pancreatic enzyme supplements, at least for several months after Whipple resection and always after total pancreatectomy. Those without vagotomy require histamine$_2$ blockers indefinitely. Patients with splenectomy must be instructed about postsplenectomy sepsis.

In view of the dismal record of chemotherapy for pancreatic cancer, one might argue that surveillance in order to discover an early recurrence is unreasonable and perhaps cruel. However, the chance of achieving a response to chemotherapy decreases as the disease progresses and performance status falls. Additionally, the patient with a good performance status gains a chance to receive new drugs with reported activity, such as gemcitabine and topotecan.

Surveillance should include images capable of discovering local, peritoneal, liver, and lung metastases in addition to CA 19-9 blood tests. The vast majority of recurrences become apparent within 2 years of initial resection.

SECONDARY TUMORS

There are no reported long-term survivors of metastatic pancreatic cancer. Solitary liver secondary tumors are the only tumors worth considering for surgical excision. We have performed three metastasectomies, two for solitary synchronous tumors and one for a metachronous tumor. All three patients died within 13 months of diffuse liver involvement.

PREVENTION

Perhaps with the exception of smoking cessation, there is no known strategy for pancreatic cancer prevention. Early detection remains the best hope for success against this neoplasm until a truly effective chemotherapeutic or immunotherapeutic agent is discovered.

FUTURE PROSPECTS

As new chemotherapeutic agents are discovered and developed, there will be many patients with metastatic pancreatic cancer on whom the drug may be tested. The more patients entered into such trials, the faster the pace of drug development. Until such time that new therapies are found, current dismal end results might be significantly improved by early detection, safe but thorough surgery, and either pre- or postoperative chemoradiotherapy. Entry of patients into adjuvant trials will speed the discovery of the optimal method and sequencing of these adjuvant therapy programs.

References

1. Cubilla AL, Fitzgerald PJ: Surgical pathology of tumors of the exocrine pancreas. In Moossa AR (ed): Tumors of the Pancreas. Baltimore: Williams & Wilkins, 1980.
2. Wingo PA, Tong T, Bolden BA: Cancer statistics 1995. CA 45:8–30, 1995.
3. Aoki K, Ogawa H: Cancer of the pancreas, international mortality trends. World Health Stat Q 31:2–27, 1978.
4. Haddock G, Carter DC: Aetiology of pancreatic cancer. Br J Surg 77:1159–1166, 1990.
5. Fontham ETH, Correa P: Epidemiology of pancreatic cancer. Surg Clin North Am 69:551–566, 1989.
6. Hirayama T: Epidemiology of pancreatic cancer in Japan. Jpn J Clin Oncol 19:208–215, 1989.
7. Krain LS: The rising incidence of carcinoma of the pancreas—real or apparent? J Surg Oncol 2:115–124, 1970.
8. Bueno de Mesquita HB, Moerman CJ, Runia S, Maisonneuve P: Are energy and energy-providing nutrients related to exocrine carcinoma of the pancreas? Int J Cancer 46:435–444, 1990.
9. Boyle P, Hsieh CC, Maisonneuve P, et al: Epidemiology of pancreas cancer (1988). Int J Pancreatol 5:327–346, 1989.
10. Gordis L, Gold EB: Epidemiology of pancreatic cancer. World J Surg 8:808–821, 1984.
11. Gold EB, Gordis L, Diener MD, et al: Diet and other risk factors for cancer of the pancreas. Cancer 55:460–467, 1985.
12. Norell SE, Ahlbom A, Erwald R, Jacobson G, et al: Diet and pancreatic cancer: A case-control study. Am J Epidemiol 124:894–902, 1986.
13. Mack TM, Yu MC, Hanisch R, Henderson BE: Pancreas cancer and smoking, beverage consumption, and past medical history. J Natl Cancer Inst 76:49–60, 1986.
14. Morgan RGH, Wormsley KG: Progress report: Cancer of the pancreas. Gut 18:580–596, 1977.
15. Wynder EL: An epidemiological evaluation of the causes of cancer of the pancreas. Cancer Res 35:2228–2233, 1975.
16. Haines AL, Moss AR, Whittemore A, Quivey J: A case-control study of pancreatic carcinoma. J Cancer Res Clin Oncol 103:93–97, 1982.
17. Hyvarinen H, Partanen S: Association of cholecystectomy with abdominal cancers. Hepatogastroenterology 34:280–284, 1987.
18. MacMahon B, Yen S, Trichopoulos D, et al: Coffee and cancer of the pancreas. N Engl J Med 304:630–633, 1981.
19. Gordis L: Consumption of methylxanthine-containing beverages and risk of pancreatic cancer. Cancer Lett 52:1–12, 1990.
20. Mills PK, Beeson WL, Abbey DE, et al: Dietary habits and past medical history as related to fatal pancreas cancer risks among Adventists. Cancer 61:2578–2585, 1988.
21. Wynder EL, Hall NEL, Polansky M: Epidemiology of coffee and pancreatic cancer. Cancer Res 43:3900–3906, 1983.
22. Heuch I, Kvale J, Jacobsen BK, Bjelke E: Use of alcohol, tobacco and coffee and risk of pancreatic cancer. Br J Cancer 48:637–643, 1983.
23. Klatsky AL, Friedman GD, Siegelaub AB: Alcohol and mortality: A ten-year Kaiser-Permanente experience. Ann Intern Med 95:139–145, 1981.
24. McLean-Ross LH, Smith MA, Anderson JR, Small WP: Late mortality after surgery for peptic ulcer. N Engl J Med 307:519–522, 1982.
25. Borch K, Kullman E, Hallhagen S, et al: Increased incidence of pancreatic neoplasia in pernicious anemia. World J Surg 12:866–870, 1988.
26. Permert J, Adrian TE, Jacobsson P, et al: Is profound peripheral insulin resistance in patients with pancreatic cancer caused by a tumor-associated factor? Am J Surg 165:61–67, 1993.
27. Kessler II: Cancer mortality among diabetics. J Natl Cancer Inst 44:673–686, 1970.
28. Wynder EL, Mabuchi K, Maruchi N, Fortner JG: Epidemiology of cancer of the pancreas. J Natl Cancer Inst 50:645–667, 1973.
29. Green A, Jensen OM: Frequency of cancer among insulin-treated diabetic patients in Denmark. Diabetologia 28:128–130, 1985.
30. Mancuso TF, El-Attar AA: Cohort study of workers exposed to betanaphthylamine and benzidine. J Occup Med 9:277–285, 1967.
31. Garabrant DH, Held J, Langholz B: DDT and pancreas cancer in a case-control study of chemical workers. Am J Epidemiol 134:755, 1991.
32. Obertop H, Bruining HA, Eeftinck M, et al: Operative approach to cancer of the head of the pancreas and the peri-ampullary region. Br J Surg 69:573–576, 1982.
33. Leadbetter A, Foster RS Jr, Haines CR: Carcinoma of the pancreas: Results from the Vermont tumor registry. Am J Surg 129:356–360, 1975.
34. Sener SF, Fremgen A, Imperato JP, et al: Pancreatic cancer in Illinois: A report by 88 hospitals on 2401 patients diagnosed 1978–84. Am Surg 57:490–495, 1991.
35. Pollard HM, Anderson WAD, Brooks FP, et al: Staging of cancer of the pancreas. Cancer 47 (Suppl):1631–1637, 1981.
36. Mallinson CN, Rake MO, Cocking JB, et al: Chemotherapy in pancreatic cancer: Results of a controlled, prospective, randomised, multicentre trial. Br Med J 281:1589–1591, 1980.
37. Hermreck AS, Thomas CY, Friesen SR: Importance of pathologic staging in the surgical management of adenocarcinoma of the exocrine pancreas. Am J Surg 127:653–657, 1974.
38. Moertel CG, Reitemeier RJ (eds): Advanced Gastrointestinal Cancer: Clinical Management and Chemotherapy. New York: Hoeber Medical Division, Harper & Row, 1969.
39. Carter SK, Comis RL: The integration of chemotherapy into a combined modality approach for cancer treatment. VI. Pancreatic adenocarcinoma. Cancer Treat Rev 2:193–214, 1975.
40. Forrest JF, Longmire WP: Carcinoma of the pancreas and periampullary region: A study of 279 patients. Ann Surg 189:129–138, 1979.
41. Nakase A, Matsumoto Y, Uchida K, Honjo I: Surgical treatment of cancer of the pancreas and the periampullary region: Cumulative results in 57 institutions in Japan. Ann Surg 185:52–57, 1977.
42. Mikal S, Campbell AJA: Carcinoma of the pancreas: Diagnostic and operative criteria based on 100 consecutive autopsies. Surgery 28:963–969, 1950.
43. Beahrs OH, Henson DE, Hutter RVP, Kennedy BJ (eds): Manual for Staging of Cancer, 4th ed. Philadelphia: JB Lippincott, 1992, pp 109–111.
44. Ishikawa O, Ohigashi H, Sasaki Y, et al: Practical usefulness of lymphatic and connective tissue clearance for carcinoma of the pancreas head. Ann Surg 208:215–220, 1988.
45. Martin J, Weinerman BH: The natural history of pancreatic cancer in Manitoba: A population based study. Can J Gastroenterol 6:201–204, 1992.
46. Freeny PC, Traverso LW, Ryan JA: Diagnosis and staging of pancreatic adenocarcinoma with dynamic computed tomography. Am J Surg 165:600–606, 1993.
47. Bakkevold KE, Arnesjø B, Kambestad B: Carcinoma of the pancreas and papilla of Vater: Presenting symptoms, signs, and diagnosis related to stage and tumour site—a prospective multicentre trial in 472 patients. Scand J Gastroenterol 27:317–325, 1992.
48. Warren KW, Christophi C, Armendariz R, Basu S: Current trends in the diagnosis and treatment of carcinoma of the pancreas. Am J Surg 145:813–818, 1983.

49. Moossa AR: Pancreatic cancer: Approach to diagnosis, selection for surgery and choice of operation. Cancer 50:2689–2698, 1982.
50. DiMagno EP, Malagelada JR, Taylor WF, Go VLW: A prospective comparison of current diagnostic tests for pancreatic cancer. N Engl J Med 297:737–742, 1977.
51. Mackie CR, Dhorajiwala J, Blackstone MO, Bowie J: Value of new diagnostic aids in relation to the disease process in pancreatic cancer. Lancet 2:385–388, 1979.
52. Moossa AR, Levin B: Collaborative studies in the diagnosis of pancreatic cancer. Semin Oncol 6:298–308, 1979.
53. Røsch T, Lorenz R, Braig C, et al: Endoscopic ultrasound in pancreatic tumor diagnosis. Gastrointest Endosc 37:347–352, 1991.
54. Dooley WC, Cameron JL, Pitt HA, et al: Is preoperative angiography useful in patients with periampullary tumors? Ann Surg 211:649–655, 1990.
55. Mackie CR, Lu CT, Noble HG, et al: Prospective evaluation of angiography in the diagnosis and management of patients suspected of having pancreatic cancer. Ann Surg 189:11–17, 1979.
56. Biehl TR, Traverso LW, Hauptmann E, Ryan JA Jr: Preoperative visceral angiography alters intraoperative strategy during the Whipple procedure. Am J Surg 165:607–612, 1993.
57. Bull DA, Hunter GC, Crabtree TG, et al: Hepatic ischemia, caused by celiac axis compression, complicating pancreaticoduodenectomy. Ann Surg 217:244–247, 1993.
58. de Roos WK, Welvaart K, Bloem JL, Hermans J: Assessment of resectability of carcinoma of the pancreatic head by ultrasonography and computed tomography. A retrospective analysis. Eur J Surg Oncol 16:411–416, 1990.
59. Mori H, Miyake H, Aikawa H, et al: Dilated posterior superior pancreaticoduodenal vein: Recognition with CT and clinical significance in patients with pancreaticobiliary carcinomas. Radiology 181:793–800, 1991.
60. Warshaw AL, Tepper JE, Shipley WU: Laparoscopy in the staging and planning of therapy for pancreatic cancer. Am J Surg 151:76–80, 1986.
61. Warshaw AL, Gu Z, Wittenberg J, Waltman AC: Preoperative staging and assessment of resectability of pancreatic cancer. Arch Surg 125:230–233, 1990.
62. Freeny PC, Marks WM, Ryan JA, Traverso LW: Pancreatic ductal adenocarcinoma: Diagnosis and staging with dynamic CT. Radiology 166:125–133, 1988.
63. Fuhrman GM, Charnsangavej C, Abbruzzese JL, et al: Thin-section contrast-enhanced tomography accurately predicts resectability of malignant pancreatic neoplasms. Am J Surg 167:104–113, 1994.
64. Jafri SZ, Aisen AM, Glazer GM, Weiss CA: Comparison of CT and angiography in assessing resectability of pancreatic carcinoma. AJR 42:525–529, 1984.
65. Soyer P, Levesque M, Elias D, et al: Preoperative assessment of resectability of hepatic metastases from colonic carcinoma: CT portography vs sonography and dynamic CT. AJR 159:741–744, 1992.
66. Karl RC, Morse SS, Halpert RD, Clark RA: Preoperative evaluation of patients for liver resection: Appropriate CT imaging. Ann Surg 217:226–232, 1993.
67. Olen R, Pickleman J, Freeark RJ: Less is better: The diagnostic workup of the patient with obstructive jaundice. Arch Surg 124:791–795, 1989.
68. Martin FM, Rossi RL, Dorrucci V, et al: Clinical and pathologic correlations in patients with periampullary tumors. Arch Surg 125:723–726, 1990.
69. Alvarez C, Livingston EH, Ashley SW, et al: Cost-benefit analysis of the work-up for pancreatic cancer. Am J Surg 165:53–60, 1993.
70. Savarino V, Mansi C, Bistolfi L, et al: Failure of new diagnostic aids in improving detection of pancreatic cancer at a resectable stage. Dig Dis Sci 28:1078–1082, 1983.
71. Kairaluoma MI, Myllyla V, Partion E, et al: Impact of new imaging techniques on survival in cancer of the head of the pancreas and the periampullary region. Acta Chir Scand 151:69–72, 1985.
72. Gudjonnson B, Livstone EM, Spiro HM: Cancer of the pancreas: Diagnostic accuracy and survival statistics. Cancer 42:2494–2506, 1978.
73. Ferrucci JT, Wittenberg J, Mueller PR, et al: Diagnosis of abdominal malignancy by radiologic fine needle aspiration biopsy. AJR 134:323–330, 1980.
74. Dickey JE, Haaga JR, Stellato TA, et al: Evaluation of computed tomography guided percutaneous biopsy of the pancreas. Surg Gynecol Obstet 163:497–503, 1986.
75. McLoughlin MJ, Ho CS, Langer B, et al: Fine needle aspiration biopsy of malignant lesions in and around the pancreas. Cancer 41:2413–2419, 1978.
76. Ferrucci JT Jr, Wittenberg J, Margolies MN, Carey RW: Malignant seeding of the tract after thin-needle aspiration biopsy. Radiology 130:345–346, 1979.
77. Bergenfeldt M, Genell S, Lindholm K, et al: Needle-tract seeding after percutaneous fine-needle biopsy of pancreatic carcinoma: Case report. Acta Chir Scand 154:77–79, 1988.
78. Smith EH: The hazards of fine-needle aspiration biopsy. Ultrasound Med Biol 10:629–634, 1984.
79. Warshaw AL: Implications of peritoneal cytology for staging of early pancreatic cancer. Am J Surg 161:26–30, 1991.
80. Hoffman JP, Weese JL, Solin LJ, et al: A single institutional experience with preoperative chemoradiotherapy for stage I-III pancreatic adenocarcinoma. Am Surg 59:772–781, 1993.
81. Nakaizumi A, Tatsuta M, Uehara H, et al: Cytologic examination of pure pancreatic juice in the diagnosis of pancreatic carcinoma: The endoscopic retrograde intraductal catheter aspiration cytologic technique. Cancer 70:2610–2614, 1992.
82. Mackie CR, Cooper MJ, Lewis MH, et al: Non-operative differentiation between pancreatic cancer and chronic pancreatitis. Ann Surg 189:480–487, 1979.
83. Wapnick S, Hadas N, Purow E, Grosberg SJ: Mass in the head of the pancreas in cholestatic jaundice: Carcinoma or pancreatitis? Ann Surg 190:587–591, 1979.
84. Hart MJ, White TT, Brown PC, Freeny PC: Potentially curable masses in the pancreas. Am J Surg 154:134–136, 1987.
85. Mansour GMI, Cucchiaro G, Niotis MT, et al: Surgical management of pancreatic lymphoma. Arch Surg 124:1287–1289, 1989.
86. Tuchek JM, DeJong SA, Pickleman J: Diagnosis, surgical intervention and prognosis of pancreatic lymphoma. Am Surg 59:513–518, 1993.
87. Cubilla AL, Fitzgerald PF: Cancer of the pancreas (nonendocrine): A suggested morphologic classification. Semin Oncol 6:285–297, 1979.
88. Kellum JM, Clark J, Miller HH: Pancreatoduodenectomy for resectable malignant periampullary tumors. Surg Gynecol Obstet 157:362–366, 1983.
89. Yamaguchi K, Taaka M: Groove pancreatitis masquerading as pancreatic carcinoma. Am J Surg 163:312–318, 1992.
90. Cattell RB, Pyrtek LJ: An appraisal of pancreatoduodenal resection: A follow-up study of 61 cases. Ann Surg 129:840–849, 1949.
91. Porter MR: Carcinoma of the pancreatico-duodenal area: Operability and choice of procedure. Ann Surg 148:711–724, 1958.
92. Longmire WP: The technique of pancreaticoduodenal resection. Surgery 59:344–352, 1966.
93. Brooks JR, Culebras JM: Cancer of the pancreas: Palliative operation, Whipple procedure, or total pancreatectomy? Am J Surg 131:516–520, 1976.
94. Herter FP, Cooperman AM, Ahlborn TN, Antinori C: Surgical experience with pancreatic and periampullary cancer. Ann Surg 195:274–281, 1982.
95. Piorkowski RJ, Blievernicht SW, Lawrence W Jr, et al: Pancreatic and periampullary carcinoma: Experience with 200 patients over a 12 year period. Am J Surg 143:189–193, 1982.
96. Malt RA: Treatment of pancreatic cancer. JAMA 250:1433–1437, 1983.
97. Trede M: The surgical treatment of pancreatic carcinoma. Surgery 97:28–35, 1985.
98. Pellegrini CA, Heck CF, Raper S, Way LW: An analysis of the reduced morbidity and mortality rates after pancreaticoduodenectomy. Am J Surg 124:778–781, 1989.
99. Gall FP, Kessler H, Hermanek P: Surgical treatment of ductal pancreatic carcinoma. Eur J Surg Oncol 17:173–181, 1991.
100. Ishikawa O, Ohigashi H, Imaoka S, et al: Preoperative indications for extended pancreatectomy for locally advanced pancreas cancer involving the portal vein. Ann Surg 215:231–236, 1992.
101. Nix GAJJ, Dubbleman C, Wilson JHP, et al: Prognostic implications of tumor diameter in carcinoma of the head of the pancreas. Cancer 67:529–535, 1991.
102. Bakkevold KE, Arnesjø B, Kambestad B: Carcinoma of the pancreas

and papilla of Vater—assessment of resectability and factors influencing resectability in stage I carcinomas. A prospective multicentre trial in 472 patients. Eur J Surg Oncol 18:494–507, 1992.
103. Geer RJ, Brennan MJ: Prognostic indicators for survival after resection of pancreatic adenocarcinoma. Am J Surg 165:68–73, 1993.
104. Cubilla AL, Fitzgerald PJ, Fortner JG: Pancreas cancer—duct cell adenocarcinoma: Survival in relation to site, size, stage and type of therapy. J Surg Oncol 10:465–482, 1978.
105. Bøttger T, Zech J, Weber W, et al: Relevant factors in the prognosis of ductal pancreatic carcinoma. Acta Chir Scand 156:781–788, 1990.
106. Willett CG, Lewandrowski K, Warshaw AL, et al: Resection margins in carcinoma of the head of the pancreas: Implications for radiation therapy. Ann Surg 217:144–148, 1993.
107. Aston SJ, Longmire WP: Pancreaticoduodenal resection: Twenty years' experience. Arch Surg 106:813–817, 1973.
108. Mannell A, van Heerden JA, Weiland LH, Ilstrup DM: Factors influencing survival after resection for ductal adenocarcinoma of the pancreas. Ann Surg 203:403–407, 1986.
109. Trede M, Schwall G, Saeger H: Survival after pancreatoduodenectomy: 118 consecutive resections without an operative mortality. Ann Surg 211:447–458, 1990.
110. Crist DW, Sitzmann JV, Cameron JL: Improved hospital morbidity, mortality, and survival after the Whipple procedure. Ann Surg 206:358–365, 1987.
111. Yamaguchi K, Nishihara K, Kolodziejczyk P, Tsuneyoshi M: Long survivors after pancreatoduodenectomy for pancreas head carcinoma. Aust NZ J Surg 62:545–549, 1992.
112. Connolly MM, Dawson PJ, Michelassi F, et al: Survival in 1001 patients with carcinoma of the pancreas. Ann Surg 206:366–373, 1987.
113. Allison DC, Bose KK, Hruban RH, et al: Pancreatic cancer cell DNA content correlates with long-term survival after pancreatoduodenectomy. Ann Surg 214:648–656, 1991.
114. Moossa AR, Levin B: The diagnosis of "early" pancreatic cancer: The University of Chicago experience. Cancer 47:1688–1697, 1981.
115. Manabe T, Miyashita T, Ohshio G, et al: Small carcinoma of the pancreas: Clinical and pathologic evaluation of 17 patients. Cancer 62:135–141, 1988.
116. Hermanek P: Staging of exocrine pancreatic carcinoma. Eur J Surg Oncol 17:167–172, 1991.
117. Mackie CR, Bowie J, Cooper MJ, et al: Ultrasonography and tumor-associated antigens: The concept of combining noninvasive tests in the screening for pancreatic cancer. Arch Surg 114:889–892, 1979.
118. Niederau C, Grendell JH: Diagnosis of pancreatic carcinoma: Imaging techniques and tumor markers. Pancreas 7:66–86, 1992.
119. Sperti C, Pasquali C, Catalini S, et al: CA 19-9 as a prognostic index after resection for pancreatic cancer. J Surg Oncol 52:137–141, 1993.
120. Tian F, Appert HE, Myles J, Howard JM: Prognostic value of serum CA 19-9 levels in pancreatic adenocarcinoma. Ann Surg 215:350–355, 1992.
121. Ozaki H, Kinoshita T, Kosuge T, et al: Evidence of effective multidisciplinary treatment for resectable pancreatic cancer from the viewpoint of the CA 19-9 level. Int J Pancreatol 9:159–163, 1991.
122. Satake K, Chung Y, Umeyama K, et al: The possibility of diagnosing small pancreatic cancer (less than 4.0 cm) by measuring various serum tumor markers. Cancer 68:149–152, 1991.
123. Frebourg T, Bercoff E, Manchon N, et al: The evaluation of CA 19-9 antigen level in the early detection of pancreatic cancer: A prospective study of 866 patients. Cancer 62:2287–2290, 1988.
124. Pollard HM, Anderson WAD, Brooks FP, et al: Staging of cancer of the pancreas. Cancer 47:1631–1637, 1981.
125. Appelqvist P, Viren M, Minkkinen J, et al: Operative finding, treatment, and prognosis of carcinoma of the pancreas: An analysis of 267 cases. J Surg Oncol 23:143–150, 1983.
126. Knight RW, Scarborough JP, Goss JC: Adenocarcinoma of the pancreas: A ten-year experience. Arch Surg 113:1401–1404, 1978.
127. Cubilla AL, Fitzgerald PJ, Fortner JG: Pancreas cancer–duct cell adenocarcinoma: Survival in relation to site, size, stage and type of therapy. J Surg Oncol 10:465–482, 1978.
128. Eskelinen M, Lipponen P: A review of prognostic factors in human pancreatic adenocarcinoma. Cancer Detect Prevent 16:287–295, 1992.
129. Eskelinen M, Lipponen P, Marin S, et al: DNA ploidy, S-phase fraction, and G2 fraction as prognostic determinants in human pancreatic cancer. Scand J Gastroenterol 27:39–43, 1992.
130. Suzuki T, Kuratsuka H, Uchida K, et al: Carcinoma of the pancreas arising in the region of the uncinate process. Cancer 30:796–800, 1972.
131. Nix GAJJ, Dubbleman C, Srivastava ED, et al: Prognostic implications of the localization of carcinoma in the head of the pancreas. Am J Gastroenterol 86:1027–1032, 1991.
132. Cubilla AL, Fortner J, Fitzgerald PJ: Lymph node involvement in carcinoma of the head of the pancreas area. Cancer 41:880–887, 1978.
133. Ozaki H, Kishi K: Lymph node dissection in radical resection for carcinoma of the head of the pancreas and periampullary region. Jpn J Clin Oncol 13:371–378, 1983.
134. Evans BP, Ochsner A: The gross anatomy of the lymphatics of the human pancreas. Surgery 36:177–191, 1954.
135. Nagai H, Kuroda A, Morioka Y: Lymphatic and local spread of T1 and T2 pancreatic cancer: A study of autopsy material. Ann Surg 204:65–71, 1986.
136. Brooks JR, Brooks DC, Levine JD: Total pancreatectomy for ductal cell carcinoma of the pancreas: An update. Ann Surg 209:405–410, 1989.
137. van Heerden JA, ReMine WH, Weiland LH, et al: Total pancreatectomy for ductal adenocarcinoma of the pancreas: Mayo Clinic experience. Am J Surg 142:308–311, 1981.
138. van Heerden JA, McIlrath DC, Ilstrup DM, Weiland LH: Total pancreatectomy for ductal adenocarcinoma of the pancreas: An update. World J Surg 12:658–662, 1988.
139. Ihse I, Lilja B, Arnesjø S, Bengmark S: Total pancreatectomy for cancer: An appraisal of 65 cases. Ann Surg 186:675–680, 1977.
140. Moossa AR, Scott MH, Lavelle-Jones M: The place of total and extended total pancreatectomy in pancreatic cancer. World J Surg 8:895–899, 1984.
141. Tryka AF, Brooks JR: Histopathology in the evaluation of total pancreatectomy for ductal carcinoma. Ann Surg 190:373–381, 1979.
142. Kloppel G, Lohse T, Bosslet K, Rückert K: Ductal adenocarcinoma in the head of the pancreas: Incidence of tumor involvement beyond the Whipple resection line. Histological and immunocytochemical analysis of 37 total pancreatectomy specimens. Pancreas 2:170–175, 1987.
143. Nakao A, Ichihara T, Nonami T, et al: Clinicohistopathologic and immunohistochemical studies of intrapancreatic development of carcinoma of the head of the pancreas. Ann Surg 209:181–187, 1989.
144. Motojima K, Urano T, Nagata Y, et al: Detection of point mutations in the Kirsten-*ras* oncogene provides evidence for the multicentricity of pancreatic carcinoma. Ann Surg 217:138–143, 1993.
145. Fortner JG: Regional pancreatectomy for cancer of the pancreas, ampulla, and other related sites. Ann Surg 199:418–425, 1984.
146. Grace PA, Pitt HA, Tompkins RK, et al: Decreased morbidity and mortality after pancreatoduodenectomy. Am J Surg 151:141–149, 1986.
147. Miedema BW, Sarr MG, van Heerden JA, et al: Complications following pancreaticoduodenectomy: Current management. Arch Surg 127:945–950, 1992.
148. Cameron JL, Pitt HA, Yeo CJ, et al: One hundred and forty-five consecutive pancreaticoduodenectomies without mortality. Ann Surg 217:430–438, 1993.
149. Bartoli FG, Arnone GB, Ravera G, Bachi V: Pancreatic fistula and relative mortality in malignant disease after pancreaticoduodenectomy. Review and statistical meta-analysis regarding 15 years of literature. Anticancer Res 11:1831–1848, 1991.
150. Prinz RA, Pickleman J, Hoffman JP: Treatment of pancreatic cutaneous fistulas with a somatostatin analog. Am J Surg 155:36–42, 1988.
151. Büchler M, Friess H, Klempa I, et al: Role of octreotide in the prevention of postoperative complications following pancreatic resection. Am J Surg 163:125–131, 1992.
152. Ishikawa O, Ohigashi H, Imaoka S, et al: Concomitant benefit of preoperative irradiation in preventing pancreas fistula formation after pancreatoduodenectomy. Arch Surg 126:885–889, 1991.
153. Bakkevold KE, Kambestad B: Morbidity and mortality after radical and palliative pancreatic cancer surgery: Risk factors influencing the short-term results. Ann Surg 217:356–368, 1993.
154. Tepper J, Nardi G, Suit H: Carcinoma of the pancreas: Review of MGH experience from 1963 to 1973: Analysis of surgical failure and implications for radiation therapy. Cancer 37:1519–1524, 1976.

155. Evans DB, Rich TA, Byrd DR, et al: Preoperative chemoradiation and pancreaticoduodenectomy for adenocarcinoma of the pancreas. Arch Surg 127:1335–1339, 1992.
156. Moore GE, Sako Y, Thomas LB: Radical pancreatoduodenectomy with resection and reanastomosis of the superior mesenteric vein. Surgery 30:550–553, 1951.
157. Fortner JG: Regional resection of cancer of the pancreas. A new surgical approach. Surgery 73:307–320, 1973.
158. Fortner JG: Surgical principles for pancreatic cancer: Regional total and subtotal pancreatectomy. Cancer 47 (Suppl):1712–1718, 1981.
159. Fortner JG: Technique of regional subtotal and total pancreatectomy. Am J Surg 150:593–600, 1985.
160. Sindelar WF: Clinical experience with regional pancreatectomy for adenocarcinoma of the pancreas. Arch Surg 124:127–132, 1989.
161. Manabe T, Suzuki T, Tobe T: Evaluation of en bloc radical pancreatectomy for carcinoma of the head of the pancreas involving the adjacent vessels. Dig Surg 2:27–30, 1985.
162. Manabe T, Ohshio G, Baba N, Tobe T: Factors influencing prognosis and indications for curative pancreatectomy for ductal adenocarcinoma of the head of the pancreas. Int J Pancreatol 7:187–193, 1990.
163. Lygidakis NJ, Brummelkamp WH, Tytgat GH, et al: Periampullary and pancreatic head carcinoma: Facts and factors influencing mortality, survival, and quality of postoperative life. Am J Gastroenterol 81:968–974, 1986.
164. Sunada S, Miyata M, Tanaka Y, et al: Aggressive resection for advanced pancreatic carcinoma. Jpn J Surg 22:74–77, 1992.
165. Nagakawa T, Konishi I, Ueno K, et al: The results and problems of extensive radical surgery for carcinoma of the head of the pancreas. Jpn J Surg 21:262–267, 1991.
166. Ishikawa O, Ohigashi H, Teshima T, et al: Clinical and histopathological appraisal of preoperative irradiation for adenocarcinoma of the pancreatoduodenal region. J Surg Oncol 40:143–151, 1989.
167. Dalton RR, Sarr MG, van Heerden JA, Colby TV: Carcinoma of the body and tail of the pancreas: Is curative resection justified? Surgery 111:489–494, 1992.
168. Nordback IH, Hruban RH, Boitnott JK, et al: Carcinoma of the body and tail of the pancreas. Am J Surg 164:26–31, 1992.
169. Miyata M, Dousei T, Tanaka Y, et al: Surgical aspect of cancer of the distal pancreas: Comparison of operative findings, mortality, morbidity, physical performance status and survival in cancer of the proximal and distal pancreas. Dig Surg 8:225–230, 1991.
170. Itani KMF, Coleman RE, Akwari OE, Meyers WC: Pylorus-preserving pancreatoduodenectomy: A clinical and physiological appraisal. Ann Surg 204:655–664, 1986.
171. Fink AS, DeSouza LR, Mayer EA, et al: Long-term evaluation of pylorus preservation during pancreaticoduodenectomy. World J Surg 12:663–670, 1988.
172. Takada T, Yasuda H, Shikata J, et al: Postprandial plasma gastrin and secretin concentrations after a pancreatoduodenectomy: A comparison between a pylorus-preserving pancreatoduodenectomy and the Whipple procedure. Ann Surg 210:47–51, 1989.
173. Sharp KW, Ross CB, Halter SA, et al: Pancreatoduodenectomy with pyloric preservation for carcinoma of the pancreas: A cautionary note. Surgery 105:645–653, 1989.
174. Roder JD, Stein HJ, Hüttl W, Siewert JR: Pylorus-preserving *versus* standard pancreaticoduodenectomy: An analysis of 110 pancreatic and periampullary carcinomas. Br J Surg 79:152–155, 1992.
175. Haslam JB, Cavanaugh PJ, Stroup SL: Radiation therapy in the treatment of irresectable adenocarcinoma of the pancreas. Cancer 32:1341–1345, 1973.
176. Komaki R, Wilson JF, Cox JD, Kline RW: Carcinoma of the pancreas: Results of irradiation for unresectable lesions. Int J Radiat Oncol Biol Phys 6:209–212, 1980.
177. Dobelbower RR Jr: Current radiotherapeutic approaches to pancreatic cancer. Cancer 47 (Suppl):1729–1733, 1981.
178. Whittington R, Dobelbower RR, Mohiuddin M, et al: Radiotherapy of unresectable pancreatic carcinoma: A six year experience with 104 patients. Int J Radiat Oncol Biol Phys 7:1639–1644, 1981.
179. Moertel CG, Frytak S, Hahn RG, et al: Therapy of locally unresectable pancreatic carcinoma: A randomized comparison of high dose (6000 rads) radiation alone, moderate dose radiation (4000 rads + 5-fluorouracil), and high dose radiation + 5-fluorouracil. Cancer 48:1705–1710, 1981.
180. Gastrointestinal Tumor Study Group: Treatment of locally unresectable carcinoma of the pancreas: Comparison of combined-modality therapy (chemotherapy plus radiotherapy) to chemotherapy alone. J Natl Cancer Inst 10:751–755, 1988.
181. Whittington R, Solin L, Mohiuddin M, et al: Multimodality therapy of localized unresectable pancreatic adenocarcinoma. Cancer 54:1991–1998, 1984.
182. Morrow M, Hilaris B, Brennan MF: Comparison of conventional surgical resection, radioactive implantation, and bypass procedures for exocrine carcinoma of the pancreas 1975–1980. Ann Surg 199:1–5, 1984.
183. Shipley WU, Wood WC, Tepper JE, et al: Intraoperative electron beam irradiation for patients with unresectable pancreatic carcinoma. Ann Surg 200:289–296, 1984.
184. Roldan GE, Gunderson LL, Nagorney DM, et al: External beam versus intraoperative and external beam irradiation for locally advanced pancreatic cancer. Cancer 61:1110–1116, 1988.
185. Mohiuddin M, Cantor RJ, Biermann W, et al: Combined modality treatment of localized unresectable adenocarcinoma of the pancreas. Int J Radiat Oncol Biol Phys 14:79–84, 1988.
186. Harter KW, Dritschilo A: Cancer of the pancreas: Are chemotherapy and radiation appropriate? Oncology 3:27–37, 1989.
187. Tepper JE, Noyes D, Krall JM, et al: Intraoperative radiation therapy of pancreatic carcinoma: A report of RTOG-8505. Int J Radiat Oncol Biol Phys 21:1145–1149, 1991.
188. Fietkau R, Sauer R: Future prospects of radiotherapy in pancreatic cancer. Eur J Surg Oncol 17:201–210, 1991.
189. Jones BA, Langer B, Taylor BR, Girotti M: Periampullary tumors: Which ones should be resected? Am J Surg 149:46–52, 1985.
190. Komaki R, Hansen R, Cox JD, Wilson JF: Phase I-II study of prophylactic hepatic irradiation with local irradiation and systemic chemotherapy for adenocarcinoma of the pancreas. Int J Radiat Oncol Biol Phys 15:1447–1452, 1988.
191. Komaki R, Wadler S, Peters T, et al: High-dose local irradiation plus prophylactic hepatic irradiation and chemotherapy for inoperable adenocarcinoma of the pancreas: A preliminary report of a multi-institutional trial (Radiation Therapy Oncology Group Protocol 8801). Cancer 69:2807–2812, 1992.
192. Pilepich MV, Miller HH: Preoperative irradiation in carcinoma of the pancreas. Cancer 46:1945–1949, 1980.
193. Kopelson G: Curative surgery for adenocarcinoma of the pancreas/ampulla of Vater: The role of adjuvant pre or postoperative radiation therapy. Int J Radiat Oncol Biol Phys 9:911–915, 1983.
194. Nguyen TD, Bugat R, Combes PF: Postoperative irradiation of carcinoma of the head of the pancreas area: Short-time tolerance and results to precision high-dose technique in 18 patients. Cancer 50:53–56, 1982.
195. Kalser MH, Ellenberg SS: Pancreatic cancer: Adjuvant combined radiotherapy and chemotherapy following curative resection. Arch Surg 120:899–903, 1985.
196. Gastrointestinal Tumor Study Group: Further evidence of effective adjuvant combined radiation and chemotherapy following curative resection of pancreatic cancer. Cancer 59:2006–2010, 1987.
197. Douglass HO Jr, Stablein DM, Kalser MH, et al: Confirmation by the Gastrointestinal Tumor Study Group that survival following potentially curative resection of pancreatic cancer is improved by multidisciplinary postoperative therapy. Adjuvant Ther Cancer 5:525–530, 1987.
198. Douglass HO Jr, Stablein DM: Ten-year follow-up of first generation surgical adjuvant studies of the Gastrointestinal Tumor Study Group. Adjuvant Ther Cancer 6:405–415, 1990.
199. Griffin JF, Smalley SR, Jewell W, et al: Patterns of failure after curative resection of pancreatic carcinoma. Cancer 66:56–61, 1990.
200. Hiraoka T: Extended radical resection of cancer of the pancreas with intraoperative radiotherapy. Baillieres Clin Gastroenterol 4:985–993, 1990.
201. Evans DB, Termuhlen PM, Byrd DR, et al: Intraoperative radiation therapy following pancreaticoduodenectomy. Ann Surg 218:54–60, 1993.
202. Whittington R, Bryer MP, Haller DG, et al: Adjuvant therapy of resected adenocarcinoma of the pancreas. Int J Radiat Oncol Biol Phys 21:1137–1143, 1991.
203. Cameron JL, Crist DW, Sitzmann JV, et al: Factors influencing

survival after pancreaticoduodenectomy for pancreatic cancer. Am J Surg 161:120–125, 1991.
204. Yeung RS, Weese JL, Hoffman JP, et al: Neoadjuvant chemoradiation in pancreatic and duodenal carcinoma: A phase II study. Cancer 72:2124–2133, 1993.
205. Jessup JM, Steele G, Mayer RJ, et al: Neoadjuvant therapy for unresectable pancreatic adenocarcinoma. Arch Surg 128:559–564, 1993.
206. Singh SM, Reber HA: Surgical palliation for pancreatic cancer. Surg Clin North Am 69:599–611, 1989.
207. Watanapa P, Williamson RCN: Surgical palliation for pancreatic cancer: Developments during the past two decades. Br J Surg 79:8–20, 1992.
208. Lucas CE, Ledgerwood AM, Bender JS: Antrectomy with gastrojejunostomy for unresectable pancreatic cancer causing duodenal obstruction. Surgery 110:583–590, 1991.
209. McGrath PC, McNeil PM, Neifeld JP, et al: Management of biliary obstruction in patients with unresectable carcinoma of the pancreas. Ann Surg 209:284–288, 1989.
210. Dowsett JF, Russell RCG, Hatfield ARW, et al: Malignant obstructive jaundice: A prospective randomized trial of by-pass surgery versus endoscopic stenting. Gastroenterology 96:A128, 1989.
211. Dowsett JF, Williams SJ, Hatfield ARW, et al: Endoscopic management of low biliary obstruction due to unresectable primary pancreato-biliary malignancy—a review of 463 consecutive cases. Gastroenterology 96:A129, 1989.
212. Speer AG, Cotton PB, Russell RCG, et al: Randomised trial of endoscopic versus percutaneous stent insertion in malignant obstructive jaundice. Lancet 2:57–62, 1987.
213. DeCaprio JA, Mayer RJ, Gonin R, Arbuck SG: Fluorouracil and high-dose leucovorin in previously untreated patients with advanced adenocarcinoma of the pancreas: Results of a phase II trial. J Clin Oncol 9:2128–2133, 1991.

Periampullary Carcinoma

John E. Meilahn, M.D.

The periampullary region is anatomically complex, including epithelia from the distal common bile duct, the pancreatic duct, the ampulla of Vater, and surrounding duodenal mucosa. Ampullary or periampullary adenocarcinoma may arise from any of these; determination of the tissue of origin is often difficult. However, the surgical treatment is similar, so identification of carcinoma is sufficient to guide subsequent treatment. This discussion centers on nonpancreatic carcinoma and excludes duodenal carcinoma except for that in the periampullary region.

EPIDEMIOLOGY

Incidence

Periampullary carcinoma that is nonpancreatic in origin is uncommon. Extrahepatic bile duct cancer occurs in 0.4% of autopsies,[1] with peak incidence in the seventh decade, and is more common in men than in women. Of these cancers, from 20% to 30% are located in the distal common bile duct. From one half to two thirds are resectable.[2–4]

Primary duodenal malignancy is rare, found in 0.035% of autopsies,[5] but the duodenum is the site for 33% to 48% of all carcinomas of the small intestine.[6] For adenocarcinoma, there appears to be a slight male preponderance, with peak incidence in the sixth, seventh, and eighth decades. From 30% to 40% are periampullary in location, 40% to 50% of those being distal to the ampulla.[7, 8] Although adenocarcinoma is most common, other tumors include lymphoma, leiomyosarcoma, carcinoid tumor, and metastases from melanoma, renal cell carcinoma, colon, or contiguous spread from adjacent lymph nodes or organs.[9]

Ampullary adenocarcinoma, also rarely encountered, is considered to be the most curable of all upper gastrointestinal malignancies. It is found in less than 0.25% of autopsies, of whom about 60% are male. The peak incidence is in the sixth and seventh decades,[10, 11] although patients as young as 30 have been seen.[12]

Risk Factors

Genetic-Familial

The vast majority of malignant ampullary adenocarcinomas appear sporadically and are considered to be multifactorial in origin and noninheritable, although a case involving three siblings has been reported.[13]

A genetic association of ampullary and duodenal carcinoma is evident in familial adenomatous polyposis (FAP), with periampullary adenomas present in 50% to 85%,[14] although adenocarcinoma develops in only 2% to 3%,[15] with average age at onset in the fifth or sixth decade. Most adenomas are clustered at or near the ampulla, suggesting an influence from exposure to bile, although bile mutagenicity has not yet been conclusively demonstrated.[16] Ampullary and duodenal adenomas are also present in 90% of those with Gardner's syndrome, the subset of FAP with osteomas and soft tissue tumors, with adenocarcinoma in the periampullary region developing in up to 12%.[17] Periampullary adenocarcinoma has recently been described in association with the hereditary flat adenoma syndrome, which is similar to FAP.[18] Since early colectomy prevents death from colon carcinoma, upper gastrointestinal screening is necessary to prevent subsequent death from periampullary malignancy.

Cholangiocarcinoma has been associated with sclerosing

cholangitis, ulcerative colitis, cholelithiasis, parasite infestation with *Clonorchis sinensis,* and choledochal cysts.[2]

Carcinoid of the ampulla is a rare lesion.[3] However, metastases may develop even with small tumors, since 50% of tumors less than 2.0 cm in diameter have had positive lymph nodes.[19] Periampullary carcinoid in association with von Recklinghausen's disease has been well recognized. In this syndrome, the majority of periampullary tumors originate in the ampulla itself, with carcinoid tumors appearing more frequently than neurofibromas.[20] It has been suggested that the tumors in this syndrome originate at an endodermal-neuroectodermal complex located near the ampulla of Vater.[21]

Most ampullary and duodenal carcinomas are believed to develop in pre-existing adenomas, with an adenoma-carcinoma sequence similar to that recognized in colon and rectal carcinoma. Residual adenomatous tissue has been found in 67% of well-differentiated adenocarcinomas of the papilla and in 30% of poorly differentiated tumors. Papillary adenomas have also been observed either to harbor or to develop into adenocarcinomas in as many as 30% of cases.[22]

Eighty percent of villous adenomas of the duodenum are periampullary in location and usually exceed 3 cm in diameter. With an incidence of malignancy from 25% to 60%, they are generally considered to be potentially malignant until proven otherwise.[23] The reason for frequent periampullary location is unknown, although some postulate the presence of carcinogens or cocarcinogens in biliary or pancreatic secretions.[24] Size is believed to be a poor predictor of malignancy, since the mean size of adenomas with atypia, carcinoma in situ, and invasion is similar.[25]

Dietary and Social

Alcohol consumption and cigarette smoking have not been implicated in the development of nonpancreatic periampullary adenocarcinoma. Pre-existing duodenal ulcer disease is not thought to pose a risk factor for development of duodenal adenocarcinoma. In 67 patients with extrahepatic cholangiocarcinoma, including cystic and hepatic duct tumors, Yen et al.[26] found no increased risk for cigarette, alcohol, or coffee use. There did appear to be an increased risk from oral contraceptives in women under 60 years of age.[26] Cholangiocarcinoma has also been reported in association with use of isoniazid[27] and methyldopa.[28]

Environmental-Occupational

Those working in the rubber, wood, and automobile industries have been thought to be at increased risk for extrahepatic cholangiocarcinoma.[26] Asbestos[29] and polychlorinated biphenyls[30] have also been associated with cholangiocarcinoma.

NATURAL HISTORY

Most patients with cholangiocarcinoma die of hepatic failure owing to biliary obstruction and cholangitis. Almost all patients currently presenting with unresectable biliary malignant obstruction are palliated with biliary stenting or surgical bypass, which extends their survival from weeks to months.

Cholangiocarcinoma presents with jaundice in more than 90% of cases. If obstruction is not relieved by stenting or surgical bypass, life expectancy is short owing to cholangitis or liver failure. In 1957, Sako and colleagues[31] reported an average survival of 23 days in five patients without definitive surgery, although jaundice preceded hospital admission by variable periods.

Periampullary duodenal adenocarcinoma is usually associated with jaundice. In 1939, Lieber and coworkers[32] reported a series of 17 patients who presented for hospital admission with unresectable disease, with subsequent survival of 2 to 42 days. Their prehospital morbidity ranged from 3 weeks to 9 months; all were jaundiced and had metastases to nodes or liver or contiguous extension to adjacent organs. In a review of the literature, they noted that 97% of patients treated nonoperatively had a survival of 6.6 months after the onset of illness.[33]

In 28 patients with ampullary adenocarcinoma, Delcore et al.[12] found that symptoms had been present for an average of 4 months (range, 1 to 24 months), with jaundice in 96%. One patient refused operation and expired shortly thereafter; three underwent bypass procedures and died within 15 months of operation.

LOCAL-REGIONAL ANATOMY AND PATHOLOGY

The papilla of Vater is located on the posteromedial wall of the retroperitoneal second portion of the duodenum, 7 to 10 cm from the pylorus, and rarely is located in the third portion of the duodenum. Within the papilla, the ampulla is a small dilated duct, representing a common pancreatobiliary channel below the junction of the distal common bile duct and the pancreatic duct. The ampulla measures 1 to 14 mm in length (75% are less than 5 mm long). Since the bile and pancreatic ducts may open near to each other on the papilla, or may open separately into the duodenum, a true ampulla is present in only 75% of individuals.[34]

The distal common bile duct usually traverses the pancreas but is uncovered on the posterior surface of the pancreas in 16% of patients. The inferior vena cava lies immediately posteriorly. Arterial blood supply to the region is rich, with a pair (anterior and posterior) of superior pancreaticoduodenal arteries from the gastroduodenal artery and a similar pair from the inferior pancreaticoduodenal arteries supplied from the superior mesenteric artery

(SMA). A replaced right hepatic artery (from the SMA) is present in 15% of patients, traveling posterior to the distal common bile duct, which may give rise to the inferior pancreaticoduodenal arteries.

Venous drainage from the second portion of the duodenum is via anterior and posterior pancreaticoduodenal venous arcades. The superior end of the anterior arcade enters the superior mesenteric vein (SMV) just inferior to the neck of the pancreas. The inferior end of the arcade also enters the SMV. The posterior pancreaticoduodenal venous arcade enters the portal vein superiorly, just above the pancreas, and enters the SMV inferiorly.

The lymphatic drainage of the second portion of the duodenum involves groups of nodes both anterior and posterior to the head of the pancreas, as well as superior and inferior. However, most lymphatics of the common bile duct and ampulla of Vater end in the posterior pancreaticoduodenal group of nodes.[34] Distal cholangiocarcinomas have been found to metastasize most frequently to the posterosuperior pancreaticoduodenal lymph nodes, with the next most common sites being nodes in the lower portion of the hepatoduodenal ligament and nodes near the SMA.[34, 35] See Figure 5–1 for the relationship of regional lymph nodes and major blood vessels to the duodenum and pancreas. Splenic lymph nodes and those at the tail of the pancreas are not regional lymph nodes but are considered metastases.[36]

TABLE 5–4
AJCC/UICC Staging for Ampullary Carcinoma (1992)

Primary Tumor (T)

TX	Primary tumor cannot be assessed
T0	No evidence of primary tumor
Tis	Carcinoma in situ
T1	Tumor limited to ampulla of Vater
T2	Tumor invades duodenal wall
T3	Tumor invades 2 cm or less into pancreas
T4	Tumor invades more than 2 cm into pancreas and/or into other adjacent organs

Regional Lymph Nodes (N)

NX	Regional lymph nodes cannot be assessed
N0	No regional lymph node metastasis
N1	Regional lymph node metastasis

Distant Metastasis (M)

MX	Presence of distant metastasis cannot be assessed
M0	No distant metastasis
M1	Distant metastasis

Stage		Grouping	
0	Tis	N0	M0
I	T1	N0	M0
II	T2	N0	M0
	T3	N0	M0
III	T1	N1	M0
	T2	N1	M0
	T3	N1	M0
IV	T4	Any N	M0
	Any T	Any N	M1

AJCC, American Joint Committee on Cancer; UICC, International Union Against Cancer.

STAGING

Although ampullary, distal common bile duct, and periampullary duodenal carcinomas resemble periampullary pancreatic carcinomas in presentation and location, each has different staging criteria. Separate TNM staging systems for ampullary and duodenal carcinomas have only recently been published by the American Joint Committee on Cancer (AJCC).[36] Currently, staging systems as published by the AJCC for ampullary, distal bile duct, and duodenal carcinomas are the same as those of the International Union Against Cancer (UICC).

Ampullary Carcinoma

The current TNM classification for ampullary carcinoma (Table 5–4) applies to all primary carcinomas that arise in the ampulla or on the papilla. Most reported series have not utilized this classification.

In 1983, Barton and Copeland[37] proposed a seven-stage system based on local extension, nodal metastases, and disseminated disease, a system used by Delcore et al.[12] in 1989.

In 1987, Yamaguchi and Enjoji[10] suggested a four-stage classification system based only on the invasive extent, without consideration of nodal or metastatic involvement. They noted that stage I tumors that were restricted to within the muscle of Oddi did not have nodal metastases and had a favorable prognosis, with a 5-year survival rate of 85% after radical resection. Stage IV tumors, which extended into the pancreas, involved nodal metastases in 78% of patients and a 5-year survival rate of 24%.

In 1988, Neoptolemos et al.[38] found that long-term survival was associated independently with tumor grade and local invasiveness. They proposed a four-stage classification based on both local invasion and nodal metastases. A scoring system obtained by adding the numeric tumor grade and stage provided a strong correlation with long-term survival.

In 1993, Willett and colleagues[39] utilized the TNM system, although survival was not reported by overall stage but by individual T and N classifications.

Distal Bile Duct Carcinoma

The current TNM classification for distal bile duct carcinoma (Table 5–5) is used for all extrahepatic bile duct carcinomas but does not include those arising within the ampulla. Extrahepatic bile duct carcinomas are reported with respect to location (upper, middle, or lower third), with most earlier series using location and histologic differentiation for reporting survival. More recent reports, both from France and the United States,[3, 4] have utilized the TNM system. However, several recent reports have used other systems.

Henson et al.,[40] in reporting the results in 1992 of the Surveillance, Epidemiology, and End Results (SEER) pro-

TABLE 5–5
AJCC/UICC Staging for Extrahepatic Bile Duct Carcinoma (1992)

Primary Tumor (T)	
TX	Primary tumor cannot be assessed
T0	No evidence of primary tumor
Tis	Carcinoma in situ
T1	Tumor invades the mucosa or muscle layer
	T1a Tumor invades the mucosa
	T1b Tumor invades the muscle layer
T2	Tumor invades the perimuscular connective tissue
T3	Tumor invades adjacent structures (pancreas, duodenum)
Regional Lymph Nodes (N)	
NX	Regional lymph nodes cannot be assessed
N0	No regional lymph node metastasis
N1	Metastasis in the cystic duct, pericholedochal and/or hilar lymph nodes
N2	Metastasis in the peripancreatic, periduodenal, periportal, celiac, superior mesenteric, and/or posterior pancreaticoduodenal nodes
Distant Metastasis (M)	
MX	Presence of distant metastasis cannot be assessed
M0	No distant metastasis
M1	Distant metastasis

Stage	Grouping		
0	Tis	N0	M0
I	T1	N0	M0
II	T2	N0	M0
III	T1	N1	M0
	T1	N2	M0
	T2	N1	M0
	T2	N2	M0
IVA	T3	Any N	M0
IVB	Any T	Any N	M1

AJCC, American Joint Committee on Cancer; UICC, International Union Against Cancer.

gram of the National Cancer Institute, defined an alternate classification in order to accommodate the various staging systems within their review. In their system, nodal metastases were included in stage II. In 1993, Kayahara and coworkers[35] investigated nodal involvement in distal bile duct carcinoma and used a classification system (N0 through N4) as proposed by the Japanese Society of Biliary Surgery.

Periampullary Duodenal Carcinoma

The current TNM classification for duodenal carcinoma (Table 5–6) was first published by the AJCC in 1992 and applies to carcinomas arising from the duodenum but not from the papilla. No recent reports have yet utilized this classification.

Most published series have used tumor location (supra-, peri-, or infra-ampullary), morphologic appearance (papillary or nonpapillary), serosal invasion, or nodal status as staging criteria; even the modified Dukes' classification for colorectal carcinoma has been used.[41]

SCREENING

The low incidence of periampullary carcinoma makes screening unrewarding. An important exception is found in those with FAP or one of its variants, in which a majority have gastroduodenal adenomas in addition to colorectal adenomas. Galandiuk et al.[23] found that duodenal adenomas were diagnosed from 14 to 33 years (mean, 24 years) after diagnosis of FAP and that colectomy preceded identification of duodenal adenomas by 2 to 32 years (mean, 17 years). While the majority were tubular adenomas, a 21% incidence of tubulovillous or villous adenomas with significant risk of invasive adenocarcinoma led to the recommendation for annual esophagogastroduodenoscopy (EGD) in polyposis patients. If adenomas were found, endoscopic biopsy or removal was performed with subsequent EGD at 6-month intervals.

In contrast, Spigelman and colleagues[42] classified gastroduodenal polyps on the basis of number, size, histologic type, and degree of dysplasia and recommended annual EGD and biopsy only for severe polyposis, with EGD performed at 3-year intervals for those with mild or moderate polyposis. However, follow-up on the incidence of malignancy was not presented.

Iida et al.[17] followed 20 patients with FAP or Gardner's syndrome for an average of 7.1 years at 1- to 3-year intervals with a side-viewing endoscope, including frequent biopsies of the papilla and ampullary orifice. Duodenal adenomas were found in 90% of patients, with tubular adenomatous change at the papilla in 55%. No malignancy was noted to occur at the papilla, but one invasive carcinoma did develop in the duodenal bulb. Noda and cowork-

TABLE 5–6
AJCC/UICC Staging for Duodenal Carcinoma (1992)

Primary Tumor (T)	
TX	Primary tumor cannot be assessed
T0	No evidence of primary tumor
Tis	Carcinoma in situ
T1	Tumor invades lamina propria or submucosa
T2	Tumor invades muscularis propria
T3	Tumor invades into subserosa or into mesentery or retroperitoneum with extension of 2 cm or less
T4	Tumor perforates visceral peritoneum or directly invades other organs or structures, including pancreas, or more than 2 cm into retroperitoneum
Regional Lymph Nodes (N)	
NX	Regional lymph nodes cannot be assessed
N0	No regional lymph node metastasis
N1	Regional lymph node metastasis
Distant Metastasis (M)	
MX	Presence of distant metastasis cannot be assessed
M0	No distant metastasis
M1	Distant metastasis

Stage	Grouping		
0	Tis	N0	M0
1	T1	N0	M0
	T2	N0	M0
II	T3	N0	M0
	T4	N0	M0
III	Any T	N1	M0
IV	Any T	Any N	M1

AJCC, American Joint Committee on Cancer; UICC, International Union Against Cancer.

ers[14] emphasized that in those with FAP, ampullary tubular adenomas developed at an average age of 31.7 years (range, 20 to 52 years), and thus found that ampullary adenomas in older patients tended to show more severe atypia than those in younger patients. In addition, biopsy of the ampullary orifice as well as the surface of the papilla was recommended, even though no gross adenomatous changes were recognized at endoscopy, since adenomas were found in this manner, and orifice (or ampullary) adenomas tended to have increased cellular atypia in comparison to surface papillary adenomas.

DIAGNOSIS

Although distal bile duct carcinoma, ampullary carcinoma, and periampullary duodenal adenocarcinoma are diverse in origin, their proximity to the distal common bile duct results in jaundice as the most common symptom (Table 5–7). For cholangiocarcinoma, jaundice is present in more than 90% of patients, whereas ampullary carcinoma is more variable, with jaundice occurring in 66% to 96%. Periampullary duodenal carcinomas produce jaundice in 50% to 80% of patients, since their origin is farther from the bile duct. Intermittent or fluctuating levels of jaundice have been observed in 10% to 50% of patients with ampullary or periampullary duodenal tumors. Jaundice is usually accompanied by dark urine and acholic stools. Pruritus is present in more than 50% of cases. Pancreatitis has occasionally been noted.

Anorexia is present in 20% to 55% of patients, with corresponding weight loss. Nausea and vomiting are more common in periampullary duodenal carcinomas than in those of ampullary or biliary origin. Abdominal pain is typically epigastric and may be exacerbated by meals. Anemia is present in less than half of cases. Occult blood in the stool has been found in 5% to 25% of patients, with melena sometimes noted with ampullary or duodenal carcinomas.

The onset of symptoms is not well recognized, with vague anorexia and gradual weight loss. Most patients have 2 to 3 months of illness before diagnosis but do not seek medical attention until after several weeks of progressive jaundice.

Laboratory studies usually show hyperbilirubinemia and an elevated alkaline phosphatase level. Anemia is present in 10% to 40% of patients.

TABLE 5–7
Symptoms and Signs of Periampullary Carcinoma

Symptom/Sign	Rate of Occurrence (%)
Jaundice	50–96
Pruritus	40–65
Abdominal pain	25–60
Anorexia	30–50
Weight loss	30–55
Nausea and vomiting	20–60
Malaise	30–45
Hepatomegaly	30
Occult blood in stool	20
Pancreatitis	0–18

Data from references 2–4, 6–8, 10–13, 31, 66, 71, 75, 77, 82, 142–149.

Diagnostic Studies

The work-up of the jaundiced patient usually begins with ultrasound or computed tomography (CT) scan to define the presence of dilated biliary ducts and the level of biliary obstruction. Ultrasound is preferred in the younger patient without weight loss, whereas the older patient with weight loss may benefit from initial CT scan, which contributes more to preoperative staging and may aid in diagnosing a more common cause, such as a pancreatic mass. The presence of intrahepatic and extrahepatic ductal dilation on ultrasound or CT scan suggests a distal bile duct, periampullary, or pancreatic cause of jaundice.

Subsequent definition of biliary pathology is accomplished by endoscopic retrograde cholangiopancreatography (ERCP), which, in experienced hands, can be used to diagnose abnormalities of the bile duct and pancreatic duct, biopsy visualized masses, obtain bile or tissue for cytologic examination, and palliate or treat through sphincterotomy or stent insertion. If ERCP is technically unsuccessful in defining the level or extent of biliary obstruction, percutaneous transhepatic cholangiography is favored with or without biliary drainage.

Ultrasonography

Ultrasonography is readily available and is the least expensive of the upper abdominal imaging techniques. However, overlying viscera with bowel gas limit complete examination of the distal bile duct and duodenum. Although the pancreas is imaged, about 20% of ultrasound examinations are technically inadequate.[43] Findings on ultrasound examination that suggest periampullary malignancy include a dilated gallbladder and common bile duct with a polypoid, intra-abdominal mass in the distal common bile duct or an abrupt termination of the duct.

The sensitivity of ultrasonography in diagnosing periampullary malignancy does not exceed 50%.[44] Since ampullary carcinoma has the same hypoechoic characteristic of pancreatic carcinoma, ultrasound may fail to distinguish between them. Liver metastases and retroperitoneal lymph node enlargement may be detected as well as tumor encasement of peripancreatic arteries and veins in some advanced cases.

Computed Tomography

A CT scan with oral and intravenous contrast agents that shows the presence of intrahepatic and extrahepatic ductal dilation suggests periampullary malignancy, although tumors less than 1 to 2 cm in diameter may not be visualized. Similarly, liver metastases less than 1 cm in diameter are usually missed on CT scan. Incremental dynamic CT with rapid intravenous injection is considered to be optimal for pancreatic evaluation, with good enhancement of the major peripancreatic blood vessels. Pancreatic involvement with carcinoma appears as a focal contrast defect relative to the surrounding enhanced parenchyma.

Warshaw et al.[45] found that 88% of ampullary carcinomas were resectable but that CT scan missed small liver metastases (1 to 3 mm in diameter), which were found by subsequent laparoscopy. Periampullary or duodenal adenocarcinoma may be detected on CT scan as an intraluminal filling defect, duodenal wall thickening, or periduodenal fat invasion.[46]

Spiral CT offers enhanced pancreatic and peripancreatic vessel imaging, which can be superior to dynamic CT scan.[47–49] With this continuous imaging technique, it takes only 30 seconds to complete scans through the pancreas and periampullary region, reducing artifact from breathing and allowing rapid intravenous contrast injection for maximal enhancement of normal pancreatic tissue and vessels.[47] Images can also be displayed in the sagittal plane for SMA imaging or in the coronal plane for visualization of the SMV, splenic vein, and portal vein. Spiral CT is not yet widely available, so its efficacy in staging periampullary malignancy has not been reported. It is likely to play a significant role in the future and may obviate the need for arteriography in evaluating peripancreatic vascular invasion.[49]

Endoscopic Retrograde Cholangiopancreatography

The papilla can usually be visualized directly by side-viewing duodenoscopy and ERCP. Early diagnostic attempts included forceps or snare biopsy of exophytic lesions. Currently, intra-ampullary tumors are detected by ERCP and confirmed by intraductal brush cytology or biopsy. After sphincterotomy, an intra-ampullary tumor may be exposed and sampled for biopsy directly. Therapeutic maneuvers include sphincterotomy, snare resection of pedunculated tumors, and insertion of biliary stents. Occasionally, laser photodestruction has been utilized.[50] The accuracy of diagnostic biopsy is about 80% to 90%.[51, 52] Ponchon and colleagues[50] found that tumors were intra-ampullary in 37% of cases, with a macroscopically normal papilla.[50] Sphincterotomy then allowed visualization and biopsy, although biopsy specimens taken at the time of sphincterotomy were incorrectly interpreted as normal in 44% of cases, whereas repeated endoscopy and biopsy 10 days later revealed ampullary tumors.

Complications of ERCP and sphincterotomy include hemorrhage, perforation, and pancreatitis.

Arteriography

A minority of periampullary tumors are seen approaching major vessels on CT scan. In these, visceral arteriography (celiac plus SMA) can assist in determining unresectability. Unresectability is strongly suggested by SMV or portal vein occlusion and may also be the case with encasement of the major veins or the SMA. However, occlusion of the gastroduodenal artery does not necessarily result in unresectability if the common and proper hepatic arteries are uninvolved. In a series of periampullary malignancies (most were pancreatic in origin), Dooley et al.[53] found that limited vessel encasement was not an absolute sign of unresectability (false-positive rate of 14%) but that none with major arterial or venous occlusion was resectable at laparotomy. In a similar but prospective study, Warshaw and coworkers[45] found similar results. Accuracy in predicting resectability was only 54%, but angiography was correct in 25 of 26 cases in predicting unresectability.

In contrast to ampullary carcinoma, distal bile duct carcinoma may require arteriography more frequently to assess invasion of the adjacent portal vein or proper hepatic artery.[54]

Laparoscopy

Laparoscopic evaluation of the liver surface and peritoneal cavity has been used to detect small implants not visualized on CT scan or ultrasound. For patients requiring laparotomy owing to duodenal obstruction, laparoscopy is unnecessary since resection or bypass will be performed. However, with availability of palliative endoscopic or percutaneous transhepatic stent placement, laparotomy may be avoided if laparoscopy discloses biopsy-proven metastases.

Warshaw et al.[45] combined CT, angiography, and laparoscopy in determining resectability and found that their results were complementary. With each modality indicating resectability, all ampullary carcinomas were found to be resectable at laparotomy. With any result positive for unresectability, two of three were unresectable at laparotomy (CT scan in one falsely showed encasement, not supported by angiography). Laparoscopy did find metastases in the only ampullary carcinoma that was metastatic. Intraoperative laparoscopic ultrasound has not yet been evaluated in determining unresectability.

Endoscopic Ultrasonography

Recently, endoscopic ultrasonography (or endosonography) has been investigated regarding its suitability for staging the depth and extent of periampullary tumors.[55–59] In addition, regional lymph nodes can be visualized and assessed for probability of metastatic involvement. This evolving technique is highly operator-dependent, with reported results from a few investigators. Therefore, at this time it does not have universal applicability.

While ERCP is effective in delineating bile and pancreatic ductal abnormalities and for biopsy of periampullary tumors, it is not as useful in assessing the extent of the disease. Conventional extracorporeal ultrasound is limited owing to overlying abdominal viscera and bowel gas.

These limitations have been overcome by introducing the echoprobe endoscopically into the duodenum and achieving acoustic contact by filling the stomach or duodenum with water and by using a water-filled balloon over the transducer in the duodenum. The individual layers of the wall of the papilla can be visualized as well as the distal bile duct and pancreatic duct. The origin of the tumor may be evident as well.

Endosonography has been used in sporadic instances to justify local resection of periampullary villous adenomas[56] and early ampullary carcinoma,[57] but this approach has not yet been validated by prospective studies. In 1990, Tio and colleagues[58] reported preoperative endosonographic TNM staging in 24 patients with ampullary carcinoma compared with the subsequently resected specimens. Most T1 and T2 carcinomas could be correctly diagnosed, but overstaging sometimes occurred owing to peritumoral inflammation or pancreatitis. Most T3 and T4 carcinomas were also identified, based on penetration into the pancreas. Overall accuracy was 87%. Lymph node involvement was more difficult to evaluate, with benign nodes often interpreted as metastases (accuracy rate of 37%). Positive nodes were better identified (accuracy rate of 80%). Distant metastases were not identified owing to the limited penetration depth of the ultrasound. As a result of incorrectly interpreting benign nodes as metastatic, no actual stage I or II ampullary carcinomas were correctly staged by preoperative endosonography, but seven of nine stage III and one stage IV carcinomas were correctly staged preoperatively.

Tio et al.[59] evaluated preoperative endosonographic staging of cholangiocarcinoma (including common bile duct and distal duct) and found an overall accuracy rate of 83% in evaluating for extent (T). As with ampullary carcinoma, overstaging could occur due to peritumoral inflammation or pancreatitis. While metastatic lymph nodes were usually correctly diagnosed, benign nodes were frequently falsely diagnosed as positive (overall accuracy rate of 55%). Peritoneal or liver metastases were not diagnosed accurately. The presence of a stent already placed at ERCP did not hinder endosonographic evaluation.

PRIMARY OPERABLE DISEASE—RESULTS OF TREATMENT

Surgical Options

Local Resection

The usual surgical treatment for resectable ampullary tumors is pancreaticoduodenectomy for all tumors with local invasion or for benign tumors thought to be locally unresectable because of involvement of the ampullary complex. However, local resection of ampullary tumors has occasionally been advocated for patients with benign adenoma or villous adenoma and for selected patients with carcinoma, including those in poor medical condition believed to be unsuitable for a radical resection. Those investigating endoscopic ultrasonography have cited local resection as possible suitable treatment for tumors with limited invasion and benign-appearing lymph nodes.[56, 57]

The technique of local resection (or ampullectomy) has varied among proponents, varying from mucosal excision to wide resection, including the entire posterior duodenal wall. The first successful resection of a periampullary tumor was performed by Halsted[60] in 1898, with an excision of duodenal wall, distal bile duct, and distal pancreatic duct. The duodenal opening was closed in an end-to-end anastomosis with reimplantation of the distal common bile duct and pancreatic duct. This patient survived the procedure but died within a year from recurrent tumor. Until the advent of the Whipple procedure, local resection was the most common surgical treatment for periampullary tumors.[61] While morbidity and mortality rates for the Whipple procedure have improved, especially in experienced hands, some authors have recently advocated that local resection be considered for selected patients.[62–65]

Local resection of benign adenomas of the papilla has been performed with acceptable results. Farouk et al.[63] reported three tubulovillous and villous adenomas that were locally excised, ranging in size from 3 to 4 cm. Pathology was suggested by endoscopic biopsy and confirmed at operation. There were no recurrences at a mean follow-up of 40 months. Asbun and coworkers[64] reported 11 patients with a preoperative diagnosis of ampullary adenoma with treatment by ampullectomy. Pathologic examination in three revealed carcinoma, with subsequent treatment by the Whipple procedure. The remaining eight patients, most of whom had villous adenomas, were treated with ampullectomy. There was no recurrence, with a follow-up of 1 to 51 months (median, 24 months). They concluded that local ampullary resection was the procedure of choice for benign ampullary tumors.

The results of local resection for periampullary carcinoma are summarized in Table 5–8. Ampullectomy for invasive carcinoma has been reported in selected patients to be associated with 5-year survival rates of 37% to 51%.[66–70] However, recent reports attest to the possibility of local recurrence. Goldberg et al.[62] reported five patients

TABLE 5–8
Results of Local Resection for Ampullary Carcinoma

Authors	No. Resected	Mortality (%)	5-Year Survival (%)
Jones et al., 1985[71]	4	0	50
Knox and Kingston, 1986[70]	25	0	51
Tarazi et al., 1986[66]	11	9	41
Robertson et al., 1987[67]	8	25	44
Delcore et al., 1989[12]	1	0	100
Farouk et al., 1991[63]	3	0	
Asbun et al., 1993[64]	1	0	100

with periampullary tumors, of which three were distal bile duct carcinomas, one a papillary ampullary carcinoma, and one an adenocarcinoma of undetermined origin. They ranged from 0.5 to 2.5 cm in diameter and were treated with wide local excision, with a sampling of regional lymph nodes negative for tumor. Morbidity included a transient biliary leak in one patient, with no mortality. The three patients with distal bile duct carcinomas died of recurrent disease at 17, 24, and 45 months. Of the other two patients, one died at 54 months with no evidence of tumor, and the other was alive at 36 months with recurrent tumor.

Farouk and colleagues[63] reported three patients with adenocarcinoma of the papilla treated by local excision, with recurrence in all ranging from 9 to 35 months. Asbun et al.[64] reported one patient with ampullary carcinoma who survived 75 months after ampullectomy with no evidence of recurrence.

With a high rate of local recurrence combined with uncertainty regarding the reliability of intraoperative frozen sections, ampullectomy for localized invasive adenocarcinoma seems to be best reserved for those thought to be at high risk for radical resection.

Radical Resection

Pancreaticoduodenectomy remains the gold standard for resection of periampullary malignancy, including adenocarcinomas of ampullary, distal bile duct, duodenal, or pancreatic ductal origin. At laparotomy, findings that preclude curative resection include local invasion of surrounding major vascular structures (inferior vena cava, SMV, portal vein, SMA), although partial resection of limited vascular invasion has occasionally been reported.[71–73] Also included is unresectable invasion into the retroperitoneum or contiguous organs or structures (transverse mesocolon), nodal metastases in regions not normally resected (portal or celiac), or evidence of peritoneal or liver metastases. Subtotal pancreatectomy is generally preferred, although total pancreatectomy has occasionally been performed to avoid pancreaticojejunostomy in the normal, friable pancreas.[11] The pylorus-preserving procedure is preferred by some owing to reported fewer late problems with dumping, diarrhea, and marginal ulceration.[74]

While perioperative mortality for radical resection has been about 25% in the past, numerous centers have demonstrated recent ability to achieve single-digit mortality rates.[67, 71, 74–76] Morbidity following pancreaticoduodenectomy ranges from 25% to as high as 60%, although some have reported improved morbidity in recent years.[75] Postoperative hemorrhage, upper gastrointestinal bleeding, intra-abdominal infection, and pancreatic fistula are the major causes of morbidity.

Ampullary Carcinoma

The results for radical pancreaticoduodenal resection for ampullary carcinoma are summarized in Table 5–9. True ampullary carcinoma is one of the more curable upper gastrointestinal malignancies, with 5-year survival rates of 23% to 55% following radical resection, including in patients with nodal metastases.[10–12, 75, 77] Resectability rates range from 64% to 89%, with nodal metastases found in 31% to 50% of those resected.

Matory et al.[78] reported 69 patients accrued over a recent 7-year period. Of 66 who were explored, 55 underwent radical resection, with an operative mortality rate of 3%. Only three had positive margins at resection; 31% had positive nodes. Complications occurred in 30%, most commonly bleeding, gastric outlet obstruction, abscess, and pancreatic fistula. Median survival after resection was 51 months.

Monson and coworkers[11] reported 104 patients with periampullary malignancy, 71% of whom had ampullary carcinoma. The remainder were of pancreatic origin in 7%, distal bile duct in 6%, duodenum in 2%, and indefinite in 14%. Radical subtotal pancreaticoduodenectomy was performed in 84% and total pancreatectomy in the remainder, with an operative mortality rate of 5.4%. Lymphatic invasion was found in 51% overall, while regional lymph nodes were positive in 31%. Median survival without lymph node involvement was 3.3 years, with a 5-year survival rate of 43%. However, positive nodes decreased median survival to 1.4 years, with a 5-year survival rate of 16%. They found that cure was not guaranteed by 5-year survival, since eight patients died of recurrent tumor more than 5 years postoperatively.

Delcore et al.[12] found that 88% of their 28 patients with ampullary carcinoma had resectable tumors, but 43% had positive lymph nodes. Tumors larger than 2.5 cm in diameter had a 54% incidence of lymph node metastases, whereas those smaller than 2.5 cm had an incidence of 25%. The 5-year survival rate for node-negative patients was 60%, while node-positive survival was 30% at 5 years and 18% at 7 years.

Dawson and Connolly[79] examined 22 cases of ampullary carcinomas and found that half actually originated from the periampullary duodenal mucosa. For true ampullary tumors, lymph node involvement was present in 36%, with an overall 5-year survival rate of 55%. Histochemical investigation of the type of mucin produced revealed a better prognosis for sialomucin-secreting tumors than for those producing sulfated mucins.

Long-term survival is dependent on the degree of local invasion (T stage), nodal metastases, and histologic grading. While various staging systems have been used to correlate tumor size and invasion with survival, only Willett et al.[39] in their recent report have utilized the TNM system. They found that Tis, T1, and T2 tumors had a 5-year local control rate of 88% and a 5-year survival rate of 70%, whereas T3 and T4 tumors (with pancreatic invasion) had a 5-year local control rate of 44% and a 5-year survival rate of 30%, with local failure defined as a recurrence in the tumor bed or para-aortic lymphatics.

TABLE 5–9
Results of Radical Resection for Ampullary Adenocarcinoma

Authors	No. Resected	Resection (%)	Mortality (%)	5-Year Survival (%)	Positive Nodes (%)
Crane et al., 1973[77]	21	81	23	29	
Warren et al., 1975[83]	109		11	23	28
Nakase et al., 1976[72]	330	77	16	5	
Forrest and Longmire, 1979[146]	21		14	24	
Williams et al., 1979[150]	27	84	11	22	55
Walsh et al., 1982[80]	44	86	16	11	36
Barton and Copeland, 1983[37]	44	79	2	23	32
Jones et al., 1985[71]	36		4	32	
Knox and Kingston, 1986[70]	24		30	27 (est)	
Tarazi et al., 1986[66]	46		13/5*	37	
Crist et al., 1987[75]	19		13/2*	36	50
Yamaguchi and Enjoji, 1987[10]	109		5	28	52
Hayes et al., 1987[149]	31	88	25/7†	39	45
Neoptolemos et al., 1988[38]	23	64		52	17
Delcore et al., 1989[12]	22	88	5	45	43
Michelassi et al., 1989[151]	23	89	22	26	50
Trede et al., 1990[76]	36		2	55	
Martin et al., 1990[153]	23			43	
Shutze et al., 1990[154]	24		13	61	21
Monson et al., 1991[11]	74		6	39 (est)	31
Willett et al., 1993[39]	41		5	54	39
Matory et al., 1993[78]	55	83	3	38	31

(est), Estimated from survival graphs.
*2% mortality during last 5-year period.
†7% mortality over last decade.

Tumor histologic grade has also been found to correlate significantly with survival.[11, 38] Others have found no correlation with tumor differentiation[12] or have noted a nonsignificant trend toward correlation.[39] Neoptolemos and coworkers[38] developed a scoring system combining grade and stage that provided strong correlation with long-term survival.

Microscopic lymphatic invasion was found to have a significant effect on survival by Monson et al.,[11] with median survivals of 8.9 years without and 1.7 years with lymphatic invasion. In their study, vascular invasion did not have a significant effect on survival.

The effect of lymph node metastases on long-term survival is demonstrated in Table 5–10, with a consistent trend toward decreased survival with positive nodes. Although some have found no statistically significant effect of nodal metastases on survival,[10, 39, 78, 80] others have demonstrated a significantly decreased survival with positive nodes.[11, 12] The presence of positive nodes in the region of potential resection should not necessarily preclude resection. A few reports exist on the effect of extent of nodal metastases, although Monson and coworkers[11] did not find any significant decrease in long-term survival from multiple nodal metastases compared with that from solitary nodal involvement.

Yamaguchi and Enjoji[10] classified the macroscopic appearance of 104 specimens of ampullary carcinoma into intramural protruding (tumor within enlarged ampulla and covered by mucosa), exposed protruding (exophytic tumor at ampulla), and ulcerating. Compared with the intramural protruding type, ulcerating tumors tended to be larger, with a higher incidence of lymphatic and venous invasion, perineural infiltration, and lymph node metastases (69% vs. 29%). The 5-year overall survival rate was 28% after pancreaticoduodenectomy but as high as 50% in the intramural protruding type.

Patterns of failure after radical resection usually include both local recurrence (tumor bed or para-aortic lymphatics) and distant metastases. Willett et al.[39] examined recurrence in 12 patients after pancreaticoduodenectomy and found local failure in only 1, both local failure and distant metastases in 5, distant metastases in only 2, and unevaluable

TABLE 5–10
Ampullary Carcinoma: Effect of Lymph Node Metastases on 5-Year Survival

Authors	5-Year Survival (%)	
	Negative Nodes	*Positive Nodes*
Warren et al., 1975[83]	40	10
Williams et al., 1979[150]	67	0
Tarazi et al., 1986[66]*	29	16
Crist et al., 1987[75]†	40	23
Hayes et al., 1987[149]	53	27
Delcore et al., 1989[12]	60	33
Shutze et al., 1990[154]	78	50
Monson et al., 1991[11]*	43	16
Willett et al., 1993[39]	80	38
Matory et al., 1993[78]	57 (est)	42 (est)

(est), Estimated from survival graphs.
*Includes periampullary biliary or duodenal carcinoma.
†50% ampullary; others biliary or duodenal carcinoma.

recurrence in 4. Sites of distant metastases included liver, peritoneum, pleura, lung, and mediastinum.

Distal Bile Duct Carcinoma

The results of radical pancreaticoduodenal resection for distal bile duct carcinoma are summarized in Table 5–11. From 50% to 67% were unresectable. Five-year survival rates of 0% to 34% were noted, with nodal metastases reported in 13% to 47%.

Nagorney and colleagues[4] found that papillary tumors predominated in the distal bile duct, whereas sclerosing tumors were more common in the hilum. For all biliary tumors, papillary morphology had a better prognosis: 44% 5-year survival rate versus 11% for nodular or sclerotic tumors. The improved prognosis of papillary morphology has also been noted by others.[40, 81]

Tumor grade and stage have also been noted to be significant predictors of outcome.[4, 40] These reports of survival versus grade and stage have grouped distal tumors with middle and proximal bile duct carcinomas; therefore, survival rate for distal tumors related to grade and stage is not reported.

While nodal metastases in these reports were present in up to 47% of cases, Kayahara et al.[35] found nodal metastases in 69% of 29 resections for distal bile duct carcinoma. Half of those without pancreatic invasion had primary group lymph node involvement (posterior pancreaticoduodenal and inferior hepatoduodenal ligament nodes). Of those patients with pancreatic invasion, approximately 35% had distant nodal involvement. The authors recommended nodal dissection around the SMA in all cases of pancreatic invasion, although no survival statistics were used to justify extended nodal dissection.

Ouchi et al.[82] found lymph node metastases to affect prognosis significantly. For 20 patients with less than 3-year survival lengths, nodal metastases were present in 70%, but they were present in only 14% of 14 patients surviving more than 3 years. Venous, lymphatic, or perineural invasion were also significant predictors, present in 85% of those surviving less than 3 years but present in 36% of those surviving more than 3 years.

Periampullary Duodenal Carcinoma

The results of radical pancreaticoduodenal resection for periampullary duodenal adenocarcinoma are summarized in Table 5–12. Various reports in the literature include distal bile duct and ampullary carcinomas with duodenal carcinomas; others include infra-ampullary duodenal tumors with periampullary tumors when reporting results. The resectability rate ranges from 43% to 81%; the 5-year survival rate ranges from 10% to 50%. Nodal metastases are found in 30% to 70% of cases.

Nodal metastases have been associated with a worse prognosis. Warren and colleagues[83] found a 50% 5-year survival rate with negative nodes but only a 22% rate with positive nodes. Ouriel and Adams[41] found a mean survival of 14.5 months with positive nodes. Lai et al.[84] emphasized that metastases to paraduodenal nodes had a significantly better prognosis than those to regional nodes, such as pancreatic, mesenteric, para-aortic, or celiac. While median survival without nodal involvement was 42 months (40% 5-year survival rate), paraduodenal nodal metastases decreased median survival to 16.5 months. Involvement of distant regional nodes decreased median survival to 6 months. In Lai and colleagues' series, such distant regional nodal metastases were present only with extraserosal tumor infiltration.

Joesting and coworkers[7] reported that histologic grade also affected survival. With Broders grade 1 tumor histology, the 5-year survival rate was 54%; with grade 2, 31%. There was only one grade 3 and no grade 4 5-year survivors.

TABLE 5–11
Results of Radical Resection for Distal Bile Duct Carcinoma

Authors	No. Resected	Resection (%)	Mortality (%)	5-Year Survival (%)	Positive Nodes (%)
Warren et al., 1975[83]	47		21	17	13
Nakase et al., 1976[72]	157	52	22	4	
Forrest and Longmire, 1979[146]	8		13	25	
Tompkins et al., 1981[81]	12	67	8	28	
Lee and Williams, 1984[152]	7	58	14	14 (est)	
Jones et al., 1985[71]	12		4	33	
Tarazi et al., 1986[66]	11		0	17	
Crist et al., 1987[75]	10			34	
Nakayama et al., 1988[140]	10	53		36 at 3 yr	
Michelassi et al., 1989[151]	9	23	22	0	25
Ouchi et al., 1989[82]	46	60	9	29	47
Martin et al., 1990[153]	18			39	
Chao and Greager, 1991[2]	4	57	25	mean, 16 mo	14
Reding et al., 1991[3]	51	51	26	median, 64 mo	
Nagorney et al., 1993[4]	22	56	0	31	16

(est), Estimated from survival graphs.

TABLE 5–12
Results of Radical Resection for Periampullary Duodenal Carcinoma

Authors	No. Resected	Resection (%)	Mortality (%)	5-Year Survival (%)	Positive Nodes (%)
Warren et al., 1975[83]	37		18	31	28
Nakase et al., 1976[72]	27	62	19	7	
Spira et al., 1977[142]	23	73	17	18	71
Forrest and Longmire, 1979[146]	5		0	40 (2 yr)	
Alwmark et al., 1980[8]	12	43	17	25 (est)	49
Joesting et al., 1981[7]	19	51	25	30	32
Ouriel and Adams, 1984[41]	11	65		50 (est)	
Jones et al., 1985[71]	12		4	17	
Tarazi et al., 1986[66]	17		0	28	
Crist et al., 1987[75]	9			33	
Lai et al., 1988[84]	8	63		median, 18 mo	64
Michelassi et al., 1989[151]	10	81	10	10	30
Dawson and Connolly, 1989[79]	11			18	55
Martin et al., 1990[153]	8			53	

(est), Estimated from survival graphs.

Second-Look Procedures

Re-exploration with intent to resect after initial laparotomy has been of benefit in selected patients. McGuire et al.[85] reported 17 patients referred with ampullary, distal bile duct, and duodenal carcinomas in which initial biliary or gastric bypasses or cholecystectomy had been performed by other surgeons at other institutions. Restaging prompted re-exploration, with CT performed for all and cholangiography and arteriography for most. Pancreaticoduodenectomy was completed in 16 (94%) and local resection in 1, with no mortality. Pathologic staging data were not presented. Mean survival was 33 months, with a 5-year survival rate of 31%. Hashimi and Sabanathan[86] reported 10 patients with nonpancreatic periampullary carcinoma; 4 patients were initially resected, with a 5-year survival rate of 50%. Of the six patients initially receiving palliative bypass, three were re-explored and resected, with one 5-year survivor.

Combination Therapy

Preoperative Radiotherapy with Chemotherapy

Recently, Yeung et al.[87] reported the results of a prospective trial of preoperative chemotherapy and radiotherapy for biopsy-proven adenocarcinoma of the pancreas and of the periampullary duodenum. Although the majority of cases were pancreatic (26), five patients with periampullary duodenal carcinoma were treated. Eligibility criteria included absence of distant metastases, no prior abdominal radiotherapy or systemic chemotherapy, and a baseline performance status (Eastern Cooperative Oncology Group) of 0, 1, or 2. All patients had biliary obstruction relieved with transhepatic or endoscopic stenting, with total bilirubin levels of 2 mg% or less at the start of neoadjuvant treatment. The prescribed total dose of radiation was 5040 cGy in 28 fractions. Chemotherapy began within 24 hours after commencement of radiotherapy and consisted of 5-fluorouracil (5-FU; 1000 mg/m^2/day by continuous infusion for two 4-day courses) as well as mitomycin C (10 mg/m^2 as a bolus at the start of chemotherapy).

Patients were re-evaluated after chemoradiation with CT scan and visceral angiogram, with subsequent surgical exploration within 6 weeks of completion of radiotherapy unless restaging revealed disease progression or distant metastases. Of the five patients with duodenal carcinoma, pulmonary metastases developed in one. Of the remaining four patients, three underwent a Whipple procedure and one had a total pancreatectomy. All of these had a complete pathologic response, with no evidence of tumor in the specimen or nodes, including one involving CT-diagnosed para-aortic lymph nodes within the radiation port. At the time of reporting, all resected patients were alive without evident disease at 8, 16, 26, and 84 months.

Postoperative Adjuvant Therapy

Patients with ampullary adenocarcinoma at high risk for recurrent disease as evidenced by positive regional lymph nodes should be considered for adjuvant treatment with postoperative 5-FU and external beam radiation therapy, although the data supporting efficacy are limited.[11] Willett et al.[39] considered patients with ampullary carcinoma to be at high risk for local recurrence, with the findings of pancreatic invasion, nodal metastases, positive resection margins, or poorly differentiated histology. Twelve such patients were treated postoperatively with radiotherapy (40 to 50.4 Gy), with 5-FU during the first and last weeks of radiotherapy. Ten of 12 were T3 or T4; 8 of 12 had positive nodes; and 3 of 12 had positive resection margins. The 5-year actuarial local control and overall survival rates were 83% and 51%, respectively. These rates were compared with those of a group of similar high-risk patients who did not receive postoperative radiotherapy, with 5-year actuarial local control and overall survival rates of 50% and

38%, respectively. However, the trend in improvement with adjuvant therapy was not statistically significant for either local control or survival. Distant metastases (liver or peritoneum) occurred in all of the six patients who died within 5 years.

Splinter and coworkers[88] reported a small, nonrandomized trial of postoperative combination chemotherapy (5-FU, doxorubicin [Adriamycin], and mitomycin C) for nine patients with pancreatic carcinoma and seven with periampullary carcinoma, most of whom had positive nodes. They found no significant survival benefit from chemotherapy but noted that half received less than 60% of the planned total dose owing to side effects, including nausea, vomiting, fatigue, and anorexia. Only one patient was able to resume normal activity during chemotherapy.

The results of adjuvant chemotherapy or radiotherapy for cholangiocarcinoma have also been disappointing. Reports of postoperative adjuvant therapy often include chemotherapy, radiotherapy, or both applied to a collected group of hilar and distal cholangiocarcinomas, making interpretation of efficacy difficult for distal, periampullary cholangiocarcinomas. No prospective trials of chemotherapy with or without radiotherapy have been reported. Minsky et al.[89] treated extrahepatic bile duct carcinoma with external beam radiation and chemotherapy (5-FU and mitomycin C). Their series of 12 patients included two gallbladder, five hilar, and five common bile duct carcinomas, with either unresectable or recurrent disease. Excluding three patients without pathologic proof of cancer, median survival was 16 months, with overall 3-year actuarial survival of 20%. Thus, the few patients and the lack of stratification to distal bile duct carcinoma preclude meaningful conclusions.

While cholangiocarcinoma is sensitive to radiation, efficacy of external beam radiation is very limited owing to the proximity of dose-limiting organs. Internal radiation using iridium-192 via biliary stents is most often applied for hilar cholangiocarcinomas but has shown benefit only for unresectable proximal tumors.[90] Intraoperative radiation therapy has also been employed, but much more commonly for proximal cholangiocarcinomas. Iwasaki et al.[91] reported three patients with distal cholangiocarcinomas treated with intraoperative radiation therapy (27.5 Gy) and the Whipple procedure: two died at 16 and 19 months, the third was alive at 80 months.

RECURRENT AND INCURABLE DISEASE—RESULTS AND COMPLICATIONS

If there is unequivocal evidence of unresectable periampullary malignancy before laparotomy, nonoperative palliation of biliary obstruction is usually selected with an endoscopically placed biliary stent or one placed by the transhepatic technique. Previously, surgical bilioenteric bypass was favored even in some unresectable patients. Endoscopically placed stents were of small diameter (5 to 8 French) and were subject to plugging, causing cholangitis and requiring repeated endoscopic changes.[92, 93] Percutaneous transhepatic stents were uncomfortable, required periodic flushing, and also required periodic changes. Currently, after transhepatic catheter insertion, metal stents (expandable to 1 cm in diameter) are routinely placed, enabling removal of the catheter.

Endoscopic stent placement has also improved. After sphincterotomy and for dilation, stents of up to 12 French diameter may be placed. The expandable metal stent has also been adapted for endoscopic insertion.

While most reports of palliative stenting apply to unresectable pancreatic carcinoma, unresectable periampullary tumors of nonpancreatic origin may be treated similarly.

Endoscopic Palliation of Biliary Obstruction

A guide wire is advanced through the obstructing tumor into the distal common bile duct, followed by a 6 to 7 French catheter. Cholangiography is done to define the proximal and distal extent of the tumor. If the ampulla appears tight, a sphincterotomy is performed. A 10 French dilator may then be used, followed by a 10 to 11.5 French stent, which is sized to protrude beyond the tumor by several centimeters to allow for tumor growth. Successful stent placement is realized in about 90% of attempts.[94] Difficulty arises with distortion or invasion of the duodenal loop by tumor or with obliteration of the ampullary orifice. Stent placement failures have usually been treated with percutaneous transhepatic stent placement or surgical bypass.

Endoscopic sphincterotomy as palliation for ampullary adenocarcinoma was reported by Bickerstaff et al.[95] In a group of 17 patients thought to be medically unfit for surgical resection, sphincterotomies were done, with 10 French stents placed in 4 of the patients. Jaundice recurred in nearly half of the patients within 4 to 11 months, requiring repeated sphincterotomies or stent changes. Surgical bypass was ultimately required in 4 of the 17 patients. Sphincterotomy alone is not typical of current palliative practice but is generally used to aid in stent placement.

Attempts to compare endoscopic stenting with surgical bypass have been difficult owing to the differences in patient selection. Those advocating endoscopic procedures often note that patients in surgical bypass series are more fit, while endoscopic stenting has been used in those thought to be poor surgical candidates. As a consequence, morbidity and mortality rates for the endoscopic procedures reflect this more gravely ill population.

At least two prospective studies have been completed that compare endoscopic stent placement with surgical biliary bypass.[96, 97] Most of these patients had pancreatic carcinoma; all were judged to be unresectable but fit for operation. However, strict criteria for unresectability were not listed.

In the first study, Shepherd and colleagues[96] prospectively randomized 52 patients to either endoscopic placement of a 10 French plastic stent or to surgical bypass (either cholecystojejunostomy or choledochojejunostomy). None had pre-existing duodenal stenosis or obstruction. Relief of jaundice was accomplished in 90% of each group; the 30-day mortality rate was 9% with stenting and 20% with surgery. Median survival was 152 days with stenting and 125 days with surgery. However, there were more readmissions in the stenting group (43%) for stent occlusion and cholangitis, requiring stent replacement. Duodenal stenosis developed in 9%.

In the second study, Andersen and coworkers[97] prospectively randomized 50 patients to endoscopic stent placement (7 or 10 French) or to surgical bypass (most of which were cholecystojejunostomies). The 30-day mortality rate was 20% with stenting and 24% with surgery. Median survival was 84 days with stenting and 100 days with surgery. Cholangitis developed in 28% of those stented and in 16% of those bypassed. Some patients required multiple re-endoscopies for stent changes; of 33 stent insertions (including three patients who had had bypass), there were 21 endoscopies required for repeated stent insertions. There was no significant difference in the length of stay. None developed duodenal obstruction.

These studies have strengthened the case for initial endoscopic palliation for unresectable malignancy with biliary obstruction, even in patients who could be considered surgical candidates for palliative biliary bypass. Duodenal stenosis or obstruction, however, is generally best treated by surgical gastrojejunostomy, even though there have been anecdotal reports of malignant duodenal obstruction palliated with the endoscopically assisted placement of a self-expanding 16-mm diameter metal stent.[98]

Patients with initial failures of endoscopic stenting have also been treated with the combined percutaneous transhepatic and endoscopic approach. In this technique, percutaneous transhepatic needle puncture of the dilated biliary tree is followed by a wire passage into the bile duct, through the malignant obstruction, and into the duodenum. The endoscopist retrieves the wire from the duodenum and uses it to place a biliary stent endoscopically, over the wire. The purported advantage over transhepatic stent placement is avoidance of the larger transhepatic tract needed for that approach. Dowsett et al.[99] reported 74 patients who failed endoscopic stent placement who then underwent the combined procedure. With distal bile duct malignant obstruction, there was successful placement of either a 10 or 11.5 French endoprosthesis in 85% of attempts.

Occlusion of the plastic stents (with resulting jaundice and cholangitis) has been recognized as the major complication, more often by internal plugging than by tumor overgrowth at the end of the stent. Plugging has been thought to result from bacterial adherence to trapped debris and deconjugated bilirubin, leading to crystal deposition and eventual lumen occlusion.[100, 101] Prophylactic stent cleaning at 2- or 3-month intervals has been suggested[102] as well as use of large-bore stents.

Using 10 and 11.5 French stents, Frakes and colleagues[103] found a 5.6% occlusion rate at 3 months and a 13.3% rate at 6 months for pancreatic carcinoma but a 0% occlusion rate at 6 months for ampullary carcinoma (with a median survival of 36 weeks). They concluded that stents could be changed at 6-month intervals. Matsuda et al.[102] examined risk factors for stent occlusion and found that age over 70 years and high serum bilirubin before stent insertion (implying more advanced carcinoma) were significant. An increased number of stent insertions was also significant, with the median duration of patency of first, second, and subsequent stents at 177, 98, and 97 days, respectively. Interestingly, gender was correlated with patency (median duration of 108 days for men and 180 days for women). This phenomenon had been reported previously.[104]

Percutaneous Transhepatic Stenting

At least three procedures have been or are being used:

1. External biliary drainage, with the end of the indwelling catheter proximal to the malignant obstruction.
2. External-internal drainage, with a catheter placed through the tumor into the duodenum, allowing bile to drain internally or externally.
3. Internal biliary percutaneous stenting, with subsequent removal of the transhepatic access catheter.[94]

If bile ducts are dilated, successful drainage is accomplished in well over 90% of patients with the main risks being bleeding (venous or arterial) and bile leakage. Intrahepatic venous bleeding is usually stopped by inserting a larger catheter to provide tamponade, whereas arterial bleeding may require arteriography and embolization. Hemorrhage into the biliary ducts can result in pain, ongoing obstruction from clots, and cholangitis.

Both external drainage and long-term insertion of an indwelling catheter for combined external-internal drainage have the advantage of established access to the bile ducts and avoidance of the need for repeated hepatic puncture for cholangiography or tube changes. Disadvantages include the constant reminder of morbidity, the possibility of tube dislodgment or inadvertent removal, localized discomfort, and the need to change the tubes periodically because of sludge buildup. The placement of effective internal biliary stents has therefore been regarded as more desirable.

In 1986, Bornman et al.[105] reported a prospective, randomized trial of transhepatic biliary stent placement (12 French plastic endoprosthesis) versus bypass surgery (cholecystojejunostomy usually performed) in 53 patients with unresectable pancreatic carcinoma. Stent placement was successful in 84% of patients, with a 30-day mortality rate of 8% after stenting and 20% after surgery. Bleeding was noted after 20% of stent insertions. While initial hospital stay after stenting was less than after surgery, recurrent jaundice developed in 38% of patients with stents, necessitating stent changes. Duodenal obstruction developed in 14% of patients after stent insertion, requiring gastrojejunostomy. The median survival was similar: 19 weeks after stenting and 15 weeks after surgery.

More recently, self-expanding flexible metal stents have been employed, with an insertion diameter of 7 French and an expanded diameter of 10 mm (30 French). Since the sides of these stents become incorporated into the bile duct wall, they are much less likely to migrate than plastic stents. Several recent reports have documented their efficacy in relieving biliary obstruction for proximal as well as distal tumors.[106–108] Biliary obstruction is relieved in 91% to 100% of patients, with a 30-day mortality rate from 0% to 9%. Stent occlusion has been noted in 9% to 24% of patients, with both tumor overgrowth at the ends and tumor ingrowth through the mesh sides. Occlusion has been treated by balloon dilatation and insertion of new stents through the lumen of the pre-existing stent.

Surgical Palliation

For effective surgical palliation of unresectable periampullary malignancy, each of the three major causes of morbidity must be addressed: (1) relief of biliary obstruction, (2) relief of actual or threatened duodenal obstruction, and (3) relief from pain. Although the techniques for palliation of each are well known, experienced judgment is required in applying them owing to the spectrum in patient presentation. Since biliary obstruction and pain from malignancy have increasingly been addressed by nonoperative techniques, a review of the recent surgical literature must take into account that patient selection may be present, with high-risk patients or those with obviously widespread disease not being referred for laparotomy and surgical palliation.

Biliary Obstruction—Cholecystojejunostomy, Choledochojejunostomy, or Choledochoduodenostomy?

Each of these procedures has been recommended for palliation of jaundice due to unresectable periampullary malignancy, but most results are gleaned from retrospective, uncontrolled reviews. Cholecystojejunostomy (CCJ) is simple to perform, does not require prolonged operating time, and may minimize blood loss. However, its long-term patency may be compromised by tumor impingement or occlusion of the cystic duct, especially with a low insertion of the cystic duct on the common bile duct (found in 10% of patients).[109]

Choledochojejunostomy (CDJ) with cholecystectomy, using either a loop or a Roux limb, is more technically demanding, requires increased operating time, and may result in increased blood loss compared with CCJ. However, it may offer increased long-term patency, since the anastomosis is farther from the tumor. CDJ is not widely performed owing to concern regarding tumor proximity and the risk of a leak that contains both biliary and gastroduodenal secretions.

In 1982, Sarr and Cameron[109] retrospectively reviewed 42 studies with 8571 patients with unresectable pancreatic carcinoma and found an operative mortality rate of 19% after biliary bypass, with a mean survival of 5.4 months. CCJ was performed with an operative mortality rate of 16% with a mean survival of 5.3 months, while CDJ had an operative mortality of 20% with a mean survival of 6.5 months. Recurrent jaundice and cholangitis occurred in 8% after CCJ but in none after CDJ. They concluded that choledochal drainage was preferred for those with prolonged expected survival or for cases with tumor near the cystic duct but that CCJ was preferred in most patients owing to its simplicity and ease of operation. This retrospective review shows mortality rates that approach those previously associated with pancreaticoduodenectomy. While occasional subsequent reports have shown similar mortality rates,[110, 111] most recent studies show improved mortality rates, ranging from 2% to 13%.[112–117] These improvements may be influenced by patient selection, with percutaneous or endoscopic biliary decompression increasingly used for higher-risk patients. Also, improvements in perioperative care may also be responsible for lower mortality rates.

In 1988, Sarfeh et al.[118] reported a prospective, randomized trial of CCJ and choledochoenterostomy (including both CDJ and choledochoduodenostomy). Limitations included the trial's small size (31 patients), the inclusion of benign disease (29% of the patients had chronic pancreatitis), and the grouping of CDJ and choledochoduodenostomy. With CCJ, the operative mortality rate was 13.3%, with both short- and long-term bypass failure in 47%; mean survival was 5.4 months. With choledochoenterostomy, the operative mortality rate was 0%, with bypass failure occurring in 12.5% and a mean survival of 6.6 months. Operating time and blood loss were significantly decreased with CCJ. They concluded that choledochoenterostomy was superior to CCJ for malignant distal biliary obstruction. However, both the study limitations and the very high CCJ failure rate should be noted.

Rappaport and Villalba[116] compared CCJ with choledochoenterostomy (the majority had had CDJ) in a retrospective review of 109 patients with unresectable pancreatic cancer. With CCJ, the mortality rate was 14%, with a mean survival of 7.8 months and a bypass failure rate of 10.9%. With choledochoenterostomy, the mortality rate was 16%, with a mean survival of 8.9 months and a bypass failure rate of 8.8%. They found no significant differences with respect to length of hospital stay or morbidity but did find decreased operative times with CCJ. In a similar retrospective review, Singh et al.[112] compared CCJ with CDJ and found increased mortality and morbidity rates with CDJ (11.7% and 38.3%, respectively) compared with those with CCJ (5.4% and 27%, respectively). Recurrent jaundice occurred in about 13% in each group.

In these studies, choledochoduodenostomy was not often used, with concerns about proximity of tumor to the anastomosis and the use of the duodenum as a drainage conduit, with the risk of subsequent duodenal obstruction. In contrast, Potts and coworkers[115] performed choledochoduodenostomy in almost half of 142 patients with unresectable pancreatic carcinoma, with the remainder receiving either CDJ or CCJ. They found that CCJ had a mortality rate of 9% and a morbidity rate of 34% due to biliary sepsis or recurrent jaundice, whereas CDJ was performed with no mortality and a morbidity rate of 16%, half that of CCJ. More impressive was their experience with choledochoduodenostomy, with no mortality and a morbidity rate (sepsis or recurrent jaundice) of only 3%, although survival periods were not specified. Singh et al.[112] found their experience with choledochoduodenostomy and cholecystoduodenostomy to be different, with a mortality rate of 8% and recurrent jaundice in 33%; they recommended anastomosis to the jejunum instead of the duodenum.

In 1993, Lillemoe and colleagues[117] also demonstrated that biliary bypass surgery, especially CDJ, could be performed with low mortality and very good long-term patency. In 118 patients with unresectable periampullary malignancy, biliary bypasses were done in 78%, with the remainder either previously bypassed or stented. Most of the bypasses (89%) were CDJ, with CCJ performed in the rest. Gastrojejunostomy was also performed in 90% of all patients. Their hospital mortality rate was only 2.5%. Morbidity included cholangitis in 8% and biliary anastomotic leakage in 4%, most of which closed spontaneously. Recurrent jaundice occurred in 2%; mean survival was 7.5 months.

Either a Roux-en-Y limb or loop of jejunum can be used for biliary bypasses. With a loop, some prefer to add a proximal jejunojejunostomy to divert the enteric contents from the biliary anastomosis[117] and to avoid intestinal obstruction if tumor extension involves the loop above the transverse mesocolon.[109] Roux diversion probably minimizes intestinal reflux into the biliary system but requires more operative time than a loop, although complication rates are similar.[115] It may therefore be more suitable for those in whom long-term survival is expected.[109, 112]

Palliation of Duodenal Obstruction

Duodenal compromise or obstruction is still managed surgically by gastrojejunostomy (GJ; either by a loop or by a Roux limb), except for those near death, who are managed by nasogastric intubation or percutaneous endoscopic gastrostomy. GJ is considered in three general classes:

1. Biliary obstruction palliated by percutaneous or endoscopic stenting, with subsequent development of duodenal obstruction.
2. At surgical bypass for biliary obstruction with therapeutic GJ if nausea, vomiting, or obstruction is present.
3. At surgical bypass for biliary obstruction with or without prophylactic GJ for those without symptoms of duodenal obstruction.

The majority of patients with periampullary malignancy present with biliary obstruction and do not have duodenal obstruction before death. However, a substantial minority do have symptoms of nausea and vomiting, leading many to recommend prophylactic GJ at initial laparotomy. While this approach adds GJ in the majority who would not require it, subsequent operation is thereby avoided in symptomatic patients less able to undergo operation. Sarr and Cameron,[109] in reviewing collected series of 1865 patients, found that 29% were treated with GJ at initial laparotomy. Of the remainder, 13% required GJ before death, with an operative mortality rate of 16%. From 10% to 20% of those never receiving GJ died with symptoms of duodenal obstruction, which might have been palliated if GJ had initially been performed. Moreover, the addition of GJ to biliary bypass did not increase operative mortality. They concluded that GJ should be performed prophylactically as well as therapeutically in those undergoing laparotomy.

Singh et al.[112] also recommended GJ, both prophylactic as well as therapeutic, in patients undergoing biliary bypass. Addition of GJ to biliary bypass did not significantly increase mortality. They found that 25% of those initially receiving only biliary bypass subsequently required GJ, all of which functioned within 10 days. An additional 24% of those receiving only biliary bypass had nausea and vomiting before death.

Lillemoe and coworkers[117] also recommended GJ at initial laparotomy. In their series of 118 patients, GJ was performed in 90% (most also had biliary bypass), with a hospital mortality rate of only 2.5%. Of those not receiving GJ, 14% subsequently had duodenal obstruction.

Delayed gastric emptying (DGE) after GJ for unresectable malignancy has been reported following both prophylactic and therapeutic procedures, leading some to question its value. Doberneck and Berndt[119] found a 26% overall incidence rate of DGE lasting a mean of 16 days. Of their patients without preoperative duodenal obstruction, 16% had DGE, while 57% of those with preoperative obstruction had DGE postoperatively. Weaver et al.[120] observed a very high morbidity and mortality rate (90%) in those with preoperative nausea and vomiting and concluded that few were effectively palliated by GJ. Proctor and Mauro[113] reported that GJ combined with biliary bypass increased mean hospital stay from 7.3 days to 24 days compared with biliary bypass alone.

Instead of GJ, Lucas and coworkers[121] performed antrectomy with antecolic GJ in 19 patients with unresectable malignancy who were symptomatic with nausea and vomiting. Most had radiographic evidence of duodenal encroachment. In this uncontrolled series, 13 patients underwent simultaneous biliary bypass and antrectomy with GJ; 5 had had previous biliary decompressive procedures. Intraluminal carcinoma was present within the pyloric channel in four patients, requiring mobilization of the lateral duodenal wall and omentum for duodenal stump closure in two patients. Length of operation ranged from 3 to 5 hours for double bypass, with no mortality and no reported major complications. Hospital stay ranged from 7 to 29 days (mean, 12 days); all patients were eating at discharge. They recommended antrectomy with GJ in all patients undergoing surgical biliary bypass, even if no symptoms of duodenal obstruction were present.

In contrast, numerous series have demonstrated a low incidence of DGE and good palliation from GJ. In performing both prophylactic and therapeutic GJ in 70 patients, Singh et al.[112] found DGE in 12.9%, with eventual functioning in 68 of 70 bypasses. DGE after GJ alone was found in 16.7% by de Rooij and colleagues[114] but in only 11% after combined biliary and duodenal bypass. In 107 patients, where preoperative vomiting was present in 22%, Lillemoe et al.[117] found overall postoperative DGE in only 8%, with a mean length of nasogastric drainage of 17 days in those patients. Prokinetic agents such as metoclopramide or erythromycin have been used in some of these patients and may be of benefit in reducing the duration of DGE. However, definitive studies are still needed. Vagotomy is not thought to be needed with GJ, since the incidence of stomal ulceration is low during the survival period and may be reduced by the prophylactic use of histamine_2 blockers.[109]

Antecolic GJ has been recommended for bypass of malignancy owing to the perceived probability that a retrocolic route would be more quickly involved by advancing tumor.[112, 119] Yet, a recent study in which 79% of GJs were placed in the retrocolic position had an incidence rate of late gastric outlet obstruction of only 4%.[117] In addition, there was a strong trend toward decreased incidence of both DGE and late gastric outlet obstruction with the use of the retrocolic position.

Laparoscopic Palliation

Laparoscopic techniques have recently been applied for palliation of both biliary and duodenal obstruction from unresectable malignancy. Hawasli[122] reported two cases of laparoscopically performed cholecystojejunostomy using a stapled and sewn anastomosis, with hospital discharge on the fourth postoperative day. Shimi et al.[123] performed laparoscopic cholecystojejunostomy in five patients after demonstrating unresectable pancreatic carcinoma at diagnostic laparoscopy. Cholecystocholangiography was first used to confirm cystic duct patency, then either a handsewn or a stapled and sewn cholecystojejunostomy was completed, without any mortality. Four of the five patients were discharged by the tenth postoperative day, and the other suffered from complications from cholangitis after endoprosthesis removal. One patient subsequently required repeated laparoscopy for treatment of anastomotic blockage due to blood clot and debris.

Laparoscopic gastroenterostomy has also been occasionally performed for duodenal obstruction. Wilson and Varma[124] reported laparoscopic antecolic gastrojejunostomy in two patients using a stapled and sewn technique, with discharge on the fourth and fifth postoperative days.

Palliation of Pain

While biliary and gastric outlet obstruction may be effectively palliated with stenting or surgical bypass, pain from unresectable periampullary carcinoma may be the most incapacitating symptom with tumor growth.

Pancreatic duct or biliary duct obstruction had previously been thought to contribute to pain, but invasion of pancreatic and peripancreatic nerves is most likely causative.[112] While surgical resection of neural tissue (splanchnic nerve resection, celiac or superior mesenteric ganglionectomy) has been attempted in the past,[125–128] most current efforts are directed toward chemical neurolysis of the celiac plexus, either by percutaneous block or by direct intraoperative injection (chemical splanchnicectomy). Ethanol in a concentration of at least 50% is typically used for celiac plexus neurolysis, with effects mediated by destruction of nerve fibers with resultant wallerian degeneration.[129] Incomplete destruction of nerve cell bodies may result in regeneration with return of abdominal pain.

Percutaneous celiac nerve block, under fluoroscopic or CT scan guidance, has been reported to achieve pain relief in 70% to 95% of patients with unresectable pancreatic carcinoma.[129–133] The block itself is painful and requires either a mixture of local anesthetic with the alcohol or parenteral analgesia. Pain that recurs after a successful initial percutaneous block may be treated with a repeated block. Brown and coworkers[131] treated 166 patients with pancreatic carcinoma and found that 85% obtained good pain relief, which lasted until death in 75%. Repeated blocks after a successful initial block were effective in 81% of those treated. Sharfman and Walsh[134] reviewed 15 series with 480 patients over a 25-year period, with a reported 87% satisfactory response to percutaneous neurolytic celiac plexus block. However, they warned of major deficiencies in many of these reports, with limited data regarding pre- and postblock analgesic requirements and duration of benefit, and concluded that available data on neurolytic celiac plexus block for pain from pancreatic carcinoma were insufficient to judge efficacy, long-term morbidity, and cost effectiveness.

Intraoperative injection of the celiac plexus (chemical splanchnicectomy) has been practiced for at least three decades, with either 6% phenol or 50% ethanol injected into the retroperitoneum on either side of the aorta in the vicinity of the celiac axis. From 70% to 88% of patients with existing pain have been reported to experience relief, with minimal morbidity.[135–138] As with reports of percutaneous celiac block, these previous reports of the success of chemical splanchnicectomy were not prospective, controlled studies and did not address the benefit of prophylactic chemical splanchnicectomy for unresectable patients who did not have significant pain at the time of laparotomy and bypass.

Lillemoe et al.[139] have recently reported the results of a prospective, randomized, double-blind study of intraoperative chemical splanchnicectomy with 50% ethanol versus a placebo injection of saline in 137 patients with unresectable pancreatic cancer. Of these, 62% were stage III and 38% were stage IV, with 75% of all carcinomas located in the pancreatic head. Two transient hypertensive events without sequelae occurred during injection (presumed adrenal injection), but no hypotensive episodes or hemorrhage occurred. In patients who had pre-existing pain, alcohol injection significantly reduced pain scores at both 2- and 4-month follow-up; these patients had a mean pain-free period of 3.3 months, compared with only 0.8 months for saline controls. Significant pain did recur before death in 65% of those receiving alcohol, while all of those receiving saline control had significant pain at the time of death. In patients who did not have pre-existing pain, alcohol injection significantly reduced pain scores at 2 and 6 months; these patients had a mean pain-free period of 7.2 months, compared with only 3.0 months for placebo. Only 46% of patients receiving alcohol required significant doses of narcotics prior to death, while 68% of placebo-treated patients required them. Percutaneous celiac plexus block was eventually given to 10% initially receiving intraoperative chemical splanchnicectomy with alcohol and to 12% receiving placebo, but the average time period between operative splanchnicectomy and percutaneous block was 11.8 months for alcohol and only 4.0 months for placebo. Interestingly, although there was no survival benefit from alcohol administered to patients without significant preoperative pain, there was a significant survival benefit in those with preoperative pain compared with placebo controls who also had preoperative pain.

Unresectable Ampullary Carcinoma

In a large series, Nakase and coworkers[72] reported 120 patients treated with biliary bypass, with an operative mortality rate of 19% and a mean survival time of 9 months. Gastrojejunostomy was performed in 12%. Knox and Kingston[70] reported 11 patients who underwent bypass, with an operative mortality rate of 36%; none survived longer than 18 months. Crane et al.[77] reported five patients treated with biliary bypass who had a mean survival of 8 months. Walsh and colleagues[80] reported seven patients treated with biliary bypass, with an operative mortality rate of 29% and one 3-year survivor. Delcore et al.[12] reported three patients who died within 15 months of palliative bypass.

Unresectable Distal Bile Duct Carcinoma

Nakase et al.[72] reported 129 patients with a 28% mortality rate from surgical palliative bypass and a mean survival length of 6.2 months. Reding and colleagues[3] reported 38 patients treated with biliary bypass, with an operative mortality rate of 18% and a median survival of 8 months. Nakayama and coworkers[140] reported 16 patients with middle and distal duct carcinoma who had a mean survival of 6.6 months after surgical bypass.

Unresectable Duodenal Carcinoma

In a report by Nakase et al.,[72] 8 of 15 patients had gastrojejunostomy, with a 7% mortality rate and a mean survival of 4 months. Lai and coworkers[84] treated nine patients with either palliative segmental resection or gastrojejunostomy and found a median survival of 6.2 months. Alwmark and colleagues[8] performed palliative bypass in 11 patients, 5 of whom left the hospital, with survivals of 4, 6, 6, 7, and 24 months. Ouriel and Adams[41] palliated nine patients with nodal metastases with a gastrojejunostomy and found a mean survival of 14 months.

CHEMOTHERAPY

Reports of chemotherapy for unresectable or recurrent ampullary carcinoma are anecdotal. Barton and Copeland[37] reported 17 patients with local extension, nodal metastases, or disseminated disease who underwent postoperative chemotherapy. Of these, 16 had previously undergone radical resection. 5-FU was most commonly used and was generally used in combination with a variety of other chemotherapeutic agents. No combination appeared to prolong life when used in either the adjuvant or the therapeutic setting.

Chemotherapy alone for cholangiocarcinoma is unpromising. Mitomycin C appears to be the most active single drug and, in combination with doxorubicin and 5-FU, has shown partial response rates of about 30% but with the risk of increased toxicity.[141] Treatment with 5-FU alone has the least toxic effects, with partial response rates of 10% to 20%.

In the past, adjuvant postoperative chemotherapy or radiotherapy for adenocarcinoma of the duodenum has been reported anecdotally,[8, 142, 143] with the impression of prolonged survival for those receiving combined chemotherapy and radiotherapy after palliative bypass, with survival from 12 to 24 months. No prospective trial of postoperative chemotherapy and radiotherapy for duodenal adenocarcinoma has been reported.

FUTURE PROSPECTS

Development of an effective adjuvant therapy for periampullary carcinoma is still needed. Willett et al.[39] have suggested that tumor dissemination during operative manipulation may be responsible for the failure of postoperative radiotherapy to provide significant improvement. They proposed low-dose preoperative external beam radiation before pancreaticoduodenectomy, with further postoperative irradiation for those patients at high risk with unfavorable tumor characteristics.

The preoperative chemotherapy and radiation given by Yeung and colleagues[87] to those with duodenal carcinoma resulted in no evidence of residual disease in resected specimens. Although it is too early for long-term results, this approach seems promising.

References

1. Cooperman AM: Cancer of the ampulla of Vater, bile duct and duodenum. Surg Clin North Am 61:99–106, 1981.
2. Chao TC, Greager JA: Carcinoma of the extrahepatic bile ducts. J Surg Oncol 46:145–150, 1991.
3. Reding R, Buard JL, Lebeau G, et al: Surgical management of 552 carcinomas of the extrahepatic bile ducts (gallbladder and periampullary tumors excluded). Ann Surg 213:236–241, 1991.
4. Nagorney DM, Donohue JH, Farnell MB, et al: Outcomes after curative resections of cholangiocarcinoma. Arch Surg 128:871–879, 1993.
5. Kleinerman J, Yardumian K, Tamaki HT: Primary carcinoma of duodenum. Ann Intern Med 32:451–465, 1950.
6. Lillemoe K, Imbembo AL: Malignant neoplasms of the duodenum. SGO 150:822–826, 1980.
7. Joesting DR, Beart RW Jr, van Heerden JA, et al: Improving survival in adenocarcinoma of the duodenum. Am J Surg 141:228–231, 1981.
8. Alwmark A, Andersson A, Lasson A: Primary carcinoma of the duodenum. Ann Surg 191:13–18, 1980.
9. Veen HF, Oscarson JE, Malt RA: Alien cancers of the duodenum. SGO 143:39–42, 1976.
10. Yamaguchi K, Enjoji M: Carcinomas of the ampulla of Vater: A clinicopathologic study and pathologic staging of 109 cases of carcinoma and 5 cases of adenoma. Cancer 59:506–515, 1987.
11. Monson JRT, Donohue JH, McEntee GP, et al: Radical resection for carcinoma of the ampulla of Vater. Arch Surg 126:353–357, 1991.
12. Delcore R Jr, Connor CS, Thomas JH, et al: Significance of tumor spread in adenocarcinoma of the ampulla of Vater. Am J Surg 158:593–597, 1989.
13. Austin JL, Organ CH Jr, Williams GR, et al: Vaterian cancer in siblings. Ann Surg 207:655–661, 1988.
14. Noda Y, Watanabe H, Iida M, et al: Histologic follow-up of ampullary adenomas in patients with familial adenomatosis coli. Cancer 70:1847–1856, 1992.
15. Beckwith PS, Van Heerden JA, Dozois RR: Prognosis of symptomatic duodenal adenomas in familial adenomatous polyposis. Arch Surg 126:825–828, 1991.
16. Spigelman AD, Crofton-Sleigh C, Venitt S, et al: Mutagenicity of bile and duodenal adenomas in familial adenomatous polyposis. Br J Surg 77:878–881, 1990.
17. Iida M, Yao T, Itoh H, et al: Natural history of duodenal lesions in Japanese patients with familial adenomatous coli (Gardner's syndrome). Gastroenterology 96:1301–1306, 1989.
18. Lynch HT, Smyrk TL, Lanspa SJ, et al: Upper gastrointestinal manifestations in families with hereditary flat adenoma syndrome. Cancer 71:2709–2714, 1993.
19. Ricci JL: Carcinoid of the ampulla of Vater. Cancer 71:686–690, 1993.
20. Klein A, Clemens J, Cameron J: Periampullary neoplasms in von Recklinghausen's disease. Surgery 106:815–819, 1989.
21. Perrone T: Duodenal gangliocystic paraganglioma and carcinoid. Am J Pathol 10:147–148, 1986.
22. Seifert E, Schulte F, Stolte M: Adenoma and carcinoma of the duodenum and papilla of Vater: A clinicopathologic study. Am J Gastroenterol 87:37–42, 1992.
23. Galandiuk S, Hermann RE, Jagelman DG, et al: Villous tumors of the duodenum. Ann Surg 207:234–239, 1988.
24. Ryan DP, Schapiro RH, Warshaw AL: Villous tumors of the duodenum. Ann Surg 203:301–306, 1986.
25. Bjork KJ, Davis CJ, Nagorney DM, et al: Duodenal villous tumors. Arch Surg 125:961–965, 1990.
26. Yen S, Hsieh CC, MacMahon B: Extrahepatic bile duct cancer and smoking, beverage consumption, past medical history and oral-contraceptive use. Cancer 59:2112–2116, 1987.
27. Lowenfels AB, Norman J: Isoniazid and bile duct cancer. JAMA 240:434–435, 1978.
28. Broden G, Bengston L: Biliary carcinoma associated with methyldopa therapy. Acta Chir Scand Suppl 500:7–12, 1980.
29. Szendroi M, Nemeth L, Vajta G: Asbestos bodies in a bile duct cancer after occupational exposure. Environ Res 30:270–280, 1983.
30. Brown OP: Mortality of workers exposed to polychlorinated biphenyls: An update. Arch Environ Health 42:333, 1987.
31. Sako K, Seitzinger GL, Garside E: Carcinoma of the extrahepatic bile ducts. Surgery 41:416–437, 1957.
32. Lieber MM, Stewart HL, Lund H: Carcinoma of the peripapillary portion of the duodenum. Part one. Ann Surg 109:219–245, 1939.
33. Lieber MM, Stewart HL, Lund H: Carcinoma of the peripapillary portion of the duodenum. Part two. Ann Surg 109:383–429, 1939.
34. Skandalakis LF, Rowe JS Jr, Gray SW, et al: Surgical embryology and anatomy of the pancreas. Surg Clin North Am 73:661–697, 1993.
35. Kayahara M, Nagakawa T, Veno K, et al: Lymphatic flow in carcinoma of the distal bile duct based on a clinicopathologic study. Cancer 72:2112–2117, 1993.
36. Beahrs OH, Henson DE, Hutter RVP, et al: Manual for Staging of Cancer, 4th ed. Philadelphia: JB Lippincott, 1992.
37. Barton RM, Copeland EM III: Carcinoma of the ampulla of Vater. SGO 156:297–301, 1983.
38. Neoptolemos JP, Talbot IC, Shaw DC, Carr-Locke DL: Long-term survival after resection of ampullary carcinoma is associated independently with tumor grade and a new staging classification that assesses local invasiveness. Cancer 61:1403–1407, 1988.
39. Willett CG, Warshaw AL, Convery K, Compton CC: Patterns of failure after pancreaticoduodenectomy for ampullary carcinoma. SGO 176:33–38, 1993.
40. Henson DE, Albores-Saavedra J, Corle D: Carcinoma of the extrahepatic bile ducts. Cancer 70:1498–1501, 1992.
41. Ouriel K, Adams JT: Adenocarcinoma of the small intestine. Am J Surg 147:66–71, 1984.
42. Spigelman AD, Williams LB, Talbot IC, et al: Upper gastrointestinal cancer in patients with familial adenomatous polyposis. Lancet 2:783–785, 1989.
43. Brambs HJ, Claussen CD: Pancreatic and ampullary carcinoma, ultrasound, computed tomography, magnetic resonance imaging and angiography. Endoscopy 25:58–68, 1993.
44. Robledo R, Prieto ML, Perez M, et al: Carcinoma of the hepaticopancreatic ampullar region: Role of US. Radiology 166:409–412, 1988.
45. Warshaw AL, Gu Z, Wittenberg J, et al: Preoperative staging and assessment of resectability of pancreatic cancer. Arch Surg 125:230–233, 1990.
46. Kazerooni EA, Quint LE, Francis IR: Duodenal neoplasms: Predictive value of CT for determining malignancy and tumor resectability. AJR 159:303–309, 1992.
47. Fishman EK, Wyatt SH, Kuhlman JE, Siegelman SS: Spiral CT of the pancreas with multiplanar display. AJR 159:1209–1215, 1992.
48. Rubin GD, Dake MD, Napel SA, McDonnell CH, Jeffrey RB Jr: Three-dimensional spiral CT angiography of the abdomen: Initial clinical experience. Radiology 186:147–152, 1993.
49. Zeman RK, Fox SH, Silverman PM, et al: Helical (spiral) CT of the abdomen. AJR 160:719–725, 1993.
50. Ponchon T, Berger F, Chavaillon A, et al: Contribution of endoscopy to diagnosis and treatment of tumors of the ampulla of Vater. Cancer 64:161–167, 1989.

51. Blackman E, Nash SV: Diagnosis of duodenal and ampullary epithelial neoplasms by endoscopic biopsy: A clinicopathologic and immunohistochemical study. Hum Pathol 16:901–910, 1985.
52. Hall TJ, Blackstone MO, Cooper MJ, et al: Prospective evaluation of endoscopic retrograde cholangiopancreatography in the diagnosis of periampullary cancers. Ann Surg 187:313–317, 1978.
53. Dooley WC, Cameron JL, Pitt HA, et al: Is preoperative angiography useful in patients with periampullary tumors? Ann Surg 211:649–655, 1990.
54. Yeo CJ, Pitt HA, Cameron JL: Cholangiocarcinoma. Surg Clin North Am 70:1429–1447, 1990.
55. Lightdale CJ, Botet JF, Woodruff JM, et al: Localization of endocrine tumors of the pancreas with endoscopic ultrasonography. Cancer 68:1815–1820, 1991.
56. Tio TL, Sie LH, Verbeek PCM, et al: Endosonography in diagnosing and staging duodenal villous adenoma. Gut 33:567–568, 1992.
57. Tio TL, Mulder CJJ, Eggink WF: Endosonography in staging early carcinoma of the ampulla of Vater. Gastroenterology 102:1392–1395, 1992.
58. Tio TL, Tytgat GNJ, Cikot RJLM, et al: Ampullopancreatic carcinoma: Preoperative TNM classification with endosonography. Radiology 175:455–461, 1990.
59. Tio TL, Cheng J, Wijers OB, et al: Endosonographic TNM staging of extrahepatic bile duct cancer: Comparison with pathological staging. Gastroenterology 100:1351–1361, 1991.
60. Halsted WS: Contributions to the surgery of the bile passages, especially of the common bile duct. Boston Med Surg J 141:645–654, 1899.
61. Hunt VC, Budd JW: Transduodenal resection of the ampulla of Vater for carcinoma of the distal end of the common bile duct. SGO 61:651–661, 1935.
62. Goldberg M, Zamir O, Hadary A, et al: Wide local excision as an alternative treatment for periampullary carcinoma. Am J Gastroenterol 82:1169–1171, 1987.
63. Farouk M, Niotis M, Branum GD, et al: Indications for and the technique of local resection of tumors of the papilla of Vater. Arch Surg 126:650–652, 1991.
64. Asbun HJ, Rossi RL, Munson JL: Local resection for ampullary tumors: Is there a place for it? Arch Surg 128:515–520, 1993.
65. Kahn MB, Rush BF Jr: The overlooked technique of ampullary excision. SGO 169:253–254, 1989.
66. Tarazi RY, Hermann RE, Vogt DP, et al: Results of surgical treatment of periampullary tumors: A thirty-five-year experience. Surgery 100:716–723, 1986.
67. Robertson JFR, Imrie CW, Hole DJ, et al: Management of periampullary carcinoma. Br J Surg 74:816–819, 1987.
68. Newman RJ, Pittman MR: Local excision in the treatment of carcinoma of the ampulla of Vater. J R Coll Surg Edinb 27:154–157, 1982.
69. Wise L, Pizzimbono C, Dehner LP: Periampullary cancer: A clinicopathologic study of 62 patients. Am J Surg 131:141–148, 1976.
70. Knox RA, Kingston RD: Carcinoma of the ampulla of Vater. Br J Surg 73:72–73, 1986.
71. Jones BA, Langer BL, Taylor BR, et al: Periampullary tumors: Which ones should be resected? Am J Surg 149:46–52, 1985.
72. Nakase A, Matsumoto Y, Uchida K, Honjo I: Surgical treatment of cancer of the pancreas and the periampullary region: Cumulative results in 57 institutions in Japan. Ann Surg 185:52–57, 1976.
73. Fortner JG: Regional pancreatectomy for cancer of the pancreas, ampulla, and other related sites. Ann Surg 199:418–425, 1984.
74. Grace PA, Pitt HA, Longmire WP: Pylorus preserving pancreatoduodenectomy: An overview. Br J Surg 77:968–974, 1990.
75. Crist DW, Sitzmann JV, Cameron JL: Improved hospital morbidity, mortality, and survival after the Whipple procedure. Ann Surg 206:358–365, 1987.
76. Trede M, Schwall G, Saeger HD: Survival after pancreatoduodenectomy: 118 consecutive resections without an operative mortality. Ann Surg 211:447–458, 1990.
77. Crane JM, Gobbel WG Jr, Scott HW Jr: Surgical experience with malignant tumors of the ampulla of Vater and duodenum. SGO 137:937–940, 1973.
78. Matory YL, Gaynor J, Brennan M: Carcinoma of the ampulla of Vater. SGO 177:366–370, 1993.
79. Dawson PJ, Connolly MM: Influence of site of origin and mucin production on survival in ampullary carcinoma. Ann Surg 210:173–179, 1989.
80. Walsh DB, Eckhauser FE, Cronenwett JL, Turcotte JG, Lindenauer SM: Adenocarcinoma of the ampulla of Vater: Diagnosis and treatment. Ann Surg 195:152–157, 1982.
81. Tompkins RK, Thomas D, Wile A, et al: Prognostic factors in bile duct carcinoma: Analysis of 96 cases. Ann Surg 194:447–457, 1981.
82. Ouchi K, Matsuno S, Sato T: Long-term survival in carcinoma of the biliary tract: Analysis of prognostic factors in 146 resections. Arch Surg 124:248–252, 1989.
83. Warren KW, Choe DS, Plaza J, Relihan M: Results of radical resection for periampullary cancer. Ann Surg 181:534–540, 1975.
84. Lai ECS, Doty JE, Irving C, Tompkins RK: Primary adenocarcinoma of the duodenum: Analysis of survival. World J Surg 12:695–699, 1988.
85. McGuire GE, Pitt HA, Lillemoe KD, et al: Reoperative surgery for periampullary adenocarcinoma. Arch Surg 126:1205–1212, 1991.
86. Hashimi H, Sabanathan S: Second look operation in managing carcinoma of the pancreas and periampullary region. SGO 168:224–226, 1989.
87. Yeung RS, Weese JL, Hoffman JP, et al: Neoadjuvant chemoradiation in pancreatic and duodenal carcinoma: A phase II study. Cancer 72:2124–2133, 1993.
88. Splinter TAW, Obertop H, Kok TC, et al: Adjuvant chemotherapy after resection of adenocarcinoma of the periampullary region and head of the pancreas. J Cancer Res Clin Oncol 115:200–202, 1989.
89. Minsky BD, Kemeny N, Armstrong JG, Reichman B, Botet J: Extrahepatic biliary system cancer: An update of a combined modality approach. Am J Clin Oncol 14:433–437, 1991.
90. Cameron JL, Pitt HA, Zinner MJ, et al: Management of proximal cholangiocarcinoma by surgical resection and radiotherapy. Am J Surg 159:91–98, 1990.
91. Iwasaki Y, Todoroki T, Fukao K, et al: The role of intraoperative radiation therapy in the treatment of bile duct cancer. World J Surg 12:91–98, 1988.
92. Cotton PB: Endoscopic methods for relief of malignant obstructive jaundice. World J Surg 6:854–861, 1984.
93. Soehendra N, Reijnders-Frederix V: Palliative bile duct drainage: A new endoscopic method of introducing a transpapillary drain. Endoscopy 12:8–11, 1980.
94. Cotton PB: Nonsurgical palliation of jaundice in pancreatic cancer. Surg Clin North Am 69:613–627, 1989.
95. Bickerstaff KI, Berry AR, Chapman RW, et al: Endoscopic sphincterotomy for the palliation of ampullary carcinoma. Br J Surg 77:160–162, 1990.
96. Shepherd HA, Royle G, Ross APR, et al: Endoscopic biliary endoprosthesis in the palliation of malignant obstruction of the distal common bile duct: A randomized trial. Br J Surg 75:1166–1168, 1988.
97. Andersen JR, Sorenson SM, Kruse A, et al: Randomized trial of endoscopic endoprosthesis versus operative bypass in malignant obstructive jaundice. Gut 30:1132–1135, 1989.
98. Keymling M, Wagner HJ, Vakil N, et al: Relief of malignant duodenal obstruction by percutaneous insertion of a metal stent. Gastrointest Endosc 39:439–441, 1993.
99. Dowsett JF, Vaira D, Hatfield ARW, et al: Endoscopic biliary therapy using the combined percutaneous and endoscopic technique. Gastroenterology 96:1180–1186, 1989.
100. Spear AG, Cotton PB, Rode J, et al: Biliary stent blockage with bacterial biofilm: A light and electron microscopy study. Ann Intern Med 108:546–553, 1988.
101. Leung JWC, Ling TKW, Kung JLS, et al: The role of bacteria in the blockage of biliary stents. Gastrointest Endosc 34:19–22, 1988.
102. Matsuda Y, Shimakura K, Akamatsu T: Factors affecting the patency of stents in malignant biliary obstructive disease: Univariate and multivariate analysis. Am J Gastroenterol 86:843–849, 1991.
103. Frakes JT, Johanson JF, Stake JJ: Optimal timing for stent replacement in malignant biliary tract obstruction. Gastrointest Endosc 39:164–167, 1993.
104. Conn M, Speer AG, Cotton PB: Factors affecting the duration of biliary stent patency in patients with pancreatic cancer. Gastrointest Endosc 35:162, 1989.
105. Bornman PC, Tobias R, Harries-Jones EP, et al: Prospective controlled trial of transhepatic biliary endoprosthesis versus bypass

surgery for incurable carcinoma of head of pancreas. Lancet 1:69–71, 1986.
106. Nicholson AA, Royston CMS: Palliation of inoperable biliary obstruction with self-expanding metal endoprostheses: A review of 77 patients. Clin Radiol 47:245–250, 1993.
107. Lee MJ, Dawson SL, Mueller PR, et al: Palliation of malignant bile duct obstruction with metallic biliary endoprostheses: Techniques, results and complications. J Vasc Int Rad 3:665–671, 1992.
108. Gordon RL, Ring EJ, LaBerge JM, et al: Malignant biliary obstruction: Treatment with expandable metallic stents—follow-up of 50 consecutive patients. Radiology 182:697–701, 1992.
109. Sarr MG, Cameron JL: Surgical management of unresectable carcinoma of the pancreas. Surgery 91:123–133, 1982.
110. Mosdell DM, Kessler C, Morris DM: Unresectable pancreatic carcinoma: What is the optimal procedure? South Med J 84:571–574, 1991.
111. Brooks DC, Osteen RT, Gray EB Jr, et al: Evaluation of palliative procedures for pancreatic cancer. Am J Surg 141:430–433, 1981.
112. Singh SM, Longmire WP Jr, Reber HA: Surgical palliation for pancreatic cancer. The UCLA experience. Ann Surg 212:132–139, 1990.
113. Proctor HJ, Mauro M: Biliary diversion for pancreatic carcinoma: Matching the methods and the patient. Am J Surg 159:67–71, 1990.
114. de Rooij PD, Rogatko A, Brennan MF: Evaluation of palliative surgical procedures in unresectable pancreatic cancer. Br J Surg 78:1053–1058, 1991.
115. Potts JR III, Broughan TA, Hermann RE: Palliative operations for pancreatic carcinoma. Am J Surg 159:72–78, 1990.
116. Rappaport MD, Villalba M: A comparison of cholecysto- and choledochoenterostomy for obstructing pancreatic cancer. Am Surg 56:433–435, 1990.
117. Lillemoe KD, Sauter PK, Pitt HA, et al: Current status of surgical palliation of periampullary carcinoma. SGO 176:1–10, 1993.
118. Sarfeh IJ, Rypins EB, Jakowatz JG, et al: A prospective, randomized clinical investigation of cholecystoenterostomy and choledochoenterostomy. Am J Surg 155:411–414, 1988.
119. Doberneck RC, Berndt GA: Delayed gastric emptying after palliative gastrojejunostomy for carcinoma of the pancreas. Arch Surg 122:827–829, 1987.
120. Weaver DW, Wiencek RG, Bouwman DL, et al: Gastrojejunostomy: Is it helpful for patients with pancreatic cancer? Surgery 102:608–613, 1987.
121. Lucas CE, Ledgerwood AM, Bender JS: Antrectomy with gastrojejunostomy for unresectable pancreatic cancer-causing duodenal obstruction. Surgery 110:583–590, 1991.
122. Hawasli A: Laparoscopic cholecysto-jejunostomy for obstructing pancreatic cancer: Technique and report of two cases. J Laparosc Surg 2:351–355, 1992.
123. Shimi S, Banting S, Cuschieri A: Laparoscopy in the management of pancreatic cancer: Endoscopic cholecystojejunostomy for advanced disease. Br J Surg 79:317–319, 1992.
124. Wilson R, Varma J: Laparoscopic gastroenterostomy for malignant duodenal obstruction. Br J Surg 79:1348, 1992.
125. Helsey WG, Dohn D: Splanchnicectomy for the treatment of intractable abdominal pain. Cleve Clin Q 34:9–25, 1987.
126. Ray BS, Console AD: The relief of pain in chronic (calcareous) pancreatitis by sympathectomy. SGO 89:1–7, 1949.
127. De Takatis G, Walter LE, Lasner J: Splanchnic nerve section for pancreatic pain: Second report. Ann Surg 131:44–49, 1949.
128. Grimson KS, Hesser FH, Kitchin WW: Early clinical results of transabdominal celiac and superior mesenteric ganglionectomy, vagotomy, or transthoracic splanchnicectomy in patients with chronic abdominal visceral pain. Surgery 22:230–233, 1947.
129. Bonica JJ, Buckley FP, Moricca G, et al: Neurolytic blockade and hypophysectomy. In Bonica JJ (ed): The Management of Pain, 2nd ed. Philadelphia: Lea & Febiger, 1990, pp 1980–2039.
130. Lebovits AH, Lefkowitz M: Pain management of pancreatic carcinoma: A review. Pain 36:1–11, 1989.
131. Brown DL, Bulley CK, Quiel EL: Neurolytic celiac plexus block for pancreatic cancer pain. Anesth Analg 66:869–873, 1987.
132. Leung JW, Bowen-Wright M, Aveling W, et al: Coeliac plexus block for pain in pancreatic cancer and chronic pancreatitis. Br J Surg 70:730–732, 1983.
133. Bridenbaugh LD, Moore DC, Campbell DD, et al: Management of upper abdominal cancer pain: Treatment with celiac plexus block with alcohol. JAMA 190:99–102, 1964.
134. Sharfman WH, Walsh TD: Has the analgesic efficacy of neurolytic celiac plexus block been demonstrated in pancreatic cancer pain? Pain 41:267–271, 1990.
135. Copping J, Willix R, Kraft R: Palliative chemical splanchnicectomy. Arch Surg 98:418–420, 1969.
136. Flanigan DP, Kraft RO: Continuing experience with palliative chemical splanchnicectomy. Arch Surg 113:509–511, 1978.
137. Sharp KW, Stevens EJ: Improving palliation in pancreatic cancer: Intraoperative celiac plexus block for pain relief. South Med J 84:469–471, 1991.
138. Gardner AM, Solomou G: Relief of the pain of unresectable carcinoma of pancreas by chemical splanchnicectomy during laparotomy. Ann R Coll Surg Engl 66:409–411, 1984.
139. Lillemoe KD, Cameron JL, Kaufman HS, et al: Chemical splanchnicectomy in patients with unresectable pancreatic cancer. A prospective randomized trial. Ann Surg 217:447–457, 1993.
140. Nakayama F, Miyazaki K, Nagafuchi K: Radical surgery for middle and distal bile duct cancer. World J Surg 12:60–63, 1988.
141. Oberfield RA, Rossi RL: The role of chemotherapy in the treatment of bile duct cancer. World J Surg 12:105–108, 1988.
142. Spira IA, Ghazi A, Wolff WI: Primary adenocarcinoma of the duodenum. Cancer 39:1721–1726, 1977.
143. Sakker S, Ware CC: Carcinoma of the duodenum; comparison of surgery, radiotherapy, and chemotherapy. Br J Surg 60:867, 1973.
144. Blumgart LH, Kennedy A: Carcinoma of the ampulla of Vater and duodenum. Br J Surg 60:33–40, 1973.
145. Spinazzola AJ, Gillesby WJ: Primary malignant neoplasms of the duodenum: Report of twelve cases. Am Surg 29:405–412, 1963.
146. Forrest JF, Longmire WP Jr: Carcinoma of the pancreas and periampullary region: A study of 279 patients. Ann Surg 189:129–138, 1979.
147. ReMine SG, Rossi RL: Management of cancer of the biliary tract. Prob Gen Surg 3:202–212, 1986.
148. Lees CD, Zapolanski A, Cooperman AM, et al: Carcinoma of the bile ducts. SGO 151:193–197, 1980.
149. Hayes DH, Bolton JS, Willis GW, et al: Carcinoma of the ampulla of Vater. Ann Surg 206:572–577, 1987.
150. Williams JA, Cubilla A, Maclean BJ, Fortner JG: Twenty-two year experience with periampullary carcinoma at Memorial Sloan-Kettering Cancer Center. Am J Surg 138:662–665, 1979.
151. Michelassi F, Erroi F, Dawson PJ, et al: Experience with 647 consecutive tumors of the duodenum, ampulla, head of the pancreas, and distal common bile duct. Ann Surg 210:544–556, 1989.
152. Lee YN, Williams MD: Clinical and laboratory findings of carcinoma of the pancreas and periampullary structures. J Surg Oncol 25:1–7, 1984.
153. Martin M, Rossi RL, Dorrucci V, Silverman ML, Braasch JW: Clinical and pathologic correlations in patients with periampullary tumors. Arch Surg 125:723–726, 1990.
154. Shutze WP, Sack J, Aldrete JS: Long-term follow-up of 24 patients undergoing radical resection for ampullary carcinoma, 1953 to 1988. Cancer 66:1717–1720, 1990.

Neuroendocrine Tumors of the Duodenum and Pancreas

Steven A. De Jong, M.D.
Richard A. Prinz, M.D.

In 1869, Paul Langerhans, a medical student at Friedrich Wilhelms University in Berlin, presented his dissertation as a candidate for the degree of Doctor of Medicine and Surgery on the microanatomy of the pancreas and described the islands of cells that now bear his name.[1] The physiologic function and importance of these cells were not known at that time. It was not until the isolation of insulin in 1922 by Banting and Best that the role of the pancreas as an endocrine organ was proven.[2] The first adenoma arising from the islets of Langerhans was described by Nicholls in 1902,[3] and the following year, Fabozzi described the first carcinoma.[4] The surgical history of pancreatic islet cell tumors dates to 1927, when a malignant insulinoma of the pancreas was found to be unresectable by W.J. Mayo. Graham is credited with the first surgical cure of a benign insulinoma, which was resected in 1929.[5] Twenty-six years later, Zollinger and Ellison described two patients with severe peptic ulceration of the upper gastrointestinal tract and an associated non–beta islet cell tumor of the pancreas.[6] In 1958, Verner and Morrison described a clinical syndrome consisting of watery diarrhea, hypokalemia, and achlorhydria. Further investigation linked this complex to a pancreatic islet cell tumor, which produces vasoactive intestinal polypeptide (VIP).[7] The glucagonoma syndrome, resulting from an alpha cell tumor of the pancreas, was described in 1966,[8, 9] and an islet cell tumor of the pancreas producing somatostatin was described in 1977.[10–12] Currently, the development and application of advanced radioimmunoassay techniques have been instrumental in clarifying our knowledge of previously known hormones and identifying many new ones. To date, 100 to 200 different gastrointestinal peptides have been isolated from approximately 40 different neuroendocrine cell types, and more than 10 hormonal syndromes have been described in association with islet cell tumors of the pancreas alone.[13–15]

Neuroendocrine tumors of the pancreas and duodenum are usually classified by the islet cell of origin and the dominant hormone produced—for example, gastrinoma, insulinoma, glucagonoma, and somatostatinoma (Table 5–13). These tumors function autonomously by overriding the normal regulatory control measures of hormone production and inhibition. The result is an overproduction and release of one dominant peptide hormone, causing an associated and distinct clinical syndrome. Conversely, the clinical presentation of some neuroendocrine tumors can be extremely subtle or even asymptomatic. A preclinical diagnosis can be obtained by screening family members at risk for development of these tumors with basal and stimulated measurements of circulating peptides. Nonfunctioning tumors can also arise from these neuroendocrine cells. They present clinically as an incidental finding during an unrelated operation or because of symptoms related to the location and mass of the tumor. These neoplasms are not as well differentiated as the functional tumors.[15] Nonfunctioning tumors may actually produce inactive or less active propeptides or peptides, or they may produce the expected peptides at undetectable levels.[16, 17]

Neuroendocrine tumors of the pancreas and duodenum are rare and account for only a small fraction of the malignant and benign neoplasms found in these organs. The knowledge gained from studying them, however, has had a wide impact on all areas of medicine and has been responsible for the development of entirely new fields of expertise. The annual incidence of neuroendocrine tumors of the pancreas and duodenum is 1 to 2 in 200,000 individuals. In contrast, the prevalence of these tumors in unselected autopsy material approaches 1 in 100, and they are usually described as an incidental finding.[18]

Prevalence, age and sex distribution, tumor size and location, malignant potential, and metastatic propensity are distinctly different for each neuroendocrine tumor type. Generally, these tumors are slow growing and well differentiated. Their associated morbidity and mortality depend as much on the type and amount of peptide produced as on their malignant potential. There is relatively little correlation between tumor size and the amount of peptide produced or the severity of the specific endocrine syndrome. The relationship between immunohistochemical findings and circulating peptide levels is relatively good but not absolute. Occasionally, an endocrine syndrome with excess peptide production may exist when specific immunohistochemical techniques fail to detect the hormone in the tumor tissue or detect an unrelated peptide.

Risk factors for the development of neuroendocrine tumors of the duodenum and pancreas are few. No dietary or social habits predict the development of these tumors, and no occupational exposures or environmental factors are linked to their origin. They do, however, occur frequently in the multiple endocrine neoplasia (MEN) syndromes, suggesting a genetic association in their etiology and development. Clinically apparent pancreatic or duodenal neuro-

TABLE 5–13
Functioning Neuroendocrine Tumors of the Pancreas and Duodenum[38, 40]

Tumor	Cell Origin	Syndrome	Malignancy (%)	Metastases (%)	Pancreatic Primary (%)	MEN I Association (%)
Insulinoma	Beta cell	Hypoglycemia	5–16	30	>95	5–10
Gastrinoma	G cell	Peptic ulcers Diarrhea	60	50–80	70–80	20–40
Glucagonoma	Alpha cell	Diabetes Dermatitis	>80	>50	100	Rare
Vipoma	Non–beta cell	Diarrhea Hypokalemia	>50 (Pancreas)	50 (Pancreas)	90	5
Somatostatinoma	D cell	Diabetes Steatorrhea	>75	75	70	Unknown

endocrine tumors occur in 50% to 80% of patients with MEN I syndrome, with insulinoma and gastrinoma being the predominant tumor types.[19]

The genetic association of neuroendocrine tumors and the MEN I syndrome has provided valuable insight into the pathogenesis of these neoplasms. Recent evidence suggests that the gene associated with the development of the MEN I syndrome is located on human chromosome 11 and codes for onco-suppressor genes.[20] Mutations at this point result in the loss of this suppressor effect and lead to the development of multicentric endocrine tumors of the duodenum and pancreas. The development of these tumors requires two separate mutations at the involved alleles. The first mutation in the hereditary form of MEN I occurs in the inherited germ cell line, while the second occurs later in the somatic cell line.[14] Sporadic occurrence of the MEN I syndrome requires that both mutations occur in the somatic cell line of the affected patient. Later in their clinical course, neuroendocrine tumors may also dedifferentiate, resulting in a loss of post-transcriptional and post-translational controls of peptide secretion to allow excessive production of single or multiple peptides.

Further genetic links to neuroendocrine cell function may be produced by the study of nondominant peptides produced by these neuroendocrine tumors. For example, alpha–human chorionic gonadotropin (αhCG) can be produced by 23% to 50% of malignant pancreatic neuroendocrine tumors but is not produced by benign tumors.[21] The absence of αhCG production, however, is no guarantee of a benign tumor. The gene that codes for α- and βhCG is located on chromosome 10 and/or 18, which is near to but distinct from chromosome 11.[22] Genetic methods to locate and characterize the production of secondary hormones may be sensitive but are not specific in predicting malignant behavior of neuroendocrine tumors. Histologic diagnosis of malignancy in neuroendocrine tumors is difficult or impossible. A diagnosis of carcinoma requires evidence of metastatic spread or gross local invasion of adjacent organs.[15] These clinical features usually require operative exploration or radiologically guided biopsy for confirmation.

Immunohistochemistry is an important tool in the histopathologic classification of neuroendocrine tumors. These techniques are useful in determining the origin and type of tumor cell and the peptide or peptides being produced. Neuron-specific enolase (NSE) is a neuronal form of the glycolytic enzyme enolase and was initially discovered in bovine brain tissue. Immunohistochemical studies have successfully localized NSE in most neuroendocrine cells.[23, 24] In the pancreas, NSE is found in the insular and extrainsular endocrine cells, the peptidergic nerves, and the neuroinsular complexes. As a result, NSE immunoreactivity has served as a useful generic marker for neuroendocrine cells of the duodenum and pancreas and is seen in many neuroendocrine tumors of these organs.[25]

Chromogranins constitute a family of glycoproteins first identified in the bovine adrenal medulla. The chromogranin family comprises three related forms, designated A, B, and C. Chromogranin A is the most abundant of the three types and is structurally similar to parathyroid secretory protein 1.[25] Immunoreactivity for chromogranins has been detected in the secretory granules of nearly all functional neuroendocrine cells, allowing their use as generic markers of normal, hyperplastic, and neoplastic neuroendocrine cells. In the pancreas, chromogranins have been localized to islet cells producing glucagon and pancreatic polypeptide as well as to the extrainsular cells located in the ductal epithelium and acinar tissues.

Monoclonal antibodies to synaptophysin, a glycoprotein isolated from bovine neurons, have localized this calcium-binding protein in adrenal medullary cells, the paraganglia, and the neuroendocrine cells of the gut, pancreas, lung, and pituitary gland. Two studies have confirmed the presence of synaptophysin in nearly all neuroendocrine tumors, making this generic marker a valuable adjunct to NSE and chromogranin detection.[26, 27] Electron microscopy can also provide vital information in characterizing these neuroendocrine neoplasms by detecting the specific type of secretory granule present in the tumor. In the future, specific methods of nucleic acid determination and gene analysis may also facilitate the identification of the cell type of origin for each specific neuroendocrine tumor.[13]

Radiologic studies are useful to determine tumor location, extent of disease, and presence of unsuspected metas-

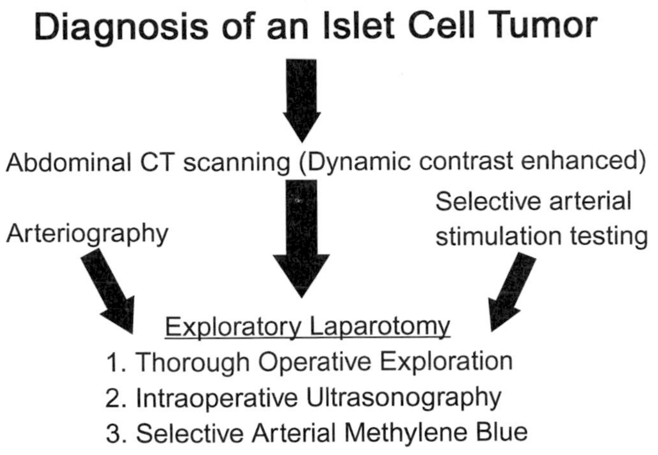

Diagnosis of an Islet Cell Tumor

Abdominal CT scanning (Dynamic contrast enhanced)

Arteriography

Selective arterial stimulation testing

Exploratory Laparotomy

1. Thorough Operative Exploration
2. Intraoperative Ultrasonography
3. Selective Arterial Methylene Blue

FIGURE 5–6. Currently recommended localization strategy for patients with islet cell tumors of the pancreas. (From Fedorak IJ, Ko TC, Gordon D, et al: Localization of islet cell tumors of the pancreas. A review of current techniques. Surgery 113:242, 1993.)

tases (Fig. 5–6). Modalities such as abdominal computed tomography (CT), magnetic resonance imaging (MRI), intraoperative ultrasonography, and arteriography have all been used successfully in localizing tumors larger than 1.5 cm in diameter (Table 5–14).[28–30] Radioimmunoassays have also been used in the localization of islet cell tumors in conjunction with selective percutaneous transhepatic catheterization of the duodenopancreatic veins.[31] Intra-arterial injection of provocative agents such as secretin or calcium, or both, into the splenic, gastroduodenal, and inferior pancreaticoduodenal arteries followed by hepatic vein sampling has been useful in localizing gastrinomas and insulinomas.[32, 33] Each artery supplies a specific area of the pancreas, and the vessel that feeds the tumor can thus be determined by which arterial injection causes a spike in hepatic vein peptide concentration. Intra-arterial methylene blue infusion into this vessel often stains these tumors blue to facilitate intraoperative localization and resection.[34]

Many common principles exist in the treatment regimens of neuroendocrine tumors. Complete surgical removal by enucleation or pancreatic resection can generally cure benign tumors. Debulking may be efficacious for patients with unresectable, recurrent, or metastatic disease to decrease peptide production.[35] Chemotherapy, administered intra-arterially or systemically, is generally palliative and frequently involves combination therapy with streptozocin and 5-fluorouracil (5-FU), doxorubicin (Adriamycin), or dimethyl triazeno imidazole carboxamide (DTIC).[36] Outcome is extremely variable, ranging from no response to complete disappearance of hepatic metastases.

TABLE 5–14
Localization Options for Neuroendocrine Tumor

Abdominal CT
  Intravenous contrast enhanced
  Dynamic scanning method
MRI with gadolinium
Ultrasonography
  Endoscopic
  Intraoperative
Angiography
  Selective arterial injections
  Digital subtraction technique
Selective arterial stimulation with hepatic vein sampling
  Intraoperative intra-arterial methylene blue injection
Percutaneous transhepatic portal venous sampling
Radionuclide scanning with radiolabeled somatostatin

Therapeutic embolization of an unresectable islet cell tumor usually has limited success because of the rich vascular supply of the tumor. Hepatic embolization of liver metastases has, however, provided effective palliation by temporarily reducing peptide production in some patients.[37] Isotopic irradiation has potential as a therapeutic option but currently lacks a reliable isotopic carrier with a specific affinity for islet or neuroendocrine cells. Radiolabeled octreotide is currently under investigation as a carrier.[38, 39] External radiation is generally ineffective, since most of these tumors are radioresistant.

Medical therapy is often directed at blocking the production or end-organ effect of the specific hormone produced by the tumor, exemplified by histamine$_2$ (H_2)-receptor blockade to control the hyperacidity of gastrinomas. Hormonal therapy using a somatostatin analogue to inhibit peptide secretion has provided effective palliation in many patients with unresectable, recurrent, or metastatic disease.[36] Long-term follow-up is essential, even after "curative operation." Periodic monitoring to detect the persistence or recurrence of peptide production is important. Secondary hormones may be produced later in the course of the disease and have substantial potential for morbidity and mortality. Provocative testing can play an important role in detecting recurrence and/or metastasis of islet cell tumors at an early stage and in the screening of family members of patients with hereditary endocrine tumors.[19]

GASTRINOMA

Epidemiology

The annual incidence of gastrinoma is estimated to be 1 in 2.5 million people; an estimated 400 new cases are reported annually in North America alone.[40] The majority of patients are men, with a mean age at presentation of 50 years. Gastrinomas are found in only 1% of patients with peptic ulcer disease and, as a result, suspicion of the Zollinger-Ellison syndrome (ZES) is certainly not warranted in all patients with an ulcer. It should be considered in patients who have severe ulcer symptoms in their early teens or initial symptoms late in life. A gastrinoma should also be suspected in patients who have recurrent peptic ulcerations after customary operations, especially when this recurrence happens early in the postoperative period (Table 5–15). It is probable that many ZES patients are treated as patients with benign peptic ulcer disease. As a result, 3 to

TABLE 5–15
Clinical Picture Prompting High Index of Suspicion for Gastrinoma

Recurrent/postoperative peptic ulcer
Multiple atypical peptic ulcerations
Intractable peptic ulcer
Jejunal ulcerations
Peptic ulcer and diarrhea
Familial history of ulcer disease
Familial history of MEN I syndrome
Hypertrophic gastric rugal folds (barium study, esophagogastroduodenoscopy)

5 years may elapse before the diagnosis of a gastrinoma is established.

Patients harboring gastrinomas should be classified as having either *sporadic* gastrinoma or *familial* gastrinoma. Sporadic gastrinomas are not inherited, and these patients have no associated endocrinopathies. In contrast, familial gastrinomas can occur in patients with the MEN I syndrome (Wermer's syndrome). An estimated 66% of gastrinomas are sporadic, while the remaining one third are associated with the MEN I syndrome. Most sporadic tumors are solitary and often malignant (60% to 75%). In contrast, gastrinomas associated with the MEN I syndrome are benign in 70% of patients, are usually smaller in size, occur at a younger age, and are often multicentric. It is important to distinguish patients with the MEN I syndrome from those with sporadic gastrinomas, as the natural history, disease process, and management can be quite different.

Life History of the Disease

Most gastrinoma patients have mild chronic symptoms that are present for some time before they seek medical attention. The ZES tumor registry has documented that nearly 30% of patients with a gastrinoma had symptoms for more than 5 years before undergoing medical evaluation and operation.[41] The mean duration of symptoms prior to proper diagnosis in another study was 32 months.[42] The clinical manifestations of gastrinoma are all related to hypergastrinemia. The most common symptom appears to be the upper abdominal pain of peptic ulcer. Episodes of recurrent severe abdominal pain secondary to the ulcer diathesis occur in 90% to 95% of patients with gastrinoma. Abdominal cramping and severe diarrhea are evident in 33% of ZES patients and may be the presenting complaint in 5% to 10%. The pathophysiology of diarrhea in ZES includes the inability of the intestinal tract to absorb the large volumes of fluid secreted by the stomach, acid-induced injury to the mucosa of the upper small intestine, precipitation of bile salts, and malabsorption via the inactivation of pancreatic lipase by the low pH.[14] The diarrhea associated with a gastrinoma can be eliminated by nasogastric suction.

Complications of peptic ulcer disease are frequent, including hemorrhage and perforation of duodenal and jejunal ulcers. The presence of jejunal ulcers in a patient without prior ulcer surgery is pathognomonic for the existence of ZES. Radiologic and endoscopic studies often reveal large gastric rugal folds and inflammation or ulceration of the duodenum, jejunum, and stomach. Acid injury to the esophagus along with severe gastroesophageal reflux has also been described.

Patients with familial gastrinomas associated with the MEN I syndrome usually have additional features in their clinical presentation to distinguish them from patients with sporadic gastrinomas. Hyperparathyroidism is seen in 15% to 25% of these patients, and they may have bone loss, nephrolithiasis, or nephrocalcinosis. Cushing's syndrome has also been described in association with ZES.[43] Excess secretion of peptide hormones, such as prolactin from pituitary hyperplasia or adenomas, can also be seen in the MEN I syndrome.

Local-Regional Anatomy and Pathology

Normally, a protein meal provokes gastrin release from the G cells of the antral mucosa into the portal system to stimulate acid secretion from the gastric parietal cells. Negative feedback inhibition of gastrin release is modulated by G-cell detection of low gastric pH and through the inhibitory effects of secretin release. In ZES, however, an excess of gastrin is continuously secreted by the pancreatic or duodenal gastrinomas. The tumor functions autonomously, leading to severe peptic ulcer disease and the classic clinical presentation.

Gastrinomas were originally described as non–beta cell tumors of the pancreas. Normal pancreatic tissue does not contain cells that release or produce gastrin. Gastrin, however, has been detected in the fetal pancreas, suggesting that activation of embryonic rests of cells may result in the development of gastrinoma.[44] In addition to the pancreas, 10% to 25% of gastrinomas may occur in the duodenal wall.[45] Other ectopic sites include the stomach, jejunum, small intestine, omentum, peripancreatic lymph nodes, ovary, and liver. Approximately 90% of gastrinomas are found within an anatomic triangle whose apices are the confluence of the cystic and common bile ducts, the border of the second and third portion of the duodenum, and the junction of the neck and body of the pancreas (Fig. 5–7).[46] Most gastrinomas are solitary tumors and may be quite small; 1- to 5-mm tumors have been found in the submucosa of the duodenum.[45]

Approximately 60% to 70% of pancreatic gastrinomas are malignant, and more than half of these have metastasized by the time of surgical intervention.[47, 48] Malignancy rates for duodenal gastrinomas vary from 25% to 70%. Other ectopic sites appear to have a much better prognosis when compared to their pancreatic counterparts.[45, 49] Metastases from pancreatic and extrapancreatic gastrinomas are predominantly to the liver. Other metastatic sites include

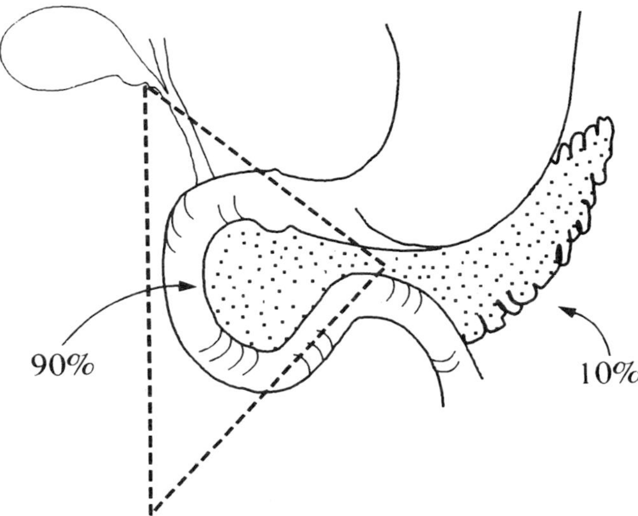

FIGURE 5–7. The majority of gastrin-producing neuroendocrine tumors of the pancreas and duodenum (90%) are found in the "gastrinoma triangle," bounded by the cystic–common bile duct confluence, the border of the second and third portions of the duodenum, and the junction of the neck and body of the pancreas. (From Stasile B, Morrow D, Passaro E: The gastrinoma triangle: Operative indications. Am J Surg 147:25, 1984.)

the lymph nodes adjacent to the pancreas and duodenum, spleen, peritoneum, lung, and mediastinum. The presence of gastrinoma in peripancreatic lymph nodes does not indicate incurability, since tumor resection may result in long-term survival with normalization of serum gastrin.[50]

Diagnosis, Screening, and Early Detection and Staging

The diagnosis of gastrinoma and ZES is based on the demonstration of an inappropriately high level of circulating gastrin for the level of gastric acidity. The initial screening study of choice is a fasting serum gastrin level. Fasting gastrin in the normal adult is less than 100 pg/ml, while levels above 500 to 1000 pg/ml are often seen in ZES. Other causes of hypergastrinemia and increased gastric acid secretion include antral G-cell hyperfunction, retained gastric antrum, short bowel syndrome, gastric outlet obstruction, and renal failure.[51] Hypergastrinemia associated with decreased gastric acid output can be seen in pernicious anemia, chronic gastritis, previous vagotomy, and gastric ulcer with associated hypochlorhydria (Table 5–16). The absolute value of fasting serum gastrin levels may have prognostic significance. In one study, patients with fasting serum gastrin levels above 1500 pg/ml had metastatic disease and patients with levels above 8000 pg/ml had massive hepatic replacement. However, absolute serum gastrin levels failed to exclude malignant disease, as 50% of patients with gastrin levels below 1500 pg/ml had metastatic disease.[52]

With the increasing use of serum gastrin as a screening test for ZES, patients are now being identified with a level of gastric acid hypersecretion and serum gastrin that is elevated but not definitely diagnostic. Forty percent of patients with ZES have gastrin levels in the intermediate range of 150 to 500 pg/ml, and the remainder have another etiology for their hypergastrinemia and increased gastric acid output.[53] Provocative testing is indicated to establish the diagnosis in these patients and to screen those with MEN I syndrome who are at high risk for development of a gastrinoma. Three provocative tests have been used to aid in the diagnosis of gastrinoma. Initially, a standardized meal was used to measure the serum gastrin response. Patients with a gastrinoma usually showed little change in the serum gastrin, whereas an exaggerated response was seen in peptic ulcer patients.[54] An intravenous calcium challenge in ZES patients causes an abrupt rise in circulating gastrin two to three times basal levels. This is usually not seen in normal subjects or in patients with simple peptic ulcer disease.[55]

Provocative testing with secretin is the most reliable way to diagnose a gastrinoma. This test is based on a paradoxical increase in serum gastrin and gastric acid secretion that occurs only in ZES patients in response to intravenous secretin (Fig. 5–8).[56] Secretin is preferred over calcium infusion because it takes less time, is more sensitive, and carries less risk to the patient.[14] A fasting patient is given an intravenous bolus of secretin using 2 IU/kg of body weight. A preinjection serum gastrin level is obtained, followed by repeated levels at 2, 5, 10, 15, and 30 minutes. If the secretin test is positive, a gastrin peak usually occurs within the first 10 minutes of testing. A rise of 200 pg/ml or greater over baseline is considered diagnostic for ZES. False-positive and false-negative results are unusual but can occur in 5% and 15% of patients, respectively.[40]

Gastric acid analysis may be helpful in patients with borderline elevations of serum gastrin. Nearly every patient with ZES displays a basal acid output of greater than 15 mEq/hour. A measured basal acid output of greater than 25 mEq/hour is pathognomonic for ZES. An hourly output of gastric juice greater than 100 ml and a 12-hour overnight volume of gastric juice exceeding 1 L are also features of the gastric analysis that favor the presence of ZES.[57–59] A basal acid output in excess of 5 mEq/hour in patients having had an acid-reducing operation supports the diagnosis of gastrinoma.[60] Some authors continue to advocate examination of the basal acid output (BAO) to maximal

TABLE 5–16
Etiology of Hypergastrinemia

High Gastric Acid Output	Low Gastric Acid Output
Gastrinoma	Pernicious anemia
Antral G-cell hyperfunction	Chronic gastritis
Retained gastric antrum	Vagotomy
Gastric outlet obstruction	Gastric ulcer (hypochlorhydria)
Antral G-cell hyperplasia	
Renal failure	
Short bowel syndrome	

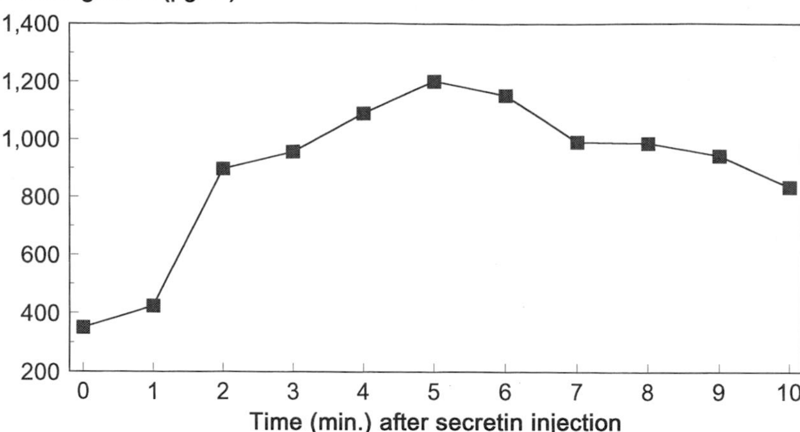

FIGURE 5–8. A paradoxical rise in the serum gastrin level results from a secretin infusion (Kabi, 2 IU/kg) in this patient with a pancreatic gastrinoma.

acid output (MAO) ratio.[57, 58] Pentagastrin is administered to stimulate gastric acid secretion. The BAO:MAO ratio is greater than 0.6 in patients with a gastrinoma because the BAO is already maximized by the excess gastrin produced by the autonomous neuroendocrine tumor. False-negative rates of 30% and false-positive rates of 2% to 10% have been reported with gastric analysis.[57–59]

Since tumor resection can be curative, the importance of accurate preoperative localization cannot be overemphasized. Even though many modalities are available, some islet cell tumors, particularly small gastrinomas and insulinomas, remain undetectable by conventional means because of tumor size or technical limitations in imaging the entire pancreas.[61] Although ultrasonography is the least expensive and most noninvasive radiologic modality available to localize gastrinomas, limited specificity and sensitivity have plagued its use. Endoscopic ultrasonography seems to have better accuracy, but this remains unproven since it has been used in only limited numbers of patients.

The initial noninvasive radiologic modality of choice for localizing gastrinomas appears to be abdominal CT utilizing bolus intravenous contrast. The CT examination should include precontrast sections of the pancreas followed by contiguous 5-mm sections through the entire gland. Dynamic incremental scanning is then performed after intravenous bolus administration of 100 to 150 ml of a 60% water-soluble contrast material. Roughly 30% to 70% of primary gastrinomas are localized accurately with this radiologic technique.[50, 62] This study is particularly useful for the preoperative detection of hepatic metastases and may detect the primary gastrinoma when its size exceeds 2 cm in diameter.[28] Extrapancreatic and multiple gastrinomas can also be localized with abdominal CT scanning.[61] A vascular blush, following the rapid injection of intravenous contrast, may assist in differentiating an islet cell tumor from a ductal carcinoma of the pancreas. The sensitivity of abdominal CT to localize these islet cell tumors accurately is dependent on the size and location of the neoplasm. This explains the wide range of accuracy rates, from 15% to 81%, that have been reported.[28, 50, 62, 63]

With the use of MRI, these tumors are typically hypointense, compared with the normal pancreas, on the T1-weighted images and hyperintense on the T2-weighted images.[28] The accuracy rate of MRI appears to be equivalent to that of CT scanning but may be improved in the future as instrumentation and technology continue to advance. The detection of hepatic metastases from gastrinomas is also possible with MRI, but it offers no specific advantage over dynamic CT scanning. Frucht et al.[64] from the National Institutes of Health found that MRI could localize only 20% of extrahepatic gastrinomas and 40% of hepatic metastases.

Selective visceral arteriography was one of the first techniques used in the localization of gastrinomas. In addition to size and location, the success of arteriography in localizing these tumors depends on their vascularity. Techniques such as digital subtraction, magnification, and biplanar views have increased the accuracy of this procedure.[65] Secretin infusion has also been used to enhance a tumor blush during the arterial and venous phases of selective arteriography.[66] The overall success rate of arteriography for visualizing primary gastrinomas is approximately 40% to 60%.[67, 68] This contrasts with an 80% accuracy rate for this modality in localizing insulinomas.[29] Hepatic metastasis is accurately detected through the use of arteriography, especially when combined with abdominal CT.[69] This combination can detect 95% of patients with hepatic metastases and provides the most accurate preoperative means for detecting liver involvement from a gastrinoma.[70]

Percutaneous transhepatic portal venous sampling (PTPVS) has been used for preoperative localization of gastrinomas.[31] Its primary role is localizing small tumors not seen with conventional, less-invasive radiologic modalities. The procedure involves the placement of a catheter through the hepatic branches of the portal vein under fluoroscopic guidance into the splenic and superior mesenteric veins. Blood is sampled from different tributaries draining different areas of the pancreas, and serum gastrin concentrations are measured. For other tumor types, the appropriate hormone can also be measured. This study places

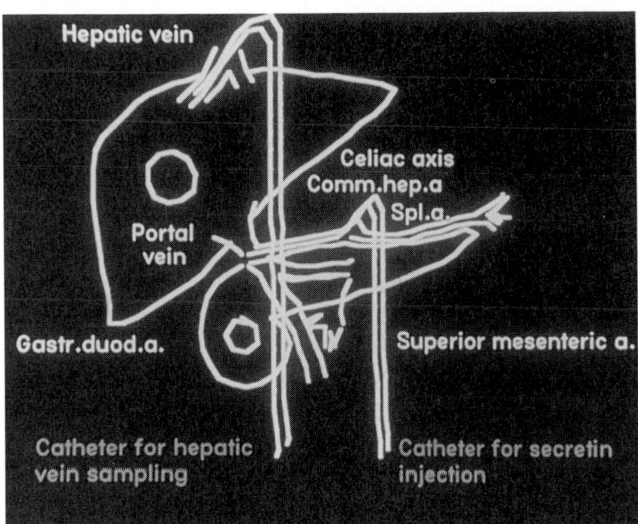

FIGURE 5–9. Selective injection of secretin into the splenic and gastroduodenal artery with hepatic vein sampling for gastrin is helpful in regionalizing gastrinomas not seen with more conventional noninvasive radiologic modalities. (From Imamura M, Takahashi K, Adachi H, et al: Usefulness of selective arterial secretin test for localization of gastrinoma in the Zollinger-Ellison syndrome. Ann Surg 205:230, 1987.)

the neuroendocrine tumor in one of three regions in the pancreas—namely, tail, body-neck, or head-uncinate process. Several authors report success rates of 73% to 90% using this method to localize gastrinomas, while others report a specificity of only 33% for this procedure in tumors occurring in the region of the pancreatic head.[31, 71, 72] While PTPVS is sensitive, the procedure requires substantial technical expertise. It is also invasive and expensive and may be difficult to interpret because of the anatomic variations of pancreatic venous drainage. As the technical sophistication and accuracy of CT and angiography increase, selective portal venous sampling does not need to be performed on a routine basis.

A selective arterial stimulation test using secretin for the localization of gastrinomas was first proposed by Imamura and colleagues[32] in 1987 (Figs. 5–9 and 5–10). An intravenous catheter is placed through the inferior vena cava into the hepatic vein to obtain blood samples at regular intervals. Following this, an arteriographic catheter is placed into the splenic, gastroduodenal, and inferior pancreaticoduodenal arteries. A 30-unit bolus of secretin is injected into each of these arteries at separate intervals. Blood samples are sequentially drawn from the hepatic vein catheter after each secretin injection. Regionalization of the gastrinoma is possible by correlating the spike in hepatic vein gastrin concentration with the area of the pancreas stimulated by the secretin injection. The accuracy of this invasive procedure has exceeded 75% in most series when used in combination with arteriography, which is routinely obtained following the selective arterial stimulation.[73] An additional modification of this procedure is the injection of methylene blue via the intra-arterial catheter during the time of operative exploration.[34] On the morning of operation, an arterial catheter is positioned into the same artery identified as feeding the tumor by preoperative selective arterial secretin stimulation. Methylene blue is injected at the time of operative exploration, and within 15 seconds the entire area fed by this artery turns blue, including the suspected vascular islet cell tumor. The bluish discoloration clears in normal tissue after 2 minutes but persists in the islet cell tumor, allowing rapid and accurate localization prior to resection. This has been successfully used in two of our patients.[34]

Another means of localization for gastrinomas is intraoperative ultrasonography (IOUS). While debate continues concerning its usefulness to identify nonpalpable pancreatic tumors, it may be helpful in localizing small, deep-seated tumors within the head of the pancreas. IOUS combined with palpation has a greater than 90% sensitivity rate for localizing pancreatic gastrinomas.[30] Most extrapancreatic gastrinomas can be detected by palpation alone. Islet cell tumors of the pancreas, including gastrinoma, appear sonolucent and are easy to distinguish from surrounding pancreatic parenchyma with IOUS. Although its use involves a

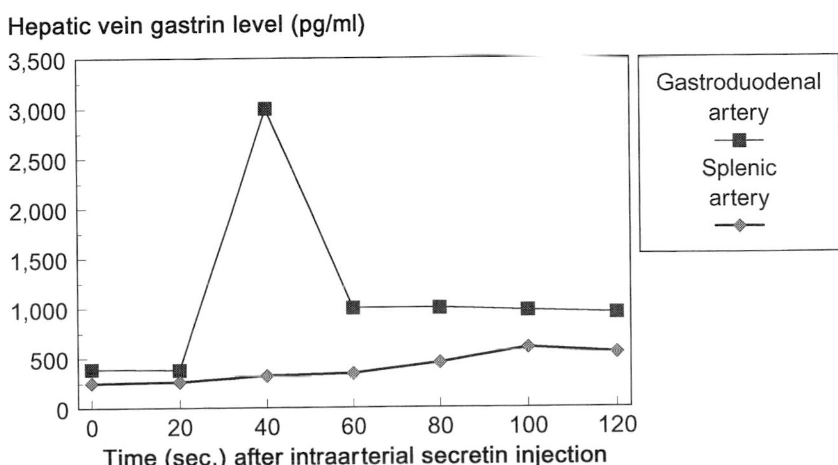

FIGURE 5–10. Selective intra-arterial secretin injection via the gastroduodenal artery and the splenic artery with hepatic vein sampling regionalizes this gastrinoma to the pancreatic head.

learning curve, IOUS appears to be a valuable tool and should be routinely used as part of the abdominal exploration for gastrinomas.[74]

Some islet cell tumors of the pancreas, including gastrinoma, have a large number of somatostatin receptors on the tumor cell surface.[39] These binding sites are thought to play a role in the inhibition of peptide production by the tumor. Octreotide acetate, a somatostatin analogue, has been modified so that it can be labeled with radioactive iodine (^{123}I) and used for localization purposes through scintigraphic techniques.[38] While the number of patients successfully localized with this technique is small, it does potentially offer a means for noninvasive preoperative localization of many neuroendocrine tumors. Intraoperative localization may also be possible with this technique using a sterile gamma probe during laparotomy.

In summary, preoperative localization of a gastrinoma should begin with a contrast-enhanced dynamic abdominal CT scan. Preoperative gastroduodenoscopy should be performed and may localize a single gastric or duodenal wall gastrinoma that is potentially curable by excision but that may be overlooked at operation. Endoscopic ultrasonography can also be added to enhance preoperative localization. This can be followed by arteriography and selective arterial stimulation testing. This should disclose or regionalize the site of the gastrinoma in more than 70% to 80% of patients. Despite the considerable experience obtained with all radiographic modalities, approximately 20% to 40% of patients with a gastrinoma have negative preoperative localization studies.[65, 70] A thorough operative exploration must still be performed in these patients. Experienced intraoperative palpation is extremely accurate in detecting the site of the pancreatic or extrapancreatic gastrinoma. IOUS is also an important adjunct for the surgeon during the initial exploration. Investigation continues into the use of selective arterial methylene blue and the use of radiolabeled somatostatin analogue with preoperative and intraoperative radionuclide scanning.

Primary Operable Disease—Results and Complications of Treatment

The treatment of ZES is controversial, and several therapeutic options exist. Initial tumor resection, total gastrectomy, vagotomy and drainage procedure, and long-term medical control may each have a place in the treatment of ZES. H_2-receptor blockers, omeprazole, and/or somatostatin analogues can adequately control the peptic ulcer diathesis in most ZES patients. Medical therapy, however, is expensive, usually requires high doses of medication, is dependent on patient compliance, and may have serious associated side effects.[75–77]

The surgical management of pancreatic and duodenal gastrinomas has evolved since the original recommendations by Zollinger and Ellison for total gastrectomy in 1955.[6] At that time, patients often presented with advanced metastatic disease and with limited options for adequate medical control of the peptic ulcer disease.[78] As a result, removal of the entire stomach was recommended and was performed with modest morbidity and mortality. When this initial recommendation for total gastrectomy was ignored, death resulted for many ZES patients.[41] Currently, the morbidity and mortality rate for total gastrectomy in these patients has decreased to 0% to 4%.[40, 79] Improved preoperative and postoperative control of the peptic ulcer disease to prevent complications and decrease emergent operations has largely been responsible for this decline.[79] Other advances in surgical care, such as intravenous hyperalimentation, are important in preventing septic complications and facilitating anastomotic healing. In the late 1960s and early 1970s, total gastrectomy with tumor excision, when feasible, was the treatment of choice for ZES. Currently, total gastrectomy is rarely indicated in the ZES patient. It is still useful for patients with no demonstrable tumor and poor preoperative medical control of the hypergastrinemia. Some patients request a total gastrectomy because of the high cost of H_2-receptor blocker administration and the necessary and expensive follow-up, such as gastric analysis and endoscopy, that is performed on a periodic basis to ensure adequate medical control.[80]

The introduction of H_2-receptor antagonists in 1977 prompted a controversy in the treatment of ZES. Their dramatic inhibitory effects on gastric acid hypersecretion provided a medical means to manage the hormonal effects of a gastrinoma. Questions concerning the morbidity and mortality of total gastrectomy and the surgeon's inability to find a single curable gastrinoma prompted a swing toward medical management in almost all ZES patients. H_2-receptor antagonists such as cimetidine, ranitidine, famotidine, the adenosine triphosphatase (ATPase) proton pump inhibitor, omeprazole, and the somatostatin analogue octreotide can effectively control acid hypersecretion, ulcer symptomatology, and diarrhea.[77, 81] Gastric acid secretion can be reduced to less than 10 mmol in patients with intact stomachs and to less than 5 mmol in patients who have had acid-reducing procedures.[80, 82] The mean dose required for each of these agents is dramatically elevated compared with that needed in peptic ulcer disease patients. The mean dose of cimetidine given in one series was 4.6 g/day, with some patients requiring up to 10 g/day for adequate control of the hypergastrinemia.[49] Failure rates with cimetidine can be as high as 50%, and large doses of this medication have resulted in impotence, gynecomastia, and other antiandrogenic effects.[76] Second- and third-generation H_2 blockers have lesser antiandrogenic side effects, but failure rates are still as high as 40%.[81, 83] Other problems, such as thrombocytopenia and altered mental status, have been reported with high-dose cimetidine use.

H_2-receptor blockers may have to be taken every 4 hours in these patients and often require combination with anticholinergic agents to enhance their effect. Omeprazole, a hydrogen-potassium ATPase inhibitor, is the drug of choice for patients with a gastrinoma because of its potency and long duration of action.[84, 85] The initial reported failure rates with omeprazole treatment for ZES have been 2% to 8%.[81, 86] However, gastric carcinoid tumors develop in rats treated long term with omeprazole, so there is some question about prolonged use in humans.[17] The ideal pharmacologic agent for inhibiting gastric acid hypersecretion in ZES patients is not available. Theoretically, this drug should be inexpensive, administered orally, have a long half-life, and be devoid of adverse effects.[87, 88]

Local excision of a gastrinoma, when possible, is now the treatment of choice in ZES patients.[50] Often these tumors are small, and enucleation is ideal.[89] Occasionally, distal pancreatectomy or a subtotal resection of the head of the pancreas is necessary. Total pancreatectomy and pancreaticoduodenal resection have had a high morbidity and mortality rate in the past. Even though the risk of these major resections has dramatically decreased, total pancreatectomy and pancreaticoduodenectomy are rarely indicated for gastrinoma.[90, 91] Gastrinomas in any location can be multiple, and the demonstration of a single gastrinoma should not dissuade the surgeon from continuing a complete exploration in search of multiple tumors. A parietal cell vagotomy has been performed in addition to tumor excision for some patients who have had difficulty with preoperative control of hypergastrinemia and gastric acid hypersecretion.[92] The pH of gastric contents recovered from the nasogastric tube in the immediate postoperative period usually provides an early clue to the effectiveness of operation.

Many important steps are involved in the conduct of operation for patients with gastrinomas that can assist in achieving successful control of hypergastrinemia and gastric hypersecretion.[40] A thorough abdominal exploration should be performed, with careful examination of the liver and bimanual palpation of the body and tail of the pancreas. An extended Kocher maneuver is performed to inspect and palpate the pancreatic head, uncinate process, and duodenum. A duodenotomy is often necessary to be certain there is no small tumor in the medial duodenal wall. Lymph nodes from the peripancreatic head, common bile duct area, and celiac axis are routinely excised or sampled, or both, for intraoperative histologic examination. Frozen section examination should be used liberally to confirm the finding and removal of a neuroendocrine tumor. Peripancreatic or capsular nodules should all be sampled for biopsy or excised to achieve successful gastrinoma localization and control. If a total gastrectomy is needed, all gastric mucosa must be removed to control gastric acid hypersecretion and prevent recurrent ulceration. Frozen section examination of the proximal and distal resection margins can be used to ensure that a total gastrectomy has indeed been performed. Blind distal pancreatectomy, when tumor is not localized at operation, is generally not recommended.

ZES may occur as part of the MEN I syndrome. This syndrome is caused by an autosomal dominant gene that manifests in the development of hyperplasia or tumors of the parathyroid glands, pancreatic islet cells, and pituitary gland.[40] Thirty percent of patients with gastrinomas have the MEN I syndrome.[93] A secretin test may be necessary to stimulate the release of gastrin in these patients and uncover a "silent" gastrinoma.[40] The vast majority of patients with pancreatic islet cell tumors have small multicentric pancreatic neoplasms as the cause for the islet cell disease.[70, 94–96] As a result, patients with familial gastrinomas and the MEN I syndrome may require different treatment than that for patients with sporadic gastrinomas.

Serum calcium and gastrin should be measured in individuals and in their family members being screened for the MEN I syndrome. Hyperparathyroidism occurs in 90% of patients and is usually the first manifestation of the syndrome. Most individuals who inherit the MEN I trait have hypercalcemia by age 30. Measurement of the serum parathyroid hormone level and a gastric acid analysis are often helpful in confirming the clinical suspicion of the MEN I syndrome. After medical therapy for gastric hypersecretion is initiated, operative treatment of the hyperparathyroidism is performed. Subtotal parathyroidectomy or total parathyroidectomy with parathyroid autotransplantation, to control hypercalcemia, should be performed before any operative procedure to correct the hypergastrinemia.[95] Decreased circulating gastrin and improved medical control of hyperacidity have been documented after parathyroidectomy. Normalization of gastrin secretion and acid production have even resulted in some patients.[97]

Continued gastric acid hypersecretion should be treated with H_2-receptor antagonists or omeprazole. Gastrinomas in patients with the MEN I syndrome are frequently multiple and small.[50, 95, 96] Preoperative or intraoperative localization of solitary gastrinomas is uncommon, and enucleation is rarely successful in achieving complete resection of the disease. Total or subtotal pancreatectomy, necessary for removing all of the disease, has a substantial risk of mortality and morbidity.[98] In light of the benign course of familial gastrinomas in 70% of patients, medical therapy using H_2-receptor blockade, octreotide acetate, or omeprazole is often the treatment of choice. Patients with a dominant or enlarging tumor mass may need resection because of the possibility of malignancy. Further information is needed to clarify the frequency of duodenal microgastrinomas in MEN I patients and whether their removal is likely to be curative.[95, 99] Total gastrectomy is reserved for complications of peptic ulcer disease and for failures of maximal medical therapy.[40, 79, 95]

Patients with the MEN I syndrome may also have islet cell tumors that produce insulin, glucagon, VIP, and pancreatic polypeptide. Measurement of these levels may be appropriate when the clinical situation suggests additional hormone excess. These patients and their families require yearly screening and follow-up with serum calcium and fasting gastrin determinations. Abdominal CT scanning is usually indicated at a 1- to 3-year interval to look for pancreatic islet cell tumors or hepatic metastases.

Recurrent and Incurable Disease—Results and Complications

Patients with metastatic gastrinoma as their initial presentation or recurrent ZES should be given a trial of medical therapy with H_2-receptor antagonists, omeprazole, and/or somatostatin. An assessment of the degree of medical control achievable with medical therapy is essential in determining the need for and extent of operative intervention for these patients.[14] Adequate medical control of the hypergastrinemia may obviate the need for surgical intervention. Several therapeutic options exist for patients who are refractory to medical therapy. A parietal cell vagotomy can be performed with minimal morbidity and mortality and can successfully facilitate medical control in these patients.[92] Unfortunately, a parietal cell vagotomy may complicate the performance of a total gastrectomy if needed in the future. Unresectable gastrinomas include large invasive tumors that involve the head of the pancreas and those with metastases that are multiple or unsafe to remove.[40] Recurrence of hypergastrinemia and peptic ulcer disease following a "curative" gastrinoma resection is indicative of persistent, recurrent, or metastatic disease. Hepatic metastases usually indicate a poor prognosis in patients with gastrinoma, but long-term survival has been reported.[93] When possible, local hepatic wedge resection for solitary hepatic metastases of gastrinoma is recommended. Anatomic hepatic resection has been reported with success for metastatic disease.[100] As a last resort, control of peptic ulcer disease and avoidance of the complications of gastric hypersecretion can be achieved through the use of total gastrectomy in ZES patients with liver metastases. Total gastrectomy may prolong survival for these patients with liver metastases because neuroendocrine tumors have a tendency for slow growth.[93] Several ZES patients with evidence of lymphatic metastases have lived 10 to 20 years with no clinical or radiologic evidence of tumor progression.[40]

Chemotherapy in patients with pancreatic or duodenal gastrinoma is largely reserved for patients with enlarging or symptomatic liver metastases. The operative finding of gastrinoma in a peripancreatic lymph node at operation is not an indication for postoperative chemotherapy. Chemotherapy for metastatic pancreatic or duodenal gastrinoma consists of streptozocin, usually in combination with 5-FU.[101] Response rates of 0% to 20% have been reported with streptozocin alone, while the addition of 5-FU increases the rates to as high as 66%.[102] Although use of streptozocin alone avoids many of the complications of myelosuppression, combination agents appear to have significant toxicity, including leukopenia, nephrotoxicity, hepatotoxicity, and immunosuppression. Response rates approaching 40% have been documented with streptozocin, 5-FU, and tubercidin.[103] Doxorubicin has been reported to achieve a 20% response rate in patients who failed to respond to streptozocin alone or in combination. While these agents decrease tumor size, they may not substantially reduce gastric acid output, so continued pharmacologic control of gastric hypersecretion is necessary. There has been no documentation of survival benefit with any of these agents. Radiation therapy has been used in patients with ZES, but only short-term palliation has been demonstrated.

Post-Treatment Care and Surveillance

ZES patients treated medically require regular follow-up to re-evaluate the efficacy of the pharmacologic control of gastric hypersecretion. Frequent endoscopy and gastric analysis should be performed at least annually and preferably every 6 months in those treated medically.[80] A careful search for antiandrogenic side effects in men taking relatively high doses of cimetidine is important. Impotence, breast tenderness, and gynecomastia can develop in 50% of these patients and may be avoided with a second- or third-generation H_2-receptor blocker.[76, 77] Fasting serum gastrin levels and secretin stimulation tests are obtained at 3- to 6-month follow-up intervals in patients with gastrinomas resected for "cure."[104] Radiologic studies and gastric analysis are obtained when persistent or recurrent gastric hypersecretion is suspected.

After total gastrectomy, ZES patients require periodic follow-up to avoid nutritional problems. Lifelong parenteral vitamin B_{12} therapy is required on a monthly basis. Folic acid, calcium, and iron supplements are important dietary additives. Total gastrectomy does not provide protection from subsequent gastrinoma growth or metastases. Serum gastrin and radiologic studies are obtained when needed to document tumor progression.

INSULINOMA

Epidemiology

Insulinoma is the most common functional neuroendocrine tumor of the pancreas. More than 1500 cases have been reported since the initial description in 1927.[105] It has an annual incidence of 1 in 1.25 million people in the United States.[106] Insulinomas have been reported in patients of all ages from newborns to nonagenarians, but their peak incidence occurs between 40 and 60 years of age. Eighty percent of patients with insulinoma are over 40 years of age, with the mean age in the mid-fifties.[107] Five percent of patients with an insulinoma have the MEN I syndrome, while 10% of MEN I patients have an insulinoma. Insulinoma associated with the MEN I syndrome seems to occur in younger patients, with a mean age of 23 years reported in one series.[108] Most studies find no sex difference in patients with insulinoma.

Life History of the Disease

The major clinical signs and symptoms of insulinoma are neuropsychiatric and result from hypoglycemia.[109] Headaches and blurred vision are common, and these patients are often unable to think coherently or remember simple details. Subtle central nervous system manifestations, such as apathy, irritability, anxiety, confusion, disorientation, and speech difficulty, can occur. Since most of these symptoms are nonspecific and more commonly due to other causes, the presence of an insulinoma may not be considered. A long interval from onset of symptoms to the diagnosis of an insulinoma is all too common.[110] As the symptoms progress, bizarre and uncharacteristic behavior becomes evident, often resulting in seizures and coma. The hypoglycemic attacks are episodic and recurrent, and they are most pronounced after periods of fasting, such as in the early morning or after exercise. Prolonged hypoglycemia is dangerous and may lead to nocturnal seizures, coma, and irreversible brain damage or death.[33]

Hypoglycemia is a stress that activates the sympathetic nervous system. Epinephrine is released, which causes symptoms such as weakness, apprehension, pronounced hunger, excessive sweating, and tachycardia.[109] Both the central nervous system and the epinephrine effects of hypoglycemia are characteristically relieved by eating. Patients with insulinomas recognize this and increase their oral intake to avoid attacks of hypoglycemia. Substantial weight gain often occurs from excessive carbohydrate consumption in patients with an insulinoma.[111, 112]

The pattern or severity of the clinical symptoms does not differentiate a benign from a malignant insulinoma. Likewise, tumor size does not correlate with the severity of symptoms. Many small insulinomas produce large amounts of insulin, whereas larger tumors may be relatively nonfunctional. Only 5% of patients with an insulinoma present with metastatic disease. The metastases are most often found in the liver or regional lymph nodes. Symptoms are usually due to excessive insulin production rather than tumor mass. Jaundice is a rare presentation.[113] Insulinomas are relatively slow-growing tumors, and most patients with an unresectable primary tumor, metastatic disease, or recurrent tumor succumb to the effects of insulin excess and not to the effects of tumor mass.

Local-Regional Anatomy and Pathology

Most insulinomas (85% to 90%) are benign. Malignancy occurs in 5% to 15% of patients, and 5% to 10% of patients have metastases at presentation. Most insulinomas (90%) are solitary and frequently small, with 70% being less than 1.5 cm in diameter.[114] Malignant insulinomas tend to be much larger, with a mean diameter of approximately 6 to 7 cm.[113] Insulinomas are evenly distributed throughout the head, body, and tail of the pancreas. Patients found to have multiple insulinomas should be evaluated for other endocrinopathies, especially the MEN I syndrome.[115] Nonpancreatic insulinomas are rare but can be found in the duodenal mucosa, the splenic hilum, or the gastrocolic ligament.

Routine histology cannot differentiate an insulinoma from another pancreatic neuroendocrine tumor. The beta cell crystal granule inclusions when seen on electron microscopy are pathognomonic for an insulinoma. Immunohistochemical techniques that reveal insulin or proinsulin immunofluorescence, or both, are diagnostic. As with other neuroendocrine tumors of the pancreas, differentiation between malignant and benign insulinomas is difficult histologically. Histologic evidence of capsular or vascular invasion may assist in the diagnosis of a malignant insulinoma, but metastases are the most reliable indicator of malignancy and are more common in men than in women. Malignant insulinomas are also more likely to secrete elevated levels of proinsulin or αhCG, or both.[113, 116]

Diagnosis, Screening, and Early Detection and Staging

Whipple's triad, consisting of the characteristic symptoms of hypoglycemia associated with blood sugar values below 50 mg/dl and immediate relief from symptoms following ingestion of glucose, was published in 1938 and remains a general guide for the suspicion of an insulinoma.[117] Insulinoma should be suspected in all patients with hypoglycemia. Modern diagnosis of an insulinoma, however, requires demonstration of plasma insulin concentrations that are inappropriately elevated in relation to plasma glucose concentrations (Table 5–17).[118] A complete evaluation is warranted for those individuals presenting with neuropsychiatric symptoms or symptoms related to excess catecholamine production, which are relieved with exogenous glucose administration. A high index of suspicion should be present in individuals with fasting hypoglycemia and in hypoglycemic patients with a family history of the MEN I syndrome.

Other, more common causes of fasting hypoglycemia include inadvertent or deliberate administration of exces-

TABLE 5–17
Clinical Evaluation for Insulinoma

Clinical suspicion with neuropsychiatric symptoms
Fasting hypoglycemia (glucose <50 mg/dl)
Normal or elevated serum insulin
Exclude exogenous insulin/sulfonylurea
Proinsulin, C-peptide, sulfonylurea levels
72-hr observed fast if needed
Insulin/glucose ratio >0.3
Tumor localization
Angiography—selective injection and subtraction
Selective intra-arterial calcium injection with hepatic vein sampling for insulin
Percutaneous portal venous sampling
Abdominal CT scanning for hepatic metastases
Intraoperative ultrasonography
Investigate familial (MEN I) possibility

sive amounts of insulin or oral hypoglycemic agents, alcohol abuse, diffuse liver disease, and large nonpancreatic tumors. Fasting hypoglycemia must be distinguished from the more common postprandial or reactive hypoglycemia.[33] Postprandial hypoglycemia occurs in patients with discoordination of glucose absorption and insulin secretion. Meals rich in carbohydrates may result in rapid absorption of glucose. This leads to an excessive and brisk rise in circulating insulin. Hypoglycemia results when no more glucose is available for absorption from the gut. This is more prevalent in females and is associated with troubling but mild symptoms of hypoglycemia. More profound difficulties can occur in some patients who have had previous gastric surgery causing symptoms of hypoglycemia and epinephrine release. This clinical presentation is often referred to as the "late dumping syndrome."[119]

When an insulinoma is suspected, the determination of fasting plasma insulin, C-peptide, and glucose levels should be made simultaneously. Factitious hypoglycemia and symptoms mimicking an insulinoma can be seen with self-administration of insulin. Measurement of circulating proinsulin and C-peptide levels are helpful in ruling out factitious hypoglycemia because these are not contained in commercially available preparations of injectable insulin but are secreted by insulinomas (Fig. 5–11).[120, 121] Measurement of insulin antibodies was helpful, since antibodies usually develop against commercially available porcine or bovine insulin and are not present in patients with an insulinoma.[122] It is less useful since the introduction of synthetic human insulin to treat diabetes. The presence of oral hypoglycemic agents causing factitious hypoglycemia can be excluded through the measurement of serum levels of sulfonylureas.

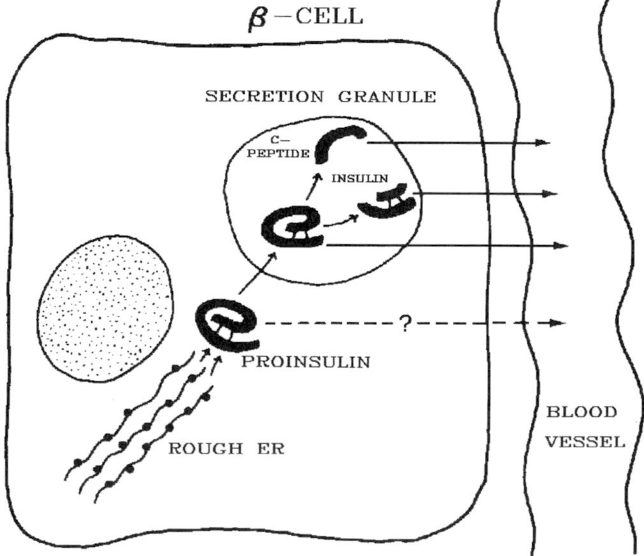

FIGURE 5–11. The pancreatic beta cell produces proinsulin as the precursor of insulin and C peptide. Elevation of the proinsulin and C-peptide serum levels may be useful in distinguishing factitious hypoglycemia from an insulinoma. (From Rubenstein AH, Kuzuya H, Horwitz DL: Clinical significance of circulating C-peptide in diabetes mellitus and hypoglycemic disorders. Arch Intern Med 137:625, 1977.)

Occasionally, it may be difficult to demonstrate an inappropriate elevation of insulin for the level of circulating glucose. Provocative testing may be needed to accentuate this difference. All provocative testing can cause dangerous hypoglycemia, so constant patient observation is required. If symptomatic hypoglycemia develops, it should be rapidly reversed with oral or intravenous glucose administration. The only provocative test we use is prolonged fasting of up to 72 hours.[33, 113, 115] Blood for glucose and insulin determinations is sampled every 4 to 6 hours during the fast and at more frequent intervals when symptoms begin to develop. Serum insulin and glucose levels are always obtained simultaneously. An elevated insulin to glucose (I/G) ratio during an episode of hypoglycemia is suspicious for insulinoma. A normal I/G ratio in the adult patient is less than 0.4 (μU insulin/mg glucose/dl). In patients with an insulinoma, this ratio is greater than 0.4 and often exceeds 1.0. The I/G ratio identifies the 33% of patients with insulinomas who have insulin levels within the normal range (<25 μU/ml).[102] During the first 24 hours of the 72-hour fast, 75% of patients have glucose levels below 40 mg/dl. The 72-hour fast is diagnostic of insulinoma in 71% of patients at 24 hours, 92% of patients at 48 hours, and 98% of patients at 72 hours.[110] C-peptide and proinsulin levels can also be obtained. Insulinomas often synthesize an excess of C peptide and proinsulin in conjunction with the hyperinsulinemia.[123, 124]

Despite the small size of most insulinomas, preoperative localization has been quite successful because of their vascular nature. Arteriography is quite sensitive in localizing insulinomas, and selective arterial injection along with digital subtraction techniques enhance our ability to image these tumors preoperatively. Tumors as small as 5 mm have been successfully imaged through arteriography. The sensitivity of arteriography in the preoperative localization of pancreatic insulinomas ranges from 84% to 87%.[125, 126] Abdominal CT scanning is limited in tumors smaller than 2 cm and demonstrates only 40% to 45% of insulinomas preoperatively. Likewise, ultrasound has difficulty in successfully localizing small insulinomas, but endoscopic ultrasonography has been successful (Fig. 5–12). CT scanning and ultrasonography almost always fail to localize insulinomas in patients with a normal arteriogram.[125] MRI has substantially improved the preoperative localization of insulinomas. Hyperintense T2-weighted MR images may demonstrate a small vascular insulinoma that was undetected by abdominal CT scanning and ultrasonography (Fig. 5–13).[28, 127] Endoscopic retrograde cholangiopancreatography (ERCP) is rarely helpful in finding insulinomas because these tumors are not ductal in origin, and it is not part of routine localization.

Transhepatic selective pancreatic vein catheterization has been used in the preoperative localization of insulinomas

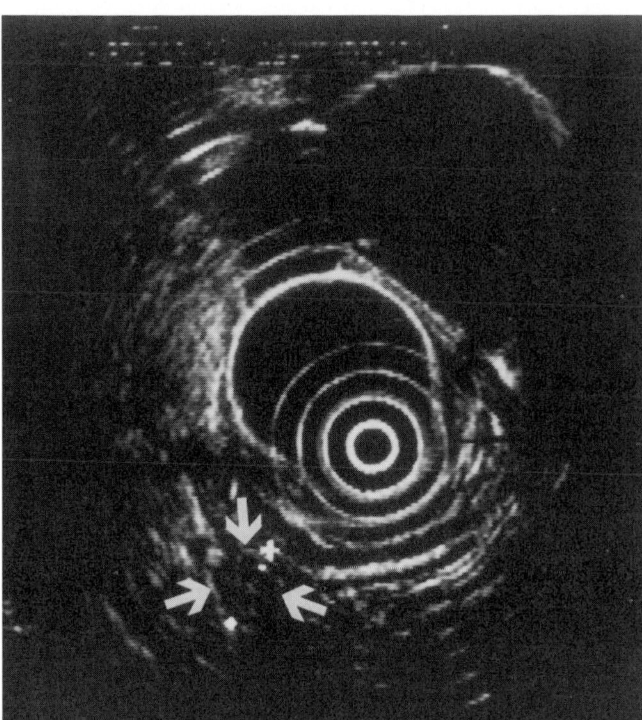

FIGURE 5–12. Endoscopic ultrasonography successfully localized an insulinoma in the pancreatic head (arrows).

that were not seen with other radiologic modalities.[128–130] An 86% sensitivity rate has been achieved using selective pancreatic vein catheterization. However, more than 15 samples had to be collected from different veins and assayed for insulin to determine accurately the region of the insulinoma. This procedure is invasive and expensive and requires the technical expertise that may not be available at all institutions. Provocative selective arterial stimulation using calcium infusion via the splenic, gastroduodenal, and inferior pancreaticoduodenal arteries and hepatic vein sampling provides similar information as portal venous sampling. It can be performed at the same time as arteriography.[131]

IOUS (intraoperative ultrasonography) appears to be of value in the operative localization of pancreatic insulinomas. The combination of IOUS and pancreatic palpation by an experienced surgeon has localized an insulinoma in 100% of explored patients in at least two series.[132] IOUS can help direct a reoperative pancreatic exploration and identify multiple pancreatic tumors in patients with the MEN I syndrome.

Preoperative localization is wise for all patients suspected of harboring an insulinoma. With an undirected pancreatic exploration, the small size of these tumors can make successful removal of the insulinoma difficult. Before the availability of preoperative localization studies, as many as 25% of pancreatic insulinomas were missed at operation despite a thorough surgical exploration of the pancreas.[126] Angiography has the best yield, but this can be increased with selective arterial calcium stimulation and IOUS.

Primary Operative Disease

Definitive therapy for a pancreatic insulinoma is operative removal of the beta cell tumor. Operative exploration of the pancreas is performed through a bilateral subcostal or an upper abdominal midline incision. The liver is examined carefully for evidence of metastases, and any and all enlarged lymph nodes along the portal triad or adjacent to the pancreas are sampled and sent for frozen section analysis to evaluate the malignant potential of the insulinoma. Bimanual palpation and exploration of the pancreas are guided by the preoperative localization studies. The entire pancreas should be explored, as multiple insulinomas occur in about 10% of patients.

Insulinomas are darker in color than the normal pancreas and usually appear reddish brown. They can also be palpated as a harder area within the pancreatic substance. Most insulinomas located in the pancreatic head are amenable to enucleation. Care must be taken not to injure the pancreatic duct when performing an enucleation, as this may result in pancreatitis or a pancreatic fistula. Pancreaticoduodenectomy is rarely necessary for small tumors, but it is appropriate for larger malignant lesions in the pancreatic head.[33] Distal pancreatectomy can be performed for insulinomas in the body or tail of the pancreas. Splenic salvage and preservation should be attempted in all cases requiring distal pancreatic resections.

If an insulinoma was not found after a complete exploration of the pancreas and duodenum, a distal pancreatectomy used to be advocated in hopes of identifying an occult tumor.[133] However, most studies have shown that a missing

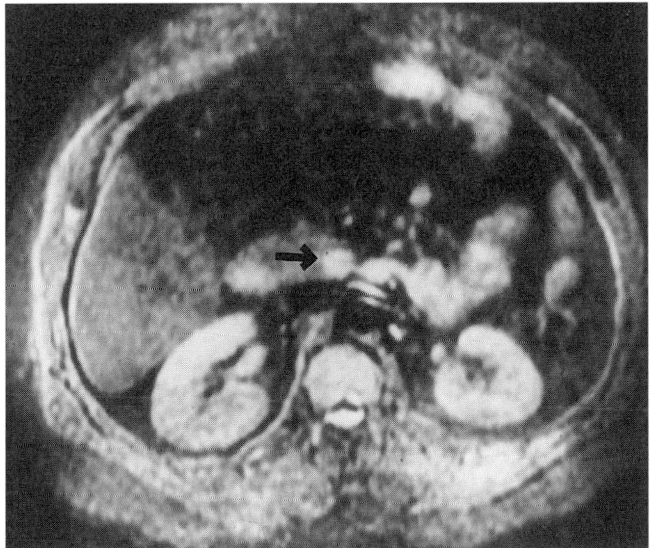

FIGURE 5–13. This insulinoma (arrow), located in the uncinate process, appears hyperintense on T2-weighted MRI scan. Abdominal CT scanning failed to visualize this tumor.

adenoma is more likely to be in the pancreatic head and uncinate process. This makes sense, since it is much easier to evaluate the tail bimanually than the head and uncinate process. If an insulinoma is not found and a distal pancreatectomy is performed, later resection of the tumor when discovered in the pancreatic head may result in a total pancreatectomy accompanied by nutritional difficulties and brittle insulin-dependent diabetes.[134] If a tumor is not found, we perform a biopsy or distal pancreatectomy to rule out nesidioblastosis, terminate the operation to reassess the diagnosis, and obtain thorough localization studies before embarking on a second exploration.[135, 136] Total pancreatectomy for insulinoma is indicated only after all medical efforts to control hyperinsulinemia have failed.[137] Operative mortality rate depends on the operative procedure and ranges from 0% to 6%; operative morbidity rate ranges from 10% to 40%.[110, 116]

Medical management of an insulinoma begins with dietary measures to minimize dangerous hypoglycemia. Judicious spacing of food intake along with an emphasis on adequate carbohydrate dietary content is extremely important in eliminating hypoglycemia. Hyperinsulinemia associated with an insulinoma can often be treated with diazoxide, an antihypertensive agent that suppresses insulin release from the pancreatic beta cells.[113] It is effective for insulinoma in oral doses of 100 to 150 mg every 8 hours. Refractory patients may require continuous intravenous glucose solutions to maintain euglycemia. Salt and water retention associated with diazoxide therapy can be ameliorated by the use of a thiazide diuretic, which can act synergistically in improving hypoglycemia. Diazoxide is also an important adjunct in preventing hypoglycemia while a patient is being prepared for operation.

Octreotide acetate (Sandostatin) lowers insulin levels in 50% to 60% of patients with an insulinoma.[138] It also blunts the insulin response to provocative stimuli such as calcium in food and secondary peptide release from insulinomas. Octreotide acetate may be the treatment of choice in patients with insulinomas who are unresponsive to diazoxide. Initial parathyroidectomy for MEN I patients with a pancreatic insulinoma may be important, as hypercalcemia may interfere with the efficacy of octreotide acetate therapy. Hypercalcemia can also promote the production and release of insulin from the insulinoma.[139] Steroids can elevate glucose concentrations, but they cause substantial side effects. Glucagon in patients with an insulinoma is of limited or short-term value.

Recurrent and Incurable Disease

Patients with unresectable insulinomas may benefit from debulking of local or metastatic disease.[33] Excellent long-term palliation can be achieved with these slow-growing tumors by lowering serum insulin levels. Formal liver resection and multiple hepatic wedge resections have been used to palliate an unresectable or metastatic insulinoma.[140] Chemotherapy with streptozocin has direct toxicity on the pancreatic beta cells. Response rates using streptozocin for advanced insulinoma range from 35% to 65%.[109] Tumor mass can be reduced in approximately 50% of patients, and survival is prolonged.[141] Unfortunately, streptozocin is toxic and can cause renal, hepatic, and bone marrow damage. Nausea and vomiting occur in nearly all patients. The addition of 5-FU augments the effect of streptozocin and increases the response rate for patients with insulinoma.[101] Octreotide acetate plays an important role in patients with metastatic or unresectable disease. It lowers insulin and normalizes glucose levels in at least 50% of patients.[138]

GLUCAGONOMA

Epidemiology

Glucagonoma is a rare neuroendocrine tumor that originates from the alpha cells in the pancreas. It is the third or fourth most common pancreatic neuroendocrine tumor. It occurs more commonly in women, with the female to male ratio ranging from 2:1 to 3:1.[142] The mean age at diagnosis is approximately 52 years, with a range of 20 to 73 years.[143] The syndrome has not been reported in children, suggesting slow tumor growth and late onset of symptoms. More than 100 glucagonomas have been reported in the world literature.[144] This neuroendocrine tumor can be found in the MEN I syndrome, and familial screening for other endocrinopathies is appropriate for these patients. Glucagonomas may be underdiagnosed because they are often asymptomatic until they have grown to a large size. Typically, the diagnosis of the glucagonoma syndrome is not considered until the characteristic typical skin rash develops in conjunction with diabetes mellitus. The diabetes in these patients is often mild and infrequently requires insulin. Sequelae related to diabetes are rare.

Life History of the Disease

The most common clinical manifestation of a glucagonoma (Table 5–18) is some form of glucose intolerance, which occurs in almost all patients.[143] Diabetes mellitus is usually mild to moderate, easily controlled with oral medication, and rarely causes ketoacidosis. There is poor correlation between serum glucagon levels in glucagonoma patients and their degree of glucose intolerance. A large

TABLE 5–18
Features of the Glucagonoma Syndrome

Clinical	Laboratory
Pancreatic tumor	Panhypoaminoacidemia
Dermatitis	Hyperglycemia
(necrolytic migratory erythema)	Hyperglucagonemia
Weight loss	Normochromic normocytic anemia
Thromboembolic disease	Increased sedimentation rate
Neuropsychiatric disorders	

insulin reserve may hide the glucose intolerance for some time, despite elevated glucagon levels.[145] Production of other hormones, such as somatostatin, may also play a role in the late onset of symptoms. Other important clinical features of the glucagonoma syndrome include the characteristic skin rash termed necrolytic migratory erythema, glossitis and stomatitis, weight loss, and weakness. Less common features include mental changes, diarrhea, arterial and venous thrombosis, anemia, and vague neurologic abnormalities.

Necrolytic migratory erythema is the most striking feature of glucagonoma (Fig. 5–14). This rash usually occurs in areas of friction or local trauma such as the feet, lower legs, hands, buttocks, perineum, perioral area, and other intertriginous areas. Local irritants, such as tape or tight-fitting shoes, may provoke the skin eruptions. When the rash is present, the additional findings of stomatitis or glossitis should further raise suspicion of a glucagonoma. The rash is commonly confused with other conditions, such as psoriasis, pemphigus, or eczema. The individual lesions involve a characteristic cycle that lasts 7 to 14 days. First, erythematous macules or papules form. These then blister, and the lesions look similar to a scald. Central erosions in the blister cause oozing and produce crusting. While the erythematous margins spread peripherally, central healing begins. Finally, the crusts fall off and the erosions heal. A distinctive bronze discoloration may remain in areas previously affected. Typically, the rash can wax and wane, making it difficult to evaluate the effect of various forms of treatment.[111]

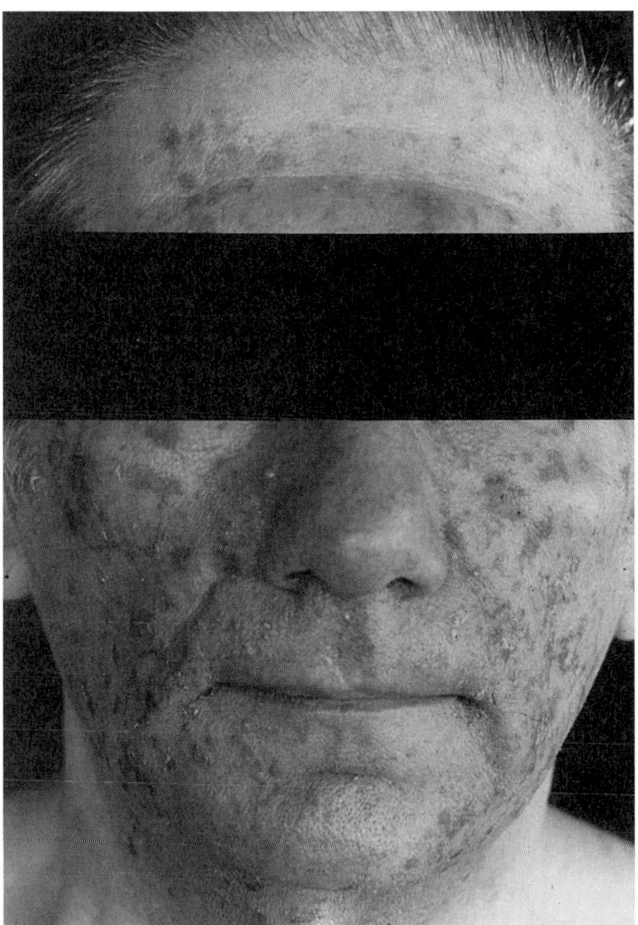

FIGURE 5–14. Necrolytic migratory erythema on the face of a patient with a glucagonoma.

A biopsy of the leading edge of the rash reveals histologic findings that are characteristic for this syndrome.[146] The dermis and lower levels of the epidermis are normal, but necrosis and lysis with bullous destruction are found in the superficial epidermis.[146] Indirect immunofluorescent techniques have failed to demonstrate any abnormal immune complexes in the dermis or epidermis in these patients.[147] The etiology of the rash is unclear.[148] Some attribute it to hypoaminoacidemia. Support for this hypothesis is based on the observation that intravenous amino acid administration has been associated with the clearing of the dermatitis.[148] Others believe that necrolytic migratory erythema is due to excess circulating glucagon or some other hormonal substance produced by the pancreatic tumor. Somatostatin analogue administration decreases circulating glucagon levels and results in rapid resolution of the rash.[149] Complete surgical removal of the glucagonoma is also quickly followed by disappearance of the rash.

Substantial weight loss is a fairly constant finding in patients with a glucagonoma. Ninety-one percent of glucagonoma patients lose more than 5 kg.[150] Malignant disease with large metastases can account for some of the extensive weight loss, but the degree of muscle wasting is often out of proportion to the amount of tumor burden. Glucagon has a direct catabolic effect on carbohydrate, protein, and fat metabolism, causing nutritional deficiency in nearly all patients. Severely depressed plasma amino acid levels are a nearly constant feature in patients with glucagonoma.

Thromboembolic disease is a common manifestation of the glucagonoma syndrome and occurs in approximately 30% of patients. Deep venous thrombosis and pulmonary emboli can be fatal.[151] Chronic warfarin or subcutaneous heparin therapy is commonly needed to prevent and treat these thromboembolic events. Cerebral and renal artery thromboses have also been reported.[152]

Episodic diarrhea occurs in about 20% of glucagonoma patients and may be related to hypersecretion of additional peptides, which induce intestinal motility disorders. Mental status alterations often accompany neuroendocrine tumors of the pancreas, and glucagonomas are no exception. Depression, disorientation, nervousness, and insomnia have all been reported.

Local-Regional Anatomy and Pathology

Primary glucagonomas are almost universally found in the substance of the pancreas. The majority of these tumors are located in the body or tail of the pancreas, while a minority are found in the head. This appears to match the normal distribution of alpha cells in the pancreas.[143] Most clinically apparent glucagonomas have been large tumors, measuring more than 5 cm in diameter at diagnosis.[153] Silent tumors can be discovered at autopsy, and these are usually less than 2 cm in diameter.

Most glucagonomas are malignant (60% to 80% of cases). Well over 50% are metastatic at the time of diagnosis. Rarely, these tumors can be multiple.[14] Lymphatic and hepatic metastases are the most common pattern of spread, but metastases have also been described to bone and the adrenal gland. These tumors are often diagnosed at an advanced stage because symptoms develop only after the tumor has reached a large size and plasma glucagon has risen to high levels.

Routine light microscopy and standard histologic techniques cannot differentiate glucagonomas from other islet cell tumors of the pancreas.[142] Immunohistochemical methods and electron microscopy can identify specific characteristics of the secretory granules in alpha cells that can distinguish a glucagonoma from other islet cell tumors. These granules stain positive for glucagon.[154]

Diagnosis, Screening, and Early Detection and Staging

The diagnosis of a glucagonoma rests on the discovery of an elevated fasting serum glucagon level. Normal values of glucagon range between 25 and 250 pg/ml. Patients with glucagon-secreting tumors generally have glucagon levels exceeding 500 to 1000 pg/ml.[143, 153] Other causes of hyperglucagonemia include renal failure, hepatic failure, or severe stress. Unfortunately, there is no reliable provocative test currently available to determine whether moderately elevated glucagon levels are due to a glucagonoma. Associated laboratory findings that may suggest the diagnosis of glucagonoma include elevated plasma glucose, depressed serum amino acid levels, hypocholesterolemia, elevated red blood cell sedimentation rate, and a characteristic normocytic and normochromic anemia (see Table 5–18).[111] This anemia is present in 85% of glucagonoma patients and is characterized by normal serum iron, vitamin B_{12}, and folate levels.[155] It is uncertain whether this anemia is due to a direct effect of hyperglucagonemia or is secondary to the catabolic state.

The localization of glucagonomas is often easy, since these tumors are usually large, solitary, and vascular. Abdominal CT scan is quite accurate and sensitive for the detection and localization of most clinically apparent glucagonomas. Angiography is reserved for those tumors not seen on abdominal CT scanning and is accurate in 80% or more of cases.[156] Percutaneous portal venous sampling has been successful but is usually not necessary.[157] A complete evaluation of the liver is necessary to determine the presence of metastatic disease and can be performed using abdominal CT scanning or hepatic arteriography.

Primary Operable Disease—Results and Complications of Treatment

Glucagonoma treatment begins with adequate preoperative preparation to control diabetes mellitus and to improve nutritional status. Preoperative intravenous hyperalimentation may be indicated in patients with extensive catabolism and weight loss. Deep venous thrombosis should be aggressively treated with heparin, and preoperative heparin prophylaxis is probably wise. The synthetic somatostatin analogue octreotide acetate may be of considerable value in the preoperative management of these patients.[158] A reduction in circulating serum glucagon levels can enhance the nutritional benefit of preoperative intravenous hyperalimentation, reverse the rash, and perhaps even lower the risk of thromboembolic disease.

The only chance for cure in patients with a glucagonoma is complete surgical extirpation, and operation is recommended in essentially all patients. Unfortunately, the majority (60% to 80%) of these tumors are malignant and are large and advanced at the time of operation. As with most neuroendocrine tumors of the pancreas, there are no reliable histologic criteria for the diagnosis of malignancy. The malignant nature of a glucagonoma is demonstrated by local spread, lymph node involvement, or hepatic metastases. If the tumor is small and presumably benign, enucleation is the best treatment. Most tumors, however, are large, involving the body or tail of the pancreas, or both, and require formal pancreatic resection, most often a distal pancreatectomy resection. While most patients with a glucagonoma are incurable, those undergoing resection can have dramatic and rapid improvement in all symptoms in the days and weeks following operation.[159] The rash disappears, weight gain occurs, and the diabetes, anemia, hypoproteinemia, and hypoaminoacidemia are reversed. Some patients undergoing an extensive pancreatic resection for glucagonoma can actually experience worsening of the diabetes as a result of the loss of pancreatic beta cell mass. Normalization of plasma glucagon serves as a reliable indicator of complete tumor removal and is useful in monitoring these patients for future recurrent or metastatic disease.[160]

Recurrent and Incurable Disease—Results and Complications

The majority of patients with a glucagonoma have preoperative or intraoperative evidence of metastatic disease. Metastases tend to involve the liver, lymph nodes, adjacent organs, bones, and adrenal glands. Preoperative demonstration of metastases during localization studies may not preclude operation, as surgical debulking can be beneficial. Glucagonomas, like the other neuroendocrine pancreatic tumors, are slow growing, and the morbidity and mortality of these tumors are often related more to the excessive hormone production than to the tumor mass. A marked decline in serum glucagon is possible with palliative surgical resection, which results in disappearance or amelioration of the preoperative manifestations of this disorder.[161] Mean response of approximately 1 year, with a mean survival of 2 years, has been shown.[35] Disease-free survival of 6 years or more has been reported with the resection of nodal metastatic spread of a glucagonoma.[162] Surgical debulking may also enhance the medical control of glucagon excess.

Systemic chemotherapy may be necessary when the primary tumor is unresectable, associated nodal or distant metastases are present, or recurrence of the syndrome is encountered. Because of its efficacy with other neuroendocrine pancreatic tumors, streptozocin combined with 5-FU has been the usual first regimen. This combination, however, has had only limited success in the small number of glucagonoma patients treated. Response rates of 30% to 35% have been reported for streptozocin with or without the addition of 5-FU.[163] Likewise, doxorubicin has been used with a 20% to 25% response rate.[164] Neither of these agents provided a survival benefit when compared to untreated controls.

We and others have favored a chemotherapy regimen using DTIC for glucagonomas.[35] Complete reversal of the glucagonoma syndrome has occurred with DTIC therapy in two of our patients.[165] Promising results have been documented in other studies, with response rates approaching 70% to 75%.[166] Currently, there are few reports of failure with DTIC in the treatment of unresectable, metastatic, or recurrent glucagonoma syndrome.[167] Further experience is obviously needed before a definitive recommendation can be made regarding the chemotherapy of choice for these patients. Chlorozotocin A is now being studied in the treatment of the glucagonoma syndrome. This new chemotherapeutic agent appears to be structurally related to streptozocin, with a lower incidence of nephrotoxicity.[164]

Hepatic artery embolization has been used to treat extensive liver metastases in patients with glucagonomas. This modality has resulted in a 50% reduction of tumor size in selected cases. Similarly, hepatic artery infusion chemotherapy with streptozocin can enhance response rates up to 50%. Both of these modalities, however, provide no proven survival advantage.[156] Likewise, neither has demonstrated reliable suppression of hyperglucagonemia.

The somatostatin analogue octreotide acetate can provide substantial symptomatic relief for patients with the glucagonoma syndrome and is the current medical modality of choice (Fig. 5–15). Resolution of the cutaneous rash, control of glucose intolerance, weight gain, and correction of hypoaminoacidemia can all occur with a marked decrease in the plasma levels of glucagon.[138] Preoperative use of octreotide acetate is advocated to reverse the catabolic effects of the hyperglucagonemia and better prepare these patients for operative exploration. Anecdotal reports exist of tumor regression or decrease in tumor growth with octreotide acetate.[168] Whether this is due to a direct effect on the tumor or is secondary to decreases in growth factors or tumor blood supply is uncertain.[168]

Glucagonoma patients refractory to octreotide acetate may benefit from a trial of human leukocyte interferon.[37] Two case reports describe dramatic clinical improvement and decreased glucagon production after administration of interferon.[169, 170] The mechanism of action remains unclear, and the beneficial effects of interferon alone, or in combination with other cytotoxic agents, need further study.

VIPOMA

Epidemiology

A syndrome of severe refractory diarrhea and hypokalemia was linked to an islet cell tumor of the pancreas by Verner and Morrison in 1958.[7] Their second review of the syndrome in 1974 described 55 patients, and currently more than 200 cases have been documented.[171, 172] The syndrome has been described as "pancreatic cholera" or the Verner-Morrison syndrome but is now best known as the watery diarrhea, hypokalemia, achlorhydria (WDHA) syndrome. The main causative agent for this syndrome appears to be VIP; prostaglandins, pancreatic polypeptide, and other intestinal hormones may also play a role.[173]

Vipomas are extremely rare, even among the functional endocrine tumors of the pancreas. They occur in adulthood at a mean age of approximately 50 years. VIP production and the vipoma syndrome have also been demonstrated in children under 10 years old with ganglioneuromas. Sixty percent of the reported vipoma patients are female and 40% are male.[174]

Life History of the Disease

VIP increases intestinal peristalsis, stimulates pancreatic fluid and bicarbonate secretion, inhibits intestinal solute absorption, promotes water and ion secretion from the intestine, and relaxes the anal sphincter. Consequently, the most prominent symptom of the vipoma syndrome is a profuse secretory diarrhea. Seventy percent of patients have more than 3 L/day of diarrhea, and more than 10 L/day is not uncommon.[175] The diarrhea is tea-colored and is unaffected by fasting or nasogastric suction, a distinguishing feature from the diarrhea of a gastrinoma.[175] Fecal fat, blood, and leukocytes are absent in the stool. The secretory diarrhea may be intermittent. It usually causes a significant metabolic acidosis and potassium deficit (200 to 300 mEq/day), resulting in weakness, lethargy, and nephropathy.[176] VIP is structurally similar to glucagon and gastric inhibitory polypeptide (GIP) and can also cause hyperglycemia and hypo- or achlorhydria.[177] Hypercalcemia should prompt a careful search for the other endocrinopathies constituting the MEN I syndrome.[171, 174] VIP also relaxes smooth muscle and can cause cutaneous flushing and dilatation of the

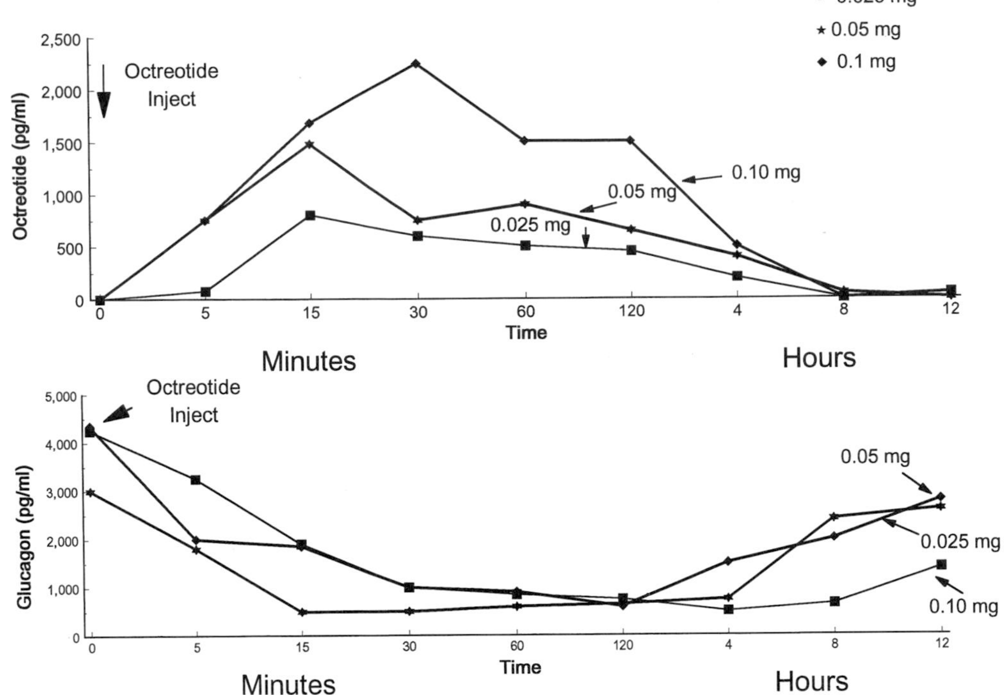

FIGURE 5–15. The circulating levels of octreotide and glucagon are shown after subcutaneous injection of octreotide doses of 0.025 mg, 0.05 mg, and 0.1 mg.

gallbladder.[178] The average duration of symptoms prior to diagnosis in these patients is 3 years. These tumors are often locally advanced or metastatic, or both, at the time of diagnosis, but death is more likely to occur from the dehydration and electrolyte abnormalities of VIP excess than from tumor mass.

Local-Regional Anatomy and Pathology

Eighty percent of patients with the WDHA syndrome have tumors located in the pancreas, while the remaining 20% have extrapancreatic tumors. These are found in ganglioneuromas, the adrenal medulla, the retroperitoneum, the stomach, the lung, and other neural crest origin tissue.[179] The cell of origin is thought to be a non–beta islet cell, but an autonomic nerve cell origin has also been postulated. The majority of pancreatic tumors (75%) are located in the body or tail, or both, but islet cell hyperplasia involving the entire gland has been reported in 10% of patients.[111, 177] The tumors range from 2 to 6 cm in diameter and are predominantly solitary.[14] Malignancy is demonstrated in half of patients, and half of these are metastatic to liver or lymph nodes at the time of diagnosis.[180] In contrast, most vipomas of neural crest origin, such as the ganglioneuromas, have a more benign course.[177]

Diagnosis, Screening, and Early Detection and Staging

The diagnosis of the WDHA syndrome is generally suspected from the clinical symptoms of profound diarrhea, severe dehydration, and significant electrolyte loss (potassium). Investigation of the diarrhea should begin with stool culture and examination to exclude the presence of an infectious etiology. Osmotic diarrhea seen in malabsorption syndromes such as celiac disease and inflammatory bowel disease resolves after a 48- to 72-hour fast. Steatorrhea, seen in the somatostatinoma syndrome, is not present in the WDHA syndrome. Diarrhea from metastatic carcinoid tumors can be diagnosed by finding elevated urinary 5-hydroxyindoleacetic acid or circulating serotonin, or bradykinin. Finally, a fasting serum gastrin and gastric acid analysis easily distinguishes the diarrhea of a gastrinoma from that of the WDHA syndrome.[14]

The diagnosis of a VIP-producing tumor requires the demonstration of an elevated fasting VIP serum level by radioimmunoassay. Episodic and erratic secretion of VIP may necessitate daily plasma measurements. Fasting VIP levels normally range from 0 to 170 pg/ml but are substantially elevated (5- to 10-fold) in vipoma patients.[181] Transient elevation of VIP has been described in acute intestinal bowel ischemia, circulatory failure, and hepatic cirrhosis, which usually does not pose diagnostic problems.[173] The major difficulty in the diagnosis of vipoma is in those patients with the clinical syndrome and a normal plasma VIP level. Other mediators might be causative in these patients, and plasma pancreatic polypeptide and prostaglandin E_2 (PGE_2), among others, should be measured.

Abdominal CT scanning is probably the initial test of choice to localize a vipoma. Imaging of the liver and adrenals is important in adults, and ganglioneuromas and retroperitoneal masses should be searched for in children with the WDHA syndrome. Angiography, intraoperative ultrasonography, and selective arterial stimulation combined with portal and splenic venous sampling have all been successful in localizing this tumor.[182, 183]

Primary Operable Disease—Results and Complications of Treatment

All patients with the clinical syndrome of WDHA and elevated plasma VIP should undergo operation to attempt total surgical extirpation. Solitary, benign-appearing, small tumors may be treated with enucleation or partial pancreatic resection. If no tumor is found, the retroperitoneum, adrenal glands, and sympathetic chains should be explored. Distal pancreatectomy may be performed in this setting, since 10% of patients with the WDHA syndrome have islet cell hyperplasia.[163] Plasma VIP levels should decrease following successful removal of all tumor or of islet cell hyperplasia.

The severe electrolyte and nutritional disturbances resulting from the secretory diarrhea must be corrected prior to operative intervention. Oral and intravenous routes of correction may be used along with control of the diarrhea. Accurate cardiovascular monitoring is required because of the large volumes of fluid and electrolytes that must be infused. Aggressive reversal of the dehydration, hypokalemia, hypomagnesemia, and metabolic acidosis can be enhanced by the preoperative use of octreotide acetate.[181] Octreotide acetate effectively decreases plasma VIP, decreases stool volume, and reverses the electrolyte and acid-base imbalance in the majority of patients.[184] Oral indomethacin (25 mg three times a day) inhibits PGE_2 and may decrease stool volume.[185]

Recurrent and Incurable Disease—Results and Complications

As with other pancreatic neuroendocrine tumors, surgical debulking, including even partial hepatic resection, may provide palliation for vipoma patients with metastatic disease by decreasing circulating VIP. Recurrent disease can occasionally be detected by a postoperative rise in plasma VIP, and localization can be performed. Nagorney et al.[186] reported the cure of a recurrent vipoma after re-exploration with pancreatic and hepatic wedge resection. Data for re-exploration on the basis of elevated VIP alone is limited, but this may be warranted in some patients.

The chemotherapeutic regimen of choice for patients with unresectable, metastatic, or recurrent disease is streptozocin combined with 5-FU.[101] Vipomas have the best response rates to streptozocin of all islet cell tumors. Response rates of 50% to 70%, with substantial decrease in tumor size and even an occasional long-term remission, have been reported.[187] Intra-arterial hepatic infusion of streptozocin may increase response rates and decrease the potential for nephrotoxicity.[188] Octreotide acetate also appears to be an effective agent in controlling the diarrhea and flushing of patients with metastatic disease; tumor regression and infarction may also occur.[189]

SOMATOSTATINOMA

Epidemiology

Somatostatin is a 14–amino acid polypeptide found widely throughout the nervous and gastrointestinal systems. In the pancreas and duodenum, it is contained in the D cells.[190] Somatostatin has widespread inhibitory actions. It decreases gastrointestinal motility, bile flow, and nearly all gut hormones involved in pancreatic endocrine and exocrine function.[191] Somatostatinomas are the rarest of all neuroendocrine tumors of the pancreas, with less than 50 reported in the world literature. There appears to be a slight female predominance with pancreatic somatostatinomas, while males predominate with intestinal and extrapancreatic somatostatinomas.[191, 192] The mean age at onset of disease is approximately 50 years, with a range of 26 to 84 years.[191] The precise incidence of this tumor is unknown, and extensive surgical experience with somatostatinoma is lacking.

Life History of the Disease

The clinical presentation of these tumors exemplifies the inhibitory action of somatostatin on neighboring neuroendocrine cells responsible for the production of insulin, cholecystokinin, glucagon, pancreatic polypeptide, and gastrin.[193] Clinical features of a somatostatinoma include diabetes mellitus, cholelithiasis, steatorrhea, indigestion, diarrhea, hypochlorhydria, jaundice, abdominal pain, and anemia.[12] Many of these abnormalities are nonspecific and can explain the difficulty of preoperative suspicion and detection. Some degree of glucose intolerance is present in all patients with a somatostatinoma, ranging from mild hyperglycemia to ketoacidosis, depending on the level of glucagon inhibition.[194, 195] Hypochlorhydria results from the inhibition of gastrin release and a decrease in gastric acid production. Diarrhea occurs in 20% to 30% of patients and is frequently multifactorial. Depressed pancreatic exocrine function results in the malabsorption of amino acids, carbohydrates, and fats and leads to an increased stool osmolarity and steatorrhea.[194]

Local-Regional Anatomy and Pathology

The majority of somatostatinomas are located in the pancreas (70%), but extrapancreatic sites such as the duodenum (20%), ampulla of Vater (<5%), and small intestine (<5%) have been described.[194, 196, 197] The majority of pancreatic somatostatinomas are located in the pancreatic head (75%), while the remainder are distributed between the body and tail (20%) and the entire gland (5%).[194] Most tumors that come to clinical attention are solitary and malignant, and 75% to 85% are metastatic to the liver at the time of diagnosis. Other metastatic sites include peripancreatic lymph nodes and bone marrow.[198] The initial case reports noted somatostatinomas as an incidental finding at the time of elective cholecystectomy.[10, 11]

Patients with small duodenal somatostatinomas can be completely asymptomatic.[196] Duodenal somatostatinomas may have a more favorable prognosis than those arising in the pancreas. While invasion of the duodenal wall can be seen, some authors suggest that distant spread of these tumors is less common.[105] Duodenal somatostatinomas have a similar histologic appearance to carcinoid tumors.[199] A new MEN syndrome has been proposed in patients with neurofibromatosis to include duodenal somatostatinomas and pheochromocytomas.[200] The duodenal tumors are located near the entry site of the biliary and pancreatic ducts, and a 40% rate of lymphatic metastasis is reported.[105]

Diagnosis, Screening, and Early Detection and Staging

The diagnosis of a somatostatinoma is suggested in the clinical setting of mild diabetes, steatorrhea, and cholelithiasis. Unfortunately, these symptoms are so nonspecific that the detection of these tumors often occurs late after distant spread has occurred.[201] Confirmation of the presence of a somatostatinoma is made by obtaining an elevated fasting somatostatin level measured by radioimmunoassay techniques or by immunohistochemical or direct measurement of tumor somatostatin content. A normal plasma somatostatin level is less than 100 pg/ml. In general, patients with somatostatinomas have a 10- to 100-fold increase in the level of polypeptide produced. A mean of 15.5 ng/ml is reported in one study.[202] Depressed levels of serum insulin and glucagon are also seen.

Provocative testing for a somatostatinoma using tolbutamide has been described in patients with normal or slightly elevated blood levels of somatostatin.[203] In somatostatinomas, tolbutamide infusion produces an increase in the serum somatostatin level. This testing, however, is rarely necessary for diagnosis in the vast majority of patients with a somatostatinoma. While most somatostatinomas are discovered intraoperatively, preoperative localization of these tumors in suspected patients is usually successful because of the large tumor size. Ultrasonography, abdominal CT scanning, angiography, upper gastrointestinal barium contrast studies, and ERCP have all been used successfully in preoperative tumor localization.[194]

Primary Operable Disease—Results and Complications of Treatment

Optimal treatment of a somatostatinoma is complete surgical resection after preoperative correction of the hyperglycemia and the nutritional deficiencies. While the majority of patients deserve operation, surgical cure may not be possible because of the malignant behavior of many of these tumors. In the absence of metastatic disease, small tumors can occasionally be enucleated whereas larger tumors require formal pancreatic resection. Pancreaticoduodenectomy may be required, as many somatostatinomas are located in the pancreatic head.[14] Even though extensive pancreatic resection can remove the somatostatin excess, hyperglycemia can persist owing to the loss of pancreatic beta cell mass. Cholecystectomy should be performed to prevent the development or complications of cholelithiasis.

Recurrent and Incurable Disease—Results and Complications

As with other neuroendocrine tumors of the pancreas, surgical debulking for somatostatinomas with advanced metastatic disease may provide palliation because of the slow growth of this tumor. The prognosis of somatostatinoma is variable, with a mean survival of months to years reported in patients with and without metastatic disease.[204] Prolonged survival is possible even in the presence of metastases.[204, 205] The optimal chemotherapy for somatostatinomas has yet to be determined, and data are limited by the rarity of this tumor. Single- or multiple-agent protocols using streptozocin, 5-FU, or doxorubicin have been reported, with a 1-year survival rate of 48% and a 5-year survival rate of 13%.[194]

NONFUNCTIONING ISLET CELL CARCINOMA

Epidemiology

Nonfunctioning islet cell tumors of the pancreas have no clinical manifestations of excess hormone production. Consequently, they can provide valuable insight into the intrinsic nature of pancreatic endocrine malignancy. These tumors are rare and account for only a small fraction of all malignant pancreatic neoplasms. In the United States, there are an estimated 125 pancreatic adenocarcinomas for every islet cell carcinoma.[15] It may be a misnomer to designate these tumors as nonfunctioning, since they may be producing undescribed hormones, inactive prohormones, or known hormones at undetectable levels. The average age of patients with nonfunctioning islet cell tumors is 60 years, and a slight female predominance is suggested. In the 1950s, 40% of all pancreatic islet cell tumors were classified as nonfunctional by clinical or laboratory criteria, or both.[206] In the last two decades, the advent of radioimmunoassay techniques, along with an increased awareness of the specific clinical syndromes of functional tumors, has led to a decrease in the number of nonfunctional tumors diagnosed.[207] Currently, 20% to 30% of all islet cell tumors are labeled nonfunctional.[208]

Life History of the Disease

The clinical presentation of nonfunctioning islet cell carcinoma, like that of pancreatic adenocarcinoma, depends on the size, location, and invasive characteristics of the primary neoplasm. Most of these nonfunctional neoplasms are difficult to recognize early and become evident only when their large size or distant metastases cause symptoms. The mass effect of these tumors can cause compression of adjacent structures, producing epigastric pain, weight loss, jaundice, nausea and vomiting, and diarrhea. The presence of a palpable abdominal mass is a common finding. Ten percent of islet cell carcinomas may be discovered incidentally through the use of abdominal CT examination for other abdominal disorders.[209] They may also be discovered during operative procedures performed for other purposes.

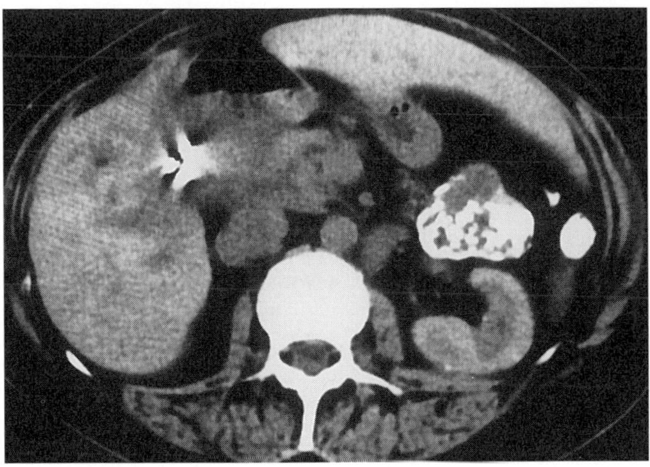

FIGURE 5–17. A nonfunctioning calcified islet cell carcinoma is located in the tail of the pancreas.

Local-Regional Anatomy and Pathology

Nonfunctioning islet cell tumors are usually located in the head of the pancreas. Whether this is a true incidence or is secondary to jaundice from biliary tract obstruction that brings lesions in the pancreatic head to attention is uncertain. Cystic and calcified body and tail lesions have been described much less frequently (Figs. 5–16 and 5–17).[15–17] These tumors are usually solitary and range in size from 2.5 to 16 cm in diameter. The vast majority (>85%) are malignant, with regional lymph node involvement or distant metastatic disease present at the time of operation. Malignancy is defined by invasion into adjacent organs, involvement of regional lymph nodes, and/or the presence of distant metastases. Gross morphologic findings of size and encapsulation are not reliable indicators of the biologic behavior of these tumors. They characteristically grow slowly, and the presence of metastatic disease does not preclude prolonged survival.

Diagnosis, Screening, and Early Detection and Staging

Preoperative diagnosis of a nonfunctioning islet cell tumor of the pancreas is rare. Abdominal CT scanning may be performed for clinical symptoms such as jaundice, epigastric pain, and a palpable abdominal mass. Abdominal CT scanning is useful for delineating the size and extent of the primary islet cell carcinoma as well as its relationship to contiguous viscera and the presence of peripancreatic or regional lymphadenopathy and liver metastases (Fig. 5–18).

Primary Operable Disease—Results and Complications of Treatment

Operative exploration for curative resection should be undertaken whenever possible for all patients with nonfunctional islet cell tumors. Resection is possible in 25% to 50% of patients, which is much more favorable than

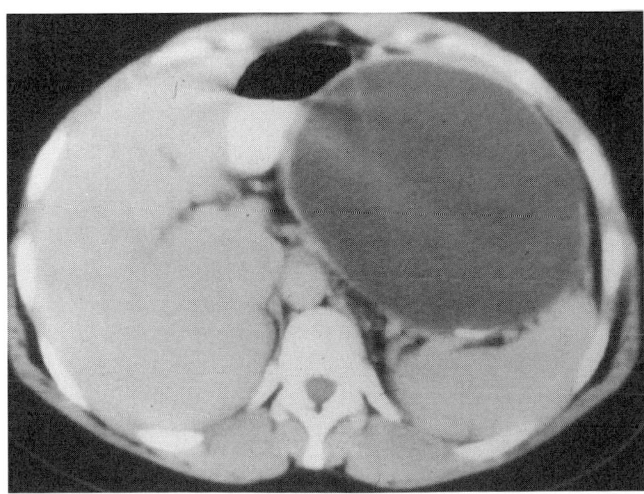

FIGURE 5–16. Abdominal CT scanning demonstrates a large cystic nonfunctional islet cell tumor of the pancreas.

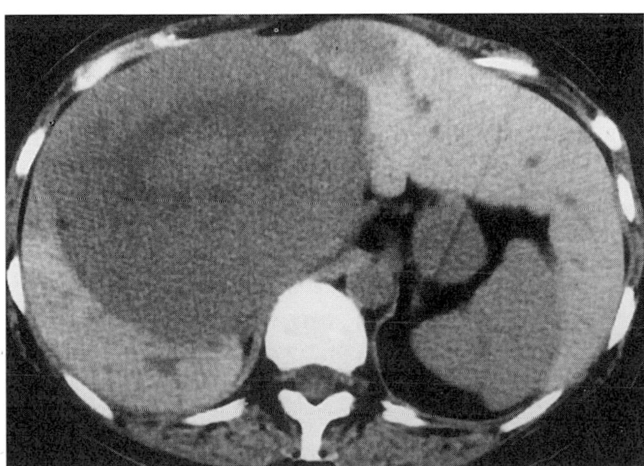

FIGURE 5–18. Extensive liver metastases from an islet cell carcinoma are noted on this abdominal CT scan.

the 10% rate for ductal adenocarcinoma of the pancreas. Nonfunctioning islet cell tumors can invade local structures, including the retroperitoneum, porta hepatis, and superior mesenteric vessels, and they can cause biliary tract or gastric outlet obstruction, or both. These features commonly prevent curative resection. Operative procedures for nonfunctional tumors include enucleation, pancreaticoduodenectomy, distal or total pancreatectomy, paraduodenal resection, and biopsy with or without gastric or biliary bypass.

Recurrent and Incurable Disease—Results and Complications

Palliative debulking may relieve the mass effect of these tumors, decrease tumor load, and facilitate postoperative chemotherapy. Biliary bypass procedures are used for patients with tumors arising from the head of the pancreas who are not candidates for curative resection. Gastric bypass procedures should be individualized, since gastroduodenal obstruction is uncommon.

The prognosis for patients with nonfunctional islet cell tumors of the pancreas is certainly more favorable than that for ductal adenocarcinoma. Three- and 5-year survival rates of 60% and 44%, respectively, have been reported for nonfunctioning islet cell carcinoma, while most patients with ductal adenocarcinoma live less than 1 year.[15, 17, 208] Prolonged survival with palliative surgery is common and is probably superior to that with functional neuroendocrine tumors. Hepatic metastases from nonfunctioning islet cell tumors can be slow growing and may remain unchanged for many years. The longest survivors appear to be patients with nonfunctional islet cell carcinomas who undergo curative pancreaticoduodenal resection.

Although no significant survival benefit has resulted from the use of chemotherapy, excellent palliation can be achieved for the complications of local or metastatic spread of these tumors. Streptozocin, doxorubicin, 5-FU, cisplatin, and chlorozotocin have been used in patients with nonfunctional islet cell carcinoma.[16, 164] While further investigation is needed, DTIC may also provide excellent palliation for these complications.[208] A 50% to 60% response rate has been described, which may double the mean survival in these patients.[165] Renal and hepatic toxicity is significant but may be decreased through the use of hepatic arterial infusion devices. Dichloromethotrexate or 5-FU and mitomycin have been infused through hepatic arterial infusion devices and may result in decreased systemic toxicity.[16]

References

1. Langerhans P: Beitrage Zur Mikroskopischen Anatomie Der Bauchspeicheldruse. Berlin: Gustar Lange, 1869.
2. Banting FG, Best CH: The internal secretion of the pancreas. J Lab Clin Med 7:251, 1922.
3. Nicholls AG: Simple adenoma of the pancreas arising from an island of Langerhans. J Med Res 8:385, 1902.
4. Fabozzi S: Uber die Histogenese des primaren Krebses des Pankres. Beitr Pathol 34:199, 1903.
5. Howland G, Campbell W, Maltby E, et al: Dysinsulinism: Convulsions and coma due to islet cell tumor of the pancreas with operation and cure. JAMA 93:674, 1929.
6. Zollinger RM, Ellison EH: Primary peptic ulcerations of the jejunum associated with islet cell tumors of the pancreas. Ann Surg 142:709, 1955.
7. Verner JV, Morrison AB: Islet cell tumor and a syndrome of refractory watery diarrhea and hypokalemia. Am J Med 25:374, 1958.
8. McGavran M, Unger R, Recant L, et al: A glucagon-secreting alpha-cell carcinoma of the pancreas. N Engl J Med 274:1408, 1966.
9. Mallinson CN, Bloom SR, Warin AP, et al: A glucagonoma syndrome. Lancet 2:1, 1974.
10. Ganda O, Weir G, Soeldner J, et al: "Somatostatinoma": A somatostatin-containing tumor of the endocrine pancreas. N Engl J Med 296:963, 1977.
11. Larsson L, Hirsch M, Holst J, et al: Pancreatic somatostatinoma: Clinical features and physiological implications. Lancet 1:666, 1977.
12. Kregs GJ, Orci L, Conlon JM, et al: Somatostatinoma syndrome—biochemical, morphologic and clinical features. N Engl J Med 301:285, 1979.
13. Friesen SR: Tumors of the endocrine pancreas. N Engl J Med 306:580, 1982.
14. Mozell E, Stenzel P, Woltering EA, et al: Functional endocrine tumors of the pancreas: Clinical presentation, diagnosis and treatment. Curr Probl Surg 27:303, 1990.
15. Thompson GB, van Heerden JA, Grant CS, et al: Islet cell carcinomas of the pancreas: A twenty-year experience. Surgery 104:1011, 1988.
16. Eckhauser FE, Cheung PS, Vinik AI, et al: Nonfunctioning malignant neuroendocrine tumors of the pancreas. Surgery 100:978, 1986.
17. Holm A, Reyes-Govea J, Aldrete JS: Diagnosis, surgical aspects, and long-term follow-up of functioning and nonfunctioning islet cell tumors of the pancreas. Contemp Surg 34:13, 1989.
18. Buchanan K, Johnston C, O'Hare M, et al: Neuroendocrine tumors: A European view. Am J Med 81:14, 1986.
19. Shepherd JJ: The natural history of multiple endocrine neoplasia type 1: Highly uncommon or highly unrecognized? Arch Surg 126:935, 1991.
20. Larsson C, Skogseid B, Oberg K, et al: Multiple endocrine neoplasia type 1 gene maps to chromosome 11 and is lost in insulinoma. Nature 332:85, 1988.
21. Kahn C, Rosen S, Weintraub B, et al: Ectopic production of chorionic gonadotropin and its subunits by islet-cell tumors: A specific marker for malignancy. N Engl J Med 297:565, 1977.
22. Bordelon-Risler M, Siciliano M, Kohler P: Necessity for two human chromosomes for human gonadotropin production in human-mouse hybrids. Somatic Cell Genet 5:597, 1979.
23. Tapia FJ, Polak JM, Barbosa AJA, et al: Neurone-specific enolase is produced by neuroendocrine tumors. Lancet 1:808, 1981.
24. Prinz RA, Marangos PJ: Use of neuron-specific enolase as a serum marker for neuroendocrine neoplasms. Surgery 92:887, 1982.
25. Dayal Y: Neuroendocrine cells of the gastrointestinal tract: Introduction and historical perspective. In Dayal Y (ed): Endocrine Pathology of the Gut and Pancreas. Boca Raton, FL: CRC Press, 1991, p 1.
26. Chejfec G, Falkmer S, Grimelius L, et al: Synaptophysin: A new marker for pancreatic neuroendocrine tumors. Am J Surg Pathol 11:241, 1987.
27. Wiedemann B, Waldherr R, Buhr H, et al: Identification of gastroenteropancreatic neuroendocrine cells in normal and neoplastic human tissue with antibodies against synaptophysin, chromogranin A, secretogranin I (chromogranin B), and secretogranin II. Gastroenterology 95:1364, 1988.
28. Stark DD, Moss AA, Goldberg HI, et al: Computed tomography and nuclear magnetic resonance imaging of pancreatic islet cell tumors. Surgery 94:1024, 1983.
29. Fulton RE, Sheedy PF, McIlrath DC, et al: Preoperative angiographic localization of insulin-producing tumors of the pancreas. Am J Roentgenol 123:367, 1975.
30. Norton JA, Cromack DT, Shawker TH, et al: Intraoperative ultrasonographic localization of islet cell tumors. Ann Surg 207:160, 1988.
31. Vinik AI, Delbridge L, Moattari R, et al: Transhepatic portal vein catheterization for localization of insulinomas: A ten year experience. Surgery 109:1, 1991.
32. Imamura M, Takahashi K, Adachi H, et al: Usefulness of selective

arterial secretin test for localization of gastrinoma in the Zollinger-Ellison syndrome. Ann Surg 205:230, 1987.
33. Kaplan EL, Rubenstein AH, Evans R, et al: Calcium infusion: A new provocative test for insulinomas. Ann Surg 190:501, 1979.
34. Ko TC, Flisak M, Prinz RA: Selective intraarterial methylene blue injection—a novel method of localizing gastrinoma. Gastroenterology 102:1062, 1992.
35. Montenegro F, Lawrence GD, Macon W, et al: Metastatic glucagonoma: Improvement after surgical debulking. Am J Surg 139:424, 1980.
36. Kvols LK, Buck M: Chemotherapy of endocrine malignancy: A review. Semin Oncol 14:343, 1987.
37. Vinik AI, Moahari AR, Pavlic I, et al: Pancreatic endocrine tumors: Medical management. In Burns GP, Banks ED (eds): Disorders of the Pancreas: Current Issues in Diagnosis and Management. New York: McGraw-Hill, 1992, p 414.
38. Lamberts SWJ, Bakker WH, Reubi JC, et al: Somatostatin-receptor imaging in the localization of endocrine tumors. N Engl J Med 323:1246, 1990.
39. Reubi JC, Maurer R, von Werder K, et al: Somatostatin receptors in human endocrine tumors. Cancer Res 47:551, 1978.
40. Wilson SD: Gastrinoma. In Howard JM, Jordan GL, Reber HA (eds): Surgical Diseases of the Pancreas. Philadelphia: Lea & Febiger, 1987, p 829.
41. Ellison EH, Wilson SD: The Zollinger-Ellison syndrome: Reappraisal and evaluation of 260 registered cases. Ann Surg 160:512, 1964.
42. Regan P, Malagelada J: A reappraisal of clinical, roentgenographic and endoscopic features of the Zollinger-Ellison syndrome. Mayo Clin Proc 53:19, 1978.
43. Maton PN, Gardner J, Jensen R: Cushing's syndrome in patients with the Zollinger-Ellison syndrome. N Engl J Med 315:1, 1986.
44. Pearse A: The cytochemistry and ultrastructure of polypeptide hormone-producing cells of the APUD series and the embryologic, physiologic, and pathologic implications of the concept. J Histochem Cytochem 17:303, 1969.
45. Thompson A, Vinik A, Eckhauser F: Microgastrinomas of the duodenum: A cause for failed operations for the Zollinger-Ellison syndrome. Ann Surg 209:396, 1989.
46. Stabile B, Morrow D, Passaro E: The gastrinoma triangle: Operative indications. Am J Surg 147:25, 1984.
47. McCarthy DM: The place of surgery in the Zollinger-Ellison syndrome. N Engl J Med 302:1344, 1980.
48. McCarthy DM: Zollinger-Ellison syndrome. Annu Rev Med 33:197, 1982.
49. Jensen R: Zollinger-Ellison syndrome: Current concepts and management. Ann Intern Med 98:59, 1983.
50. Deveney CW, Deveney KE, Stark D, et al: Resection of gastrinomas. Ann Surg 198:546, 1983.
51. Vinik AI, Strodel WE, Lloyd RV, et al: Unusual gastroenteropancreatic (GEP) tumors and their hormones. In Thompson NW, Vinik AI (eds): Endocrine Surgery Update. New York: Grune & Stratton, 1983, p 293.
52. Stabile B, Braunstein G, Passaro E: Serum gastrin and human chorionic gonadotropin in the Zollinger Ellison syndrome. Arch Surg 115:1090, 1980.
53. Creutzfeldt W, Arnold R, Creutzfeldt C, et al: Pathomorphologic, biochemical and diagnostic aspects of gastrinomas (Zollinger-Ellison syndrome). Hum Pathol 6:47, 1975.
54. Greider MH, Rosai J, McGuigan JE: The human pancreatic islet cells and their tumors. II. Ulcerogenic and diarrheogenic tumors. Cancer 33:1423, 1974.
55. Passaro E Jr, Basso N, Walsh JH: Calcium challenge in the Zollinger-Ellison syndrome. Surgery 72:60, 1972.
56. Isenberg JI: Unusual effect of secretin on serum gastrin, serum calcium and gastric acid secretions in a patient with suspected Zollinger-Ellison syndrome. Gastroenterology 62:626, 1972.
57. Deveney C, Deveney K: Zollinger-Ellison syndrome (gastrinoma): Current diagnosis and treatment. Surg Clin North Am 67:411, 1987.
58. Faye M, Rhodes J, Beck P: Gastric secretion in duodenal ulcer with particular reference to the diagnosis of Zollinger-Ellison syndrome. Gastroenterology 58:476, 1970.
59. Lewin M, Stagg B, Clark C: Gastric acid secretion and diagnosis of Zollinger-Ellison syndrome. Br Med J 2:139, 1973.
60. Aoyagi T, Summerskill W: Gastric secretion with ulcerogenic islet cell tumor: Importance of basal acid output. Arch Intern Med 117:667, 1966.
61. Wank S, Doppman J, Miller D, et al: Prospective study of the ability of computerized axial tomography to localize gastrinomas in patients with Zollinger-Ellison syndrome. Gastroenterology 92:905, 1984.
62. Dunnick N, Doppman J, Mills S, et al: Computed tomographic detection of non-beta pancreatic islet cell tumors. Radiology 135:117, 1980.
63. Fedorak IJ, Ko TC, Gordon D, et al: Localization of islet cell tumors of the pancreas: A review of current techniques. Surgery 113:242, 1993.
64. Frucht H, Doppman JL, Norton JA, et al: Gastrinomas: Comparison of MR imaging with CT, angiography. Ultrasound Radiol 171:713, 1989.
65. Mills S, Doppman J, Dunnick N, et al: Evaluation of angiography in Zollinger-Ellison syndrome. Radiology 131:317, 1979.
66. Debas HT, Soon-Shiong P, McKenzie AD, et al: Use of secretin in the roentgenologic and biochemical diagnosis of duodenal gastrinoma. Am J Surg 145:408, 1983.
67. Wilson SD: Z-E Tumor Registry. Medical College of Wisconsin, 8700 W. Wisconsin Avenue, Milwaukee, WI 53226.
68. Broughan TA, Leslie JD, Soto JM, et al: Pancreatic islet cell tumors. Surgery 99:671, 1986.
69. Deveney C, Deveney K, Jaffe B, et al: Use of calcium and secretin in the diagnosis of gastrinoma. Ann Intern Med 87:680, 1977.
70. Norton J, Collin M, Gardiner J, et al: Prospective study of gastrinoma localization and resection in patients with Zollinger-Ellison syndrome. Ann Surg 204:468, 1986.
71. Fraker DL, Norton JA: Localization and resection of islet cell tumors of the pancreas. JAMA 259:3601, 1988.
72. Roche A, Raisonnier A, Gillon-Savouret MC: Pancreatic venous sampling and arteriography in localizing insulinomas and gastrinomas: Procedure and results in 55 cases. Radiology 145:621, 1982.
73. Doppman JL, Miller DL, Chang R, et al: Gastrinomas: Localization by means of selective intraarterial injection of secretin. Radiology 174:25, 1990.
74. Sigel B, Coelho JCU, Nyhus LM, et al: Detection of pancreatic tumors by ultrasound during surgery. Arch Surg 117:1058, 1982.
75. Johnson L: New aspects of the trophic actions of gastrointestinal hormones. Gastroenterology 72:788, 1977.
76. Jensen R, Collen M, Pandol S: Cimetidine-induced impotence and breast changes in patients with gastric hypersecretory states. N Engl J Med 308:883, 1983.
77. Collen M, Howard J, McArthur K, et al: Comparison of ranitidine and cimetidine in the treatment of gastric hypersecretion. Ann Intern Med 100:52, 1984.
78. Zollinger RM: The ulcerogenic (Zollinger-Ellison) syndrome. In Friesen SR (ed): Surgical Endocrinology: Clinical Syndromes. Philadelphia: JB Lippincott, 1982, p 203.
79. Thompson JC, Lewis BG, Wiener I, et al: The role of surgery in the Zollinger-Ellison syndrome. Ann Surg 197:594, 1983.
80. Raufman JP, Collins S, Pandol S, et al: Reliability of symptoms in assessing control of gastric acid secretion of patients with Zollinger-Ellison syndrome. Gastroenterology 84:108, 1983.
81. Lloyd-Davies KA, Rutgersson K, Lovell S: Omeprazole in Zollinger-Ellison syndrome: Four year international study. Gastroenterology 90:1523, 1986 (abstract).
82. Maton PN, Frucht H, Vinayek R, et al: Medical management of patients with Zollinger-Ellison syndrome who have had previous gastric surgery: A prospective study. Gastroenterology 94:294, 1988.
83. Mignon M, Vallot T, Hervoir P, et al: Ranitidine versus cimetidine in the management of Zollinger-Ellison syndrome. In Riley A, Salmon PR (eds): Ranitidine. Amsterdam: Excerpta Medica, 1982, p 169.
84. Lamers CBHW, Lind T, Moberg S, et al: Omeprazole in Zollinger-Ellison syndrome. N Engl J Med 310:758, 1984.
85. McArthur KE, Collen MJ, Maton PN, et al: Omeprazole: Effective, convenient therapy for Zollinger-Ellison syndrome. Gastroenterology 88:939, 1985.
86. Ekman L, Hansson E, Havu N, et al: Toxicologic studies on omeprazole. Scand J Gastroenterol 108(Suppl):53, 1985.
87. Wilson SD: The role of surgery in children with the Zollinger-Ellison syndrome. Surgery 92:682, 1982.

88. Wolfe MM, Alexander RW, McGuigan JE: Extrapancreatic, extraintestinal gastrinoma: Effective treatment by surgery. N Engl J Med 306:1533, 1982.
89. Bonfils S, Landor J, Mignon M, et al: The results of surgical management in 92 consecutive patients with Zollinger-Ellison syndrome. Ann Surg 194:692, 1981.
90. Herter F, Cooperman A, Ahlborn T: Surgical experience with pancreatic and periampullary cancer. Ann Surg 195:274, 1982.
91. Crist D, Sitzmann J, Cameron J: Improved hospital morbidity, mortality, and survival after the Whipple procedure. Ann Surg 206:358, 1987.
92. Richardson C, Peters M, Feldman M, et al: Treatment of Zollinger-Ellison syndrome with exploratory laparotomy, proximal gastric vagotomy, and H_2-receptor antagonists. Gastroenterology 89:357, 1985.
93. Fox PS, Hofmann JW, Wilson SD, et al: Surgical management of the Zollinger-Ellison syndrome. Surg Clin North Am 54:395, 1974.
94. Thompson NW, Lloyd RV, Nishiyama RH, et al: MEN I pancreas: A histologic and immunohistochemical study. World J Surg 8:561, 1984.
95. van Heerden JA, Smith SL, Miller LJ: Management of the Zollinger-Ellison syndrome in patients with multiple endocrine neoplasia type I. Surgery 100:971, 1986.
96. Stabile BE, Passaro E Jr: Benign and malignant gastrinoma. Am J Surg 149:144, 1985.
97. Norton J, Cornelius M, Doppman J, et al: Effect of parathyroidectomy in patients with hyperparathyroidism, Zollinger-Ellison syndrome, and multiple endocrine metaplasia type I: A prospective study. Surgery 102:958, 1987.
98. Tisell LE, Ahlman H, Jansson S, et al: Total pancreatectomy in the MEN I syndrome. Br J Surg 75:154, 1988.
99. Malagelada JR, Edis AJ, Adson MA, et al: Medical and surgical options in the management of patients with gastrinoma. Gastroenterology 84:1524, 1983.
100. Norton J, Doppman J, Gardner J, et al: Aggressive resection of metastatic disease in selected patients with malignant gastrinoma. Ann Surg 203:352, 1986.
101. Moertel C, Hanley J, Johnson L: Streptozotocin alone compared to streptozotocin and fluorouracil in the treatment of advanced islet cell carcinoma. N Engl J Med 303:1189, 1980.
102. Broder L, Carter S: Pancreatic islet cell carcinoma. II. Results of treatment with streptozotocin in 52 patients. Ann Intern Med 79:108, 1973.
103. Awrich A, Fletcher W, Klotz J, et al: 5-FU versus combination therapy with tubercidin, streptozotocin, and 5-FU in the treatment of pancreatic carcinomas: COG protocol 7230. J Surg Oncol 12:267, 1979.
104. Zollinger RM: Gastrinoma: Factors influencing prognosis. Surgery 97:49, 1985.
105. Jaffe B: Surgery for gut hormone-producing tumors. Am J Med 82:68, 1987.
106. Koolie H, White T: Pancreatic islet beta cell tumors and hyperplasia: Experience in 14 Seattle hospitals. Ann Surg 175:326, 1972.
107. Broder L, Carter S: Pancreatic islet cell carcinoma. Clinical features of 52 patients. Ann Intern 79:101, 1973.
108. Service F, van Heerden J, Sheedy P: Insulinoma. In Service F (ed): Hypoglycemic Disorders—Pathogenesis, Diagnosis, and Treatment. Boston: GK Hall Medical Publishers, 1983, p 111.
109. Stefanini P, Carboni M, Patrassi N, et al: Beta-islet cell tumors of the pancreas: Results of a study on 1,067 cases. Surgery 75:597, 1974.
110. Kaplan E, Arganini M, Kang S: Diagnosis and treatment of hypoglycemic disorders. Surg Clin North Am 67:395, 1987.
111. Prinz R: Islet-cell tumors of the pancreas. Res Medica 3:3, 1986.
112. Kavlie H, White TT: Pancreatic islet beta-cell tumors and hyperplasia. Ann Surg 175:326, 1972.
113. Danforth D, Gordon P, Brennan M: Metastatic insulin secreting carcinoma of the pancreas: Clinical course and the role of surgery. Surgery 96:1027, 1984.
114. Service F, Dale A, Elveback L, et al: Insulinoma—clinical and diagnostic features of 60 consecutive cases. Mayo Clin Proc 51:417, 1976.
115. Rasbach D, van Heerden J, Telander R, et al: Surgical management of hyperinsulinism in the multiple endocrine neoplasia type I syndrome. Arch Surg 120:584, 1985.
116. Proye C: Surgical strategy in insulinoma: Clinical review. Acta Chir Scand 153:481, 1987.
117. Whipple AO, Frantz VK: Adenoma of islet cells with hyperinsulinism: A review. Ann Surg 101:1299, 1935.
118. Harrison TS: Hyperinsulinism and its surgical management. In Hardy JD (ed): Rhoad's Surgery, Principles and Practice. Philadelphia: JB Lippincott, 1977.
119. Moss NH, Kaplan EL: Insulinoma and nesidioblastosis. In Howard JM, Jordan GL Jr, Reber HA (eds): Surgical Diseases of the Pancreas. Philadelphia: Lea & Febiger, 1987.
120. Rubenstein AH, Kuzuya H, Horwitz DL: Clinical significance of circulating C-peptide in diabetes mellitus and hypoglycemic disorders. Arch Intern Med 137:625, 1977.
121. Turner RC, Heding LG: Plasma proinsulin, C-peptide and insulin in diagnostic suppression tests for insulinomas. Diabetologia 13:571, 1977.
122. Klein RF, Seino S, Sanz N, et al: High-performance liquid chromatography used to distinguish the autoimmune hypoglycemia syndrome from factitious hypoglycemia. J Clin Endocrinol Metab 61:571, 1985.
123. Berger M, Bordi C, Cuppers H, et al: Functional and morphologic characterization of human insulinomas. Diabetes 32:921, 1983.
124. Service F, Horowitz D, Rubenstein A, et al: The C-peptide suppression test for insulinoma. J Lab Clin Med 90:180, 1977.
125. Dunnick N, Long J, Krudy A, et al: Localizing insulinomas with combined radiographic methods. AJR 135:747, 1982.
126. Fulton R, Sheedy P, McIlrath D, et al: Preoperative angiographic localization of insulin-producing tumors of the pancreas. AJR 123:367, 1975.
127. Gunther RW, Klose KJ, Ruckert K, et al: Localization of small islet-cell tumors. Preoperative and intraoperative ultrasound, computed tomography, arteriography, digital subtraction angiography, and pancreatic venous sampling. Gastrointest Radiol 10:142, 1985.
128. Cho KJ, Vinik AI, Thompson NW, et al: Localization of the source of hyperinsulinism: Percutaneous transhepatic portal and pancreatic vein catheterization with hormone assay. Am J Roentgenol 139:237, 1982.
129. Doppmann JL, Brennan MF, Dunnick NR, et al: The role of pancreatic venous sampling in the localization of occult insulinomas. Radiology 138:557, 1981.
130. Ingemansson S, Kuhl C, Larson LI, et al: Localization of insulinomas and islet cell hyperplasias by pancreatic vein catheterization and insulin assay. Surg Gynecol Obstet 146:725, 1978.
131. Doppmann JL, Miller DL, Chang R, et al: Insulinomas: Localization with selective intraarterial injection of calcium. Radiology 178:237, 1991.
132. Gorman B, Charboneau J, James E, et al: Benign pancreatic insulinoma: Preoperative and intraoperative sonographic localization. AJR 147:929, 1986.
133. Laroche GP, Ferris DO, Priestley JT, et al: Hyperinsulinism: Surgical results and management of occult functioning islet cell tumors: Review of 154 cases. Arch Surg 96:763, 1968.
134. Fonkalsrud EW, Dilley RB, Longmire WP: Insulin secreting tumors of the pancreas. Ann Surg 159:730, 1964.
135. Stringel G, Dalpe-Scott M, Perelman AH, et al: The occult insulinoma—operative localization by quick insulin radioimmunoassay. J Pediatr Surg 20:734, 1985.
136. Tutt GO Jr, Edis AJ, Service FJ, et al: Plasma glucose monitoring during operation for insulinoma: A critical reappraisal. Surgery 88:351, 1980.
137. Filipi CJ, Higgins GA: Diagnosis and management of insulinoma. Am J Surg 125:231, 1973.
138. Woltering E, Mozell E, O'Dorisio T, et al: Suppression of primary and secondary peptides with somatostatin analog in the therapy of functional endocrine tumors. Surg Gynecol Obstet 167:453, 1988.
139. Sardi A, Singer J: Insulinoma and gastrinoma in Wermer's disease (MEN I). Arch Surg 122:835, 1987.
140. Howard T, Stabile B, Zinner M, et al: Anatomic distribution of pancreatic endocrine tumors. Am J Surg 159:258, 1990.
141. Schein P, Kahn R, Gordon P, et al: Streptozotocin for malignant insulinoma and carcinoid tumor: Report of eight cases and review of the literature. Arch Intern Med 132:555, 1973.
142. Bloom S, Polak J: Glucagonoma syndrome. Am J Med 82:25, 1987.
143. Leichter S: Clinical and metabolic aspects of glucagonoma. Medicine 59:100, 1980.

144. Guillausseau PJ, Guillausseau C, Villet R, et al: Les glucagonomes. Aspects cliniques, biologiques, anatomo-pathologiques et therapeutiques (revue generale de 130 cas). Gastroenterol Clin Biol 6:1029, 1982.
145. Ohneda A, Otsuki M, Fujiya H, et al: A malignant insulinoma transformed into a glucagonoma syndrome. Diabetes 28:962, 1979.
146. Kahan R, Perez-Figaredo M, Neimanis A: Necrolytic migratory erythema. Distinctive dermatosis of the glucagonoma syndrome. Arch Dermatol 113:792, 1977.
147. Mallison CN, Kahn CR, Schieberger R, et al: A glucagonoma syndrome. Lancet 2:1, 1974.
148. Norton JA, Jaspan J, Kasselberg T, et al: Amino acid deficiency and the skin rash associated with glucagonoma. Ann Intern Med 91:213, 1979.
149. Stacpoole PW, Jaspan J, Kasselberg T, et al: A familial glucagonoma syndrome. Am J Med 70:1017, 1981.
150. Prinz RA, Sugimoto J, Lorincz A, et al: Glucagonoma. In Howard JM, Jordan GL Jr, Reber HA (eds): Surgical Diseases of the Pancreas. Philadelphia, Lea & Febiger, 1987, p 848.
151. Roggli VI, Judge DM, McGavran MH: Duodenal glucagonoma: A case report. Hum Pathol 10:350, 1979.
152. O'Dorisio T, O'Dorisio M: Endocrine tumors of the gastroenteropancreatic (GEP) axis. In Mazzaferri E (ed): Endocrinology. New York: Elsevier Science Publishing, 1985, p 764.
153. Holst J: Glucagon-producing tumors. In Cohen S, Soloway R (eds): Hormone-Producing Tumors of the Gastrointestinal Tract. New York: Churchill Livingstone, 1985, p 57.
154. Warn T, Block M, Hafiz G, et al: Glucagonomas. Ultrastructure and immunocytochemistry. Cancer 51:1091, 1983.
155. Naets J, Gans M: Inhibitory effect of glucagon on erythropoiesis. Blood 55:997, 1980.
156. Friesen S: Update on the diagnosis and treatment of rare neuroendocrine tumors. Surg Clin North Am 67:2, 1987.
157. Ingemansson S, Holst J, Larsson L, et al: Localization of glucagonomas by pancreatic vein catheterization and glucagon assay. Surg Gynecol Obstet 145:509, 1977.
158. Zollinger R, Ellison E, Carey L, et al: Observations on the postoperative tumor growth of certain islet cell tumors. Ann Surg 184:525, 1976.
159. Higgins G, Recant C, Fischman A: The glucagonoma syndrome. Surgically curable diabetes. Am J Surg 137:142, 1979.
160. Prinz RA: Glucagonoma syndrome. Surg Rounds 10:63, 1987.
161. Valverde I, Lemon HM, Kessinger A, et al: Distribution of plasma glucagon immunoreactivity in a patient with suspected glucagonoma. J Clin Endocrinol Metab 42:804, 1976.
162. Hendry WS, Munro A: Pancreatic glucagonoma with lymph node metastases: Disease-free survival six years after resection. J R Coll Surg Edinb 31:115, 1986.
163. Danforth DN, Triche T, Doppman JL, et al: Elevated plasma proglucagon-like component with a glucagon secreting tumor: Effect of streptozotocin. N Engl J Med 295:242, 1976.
164. Kvols L, Buck M, Fischman A: Chemotherapy of metastatic carcinoid and islet cell tumors. Am J Med 82:77, 1987.
165. Prinz RA, Badrinath K, Banerji M, et al: Operative and chemotherapeutic management of malignant glucagon-producing tumors. Surgery 90:713, 1981.
166. Kessinger A, Foley J, Lemon H: Treatment of malignant APUD cell tumors. Effectiveness of DTIC. Cancer 51:790, 1983.
167. Hallengren B, Dymling JF, Manhem P, et al: Unsuccessful DTIC treatment of a patient with glucagonoma syndrome. Acta Med Scand 213:317, 1983.
168. Boden G, Ryan I, Eisenschmid B, et al: Treatment of inoperable glucagonoma with the long-acting somatostatin analog SMS 201-995. N Engl J Med 315:1686, 1986.
169. Sheehan-Dare RA, Simmons AV, Cotterill JA, et al: Hepatic tumors with hyperglucagonemia. Cancer 62:912, 1988.
170. Jones DV Jr, Samaan NA, Sellin RV, et al: Metastatic glucagonoma: Clinical response to a combination of 5-fluorouracil and α-interferon. Am J Med 93:348, 1992.
171. Verner JV, Morrison AB: Endocrine pancreatic islet disease with diarrhea: Report of a case due to diffuse hyperplasia of non-beta islet tissue with a review of 54 additional cases. Arch Intern Med 133:492, 1974.
172. Fausa O, Fretheim B, Elgjo K, et al: Intractable watery diarrhea, hypokalemia, and achlorhydria associated with nonpancreatic retroperitoneal neurogenic tumor containing VIP. Scand J Gastroenterol 8:713, 1973.
173. Bloom SR: Vasoactive intestinal polypeptide, the major mediator of the WDHA (pancreatic cholera) syndrome: Value of measurement in diagnosis and treatment. Am J Dig Dis 23:373, 1978.
174. Long RG, Bryant MG, Mitchell SJ, et al: Clinicopathologic study of pancreatic and ganglioneuroblastoma tumors secreting vasoactive intestinal polypeptide (VIPomas). Br Med J 282:1767, 1981.
175. Krejs G: VIPoma syndrome. Am J Med 82:37, 1987.
176. Telling M, Smiddy FG: Islet tumors of the pancreas with intractable diarrhea. Gut 2:12, 1961.
177. Bloom S, Long R, Bryant M, et al: Clinical, biochemical, and pathological studies on 62 vipomas. Gastroenterology 78:1143, 1980.
178. Zollinger RM, Tompkins RK, Amerson JR, et al: Identification of the diarrheogenic hormone associated with non-beta islet cell tumors of the pancreas. Ann Surg 168:502, 1968.
179. McGill DB, Carney JA, Phillips SF, et al: Hormonal diarrhea due to pancreatic tumor. Gastroenterology 79:571, 1980.
180. Daggett P, Goodburn E, Kurtz A, et al: Is preoperative localization of glucagonomas necessary? Lancet 1:483, 1981.
181. O'Dorisio T, Mekhjian H: VIPoma syndrome. In Cohen S, Soloway R (eds): Hormone-Producing Tumors of the Gastrointestinal Tract. New York: Churchill Livingstone, 1985, p 101.
182. Rosch J, Holman D: Superselective arteriography of the pancreas. In Anacker H (ed): Efficacy and Limitations of Radiologic Diagnosis of the Pancreas. Stuttgart: Georg Thieme, 1975, p 159.
183. Kingham J, Dick R, Bloom S, et al: Vipoma: Localization by percutaneous transhepatic portal venous sampling. Br Med J 2:1682, 1978.
184. Ellison E, O'Dorisio T, Benson G: Modulation of functional gastrointestinal endocrine tumors by endogenous and exogenous somatostatin. Am J Surg 151:668, 1986.
185. Jaffee B, Kopen D, De Schryver-Kecskemeti K, et al: Indomethacin-responsive pancreatic cholera. N Engl J Med 297:817, 1977.
186. Nagorney DM, Bloom SR, Polak JM, et al: Resolution of recurrent Verner-Morrison syndrome by resection of metastatic VIPoma. Surgery 93:348, 1983.
187. Gagel R, Costanza M, DeLellis R, et al: Streptozotocin-treated Verner-Morrison syndrome: Plasma vasoactive intestinal polypeptide and tumor response. Arch Intern Med 136:1429, 1976.
188. Kahn C, Levy A, Gardner J, et al: Pancreatic cholera: Beneficial effect of treatment with streptozotocin. N Engl J Med 292:941, 1975.
189. Raskone A, Rue E, Chavialle J, et al: Effect of somatostatin on small bowel water and electrolyte transport in a patient with pancreatic cholera. Dig Dis Sci 27:459, 1982.
190. Thompson JC, Marx M: Gastrointestinal hormones. Curr Probl Surg 21:1, 1984.
191. Crain EL Jr, Thorn GW: Functioning pancreatic islet cell adenomas. Medicine 28:427, 1949.
192. Vinik AI, Strodel WE, Eckhauser FE, et al: Somatostatinomas, PPomas, and neurotensionomas. Semin Oncol 14:263, 1987.
193. Vale W, Rivier C, Brown M: Regulatory peptides of the hypothalamus. Annu Rev Physiol 39:473, 1977.
194. Harris G, Tio F, Cruz A: Somatostatinoma: A case report and review of the literature. J Surg Oncol 36:8, 1987.
195. Jackson J, Raju U, Fachnie JD, et al: Malignant somatostatinoma presenting with diabetic ketoacidosis. Clin Endocrinol 26:609, 1987.
196. Somers G, Pipeleers-Marichal M, Gepts W, et al: A case of duodenal somatostatinoma: Diagnostic usefulness of calcium-pentagastrin test. Gastroenterology 85:1192, 1983.
197. Kaneko H, Yanaihara N, Ito S, et al: Somatostatinoma of the duodenum. Cancer 44:2273, 1979.
198. Reynolds C, Pratt R, Chan-yan C, et al: Somatostatinoma—the most recently described pancreatic islet cell tumor. West J Med 142:393, 1985.
199. Dayal Y, Tallberg K, Nunnemacher G, et al: Duodenal carcinoids in patients with and without neurofibromatosis. Am J Surg Pathol 10:348, 1986.
200. Griffiths D, Williams G, Williams E: Duodenal carcinoid tumors, pheochromocytoma and neurofibromatosis. Islet cell tumor, pheochromocytoma and the Von Hippel–Lindau complex: Two distinctive neuroendocrine syndromes. Q J Med 64:769, 1987.
201. Bloom SR, Polak JM: Glucagonomas, VIPomas, and somatostatinomas. Clin Endocrinol Metab 9:285, 1980.

202. Boden G, Shimoyama R: Somatostatinoma. In Cohen S, Soloway R (eds): Hormone-Producing Tumors of the Gastrointestinal Tract. New York: Churchill Livingstone, 1985, p 85.
203. Rouiller D, Schusdziarra V, Harris V, et al: Release of pancreatic and gastric somatostatin-like immuno-reactivity in response to the octapeptide of cholecystokinin, secretin, gastric inhibitory polypeptide and gastrin-17 in dogs. Endocrinology 107:524, 1980.
204. Sakazaki S, Umeyama K, Nakagawa H, et al: Pancreatic somatostatinoma. Am J Surg 146:674, 1983.
205. Kelly TR: Pancreatic somatostatinoma. Am J Surg 146:671, 1983.
206. Howard JM, Moss NH, Rhoads JE: Hyperinsulinism and islet cell tumors. Surg Gynecol Obstet 90:417, 1950.
207. Kent RB III, van Heerden JA, Weiland LH: Nonfunctioning islet cell tumors. Ann Surg 193:185, 1981.
208. Prinz RA, Badrinath K, Chejfec G, et al: "Nonfunctioning" islet cell carcinoma of the pancreas. Am Surg 49:345, 1983.
209. Legaspi A, Brennan MF: Management of islet cell carcinoma. Surgery 104:1018, 1988.

6

Cancer of the Colon, Rectum, and Anus

Colorectal Cancer

Catherine Mahut, M.D. • Hartley S. Stern, M.D.

INCIDENCE

Colorectal cancer is a leading cause of death in Western societies. It now represents nearly 11% of all cancer diagnoses and is the second most common cause of cancer mortality in the United States.[1] Approximately 55,000 deaths from colorectal cancer are predicted in the United States in 1995, with 138,000 new cases diagnosed.[2]

A review of recent data shows a steadily rising incidence from 1950 to a peak of 67 in 100,000 in 1986. (Since that time, there has been a steady, as of yet unexplained, slight decline.) Mortality remained steady during this interval. When colon and rectal cancer statistics are reviewed separately, it is apparent that the increase has occurred owing to a rising incidence of colon cancer, while the incidence of rectal cancer has remained stable (Table 6–1).

Discrepancies persist in both incidence and mortality in black versus white populations. The incidence of colon cancer increased in blacks by 30.6% over the 15 years preceding 1988, while there was only a 5.4% increase in whites during the same period.[1] Mortality for blacks also increased during this period, to 22.4% for colon and rectum cancers combined. Mortality for whites decreased to 19.4% during the same period.

ETIOLOGY

Genetics

The etiology of colorectal cancer is complex and multifactorial. A great deal of work has been done to elucidate risk factors that play a role in the development of this disease.

The genetics of colorectal carcinoma, and the development of preceding adenomas, have also been studied extensively. Three clinical patterns of inheritance have been described: (1) the familial adenomatous polyposis (FAP) syndrome, (2) the hereditary nonpolyposis colorectal cancer (HNPCC) syndrome, and (3) sporadic adenomatous polyps.[3]

TABLE 6–1
Age-Adjusted Cancer Incidence Rates from the Surveillance, Epidemiology, and End Results Program 1973–88 (Men and Women)*

Site	Average Rate (%)†		Percent Change 1973–88	EAPC 1973–88 (%)
	1973–74	*1987–88*		
Whites				
Colon/rectum	47.5	48.5	2.1	0.3
Colon	32.6	34.4	5.4	0.6
Rectum	14.9	14.2	−5.0	−0.3
All sites	325.7	380.2	16.8	1.1
Blacks				
Colon/rectum	41.3	50.7	22.7	1.4
Colon	29.9	39.0	30.6	1.8
Rectum	11.4	11.6	2.1	0.4
All sites	347.5	404.2	16.3	1.3

Adapted from Greenwald P: Colon Cancer Overview. Cancer 70(5): 1206–1215, 1992.

EAPC, Estimated annual percent change during the 16-year period.

*Rates are per 100,000 and are age-adjusted to the 1970 United States standard population.

†Average annual rate during the specified 2-year period.

Familial Adenomatous Polyposis

The FAP syndrome is characterized by autosomal dominant transmission, typified by the development of hundreds of adenomatous polyps of the colon.[4] These commonly begin to occur during late childhood or early adulthood. Colon cancer is an inevitable outcome if a prophylactic colectomy is not performed. These cancers are predominantly left-sided, with an average age at diagnosis of 39 years.

Affected individuals also have an increased incidence of polyps within the remainder of the gastrointestinal tract. Up to 50% of subjects have hyperplastic gastric polyps that are benign and can be ignored.[5] Duodenal adenomatous polyps are even more common, being present in almost all cases. These carry a lifetime risk of 10% to 12% for periampullary cancer and may also cause symptoms due to biliary or pancreatic obstruction. Periampullary cancer is now replacing colon cancer in these individuals as the major cause of death.[6] The remainder of the small intestine also harbors occasional adenomatous polyps, although these have very low malignant potential and are rarely symptomatic. Additionally, other benign, extracolonic tumors, including osteomas, epidermal inclusion cysts, and fibromas, represent a separate phenotype, previously referred to as Gardner's syndrome. Desmoid tumors and mesenteric fibromatosis are potentially troubling manifestations owing to their propensity for local recurrence and encroachment on the mesenteric vascular supply, and they are currently the second leading cause of death in these individuals.[6]

Recent advances in the field of molecular genetics have resulted in the identification of the gene mutation responsible for adenomatous polyposis coli (APC). The APC gene is on the long arm of chromosome 5, and any one of several observed mutations results in the clinical syndromes under discussion.[7] Linkage analysis can identify those individuals who have inherited the mutated APC gene.[8, 9] An accumulation of several molecular genetic mutations is required to produce colorectal carcinoma in FAP and sporadic colon cancers.

Hereditary Nonpolyposis Colorectal Cancer

HNPCC encompasses two distinct clinical presentations of colorectal cancer. In both, there is autosomal dominant inheritance of predominantly right and transverse colon cancers, with an average age at diagnosis of 45 years.[10] Adenomatous polyps are present, but polyposis is not. An increased risk of metachronous and synchronous colonic cancers is recognized, with a risk of up to 40% at 10 years following the initial colon cancer.[11] One of these clinical scenarios is associated with an elevated incidence of extracolonic carcinomas, most notably endometrial carcinoma, while the other is not.[12] Other carcinomas found more frequently in this syndrome include gastric, urologic, laryngeal, ovarian, pancreatic, and bile duct carcinomas.[13] The gene mutation or mutations responsible for this syndrome have not yet been identified, although several laboratories are actively pursuing this. Thus, an increased emphasis is placed on an accurate, complete family history, as this is the only method available to differentiate HNPCC cases from sporadic ones.

Recently, a working definition of HNPCC was proposed by the International Collaborative Group on Hereditary Nonpolyposis Colorectal Cancer,[14] to include:

1. At least three relatives in a family must have histologically verified colorectal cancer, and one of the relatives should be a first-degree relative to the other two; FAP should be excluded.
2. At least two successive generations should be affected.
3. In one of the affected patients, colorectal carcinoma should be diagnosed when the patient is younger than 50 years of age.

"Clustered" Colon Cancer

Although FAP and HNPCC have received much attention, more than 90% of cases of colonic adenomatous polyps are "sporadic" in nature.[3] In spite of this label, a careful family history remains of paramount importance, as familial clustering of these neoplasms has been documented. Population studies have revealed an increased two- to threefold risk for colon cancer in first-degree relatives of those with colon cancer.[15–17] This risk persists when those with HPNCC or FAP are excluded from the analysis.

A recent study of a large Utah kindred of more than 5000 individuals related to a pair of siblings and a nephew with colon cancer was carried out, with spouses as the control group.[18] An increased number of adenomatous polyps (21% vs. 9%, $P < .005$) was found in the members of the kindred. An analysis of the pedigree strongly suggested that the adenomatous polyps and colon cancer were inherited in an autosomal dominant pattern with variable penetrance.

Gene Mutations

Further work is ongoing to elucidate other gene mutations that play a role in the development of colorectal cancer. It is recognized that a series of genetic alterations must occur for colorectal carcinoma to develop.[19–21]

EPIDEMIOLOGY

Major geographic differences exist in colon cancer incidence and prevalence rates around the world, with the highest rates occurring in the developed world (except Japan), intermediate rates in Eastern Europe, and low rates in Asia and Africa.[22] These differences diminish within one generation in migrants moving from countries of low incidence to North America.[23, 24] Such data provide support for the importance of environmental factors in this disease. From population studies, a number of dietary factors have been implicated as showing a positive correlation with colon cancer incidence—namely, high calories, meat, and fat.[25, 26] Others appear to have a protective effect, such as cruciferous vegetables, starch, fiber, calcium, selenium, and vitamins A, C, and E.[27, 28]

Case-control studies based on diet records have been performed to further evaluate the findings of the population studies. There has been a lack of agreement among the published results. Although the results of several earlier studies suggested that dietary fat exerted an important effect on colon cancer risk,[25, 26] others indicated simple sugars, total calories, or complex carbohydrates to be of greater importance.[29, 30]

Fiber

The role of dietary fiber in the pathogenesis of colorectal cancer has been the focus of intensive research ever since Burkitt postulated a link in 1971.[22] Many studies have linked a high-fiber diet with a decreased risk of developing colon cancer, but these findings have not been unanimous. A recent critical review of epidemiologic studies published since 1970 identified 43 papers, of which 37 were subsequently analyzed.[31] Twenty-one of the studies strongly or moderately supported the hypothesis that fiber was protective against colon cancer. Only two studies were definitive in not showing such a protective effect.

Although such agreement is impressive, many questions remain unanswered. The mechanism by which dietary fiber exerts its protective effects has not been positively identified. Postulated mechanisms include a secondary change of gut flora,[32] increased stool bulk with subsequent dilution of potentially harmful substances, and a primary impact on bile acid metabolism, including the production, absorption, and enterohepatic circulation of bile acids.[33] Fecal secondary bile acids have been shown to be colonic tumor promoters, and studies have documented a decrease in the concentration of fecal bile acids in humans on a high wheat bran diet.[34] The prevalence of fecal mutagens is increased in populations at increased risk for colon cancer.[35] Human studies have documented a reduction in fecal mutagenic activity in individuals taking supplemental fiber in the form of 11 g of cereal fiber daily for 4 weeks.[36] The actual implications of such results, and the extent of the role these mutagens play in the development of human colorectal cancer, remain to be further elucidated.

Other areas of controversy are the relative importance of soluble versus insoluble fiber in providing a protective effect, as well as the actual source of the fiber.[37] Much of the data do not permit differentiation of cereal and grain sources of fiber from vegetable sources, and it is unclear whether other unidentified variables are at play in providing this protective effect. The Second National Health and Nutrition Examination was conducted in the United States from 1976 to 1980, revealing that vegetables are the population's primary source of fiber, followed by bread and fruit.[38] It was also found that Americans consume only 10 g of fiber daily, on average, in contrast to the 20 to 30 g of daily fiber recommended by the National Cancer Institute (NCI).[39]

Fat

The evidence that persons consuming large amounts of fat are at high risk for colorectal cancer is based mainly on international epidemiologic and case-control studies.[22, 26] Also, several experimental animal studies have supported this assumption.[40, 41] Dietary fat has been suggested to be a promoter of colorectal cancer by being a source of free fatty acids and by increasing the concentration of bile acids in the feces.[42] In a typical high-fat Western diet, dietary fat is the source of about 75% of the fecal fatty acids.[43] Soluble fatty acids damage the colonic mucosa in humans, while animal studies have shown that secondary bile acids also cause mucosal damage.[44] In each case, the damage is repaired by rapid cell proliferation, providing an opportunity for hyperplasia and neoplasia. Thus, cell proliferation may be considered to be due to the promoting effect of dietary fat.

Stadler et al.[45] have demonstrated that consumption of 90 g of corn oil per day increases colonic proliferation indices.[45] In light of this, analysis of international data has led to a recommendation that daily fat intake be limited to 15% to 25% of total calories.[46] Several other studies have suggested that a high saturated fat intake is associated with a higher risk of colon cancer, while such correlations with monounsaturated or polyunsaturated fats (such as olive oil or fish oil) have not been documented.[47] Intervention studies in high-risk populations with low-fat, high-fiber diets have failed to demonstrate an overall protective effect for colon cancer risk based on proliferation indices.[48]

Calcium

Calcium reacts with soluble fatty and bile acids to form insoluble bile salts and thus reduces the concentration of bile acids in the stool.[49] When rat colons were perfused with graded doses of deoxycholic acid, a secondary bile acid, there was epithelial damage and loss of DNA in the perfusion stream. This damage was inhibited if the bile acid was mixed with a calcium salt solution.[50]

Lipkin and Newmark[51] showed a significant reduction in proliferation indices of persons from nonpolyposis cancer families after calcium supplementation for 2 to 3 months. Rozen and colleagues[52] have shown that calcium suppresses increased rectal epithelial proliferation found in asymptomatic first-degree relatives of colorectal cancer patients. However, Gregoire et al.[53] and Stern and coworkers[54] have demonstrated no reduction in proliferative indices with calcium. Thus, calcium supplementation for colon cancer risk reduction remains controversial.

Alcohol, Fecal pH, and Vitamins

Rectal cancer has not been demonstrated to be associated with the same environmental factors associated with colon cancer. There is, however, some evidence suggesting a link between rectal cancer and alcohol consumption.[55, 56]

Reduced fecal pH is thought to have a protective effect by possibly precipitating bile acids, taking them out of solution and thus rendering them unavailable for inducing colonic damage. However, intervention studies with stool acidification have not confirmed this.[57]

Vitamins A, C, E, and selenium are thought to have a protective effect via possible antioxidant effects. Long-term intervention studies have not confirmed these results.[27, 28]

Inflammatory Bowel Disease

A history of inflammatory bowel disease is a well-recognized risk factor for the development of colorectal carcinoma. Since the first reports of colon cancer in a patient with ulcerative colitis in 1925,[58] numerous studies have confirmed the link.[59–61] An increased incidence of colon cancer in patients with Crohn's disease has more recently been established.[61, 62]

The underlying pathogenetic mechanisms have not been clearly demonstrated, but chronic inflammation is presumed to play a major role. Molecular genetic studies have recently shown that these carcinomas are less commonly associated with a common mutation of the K-*ras* proto-oncogene than carcinomas in the general population.[63]

Ekbom et al.[64] published results of a population-based study in 1990. More than 3000 patients with ulcerative colitis were followed through 1984; follow-up ranged from 1 to 60 years after diagnosis. As expected, this cohort demonstrated an increased incidence of colorectal cancer, with a standardized incidence ratio of 5.7. Independent risk factors for colorectal cancer were extent of disease at diagnosis and the patient's age at diagnosis. The absolute risk of colorectal cancer was 30% 35 years after a diagnosis of pancolitis and 40% for those initially diagnosed when younger than 15 years old. Other authors have suggested lower rates.[60, 65, 66] The optimal interval between surveillance colonoscopies and the timing and indications for prophylactic colectomy persist as areas requiring further delineation.

ANATOMY

Colon

The colon begins at the ileocecal valve and ends at the rectum. The right and left colon are fixed, while the transverse and sigmoid colon are more mobile owing to their mesocolons. The appendix arises from the inferior aspect of the cecum, and the greater omentum is attached to the anterosuperior edge of the transverse colon.

Four layers compose the colonic wall: mucosa, submucosa, muscularis, and serosa. The mucosa is composed of closely apposed, straight, tubular glands throughout the length of the colon. There are two muscle layers: an inner circular layer and an outer longitudinal layer, which actually consists of three distinct bands, the teniae coli, spaced at equal intervals along the circumference of the bowel. The teniae converge at the base of the appendix and become indistinct at the rectosigmoid junction, where they splay out, becoming evenly distributed around the bowel. Between the teniae, the bowel wall forms sacculations called haustra, which are separated by folds of the bowel wall, the plicae semilunares. The appendices epiploicae are fatty appendages on the serosal surface.

The luminal diameter of the colon is widest in the cecum, averaging 8 cm, and then steadily decreases to 2 to 3 cm in the sigmoid colon.

Rectum

The rectum spans 12 to 15 cm, from the rectosigmoid junction to the anal canal, at the level of the levator ani muscles to the pelvic floor. The peritoneum covers the proximal third of the rectum anteriorly and along both sides. The middle third is covered by peritoneum only anteriorly, while the distal third is entirely extraperitoneal.

The peritoneal reflection anteriorly lies approximately 7 cm from the anal verge, delineating the rectouterine pouch of Douglas in females. In males, the anterior peritoneal reflection lies posterior to the bladder. The valves of Houston are three mucosal folds present at varying distances from the anal verge. Typically, two of these folds arise on the left side and one on the right.

The extraperitoneal rectum is attached to the sacrum by way of rectosacral fascia, also known as Waldeyer's fascia. Denonvilliers' rectovesical fascia is found anteriorly. The lateral stalks of the rectum are thickened bands of the endopelvic fascia.

Blood Supply

The superior mesenteric artery, via its ileocolic, right colic, and middle colic branches, supplies the right colon from the ileocecal valve to the midtransverse colon. The aorta gives rise to the inferior mesenteric artery at the level of L-3. Its first branch, the left colic artery, supplies the splenic flexure and descending colon. The sigmoid arteries supply the sigmoid colon, and then the inferior mesenteric artery terminates as the superior rectal artery. The marginal artery of Drummond courses along the mesenteric aspect of the colon, providing an anastomosis between the superior and the inferior mesenteric arterial territories (Fig. 6–1). The superior rectal artery supplies the superior aspect of the rectum and anastomoses with the two middle rectal arteries, branches of the internal iliac artery. The inferior rectal artery arises from the internal pudendal artery and traverses Alcock's canal before reaching the inferior rectum and anal canal.

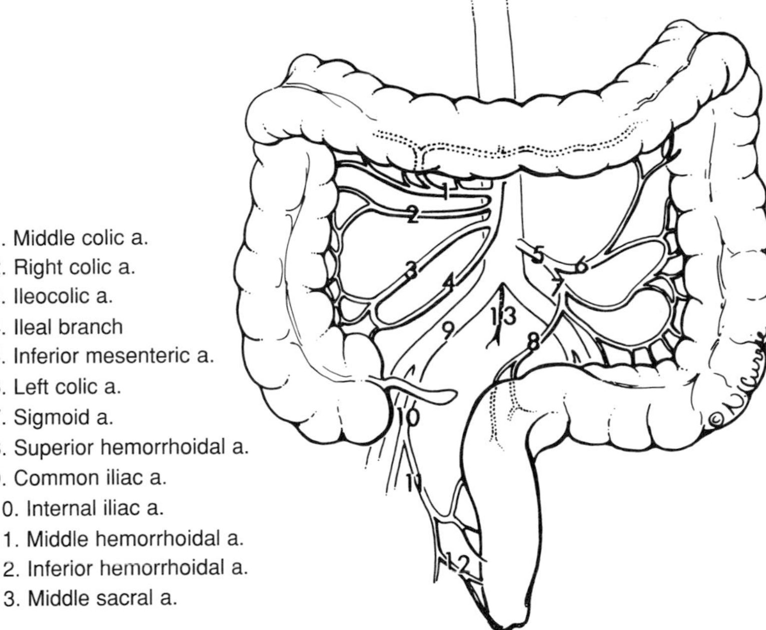

FIGURE 6–1. Vascular supply of the colon and rectum.

The venous drainage of the colon and rectum essentially follows the arterial supply. Venous blood from the colon and superior rectum drains into the liver through the portal vein, while the remainder of the rectum is drained into the internal iliac veins and thus directly into the systemic circulation.

Lymphatic Drainage

Lymphatics within the colon originate as an intramural plexus within the muscularis mucosa. These then empty into epicolic nodes found immediately adjacent to the bowel wall. The next echelon of nodes, the paracolic nodes, are found in the mesentery, while the intermediate nodes lie alongside the main arterial branches of the superior and inferior mesenteric arteries. The main nodes are at the origins of these arteries.

Generally, the lymphatics of the colon follow the arterial supply. The upper rectum is drained by lymphatics, which enter the inferior mesenteric nodes. Lymph from the middle rectum flows into the internal iliac nodes as well as superiorly to the inferior mesenteric nodes. The lower rectum

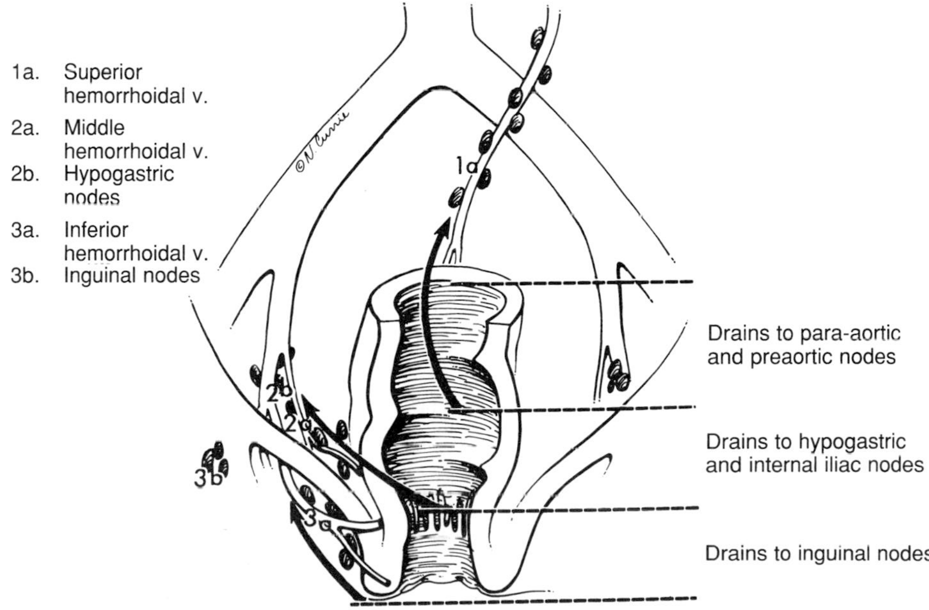

FIGURE 6–2. Lymphatic drainage of the rectum.

has extensive lymphatics, which drain into both the internal iliac and the inferior mesenteric chains (Fig. 6–2).

Nerve Supply

The colon is supplied by both sympathetic and parasympathetic nerves. The sympathetic supply from the T10-12 levels proceeds via the celiac, preaortic, and superior mesenteric plexuses to the right colon. The sympathetic nerves to the left colon and rectum arise from L1-3 and travel with the inferior mesenteric artery. Sympathetic stimuli inhibit peristalsis of the colon and rectum.

The parasympathetic nerves promote peristalsis of the large bowel. The right vagus sends fibers to the right colon, while the left colon and rectum are supplied by fibers from S2-4.

The pelvic autonomic nerves are at significant risk of injury during dissection of the rectum. The nervi erigentes emerge from the spinal cord at S2-4. These nerves join with the sympathetic fibers from L1-3 to form the pelvic plexuses, as well as the periprostatic plexus in men. The normal function of the lower genitourinary system, the rectum and anal canal, and, in particular, sexual function is dependent on these nerves. Injury to these nerves is a major source of postoperative morbidity following rectal cancer surgery.

ADENOMA-CARCINOMA SEQUENCE

Prevalence and Distribution

Colorectal adenomas (or polyps) are very common benign neoplasms increasing in occurrence with advancing age.[67] Their prevalence varies significantly in reported studies and ranges between 20% and 70%.[68–71] Differences in reported figures are explained by geographic and ethnic variations as well as different methodology, population groups included, and techniques employed in these studies.[69] International autopsy studies indicate that, with some rare exceptions, adenoma prevalence and distribution patterns are similar to those of colorectal cancer in the same region, suggesting common etiologic factors and mechanisms leading to both diseases.[67, 72, 73]

Current autopsy data suggest that geographic variations are among the most significant in determining adenoma prevalence in different population groups. However, some exceptions to these parallel patterns for colorectal adenoma and carcinoma were reported in South African Bantu populations, in which carcinoma incidence was reported to be very low.[74]

Specific Associations

Race

Both adenoma and carcinoma incidence rates were reported in different ethnic groups in Israel, being low among Arab populations and Sephardic Jews and significantly higher among Ashkenazi Jews.[75, 76] In a New Orleans study, blacks appear to have lower polyp prevalence than do whites from the same area.[72]

Socioeconomics

Both polyp and cancer rates appear to be significantly higher among higher-class populations as compared to among the lower class in Cali, Columbia.[72]

Age

Polyps are very uncommon under age 50, increase with age, and reach a peak incidence in the seventh and eighth decades.[77, 78] Prevalence rates are as low as 0.06% in men in age groups below 50 but increase almost nine-fold in the seventh and eighth decades.[79]

Gender

Sex differences have been noted in most autopsy studies, with a slight male predominance of 1.4 to 1.6:1.[79] The ratio is much higher in Japan, with a male to female ratio of 2.5:1.[68, 78]

Anatomic Distribution

Overall, adenomas are distributed equally throughout the colon, with a slightly increased frequency in the cecum, ascending colon, and left colon.[68] These findings are different from the distribution of large bowel cancer, which is still more frequent in the distal colon despite a recent trend to a right shift in distribution.[80] However, more recently, the National Polyp Study found that larger and more dysplastic polyps occurred more frequently in the left colon.[81]

The introduction of the fiberoptic flexible colonoscopy has resulted in an increase in frequency of polyps detected in asymptomatic patients (range, 5–22%).[82, 83] The relative risk for metachronous tumors was also increased in other studies: 2.7 for patients with polyps larger than 1 cm at the initial examination as compared to the expected risk ratio. The distribution of subsequent carcinomas was not related to the initial findings, where most polyps were distributed in the distal colon and carcinomas were not.[84]

Carcinoma in Adenomas

There is convincing evidence that many carcinomas arise from adenomatous polyps. However, it is still uncertain whether all carcinomas arise from their precancerous precursors. Foci of residual adenoma are occasionally found in carcinoma specimens. The frequency of this finding is related to the extent of carcinoma invasion through the bowel wall.[85]

In one study, remnants of adenoma were identified in

almost one in four cancers.[86] In general, however, the malignant potential of an adenoma was related to size and progressively dysplastic histology.[87, 88] Although polyps larger than 2 cm are commonly regarded as the "high-risk" lesions, occasionally even smaller adenomas do contain malignant tissue.

Synchronous Lesions

Several studies have examined the coexistence of polyps and carcinomas. The incidence of polyps in surgical specimens of the large bowel resected for carcinoma is several times higher than in operated matched controls. Retrospective studies with different inclusion criteria in patients with colorectal cancer have shown a rate of synchronous polyps of up to 62%.[71, 85, 89]

Metachronous Lesions

Patients with adenomatous polyps are at increased risk for both metachronous adenomas and carcinomas.[90–92] Although some of them may represent lesions missed at the initial study, the findings could not be explained solely on this basis.[70]

The suggested cumulative rate for developing further adenomas and cancer increased steadily over 15 years.[91] The figures varied with increasing numbers of polyps at the initial examination, approaching 50% for further adenoma and 5% for carcinoma in patients after 15 years of follow-up when a single adenoma was initially found as compared to 4 in 5 for polyps and 1 in 8 for cancer risk in patients with multiple initial lesions.[91] In the National Polyp Study, there was a 35% recurrence rate of adenomas after 3-year follow-up, with a tendency toward smaller size and more proximal distribution at 1 year follow-up and more equal distribution at 3 years.[93]

Age of Onset

Adenomas are found at an earlier age than carcinomas. The mean age for adenomas is in the sixth decade, while the mean age for carcinomas is several years older.[94, 95]

Natural History

The strongest indirect evidence for the polyp-cancer sequence would be presumed reduction in cancer incidence following the intervention of polypectomy. Several polyp intervention studies aimed at reducing colorectal cancer–related mortality have been carried out.[96–98]

In one study of more then 21,000 asymptomatic participants, the results showed a significant reduction of 85% of expected cancers after long-term follow-up of at least 25 years. Although 13 rectosigmoid cancers were not prevented, most of them were detected at the earlier stages.[96]

That removal of an adenomatous polyp can influence rectal cancer incidence was recently demonstrated in a long-term follow-up study of patients who had polypectomy but did not undergo surveillance. After polypectomy, the incidence of rectal cancer approached the incidence in the general population.[99]

Natural history and future risk of malignant transformation were studied in two retrospective studies. The risk of cancer diagnosis from diagnosis of polyps was 8% at 10 years and 24% at 20 years. The results support excision of all adenomatous polyps that are 1 cm or larger.[100]

The hypothesis that some polyps have selective malignant potential but most do not is supported by autopsy series that demonstrated high prevalence rates of adenomatous polyps of up to 70%, whereas the incidence of carcinomas in Western countries (United States and Canada) is approximately 5% to 7%.[100]

Histologic Variations

Three major histologic and morphologic findings related to increased risk of malignant potential in adenomas are the size, severity of dysplasia, and degree of villous component ("villosity") of the adenoma.

Adenoma Size

Histologically, all adenomas are classified according to the tubular and villous component into villous, tubular, and intermediate types. The most frequently seen histologic type in adenomas of all sizes is the tubular type, while the villous type is the most uncommon.

Dysplasia and Extent of Villous Component

Dysplastic changes, or mucosal atypia, describe the degree of cell differentiation, architectural distortion, and nuclear abnormalities and are classified as mild, moderate, or severe dysplasia. Severe dysplasia was previously termed carcinoma in situ; however, more recently the World Health Organization has recommended avoidance of this term to reduce misinterpretations of the clinical significance associated with the use of the term carcinoma.

It appears that adenoma size and the extent of villous component are the two major and independent risk factors associated with severity of dysplasia found in adenomas.[81] Another independent variable associated with risk of high-grade dysplasia is increasing age. Both high-grade dysplasia and larger adenomas showing predominantly villous components are seen more frequently in elderly patients, with an almost doubled frequency after age 60.[81]

Similarly, the frequency of malignant changes seen within adenomas varies significantly with the histologic pattern, size, and degree of dysplasia. Carcinoma was found in 5.7% of adenomas with mild dysplasia, 18% with moderate, and 34.5% with severe.[88] Severe atypia is very uncommon in small polyps with a tubular pattern, but, when found, it is associated with a high likelihood of carcinoma being present in those lesions. However, in large (>2 cm) lesions, cancer rates were not influenced by severity of dysplasia.[88]

Process of Stepwise Evolution

Implicit in the concept of the adenoma-carcinoma sequence is the process of stepwise evolution of a malignant tumor within its benign precursor, the adenomatous polyp. According to our current understanding of this evolution, the process occurs as a result of an accumulation of mutations that transform a normal cell to a malignant phenotype. Subsequently, the transformed cell loses the control of growth regulation and differentiation and becomes clonally expanded, giving rise to a neoplastic cell cluster.[101] However, direct and thus definitive proof of an adenoma-carcinoma sequence is difficult to obtain, since the natural history of a polyp is interrupted by excision. Moreover, biopsy specimens do not necessarily represent the whole histology of the polyp. Most previous studies investigating the polyp-carcinoma sequence employing either autopsy material, surgical specimens, or rigid proctosigmoidoscopy were limited to collection of data on lesions having polypoid appearance. Some early studies in the 1960s, however, demonstrated a lack of histologic evidence of adenomatous tissue within small cancers, suggesting possible de novo malignant formation.

Aberrant Crypt Foci and Microadenoma

Unifying phenomena may come from the work of McLellan and Bird[102] who have defined a method of identifying aberrant crypt foci (ACF) and microadenoma (MA) in animals and humans in large sections of colon by studying the mucosa in the direction of the lumen as opposed to vertical sectioning. It appears that MA may develop by fission from a single aberrant crypt. A carcinoma may go through a gross adenoma stage or, rarely, come directly from an MA too small to be readily seen on standard histology. Our own animal model work supports this hypothesis.[103]

The significance of these findings was further reinforced by recent detection of ACF in human colon mucosa in patients with colorectal cancer and colonic polyposis, suggesting that they represent the earliest preneoplastic lesions (Fig. 6–3).[104–106]

The authors are currently assessing the natural history of microadenoma in an animal model (Fig. 6–4).

Familial Adenomatous Polyposis

As discussed earlier, FAP is an autosomal dominant inherited disorder of colonic epithelium that, if left untreated, leads to the development of colonic cancer in 100% of cases.[107] The phenotypic hallmark of the disease is the occurrence of hundreds to thousands of adenomas in the colon, usually in childhood or adolescence.

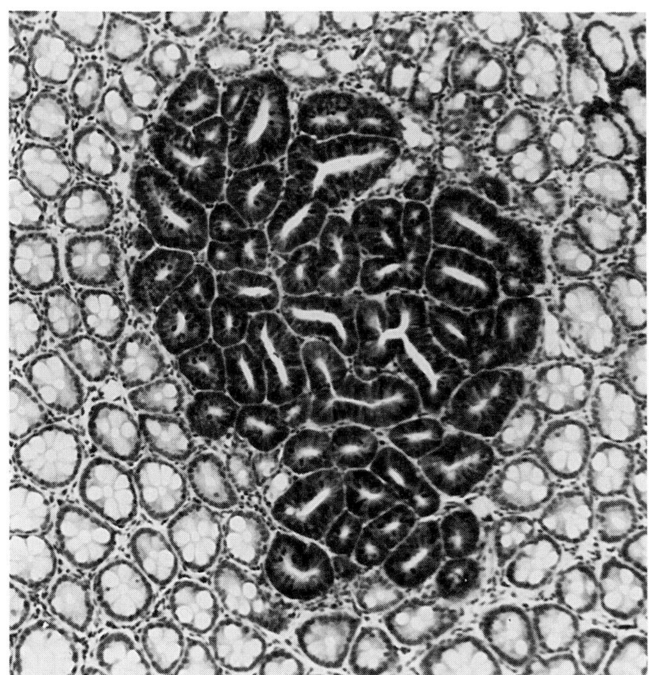

FIGURE 6–3. Aberrant crypt foci.

Genetic Mutations in Colon Carcinogenesis

The K-*ras* Oncogene

As discussed earlier, it is now clear that an accumulation of genetic mutations is required for the progression of normal epithelium to adenoma to carcinoma.

The three *ras* genes, N-*ras,* H-*ras,* and K-*ras,* code for highly conserved G proteins, which are located on the inner surface of the plasma membrane and appear to be important in signal transduction. Mutational activation of *ras* genes, primarily by single base pair substitutions, results in a loss of intrinsic GTP-ase activity. The mutated *ras* protein remains constitutively activated and participates in malignant transformation of the cell.[108]

Mutations of the *ras* gene occur early in experimental and human carcinogenesis.[109] In premalignant colorectal adenomas from both FAP patients and normal individuals, *ras* mutations can be found in up to 60% of lesions. The majority of these mutations are single nucleotide substitutions in codon 12 of the K-*ras* gene.[108, 110] These mutations are also present in many other common human cancers, including pancreatic and lung cancer, and are probably

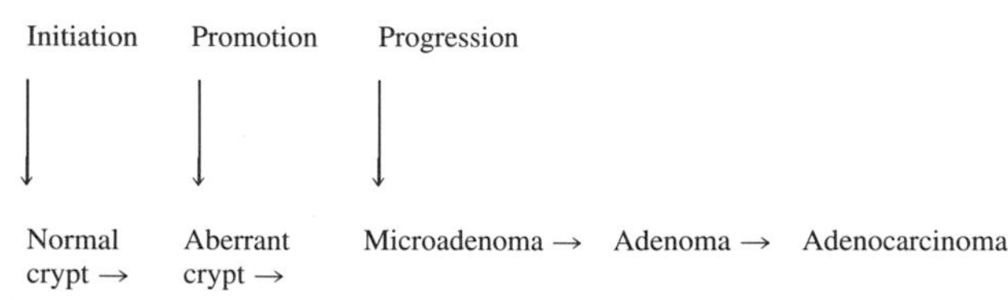

FIGURE 6–4. Proposed sequential development of colon cancer.

important in their pathogenesis.[108] In fact, it has been shown recently that the presence of *ras* mutations was predictive of a worse outcome in non–small cell lung cancer patients irrespective of treatment intent.[111]

Tumor Suppressor Genes At the Chromosome 5q21-22 Locus

Genetic alterations involving allelic deletions of the chromosome 5q21-22 region are observed in both familial and sporadic colon cancer and are thought to be one of the earliest events in colorectal tumorigenesis. With the use of cytogenetic and restriction fragment-length polymorphism (RFLP) linkage technique, the genetic locus for the inherited disorder of FAP was localized to the same chromosomal region.[7] In patients without polyposis, via the loss of heterozygosity (LOH) technique, allelic losses of chromosome 5q have been observed in 20% to 50% of colorectal carcinomas and in 30% of colorectal adenomas.[110, 112, 113] Recently, in a series of 65 colorectal carcinomas, 54% of tumors exhibited allelic losses in the FAP locus region.[112] In FAP patients with one inherited germline mutation, allelic deletions of chromosome 5q21-22 were found to be rare in adenomas.[110, 112, 113] However, a preferential loss of the normal allele inherited from an unaffected parent as seen in 25% to 40% of colorectal tumors in FAP patients.[114] These studies provide evidence that (1) the chromosome 5q21-22 region harbors a tumor suppressor gene or genes, one of which is involved in causing the inherited disorder of FAP, and (2) molecular alterations at 5q were one of the earliest events in the mutational pathway leading from normal colonic epithelium to colon carcinoma.

Recently, in an attempt to clone the gene responsible for causing FAP, several candidate genes, including two tumor suppressor genes were isolated by positional cloning.[115, 116] Germline mutations of the adenomatous polyposis coli (APC) gene have been demonstrated in several unrelated FAP patients, and somatic mutations of APC have been observed in hereditary and nonhereditary colon cancers.[116–121]

The Adenomatous Polyposis Coli Gene

The APC gene consists of 15 exons spanning a 10-kb region. The last exon is unusually long and contains more than 6000 nucleotides. The majority of germline as well as somatic APC mutations are found in the first half of this exon. Mutations in the APC gene are reported to be deletions, small (one to two nucleotides) insertions, nonsense and missense mutations, and most of them are predicted to result in a truncated gene product.

Mutation in the APC gene is thought to be a rate-limiting step in the development of colorectal neoplasia, since it is one of the earliest genetic events in this pathway as evidenced by the FAP phenotype. Recent analyses of colorectal tumors have shown that the APC mutations occur at a high frequency in adenomas and carcinomas.[121, 122] Approximately 60% to 80% of tumors have mutation of one APC allele, and 60% have loss or inactivation of both APC alleles. Somatic mutations of APC are observed in benign adenomas as small as 0.5 cm in diameter. The frequency of APC mutations is uniform (60%) in early (benign adenomas) versus late (carcinomas) events of colorectal tumorigenesis. In one study, the colorectal tumors with APC mutations were also analyzed for the presence of *ras* mutations, and only 20% were found to have an additional *ras* mutation. These observations provide important in vivo evidence that (1) the same molecular event (i.e., genetic aberrations of APC) can cause the initiation and early progression to colon cancer, and (2) the APC mutations precede *ras* mutations, which heretofore were the only known specific mutations in early stages of colon cancer.

PATHOLOGY

Adenocarcinoma accounts for the vast majority of malignant neoplasms of the colon and rectum. Grossly, these are either polypoid or infiltrating. In general, the microscopic extent of disease correlates well with the gross disease, and extensive local microscopic spread beyond the palpable lesion is uncommon. An understanding of this local growth characteristic has led to revision of the acceptable distal resection margin down to 2 cm for rectal cancers.

A histologic grading system has been devised based primarily on the degree of differentiation of the lesion, as evidenced by gland formation, and by the cytologic features of individual cells. The majority of colorectal cancers fall into the intermediate, grade II, category. Grade I, well-differentiated, and grade III or high-grade tumors each account for approximately 10% to 25% of all primary lesions.

The presence or absence of mucin production is also specifically commented on. While most adenocarcinomas of the large intestine produce some mucin, the presence of mucin involving 50% or more of the tumor area results in the lesion being classified as a colloid or mucinous carcinoma.[123] This mucin is usually extracellular, but signet-ring cell carcinomas contain the mucin in an intracellular location. The prognostic implications of mucinous tumors have been studied by several groups.[123–125] Symonds and Vickery[123] found that mucinous rectal cancers had a significantly worse 5-year survival than similar-stage nonmucinous tumors (18% vs. 49%, $P < .0005$), while Sasaki et al.[125] did not find any independent prognostic significance to the presence of mucin. The rare signet-ring cell cancers, however, have been found to have a significantly poorer prognosis in reviews comparing these to other, comparable-stage cancers.[125, 126]

When carcinoma is identified in an endoscopically resected polyp, its histologic characteristics are graded according to the aforementioned classification. Other microscopic features of importance to the clinician are the status of the resection margin (base of stalk), and the presence or absence of lymphatic invasion. These criteria are used in determining whether further intervention is warranted or whether polypectomy alone is considered adequate treatment.

Other, much less common malignancies of the colon and rectum include carcinoid tumors, lymphoma, and various connective tissue tumors, the most common of which is leiomyosarcoma.

DIAGNOSIS, SCREENING, AND EARLY DETECTION

Diagnosis

Symptoms

The majority of patients with colorectal cancer present with symptoms. The nature of the symptoms depends in part on the location of the primary lesion in the colon. Patients with rectal tumors present most commonly with hematochezia or constipation.[127, 128] Symptoms of left-sided cancers are bleeding, constipation, and abdominal pain, while splenic flexure lesions have the highest incidence of obstruction.[129] Tumors in the ascending colon bleed in an occult manner until weakness secondary to anemia produces symptoms. Other manifestations are abdominal pain and nausea. Colonic perforation is the mode of presentation in 7% of cases of colorectal carcinoma. This is least likely if the primary tumor is in the rectum or rectosigmoid (3%), while the other sites have a 10% to 12% likelihood of this complication.[129]

Evaluation

Once a patient presents with symptoms suggestive of colorectal carcinoma, a thorough work-up is indicated. Physical examination should focus on evaluation of lymph nodes, careful abdominal examination, digital rectal examination, as well as assessment of any extracolonic manifestations of primary or metastatic disease. Enlarged lymph nodes should be sought out in the inguinal region as well as the left supraclavicular region (Virchow's node). Abdominal examination may reveal a palpable primary tumor, hepatomegaly, or signs of impending obstruction. A careful rectal examination may reveal the primary lesion, which must be assessed for mobility, location, size, extent of rectal circumference involved, and direct extension into prostate or vagina. Transperitoneal seeding into the pouch of Douglas may be palpated as a Blumer's shelf.

Extracolonic manifestations of colorectal carcinoma have been well described. These include thrombophlebitis, acanthosis nigricans, hypokalemia secondary to a rectal villous tumor, dermatomyositis, Cushing's syndrome secondary to ectopic adenocorticotropic hormone, hypertrophic osteoarthropathy, and hypercalcemia. These are uncommon presenting manifestations of colorectal carcinoma.

Laboratory tests are of limited use in assisting with the diagnosis of colorectal cancer. Documentation of an elevated carcinoembryonic antigen (CEA) level is suggestive of a malignant lesion, and microcytic anemia supports a possible right-sided lesion, but neither of these is highly specific.

Further work-up involves visualization of the colon, and biopsy of the lesion provides definitive diagnosis. Rigid sigmoidoscopy to 25 cm should allow for identification of approximately 30% of adenomas and cancers.[130] A full colonoscopy is also indicated, even if a tumor is identified and sampled for biopsy on rigid sigmoidoscopy, as 5% of individuals are found to have a synchronous primary lesion elsewhere in the colon. Air-contrast barium enema may be combined with flexible sigmoidoscopy in place of colonoscopy.

Screening and Early Detection

Controversy abounds regarding the role and benefits of screening for colorectal cancer in the general population. Several issues are being debated, among them (1) whether one must demonstrate a definitive reduction in mortality or incidence of invasive disease to justify implementation of a screening procedure, (2) the cost effectiveness of any proposed screening test, and (3) the acceptable sensitivity, specificity, and positive predictive value for a given test. Also in question is the optimal combination of tests, as well as the appropriate interval between negative screens, and whether the general population or only those deemed to be at high risk should be assessed. The presence of lead-time bias and length-biased sampling (the increased likelihood of screening detecting slow-growing, and therefore more favorable, tumors) complicates statistical evaluation of any proposed screening maneuver.[131]

Although uncertainty persists, there is general agreement that ongoing evaluation of the two most commonly used screening tests—fecal occult blood testing and sigmoidoscopy—is essential.

Fecal Occult Blood Testing

The testing of stool for the presence of occult blood has been widely used since 1967.[132] Its ease of use, low cost, and wide availability have been instrumental in its rapid and wide acceptance by physicians. Until recently, however, this modality had not been carefully scrutinized to determine its true impact on mortality from colorectal cancer.

Since 1975, a number of large, controlled clinical trials have been undertaken to study fecal occult blood testing. From 1975 to 1991, 21,756 individuals over the age of 40 entered the trial at the Memorial Sloan-Kettering Cancer Center and the Preventive Medicine Institute–Strang Clinic in New York.[133] Following a physical examination and rigid sigmoidoscopy to 25 cm, patients were randomized to fecal occult blood testing or no testing. Although final results have not been published, a preliminary report in 1988 indicated a compliance of approximately 75% for the fecal occult blood test and a 1.7% positivity of the nonhydrated slides. Analysis of the screen-detected cancers revealed a shift to earlier stage, with Dukes stage A and B accounting for 65% of them, compared to only 33% in the control group ($P < .05$). After a 10-year follow-up, the screened group had a 43% lower mortality rate from colorectal cancer, consistent across all age groups.

Another trial, conducted at the University of Minnesota, also began in 1975. Its preliminary report, published in 1980, revealed that 48,000 persons age 50 to 80 years old were randomized to one of three study groups.[134] One group underwent fecal occult blood testing annually for 5 years, the second group was tested biannually for 5 years, and the control group received usual medical care. Of 873 individuals who underwent evaluation following a positive fecal occult blood test, 74 have been found to have 77 gastrointestinal tract cancers: 56 colon cancers, 16 rectal cancers, 3 gastric cancers, 1 pancreatic cancer, and 1 secondary colon cancer. Furthermore, another 31% of those with positive fecal occult blood studies were found to have gastrointestinal polyps. More than 75% of the identified cancers were early, either Dukes stage A or B lesions. Mortality data have not yet been released.

Three large European studies are also under way. An English study still undergoing accrual had entered 107,349 people age 50 to 74 at date of last publication.[135] Fifty-three percent of the 52,258 eligible study group has undergone the first of the planned biannual screens, and 52% of the 63 cancers diagnosed in this group were Dukes stage A. While this reveals a promising stage shift in comparison to the control group, in whom only 10.6% of cancers were stage A, documentation of affect on mortality will take many more years. Similarly large trials in Sweden and Denmark are also ongoing.

In spite of the concerted effort to definitively document the efficacy of fecal occult blood testing as a screening procedure, many criticisms of this test persist. In a recent review, Alquist[136] cited the low compliance rates in the general population, the inherently low specificity of blood as a marker for colorectal cancer, the limitations of the common guaiac-based test, the potential for error due to improper fecal sampling, the remarkably low rates of cancer detection found in some studies for both the Hemoccult (<26%) and the HemoQuant (<33%) tests, and the high cost and associated risks of diagnostic evaluation of individuals with a positive test.

Whatever the results of the randomized trials under way, the search for a better screening test will continue.

Sigmoidoscopy

In light of the shortcomings of fecal occult blood testing, sigmoidoscopy continues to be advocated as an alternative screening procedure. To date, no randomized, controlled trial of sigmoidoscopy alone has been completed.

Rigid sigmoidoscopy, when performed to 25 cm, should be able to detect 35% to 45% of colorectal cancers.[131] This procedure was included as part of the multiphasic health checkup for one of the groups participating in the Kaiser Foundation Health Plan study. The final analysis of this study revealed that although there was a significant reduction in mortality from colorectal cancer, this could not be attributed to the use of sigmoidoscopy.

More recently, the results of a case-control study of screening sigmoidoscopy and mortality from colorectal cancer were published.[137] The exposure to screening rigid sigmoidoscopy during the 10 years prior to diagnosis of fatal cancer of the distal colon or rectum in 261 members of the Kaiser Permanente Health Plan was compared to 868 matched controls. After adjusting for potential confounding factors, a statistically strong protective effect of screening rigid sigmoidoscopy was demonstrated, with mortality from colorectal cancer within the distal 20 cm being reduced by 50% to 70%.

Rigid sigmoidoscopy is an uncomfortable procedure, and the scope cannot reliably be passed for its full length in many patients.[131] As such, the flexible sigmoidoscopes are becoming more commonly used in the screening setting. When compared with the rigid scopes, the flexible ones have been shown to be more acceptable to patients and to detect significantly more malignancies.[138] The disadvantages of flexible sigmoidoscopy include its increased cost and the higher risk of perforation, estimated to be 0.02% for the 35-cm scope and 0.045% for the 60-cm scope.[130]

In an attempt to address the outstanding questions regarding the role of sigmoidoscopy in screening for colorectal cancer, the NCI has undertaken a large, prospective, randomized, controlled trial evaluating the impact of 60-cm flexible sigmoidoscopy on mortality from colorectal cancer in men and women age 60 to 74.[139] Accrual has been targeted at 148,000 participants.

Colonoscopy

Colonoscopy is not currently advised as a screening test for the general population, owing in part to its cost and increased risk of colon perforation, estimated to be 0.2%.[130] However, it is recommended for the surveillance of individuals at high risk for the development of colorectal carcinoma.[140]

Recommendations

Screening recommendations by national policy-making bodies are not uniform among developed nations, reflecting the ongoing controversies in this field.

The American Cancer Society and the NCI recommend an annual digital rectal examination after the age of 40 and annual fecal occult blood testing and sigmoidoscopy every 3 to 5 years after the age of 50.[139] This is in contradistinction to the findings of the Canadian Periodic Health Examination Task Force, which does not recommend screening for the general population.[141] A neutral approach has been advocated by the U.S. Preventive Services Task Force, which neither recommends screening nor actively advises against it.[142]

These recommendations will continue to evolve as existing trials mature and new data come to light.

STAGING

Once a malignancy of the colon or rectum is diagnosed, the extent of disease is assessed. This comprises two phases: clinical staging and pathologic staging.

Clinical Staging

The clinical stage is evaluated by a thorough workup, including careful physical examination for local tumor characteristics and lymphadenopathy, colonoscopy, and biopsy, as well as imaging of the pelvis, liver, lungs, or any other relevant organs.

Further evaluation is carried out intraoperatively: the primary lesion is carefully inspected for resectability: peritoneal seeds or other signs of distant spread are searched for: and the liver is thoroughly palpated, with intraoperative ultrasound being available for assessment of areas of concern.

Pathologic Staging

The most widely used pathologic classification of these tumors has been based on Dukes' original description of rectal tumors in 1932.[143] This was subsequently applied to colon tumors as well. In Dukes' original paper, only three stages were described:

A: Involvement of the muscularis mucosa, with invasion into, but not through, the muscularis propria; lymph nodes are not involved

B: Invasion through the full thickness of the bowel wall (muscularis propria), but lymph nodes remain uninvolved

C: Regardless of the depth of invasion of the tumor through the bowel wall, the lymph nodes are found to contain metastatic tumor

This classification was shown to be predictive of outcome, was straightforward, and gained wide acceptance. It did not, however, provide for description of any metastatic disease present or direct extension into adjacent organs, perforation, or other noteworthy features.

Since then, several modifications of this original classification have been popularized. Many of them include a "D" stage, signifying disease metastatic to distant viscera. The Aster-Coller modification has been one of the more widely used versions:

A: Lesion does not extend through mucosa

B1: Lesion extends into, but not through muscularis propria; lymph nodes are not involved

B2: Lesion extends through the muscularis propria; lymph nodes are not involved

C1: Lesion extends into, but not through, muscularis propria; lymph nodes are involved with tumor

C2: Lesion extends through the muscularis propria; lymph nodes are involved with tumor

In recent years, attempts have been made to achieve worldwide standardization of the reporting of colorectal cancer staging. The American Joint Committee on Cancer (AJCC) and the TNM Committee of the International Union Against Cancer (UICC) have reached a consensus on a TNM-based staging system intended to supplant the many other systems in use for carcinoma of the colon and rectum (Table 6–2). It was intentionally created to closely follow the well-known Dukes classification.

PRIMARY OPERABLE DISEASE

Several treatment options exist for a patient with colorectal cancer. The overall health of the patient as well as

TABLE 6–2
AJCC/UICC TNM Staging System for Carcinoma of the Colon and Rectum

Stage	Primary Tumor	Regional Lymph Nodes	Distant Metastasis	Dukes Stage
0	Tis	N0	M0	
I	T1	N0	M0	
	T2	N0	M0	A
II	T3	N0	M0	
	T4	N0	M0	B
III	Any T	N1	M0	
	Any T	N2, N3	M0	C
IV	Any T	Any N	M1	

Primary Tumor (T)

Tx	Primary tumor cannot be assessed
T0	No evidence of primary tumor
Tis	Carcinoma in situ
T1	Tumor invades submucosa or tumor invades the stalk of a resected polyp
T2	Tumor invades muscularis propria
T3	Tumor invades through the muscularis propria into the subserosa or nonperitonealized pericolic or perirectal tissues
T4	Tumor perforates the visceral peritoneum or directly invades other organs or structures

Regional Lymph Nodes (N)

Nx	Regional lymph nodes cannot be assessed
N0	No regional lymph node metastasis
N1	Metastasis in one to three pericolic or perirectal lymph nodes
N2	Metastasis in four or more pericolic or perirectal lymph nodes
N3	Metastasis in any lymph node along the course of a named vascular trunk

Distant Metastasis (M)

Mx	Presence of distant metastasis cannot be assessed
M0	No distant metastasis
M1	Distant metastasis present

AJCC, American Joint Committee on Cancer; UICC, International Union Against Cancer.

the local and distant extent of disease have an impact on which treatment is proposed. Although surgical excision of the primary lesion remains the treatment of choice in the majority of situations, there is an ever-increasing role for both radiotherapy and chemotherapy.

Surgical Options

Colon

Wide excision of the primary tumor with a regional lymphadenectomy remains the treatment of choice for uncomplicated primary tumors of the colon. These standard surgical procedures are well described in many texts. In brief, for a lesion in the right colon, the ileocolic and right colic arteries are divided, with a resulting ileotransverse colostomy. A lesion at the hepatic flexure is treated by excision of the ascending and transverse colon, with ligation of the ileocolic, right colic, and middle colic arteries and reconstruction with an ileodescending colon anastomosis. Tumors of the splenic flexure and the transverse colon are both managed with subtotal colectomy and ileosigmoid anastomosis. For a malignancy of the descending or sigmoid colon, the inferior mesenteric artery is ligated, facilitating a left hemicolectomy. Lesions of the rectosigmoid and upper rectum are excised following division of the inferior mesenteric artery as well, with subsequent descending colorectal anastomosis.

The major vessels are to be divided near their origin to facilitate a wide lymphatic dissection. "High ligation" of the inferior mesenteric artery at its aortic origin has been proposed as a technique providing superior long-term outcome following left colon resection,[144] but more recent data do not support this concept unequivocally.[145] The true impact of high ligation of the inferior mesenteric artery remains unresolved.

The optimal length of clear resection margins has also been debated in the literature. While it was believed and practiced for many years that a 5-cm length of microscopically uninvolved bowel was required, more recent studies have evaluated the patterns of distal mucosal spread.[146] The finding that fully 98% of well-differentiated tumors spread less than 2 cm has led to the recommendation that distal margins need not exceed this length. When a colonic neoplasm is found at laparotomy to be invading an adjacent organ, en bloc resection of the primary lesion with the adherent viscus is indicated to provide for a curative resection. Adhesions to the tumor should not be dissected off, as this may result in the microscopic seeding of malignant cells into the peritoneal cavity.

The role of subtotal colectomy and primary anastomosis in the management of colon cancer is being increasingly advocated as an oncologically sound procedure with minimal morbidity and mortality.[147] Several widely accepted indications for this operation include the presence of multiple polyps associated with a primary tumor, the presence of synchronous carcinomas, carcinoma associated with ulcerative colitis, and FAP coli. Other relative indications include the occurrence of a metachronous colon cancer, the presence of a colorectal neoplasm in a young person with a positive family history of colon cancer, and the presence of significant diverticular disease in conjunction with a right-sided tumor. The role of subtotal colectomy in the setting of colon obstruction remains a contentious issue and is addressed more fully later.

One concern with subtotal colectomy has been the increased frequency of bowel movements postoperatively as a source of long-term morbidity. A review of 72 patients who underwent subtotal colectomy in both the elective and the emergency setting found 56% of patients having less than three bowel movements daily at 2-month follow-up.[147] A further 25% were having between three and five movements daily, while 5% were constipated. Of the 13% having more than five bowel movements daily, nearly two thirds had more than 10 cm of terminal ileum resected, suggesting that bile salt malabsorption may play an important role in the pathophysiology of this problem.

Rectum

The principles of surgical management of rectal malignancies are the same as those of colonic tumors. There are, however, certain anatomic differences that necessitate special attention. The long-term outcome following excision of rectal cancer has been marred by a local recurrence rate approaching 30% for stage II disease and 50% for stage III lesions.[148] Studies into possible causes for this finding have led to an appreciation of the importance of the lateral margins during the pelvic dissection. Quirke et al.[149] demonstrated a strong inverse relationship between the extent of the lateral margins excised and local recurrence rates. This association persisted independent of the degree of histologic differentiation, type of resection, or stage of the tumor. This wide excision of the mesorectum en bloc with the rectum is associated, however, with a higher morbidity, particularly genitourinary complications.

Much effort has been directed toward the development of sphincter-saving procedures for tumors of the distal rectum. The low anterior resection, most often with a stapled anastomosis, remains the most commonly performed resection of these lesions. Several other operative approaches exist, however, and these have reached variable acceptance among American surgeons. A coloanal anastomosis may be utilized following resection of tumor in the distal third of the rectum.[150] After the mucosa of the distal rectum is stripped, the end of the rectum is anastomosed to the sigmoid colon. This may be accomplished with either a hand-sewn technique or an endoluminal stapling device. A combined abdominosacral procedure has been advocated as an alternative approach to a lesion of the middle rectum.[151] This technique never gained widespread popularity, however, perhaps because of its perceived technical difficulty.

With the widely accepted indications for adjuvant radiotherapy following excision of stage II and III rectal tumors, there is increasing interest in means of protecting the small bowel from the effects of radiation. An initial step is to reperitonealize the pelvis following a low anterior resection. The small bowel may also be suspended in a sling of absorbable mesh tacked to the retroperitoneum.[152, 153] The placement of an inflatable prosthesis into the pelvis also achieves the intended effect, and it can be easily removed following completion of the radiation course in its deflated state.

Lesions of the lower and middle rectum are uniquely accessible by the transanal route, facilitating local excision. This has proved feasible in appropriately selected patients, avoiding an almost certain colostomy. The accepted criteria that a lesion must meet include small size (<3 to 4 cm), lying within 8 cm of the anal verge, mobile, not ulcerated, polypoid, and well- or moderately well differentiated histology.[154] An important adjunct to local excision is the careful pathologic evaluation of the appropriately oriented specimen postoperatively, with special attention paid to depth of invasion, status of margins, and presence of any negative prognostic histologic factors. Complete local excision is acceptable for a T1 tumor without any negative prognostic factors. A T2 lesion, extending into the muscularis propria, is at higher risk of recurring locally. Thus, while subsequent management is individualized, adjuvant radiotherapy may be administered if further, more radical surgery is not undertaken. A more advanced lesion should be managed with radical, extirpative surgery. A recent report on the outcome of 57 patients following transanal excision of rectal cancer for cure revealed an 82.5% 5-year survival rate.[155]

Other transanal procedures are fulguration with electrocautery and eradication with a laser. Although effective in controlling local symptoms, both of these methods have the distinct disadvantage of not providing a specimen for histologic review. These procedures are usually recommended for treatment of medically unfit patients or for palliative procedures.[156, 157]

Emergency Surgery for Colon Cancer

In spite of increasing attention to the early detection and treatment of colorectal cancer, up to 15% of such patients still present emergently with signs of obstruction or perforation, or both.[158] In a recently published review of the outcome of 77 such patients, Runkel and colleagues[158] found that 74% had obstruction, most commonly in the left colon, while 26% had perforation, which was most common in the right colon. It was uncommon for rectal cancers to present emergently.

Perforated cancers are most commonly managed by primary resection. The decision to anastomose or not depends on the extent of peritoneal soiling and the proposed site of the anastomosis. Ileocolonic anastomoses in the presence of localized peritonitis can be carried out with relative safety, while a colocolonic anastomosis, even in the presence of limited peritonitis, is associated with a higher morbidity. Strong consideration should then be given to a Hartmann procedure. Perioperative mortality rate for all perforated cancers was 30%, with intra-abdominal sepsis being the leading cause of death.[156]

Obstruction is the more common emergency presentation of advanced colorectal cancer. While the standard method for dealing with this situation has been a staged procedure, with proximal decompression being the first step, the associated morbidity and mortality have remained high, and there has been increasing interest in more aggressive initial management. One of the issues has been the high incidence of left-sided lesions producing this complication and the reluctance to perform a colocolonic anastomosis in unprepared colon. This has led to renewed interest in the role of emergency extended right hemicolectomy, or subtotal colectomy, as definitive management in selected patients.

Brief et al.[147] reviewed the expanding role of subtotal colectomy. Included in their 72 patients were 23 with acute or subacute obstruction of the descending or sigmoid colon, all of whom underwent subtotal colectomy and ileocolonic anastomosis. One postoperative death occurred in this group, a figure comparable to the published results of other groups.[159, 160] An interesting finding is that the long-term functional result may well be related to the length of retained terminal ileum, with 62% of those patients with more than five bowel movements daily having had more than 10 cm resected. Even in the unstable patient in whom a proximal diversion is deemed necessary, subtotal colectomy should be considered for the next stage, obviating the need for a third operation.

Of note, the postoperative morbidity and mortality following surgery for obstruction or perforation seem most highly related to the stage of the disease.[158] In patients with metastatic disease, there was a 50% mortality rate, compared to 13% among those with localized disease.

One of the most difficult operative situations arises when one is faced with a locally advanced rectal tumor in the absence of distant disease. If an aggressive local approach is not undertaken, there is a high likelihood that the patient will suffer a prolonged, debilitating course with unrelenting pelvic pain. Several specialized centers have published their results following pelvic exenteration for primary rectal cancer.[161–163] Operative mortality and morbidity were reasonable, and a 5-year survival rate of 40% to 50% for node-negative patients was achieved.

For tumors adherent posteriorly in the midline, en bloc resection of the coccyx and sacrum to the level of S-5 has been described.[164] This may provide for disease-free margins and should be considered for selected patients, although morbidity is high.

Oophorectomy

The role of oophorectomy at the time of resection of a primary colorectal cancer remains unclear. Up to 10% of women undergoing such surgery have been found to have microscopic metastases in their ovaries, with the deposits being bilateral at least 50% of the time.[165] While a bilateral oophorectomy in postmenopausal women adds little to operative time and morbidity, its true impact on survival is questionable, as ovarian metastases are associated with a poor prognosis and 5-year survival is uncommon.[166]

The role of oophorectomy in premenopausal women sparks even greater controversy. McKeigan and Ferguson[167] found that 25% of premenopausal women had ovarian metastases, and the prognosis seemed to be improved in those who underwent oophorectomy.[167] Although there are data supportive of prophylactic oophorectomy in women undergoing excision of colorectal carcinoma, this is not widely accepted.

Radiotherapy

Radiotherapy is now established in the adjuvant setting following excision of locally advanced rectal carcinoma. It has also been utilized as a primary therapeutic modality in specific cases.

Neoadjuvant Radiotherapy

Numerous studies have been done of the effects of radiation in the preoperative setting in rectal cancer. Difficulty in drawing conclusions from the many reports has been due in part to the wide variations in dose and protocol. Preoperative doses have ranged from one dose of 500 cGy[168] to 2000 cGy over 2 weeks[169] to 3450 cGy administered in 15 fractions.[170] The trials using low-dose radiation (<20 cGy) have not shown measurable benefits.[168, 171]

More favorable results have occurred following high-dose preoperative radiation therapy. Several recent studies have been published revealing a consistent improvement in local-regional control in the radiation arms as compared to the control arms. A Swedish study found a statistically significant reduction in local recurrence following preoperative radiation, with long-term survival unchanged.[172] The final results of a European Organization for Research and Treatment of Cancer (EORTC) trial have also identified a marked improvement in local-regional control in patients who received 3450 cGy in 15 fractions preoperatively.[170] Those receiving the combined treatment had a local recurrence rate of only 15%, versus 35% for those treated with surgery alone ($P < .001$).

In April 1990, the National Institutes of Health (NIH) published the results of a Consensus Conference, stating that moderate- to high-dose preoperative radiotherapy resulted in significantly decreased local recurrence rates, without a survival benefit.[173]

There remain some drawbacks to high-dose preoperative radiotherapy. It is contraindicated in the elderly and in those with atherosclerosis, cardiac disease, or at risk for thromboembolic disease.[170] Many surgeons remain hesitant to operate in a radiated field. Data from high-dose preoperative radiation studies reveal no increase in postoperative morbidity in some trials,[170] while others found a significant increase in incidence of both wound infections and mortality.[174]

Adjuvant Radiotherapy

Postoperative radiotherapy has the advantage of being administered after pathologic staging is completed, allowing those with stage II or III lesions to be identified and selected for treatment. It also allows surgery to proceed in a nonirradiated field without preoperative delay. There is also the potential for directing a boost of radiation to a specific area of concern, which may be marked intraoperatively with clips.

Several large multicenter trials have been undertaken in recent years to evaluate optimal adjuvant therapy following surgery for rectal cancer (Table 6–3). They have included chemotherapy as well as radiation, both singly and in combination.

In evaluations of the use of radiation alone following excision of stage II and III rectal tumors, the results are variable. The Gastrointestinal Tumor Study Group (GITSG) found no change in local recurrence following surgery alone or surgery and a course of 40 or 48 Gy over 4½ to 5½ weeks.[175] The reported results from the North Central Cancer Treatment Group (NCCTG), the Mayo Clinic, and Duke University found a local recurrence rate of 25% after 50 Gy were given in 28 fractions following surgery.[176] This trial did not include a surgery-only arm. The National Surgical Adjuvant Breast and Bowel Project R01 trial demonstrated a decrease in local recurrence with 46 to 47 Gy given in 26 to 27 fractions and a perineal boost to post–abdominoperineal resection patients.[177] The

TABLE 6–3
Local Recurrence and Survival in Published Randomized Postoperative Adjuvant Trials in Rectal Cancer

Trial/Arms	No. of Patients	Local Recurrence (%)	5-Year Survival Rate (%)
GITSG	202		
S alone	58	24	47
XRT	50	20	58
CT	48	27	56
XRT + CT	46	11	72
NCCTG	204		
XRT	101	25	49
XRT + CT	103	13	55
NSABP R01	555		
S alone	184	25	43
XRT	184	16	41
CT	187	21	53

Adapted from Coia LR, Hanks GE: The role of adjuvant radiation in the treatment of rectal cancer. Semin Oncol 18:571–584, 1991.

GITSG, Gastrointestinal Tumor Study Group; S, surgery; XRT, radiation; CT, chemotherapy; NCCTG, North Central Cancer Treatment Group; NSABP-R01, National Surgical Adjuvant Breast and Bowel Project—R01.

16% local recurrence rate following surgery and radiation, when compared to the 25% local recurrence rate after surgery alone, just failed to reach statistical significance ($P = .06$).

In none of these major trials did the addition of radiation make a significant impact on overall survival.

Adjuvant radiation alone is tolerated well by most patients. The GITSG paper reported severe reactions in 16% of the radiation-only arm, and 5% of this arm developed severe radiation enteritis.[78]

Chemotherapy

Colon Cancer

Until quite recently, demonstration of a significant benefit from adjuvant therapy following excision of colon cancer was lacking. In 1989, a study was published revealing a significant improvement in disease-free survival in patients with stage C carcinoma of the colon or rectum receiving 5-fluorouracil (5-FU) and levamisole for 1 year ($P = .003$) following surgical excision.[179] An overall survival benefit was also demonstrated with the same combination of chemotherapeutic agents ($P = .03$).

This prompted the initiation of a much larger study evaluating the impact of adjuvant chemotherapy on 1296 patients with resected carcinomas of the colon only, with pathologic staging revealing stage B2 or C disease.[180]

While follow-up has not been long enough to demonstrate any significant benefits in the stage B2 group, the 304 patients with stage C disease who received both 5-FU and levamisole had a significantly improved local recurrence rate when compared to the control arm ($P = .0002$). No such improvement was found in the 310 stage C patients who received levamisole alone.

Evaluation of the survival data at 3½ years found an equally impressive benefit for those stage C patients on the combination chemotherapy arm ($P = .0064$) (Fig. 6–5).

Toxicity related to this combination protocol seemed mainly related to 5-FU, with most of the side effects being of mild or moderate severity. While only 3.5% of patients receiving levamisole alone stopped their therapy early due to toxicity, 12% of those on the combination arm discontinued therapy early primarily because of drug toxicity.

The NIH Consensus Conference in April 1990 recognized the clinical significance of these studies and, while recognizing the need for further follow-up, advocated the recommendation of 5-FU and levamisole to all stage III patients.[173]

Several multicenter studies have evaluated other combinations of chemotherapeutic agents. Many of these protocols have included methyl-CCNU (chloroethyl-cyclohexyl-nitrosourea) as one of the drugs, and there are significant concerns about the long-term toxicity of this particular agent, in particular its leukemogenic properties.[175, 181]

Portal Vein Infusion

Chemotherapeutic agents have been infused directly into the portal vein in an effort to reduce the incidence of subsequent hepatic metastases. One such randomized study found that continuous infusion of high-dose 5-FU for 7 days following resection of the primary colorectal tumor resulted in fewer liver metastases developing in these patients.[182] These results have not been reproduced by other groups, and this mode of adjuvant therapy remains investigational.

Combined Radiotherapy and Chemotherapy

The benefits of combination radiotherapy and chemotherapy in the adjuvant treatment of rectal cancer have

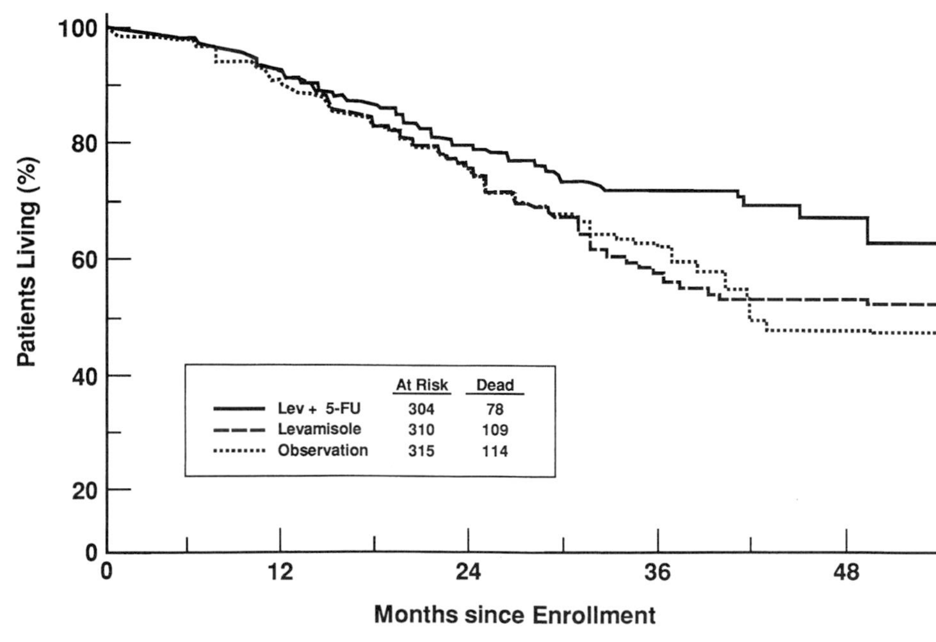

FIGURE 6–5. Intergroup study of adjuvant levamisole (Lev) and 5-fluorouracil (5-FU) on curable colon cancer. (Adapted from Moertel CG, Fleming TR, MacDonald JS, et al: Levamisole and fluorouracil for adjuvant therapy of resected colon carcinoma. N Engl J Med 322:352–358, 1990.)

been well documented. Several well-designed multicenter trials have addressed this mode of therapy in one or more arms of their protocols (Table 6–4).

The NCCTG study found that 4500 to 5040 cGy administered to the pelvis, in combination with 5-FU and methyl-CCNU, reduced the recurrence of rectal cancer by 34% (P = .0016) to 41.5% when compared with surgery plus radiation alone.[176] The initial local recurrence rate was significantly improved (P = .036), as was the incidence of distant metastases (P = .011). Overall survival was improved by 29% to an absolute figure of 53% (P = .043) after a median follow-up of more than 7 years.

The results of the GITSG-7175 study revealed similarly promising results.[175] The combination of 4000 to 4400 cGy with simultaneous 5-FU, followed by 5-FU and methyl-CCNU for 18 months, resulted in a survival improvement of 42% after 10 years of follow-up. The local recurrence rate decreased to 24%, compared to 41% in the surgery-only arm.

The above results led the NIH Consensus Conference to remark that postoperative radiotherapy and chemotherapy formed the best available adjuvant treatment for rectal cancer. The need for clarification of the role of methyl-CCNU in the chemotherapy protocols was reiterated.

FOLLOW-UP SURVEILLANCE

A regular follow-up regimen plays an integral role in the comprehensive care of the patient with colorectal cancer. The aim is to detect recurrences at the earliest possible time, thus maximizing the likelihood of a good outcome. Surveillance is also carried out to detect the development of any metachronous tumors.

Clinical Evaluation

The majority of recurrences of colorectal cancer occur within the first 2 years following excision of the primary tumor.[183] Thus, follow-up is most intensive during this time. During these first 2 years, patient visits are scheduled for every 2 to 4 months, at which time any new symptoms are sought out and a physical examination is performed. The interval between visits may be extended to 6 months for the subsequent 3 years, and then annually. The role of fecal occult blood testing at these visits is debatable, as most local recurrences are extraluminal with late mucosal involvement. This test may, however, detect an asymptomatic metachronous tumor and therefore is often performed. A similar line of thought applies to rigid sigmoidoscopy performed in patients with low anastomoses.

Laboratory Investigations

The performance of regular laboratory tests at these visits is a common practice, albeit an imperfect one.

Liver Enzymes

The monitoring of liver enzymes is done to detect asymptomatic metastatic disease. An elevated serum alkaline phosphatase level was found in one study to have a sensitivity of 77% for detecting liver metastases but a specificity of only 66%.[184] The utility of other liver enzymes in screening is less clear.

TABLE 6–4
Design of Trials of Postoperative Adjuvant Treatment of Rectal Cancer

Trial	Arm	Radiation Total Dose (Gy)	Chemotherapy		Interval from Surgery to Adjuvant Treatment (days)
			Agents	*Sequence*	
GITSG 7175					
	S alone	—	—	—	—
	XRT	40 or 48	—	—	60
	CT	—	5-FU, mCCNU	—	60
	XRT + CT	40 or 44	5-FU, mCCNU	C, PT	60
Mayo/NCCTG 794751					
	XRT	50.4	—	—	21–70
	XRT + CT	50.4	5-FU, mCCNU	PR, C, PT	21–70
NSABP R01					
	S alone	—	—	—	—
	XRT	46–47	—	—	<75
	CT	—	5-FU, mCCNU, VCR	—	21–42
ECOG 4276					
	XRT	45 or 51	—	—	
	XRT + CT	45 or 51	5-FU, mCCNU	PT	
	CT	—	5-FU, mCCNU	—	
GITSG 7180					
	XRT + CT	43.2	5-FU	C, PT	
	XRT + CT	43.2	5-FU, mCCNU	C, PTC, PT	

Adapted from Coia LR, Hanks GE: The role of adjuvant radiation in the treatment of rectal cancer. Semin Oncol 18:571–584, 1991.

GITSG, Gastrointestinal Tumor Study Group; S, surgery, XRT, radiation; CT, chemotherapy; 5-FU, 5-fluorouracil; mCCNU, methyl-chloroethyl-cyclohexyl-nitrosourea; C, concurrent; PT, postradiation; NCCTG, North Central Cancer Treatment Group; PR, preradiation; NSABP-R01, National Surgical Adjuvant Breast and Bowel Project—R01; VCR, vincristine; ECOG, Eastern Cooperative Oncology Group.

Carcinoembryonic Antigen

The serial measurement of plasma CEA is the most common of colorectal cancer follow-up studies. A preoperative level should be determined and is found to be elevated in 50% of those with stage B or C disease.[185] A curative resection should be followed by a fall to the normal range within 1 to 4 months of surgery.[186] While the frequency of CEA testing in the early postoperative period varies from monthly[187] to every 2 to 3 months,[188] the principle of regular, frequent CEA determinations is firmly established. The interpretation of these serial levels, and the determination of what constitutes a positive result, is less well defined.

Dentsman et al.[189] prepared a statistical analysis of seven published decision rules to predict tumor recurrence. This was predicated on the assumption that a positive test result would trigger a series of expensive investigations to localize the presumed recurrence and would possibly lead to a second-look laparotomy. The analysis revealed that a cutoff value of 6.0 ng/ml was the single value with the maximal agreement between predicted and observed tumor recurrences. A proposal that an increase in the slope of the plotted CEA values of greater than 12.6% per month might lead to an even higher correlation between predicted and actual tumor recurrences was put forth. It was also found in this study that late recurring tumors were less likely to present with elevations of CEA levels. A confounding factor is the number of benign conditions that may also elevate the CEA level. These include many inflammatory conditions, including diverticulitis, pancreatitis, peptic ulceration, and hepatitis, as well as cholelithiasis and smoking. In spite of its limitations, the serial measurement of this antigen represents the best noninvasive technique currently available for early detection of recurrent disease.[184]

Radiologic Tests

A variety of radiologic investigations have been proposed as part of the routine postoperative care of these patients.[185] A chest radiograph may detect a solitary metastasis amenable to surgical excision. Commonly, this is performed on an annual basis.

The role of computed tomography (CT) scanning to detect asymptomatic tumor recurrence has been evaluated by several investigators and has been found lacking in sensitivity.[187] Sugarbaker and colleagues[187] found it was the initial positive test leading to the diagnosis of recurrent disease in only 2 of the 28 patients found ultimately to have intra-abdominal recurrence. CT scanning is, however, included in the battery of tests performed once local recurrence is suspected on some other basis, and, in this situation, its sensitivity is a much higher 85%.

This same study evaluated the role of several other imaging tests, including full lung tomograms, liver and spleen scans, intravenous pyelograms, and bone scans. These were also found not to be indicated in the routine postoperative regimen, but bone scans and lung tomograms were recommended as part of the work-up once recurrent disease was suspected.

The utility of magnetic resonance imaging (MRI) in evaluating the abdominal cavity for suspected recurrences is being evaluated. T1-weighted MR images have been found to be as effective as CT in the identification of hepatic metastases, and the false-positive rate is only 3%, as compared to 16% for CT.[190] As MRI technology continues to improve and expand, new applications for it may arise in the postoperative care of colorectal cancer patients.

Colon Imaging

One of the goals in following resected colorectal cancer patients is to detect the presence of a metachronous colon or rectal tumor. This occurs in 5.4% of all patients within 20 years of the first resection.[191] Thus, imaging of the colon forms an important part of their care. Either colonoscopy or air-contrast barium enema combined with flexible sigmoidoscopy should be performed on a regular basis. The choice of procedure depends in part on local availability and expertise and is somewhat controversial. Colonoscopy is undeniably more sensitive in detecting polyps[192] and permits simultaneous therapeutic or diagnostic interventions to be performed. The optimal interval for imaging of the colon has not been definitively identified, but annual examination during the first 2 years, and then repeated examinations every 2 to 3 years, constitute a common protocol.[193]

Summary

The goal of close follow-up of patients following complete excision of a colorectal carcinoma is to detect recurrences early, with the intent of providing further potentially curative intervention. The documented long-term survivors of hepatic resection of colorectal cancer metastases and following aggressive surgical resection of localized pelvic recurrences cannot be ignored. Several issues come into play when the true impact of a surveillance protocol is evaluated, including lead-time bias, emotional cost to patients found to have unresectable recurrences, and overall cost effectiveness. The relative importance of these concepts may never be agreed on unanimously, and personal attitudes will doubtless continue to be a major factor in the comprehensiveness of follow-up regimens.

DISTANT DISEASE

While the percentage of resectable primary colorectal tumors is high, overall survival has remained stable, with approximately 50% of patients eventually succumbing to this disease. Increasing volumes of literature support resection of selected metastatic sites in the absence of other disease, but the majority of patients with metastatic disease do not qualify for such potentially curative surgery. This leaves chemotherapy for palliation of widespread metastases and radiotherapy for management of localized, symptomatic disease.

Liver Metastases

Approximately 10% of patients presenting for treatment of a primary colorectal cancer are found to have hepatic metastases at the time of surgery.[194] Of patients with more widely disseminated disease, in up to 40% the liver is the primary site of involvement.[195] In 20% of those with metastases, the liver is the only site of identified disease.[196] These data underscore the important role the liver plays in the natural history of colorectal cancer.

Surgical Resection

The natural history of unresected solitary hepatic metastases proven by biopsy was reported in an early retrospective review in 1976.[197] The median survival was 20 months with no 5-year survivors.

A multi-institutional review of 859 patients who underwent hepatic resection of colorectal metastases included 509 who had solitary lesions.[198] Their 5-year actuarial survival was 37%, and 5-year actuarial disease-free survival was 25%. Analysis of prognostic factors found the presence of positive hepatic nodes and extrahepatic metastases to be contraindications to liver resection. Other, less significant negative features included hepatic resection margins of less than 1 cm, a disease-free interval of less than 1 year, and stage C disease in the primary colon or rectal tumor.

A less clear situation arises when there are several metastases within the liver without evidence of extrahepatic disease. Several studies have addressed this issue without achieving unanimous agreement on clear surgical guidelines. Fegiz et al.[199] found that 3-year survival was significantly better following resection of solitary metastases (33.8%) as compared to multiple metastases (17%). This difference was no longer apparent at 5 years. Vogt and coworkers[200] found no difference in 5-year survival data for those with solitary versus multiple lesions. Two other studies have found the number of metastatic lesions to make a difference. A study from Sweden involving 72 hepatic resections reported a significant survival difference at 5 years when three or fewer lesions were compared to four or more,[201] and the large series reported by Hughes and colleagues[202] found a statistically better actuarial 5-year survival among those having had resection of a solitary metastasis rather than multiple lesions.

Other issues remain unresolved. The prognostic significance of satellite lesions surrounding an otherwise solitary metastasis is unclear.[203] The presence of synchronous versus metachronous disease, the stage of the primary tumor, the extent of hepatic resection, and the minimal acceptable disease-free microscopic margin are other contentious points.

Regional Therapy

Regional infusion of chemotherapeutic agents, most commonly via the hepatic artery, is under active investigation. The intent is to achieve high local tissue concentrations while reducing the systemic concentrations and associated toxicity. This modality has been applied both following resection of hepatic metastases and in those with unresectable hepatic secondary tumors.

Wagman et al.[204] found no survival advantage following hepatic artery infusion of fluorodeoxyuridine (FUdR) among patients with resected and unresected hepatic metastases. This therapeutic regimen is associated with significant hepatic and biliary toxicity. Other randomized studies of hepatic arterial infusion of FUdR or 5-FU have had similarly disappointing results, with a marginal impact on overall survival, although the disease in the liver did show evidence of regression.[205, 206] At present, this form of treatment remains experimental.

Pulmonary Metastases

Although less common than hepatic metastases, the lung is a site of metastatic disease in up to 15% of patients having undergone complete excision of a primary colorectal cancer.[207] This is seen more commonly following tumors in the rectum, and the lesions are often multiple.[124]

Resection of a solitary pulmonary metastasis was reported in the literature as early as 1947.[208] Goya and colleagues[209] recently published data from 62 thoracotomies for resection of solitary and multiple colorectal cancer metastases. The patients with solitary metastases with a maximum diameter of less than 3.0 cm had the best outcome. There was a significant difference in survival figures between those with solitary lesions, with a 5-year survival rate of 53.1%, and those with two or more lesions, whose 5-year survival rate was 12.6% ($P < .05$). Overall, the 5-year survival rate was 42% and the 10-year survival rate was 22%. This included three patients with incomplete resections of their pulmonary lesions. The persistent decline in survival was due to progressive systemic disease in most patients. Numerous factors found not to be significant variables with respect to survival included disease-free interval, stage or location of the primary tumor, and extent of the pulmonary resection.

Others have published similar data. Mansel et al.[210] reviewed 66 patients who underwent thoracotomy for solitary and multiple lesions. The 5-year survival rate was 38%, and there was a significantly better survival following resection of solitary versus multiple metastases ($P < .001$).

It has been postulated that operable metastatic disease has a slower natural rate of growth and that long-term survivors following thoracotomy for metastases merely reflect this difference in the natural history of their disease.

The true impact and role of resection of pulmonary metastases remain to be elucidated.

Systemic Therapy

Chemotherapy

For the majority of patients presenting with metastatic colorectal cancer, systemic chemotherapy is the mainstay of available treatment. In spite of ongoing efforts to develop more effective regimens, patients with unresectable metastatic disease have a median survival of 6 to 10 months.[211]

5-FU remains the backbone of systemic chemotherapeutic regimens in metastatic colorectal cancer. Initially, 5-FU was administered alone and attention was focused on ideal dosing schedules as well as mode of administration. Studies have documented that intravenous dosing is more effective than oral administration.[212] The optimal dosing schedule remains unclear, with once-weekly administration, 5-day bolus infusions, and prolonged continuous infusion all being utilized at present.[213] Results have been disappointing, with only 20% of patients sustaining a partial response.[214]

Many chemotherapeutic drugs have been combined with 5-FU in an attempt to improve outcome. None of them have been shown to significantly improve survival.[215] The favorable impact of 5-FU with levamisole in the adjuvant treatment of stage III colon cancer led to interest in the role of this combination in the management of metastatic disease. This was addressed by Buroker and coworkers,[216] who found no significant improvement in response rates and survival with this regimen.

Modulation of 5-FU activity by the addition of various substances has also been studied. There has been an apparent improvement in response from combining phosphonoacetyl-L-aspartate (PALA) with 5-FU.[217]

5-FU has also been combined with leucovorin, a drug that increases the cytotoxic potential of 5-FU by enhancing the binding of 5-FU to thymidylate synthetase. Erlichman et al.[218] found a significantly improved response rate in patients given 5-FU and leucovorin (33%) compared with the 5% response rate in the 5-FU–only group ($P < .0005$). This has been the most promising avenue of investigation to date and has been evaluated by several other groups as well (Table 6–5). The optimal dose of leucovorin has not been definitively identified, and further research into this regimen is ongoing.[211]

Immunotherapy

Immunotherapy treatments generally depend on modulation of the host immune system to improve response rates, and hopefully survival, of patients with metastatic colorectal cancer. Active specific therapies, as exemplified by tumor vaccines, and passive therapies, including monoclonal antibodies, have been evaluated.[219] Results have been disappointing in colon cancer. This treatment remains experimental at present.

LOCAL-REGIONAL RECURRENT AND INCURABLE DISEASE

While many patients present with colorectal cancer at a stage at which it can be excised, up to 30% of individuals still present with disease that is not resectable for cure.[183] This may be caused by locally advanced disease or distant metastases. Unresectability may be due to local characteristics or distant metastases that preclude a curative resection. Another clinical problem is local-regional recurrence, most commonly occurring in the pelvis after excision of rectal cancer, which is a source of great morbidity.

Advanced Local Disease

When an unresectable primary tumor is encountered, the surgeon's intraoperative decision-making skills are called to task. The decision as to which procedure to perform for palliation depends on the specific clinical situation.

A low-lying rectal tumor with a propensity to bleed may be left in situ, and a plan for intermittent transanal fulguration would be appropriate. A nearly obstructing lesion of the rectosigmoid, made incurable by metastatic liver disease, might be best managed by excision and a Hartmann procedure if a low anterior resection were thought to be too difficult or to carry too high a potential morbidity. A locally advanced rectal tumor with fixation to the pelvic sidewall may be best managed with a diverting proximal colostomy.

When palliative stomas are created, special attention should be paid to operative technique and siting to facilitate the best possible palliation.[220] The use of fascial bridge to support a loop colostomy obviates the need for a rod, providing a more manageable stoma. In patients expected to live for up to 1 to 2 years, the longer-term complications of a loop colostomy, including prolapse and herniation, become relevant considerations. An end-loop stoma has a lower rate of prolapse and is less bulky, allowing for a more discrete appliance and better patient acceptance. A "hidden" loop colostomy may be placed in a subcutaneous position in a patient who has the potential for obstruction in the future. This can then be easily opened under local anesthesia if obstruction should occur, preventing the need for another operation.

Symptomatic bony invasion may respond to radiotherapy. However, it has been shown that symptom control is achieved only for an average of 4 months. Thus, this modality is administered once clinically warranted, not on immediate diagnosis of the situation. Radiotherapy may also be given in the neoadjuvant setting when a locally advanced lesion is first discovered. High-dose, preoperative radiation may significantly minimize bulky disease, reduce the degree of lymph node involvement, and allow for a potentially curative resection to proceed subsequently.[221]

Recurrent Disease

Local recurrence occurs in up to 76% of patients who have recurrent colon cancer, and up to 35% of all patients

TABLE 6–5
Randomized Studies of 5-Fluorouracil (5-FU) Modulated by Leucovorin (LV)

Study	Design	Results
Erlichman et al.[218]	5-day schedule of 5-FU (370 mg/m²/day) vs. 5-FU (370 mg/m²/day) + LV (200 mg/m²/day); 125 evaluable patients with metastatic colorectal cancer	5-FU + LV produced significant improvement in response rate (33% vs. 7%), time to progression of disease, and median survival (1.26 vs. 9.6 mo)
Doroshow et al.[228]	5-day schedule of bolus 5-FU (370 mg/m²/day) + high-dose LV (500 mg/m²/day) by continuous infusion vs. 5-FU (370 mg/m²/day) alone; crossover design; 76 evaluable patients	5-FU + LV was superior for time to progression; response rate 44% versus 13%; trend toward prolonged survival
Petrelli et al.[229]	Three treatment arms; 5-day schedule of 5-FU alone (500 mg/m²/day); weekly 5-FU (600 mg/m²) + high-dose LV (500 mg/m²); weekly 5-FU (600 mg/m²) + low-dose LV (25 mg/m²); 328 evaluable patients	Response rate, 30.3% for high-dose LV regimen, 18.8% for low-dose regimen, 12.1% for 5-FU alone; trend toward longer survival in high-dose LV group
Poon et al.[230]	Treatment arms (5-day schedule); 5-FU alone (500 mg/m²/day); 5-FU (370 mg/m²/day) + intermediate-dose LV (200 mg/m²); 5-FU (425 mg/m²/day) + low-dose LV (20 mg/m²); 5-FU (325 mg/m²/day) + cisplatin (20 mg/m²/day); sequential MTX (200 mg/m² over 4 hr) followed at hour 7 by 5-FU (900 mg/m²) and at hour 24 by oral LV (14 mg/m² q6h × 8) q3wk; low-dose MTX (40 mg/m²) followed at hour 24 by 5-FU (700 mg/m²) on days 1 and 8 q4wk; 429 evaluable patients with metastatic colorectal cancer	Both LV regimens produced significant survival advantage (12 vs. 7.7 mo) compared with 5-FU alone; tumor response rate was highest in low-dose LV regimen (43%); improved interval-to-tumor-progression rates in 5-FU + LV arms
Petrelli et al.[231]	Three treatment arms; loading course of 5-FU alone (450 mg/m²/day, then 200 mg/m² qod for six doses); weekly 5-FU (600 mg/m²) + high-dose LV (500 mg/m²); weekly MTX (50 mg/m² over 4 hr) immediately followed by 5-FU (600 mg/m²); 65 evaluable patients	Response rate, 11% for 5-FU alone, 5% for 5-FU + MTX, 48% for 5-FU + LV; median duration of response was 10 mo for 5-FU + LV; no significant differences in overall survival
NCOG[232]	Three treatment arms; 5-day loading course of 5-FU alone (12 mg/kg/day) followed by weekly treatment (15 mg/kg) with maximum dose of 800 mg; 5-day schedule of 5-FU (400 mg/m²) + high-dose LV (200 mg/m²/day); sequential MTX (50 mg/m² q6h × 5) followed at hour 24 by 5-FU (500 mg/m²) and LV (10 mg/m² q6h × 6)	No differences in response rates among treatment groups; median time to failure was significantly different between 5-FU alone and sequential MTX, 5-FU, and LV (138 vs. 182 days, $P = .04$); no differences in median survival

Adapted from Grem JL: Current treatment approaches in colorectal cancer. Semin Oncol 18(Suppl 1):17–26, 1991.
MTX, Methotrexate.

who have undergone excision of rectal cancer suffer the same fate.[222] While the development of adjuvant therapy protocols has been aimed at decreasing the incidence of local failure, as well as systemic relapse, locally recurrent tumor remains a clinical problem of significant proportions.

Local recurrence of colon cancer in the tumor bed or involving other intra-abdominal viscera is often asymptomatic, and its true extent may not be fully appreciated until autopsy.[223] Anastomotic recurrence occurs in 5% to 15% of patients following excision of colorectal cancers.[224] The mode of development of this form of recurrent disease remains under debate. Studies have demonstrated a definite propensity for these recurrences to develop at colocolic and colorectal anastomoses, with only a very small percentage occurring at ileocolic anastomoses.[225] With exploration for possible reresection as the only hope of cure, the importance of regular follow-up endoscopy is reiterated, with improved complete reresection rates in those studies employing this in routine follow-up.[226]

TABLE 6–6
Survival After Resection of Regional Tumor Recurrence

Authors (Year)	Operation	No.	Median Survival Time (mo)	5-Year Survival Rate (%)
Wanebo et al. (1987)[233]	Abdominosacral resection	28	36	20
Pearlman et al. (1987)[234]	Sacropelvic exenteration	15	18	60*
Schiessel et al. (1986)[235]	Resections for local recurrence	109	14	30*
Gunderson et al. (1988)[236]	Resections for radiograph	36	16	17
Polk et al. (1971)[237]	Curative resection	11	21	25
Vassilopoulos et al. (1981)[226]	Reresection of abdominal recurrence	12	41	34

Adapted from Benotti P, Steele G Jr: Patterns of recurrent colorectal cancer and recovery surgery. Cancer 70:1409–1413, 1992.
*Projected.

Locally recurrent rectal cancer presents a clinical challenge. Historically, pelvic recurrences have not been amenable to curative reoperation, committing the patient to progressive, unremitting pain. However, radiotherapy and chemotherapy have had limited success in palliating these patients. This has led to renewed interest in aggressive surgical techniques in the search for the best palliative intervention in patients with isolated pelvic recurrences.

Benotti and Steele[227] have reviewed their experience with radical excision of isolated pelvic recurrences in 51 patients, of whom 38 had recurrent colorectal cancer. Surgical procedures included "completion" abdominoperineal resection, radical resection of tumor recurrence, and pelvic exenteration. Major exenteration was indicated only if all tumor could be resected, not as a planned palliative procedure. Piecemeal excision was not performed, as it was followed by early recurrence and did not provide adequate palliation. Intraoperative radiotherapy was used only shortly before or after a course of conventional external beam radiotherapy as a boost. Its role remains to be better defined. At laparotomy, seven patients were found to have clearly unresectable disease, and only biopsy or diversion was performed. Of those with colorectal cancer, overall survival is 35% after median follow-up of more than 24 months.[228] In the group who underwent palliative resection, median survival was 12 months. Of the 26 patients with colorectal cancer recurrence who underwent a curative procedure, 5 remain disease-free at a median follow-up of 39 months, and median survival was 22 months for the 17 who died. Only two postoperative deaths occurred, and median hospital stay was 2 to 3 weeks.

While similar results have been obtained by some other groups (Table 6–6), not all have had even this modest degree of success. In the personal experience of the authors, excision of pelvic recurrences involving the sacrum in nine consecutive patients has not led to any long-term survivors. Further work is needed to better define preoperatively those who stand to benefit from radical extirpative procedures. The efficacy of adjuvant therapies must also be improved.

References

1. National Cancer Institute Division of Cancer Prevention and Control Survey. National Institutes of Health Publication No. 91-2789.
2. Wingo PA, Tong T, Bolden S: Cancer statistics, 1995. CA 45:8–30, 1995.
3. Burt RW, Bishop DT, Cannon-Albright L, et al: Hereditary aspects of colorectal adenomas. Cancer 70:1296–1299, 1992.
4. Bussey HJR: Familial Polyposis Coli: Family Studies, Histopathology, Differential Diagnosis and Results of Treatment. Baltimore: Johns Hopkins University Press, 1975.
5. Sivak MV, Jagelman DG: Upper gastrointestinal endoscopy in polyposis syndromes: Familial polyposis coli and Gardner's syndrome. Gastrointest Endosc 30:102–194, 1984.
6. Berk T, Cohen Z, McLeod R, Stern HS: Management of mesenteric desmoid tumours in familial adenomatous polyposis. CJS 35:393–395, 1992.
7. Leppert M, Dobbs P, Scambler P, et al: The gene for familial polyposis maps to the long arm of chromosome 5. Science 238:1411–1413, 1987.
8. Nishisho I, Nakamura Y, Miyoshi Y, et al: Mutations of chromosome 5q21 genes in FAP and colorectal cancer patients. Science 53:665–669, 1991.
9. Petersen GM, Slack J, Nakamura Y: Screening guidelines and premorbid diagnosis of familial adenomatous polyposis using linkage. Gastroenterology 100:1658–1664, 1991.
10. Lynch HT, Watson P, Kriegler M, et al: Differential diagnosis of hereditary nonpolyposis colorectal cancer (Lynch syndrome I and Lynch syndrome II). Dis Colon Rectum 31:373–377, 1988.
11. Fitzgibbons RJ Jr, Lynch HT, Stanislav GV, et al: Recognition and treatment of patients with hereditary nonpolyposis colon cancer (Lynch syndromes I and II). Ann Surg 206:289–295, 1987.
12. Lynch PM, Lynch HT, Harris RE: Hereditary proximal colonic cancer. Dis Colon Rectum 23:661–668, 1977.
13. Lynch HT, Watson P, Smyrk TC, et al: Colon cancer genetics. Cancer 70:1300–1312, 1992.
14. Vasen HFA, Mecklin JP, Meera Khan P, Lynch HT: The International Collaborative Group on Hereditary Non-Polyposis Colorectal Cancer (ICG-HNPCC). Dis Colon Rectum 34:424–425, 1991.
15. Lovett E: Family studies in cancer of the colon and rectum. Br J Surg 63:13–18, 1976.
16. Duncan JL, Kyle J: Family incidence of carcinoma of the colon and rectum in north east Scotland. Gut 23:169–171, 1982.
17. Guillem JG, Neugut AI, Forde KA, et al: Colonic neoplasms in asymptomatic first-degree relatives of colon cancer patients. Am J Gastroenterol 83:271–273, 1988.
18. Burt RW, Bishop T, Cannon L, et al: Dominant inheritance of adenomatous colonic polyps and colorectal cancer. N Engl J Med 312:1540–1544, 1985.
19. Vogelstein B, Fearon ER, Hamilton SR, et al: Genetic alterations during colorectal-tumor development. N Engl J Med 319:525–532, 1988.
20. Fearon ER, Cho KR, Nigro JM, et al: Identification of a chromosome 18q gene which is altered in colorectal cancers. Science 247:49–56, 1990.
21. Sidransky D, Tokino T, Hamilton SR, et al: Identification of *ras* oncogene mutations in the stool of patients with curable colorectal tumours. Science 256:102–105, 1992.
22. Burkitt DP: Epidemiology of cancer of the colon and rectum. Cancer 28:3–13, 1971.
23. Haenszel W, Kurihara M: Studies of Japanese migrants; mortality from cancer and other diseases among Japanese in the United States. J Natl Cancer Inst 40:43–68, 1967.
24. Doll R, Peto R: The causes of cancer; quantitative estimates of avoidable risks of cancer in the United States. J Natl Cancer Inst 66:1197–1312, 1981.
25. McKeown-Eyssen G, Bright-See E: Dietary factors in colon cancer: International relationships. Nutr Cancer 6:160–170, 1984.
26. Jain M, Cook GM, Davis FG, et al: A case-control study of diet and colorectal cancer. Int J Cancer 26:757–768, 1980.
27. Bruce WR: Recent hypothesis for the origin of colon cancer. Cancer Res 47:4237–4242, 1987.
28. Kashtan H, Stern HS: Colonic proliferation and colon cancer risk. Isr J Med Sci 28:813–819, 1992.
29. Bristol, HB, Emmett PM, Heaton KW, et al: Sugar, fat and the risk of colorectal cancer. Br Med 291:1467–1470, 1985.
30. Miller AB, Howe GR, Jain M, et al: Food items and food groups as risk factors in a case-control study of diet and colorectal cancer. Int J Cancer 32:155–161, 1983.
31. Trock B, Lanza E, Greenwald P: Dietary fiber, vegetables, and colon cancer: Critical review and meta-analyses of the epidemiologic evidence. J Natl Cancer Inst 82:650–661, 1990.
32. Salyers AA: Diet and the colonic environment: Measuring the response of human colonic bacteria to changes in the host's diet. In Vahouny GV, Kritchevsky D (eds): Dietary Fiber: Basic and Clinical Aspects. New York: Plenum Press, 1986, pp 119–130.
33. Story JA, Thomas JN: Modification of bile acid spectrum by dietary fiber. In Vahouny GV, Kritchevsky D. (eds): Dietary Fiber: Basic and Clinical Aspects. New York: Plenum Press, 1982, pp 193–201.
34. Cummings JH, Southgate DAT, Branch W, et al: Colonic response to dietary fiber from carrot, cabbage, apple, bran and guar gum. Lancet 1:5–9, 1978.
35. Mower HF, Ichinotsubo D, Wang LW, et al: Fecal mutagens in two Japanese populations with different colon cancer risks. Cancer Res 42:1164–1169, 1982.
36. Reddy BS, Sharma C, Simi B, et al: Metabolic epidemiology of colon cancer: Effect of dietary fiber on fecal mutagens and bile acids in healthy subjects. Cancer Res 47:644–648, 1987.
37. Freudenheim JL, Graham S, Horvath PJ, et al: Risks associated with source of fiber and fiber components in cancer of the colon and rectum. Cancer Res 50:3295–3300, 1990.
38. Block G, Lanza E: Dietary fiber sources in the United States by demographic group. J Natl Cancer Inst 79:83–91, 1987.
39. Smigel K: Experts review NCI's Dietary Guidelines. J Natl Cancer Inst 82:344–345, 1990.
40. Reddy BS, Maeura Y: Tumour promotion by dietary fat in azoxymethane-induced carcinogenesis in female F344 rats: Influence of amount and source of dietary fat. J Natl Cancer Inst 72:745–750, 1984.
41. Nigro ND, Singh DV, Campbell RL, et al: Effect of dietary beef fat on intestinal tumour formation by azoxymethane in rats. J Natl Cancer Inst 54:439–442, 1975.
42. Bull AW, Soullier BK, Wilson PS, et al: Promotion of azoxymethane-induced intestinal cancer by high-fat diet in rats. Cancer Res 39:4956–4959, 1979.
43. Phillips RL: Role of lifestyle and dietary habits in risk of cancer among Seventh-Day Adventists. Cancer Res 35:3513–3522, 1975.

44. Georg KJ, Specht W, Nell G, et al: Effect of deoxycholate on the perfused rat colon. Digestion 25:145–154, 1982.
45. Stadler J, Stern HS, Yeung KS, et al: Effect of high fat consumption on cell proliferation activity of colorectal mucosa and on soluble fecal bile acids. Gut 29:1326–1331, 1988.
46. Wynder EL, Reddy BS, Wiesburger JH: Environmental dietary factors in colorectal cancer. Cancer 70:1222–1228, 1992.
47. Hursting SD, Thornquist M, Henderson M: Types of dietary fat and the incidence of cancer at five sites. Prev Med 19:242–253, 1990.
48. Gregoire R, Yeung KS, Stadler J, et al: Effect of high fat and low fiber meals on the cell proliferation activity of colorectal mucosa. Nutr Cancer 15:21–26, 1991.
49. Graham DY, Sackman JW: Solubility of calcium soaps of long-chain fatty acids in simulated intestinal environment. Dig Dis Sci 28:733–736, 1983.
50. Rafter JJ, Eng VWS, Furrer R, et al: Effects of calcium on the mucosal damage produced by deoxycholic acid in the rat colon. Gut 27:1320–1329, 1986.
51. Lipkin M, Newmark HL: Effect of added dietary calcium on colonic epithelial cell proliferation in subjects at high risk for familial colonic cancer. N Engl J Med 313:1381–1384, 1985.
52. Rozen P, Fireman Z, Fine N, et al: Oral calcium suppresses increased rectal epithelial proliferation of persons at risk of colorectal cancer. Gut 30:650–655, 1989.
53. Gregoire RC, Stern HS, Yeung KS, et al: Effect of calcium supplementation on mucosal cell proliferation in high risk patients for colon cancer. Gut 30:376–382, 1989.
54. Stern HS, Gregoire RC, Kashtan H, Stadler J, Bruce WR: Long term effects of dietary calcium on risk markers for colon cancer in patients with familial polyposis. Surgery 108:528–533, 1990.
55. Wynder EL, Shigematsu T: Environmental factors of cancer of the colon and rectum. Cancer 20:1520–1561, 1967.
56. Pollack ES, Nomura AMY, Heilbrun LK, et al: Prospective study of alcohol consumption and cancer. N Engl J Med 310:617–621, 1984.
57. Stern HS, Gregoire R, Kashtan H, et al: A randomized controlled trial of sodium sulfate and dietary fiber on fecal pH and mucosal risk factors for colon cancer. J Natl Cancer Inst 82:950–952, 1990.
58. Crohn BB, Rosenberg M: Sigmoidoscopic picture of chronic ulcerative colitis. Am J Med Sci 170:220–225, 1925.
59. Edwards FC, Truelove SC: The course and prognosis of ulcerative colitis. IV. Gut 5:15–21, 1964.
60. Gilat T, Fireman Z, Grossman A, et al: Colorectal cancer in patients with ulcerative colitis: A population study in central Israel. Gastroenterology 94:870–877, 1988.
61. Ekbom A, Helmick C, Zack M, et al: Increased risk of large bowel cancer in Crohn's disease with colon involvement. Lancet 336:357–359, 1990.
62. Savoca PE, Ballantyne GH, Cahow CF: Gastrointestinal malignancies in Crohn's disease: A 20-year experience. Dis Colon Rectum 33:7–11, 1990.
63. Burmer GC, Levine DS, Kulander BJ, et al: c-Ki-*ras* mutations in chronic ulcerative colitis and sporadic colon carcinoma. Gastroenterology 99:416–420, 1990.
64. Ekbom A, Helmick C, Zack M, et al: Ulcerative colitis and colorectal cancer: A population-based study. N Engl J Med 323:1228–1233, 1990.
65. Madjilessi SH, Farrer RG, Easley KA, et al: Colorectal and extra-colonic malignancy in ulcerative colitis. Cancer 58:1569–1574, 1986.
66. Gyde SN, Prior P, Allan RN, et al: Colorectal cancer in ulcerative colitis: A cohort study of primary referrals from three centers. Gut 29:206–217, 1988.
67. Correia P, Strong JP, Reif A, et al: The epidemiology of colorectal cancer. Cancer 39:2258–2264, 1977.
68. Sato E, Ouchi A, Sasano N, et al: Polyps and diverticulosis of large bowel in autopsy population of Akita prefecture, compared with Miyagi. Cancer 37:1316–1321, 1976.
69. Burt RW, Samowitz WS: The adenomatous polyp and the hereditary polyposis syndromes. Gastroenterol Clin North Am 17L:657–678, 1988.
70. Eide TJ: Prevalence and morphologic features of adenomas of the large intestine in individuals with and without colorectal carcinoma. Histopathology 10:111–118, 1986.
71. Williams AR, Balasooriya BAW, Day DW: Polyps and cancer of the large bowel: A necropsy study in Liverpool. Gut 23:835–842, 1982.
72. Correia P, Haenszel W: The epidemiology of large-bowel cancer. Adv Cancer Res 26:2–141, 1978.
73. Hill M: Metabolic epidemiology of large bowel cancer. In De Cose JJ, Sherlock P (eds): Gastrointestinal Cancer I. Boston: Martinus Nijhoff, 1981, pp 187–226.
74. Bremner CG, Ackerman LV: Polyps and carcinoma of the large bowel in the South African Bantu. Cancer 26:991–999, 1989.
75. Bat L, Pinesw A, Ron E, et al: Colorectal adenomatous polyps and carcinoma in Ashkenazi and non-Ashkenazi Jews in Israel. Cancer 58:1167–1171, 1986.
76. Niv Y: Colorectal polyps in the upper Gallilee. Isr J Med Sci 25:313–317, 1989.
77. Vatn M, Stalsberg H: The prevalence of polyps of the large intestine in Oslo: An autopsy study. Cancer 49:819–925, 1982.
78. Hoff G, Foester A, Vatn MH, et al: Epidemiology of polyps in the rectum and colon. Scand J Gastroenterol 21:853–862, 1986.
79. Clark JC, Collan Y, Eide TJ, et al: Prevalence of polyps in an autopsy series from areas with varying incidence of large-bowel cancer. Int J Cancer 36:179–186, 1985.
80. Rhodes JB, Holmes C: Changing distribution of colorectal cancer. JAMA 238:1641–1643, 1977.
81. O'Brien MJ, Winawer SJ, Zauber AN, et al: National Polyp Study Workgroup. The National Polyp Study. Gastroenterology 98:371–379, 1990.
82. Neugut AI, Pita S: Role of sigmoidoscopy in screening for colorectal cancer. Gastroenterology 95:492–499, 1989.
83. Selby JV, Friedman GD: Sigmoidoscopy in the periodic health examination of asymptomatic patients. JAMA 261:595–561, 1989.
84. Rex DK, Lehman GA, Hawes RH, et al: Screening colonoscopy in asymptomatic average-risk persons with negative fecal occult blood tests. Gastroenterology 100:64–67, 1991.
85. Lev R: Malignant potential of adenomatous polyps. In Lev R (ed): Adenomatous Polyps of the Colon. New York: Springer-Verlag, 1980, pp 52–88.
86. Eide TJ: Remnants of adenomas in colorectal carcinomas. Cancer 51:1866–1872, 1983.
87. Enterline HT, Evans GW, Mercudo-Lugo R, et al: Malignant potential of adenoma of colon and rectum. JAMA 179:322–330, 1962.
88. Muto T, Bussey HJR, Morson BC: The evolution of cancer of the colon and rectum. Cancer 36:2251–2270, 1975.
89. Tierney RP, Ballantyne GH, Modlin IM: The adenoma to carcinoma sequence. SGO 171:81–94, 1990.
90. Bussey HJR, Wallace MH, Morson BC: Metachronous carcinoma of the large intestine and intestinal polyps. Proc R Soc Med 60:208–210, 1967.
91. Morson BC, Bussey HJR: Magnitude of risk for cancer in patients with colorectal adenomas. Br J Surg 72(Suppl):S23–S28, 1985.
92. Lofti AM, Spencer RJ, Ilstrup DM, Melton MS III: Colorectal polyps and the risk of subsequent carcinoma. Mayo Clin Proc 61:337–343, 1986.
93. Winawer SJ, Zaumber Z, Diaz B, et al: The National Polyp Study: Overview of program and preliminary report of patient and polyp characteristics. In Steele GI, Burke RW, Winawer SJ, Kerr GP (eds): Basic and Clinical Perspectives of Colorectal Polyps and Cancer. Progress in Clinical and Biological Research, Vol. 279. New York: Alan R. Liss, 1988.
94. Bech K, Kronberg O, Fenger C: Adenomas and hyperplastic polyps in screening studies. World J Surg 15:7–13, 1991.
95. Cannon-Albright LA, Skolnik MH, Bishop DT, et al: Common inheritance of susceptibility to colonic adenomatous polyps and associated colorectal cancers. N Engl J Med 319:533–537, 1991.
96. Gilbertsen VA, Nelms JM: The prevention of invasive cancer of the rectum. Cancer 41:1137–1139, 1978.
97. Friedman GD, Collen MF, Fireman BH: Multiphasic health check up evaluation: A 16 year follow up. J Chronic Dis 39:453–463, 1986.
98. Selby JV, Friedman GD, Quesenberry CP, Weiss NS: A case-control study of screening sigmoidoscopy and mortality from colorectal cancer. N Engl J Med 326:653–657, 1992.
99. Winawer SG, Zauber AG, Gerdes H, National Polyp Study Workgroup: Reduction in colorectal cancer incidence following colonoscopic polypectomy: Report from the National Polyp Study. Gastroenterology 100:410, 1991.
100. Stryker SJ, Wolff BG, Culp CE, et al: Natural history of untreated colonic polyps. Gastroenterology 93:1009–1013, 1987.
101. Fearon ER, Hamilton SR, Vogelstein B: Clonal analysis of colorectal tumours. Science 238:193–197, 1987.

102. McLellan EA, Bird RP: Aberrant crypts: Potential preneoplastic lesions in the murine colon. Cancer Res 48:6187–6192, 1988.
103. Vivona AA, Shpitz B, Medline A, et al: K-*ras* mutations in aberrant crypt foci, adenomas and adenocarcinomas during azoxymethane-induced colon carcinogenesis. Carcinogenesis 14:1777–1781, 1993.
104. Ponz de Leon M, Roncucci L, Di Donata P, et al: Pattern of epithelial cell proliferation in colorectal mucosa of normal subjects and of patients with adenomatous polyps or cancer of the large bowel. Cancer Res 48:4121–4126, 1988.
105. Pretlow TP, Barrow BJ, Scott Ashton W, et al: Aberrant crypts: Putative pre-neoplastic foci in human colonic mucosa. Cancer Res 51:1564–1567, 1991.
106. Roncucci L, Medline A, Bruce R: Classification of aberrant crypt foci and microadenomas in human colon. Cancer Epidemiol Biomarkers Prev 1:57–60, 1991.
107. Watne A, Sohrabi A: Criteria for diagnosis of inherited colonic polyposis syndromes. In Herrera L (ed): Familial Adenomatous Polyposis. New York: Alan R. Liss, 1990, pp 23–31.
108. Bos JL, Fearon ER, Hamilton SR, et al: Prevalence of *ras* gene mutations in human colorectal cancers. Nature 327:293–297, 1987.
109. Barbacid M: *Ras* genes. Annu Rev Biochem 56:779–827, 1987.
110. Vogelstein B, Hamilton SR, Kern SE, et al: Genetic alterations during colorectal-tumour development. N Engl J Med 319:525–532, 1988.
111. Mitsudomi T, Steinberg SM, Oie HK, et al: *Ras* gene mutations in non–small cell lung cancers are associated with shortened survival irrespective of treatment intent. Cancer Res 51:4999–5002, 1991.
112. Solomon E, Voss R, Bodmer WF, et al: Chromosome 5 allele loss in human colorectal carcinomas. Nature 328:616–619, 1987.
113. Sasaki M, Okamoto M, Sato C, et al: Loss of constitutional heterozygosity in colorectal tumors from patients with familial polyposis coli and those with nonpolyposis colorectal carcinoma. Cancer Res 49:4402–4406, 1989.
114. Okamoto M, Saska M, Sugio K, et al: Loss of constitutional heterozygosity in colon carcinoma from patients with familial polyposis coli. Nature 331:273–277, 1988.
115. Groden J, Thliveris A, Samowitz W, et al: Identification and characterization of the familial adenomatous polyposis coli gene. Cell 66:589–600, 1991.
116. Kinzler KW, Nilbert MC, Su LK, et al: Identification of FAP locus genes from chromosome 51q21. Science 253:661–665, 1991.
117. Joslyn G, Carlson M, Thliveris A, et al: Identification of deletion mutations and three new genes at the familial polyposis locus. Cell 66:601–613, 1991.
118. Miyoshi Y, Nagase H, Ando H, et al: Somatic mutations of the APC gene in colorectal tumors: Mutation cluster region in the APC gene. Hum Mol Genet 1:229–233, 1992.
119. Nagase H, Miyoshi Y, Horii A, et al: Correlation between the location of germ-line mutations in the APC gene and the number of colorectal polyps in familial adenomatous polyposis patients. Cancer Res 52:4055–4057, 1992.
120. Fodde R, van de Luijt R, Wijnen J, et al: Eight novel inactivating germ line mutations at the APC gene identified by denaturing gradient gel electrophoresis. Genomics 13:1162–1168, 1992.
121. Powell SM, Zilz N, Beazer-Barclay Y, et al: APC mutations occur early during colorectal tumorigenesis. Nature 359:235–237, 1992.
122. Miyoshi Y, Ando H, Nagase H, et al: Germ-line mutations of the APC gene in 53 familial adenomatous polyposis patients. Proc Natl Acad Sci USA 89:4452–4456, 1992.
123. Symonds DA, Vickery AL Jr: Mucinous carcinoma of the colon and rectum. Cancer 37:1891–1900, 1976.
124. Pihl E, Hughes ESR, McDermott FT, et al: Lung recurrence after curative surgery for colorectal cancer. Dis Colon Rectum 30:417–419, 1987.
125. Sasaki O, Atkins WS, Jass JR: Mucinous carcinoma of the rectum. Histopathology 11:254–257, 1982.
126. Bonello JC, Sternberg SS, Quan SHQ: The significance of signet cell variety of adenocarcinoma of the rectum. Dis Colon Rectum 23:180–183, 1980.
127. Bear HD, MacIntyre J, Burns HJG, et al: Colon and rectal carcinoma in the west of Scotland. Symptoms, histologic characteristics, and outcome. Am J Surg 147:441–446, 1984.
128. Sugarbaker PH: Clinical evaluation of symptomatic patients. In Steele G Jr, Osteen RT (eds): Colorectal Cancer: Current Concepts in Diagnosis and Treatment. New York: Marcel Dekker, 1986, pp 59–98.
129. Aldridge MC, Phillips RKS, Hittinger R, et al: Influence of tumour site on presentation, management and subsequent outcome in large bowel cancer. Br J Surg 73:663–670, 1986.
130. Eddy DM: Screening for colorectal cancer. Ann Intern Med 113:373–384, 1990.
131. Winawer SJ, Schottenfeld D, Flehinger BJ: Colorectal cancer screening. J Natl Cancer Inst 83:243–253, 1991.
132. Greegor DH: Diagnosis of large bowel cancer in the asymptomatic patient. JAMA 201:943–945, 1967.
133. Flehinger BJ, Herbert E, Winawer SJ, et al: Screening for colorectal cancer with fecal occult blood test and sigmoidoscopy: Preliminary report of the colon project of Memorial Sloan-Kettering Cancer Center and PMI–Strang Clinic. In Chamberlain J, Miller AB (eds): Screening for Gastrointestinal Cancer. Toronto: Huber, 1988, pp 9–16.
134. Gilbertsen VA, McHugh R, Schuman L, et al: The early detection of colorectal cancers: A preliminary report of the results of the occult blood study. Cancer 45:2899–2901, 1980.
135. Hardcastle JD, Thomas WB, Chamberlain J, et al: Randomized controlled trial of faecal occult blood screening for colorectal cancer. Lancet 1:1160–1164, 1989.
136. Alquist DA: Occult blood screening—obstacles to effectiveness. Cancer 70(Suppl):1259–1265, 1992.
137. Selby J, Friedman GD, Quesenbery CP, et al: A case control study of screening sigmoidoscopy and mortality from colorectal cancer. New Engl J Med 326:653–657, 1992.
138. Bohlman TW, Katon RM, Lipschutz GR, et al: Fiberoptic pansigmoidoscopy. An evaluation and comparison with rigid sigmoidoscopy. Gastroenterology 72:644–649, 1977.
139. Smart CR: Screening and early diagnosis. Cancer 70(Suppl):1246–1251, 1992.
140. Patel D: Is screening for colorectal cancer worthwhile? Can J Oncol Suppl Colorectal Cancer 2:2–5, 1992.
141. Canadian Task Force on the Periodic Health Examination: The periodic health examination. 2. 1989 Update: Early detection of colorectal cancer and problem drinking. Can Med Assoc J 141:209–216, 1989.
142. U.S. Preventive Services Task Force: Guide to Clinical Preventive Services. Baltimore: William & Wilkins, 1989.
143. Dukes CE: The classification of cancer of the rectum. J Pathol 35:323–332, 1923.
144. Moynihan BGA: Cancer of the sigmoid flexure and rectum. Surg Gynecol Obstet 6:463–468, 1908.
145. Pezim ME, Nichols RJ: Survival after high or low ligation of the inferior mesenteric artery during curative surgery for rectal cancer. Ann Surg 200:729–733, 1984.
146. Williams NS, Dixon MF, Johnston D: Re-appraisal of the 5 cm rule of distal excision for carcinoma of the rectum: A study of distal intramural spread and of patients' survival. Br J Surg 70:150–154, 1983.
147. Brief DK, Brener BJ, Goldenkranz R, et al: Defining the role of subtotal colectomy in the treatment of carcinoma of the colon. Ann Surg 213:248–252, 1991.
148. Gunderson LL, Sosin H: Areas of failure found at re-operation (second or symptomatic look) following "curative surgery" for adenocarcinoma of the rectum: Clinicopathologic correlation and implications for adjuvant therapy. Cancer 34:1278–1292, 1974.
149. Quirke P, Dixon MF, Durdey P, et al: Local recurrence of rectal adenocarcinoma due to inadequate surgical resection: Histo-pathologic study of lateral tumour spread and surgical excision. Lancet 2:996–998, 1986.
150. Parks AG, Percy JP: Resection and sutured col-anal anastomosis for rectal carcinoma. Br J Surg 69:301–304, 1982.
151. Localio SA, Eng K, Coppa GF: Abdominosacral resection for midrectal cancer: A fifteen year experience. Ann Surg 193:320–324, 1983.
152. Devereaux DF, Eisenstat, T, Zinkin L: The safe and effective use of postoperative radiation therapy in modified Astler-Coller stage C3 rectal cancer. Cancer 63:2393–2396, 1989.
153. Deutsch AA, Stern HS: Technique of insertion of pelvic Vicryl mesh sling to avoid postradiation enteritis. Dis Colon Rectum 32:628–630, 1989.
154. Lavery IC: Curative local procedures for rectal cancer. Semin Colon Rec Surg 1:25–31, 1990.
155. Decosse JJ, Wong RJ, Quan SHQ, et al: Conservative treatment of distal rectal cancer by local excision. Cancer 63:219–223, 1989.

156. Salvati EP, Rubin RJ, Eisenstat TE, et al: Electro-coagulation of selected carcinoma of the rectum. Surg Gynecol Obstet 166:393–396, 1988.
157. Kashtan H, Stern H: The use of lasers in colorectal cancer. Cancer Invest 11:33–35, 1993.
158. Runkel NS, Schlag P, Schwarz C, et al: Outcome after emergency surgery for cancer of the large intestine. Br J Surg 78:183–188, 1991.
159. Morgan WP, Jenkins N, Lewis P, Aubrey DA: Management of obstructing carcinoma in the left colon by extended right hemicolectomy. Am J Surg 149:327–329, 1985.
160. Halevy A, Levi J, Orda R: Emergency subtotal colectomy: A new trend for treatment of obstructing carcinoma of the left colon. Ann Surg 210:220–223, 1989.
161. Ledesma EJ, Bruno S, Mittelman A: Total pelvic exenteration in colorectal disease. Ann Surg 194:458–471, 1981.
162. Lopez MJ, Kraybille WG, Downey RS, Johnston WD, Bricker EM: Exenterative surgery for locally advanced rectosigmoid cancers. Is it worthwhile? Surgery 102:644–651, 1987.
163. Boey J, Wong J, Ong GB: Pelvis exenteration for locally advanced colorectal carcinoma. Ann Surg 195:513–518, 1982.
164. Sugarbaker PH: Partial sacrectomy for en bloc excision of rectal cancer with posterior fixation. Dis Colon Rectum 25:708–711, 1982.
165. Graffner HOL, Alm POA, Oscarson JEA: Prophylactic oophorectomy in colorectal carcinoma. Am J Surg 146:233–235, 1983.
166. Blamey S, McDermott F, Pihl E, et al: Ovarian involvement in adenocarcinoma of the colon and rectum. Surg Gynecol Obstet 153:42–44, 1981.
167. McKeigan JM, Ferguson JA: Prophylactic oophorectomy and colorectal cancer in premenopausal patients. Dis Colon Rectum 22:401–405, 1979.
168. Medical Research Council Working Party: The evaluation of low dose pre-operative xray therapy in the management of operable rectal cancer; Results of a randomly controlled trial. Br J Surg 71:21–25, 1984.
169. Roswit B, Higgins GA, Keehn R: Pre-operative irradiation for carcinoma of the rectum and rectosigmoid colon: Report of a national Veterans Administration randomized study. Cancer 35:1597–1602, 1975.
170. Gerard A, Buyse M, Nordlinger B, et al: Pre-operative radiotherapy as adjuvant treatment in rectal cancer—final results of a randomized study of the European Organization for Research and Treatment of Cancer (EORTC). Ann Surg 208:606–614, 1988.
171. Stearns MW, Deddish MR, Quan SH, et al: Pre-operative roentgen therapy for cancer of the rectum and rectosigmoid. Cancer 37:2866–2874, 1974.
172. Pahlman L, Glimelius B: Pre or postoperative radiotherapy in rectal and rectosigmoid carcinoma. Ann Surg 211:187–195, 1990.
173. NIH Consensus Conference: Adjuvant therapy for patients with colon and rectal cancer. JAMA 264:1444–1450, 1990.
174. Stockholm Rectal Cancer Study Group: Pre-operative short term radiation therapy in operable rectal carcinoma—a prospective randomized trial. Cancer 66:49–55, 1990.
175. Thomas PR, Linblad AS: Adjuvant postoperative radiotherapy and chemotherapy in rectal carcinoma: A review of the Gastro-Intestinal Tumor Study Group experience. Radiother Oncol 13:245–252, 1988.
176. Krook JE, Moertel CG, Gunderson LL, et al: Effective surgical adjuvant therapy for high risk rectal carcinoma. N Engl J Med 324:709–715, 1991.
177. Fisher B, Wolmark N, Rockette H, et al: Postoperative adjuvant chemotherapy or radiation therapy for rectal cancer. Results from NSABP R-01. J Natl Cancer Inst 80:21–29, 1988.
178. Gastrointestinal Tumor Study Group: Prolongation of the disease-free interval in surgically treated rectal carcinoma. N Engl J Med 312:1465–1472, 1985.
179. Laurie JA, Moertel CG, Fleming TR, et al: Surgical adjuvant therapy of large bowel carcinoma: An evaluation of levamisole and the combination of levamisole and fluorouracil. J Clin Oncol 7:1447–1456, 1989.
180. Moertel CG, Fleming TR, Macdonald JS, et al: Levamisole and fluorouracil for adjuvant therapy of resected colon carcinoma. N Engl J Med 322:352–358, 1990.
181. Wolmark N, Fisher B, Rockette H, et al: Postoperative adjuvant chemotherapy or BCG for colon cancer: Results from NSABP Protocol C-01. J Natl Cancer Inst 80:30–36, 1988.
182. Taylor I, Michin D, Mullee M, et al: A randomized controlled trial of adjuvant portal vein cytotoxic perfusion in colorectal cancer. Br J Surg 72:359–363, 1985.
183. Sardi A: Multiple operations for recurrent colorectal cancer. Semin Surg Oncol 7:146–156, 1991.
184. Tartter PI, Slater G, Gelernt I, Ausfses AH: Screening for liver metastases from colorectal cancer with CEA and alkaline phosphatase. Ann Surg 193:357–360, 1981.
185. Kagan AR, Steckel RJ: Routine imaging studies for the post treatment surveillance of breast and colorectal carcinoma. J Clin Oncol 9:837–842, 1991.
186. Kelly CJ, Daly JM: Colorectal cancer—principles of postoperative follow up. Cancer 70:1397–1408, 1992.
187. Sugarbaker PH, Gianola FJ, Dwyer A, Neuman NR: A simplified plan for follow up of patients with colon and rectal cancer supported by prospective studies of laboratory and radiologic test results. Surgery 102:79–87, 1987.
188. Steele G Jr: Follow up plans after "curative" resection of primary colon or rectal cancer. In Steele G Jr, Osteen RT (eds): Colorectal Cancer: Current Concepts in Diagnosis and Treatment. New York: Marcel Dekker, 1986, pp 247–279.
189. Dentsman F, Rosen L, Khubchandani T, et al: Comparing predictive decision rules in postoperative CEA monitoring. Cancer 58:2089–2095, 1986.
190. Ward BA, Miller DL, Frank JA, et al: Prospective evaluation of hepatic imaging studies in the detection of colorectal metastases: Correlation with surgical findings. Surgery 105:180–187, 1989.
191. Morson BC: The evolution of colorectal carcinoma. Clin Radiol 35:425–431, 1984.
192. Gilbertsen VA: Proctosigmoidoscopy and polypectomy in reducing the incidence of rectal cancer. Cancer 334:936–939, 1974.
193. Brady PG, Straker RJ, Goldschmidt S: Surveillance colonoscopy after resection for colon carcinoma. South Med J 83:765–768, 1990.
194. Decosse JJ, Cennerazzo W: Treatment options for the patient with colorectal cancer. Cancer 79:1342–1345, 1992.
195. Weiss L, Grundmann E, Torhorst J, et al: Hematogenous metastatic patterns in colonic carcinoma: An analysis of 1541 necropsies. J Pathol 150:195–203, 1986.
196. Wood CB, Gillis CR, Blumgart LH: A retrospective study of the natural history of patients with liver metastases from colorectal cancer. Clin Oncol 2:285–288, 1976.
197. Wilson SM, Adson MA: Surgical treatment of hepatic metastases from colorectal cancers. Arch Surg 111:330–334, 1976.
198. Hughes KS, Simon R, Songhorabdo S, et al: Resection of the liver for colorectal carcinoma metastases: A multi-institutional study of indications for resection. Surgery 103:278–279, 1988.
199. Fegiz G, Ramacciaato G, Gennari L, et al: Hepatic resections for colorectal metastases: The Italian Multicenter Experience. J Surg Oncol 2(Suppl):144–154, 1991.
200. Vogt P, Raab R, Ringe B, Pichlmayr R: Resection of synchronous liver metastases from colorectal cancer. World J Surg 15:62–67, 1991.
201. Ekberg H, Tranberg KG, Andersson R, et al: Determinants of survival in liver resection for colorectal secondaries. Br J Surg 73:727–731, 1986.
202. Hughes KS, Rosenstein RB, Songhorabodi S, et al: Resection of the liver for colorectal carcinoma metastases: A multi-institutional study of long term survivors. Dis Colon Rectum 31:1–4, 1988.
203. Cobourn CS, Makowka L, Langer B, et al: Examination of patient selection and outcome for hepatic resection for metastatic disease. Surg Gynecol Obstet 165:239–246, 1987.
204. Wagman LD, Kemeny MM, Leong L, et al: A prospective, randomized evaluation of the treatment of colorectal cancer metastases to the liver. J Clin Oncol 8:1885–1893, 1990.
205. Chang AE, Schneider PD, Sugarbaker PH, et al: A prospective randomized trial of regional versus systemic continuous 5-fluorodeoxyuridine chemotherapy in the treatment of colorectal liver metastases. Ann Surg 206:685–693, 1987.
206. Martin JK, O'Connell MJ, Wieand HS, et al: Intra-arterial floxuridine vs. systemic fluorouracil for hepatic metastases from colorectal cancer. Arch Surg 125:1022–1027, 1990.
207. Murray KD: Excision of pulmonary metastasis of colorectal cancer. Semin Surg Oncol 7:157–161, 1991.
208. Alexander J, Haight C: Pulmonary resection for solitary metastatic sarcomas and carcinomas. Surg Gynecol Obstet 85:129–146, 1947.

209. Goya T, Miyazawa N, Kondo H, et al: Surgical resection of pulmonary metastases from colorectal cancer—10 year follow up. Cancer 64:1418–1421, 1989.
210. Mansel JK, Zinsmeister AR, Pairolero PC, Jett JR: Pulmonary resection of metastatic colorectal adenocarcinoma—a ten year experience. Chest 89:109–112, 1986.
211. Grem JL: Current treatment approaches in colorectal cancer. Semin Oncol 18(Suppl):17–26, 1991.
212. Hahn RG, Moertel CG, Schutt AJ, et al: A double-blind comparison of intensive course 5-fluorouracil by oral versus intravenous route in the treatment of colorectal carcinoma. Cancer 35:1031–1035, 1975.
213. Mayer RJ: System therapy for colorectal cancer: An overview. Semin Oncol 18(Suppl):62–66, 1991.
214. Carter SK, Friedman M: Combined modality treatment of large bowel carcinoma. Cancer Treat Rev 1:114–128, 1974.
215. Mayer RJ: Chemotherapy for metastatic colorectal cancer. Cancer 70:1414–1424, 1992.
216. Buroker TR, Moertel CG, Fleming TR, et al: A controlled evaluation of recent approaches to biochemical modulation or enhancement of 5-fluorouracil therapy in colorectal carcinoma. J Clin Oncol 3:1624–1631, 1985.
217. Ardalan B, Singh G, Silverman H: A randomized phase I and II study of short term infusion of high dose fluorouracil with or without *N*-(phosphonoacetyl)-L-aspartatic acid in patients with advanced pancreatic and colorectal cancer. J Clin Oncol 6:1053–1058, 1988.
218. Erlichman C, Fine S, Wong A, et al: A randomized trial of fluorouracil and folinic acid in patients with metastatic colorectal carcinoma. J Clin Oncol 6:469–475, 1988.
219. Wadler S: The role of immunotherapy in colorectal cancer. Semin Oncol 18(Suppl):27–38, 1991.
220. Stern HS: Choices of stomas in intestinal surgery. Ann R Coll Phip Surg Can 23:341–344, 1990.
221. Poulter C: Radiation therapy for advanced colorectal cancer. Cancer 70(Suppl):1434–1437, 1992.
222. Mohiuddin M, Marks G: Adjuvant radiation therapy for colon and rectal cancer. Semin Oncol 18:411–420, 1991.
223. Russell AH, Tong D, Dawson LE, et al: Adenocarcinoma of the proximal colon. Sites of initial dissemination and patterns of recurrence following surgery alone. Cancer 53:360–367, 1984.
224. Umpleby HC, Williamson RCN: Anastomotic recurrence in large bowel cancer. Br J Surg 74:873–878, 1987.
225. Wright HK, Thomas WH, Cleveland JC: The low recurrence rate of colonic carcinoma in ileocolic anastomoses. Surg Gynecol Obstet 129:960–962, 1969.
226. Vassilopoulos PP, Yoon JM, Ledemas EJ, et al: Treatment of recurrence of adenocarcinoma of the colon and rectum at the anastomotic site. Surg Gynecol Obstet 157:777–780, 1981.
227. Benotti P, Steele G Jr: Patterns of recurrent colorectal cancer and recovery surgery. Cancer 70:1409–1413, 1992.
228. Doroshow JH, Multhauf P, Leong L, et al: Prospective randomized comparison of fluorouracil versus fluorouracil and high-dose continuous infusion leucovorin calcium for the treatment of advanced measurable colorectal cancer in patients previously unexposed to chemotherapy. J Clin Oncol 8:491–501, 1990.
229. Petrelli N, Douglass HO Jr, Herrera L, et al: The modulation of fluorouracil with leucovorin in metastatic colorectal carcinoma: A prospective randomized phase III trial. J Clin Oncol 7:1419–1426, 1989.
230. Poon MA, O'Connell MJ, Moertel CG, et al: Biochemical modulation of fluorouracil: Evidence of significant improvement of survival and quality of life in patients with advanced colorectal carcinoma. J Clin Oncol 7:1407–1418, 1989.
231. Petrelli N, Herrera L, Rustum Y, et al: A prospective randomized trial of 5-fluorouracil versus 5-fluorouracil and high-dose leucovorin versus 5-fluorouracil & methotrexate in previously untreated patients with advanced colorectal carcinoma. J Clin Oncol 5:1559–1565, 1987.
232. Valone FH, Friedman MA, Wittlinger FS, et al: Treatment of patients with advanced colorectal carcinomas with fluorouracil alone, high-dose leucovorin plus fluorouracil, or sequential methotrexate, fluorouracil, and leucovorin: A randomized trial of the Northern California Oncology Group. J Clin Oncol 7:1427–1436. 1989.
233. Wanebo HJ, Gaker DL, Whitehill R, Morgan RF, Constable WC: Pelvic recurrence of rectal cancer: Options for curative resection. Ann Surg 205:482–495, 1987.
234. Pearlman NW, Donohue RE, Stiegmann GV, Ahnen DJ, Sedlacek SM, Braun TJ: Pelvic and sacropelvic exenteration for locally advanced or recurrent anorectal cancer. Arch Surg 122:537–541, 1987.
235. Schiessel R, Wunderlich M, Herbst F: Local recurrence of colorectal cancer: Effect of early detection and aggressive therapy. Br J Surg 73:342–344, 1986.
236. Gunderson LL, Martin JK, Beart RW, et al: Intraoperative and external beam irradiation for locally advanced colorectal cancer. Ann Surg 207:52–60, 1988.
237. Polk HC, Spratt JS: Recurrent colorectal carcinoma: Detection, treatment, and other considerations. Surgery 69:9–23, 1971.

Cancer of the Anal Canal

Catherine Mahut, M.D. • Hartley S. Stern, M.D.

ANATOMY

The term "anal canal" has unfortunately been defined in many different ways, creating confusion where none ought to exist. Anatomists generally consider the anal canal to encompass the area between the dentate line and the anal verge. Surgeons consider the anal canal to run from the upper border of the anorectal muscular ring to the palpable groove between the lower edge of the internal sphincter and the subcutaneous portion of the external sphincter, measuring 3.5 to 4.5 cm in length in women and 4.0 to 5.0 cm in men.[1] For the purpose of this chapter, we have adopted the use of the surgical anal canal definition and refer to tumors entirely below the dentate line extending onto anal skin as anal margin tumors. This is in essence what the American Joint Committee on Cancer has done.

The importance of clarifying which definition is being utilized cannot be overstated, since in most but not all series the predisposition to lymph node or hematogenous metastases appears to be greater in tumors arising in the anal canal.[2]

TABLE 6–7
Anal Cancer—Selected Results of Concurrent Radiation, 5-Fluorouracil (5-FU), and Mitomycin

Reference	Chemotherapy		Radiation (Gy/Fraction/ Time)	Primary Tumor Control		Regional Node Control	5-Year Survival Rate
	*5-FU**	*Mitomycin*					
Leichman[14]	1000 mg/m²/24 hr IVI days 1–4 and 29–32	15 mg/m² IVB day 1	30 Gy/15/days 1–21	31/34 (91%) (≤5 cm)	7/10 (70%) (<5 cm)	NS	80%, crude
Sischy[15]	1000 mg/m²/24 hr IVI days 2–5 and 28–31	10 mg/m² IVB day 1	40.8 Gy/24/days 1–35	22/26 (85%) (<3 cm)	32/50 (64%) (≥3 cm)	NA	73%, 3-yr actuarial
Cummings[7]	1000 mg/m²/24 hr IVI days 1–4 and 43–46	10 mg/m² IVB days 1 and 43	48–50 Gy/24–20/ days 1–58 (split course)	25/27 (93%) (≤5 cm)	16/20 (80%) (>5 cm or T4)	4/5	65%, actuarial
Schneider[16]	1000 mg/m²/24 hr IVI days 1–4 and 29–32	10 mg/m² IVB days 1 and 29	50 Gy/25–28/ days 1–35 ± boost	21/22 (95%) (≤5 cm)	14/19 (74%) (>5 cm or T4)	3/4	77%, actuarial
Papillon[17]	600 mg/m²/24 hr IVI (120 hr) days 1–5	12 mg/m² IVB day 1	42 Gy/10/days 1–19 plus interstitial boost 20 Gy day 78	—	57/70 (81%) (≤4 cm)	NS	NS
Tanum[18]	1000 mg/m²/24 hr IVI days 1–4	10–15 mg/m² IVB day 1	50–54 Gy/25–27/ days 1–35	28/30 (93%) (≤5 cm)	42/56 (75%) (>5 cm or T4)	NS	72%, actuarial
Cummings[7]	1000 mg/m²/24 hr IVI days 1–4	10 mg/m² IVB day 1	50 Gy/20/days 1–28	3/3 (100%) (≤5 cm)	11/13 (85%) (>5 cm or T4)	3/3	75%, actuarial
Doci[19]	750 mg/m²/24 hr IVI days 1–5/ 43–47/85–89	15 mg/m² IVB days 1/43/85	54–60 Gy/30–33/ days 1–53 (split course)	28/38 (74%) (≤5 cm)	9/17 (53%) (>5 cm)	8/8	81%, actuarial

Adapted from Cohen A, Cummings B, et al: Cancer of the Colon, Rectum & Anus. New York, McGraw-Hill, 1994.
IVI, Continuous intravenous infusion; IVB, intravenous bolus injection; NS, not stated; NA, not applicable; T4, invading adjacent organs.
*All infusions 96 hours except where shown.

HISTOPATHOLOGY

Epidermoid cancer is the most frequent cancer in the anal canal, accounting for 80% of all primary tumors in this region.[3] Melanoma, adenocarcinoma, lymphoma, carcinoid tumors, and sarcomas make up the remaining 20% of tumors. Epidermoid cancer may be further subclassified into squamous, basaloid, mucoepidermoid, and the rare small cell anaplastic tumors. For practical purposes, except for the poor prognosis in anaplastic tumors, the remainder have similar behavior patterns and are thus treated similarly.[4]

ETIOLOGY

The transmission of specific human papillomaviruses (HPVs) is associated with a spectrum of anogenital neoplasia.[5] Palmer et al.[6] as well as others have demonstrated a correlation with HPV 16 and 18 in the development of squamous carcinoma of the anus.[6]

NATURAL HISTORY

Hematogenous spread is less common in anal tumors than lymphatic and direct local extension.[7] The major lymphatic pathways are shown in Figure 6–2. At the time of diagnosis, pelvic or inguinal node metastases are present in 15% to 30% of patients.[4, 8, 9] After any form of radical treatment, relapse is more common in the pelvis than outside the pelvis.[4, 10]

TREATMENT

In the last 20 years, there has been tremendous change in the overall approach to the management of anal tumors with the introduction of treatment with combined chemotherapy and radiation. These changes in approach have come about because the evidence of consistently high cure rates and sphincter preservation have by and large pushed surgery to the realm of salvage treatment. Current survival data suggest that about 70% of patients are cured with this approach and that anal function is preserved in 90%.[11]

Although there is no controversy that the nonoperative approach is preferred, a number of questions are still to be resolved. They include determining

1. The relative merits of combined radiation and chemotherapy versus radiation alone.
2. The type and dose of chemotherapy.
3. The most effective radiation technique and dose.

The most common approach is the one originally described by Nigro and colleagues.[12] Originally intended as an adjuvant treatment, they ultimately established a protocol that combined 30 Gy in 15 treatments in 3 weeks together with a bolus injection of mitomycin (15 mg/m^2) on the first day of radiation and a continuous infusion of 5-fluorouracil (5-FU; 1000 mg/m^2/24 hours for 96 hours) on days 1 to 4 of radiation, the 5-FU infusion being repeated on days 29 to 32. A number of modifications have evolved to exploit the potential synergistic interactions and to reduce toxicities (Table 6–7).

Surgery for salvage of failures after combination of chemotherapy and radiation therapy generally has a poor prognosis. Zelnick and coworkers[13] reviewed their own as well as published series of abdominoperineal resection in this setting and found 17 of 24 patients (71%) dead of disease within 3 years. Thus, treatment of these failures remains a complex problem.

References

1. Nivatvongs S, Stern HS, Frych DS: The length of the anal canal. Dis Colon Rectum 24:600, 1981.
2. Greenall MS, Quan SHG, DeCosse JJ: Epidermoid cancer of the anus. Br J Surg 149:95, 1985.
3. Morson BC, Sobin JH: Histologic typing of intestinal tumours. In International Histologic Classification of Tumors, No. 15. Geneva: World Health Organization, 1976.
4. Boman BM, Moertel CG, O'Connell MJ, et al: Carcinoma of the anal canal. A clinical and pathologic study of 188 cases. Cancer 54:114, 1984.
5. Gross G, Ikenberg H, Gissman L, et al: Papillomavirus infection of the anorectal region: Correlation between histology, clinical picture and virus type: Proposal of a new nomenclature. J Invest Dermatol 88:147–152, 1985.
6. Palmer JG, Scholefield JH, Coates PJ, et al: Anal cancer and human papillomaviruses. Dis Colon Rectum 32:1016–1022, 1989.
7. Cummings BJ, Keane TJ, Thomas GM, et al: Results and toxicity of the treatment of anal carcinoma by radiation therapy or radiation therapy and chemotherapy. Cancer 54:2062, 1984.
8. Golden GT, Horsley JS: Surgical management of epidermoid cancer of the anus. Am J Surg 131:275, 1976.
9. Stearns MW, Uronacher C, Sternberg SS, et al: Cancer of the anal canal. Cancer 4:1, 1980.
10. Cummings BJ, Thomas GM, Keane TJ, et al: Primary radiation therapy in the treatment of anal canal carcinoma. Dis Colon Rectum 25:778, 1982.
11. Cummings BJ: Current management of epidermoid carcinoma of the anal canal. Gastroenterol Clin North Am 16:125–142, 1987.
12. Nigro ND, Vaitkevicious UK, Considene B: Combined therapy for cancer of the anal canal: A preliminary report. Dis Colon Rectum 17:354, 1974.
13. Zelnick RS, Haas PA, Ajlouni M, et al: Results of abdominoperineal resections for failures after combination chemotherapy and radiation therapy for anal canal cancers. Dis Colon Rectum 35:574–578, 1992.
14. Leichman L, Nigro N, Vaitkevicius VK, et al: Cancer of the anal canal. Model for preoperative adjuvant combined modality therapy. Am J Med 78:211, 1985.
15. Sischy B: The use of radiation therapy combined with chemotherapy in the management of squamous cell carcinoma of the anus and marginally resectable adenocarcinoma of the rectum. Int J Radiat Oncol Biol Phys 11:1587, 1985.
16. Schneider IHF, Grabenbauer GG, Rech T, et al: Combined radiation and chemotherapy for epidermoid carcinoma of the anal canal. Int J Colorectal Dis 7:192–196, 1992.
17. Sischy B, Doggett RLS, Krall JM, et al: Definitive irradiation and chemotherapy for radiosensitization in management of anal carcinoma: Interim report on Radiation Therapy Oncology Group Study No 8314. J Natl Cancer Inst 81:850–856, 1989.
18. Tanum G, Tveit K, Karlsen KO, et al: Chemotherapy and radiation therapy for anal carcinoma. Cancer 67:2462–2466, 1991.
19. Doci R, Zucoli R, Bombelli L, et al: Combined chemoradiation therapy for anal cancer. Ann Surg 215:150–156, 1992.

7

Lung Cancer

Primary Lung Tumors

James C. Harvey, M.D. • Julianna Pisch, M.D.
Christopher Erdman, B.A. • Eva Rubin, M.D.
Edward J. Beattie, M.D.

Lung cancer, a disease of relatively modern times, has been increasing in incidence for six decades. However, only since the 1950s have convincing epidemiologic studies linked an increase in smoking, especially cigarette smoking, to the increasing death rate attributed to lung cancer.[1, 2] In 1995, approximately 170,000 new cases of lung cancer will be diagnosed, accounting for 14% of new cancers for men and 13% for women.[3] There will be approximately 157,000 deaths from lung cancer during the year, or 33% total cancer deaths for men and 24% for women. The incidence rate has increased from 4 cases per 100,000 patient-years in men and women in 1930 to 74 cases in men and 27 cases in women in 1987. The death rate in men has recently seemed to reach a plateau, which may be attributed to a decrease in cigarette smoking among men that began in 1965,[4] following the first Surgeon General's report (Fig. 7–1). An upward trend continues among women. These statistics may be improved only by

1. Discovering and implementing preventive measures (i.e., methods of discouraging smoking initiation and helping with smoking-cessation measures).
2. Detecting the disease "early," which could involve either newer cost-efficient means (such as searching for markers in sputum cytology) or making screening measures that we already have (i.e., chest radiographs) more cost efficient.
3. Discovering means of extending treatment to patients who have not been candidates for major surgical resections in the past (i.e., improvements in systemic therapy and in internal radiation [brachytherapy]).

Modern operative technique of individual ligation of hilar vessels was described as early as 1912, but the patient died as a result of failure to understand principles of managing pleural spaces.[5, 6] Most subsequent pulmonary resections were performed by a "mass" ligature of hilar structures until 1932, when Churchill reintroduced individual dissection and ligation.[7] The next technical landmark in the history of lung cancer surgery was Graham's successful pneumonectomy in 1933.[8] For most of the time since then, only that minority of patients who presented with tumors that could be completely removed surgically and who could withstand the required loss of pulmonary parenchyma had even a chance of survival.

EPIDEMIOLOGY

Smoking

An increasing frequency of lung cancer was first observed during the 1930s, probably as a result of a gradual change in preference for cigarettes over pipe smoking. This was suspected at least as early as 1941, when Ochsner and DeBakey[9] called attention to the similarity of the rate of increase in cigarette sales in the United States and the rate of increase in prevalence of lung cancer.

In 1947, the Medical Research Council of Great Britain held a conference to discuss whether or not the dramatic increase in lung cancer deaths was "real" and if it was, to attempt to discover an explanation for its cause. A committee was organized to design a study to investigate possible

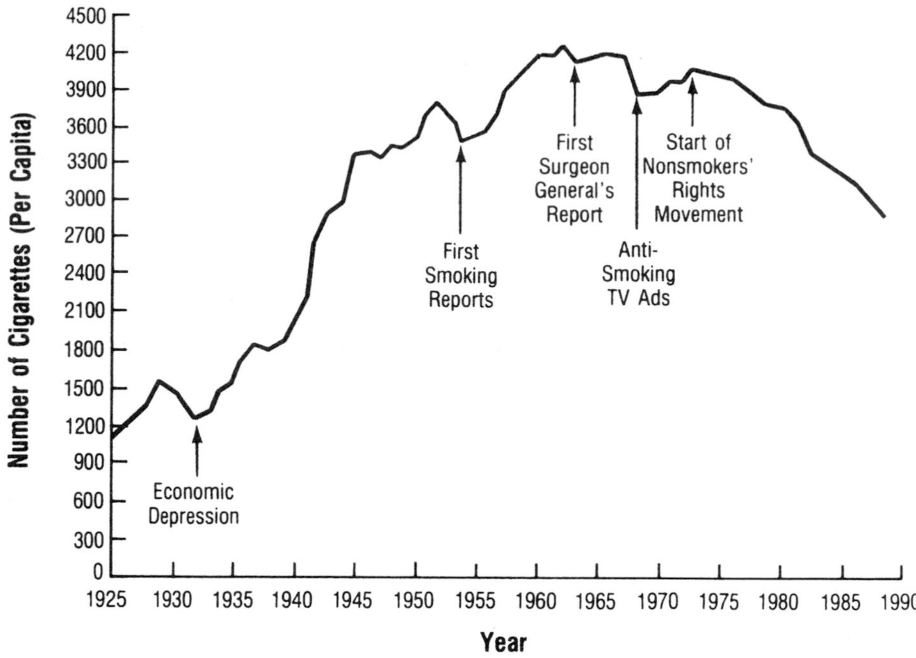

FIGURE 7–1. Annual per capita cigarette consumption. An overall decline began following the first Surgeon General's report and is continuing. The plateau in the male death rate has been attributed to this decline. (From Garfinkel L, Silverberg E: Lung cancer and smoking trends in the United States over the past 25 years. CA 41:140, 1991.)

associations, including coal smoke and general urban atmospheric pollution, arsenicals (increasingly used at that time in the treatment of syphilis), tobacco smoking, and other possibly relevant exposures that were thought to have increased during the previous 50 years. Interestingly, neither of the investigators who ultimately carried out the study (Richard Doll and A. Bradford Hill) had an a priori belief that cigarette smoking would be found of paramount importance. In Doll's words, "cigarette smoking was such a normal thing and had been for such a long time that it was difficult to think that it could be associated with any disease." At the onset of Doll and Hill's studies, general urban atmospheric pollution was at the top of the list of probable causes. Coal smoke had been prevalent in urban areas for decades and therefore was not, alone, a likely causal factor for an increasing incidence of disease. However, the additional elements of automobile exhaust fumes and known carcinogens in coal tars used to pave roads were thought to be the most likely contributors at the start of their investigations. This initial skepticism regarding tobacco may seem strange, in retrospect, because the association of pipe smoking with carcinomas of the lip and tongue was already appreciated; however at that time, these tumors were more often thought to be due to heat from the pipe stem than from the tobacco.[10]

Doll and Hill's initial study involved interviews of patients with cancers of the lung, stomach, and colon carried out in 20 London hospitals. Interviews were actually performed by medical social workers who, it was supposed, would not know the subject's disease. This was an attempt to avoid bias attributable to that knowledge. Other reasons patients with nonlung cancers were interviewed were to discover whether incriminating factors were specific for lung cancer or were more generally associated with cancers and to have them serve as a "control" group—a "case-control" study. In addition, a group of patients with diseases other than cancer, each chosen to "match" ("matched controls") a lung cancer patient in sex, age, and same time in the same hospital, was interviewed.

Every diagnosis of "query lung cancer, stomach cancer or large bowel cancer" was checked after the interviewee was discharged from hospital. At this stage, it was observed that many patients interviewed in the belief that they had lung cancer *did not have it.* It was further observed that the diagnosis was only infrequently changed in the case of heavy smokers, while it was frequently the case that nonsmokers originally classified in the "lung cancer" group had their diagnosis changed. The data were so striking that by the beginning of 1949 Doll and Hill were convinced that the association of lung cancer with cigarette smoking was strong, and there did not seem to be a strong association with any of the other factors suspected at the study's inception.[2, 10]

By the time the data for 650 men with lung cancer diagnosed in London hospitals had been studied, the investigators believed that a cause-and-effect relationship had been revealed, but they refrained from publishing such an important and unanticipated conclusion until they could duplicate the results in other British cities, eliminating the possibility "that something special about London . . . produced the result."[10] While Doll and Hill were collecting data from patients in Bristol, Cambridge, Leeds, and Newcastle, Wynder and Graham published their study of 684 cases.[1] Doll and and Hill's case-control study was published later in the same year.[2] By 1952, Doll and Hill had studied 1465 lung cancer patients.[11] A few earlier small studies had found an association of lung cancer with cigarette smoking, but the papers of Wynder and Graham and of Doll and Hill were not only larger but noteworthy for high standards in case-control methodology. Either in the design of these studies or in their analyses, a broad range of potentially important factors were examined: age; sex; urban or rural residence; social class; occupation; exposure to air pollutants; forms of domestic heating; place of interview; interview bias; diagnostic bias; and an exhaustive smoking history, which included age at which interviewee started (and stopped) smoking and age at which principle changes in the history occurred, whether or not inhaling was part of the habit, and cigarette versus pipe preference.[12]

In October 1951, Doll and Hill initiated a cohort study of physicians on the *Medical Register* in the United Kingdom. More than 40,000 sufficiently complete replies were received from 59,600 questionnaires. By March 1956, 1854 deaths had been ascertained and classified with respect to cause—86 confirmed lung cancers. Analysis of the data retrieved revealed "a marked and steady increase in the death rate from lung cancer as the amount smoked increases . . . the death rate of the heavy smokers is approximately twenty times the death rate of the non-smokers." Furthermore, the mortality was "significantly greater in cigarette than in pipe smokers . . . for each of the smoking categories, light, medium, and heavy, and therefore appears to be a function of the method of smoking irrespective of the amount." When death rates of smokers were compared with those of individuals who had given up the habit 10 years or more previously, "a progressive and significant reduction in mortality with the increase in the length of time over which smoking has been given up" was found.[13]

Doll and Hill then demonstrated both in a retrospective (case-control)[2] and in a prospective (cohort)[13] study that

1. Smokers had a higher mortality from lung cancer than nonsmokers.
2. Heavy smokers had a higher mortality from lung cancer than light smokers.
3. Cigarette smokers had a higher mortality than pipe smokers.
4. Excess mortality of cigarette smokers could be decreased by giving up the habit.

Up until that time, epidemiologic methods had not been commonly applied toward the investigation of chronic disease; in fact, the methodology developed during the 1950s to analyze the risks of cigarette smoking was to become the methodology of chronic disease. White[12] calls attention to important publications of the 1950s describing improvements in methodology of the study of chronic disease in general and of lung cancer in particular. The powerful techniques of case-control methodology developed in this decade permitted the revelation of possible causal relationships even before specific carcinogens were identified or possible mechanisms proposed. In White's words, "the method is well adapted to etiologic studies whenever the risk factor can be assessed by taking a subject's history, and it is especially effective, relative to other methods, when the disease has a long latent period, as is typical of chronic diseases." The cohort studies of Doll and Hill and of others were landmarks not only in the epidemiology of cancer but of chronic disease in general and in the study of the etiology of noninfectious disease.

The epidemiologic work that began in the 1950s and is continuing today has generated data that suggest a causal association of smoking with lung cancer, including the following observations:

1. The rarity of lung cancer in lifetime nonsmokers.
2. The large magnitude of the association with smoking, generally a 10-fold increased risk for current smokers relative to never smokers.
3. The dose-response relationship between amount smoked and relative risk of lung cancer, which can exceed 40-fold in heavy smokers.
4. The fact that relative risk increases with duration of smoking and with earlier age of starting smoking.
5. The progressive reduction in the relative risk with increasing years after quitting smoking.
6. The correlation between prevalence of smoking and lung cancer mortality rates in successive birth cohorts of men and women in the United States.

In the 1950s, some distinguished scientists had difficulty accepting the causal relationship of cigarette smoking to lung cancer because the "observational" methods of epidemiology were thought to be less than compelling evidence in the absence of any known carcinogen (at that time) in cigarette smoke and in the absence of any experimental studies demonstrating the induction of tumors following exposure to tobacco smoke.[14, 15] Since then, carcinogens have been discovered in tobacco smoke, and the mutagenicity of experimentally inhaled tobacco smoke has been confirmed.[16]

In the original studies, the association was convincing only for squamous cell and small cell lung cancer, but subsequent studies have been able to demonstrate a strength of association, though of a lesser magnitude, for glandular tumors, including the bronchioalveolar and anaplastic large cell varieties.[17]

Environmental Tobacco Smoke

It is biologically plausible that if inhaled cigarette smoke induces airway cancers, then "sidestream smoke" or environmental tobacco smoke should also increase the risk of lung cancer. In the early 1980s, two reports suggested that nonsmoking wives of smoking husbands had a significantly increased risk of lung cancer compared with nonsmoking women married to nonsmoking men. In the subsequent decade, more than 30 studies have addressed the problem, but there have been inconsistencies relating to the presence or absence of an association.[18] The largest published study of lung cancer in nonsmoking women did demonstrate that women whose husbands smoked had an increased relative risk for lung cancer, especially for adenocarcinoma. This risk tended to increase with the increasing number of pack-years of the smoking husbands.[19] Other environmental tobacco smoke exposures in adult life, such as occupational and social settings, also seemed to be associated with an increased risk. Exposure in childhood has not always been found to be a risk.[19]

Studies of passive smoking must overcome many challenges, including difficulties in obtaining accurate exposure histories; the lack of biologic markers for long-term exposures; and the possibility of confounding by dietary, household, and occupational exposures. A meta-analysis carried out by the National Research Council in 1986 combining the results of more than 30 studies found the relative risk for lung cancer of nonsmoking women whose husbands smoked to be 1.34 compared with nonsmoking women whose husbands were also nonsmokers.[20] Generally, an association is considered weak if the odds ratio is less than 3.0 and particularly so when it is less than 2.0 (as is most often the case in reports attempting to link environmental tobacco smoke with lung cancer), but it has been noted that there are many situations in medicine in which associations appear slight (e.g., "few persons harboring the meningococcus fall sick of meningococcal meningitis"[21]). Wynder and Kabat[22] have noted that the "association of environmental tobacco smoke and lung cancer risk, even if weak, would still be of concern as a public health problem and that most people are at one time or another exposed to smoke from burning tobacco products and the exhaled pollutants of tobacco smokers." Because of the special association noted with glandular tumors rather than squamous cell cancers, the investigations may be more fruitful if the emphasis is devoted to analyzing the specific relationship of adenocarcinomas to exposure to environmental tobacco smoke.[18, 22]

Environmental and Occupational Exposures

Air Pollution

There is an "urban factor" associated with lung cancer—a 1.5- to 2.0-fold greater incidence of lung cancer in cities than in rural areas. It is difficult to be confident that this effect is related to air pollution, a complex mixture of factors that has varied over time and is different from place to place, rather than to increased urban cigarette smoking and occupational exposures. However, it is known that populations exposed to point sources of pollution such as smelters suffer an increased incidence of lung cancer even after adjustment for smoking and occupational differences.

Studies examining relative lung cancer risks related to urban versus rural residence have found that for both smokers and nonsmokers, urban residence is associated with an increased risk of lung cancer. Compared with cigarette smoking, however, the percentage increase in lung cancer risk is calculated to be only modest.[18]

Asbestos Exposure

Exposure to asbestos fibers has been clearly linked to an excess of lung cancer deaths. Asbestos-induced lung cancer is characterized by an interval of 20 or more years between exposure to asbestos and subsequent development of lung cancer. The exposure itself need not have been lengthy, as evidenced by a cohort of workers in an amosite factory whose risk for development of lung cancer was doubled after working only 9 months or less in the factory. Also, a persisting excess risk of lung cancer has been observed among former shipyard workers of the World War II era.

The carcinogenicity of asbestos exposure is synergistic with cigarette smoking. The relative risk for development of lung cancer with asbestos exposure alone is about 5 times that of the "normal" population, 10 times for cigarette smokers alone, but 50 times for smoking asbestos workers.[23] Typical occupational risks for asbestos exposure include mining, milling, and textile, insulation, shipyard, and cement work.

Other Occupational Exposures

Other occupational groups with suspected higher risks of lung cancer include those exposed to radiation, including radon; polycyclic aromatic hydrocarbons; mustard gas; chloromethyl ethers; chromium; nickel; inorganic arsenic; and vinyl chlorides. Other suspected agents include acrylonitrile exposures encountered by rubber workers; beryllium; ferric oxide dust; and lead and cadmium.[16, 24–26]

For radon exposure,[16, 18] an increased risk for lung cancer has been established among uranium miners in Colorado, Canada, and the former Czechoslovakia and among other miners in Britain and the United States. Experimentally, respiratory tumors have been induced by inhaled radon daughters in laboratory animals. Radon is known to act synergistically with cigarette smoking, but the risk is less than the multiplicative risk associated with asbestos exposure.

The knowledge of the increased risk of lung cancer associated with radon exposure in the occupational setting has led to public concern regarding even the lower level of radon exposure in some homes. Results regarding the risk of residential radon exposure are inconclusive, with little or no effect found attributable to radon exposure in studies performed in New Jersey and China. A study from Sweden showed not only an increased risk associated with radon exposure but synergism with cigarette smoking. Prospective studies might reveal the threshold of radon exposure that places the residents of a dwelling at risk and clarify the interaction between radon exposure and cigarette smoking.[27]

Diet

Vegetables

A high intake of vegetables has been found to be protective in epidemiologic studies of diet and lung cancer.[18] Some studies have demonstrated protective effects of dietary vitamin A intake from vegetable sources.[28] Others have found a strong protective effect of (variously) all vegetables, dark-green vegetables, cruciferous vegetables, and tomatoes. It has been hypothesized that the antioxidant effect of beta carotene, vitamin C, and vitamin E, free radical scavengers, explains the protective effect of dietary vegetable consumption. Clinical trials are under way to test the protective effects of vitamin A, beta carotene, synthetic retinoids, vitamin E, and selenium in high-risk persons, including smokers and asbestos-exposed workers.[29–32]

Fat Intake

In general, there is a higher incidence of lung cancer in countries where there is higher animal fat consumption. Case-control studies have revealed a dietary association of fat and cholesterol intake with lung cancer even after adjustment for smoking.[18]

Hormones

Data exist that suggest that endocrine factors influence the development of adenocarcinoma of the lung in women. Estrogen receptors are found with a high incidence in adenocarcinomas but not in squamous cell lung tumors, and there is known to be a higher risk of adenocarcinoma of the lung among 10-year survivors of endometrial cancer as well as among women seeking estrogen replacement therapy. There is also a high risk of adenocarcinoma of the lung among Chinese women with short menstrual cycles (<26 days) in spite of a low prevalence of smoking in this population.[18]

Genetic Association

Case-control studies and pedigree analyses have discovered familial aggregations of lung cancers that persist even after adjustment for varying smoking habits and environmental exposures. The fact that adenocarcinomas are more common in families with other cancers and inherited lung disorders suggests a genetic propensity for adenocarcinoma.[18]

Behavioral scientists have demonstrated that there may be a genetic predisposition to smoking,[33] which is manifested not by initiation of the habit but by its continuance once initiated.[34]

LIFE HISTORY OF LUNG CANCER

Early (stage I) lung cancer, usually diagnosed after a routine chest radiograph reveals a shadow in an asymptomatic patient, is compatible with prolonged survival when complete resection is performed. Most patients, however, have symptoms at the time of diagnosis and are already in an advanced stage.[35] The symptoms may be related to airway obstruction, invasion of adjacent thoracic structures, pleural irritation, or systemic manifestations. The most common symptom is a cough, or perhaps more frequently a change in cough, since most cigarette smokers already have a "smoker's cough." An obstructing tumor may reveal itself with symptoms of wheezing, stridor, or pneumonia with fever, cough, and purulent sputum production. An occasional sequela is lung abscess formation. Blood-streaked sputum occurs in about 25% of lung cancer patients, but massive hemoptysis is rare. Dyspnea has been commonly reported among lung cancer patients, but it is often a consequence of emphysematous changes secondary to prolonged cigarette smoking rather than specific for lung cancer. A change in baseline exercise tolerance may be due to airway obstruction or a pleural effusion, which can greatly handicap exercise tolerance. Pain is a serious prognostic sign, since it may indicate pleural, chest wall, spinal, or mediastinal involvement. Hoarseness may arise from involvement of the recurrent laryngeal nerve, especially on the left side, where the nerve descends to the ligamentum arteriosum. A paralyzed diaphragm suggests involvement of the phrenic nerve, due to either direct invasion or metastasis to the mediastinum.

Systemic changes such as pulmonary osteoarthropathy can occur, as can generalized abnormality secondary to abnormal hormone production or biochemical changes. Peculiar myoneuropathies such as Eaton-Lambert syndrome along with other neurologic and endocrine conditions are uncommon but are important to distinguish from musculoskeletal and neurologic complaints due to metastatic disease. Symptoms due to abnormal secretory products of the primary lung tumor may be relieved by treating the tumor. Occasionally, central nervous system symptoms are the first manifestation of an occult primary lung cancer with brain metastases. New musculoskeletal complaints or bone pain may also be a symptom of metastatic disease due to an occult lung cancer.

Tumors of the lung may invade locally, crossing fissures into adjacent lobes or extending into pleura, chest wall, and mediastinal structures. Tumor cells also migrate via lymphatic channels of the tracheobronchial tree into nodes that communicate with lymphatics accompanying major pulmonary vessels into the mediastinum. In the mediastinum, metastatic tumors may grow within nodes (see Color Fig. 7–2) ranging from the paratracheal area (levels 1 to 4), arch of the aorta (levels 5 and 6), and subcarinal area (level 7), through the inferior pulmonary ligament (levels 8 and 9). From the upper paratracheal area, lymphatics may drain into supraclavicular nodes. Systemic metastases arise from exfoliated tumor cells carried through pulmonary veins and distributed by hematogenous spread. Metastases to brain, bone, liver, adrenal glands, and other organs

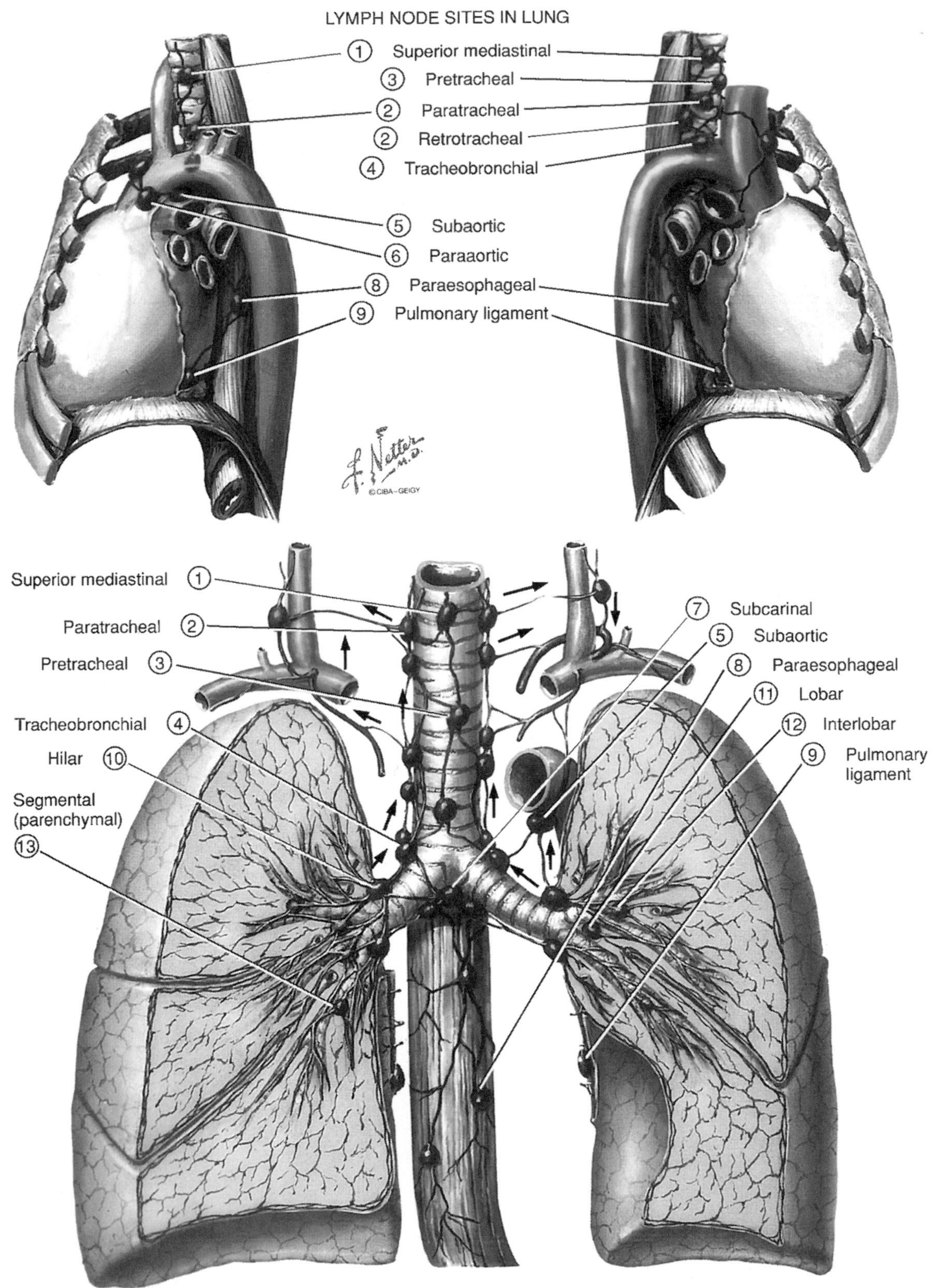

FIGURE 7–2. Staging map for lung cancer. Single-digit numbers designate mediastinal nodes; double-digit numbers designate thoracic nodes. (From Harvey JC, Beattie EJ: Lung cancer. CIBA-GEIGY Clin Symp 45:6, 1993. © Copyright 1993, CIBA-GEIGY Corporation. Reprinted with permission from Clinical Symposia, illustrated by Frank H. Netter, M.D., John A. Craig, and David Mascaro. All rights reserved.)

roughly parallel cardiac output distribution. Death is most often related to distant spread of tumor. Either surgery or radiotherapy most often provides local control, but only the development of more effective combinations of systemic treatment will truly result in a great impact on survival.

LOCAL-REGIONAL ANATOMY

Figures 7–3 and 7–4 clearly demonstrate the anatomy of the hemithoraces, with the lungs removed for clarity of exposure. The mediastinum is lined by pleura continuous with that of the chest wall and diaphragm. The phrenic nerve is seen accompanying the vena cava in the right chest. On the left side it enters the chest lateral to the innominate vein.[36]

The vagus nerves enter the chest in the midmediastinum, turning posteriorly to the hila to accompany the esophagus. On the right side, the recurrent nerve is given off high in the chest, passing posteriorly and medially under the subclavian artery; on the left, the recurrent nerve passes beneath the ligamentum arteriosum. The main hilar relationships are appropriately labeled. In the midmediastinum, the trachea descends posterior to the superior vena cava and bifurcates into right and left main bronchi below the azygos vein. The esophagus runs posterior to the trachea and anterior to the vertebral bodies. The esophagus is more to the right in its midportion and more to the left as it progresses distally.

The lateral view of the right lung (Fig. 7–5) reveals the oblique fissure, separating the upper and middle lobes from the lower, and the horizontal fissure, separating the upper lobe from the middle. The oblique fissure follows the course of the sixth rib, while the horizontal fissure originates at a point of intersection of a midaxillary line and the oblique fissure, continuing anteriorly toward the sternum at

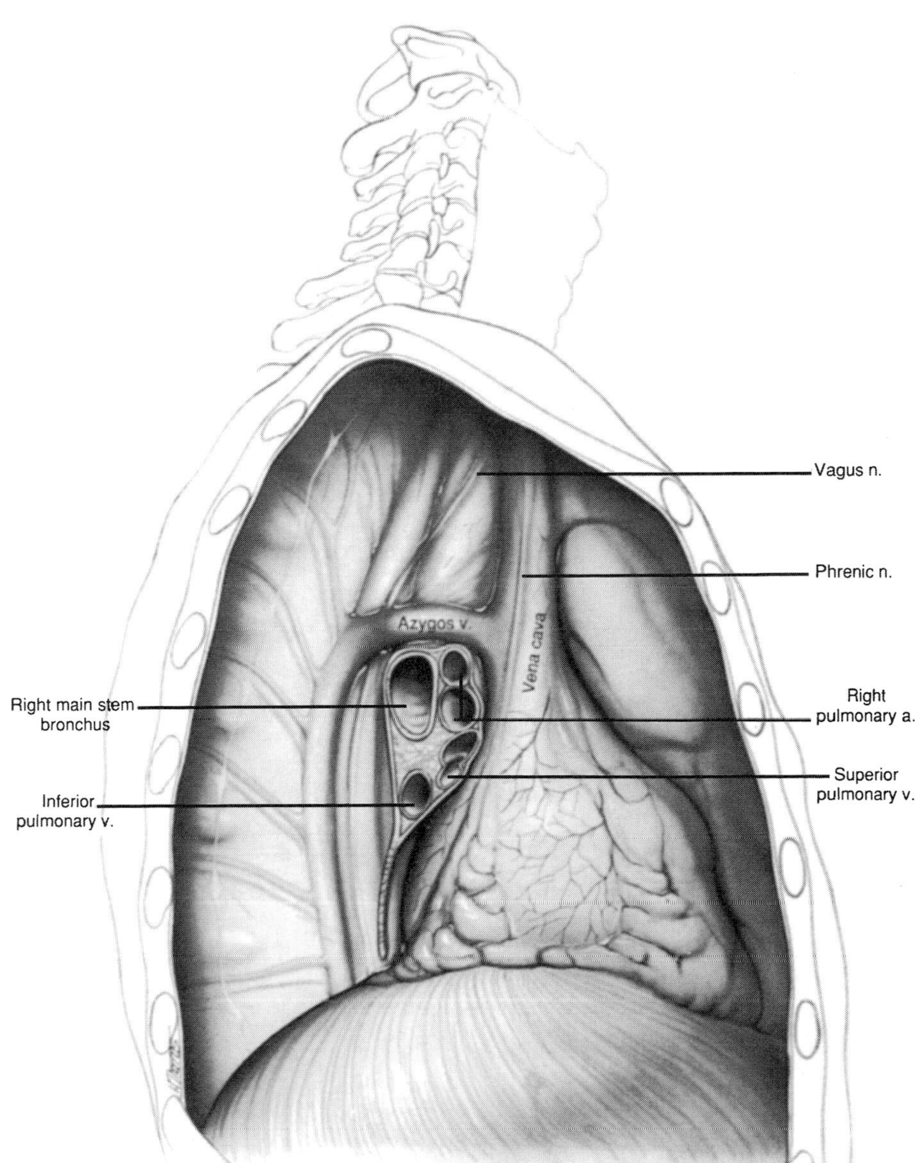

FIGURE 7–3. Medial right chest. (From Beattie EJ, et al: Atlas of thoracic surgery. In Beattie EJ, et al [eds]: Thoracic Surgical Oncology. New York: Churchill Livingstone, 1992, p 67.)

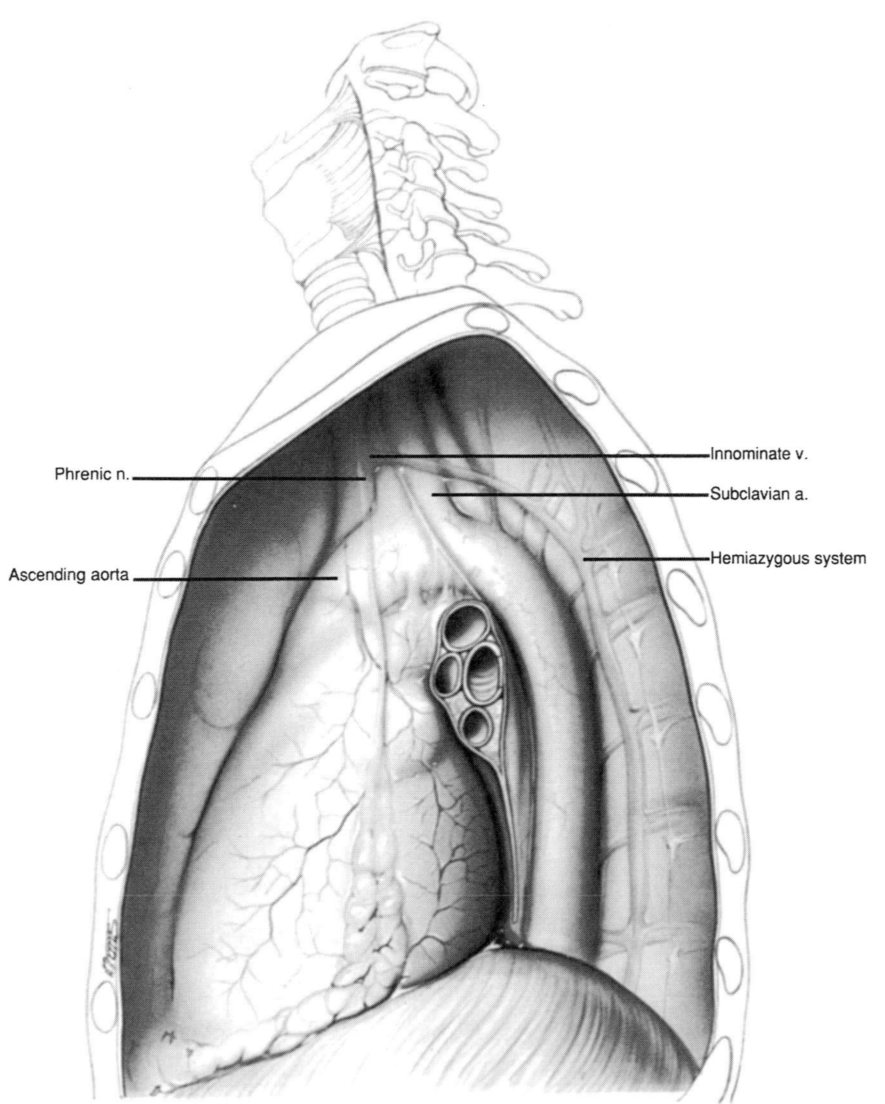

FIGURE 7–4. Medial left chest. (From Beattie EJ, et al: Atlas of thoracic surgery. In Beattie EJ, et al [eds]: Thoracic Surgical Oncology. New York: Churchill Livingstone, 1992, p 75.)

the fourth interspace. The bronchi and their branches are the key to the various subdivisions of the lung. Anatomic variations occur, but generally the right upper lobe orifice originates shortly below the carina and trifurcates into apical, anterior, and posterior segments. The bronchus intermedius continues caudad, bifurcating into the middle and lower lobes. There are two segments (lateral and medial) of the middle lobe and five segments (one superior and four basal—posterior, lateral, anterior, and medial) of the lower lobe. The pulmonary artery branches are for the most part anterior and slightly cephalad of each accompanying segment. Intrapulmonary veins drain into intersegmental veins and lead to superior or inferior pulmonary veins. The middle lobe most often drains into the superior pulmonary vein, but occasionally there is a middle lobe tributary draining into the inferior pulmonary vein.

The major blood supply to the lung is as described above. However, the lung, like the liver, has two blood supplies. The major nutrient vessels to the lung parenchyma, especially the bronchi, are bronchial arteries, branches of the aorta, or intercostal arteries. Systemic veins drain along the bronchi into the azygos system on the right, the hemiazygos on the left.

In the lateral view of the left lung (Fig. 7–6), the artist has drawn the standard anatomy with which the surgeon should be familiar. As one opens the oblique fissure, the first important structure seen is the main pulmonary artery. One can see the lingular artery branch, which runs anteriorly in the lowest portion of the left upper lobe. There is a more proximal arterial branch going up to the anterior segment and a branch to the posterior segment. These branches are variable. The superior segment branch can be seen running to the superior segment of the left lower lobe. The bronchus is sometimes difficult to expose until the necessary branches of the pulmonary artery are divided. The left upper lobe bronchus with its inferior division, the lingula, and its superior division containing the rest of the upper lobe segments is clearly seen. The superior segmental bronchus and the continuation into the left lower lobe basal segmental bronchi are also visible. The inferior pul-

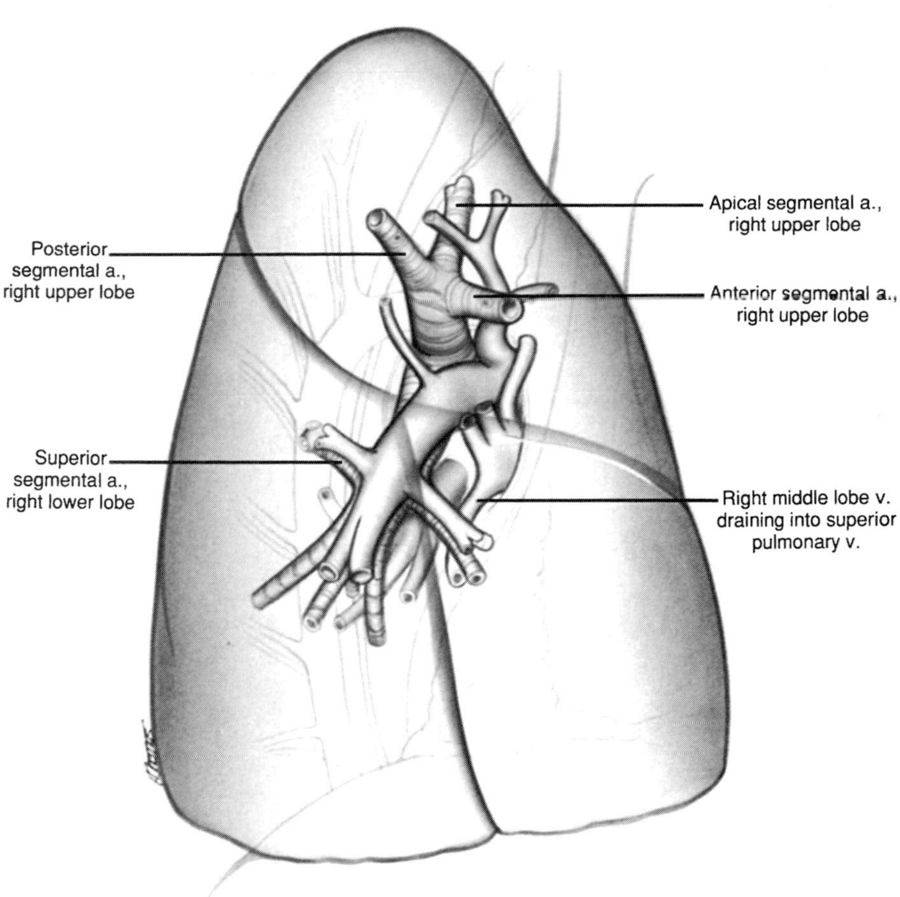

FIGURE 7–5. Lateral view of right lung. (From Beattie EJ, et al: Atlas of thoracic surgery. In Beattie EJ, et al [eds]: Thoracic Surgical Oncology. New York: Churchill Livingstone, 1992, p 71.)

monary vein is hidden and thus is not readily apparent in this approach, although some of it is seen slightly anterior and caudal to the bronchus, a relationship that can be appreciated in Figure 7–4.

The lymphatic system is the important scavenging system in the lung. There are no lymphatics in alveoli. Lymph vessels originate in the central acinar area and in interlobar septa. They generally accompany blood vessels to the hilum, passing through lymph nodes in a cephalad course. On the left side, lymphatics join the thoracic duct, which itself arches to the neck and enters the venous system at the junction of the left subclavian and internal jugular veins. The lymphatic chain system on the right is smaller but ultimately enters the venous system in the right neck in the region posterior to the right internal jugular-subclavian vein junction. Cancer can be spread contralaterally through communications between left and right systems. Color Figure 7–2 illustrates the location of thoracic and mediastinal lymph nodes with the official American Joint Committee on Cancer (AJCC) numbering system.

PATHOLOGY

Lung tumors are broadly classified as non–small cell lung carcinomas (NSCLCs), small cell lung carcinomas (SCLCs), and miscellaneous tumors.[37, 38] The proportion of cases is approximately 75% to 85% non–small cell, 15% to 25% small cell, and 2% to 3% others.

Classification of tumors by cell type is complicated by the fact that there is often a mixture of cell types within a tumor. Most of the time, the classification of a tumor is determined by the predominant cell type or is reported as of mixed cellularity. A non–small cell tumor that also contains evidence of a small cell component has a worse prognosis by virtue of detection of small cell elements. For NSCLCs, correct staging of the tumor is a more important factor in treatment and survival than cell type.

NSCLCs and SCLCs have different life histories and treatments. Surgical excision remains the predominant treatment in the former, but chemotherapy plus radiotherapy without surgical excision is standard care in the latter. Ideally, we would like better ways to determine tumor virulence and curability. Flow cytometry may prove helpful in that increase in DNA seems more unfavorable. The presence of a K-*ras* oncogene in adenocarcinomas seems to identify a less favorable group.[39]

Non–Small Cell Lung Carcinomas

Adenocarcinoma

In recent years, adenocarcinoma has become the most common NSCLC in the United States. Characteristically,

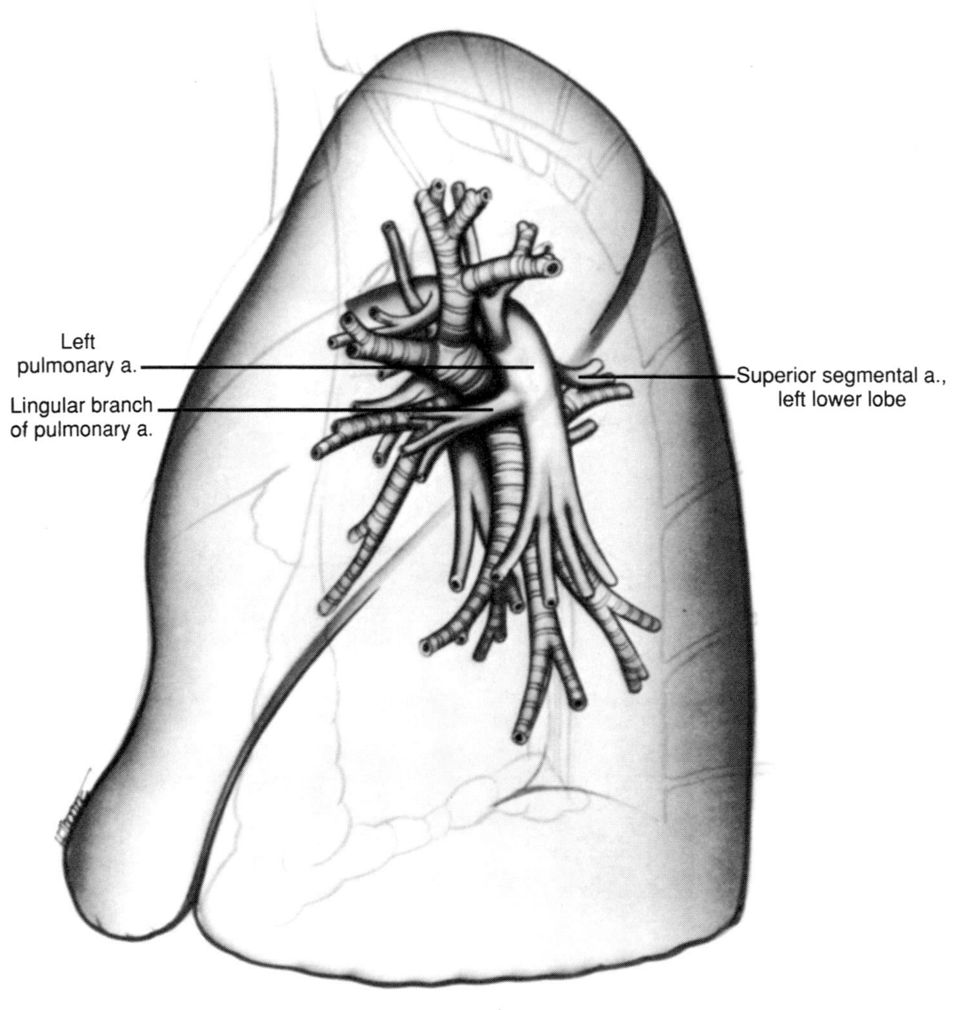

FIGURE 7–6. Lateral view of left lung. (From Beattie EJ, et al: Atlas of thoracic surgery. In Beattie EJ, et al [eds]: Thoracic Surgical Oncology. New York: Churchill Livingstone, 1992, p 78.)

adenocarcinomas are glandular cancers recognized by mucin production and the formation of tubular or papillary structures. The World Health Organization (WHO) classification recognizes four subtypes—namely, adenocarcinoma (acinar, tubular), papillary, bronchioalveolar, and solid (Table 7–1). The intercellular mucin is visualized by special stains, such as periodic acid–Schiff, Alcian blue, and mucicarmine, as droplets or vacuoles. Since many other kinds of adenocarcinoma tumors originate outside the thorax, it may be difficult to ascertain that the adenocarcinoma in the chest is a primary rather than a metastatic tumor. Pathologic expertise and careful clinical evaluation may be necessary before the tumor's primary status can be determined. Occasionally, primary pulmonary adenocarcinoma resembles colon carcinoma with signet-ring cells. Some cells may resemble Clara cells or type II pneumocytes.

Adenocarcinomas tend to develop in peripheral sites and frequently contain scarring. At times, it is very difficult to determine whether the adenocarcinoma has developed in a scar and is a true "scar carcinoma" or whether the lung scar is secondary to tumor growth. Frequently, this matter is resolved only by serial review of chest radiographs showing that a scar had been present for some time and that a tumor developed within the scar.

A subtype of adenocarcinoma is the so-called bronchioalveolar carcinoma. In this type of cancer, the tumor grows along the alveolar septa and may leave the alveolar architecture quite intact. This tumor is often multifocal, either developing throughout the involved lobe or spreading to other lobes of the lung. Bronchioalveolar carcinoma may produce a considerable amount of mucin and, in advanced stages, has a worse prognosis. The non–mucin-producing form of bronchioalveolar carcinoma is more likely to consist of Clara cells or type II pneumocytes.

Squamous Cell Carcinoma

Squamous cell carcinoma is now less common in the United States than adenocarcinoma, representing some 30% to 40% of NSCLCs. Squamous cell carcinoma tends to be located in a more central position in the lung, frequently in a main or lobar bronchus. More often the upper lobes are involved. Occasionally, small in situ squamous

TABLE 7–1
World Health Organization Histologic Classification of Malignant Epithelial Tumors of the Lung (1981)

1. Squamous cell carcinoma (epidermoid carcinoma)
   Variant:
   a. Spindle cell (squamous) carcinoma
2. Small cell carcinoma
   a. Oat cell carcinoma
   b. Intermediate cell type
   c. Combined oat cell carcinoma
3. Adenocarcinoma
   a. Acinar adenocarcinoma
   b. Papillary adenocarcinoma
   c. Bronchioalveolar carcinoma
   d. Solid carcinoma with mucus formation
4. Large cell carcinoma
   Variant:
   a. Giant cell carcinoma
   b. Clear cell carcinoma
5. Adenosquamous carcinoma
6. Carcinoid tumor
7. Bronchial gland carcinomas
   a. Adenoid cystic carcinoma
   b. Mucoepidermoid carcinoma
   c. Others
8. Others

cell carcinomas can be detected by desquamated cancer cells in the sputum but are not visible on a standard chest radiograph. These early forms of tumor are highly curable.

Central squamous cell tumors are more likely to produce symptoms of bronchial obstruction, pneumonia, and bleeding than are peripheral adenocarcinomas, which tend to be more silent coin lesions, at least initially. Occasionally, squamous cell carcinomas have a malignant spindle cell appearance and may look somewhat like a sarcoma. The presence of keratin in the tumor is a relatively reliable indicator that the tumor cell is squamous cell carcinoma. Microscopically, the presence of intercellular bridges is also an indication of squamous cell carcinoma.

Large Cell Carcinoma

Large cell carcinomas constitute approximately 10% of NSCLCs. Large cell carcinomas examined by electron microscopy reveal evidence of squamous glandular or neuroendocrine differentiation, or a combination of these, and thus seem to be a collection of poorly differentiated epithelial tumors. This matter is currently under debate. It is important to have sufficient tissue for the pathologist to examine in order to be certain of the diagnosis of a large cell carcinoma.

The WHO has recognized two subgroups of large cell carcinoma—namely, giant cell carcinoma, which usually occurs in heavy smokers, and clear cell carcinoma. Large cell carcinomas are characterized by rapid growth, and carcinoembryonic antigen (CEA) is often present. It may be difficult to distinguish these from metastatic tumors.

Small Cell Lung Carcinomas

Small cell carcinomas of the lung are subdivided, in the WHO classification, as oat cell carcinoma, intermediate cell type, or combined small cell carcinoma. It is not clear that these subdivisions have any important clinical prognostic features. The small cell carcinomas generally are centrally located, with extensive mediastinal nodal involvement. They tend to grow rapidly and to disseminate early. Although they are initially very sensitive to radiotherapy and chemotherapy, long-term survival remains a challenge.

Paraneoplastic syndromes are common. The most common of these syndromes is the syndrome of inappropriate antidiuretic hormone (SIADH). A myasthenic syndrome caused by an antibody that interferes with acetylcholine production and transmission across synapses—the Eaton-Lambert syndrome—is found in as many as 6% of patients with these tumors. Adrenocorticotropic hormone (ACTH), growth hormone, and calcitonin may also be produced, giving rise to glucose intolerance, severe hypocalcemic alkalosis, hypercalcemia, and other difficult-to-treat symptoms.

The distinguishing pathologic feature of these tumors, aside from their small size, is the fact that their histologic arrangement resembles a spread of oats. Electron microscopy reveals neuroendocrine granules that vary from 50 to 200 nm in diameter but average about 100 nm. Immunohistochemistry has been used in an attempt to distinguish more accurately between SCLCs and NSCLCs, but a completely specific marker has not been found.

Miscellaneous Tumors

Carcinoid Tumor

Carcinoid tumors (bronchial carcinoids) are neuroendocrine tumors histologically similar to those seen in the gastrointestinal tract. Bronchial carcinoids are relatively rare, representing only 1% to 2% of all primary lung tumors. Usually, they are centrally located in the tracheobronchial tree, but they can be peripheral. They probably arise from specialized Kulchitsky-like cells in the basal layer of bronchial epithelium and mucous glands. Neurosecretory-type granules and argyrophylic stains distinguish carcinoid tumors from SCLCs, as does the lack of focal squamous or glandular differentiation.

Formerly, carcinoid tumors were called bronchial adenomas, but this term should be abandoned since they are malignant tumors. The degree of malignancy for so-called typical carcinoids, which constitute 90% of bronchial carcinoids, is usually low grade, with little mitotic activity, pleomorphism, necrosis, or loss of organoid pattern. Regional metastases do occur but only at a rate of about 5%.[40]

The remaining 10% of bronchial carcinoid tumors are called atypical carcinoids. Histologically, these tumors are characterized by a relative increased cellularity, moderate nuclear hyperchromasia, variation in size and shape of cells, and increased mitotic activity. Approximately 40% of atypical carcinoid tumors have lymph node metastases when diagnosed.[41]

Among the important features of carcinoid tumors is their tendency to occur in a younger population than do bronchogenic carcinomas. Their cause is unknown but is unrelated to cigarette smoking. Symptoms are those of airway obstruction, since they tend to occur in proximal bronchi or the trachea. Ulcerations may produce hemoptysis as a presenting complaint. These tumors are often quite vascular, so hemoptysis can be life threatening. Caution is recommended in the biopsy of carcinoid tumors. The carcinoid syndrome occurs in only 5% of patients.

Patients with bronchial carcinoid tumors less than 3.0 cm in diameter, without metastasis to regional lymph nodes, have a 5-year survival rate of 90% to 95% following surgical resection. Long-term survival is possible even in case of positive lymph nodes,[42] atypical histology being perhaps a more ominous prognostic indicator.

Adenoid Cystic Carcinoma

In the older literature, the adenoid cystic carcinoma was also referred to as a cylindroma. This tumor occurs in both sexes, usually in middle age. Most of the tumors occur in main bronchi, and they may extend into the trachea. They tend to be slow-growing tumors. Since they have a tendency to submucosal and perineural spread, it is difficult to treat these tumors effectively with an adequate surgical margin. Therefore, they may recur locally after a period of years. When they occur in the tracheobronchial tree, metastasis is uncommon.

These tumors should be treated with relatively wide local excision and with preservation of as much lung tissue as possible. They tend to be relatively resistant to radiotherapy and to chemotherapy.

Mucoepidermoid Carcinoma

Mucoepidermoid carcinomas of the tracheobronchial tree tend to be more malignant than bronchial carcinoids and adenoid cystic carcinomas, behaving more like NSCLCs. Mucoepidermoid tumors contain glandular and squamous elements. Low-grade tumors with little atypia or few mitoses rarely metastasize, and resection is usually curative. In high-grade tumors, metastasis to lymph nodes can occur. The surgical treatment of mucoepidermoid carcinomas is the same as that of lung carcinomas. As is the case with carcinoid tumors, mucoepidermoid tumors have been reported in childhood.[43]

DIAGNOSIS, SCREENING, AND EARLY DETECTION

Diagnosis

Four ways to confirm the diagnosis of lung cancer are in common use. The first and simplest way is to collect sputum for cytopathology. In the case of a patient who already has a productive cough, a sample fixed in 50% alcohol for cytologic study may easily be collected. For a patient whose sputum production is scanty, a pooled collection may be obtained by instructing the patient to raise whatever sputum is possible first thing in the morning and to expectorate it directly into alcohol. A 3-day collection obtained in this manner improves the results over a solitary sample.

The second major diagnostic technique is fiberoptic bronchoscopy. A tumor directly visible may be sampled. Peripheral lesions may yield a diagnosis through brushings and washings directed into the appropriate segment or subsegmental bronchus. Fluoroscopy is often valuable in guiding a brush or needle for biopsy into the lesion. When there is evidence of hilar or mediastinal adenopathy, a transbronchial needle biopsy may be performed to obtain the diagnosis from nodal tissue.

The third technique is percutaneous needle biopsy. For lesions visible with the fluoroscope, especially when they are close to the surface of the lung, interventional radiologists may obtain needle biopsy samples with a "skinny needle" (see Color Fig. 7–7). Skilled cytopathologists can often provide a specific diagnosis, sometimes even confident of the cell type of a lung tumor. Only a minority of patients have significant pneumothoraces after needle biopsy, with fewer than 5% of our patients requiring chest tube drainage for this problem. Hemothorax or hemoptysis is seldom a result of skinny-needle biopsy unless lesions are hilar or near major blood vessels.

Fourth and finally, a diagnosis may be established by excision of the lesion. Excision of the lesion may be accomplished through a small "diagnostic" incision, reserving the full posterolateral thoracotomy for thorough cancer operations after the diagnosis is established. Thoracoscopy, or video-assisted thoracic surgery, is proving very useful in accomplishing small diagnostic wedge excisions using either mechanical staplers or lasers (Figs. 7–8 to 7–11).

Screening and Early Detection

The American Cancer Society in its most recent recommendations for cancer detection did not advise that an annual chest radiograph be performed for lung cancer screening.[45]

Boucot and Weiss[46] in 1973 reported 6136 smoking males recruited in 1959 in Philadelphia who had semiannual chest photofluorograms for 10 years. A total of 121 lung cancers were found; 33 tumors were resected, but only 8% of the cancer patients survived for 8 years. Largely because of this study, screening chest radiographs were deemed not valuable in detecting lung cancer for cure.

In the early 1970s, the National Cancer Institute embarked on a National Lung Project to study the value of sputum cytology in screening high-risk individuals for curable lung cancer. Johns Hopkins Hospital, the Mayo

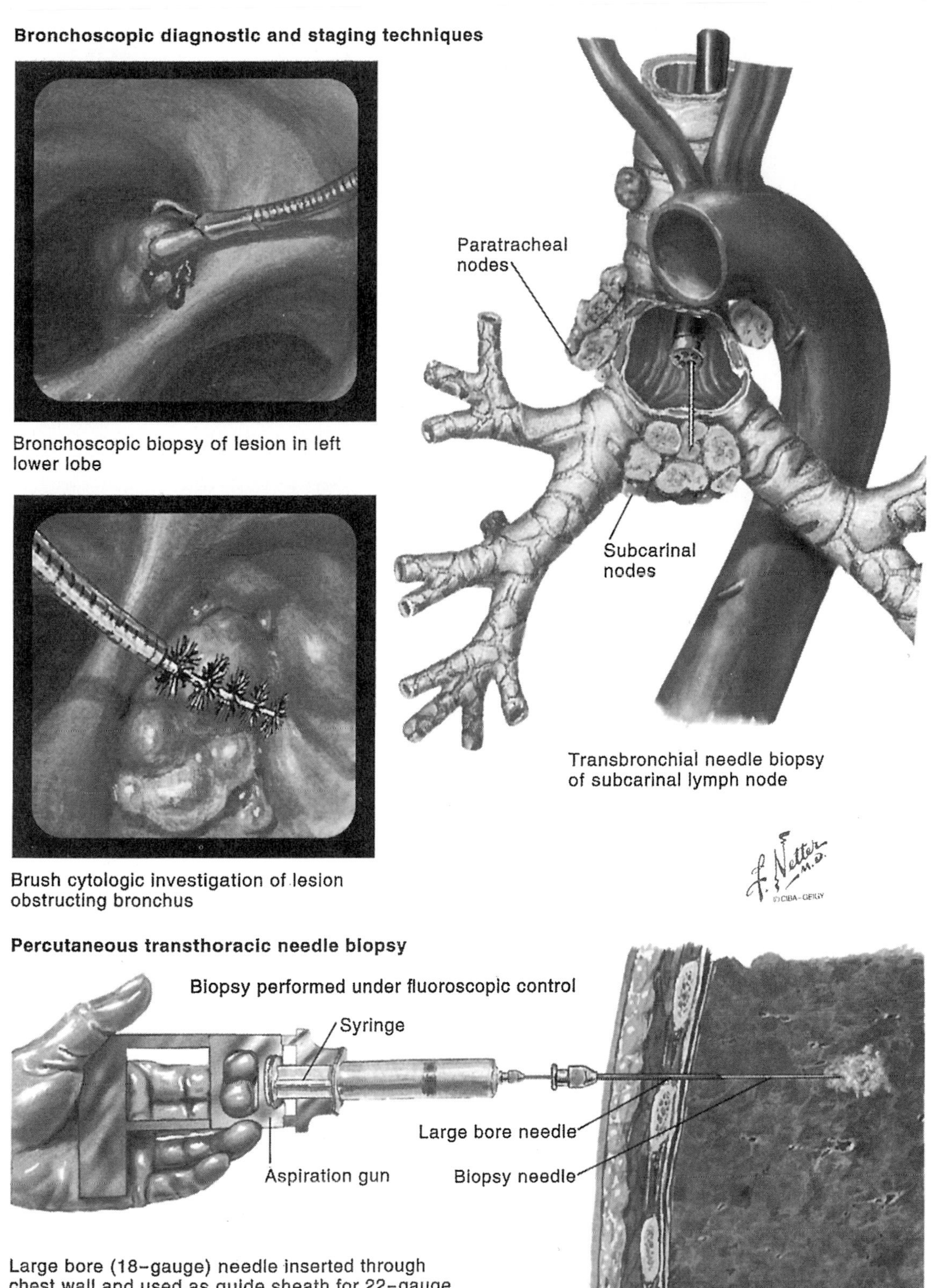

FIGURE 7–7. Bronchoscopy and percutaneous needle biopsy in the diagnosis of lung cancer. (From Harvey JC, Beattie EJ: Lung cancer. CIBA-GEIGY Clin Symp 45:14, 1993. © Copyright 1993 CIBA-GEIGY Corporation. Reprinted with permission from Clinical Symposia, illustrated by Frank H. Netter, M.D., John A. Craig, and David Mascaro. All rights reserved.)

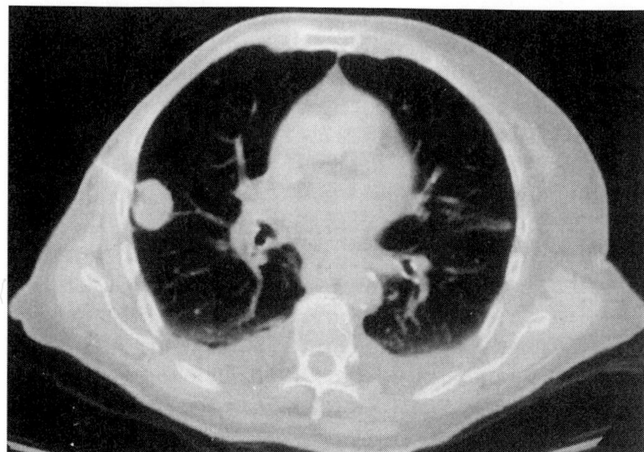

FIGURE 7–8. CT scan revealing a 2.5-cm tumor in lateral segment of right middle lobe. (From Harvey JC, et al: Choice of procedure for surgical treatment of non–small cell lung cancer. Semin Surg Oncol 9:92–98, 1993.)

Clinic, and Memorial Sloan-Kettering Cancer Center were invited to participate in this project. Each institution recruited 10,000 males who were older than 45 years of age and who had smoked at least one pack of cigarettes a day for more than 20 years. The project designs of the Johns Hopkins and Memorial Sloan-Kettering studies were similar. The 10,000 males in each group were subdivided into a "control" group of approximately 5000 members who received an annual posteroanterior (PA) and lateral chest radiograph, and an "experiment" group of 5000 members who received an annual PA and lateral chest radiograph plus sputum cytology performed every 4 months. The Mayo Clinic project differed in that two cohorts were to be (1) an intensely screened group receiving both PA stereo chest radiographs and sputum cytology every 4 months ("experiment") and (2) a group who were recommended to have annual chest radiographs plus sputum cytology not monitored at the Mayo Clinic ("control").

In the first screen at the three institutions, 79 lung cancer patients were found at Johns Hopkins, 91 at the Mayo Clinic, and 53 at Memorial Sloan-Kettering, for a total of 223 *prevalence* lung cancers. Of these patients, 105 (47%) were stage I, and the 5-year survival rate for this group was greater than 75%.[47]

In the subsequent *incidence* lung cancers at Johns Hopkins, 194 lung cancers were found in the experiment group and 202 in the control group.[48] At Memorial Sloan-Kettering, 114 patients were found with lung cancer in the experiment group and 121 in the control group.[49] At the Mayo Clinic, 202 patients were found in the experiment group and 160 in the control group.[50]

Johns Hopkins reported that their *incidence* patients had a 20% survival at 8 years in both the control and the experiment groups. In the Memorial Sloan-Kettering study, of a total of 288 lung cancers (*prevalence* plus *incidence,* 117 were stage I lung cancers, and 76% of these patients were alive 5 years later. The overall 5-year survival rate in the Memorial Sloan-Kettering screen was 35%. In both the Johns Hopkins and the Memorial Sloan-Kettering studies, there was no statistical difference in survival between the control and the experiment groups. Thus, the conclusion should be that in these two studies, sputum cytology added to annual chest radiographs did not help in finding addi-

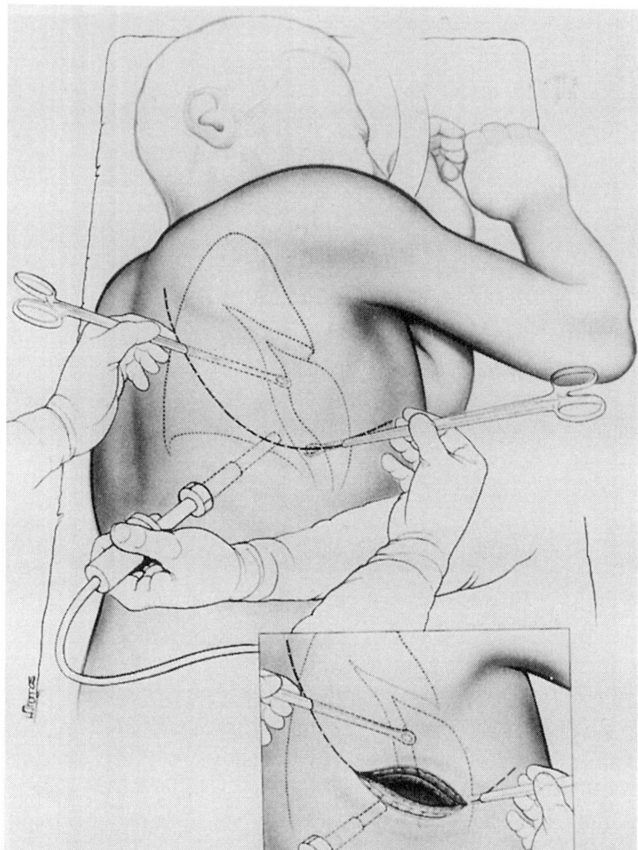

FIGURE 7–9. Patient positioned for video-assisted thoracic surgery incision. A mini-incision is required for safe extraction of the specimen. (From Harvey JC, et al: Choice of procedure for surgical treatment of non–small cell lung cancer. Semin Surg Oncol 9:92–98, 1993.)

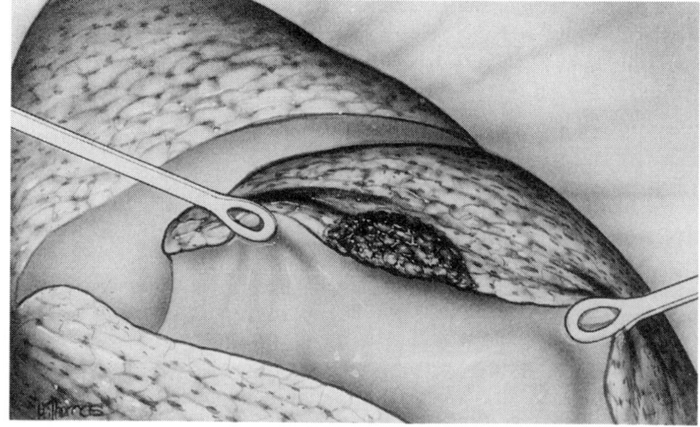

FIGURE 7–10. Tumor visible at the fissure. (From Harvey JC, et al: Choice of procedure for surgical treatment of non–small cell lung cancer. Semin Surg Oncol 9:92–98, 1993.)

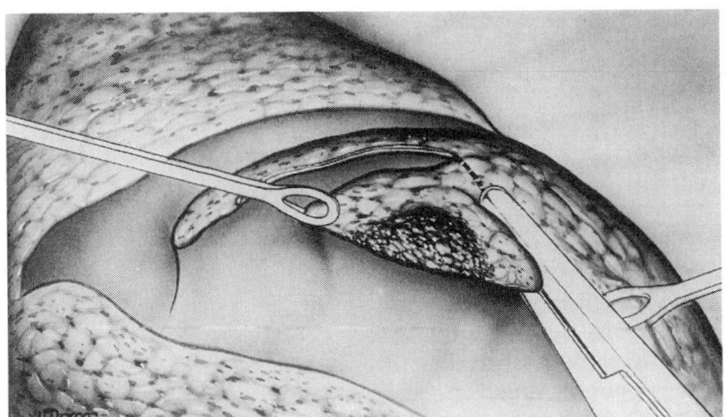

FIGURE 7–11. A linear mechanical stapling device may be used for diagnostic wedge incision. (From Harvey JC, et al: Choice of procedure for surgical treatment of non–small cell lung cancer. Semin Surg Oncol 9:92–98, 1993.)

tional curable lung cancer. It is important to note that there was no control group not receiving chest radiographs.

The Mayo Clinic reported that, in their frequently dual-screened (experiment) cohort, there was a 40% 5-year survival rate for the lung cancers detected. In the cohort recommended for yearly dual screening, the so-called "unscreened" (control) group, the 5-year survival rate was 15%. Thus, in the Mayo Clinic study there was a decreased number of lung cancers found in the control group. Some epidemiologists make much of the fact that deaths from lung cancer were reported to be the same in both Mayo Clinic groups. From this observation they concluded that early detection did not reduce deaths from lung cancer.[47–50]

In a recent update of the data reported by the three participating institutions, Flehinger and Melamed[51] attempted to develop a mathematic model for drawing conclusions about radiographic screening.[51] They assumed that in individuals in a disease-free cohort, lung cancer develops "at some unobservable time" and that it is "initially stage I." If an individual is enrolled in a screening program, he or she undergoes an examination shortly after the onset of disease, which may or may not detect the disease; if detection occurs, treatment is initiated. Successful treatment results in unimpaired health; unsuccessful treatment results in rapid death. Using this model and data from the early detection studies, they concluded that

1. The mean duration of stage I NSCLC is 4 years.
2. The probability of detecting stage I NSCLC by chest radiograph is 16% or less.
3. The probability of curing stage I NSCLC is 50% or less.
4. Annual examination of a high-risk population from age 45 to 80 years would reduce mortality by only 18% or less.

Flehinger and Melamed calculate that these far from optimal results would still prevent 25,000 NSCLC deaths per year.

Mulshine et al.[52] reviewed the current status of screening for lung cancer: "Randomized trials that use a mortality endpoint eliminate the need for considering selection, lead time, and length bias in evaluating benefit." Improvement in lung cancer control can come from prevention, early detection, or improved treatment. By the year 2000, a million more lung cancer deaths are predicted in the United States, even if not one more cigarette were lit. On theoretic grounds, markers in serum would not be expected to diagnose localized stage I lung cancer. Tockman[48] reported on two cancer-associated monoclonal antibodies used to stain sputum samples in the Johns Hopkins National Lung Project. In 8 years of clinical studies, 626 individuals showed moderate or greater atypia in sputum cytology. Sensitivity was 91% in those in whom lung cancers developed, and specificity was 88% among those who remained free of cancer.

Since the Lung Cancer Study Group has shown a 3% per year rate of new primary lung cancers in the cured stage I patients, patients with a previous lung cancer are a good cohort for the Tockman monoclonal antibody sputum study.

A case-control study undertaken by the Japanese Lung Cancer Screening Research Group compared survival rates of 1297 "screen-detected" and 1297 "symptom-detected" patients with lung cancer. This study showed improved survival among screen-detected patients whose cancers were diagnosed at an earlier stage and had a better resectability rate (Fig. 7–12). It was possible to show improved survival of screen-detected patients versus symptom-detected patients out to 10 years from diagnosis.[53]

STAGING

The TNM staging system (Table 7–2) has been adopted by most authorities in the care of the lung cancer patient.[54] "T" pertains to the size and extent of the primary tumor. A tumor less than 3 cm in diameter surrounded by lung tissue is T1; a tumor that either is greater than 3 cm in diameter or involves visceral pleura is T2. A tumor involving parietal pleura is T3. It is also T3 if it is within 2 cm of the carina without involving the carina. It is T3 if it directly extends into the chest wall (including, therefore, most superior sulcus tumors), diaphragm, mediastinal pleura, or pericardium, as long as it does not invade the heart, great vessels, trachea, esophagus, or vertebral bodies. A T4 tumor is one of any size with invasion into the mediastinum (beyond pleura) involving the heart, great vessels, trachea, esophagus, vertebral body, or carina; therefore, some superior sulcus tumors are T4. Malignant pleural effusions are also T4 tumors.

"N" denotes nodal involvement. N0 tumor has no metastases to regional lymph nodes, and N1 tumor has metastases to lymph nodes in the peribronchial or ipsilateral hilar region, or both. N2 tumors are metastatic to ipsilateral, mediastinal lymph nodes, including subcarinal nodes. N3 designates metastases to contralateral lymph nodes and to ipsilateral or contralateral supraclavicular lymph nodes.

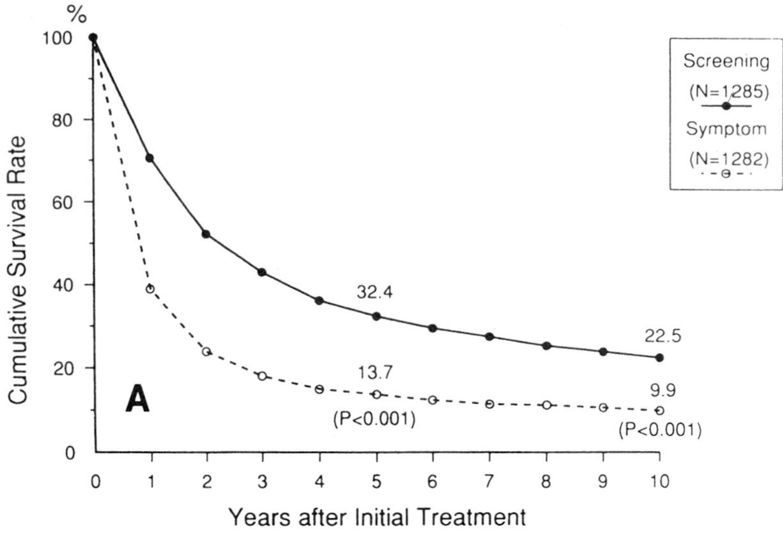

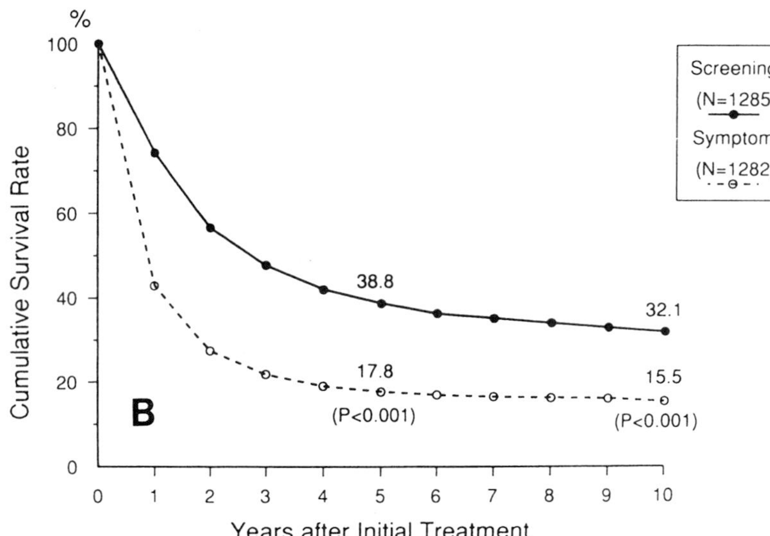

FIGURE 7–12. *A,* Survival curves of screen-detected versus symptom-detected non–small cell lung carcinomas (NSCLCs). *B,* Survival curves excluding deaths not due to NSCLC. (From Naruke T, et al: Comparative study of survival of screen-detected compared with symptom-detected lung cancer cases. Semin Surg Oncol 9:80–84, 1993.)

"M" designates either no known distant metastases (M0) or distant metastases present (M1). The most common site for metastases from lung cancer is the brain, followed by skeleton, liver, and adrenal gland. One should note where the metastases are located, such as M1 (brain).

There has been controversy regarding staging when multiple nodules are present in lungs. Synchronous lung cancers have been believed by some to represent metastatic disease (M1), although in fact it is often difficult to distinguish this situation from double primary tumors. Survival following resection in this situation is less than would be expected from two separate primary tumors but more than expected if this were truly a manifestation of metastatic disease, indicating that synchronous nodules are probably a mixed population comprising metastases (M1) as well as separate primary tumors.[55] The most recent AJCC staging manual suggests a T4 designation for the situation in which an intrapulmonary, ipsilateral metastasis is found in another lobe, reserving the M1 designation for contralateral metastasis. Multiple tumors in the same lobe otherwise meeting T1 criteria are designated T2. A T2 primary tumor with another mass in the same lobe is upgraded to T3. All other multiple ipsilateral tumors are designated T4 tumors.[54]

Diagnostic Imaging

Diagnostic imaging techniques employed to assist in clinical staging of a lung cancer[56] commonly include PA and lateral chest radiographs and computed tomography (CT) or magnetic resonance imaging (MRI) scans. For determination of the "T" component of staging, we must assess tumor size, extension to adjacent structures, signs of obstruction such as atelectasis or pneumonia, and pleural effusions. Conventional PA and lateral chest radiographs often accurately assess tumor size, especially peripheral lesions. The presence of atelectasis or pneumonia may

TABLE 7–2
TNM Staging System

Primary Tumor (T)
TX Primary tumor cannot be assessed, or tumor proven by the presence of malignant cells in sputum or bronchial washings but not visualized by imaging or bronchoscopy
T0 No evidence of primary tumor
Tis Carcinoma in situ
T1 Tumor 3 cm or less in greatest dimension, surrounded by lung or visceral pleura, without bronchoscopic evidence of invasion more proximal than the lobar bronchus (i.e., not in the main bronchus)*
T2 Tumor with any of the following features of size or extent: more than 3 cm in greatest dimension; involving main bronchus, 2 cm or more distal to the carina; invading the visceral pleura; associated with atelectasis or obstructive pneumonitis that extends to the hilar region but does not involve the entire lung
T3 Tumor of any size that directly invades any of the following: chest wall (including superior sulcus tumors), diaphragm, mediastinal pleura, or parietal pericardium; or tumor in the main bronchus less than 2 cm distal to the carina but without involvement of the carina; or associated atelectasis or obstructive pneumonitis of the entire lung
T4 Tumor of any size that invades any of the following: mediastinum, heart, great vessels, trachea, esophagus, vertebral body, carina; or tumor with a malignant pleural effusion†

Regional Lymph Nodes (N)
NX Regional lymph nodes cannot be assessed
N0 No regional lymph node metastasis
N1 Metastasis in ipsilateral peribronchial and/or ipsilateral hilar lymph nodes, including direct extension
N2 Metastasis in ipsilateral mediastinal and/or subcarinal lymph node(s)
N3 Metastasis in contralateral mediastinal, contralateral hilar, ipsilateral or contralateral scalene, or supraclavicular lymph node(s)

Distant Metastasis (M)
MX Presence of distant metastasis cannot be assessed
M0 No distant metastasis
M1 Distant metastasis

Stage Grouping

Occult	TX	N0	M0
Stage 0	Tis	N0	M0
Stage I	T1	N0	M0
	T2	N0	M0
Stage II	T1	N0	M0
	T2	N1	M0
Stage IIIA	T1	N2	M0
	T2	N2	M0
	T3	N0	M0
	T3	N1	M0
	T3	N2	M0
Stage IIIB	Any T	N3	M0
	T4	Any N	M0
Stage IV	Any T	Any N	M1

*The uncommon superficial tumor of any size with its invasive component limited to the bronchial wall, which may extend proximal to the main bronchus, is also classified as T1.

†Most pleural effusions associated with lung cancer are due to tumor. However, there are a few patients in whom multiple cytopathologic examinations of pleural fluid are negative for tumor. In these cases, fluid is nonbloody and is not an exudate. When these elements and clinical judgment dictate that the effusion is not related to the tumor, the effusion should be excluded as a staging element and the patient should be staged as T1, T2, or T3.

obscure the size of the underlying mass, but CT or MRI can frequently distinguish underlying mass from surrounding atelectasis or inflammation. Contrast-enhanced CT is superior to MRI for these distinctions with present-day instrumentation.

Chest wall invasion can frequently be distinguished on chest radiographs without additional studies. It is important to remember that although chest wall invasion is present in approximately 8% of patients with peripheral pleural-based tumors, this is not in itself a sign of inoperability. Furthermore, history of localized pain is more reliable than CT for predicting chest wall invasion. MRI is superior to CT for evaluation of chest wall invasion.

Distinguishing visceral (T2) from parietal (T3) pleural involvement is not always possible with present-day imaging techniques (Fig. 7–13), but, again, the presence of localized pain is strong evidence of parietal pleural involvement. Invasion of the mediastinum is often overestimated by CT and MRI, such that invasion is frequently suggested when the tumor simply abuts rather than invades a mediastinal structure. Linear or nodular extensions and interdigitations of tumor into mediastinal fat are considered reliable indications of mediastinal invasions. Demonstration of invasion of specific structures in the mediastinum, such as esophagus, phrenic nerve, and major pulmonary vessels, requires contrast or endoscopic evaluation of the esophagus, fluoroscopy of the diaphragm, and pulmonary angiography, respectively.

Malignant pleural effusions are generally thought to indicate inoperability (T4). CT frequently shows small pleural effusions not identifiable on conventional chest radiographs. Such effusions may be unrelated to the primary tumor, such as those due to congestive heart failure. Some effusions are due to obstruction of hilar lymphatics or are secondary to postobstructive atelectasis or pneumonia. We insist on the documentation of malignant cells in the pleural effusion before we categorically consider the patient unresectable. Cell samples for cytologic confirmation may be obtained by thoracentesis. In ambiguous situations, it is wise to perform thoracoscopy to search for pleural seeding (Fig. 7–14).

Evaluation of Nodal Metastasis

At the time of diagnosis, most studies show that more than 70% of lung cancer patients already have at least

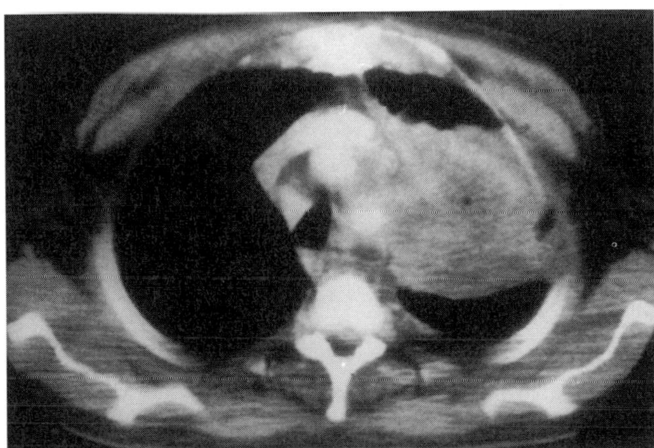

FIGURE 7–13. Contrast-enhanced CT scan showing tumor abutting chest wall. Although findings suggested chest wall invasion, they were not definitive. Study of the surgical specimen showed only parietal pleural invasion.

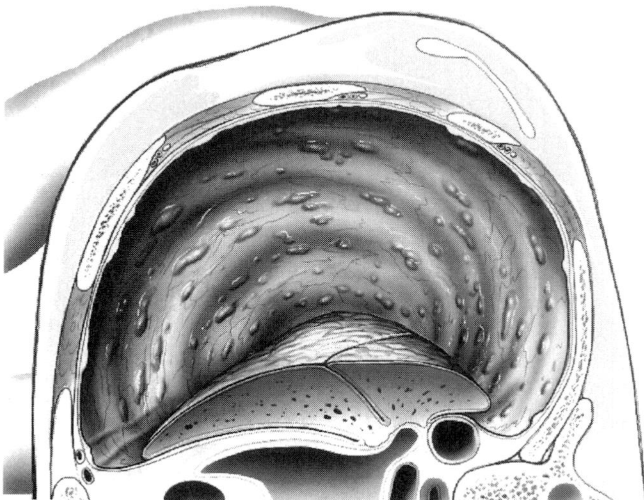

FIGURE 7–14. Drawing of the thoracoscopic view of seeding of parietal pleura.

regionally advanced disease. Conventional chest radiographs are neither accurate nor sensitive for revealing hilar or mediastinal nodal enlargement. CT and MRI have greater accuracy, depending on thresholds accepted as positive. Generally, nodes of less than 1 cm in diameter are considered normal in size, while those greater than 2 cm are considered abnormally enlarged. However, micrometastases may exist in small nodes, and larger nodes may be found without tumor. In areas of endemic granulomatous disease (such as histoplasmosis), enlarged nodes may still be benign. It is our opinion that, at present, there are no imaging techniques sensitive or specific enough to justify dispensing with node sampling procedures if accurate staging is the goal.[57]

CT or MRI is important in the pretreatment evaluation of patients receiving primary radiotherapy. Evaluation with these methods has been shown to improve dosimetry compared with conventional radiographs. They are also useful in post-treatment follow-up. There is no advantage to MRI compared with CT for these purposes.

Evaluation of Distant Metastases

A complete history, physical examination, and review of routine laboratory profiles identify patients with a high likelihood of distant metastatic disease. Bone scans and brain scans are not routinely ordered unless review of systems suggest unexplained new musculoskeletal complaints, bone pain, or new neurologic problems. Liver metastases are carefully sought if alkaline phosphatase is elevated, but the liver and adrenals are usually seen in computed tomograms of the chest and upper abdomen. The most frequent sites of metastatic disease are the central nervous system, liver, bone, bone marrow, adrenal glands, and lung. We have learned that adrenal masses larger than 2 cm in size, even if atypical for adrenal adenomas, must be sampled for biopsy before metastasis is assumed. Many prove to be benign adenomas or adrenal hyperplasia.

Thoracentesis

Thoracentesis is routinely performed in the presence of a pleural effusion. As much fluid as possible up to 1 L is retrieved, and a representative sample mixed with 50% alcohol should be studied by the cytopathologist.

Thoracoscopy

Thoracoscopy is useful to evaluate for pleural seeding and also for evaluating mediastinal nodes in the subaortic (levels 5 and 6) regions (Fig. 7–15).

Mediastinoscopy

Mediastinoscopy (see Color Fig. 7–16) is part of our routine staging for otherwise operable patients. It is more sensitive and specific than CT or MRI.[57] As neoadjuvant chemotherapy or chemotherapy and radiotherapy protocols improve, accurate presurgical treatment will become mandatory. Already, preliminary studies have demonstrated superior survival among patients with positive mediastinal nodes treated with preoperative chemotherapy compared with those randomized into a postoperative chemotherapy treatment plan.[58]

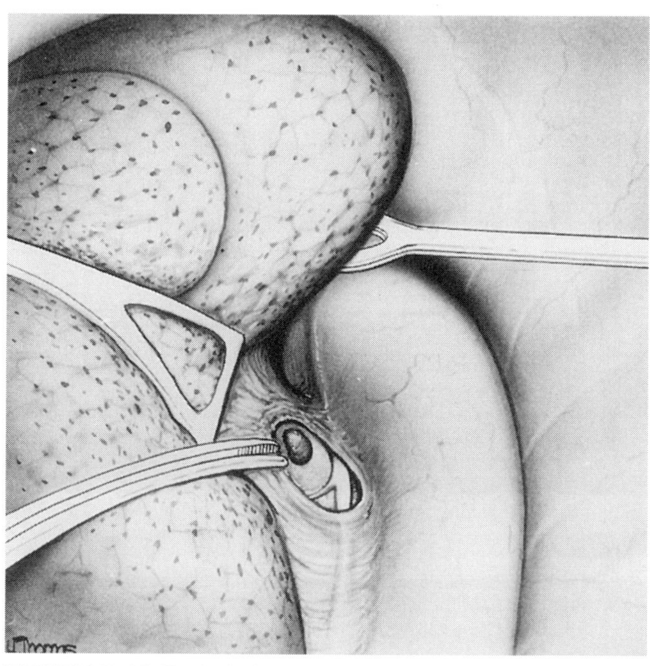

FIGURE 7–15. Typical video-assisted thoracic surgery view of a level 5 node exposed with an endodissector. A lung clamp and ring forceps retract the lung. (From Harvey JC, et al: Choice of procedure for surgical treatment of non–small cell lung cancer. Semin Surg Oncol 9:92–98, 1993.)

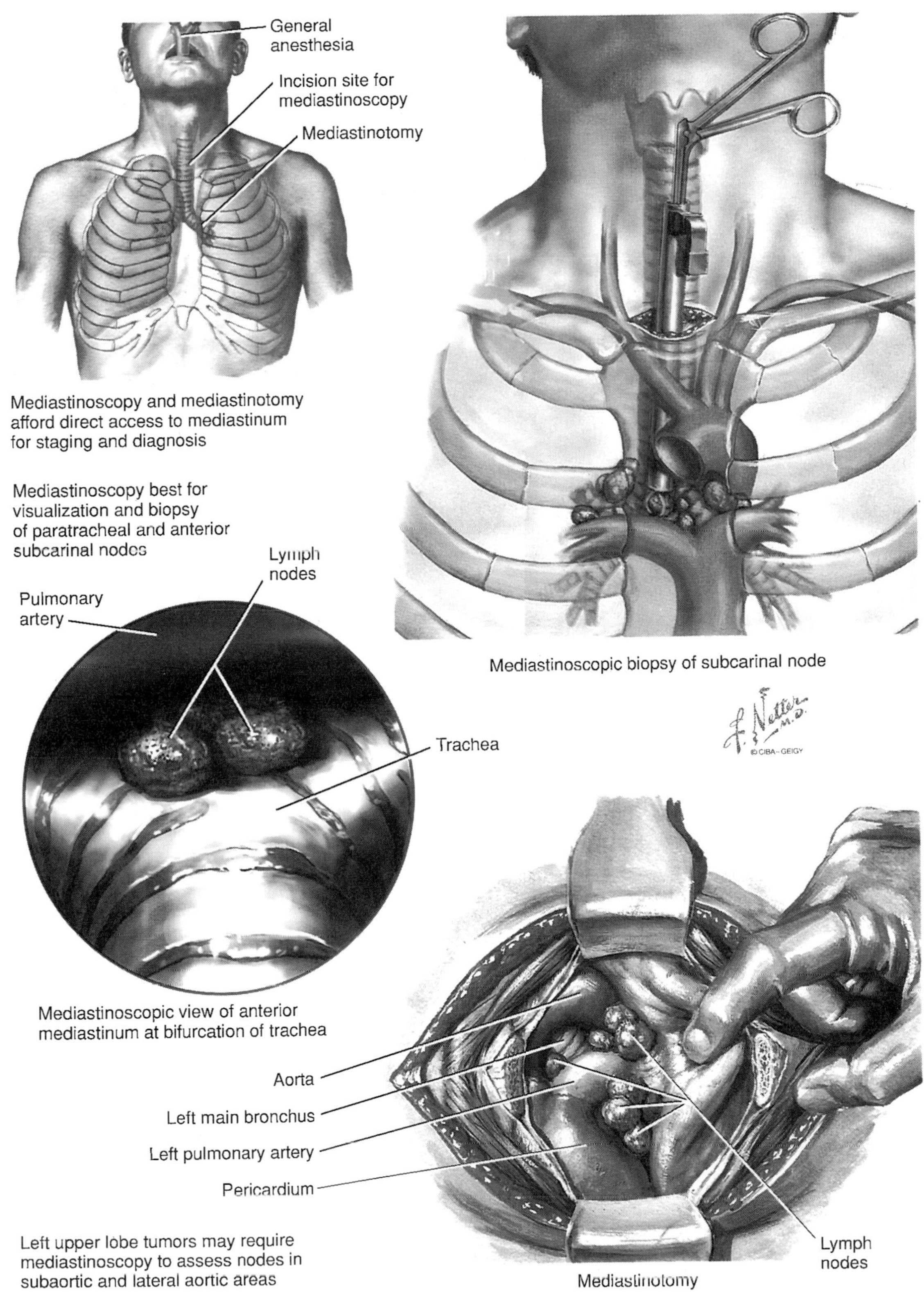
General
anesthesia
Incision site for
mediastinoscopy
Mediastinotomy
Mediastinoscopy and mediastinotomy
afford direct access to mediastinum
for staging and diagnosis
Mediastinoscopy best for
visualization and biopsy
of paratracheal and anterior
subcarinal nodes
Lymph
nodes
Pulmonary
artery
Trachea
Mediastinoscopic biopsy of subcarinal node
F. Netter M.D.
© CIBA-GEIGY
Mediastinoscopic view of anterior
mediastinum at bifurcation of trachea
Aorta
Left main bronchus
Left pulmonary artery
Pericardium
Left upper lobe tumors may require
mediastinoscopy to assess nodes in
subaortic and lateral aortic areas
Lymph
nodes
Mediastinotomy

FIGURE 7–16. Mediastinoscopy and mediastinotomy. (From Harvey JC, Beattie EJ: Lung cancer. CIBA-GEIGY Clin Symp 45:22, 1993. © Copyright 1993 CIBA-GEIGY Corporation. Reprinted with permission from Clinical Symposia, illustrated by Frank H. Netter, M.D., John A. Craig, and David Mascaro. All rights reserved.)

Mediastinotomy (Chamberlain Procedure)

Mediastinotomy involves resection of the medial anterior second rib, which permits easy sampling of subaortic nodes (see Color Fig. 7–16). We more often use thoracoscopy to accomplish inspection of this area at present (see Fig. 7–15).

PRIMARY OPERABLE NON–SMALL CELL LUNG CARCINOMA

Best results are obtained for stage I to stage IIIA tumors if complete resection is performed, preferably a lobectomy but up to a pneumonectomy, along with adjacent locally invaded structures. Lesser procedures (wedge or segmental resection) have not proven as effective as lobectomy[58] but are acceptable procedures in the cases of limited pulmonary reserve.[59–62] After it is determined that the patient is a candidate for resection by virtue of stage of disease, an evaluation of the overall risks of surgery for each particular patient is the next step.

Risk Factors for Pulmonary Resection

The four generally accepted incremental risk factors for morbidity and mortality of pulmonary resection are

1. Age.
2. Diminished pulmonary reserve.
3. Cardiovascular disease.
4. Need for pneumonectomy for complete excision.

Age

Most studies have found age to be an incremental risk factor for any pulmonary resection. Mortality and morbidity of pulmonary resection have been found to increase even in carefully selected patients over 70 years of age in most studies.[63, 64]

Diminished Pulmonary Reserve

Arterial blood gases and pulmonary function tests are generally performed as part of the preoperative evaluation.[64] Smoking is prohibited in the preoperative period. Reversible airway disease is treated with bronchodilators, and chronic bronchitis is treated with antibiotics in order to optimize pulmonary performance. Baseline levels can be dramatically improved by weeks of smoking cessation,[65, 66] but this is not always practical or even possible.

Arterial Blood Gases

Even minimal elevation of Pco_2 is indicative of severe disturbance in alveolar ventilation, so a preoperative Pco_2 greater than 45 mm Hg is usually considered an indication of inoperability. An arterial Po_2 less than 60 is usually indicative of high risks for pulmonary resection; an exception is the circumstance of complete airway obstruction resulting in desaturated blood entering the pulmonary veins arising from perfused but nonventilated lungs.

Pulmonary Function Tests

Pulmonary function testing is useful in evaluating the risk of pulmonary resection. Many threshold guidelines have been calculated as high risk for resection, but it must be remembered that the problems associated with pulmonary resection depend not only on loss of functioning alveoli but also on an interaction of complex cardiopulmonary alterations (sometimes transient alterations) in pulmonary artery pressure and cardiac output. Special studies, including perfusion scans (xenon radiospirometry and technetium microaggregate lung scanning) and exercise testing, may be useful in borderline reserve candidates with resectable disease.

It is generally agreed that a predicted postoperative FEV_1 greater than 800 ml is required in most adults. It has also been determined that patients with a postoperative FEV_1 greater than 40% of predicted are at low risk of mortality and morbidity for pneumonectomy, while a predicted postoperative FEV_1 less than 30% should usually be considered a prohibitive risk for pneumonectomy.[67] These parameters serve as useful guidelines but cannot be regarded as absolute, since there are exceptions and it has been asked whether there is such a thing as an unacceptable surgical risk in treating a disease with a mortality approaching 100%.[68]

Cardiovascular Disease

The prevalence of cardiovascular disease increases with age and therefore represents a major risk factor among patients in the lung cancer age group. Coronary artery disease is present in about 80 in 1000 patients older than 65.[69, 70]

Previous Myocardial Infarction

Previous myocardial infarction is the most consistently reported risk factor for cardiac death following pulmonary resection, especially at an interval of less than 6 months from the infarction.[71] If it is necessary to operate within 6 months of a myocardial infarction, the risk may be substantially reduced by intensive perioperative monitoring using measurements obtained with a Swan-Ganz catheter and appropriate interventions to optimize cardiac performance.[72]

Left Ventricular Dysfunction

Evidence of left ventricular dysfunction, including clinical or radiographic signs of congestive heart failure, has been found to be a high risk for cardiac mortality following pulmonary resection. The relative values of specific signs remains a subject of dispute, but it seems that third heart sounds and left ventricular wall dysfunction are more important than cardiomegaly.[69]

Unstable Angina

Unstable angina must be controlled prior to pulmonary resection, but chronic stable angina has not been found to be a substantial risk factor for pulmonary resection.[70]

Hypertension

Hypertension is the most common cardiovascular disease in the United States, and most studies find it to be a predictor of perioperative cardiovascular mortality.[72] Its presence should be discovered in the perioperative screening interval, and surgery should be delayed until treatment is optimized.

Cardiac Arrhythmias

Frequent premature ventricular contractions (PVCs) are associated with increased perioperative complications and death. Although death is often not due to the arrhythmia per se, frequent PVCs should be considered indicative of severe heart disease. Other arrhythmias detected preoperatively have not been convincingly associated with perioperative complications.[69, 70, 73]

Other Cardiovascular Risk Factors

Cerebrovascular disease has been identified as a risk factor for cardiovascular morbidity in some studies.[74] Peripheral vascular disease has not been found to contribute significantly to the risk of pulmonary resection.[69]

Need for Pneumonectomy

Pneumonectomy, especially right pneumonectomy and especially in the case of patients older than 70 years of age, is associated with significant incremental risk compared with lesser resections.[63]

Surgical Procedures

Pneumonectomy or Lobectomy

The first successful pneumonectomy for lung cancer was performed in 1933. By the end of that decade, it was considered by many authorities as the only acceptable procedure for cure of lung cancer.[8] Lesser procedures (lobectomies, segmentectomies, and wedge excisions) were believed to result invariably in higher recurrence rates. The mortality of pneumonectomy (primarily due to pulmonary and cardiac insufficiency), as well as the problems associated with management of the pneumonectomy space, was discouraging enough to overcome eventually the bias that only pneumonectomy was an adequate operation. It is now generally accepted that lobectomy, when all tumor is removed, is the standard operation for NSCLC. Equal cure rates are achievable with lobectomy, at greatly diminished risk, compared with pneumonectomy.[5, 75–80] Pneumonectomy is reserved for those patients whose tumor necessitates it for complete excision, and then only if their general medical condition permits.

Technical details regarding pulmonary resections should be reviewed in an atlas of thoracic surgery.[36] Results following complete resection are presented in Table 7–3.

Wedge or Segmental Resection

As early as 1939, Churchill and Belsey[81] applied segmental resections to treatment of pulmonary problems and hypothesized that "the segment may replace the lobe as the surgical unit of the lung." Other surgeons have believed that anatomic "wedge" excisions would prove an adequate cancer operation for stage I disease. The development of mechanical stapling devices has simplified the technical problems of conservative lung surgery. We have performed conservative resection, using these devices, as procedures of choice in situations in which pulmonary reserve is limited or other medical factors dictate the advisability of a rapidly performed, less extensive procedure. Even when complete resection with "adequate" margins is obtained by such conservative surgery, it has been found that the survival is considerably less than that obtained by standard lobectomy.[82]

A recently completed Lung Cancer Study Group protocol prospectively compared lobectomy with wedge or segmental resections among patients who could have physiologically tolerated lobectomy. Preliminary reports have described increased rates of local recurrence and of brain metastases among the wedge or segmental resection cohort compared with lobectomy controls.[83] We therefore recommend complete anatomic resection and node dissection for all patients whose pulmonary reserve and general performance status permit.

Video-Assisted Resection

In the past few years, it has become possible to perform surgical procedures with remote video imaging techniques via appropriately chosen "mini-incisions" of approximately 1 cm. Numerous reports have documented the feasibility of video-assisted thoracic surgery (VATS) for diagnostic excisions of pulmonary nodules and for mediastinal node sampling, which allows diagnosis of cancer (or its exclusion if the nodule is completely excised) and staging.[44, 84] In the case of cancer exclusion, the patient is

TABLE 7–3
Five-Year Survival Rate Following Complete Resection

Stage	TNM	5-Year Survival Rate (%)
I	T1, N0, M0	80
	T2, N0, M0	60
II	T1–2, N1	40–50
IIIa	T3, N0	40
	T1–2, N2	25
	T3, N1–2	10

spared a major procedure. In the case of node sampling "upstaging," better treatment planning can be derived.

The major anatomic resections have also been accomplished with VATS. Critical collection of data allowing evaluation of risks associated with major resections by this technique have not yet been reported, and there are not yet sufficient numbers of patients to report long-term results. In our view, the technique remains experimental. We continue to consider open lobectomy the procedure of choice for patients whose performance status permits it. We have been pleased with VATS using either Nd:YAG laser or mechanical staplers to perform wedge resections for people who cannot tolerate lobectomy, an acceptable compromise for those patients. "Consumer-driven" marketing for lesser surgery should be resisted until such time as equal efficacy with standard techniques is proven.

Chest Wall Resection

A tumor is classified T3 whenever parietal pleura is involved whether or not tumor extends into the chest wall. It has long been appreciated that long-term survival is achievable with full-thickness chest wall resection whenever tumor invades ribs or chest wall muscles[85] unless mediastinal nodes are involved.[86, 87] Whether such an extensive resection is required for T3 tumors in which the surgeon believes that a tumor-free plane can be achieved with extrapleural dissection is still in dispute.[77, 87] There are data from the Mayo Clinic indicating that survival is very significantly improved when en bloc chest wall resection is performed as compared to an extrapleural resection (75% vs. 28%).[88] If regional nodes are involved in this situation (T3, N2), survival is reduced to 10% to 20% regardless of the extent of treatment.

The resulting chest wall defects may be reconstructed using a variety of prosthetic mesh materials,[89] but some authorities believe that small defects do not need to be closed, especially if they lie beneath the scapula.[90]

Sleeve Resection

Some airway tumors are located in areas that permit resection of involved airway while conserving lung parenchyma. Examples are tumors of the carina (T4 tumors) and tumors of the right upper lobe orifice.

Most often, tumors of the carina are considered unresectable and are palliated in various ways, including external or internal radiotherapy,[91, 92] laser ablation,[93] and dilatation and stenting.[94, 95] In rare circumstances, it is possible to resect the carina completely. A variety of airway mobilizations and plastic reconstructions re-establish airway continuity (Fig. 7–17). Long-term results of these efforts are superior compared with those of alternative treatments for squamous cell carcinomas and miscellaneous tumors (e.g., carcinoid tumors).[96–99]

For tumors of the upper lobes extending into orifices of the main bronchi or into bronchus intermedius, it is sometimes technically feasible to excise the lobe in continuity with a "sleeve" of proximal airway, thereby avoiding pneumonectomy (Fig. 7–18). It is well established that long-term cure rates are not compromised by this conservative surgery, so its use need not be restricted to patients with prohibitive risk for a pneumonectomy. Increasingly, it is becoming accepted that sleeve lobectomy should be employed whenever complete resections can be accomplished by this technique.[99–101]

Preoperative evaluation includes a bronchoscopy, performed by the surgeon, as a critical procedure to estimate the feasibility of sleeve resection. We recommend mediastinoscopy regardless of CT scan interpretation because it is our preference to proceed with pneumonectomy whenever nodes at the tracheobronchial angle (level 4) contain tumor, unless pulmonary reserve is inadequate.

Pulmonary angiography is selectively employed to identify pulmonary artery involvement at the lobar level. Angioplasty has sometimes been performed along with bronchoplasty but the mortality rate for this combination has been greater than 15% in experienced hands.[102]

Frozen section evaluation of resection margins is essential if incomplete resections are to be avoided. Another important intraoperative concern is protection of the bronchial anastomosis with a pleural pedicle—in this case not only to augment development of systemic circulation but also to cushion the anastomosis from pulmonary artery branches, reducing the risk of fatal bronchovascular fistula.

The operative mortality rate for sleeve resection is reported to be less than 10%.[99–102] Actuarial 5-year survival greater than 60% has been reported in the absence of involved lymph nodes. For resections involving positive N1 lymph nodes, most have found greatly diminished survival, but DesLauriers and colleagues[101] reported a 60% 5-year survival rate for 31 patients with N1 disease.

Nonsurgical Options

Chemotherapy

Only a few drugs have been proven capable of inducing significant responses as single agents (defined as complete and partial responses in the range of 15% to 25%) in NSCLC. The most effective agents have been cisplatin, vindesine, mitomycin C, etoposide, and ifosfamide, given in combination form so that the dose and toxicity of each drug may be reduced. Several combinations, usually cisplatin-based, have demonstrated that synergy may be achieved (response rates up to 60%) with manageable toxicity. However, at present there are no combinations of drugs that may substitute for surgical resection.[103]

Radiotherapy

Ionizing radiation may be delivered in either electromagnetic or particulate form. Electromagnetic radiation comprises roentgen rays, produced by electrons interacting on the outer structures of atoms, and gamma rays, the effect of changes in the nucleus of the atom. Radioisotopes, such

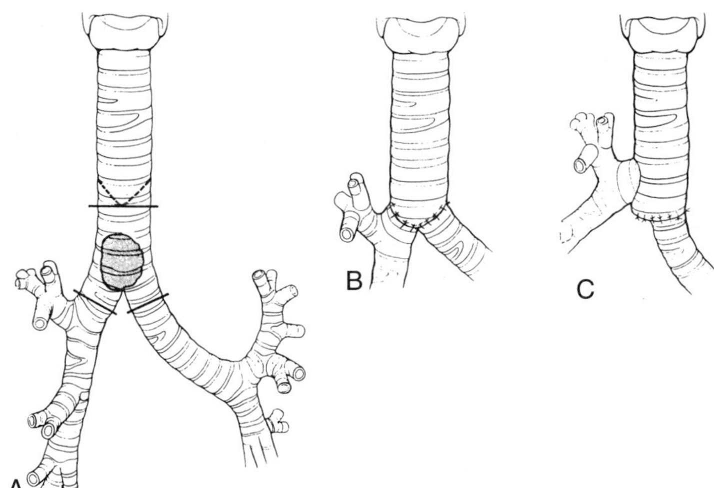

FIGURE 7–17. *A,* A tumor of the carina. *B,* Primary reconstruction with end-to-end anastomosis. Reconstruction is also possible by anastomosing left bronchus to end trachea stump and right bronchus to a lateral bronchotomy *(C).*

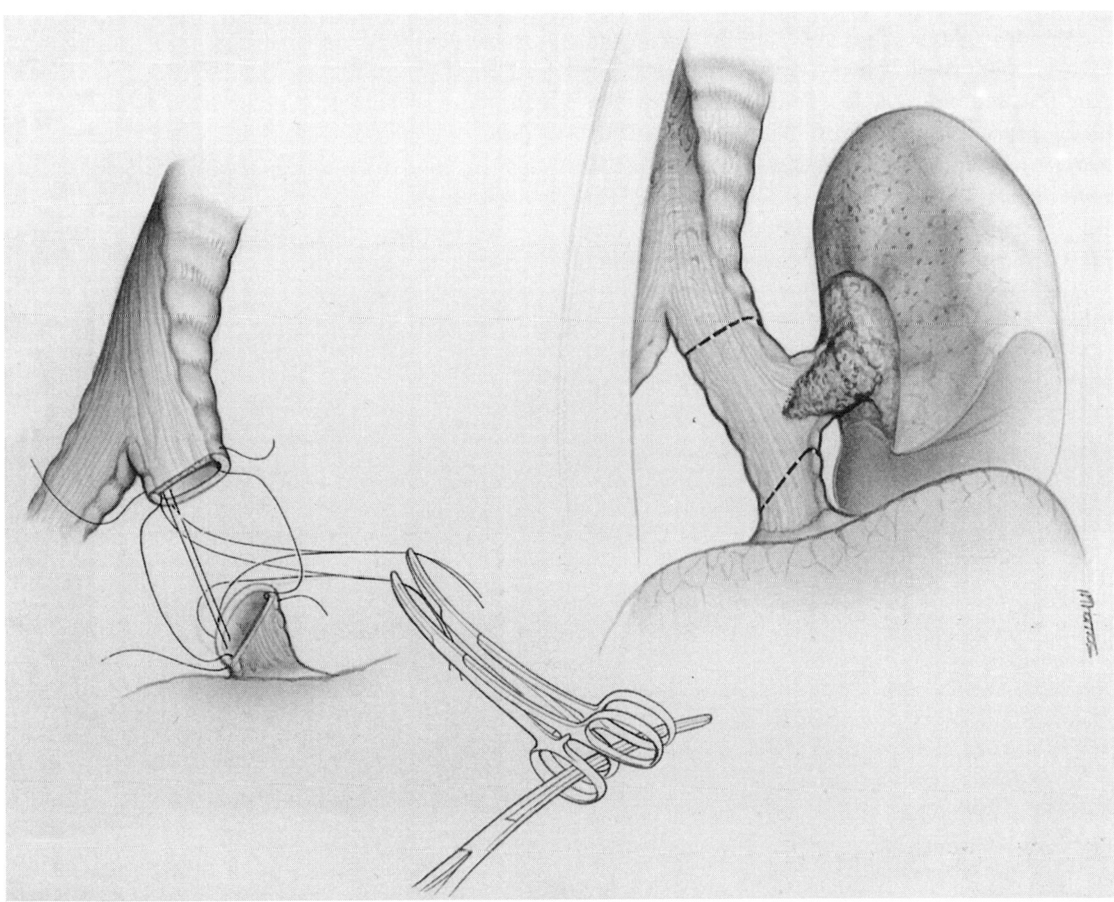

FIGURE 7–18. A right upper lobe tumor extending into orifice of bronchus intermedius. The lobe with a "sleeve" of right main bronchus and bronchus intermedius is resected, and bronchus intermedius is anastomosed to the main bronchial stump. (From Beattie EJ, et al: Atlas of thoracic surgery. In Beattie EJ, et al [eds]: Thoracic Surgical Oncology. New York: Churchill Livingstone, 1992, p 111.)

as iodine 125, iridium 192, and cesium 137, are gamma emitters by way of decay.[104, 105] Heavy particle beams (fast neutrons, protons, helium ions, neon, argon, and pions) are capable of providing higher tumor dose relative to normal tissue.[106, 107]

Modern radiotherapy, with the help of recent developments in computer technology and linear accelerators, possesses the tools for precise targeting of tumor volume with high doses of ionizing radiation, which compromises the reproductive integrity of targeted cells. Such cells may appear undamaged until their first division. A tumor's radiosensitivity depends on its capacity to repair itself after radiation injury and varies for different cell types and for tumor volume. A total dose of 5000 cGy is sufficient to eradicate subclinical disease; however, for tumors 5.0 cm in diameter, calculated doses of up to 10,000 cGy theoretically achieve only 70% to 80% control, with a high incidence of radiation side effects.[91–109]

External Radiotherapy

Patients referred for external radiotherapy usually have conditions that are nonresectable because of either the extent of the tumor or the medical condition of the patient. When disease is confined to the chest, these patients may be considered for curative treatment under special circumstances. Histologic confirmation of malignant tumor by means of biopsy or cytology is always required.

Patients with severe obstructive lung disease, congestive heart failure, or recent myocardial infarction need a very careful design of radiation treatment because of the high risk of acute and late complications, but they can be treated with curative intent. In designing treatment portals, diagnostic or planning CT scans are used for the precise delineation of tumor volume. Custom-made blocks are created for each patient to exclude as much normal tissue as possible from the high-dose radiation field. To ensure a homogeneous dose distribution, computer-generated isodose curves are used to prescribe the daily and total doses. The spinal cord dose is calculated by using lateral x-ray films. The dose to the cord is kept under 4500 cGy by using special wedges or tissue-equivalent compensators. Treatment is started with anteroposterior and posteroanterior fields. These fields cover the primary tumor and the relevant lymph node–bearing areas, such as the ipsilateral hilum, mediastinum, and paratracheal lymph nodes. If the tumor is located in the upper lobes, the supraclavicular areas are included in the treatment field. In selected cases, the contralateral hilum also is included in the treatment field.

Approximately 3600 cGy is given with 180- to 280-cGy daily fractions to the anteroposterior and posteroanterior portals, and then the beam direction is changed to avoid the spinal cord. This arrangement also includes less lung tissue within the zone of high-dose radiation. A total dose of 5000 cGy to the mediastinum is usually prescribed, but the primary tumor receives 6400 to 6600 cGy. With this dose, complete responses of 35% for stages I, II, and IIIA patients and a 7% 5-year recurrence-free survival rate have been reported.[110–113]

Acute side effects of radiotherapy include esophagitis, bronchitis, and erythema of the skin. Bronchitis secondary

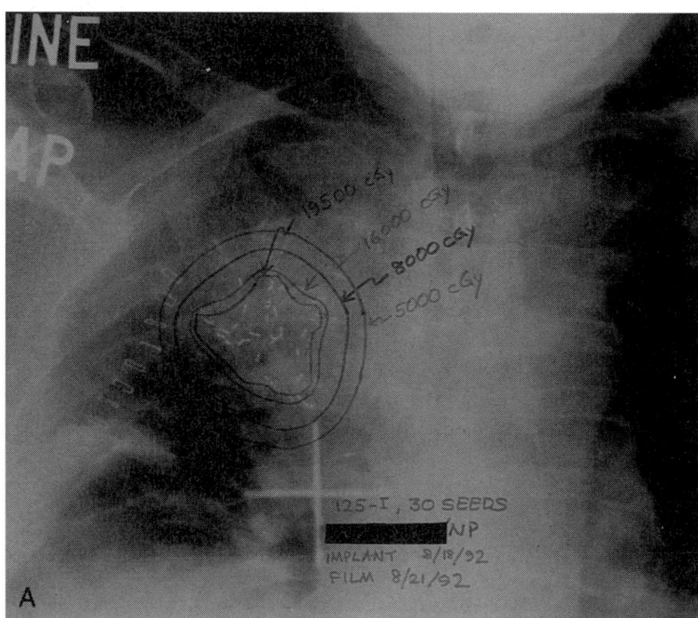

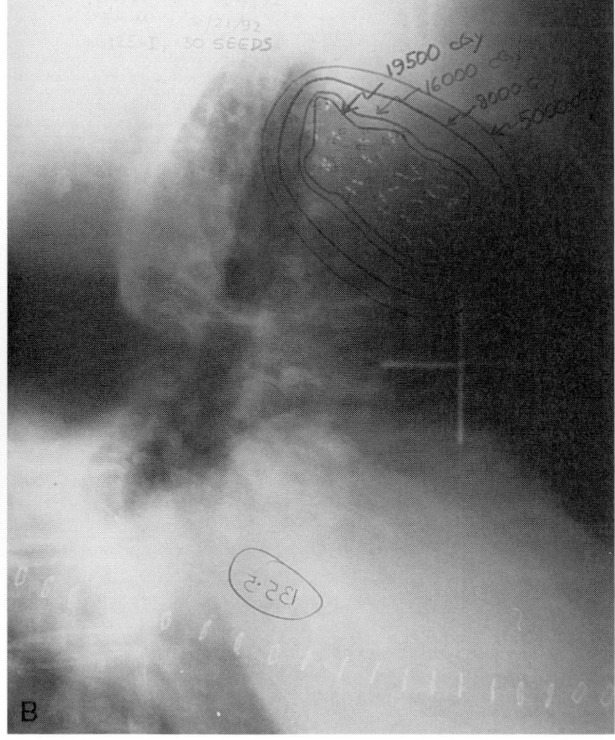

FIGURE 7–19. Posteroanterior *(A)* and lateral *(B)* views of tumor implanted with iodine 125 seeds. Isodose curves have been computed and marked on the radiographs.

to irradiation or infection may require antibiotics and cough medication. Dysphagia is well controlled with simple analgesics and lidocaine (Xylocaine Viscous) 2%.

Internal Radiotherapy (Brachytherapy)

To improve local control in an unresectable or incompletely resected tumors, intraoperative radiotherapy with artificial isotopes as radioactive sources was pioneered by Henschke[114] at Memorial Hospital in New York. He postulated that a much higher dose can be delivered to the tumor with less damage to normal tissues with implantation than with external radiation alone. A combination of surgery, brachytherapy, and external radiation was promoted and further refined by Hilaris and coworkers[115] and Greenblatt and colleagues.[116]

Internal radiotherapy provided by implantation of iodine 125 seeds has been employed by us when predicted risks of lobectomy or pneumonectomy are prohibitive and wedge or segmental excisions are not technically feasible. Chest wall invasion is not a contraindication. Iodine 125 has a low-energy gamma emission (30 kV) and long half-life (60 days), making it safe for handling in the operating room and possible to store for easy availability on short notice. Nomograms permit intraoperative calculations of the number and spacing of sources of given energy per volume of tumor.

Fleischman and coworkers[117] found local control of tumors less than 5.0 cm in diameter to be 83%, the same as that of limited resection in surgical series and superior to that achieved by external beam therapy (with which local failures range up to 70%). Successful local control is attributed to two factors: (1) interstitial brachytherapy allows much higher doses (8000 to 20,000 cGy) to be delivered to a smaller volume of lung than is capable with external beam radiation (5000 to 7000 cGy) and (2) more accurate coverage of the tumor is possible due to open operative source placement within the mass.[117] With sources placed only 1.0 cm beyond the mass, no significant pneumonitis is seen because the volume of normal lung exposed to high-dose radiation is limited (Fig. 7–19*A* and *B*). This technique is especially useful in treating older patients, avoiding the morbidity and mortality of a high-risk resection, especially completion pneumonectomy.

A second form of internal radiotherapy is provided by afterloading catheters sutured to a mediastinal bed, following a dissection in which nodes are found to be positive or near chest wall resections with close margins.[118, 119] Iridium 192 sources may be inserted into the catheter at the end of the first postoperative week (Fig. 7–20*A* and *B*). The radioactive energy, delivered either at high dose rate or low dose rate, is generally supplemented by external beam radiation. Internal radiotherapy has not been able to achieve survival equal to complete resection but has resulted in 3-year survival greater than 30% among unresectable tumors less than 5.0 cm in diameter and has improved local control for locally advanced unresectable patients.

Color Figure 7–21 illustrates radiation options.

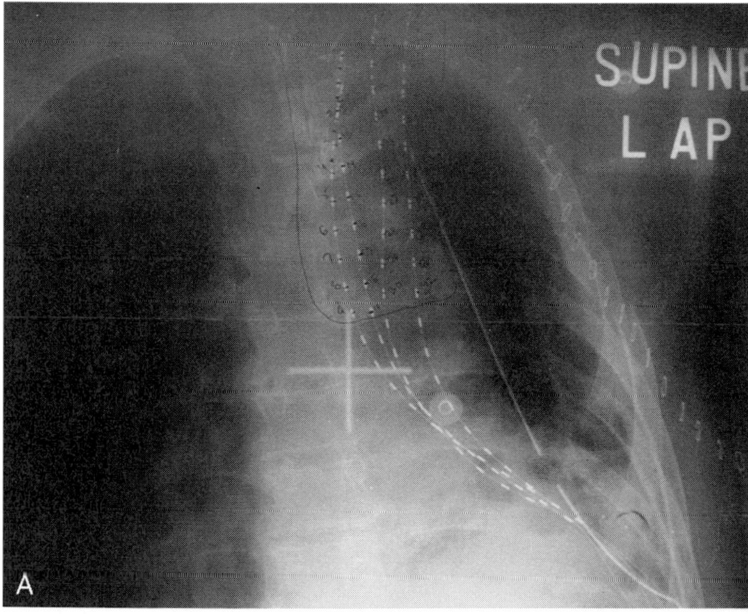

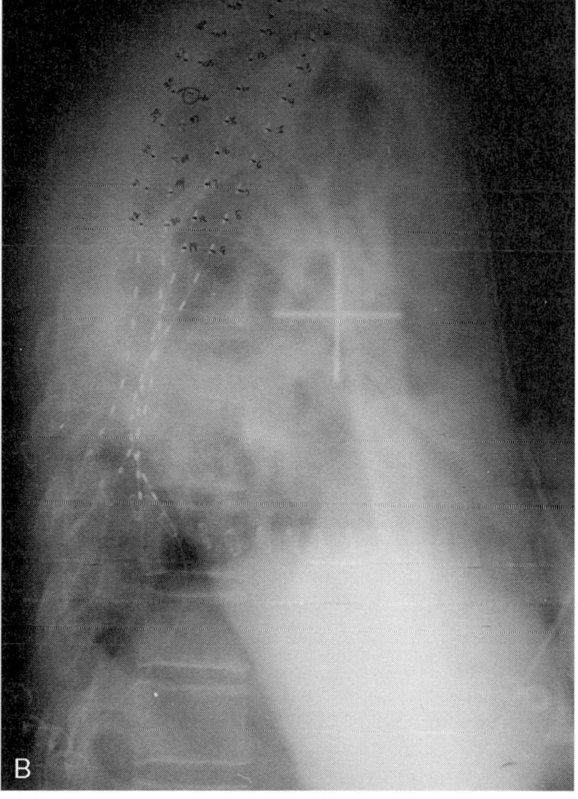

FIGURE 7–20. Posteroanterior *(A)* and lateral *(B)* views of afterloading catheters that have been secured with absorbable mesh sewn into place.

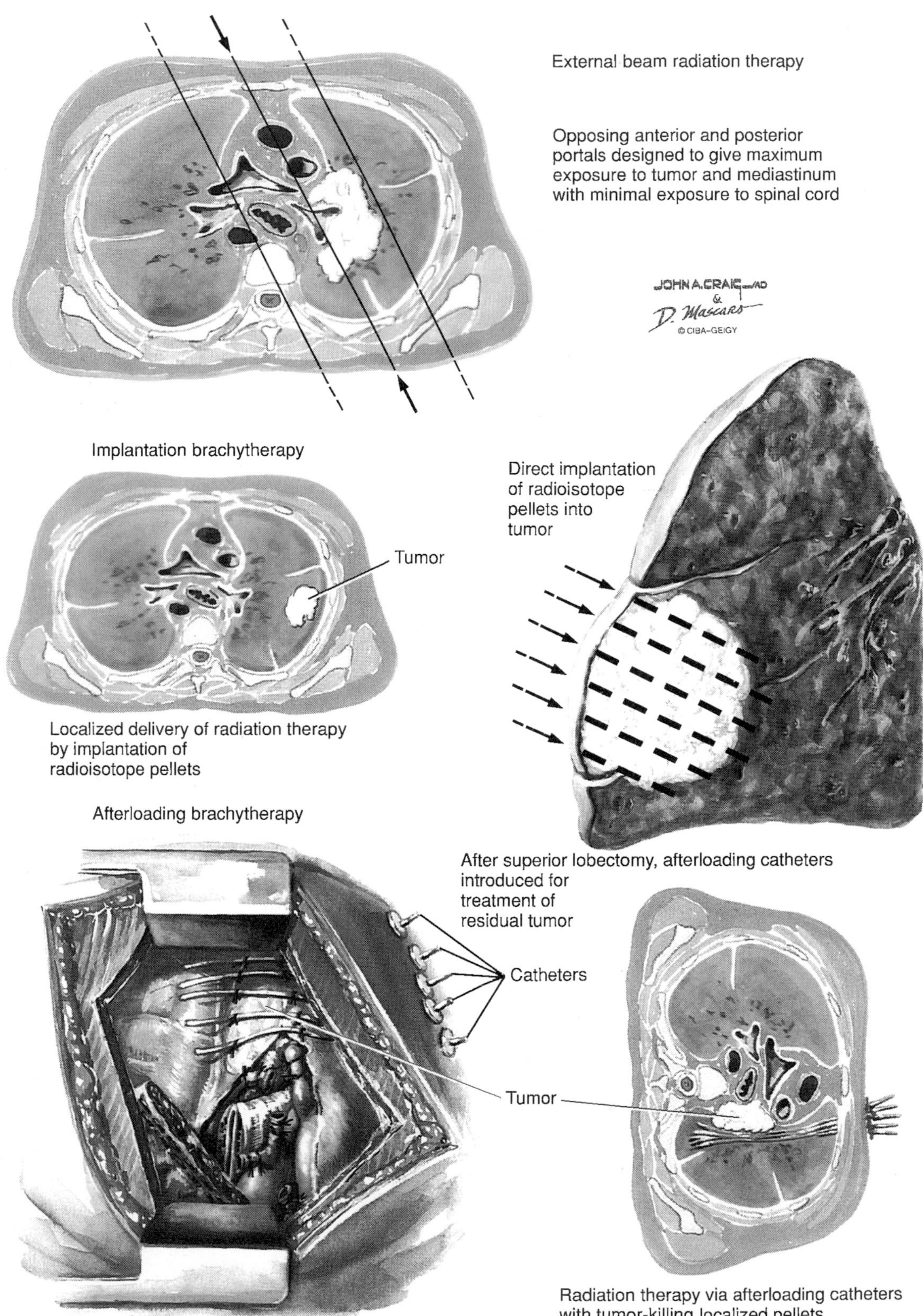
External beam radiation therapy
Opposing anterior and posterior portals designed to give maximum exposure to tumor and mediastinum with minimal exposure to spinal cord
JOHN A.CRAIG
&
D. Mascaro
© CIBA-GEIGY
Implantation brachytherapy
Tumor
Direct implantation of radioisotope pellets into tumor
Localized delivery of radiation therapy by implantation of radioisotope pellets
Afterloading brachytherapy
After superior lobectomy, afterloading catheters introduced for treatment of residual tumor
Catheters
Tumor
Radiation therapy via afterloading catheters with tumor-killing localized pellets

FIGURE 7–21. Radiotherapy options. (From Harvey JC, Beattie EJ: Lung cancer. CIBA-GEIGY Clin Symp 45:27, 1993. © Copyright 1993 CIBA-GEIGY Corporation. Reprinted with permission from Clinical Symposia, illustrated by Frank H. Netter, M.D., John A. Craig, and David Mascaro. All rights reserved.)

Combination Therapies

Postoperative Radiotherapy

Because most patients with stage II or III disease die of tumor, even when the the surgeon's assessment was that all tumor had been removed, it seemed rational to supplement surgical resection with postoperative radiation. A prospective, randomized trial conducted by the Lung Cancer Study Group investigated the efficacy of postoperative external radiation to the mediastinum for completely resected stage II to III NSCLC. Patients receiving other therapies were excluded from this study.

Patients in the treatment limb of the study were given 5000 cGy over a 5-week period and compared with a control group given no treatment. At a mean follow-up time of 3.5 years, it was not possible to detect a significant difference in disease-free survival in the treatment group, but significant radiation toxicity among the treatment cohort included esophagitis, dermatitis, and neurotoxicities (including one case of paraplegia 2 years after treatment). Radiation did decrease the incidence of local recurrence but could not effect long-term survival because 75% of recurrences were outside of the radiation fields. Although no update of this powerful study has been published, no survival benefit will occur with postoperative radiotherapy if previously reported trends persist.[120]

Preoperative Radiotherapy

The observation that radiotherapy can induce significant responses among inoperable patients is the historical reason for attempts to employ it preoperatively to improve resectability. It has been observed that preoperative radiation might result in increased resectability but at the expense of increased complications and with no increase in long-term survival.[121, 122]

Superior sulcus tumors (Pancoast's tumors) are exceptions to the observation that preoperative irradiation provides no survival benefit. These tumors, located in the posteromedial apex of the chest, typically present with symptoms of pain and paresthesia in the shoulder, arm, or hand related to compression of the eighth cervical and first two thoracic nerve roots of the brachial plexus. There may also be atrophy of muscles of the hand. If the sympathetic chain is invaded, there may be Horner's syndrome (see Color Fig. 7–22).[123] Roentgenograms confirm the location of the tumor and may also reveal destruction of ribs, transverse processes, or vertebral bodies (Figs. 7–23 to 7–25). In the absence of bone destruction, the tumor may appear as "pleural thickening," but the diagnosis must be ruled out in symptomatic cases (Fig. 7–26).

Early attempts at treatment by either surgery or irradiation were unsatisfactory. The first encouraging results were attained by surgical resection following a course of external beam irradiation and a rest period. Standard care now involves treatment with 3000 cGy, a 3-week rest, and en bloc resection. The resected tumor mass typically includes upper lobe of lung, chest wall, transverse processes, portions of vertebral body, inferior portions of brachial plexus, and, in some cases, portions of subclavian artery.[124] Darteville et al.[125] have described the advantages of an anterior approach, especially in cases requiring resection of subclavian artery, but most continue to employ the more familiar posterolateral thoracotomy. Patients were treated in this fashion by Paulson[126, 127] with a 2.6% operative mortality rate and 5-, 10-, 15-year survival rates of 31%, 26%, and 22%, respectively, for 131 patients completing treatment. No patients with either hilar or mediastinal nodal involvement survived 2 years.

In cases of inoperability, the dose of irradiation is increased as tolerated.[128] Whenever operative findings preclude complete resection, brachytherapy may be employed, but our preferred treatment is "standard," as described above.[129]

Induction Chemotherapy or Chemoradiotherapy Followed by Surgery

Induction chemotherapy (adjuvant chemotherapy) using combinations of drugs of proven single-agent efficacy—usually cisplatin-based—is employed with the intention of converting bulky N2, stage IIIa NSCLC to resectable disease. The combination of cisplatin and vindesine with or without mitomycin C has been reported from the Memorial Sloan-Kettering Cancer Center.[130–132] Response rates greater than 70% have been reported, but most are in the neighborhood of 50%. Complete surgical resections were performed in more than half of these patients. Approximately 14% had a complete response to chemotherapy as determined by surgical specimens, including primary tumor and mediastinal nodes. Median survival of these patients has been 19 months, compared with 12 months for historical controls. Similar results have been reported from the University of Toronto.[103] Toxicity has included mitomycin lung toxicity, early and late; chemotherapy-induced sepsis; and increased incidence of postpneumonectomy bronchopleural fistulas, sometimes of lethal consequence. However, most surgery has been uneventful.

Shepherd[133] has reviewed 15 phase II pilot trials of various chemotherapy regimens: 5 with chemotherapy alone, 4 with chemotherapy and subsequent radiation, and 6 with chemotherapy and concurrent radiation. Response rates were in the neighborhood of 50%, but complete remissions were less than 15%. Pathologic complete response rates were most often less than 10%. Of the 70% of such patients eligible for resection, complete resections were possible in 60%. Median survival was about 1.5 years. Shepherd cautiously concluded that any survival benefit observed may be explained by selection bias and that, until randomized trials are concluded, such trials must be regarded as investigational.

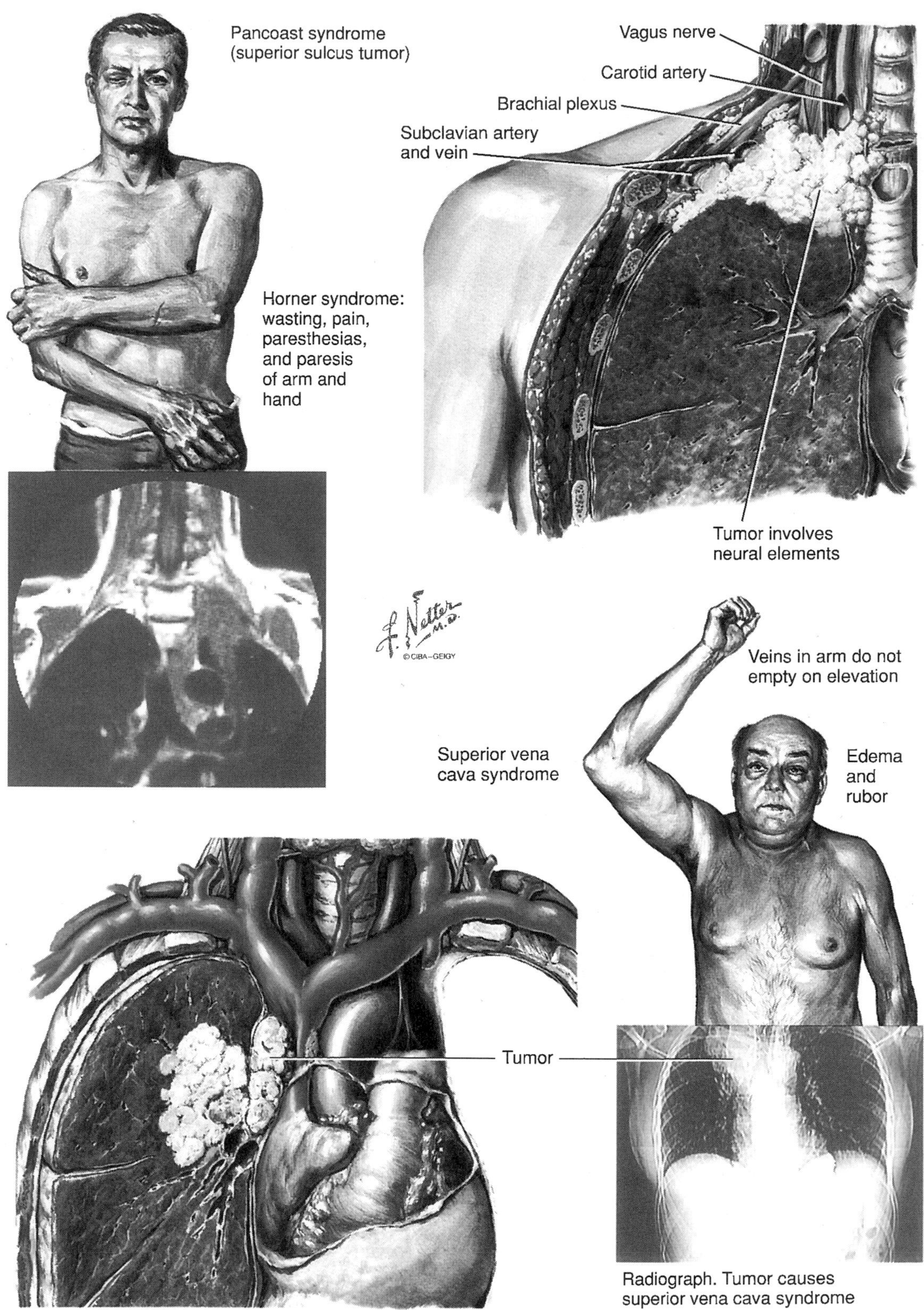

FIGURE 7–22. Superior sulcus tumor and superior vena cava syndrome. (From Harvey JC, Beattie EJ: Lung cancer. CIBA-GEIGY Clin Symp 45:12, 1993. © Copyright 1993 CIBA-GEIGY Corporation. Reprinted with permission from Clinical Symposia, illustrated by Frank H. Netter, M.D., John A. Craig, and David Mascaro. All rights reserved.)

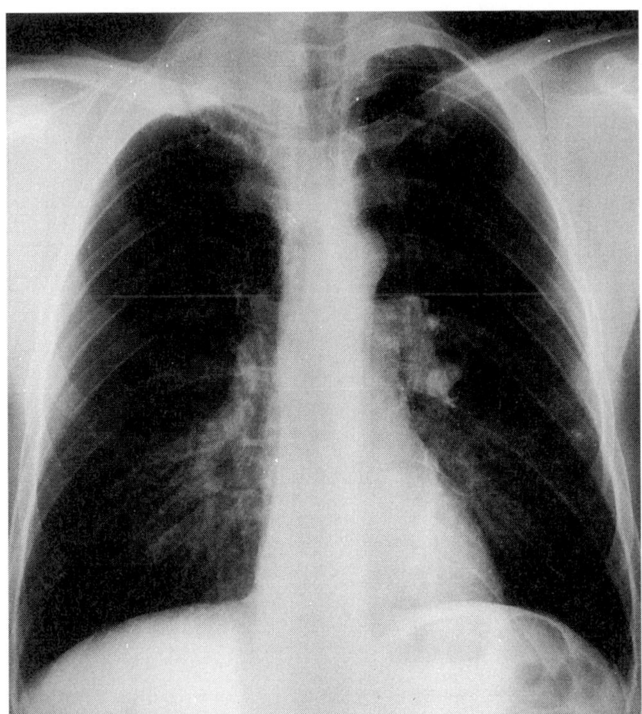

FIGURE 7–23. Chest radiograph of a 40-year-old man with right shoulder and arm pain showing a right apical mass and destruction of the second and third ribs.

Pisch and coworkers[134] have reported the experience with simultaneous chemotherapy and radiation with or without subsequent resection (i.e., whenever feasible) for stage IIIA (18 patients) and IIIB (23 patients) tumors. Updated actuarial survivals are 49% at 2 years and 28.2% at 4 years. The results of some multidisciplinary management programs for locally-regionally advanced disease are shown in Table 7–4.[134–140]

The goal in such aggressive experimental treatments is not only to convert unresectable disease to resectable but also to control distant micrometastases. An advantage of giving chemotherapy preoperatively rather than postoperatively to achieve the same goal is that preoperative treatment provides an in vivo test of efficacy for the specific patient's tumor and guides the clinician in deciding whether to continue the treatment postoperatively. Generally, adjuvant treatment has not yielded as encouraging results as neoadjuvant treatment plans.[58, 141]

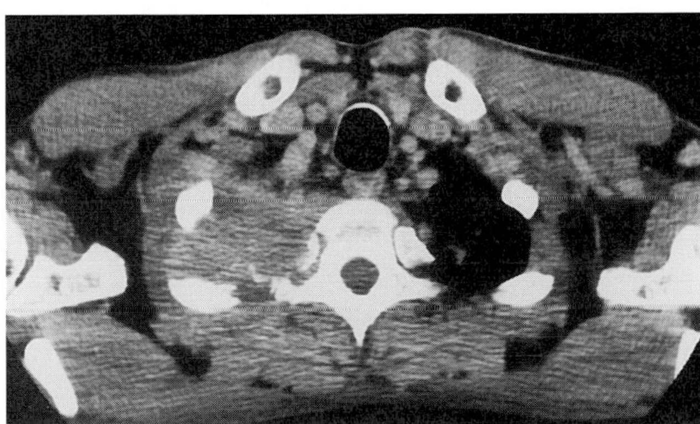

FIGURE 7–24. CT scan confirming destruction of posterior ribs and costovertebral junction.

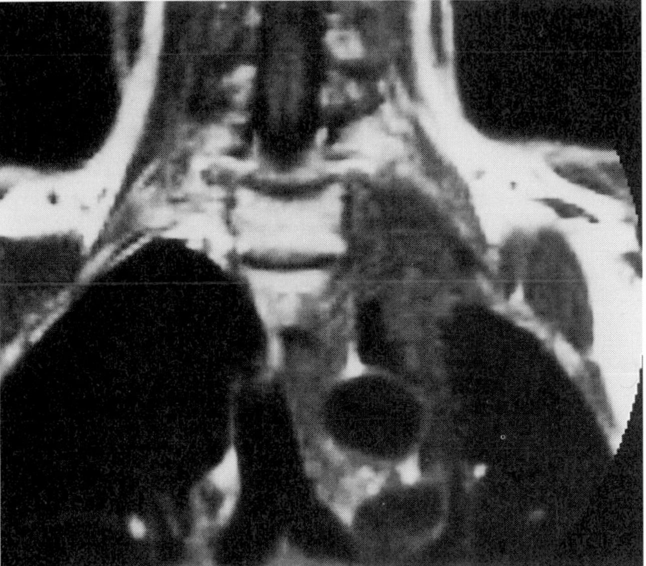

FIGURE 7–25. MRI scan showing mass in upper lobe extending into soft tissues above apex, extending along inferior aspect of the brachial plexus, and encroaching on lateral vertebral body.

National trials are ongoing to test irradiation with various chemotherapy combinations (some constituents of which are radiopotentiators) in attempts to achieve significant local-regional responses while improving on the disappointing distant failure rates.

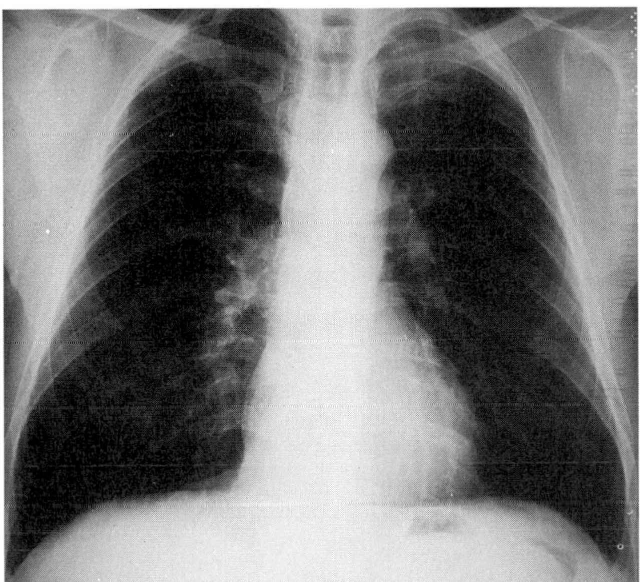

FIGURE 7–26. Chest radiograph of a 60-year-old man with left shoulder pain. An opacity is faintly visible at the left apex. Biopsy confirmed adenocarcinoma.

TABLE 7–4
Multimodality Treatment of Locally Advanced Lung Cancer

Authors	Radiation Therapy: *No. of Patients*	Radiation Therapy: *Gy*	Chemotherapy	Schedule	Response (CR + PR) (%)	Resected (%)	Survival Rate (%): *1 yr*	Survival Rate (%): *2 yr*
Pisch et al.[134]	50	40–60	Cisplatin + 5-FU VP16	Simultaneous	48	42	—	49
Bonomi et al.[135]	20	50	Mitomycin Cisplatin 5-FU	Sequential	60	20	—	15
Farley et al.[136]	13	50–60	Vincristine Mitomycin + 5-FU	Simultaneous	92	—	—	—
Johnson et al.[137]	107	60	Vindesine	Simultaneous	34	—	36	14
Taylor et al.[138]	64	40	Cisplatin + 5-FU	Simultaneous	56	61	49	—
Strauss et al.[139]	22	55–60	Vindesine + cisplatin	Sequential	55	59	—	—
Le Chevalier et al.[140]	176	65	Vindesine Cyclophosphamide Cisplatin	Sequential	31	Not attempted	50	21

CR, Complete response; PR, partial response; 5-FU, 5-fluorouracil; VP16, etoposide.

METASTATIC OR RECURRENT DISEASE

For the most part, only palliative options are available for symptomatic relief of metastatic and recurrent disease. However, quality of life may be improved by prompt initiation of treatment at onset of symptoms. Durable relief of troublesome symptoms is achievable, but long-term survival is exceptional.

Surgery

The only situation in which surgery has an important role in the treatment of tumors metastatic beyond the thorax is that of *solitary brain metastasis* accompanying otherwise resectable disease.

About 30% of patients with NSCLC ultimately have brain metastases, which amounts to a problem of magnitude comparable to the number of new cases of cancer of the rectum, pancreas, stomach, and esophagus. Untreated brain metastases result in progressive deterioration, with a median survival of approximately 1 month. Corticosteroids may yield a rapid, dramatic relief of neurologic symptoms, but survival is only about 2 months. Whole brain irradiation palliates approximately 80% of patients, but the survival benefit has been unimpressive, with median survival time generally less than 6 months.

Surgical resection of the primary brain metastasis followed by resection of the primary tumor and whole brain irradiation improves median survival to 14 months, with a 1-year survival rate of 58% and a 5-year survival rate of 13%. This is true whether the tumors are synchronous or metachronous and depends on complete resection rather than TNM stage of the primary lung cancer. These data suggest that even in the presence of extensive disease, complete resection of the brain metastasis and local-regional disease is recommended whenever possible. The decision about which tumor should be approached first generally depends on symptoms. Symptomatic brain metastases are the first to be resected in cases of discovery simultaneously with "incidentally" discovered primary lung tumors.[142]

Radiotherapy

External Beam Irradiation

External beam irradiation is sometimes beneficial in relieving local symptoms of advanced or metastatic disease.[91, 104–113]

Endobronchial Internal Radiotherapy

Afterloading catheters may be positioned endobronchially for palliation of unresectable airway tumors. Under direct vision combined with remote video imaging, afterloading catheters are passed over a guide wire inserted through an operating port of a 4.9-mm-diameter flexible bronchoscope. The longitudinal dimension of the tumor is measured by passing the endoscope beyond the visible tumor. When this is not possible, the approximate length is estimated from the pretreatment computed tomograms. Positioning is confirmed fluoroscopically, the bronchoscope is removed, and the patient is transferred to the radiotherapy suite for treatment planning (Fig. 7–27).

With a high-activity iridium 192 radiation source, a dose of 500–750 cGy is given at a 0.5- to 1.0-cm depth from the center of the source. The treatment is administered over 10 to 15 minutes, and the patient is discharged the same day. Some patients have had a repeated treatment in 2 weeks.[92, 143, 144]

Excellent palliation has been obtained for hemoptysis, with 93% of patients relieved for the duration of their lives. Among patients treated with cough, 80% were able to reduce cough suppression medications or were completely relieved, but 20% had no relief. Atelectasis and pneumonia cleared completely in 20%.[92]

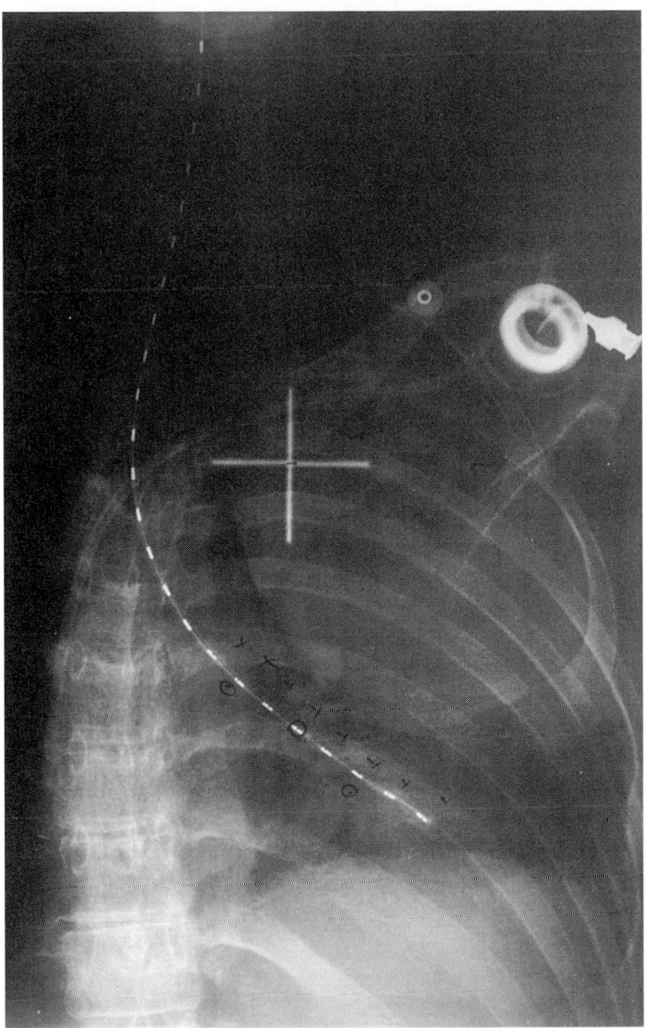

FIGURE 7–27. Treatment planning radiograph demonstrating position of endobronchial afterloading catheter.

We believe this to be a useful palliative modality with a low rate of complications. A major advantage is the ability to provide a tumor-site dose of radiation in a few minutes of outpatient time for patients with generally very limited life expectancy and troublesome symptoms.

Chemotherapy

Chemotherapy combinations similar to those employed in neoadjuvant therapy have been demonstrated to prolong survival among previously untreated patients with NSCLC when compared with supportive care alone.[145–147] Furthermore, costs of supportive care alone exceed those of an aggressive treatment policy because a major contribution to cost is the hospitalization rather than the chemotherapeutic agents.[148]

Superior Vena Cava Syndrome

Extensive compression of the superior vena cava due to encroachment of paratracheal nodes (N2) results in a syndrome of facial edema and rubor with bulging neck veins and development of extensive collateral venous return via the upper torso and arms. The clinical diagnosis is confirmed by x-ray (see Color Fig. 7–22) or scans.

Formerly, urgent irradiation without tissue diagnosis was frequently used in treatment of this syndrome, but it is now known that mediastinoscopy can be safely employed to achieve specific tissue diagnosis.[149] Tumor-specific therapy is far superior to the results achieved through urgent irradiation without a diagnosis. Gauden[150] has described the results of irradiation for NSCLC as "poor," with only 19% of patients achieving complete relief of symptoms. The 2-year survival rate was only 2%, and 30% of patients had no demonstrable response. No deaths occurred due to venous compression, but deaths did occur as a result of associated tracheal compression.

Various stents[151–153] and bypasses[154, 155] have been used to palliate the venous and airway[95] obstructions.

Post-treatment Surveillance

Each year, second primary tumors arise among 2% to 3% of patients surviving previous treatment of tumors of the aerodigestive tract. Therefore, lung cancer patients must be followed closely to detect second primary cancers of the head and neck and the esophagus as well as those of the lung. Patients are evaluated with a complete history, review of systems, physical examination, chest radiographs, and complete blood counts and blood chemistries (including selected tumor markers) every 2 to 3 months of the first 2 postoperative years and every 4 to 6 months thereafter. Second primary lung cancers are treated using the same selection criteria initially employed. Previous treatment has resulted in more than usual compromise of pulmonary reserve in these patients, so conservative resections or internal irradiation is frequently indicated.

Faber[156] has reported results of surgical treatment of 114 patients with a second primary lung cancer and 18 with third primary tumors. All patients had (1) a different cell type, (2) a tumor-free interval of 24 months, (3) a second primary tumor in the contralateral lung, or (4) a new tumor in a separate ipsilateral lobe. The operative mortality rate was 8.8% (10 of 114) for the second resection and 5.5% (1 of 18) for the third resection. Cumulative survival following second resection was 33% at 5 years and 20% at 10 years. Results were similar whether or not the second tumor was of the same cell type as the first.

TREATMENT OF SMALL CELL LUNG CARCINOMA

SCLC constitutes 15% to 25% of lung cancers in the United States. It is recognized as a tumor that remains particularly aggressive in spite of being initially responsive to a variety of therapeutic attacks. High response rates, including complete responses during 2 to 3 years, have not yet resulted in the long-term disease-free survivals achieved with other solid tumors whose therapies have achieved durable 2- to 3-year survivals. Furthermore, long-term combined-modality therapies are associated with severe toxicities.

Recent reviews suggest that only 7% of patients with limited disease (LD) and 1% of patients with extensive disease (ED) survive 5 years. LD (approximately one third of cases) is defined as disease confined to one hemithorax, mediastinum, and supraclavicular fossa; ED comprises all other situations. It must be emphasized that even LD is almost always very extensive, "limited" only in the sense that it can be encompassed in a single radiotherapy portal.[157]

Radiotherapy

It was not until the 1960s that the propensity of SCLC for distant metastases, even greater than that of NSCLC, was recognized. By the end of that decade, radiotherapy became established as the local treatment modality. It was soon discovered that the addition of chemotherapy improved local control and, in some instances, survival. Now, combination chemotherapy is the treatment of choice for extensive SCLC, but radiotherapy remains important in palliation of local complications.[105]

Improvement in local control is achieved when radiotherapy is added to chemotherapy regimens for LD because many important drugs are radiosensitizers. However, they also radiosensitize normal tissue and are consequently associated with increased rates of esophagitis, pneumonitis, and myelosuppression in some trials, especially when radiation (which we avoid) was administered simultaneously with doxorubicin.[158–160]

A great variety of doses, fractionations, and durations of radiotherapy are in use.

Prophylactic Cranial Irradiation

Prophylactic cranial irradiation (PCI) has been employed because brain metastases are common in SCLC, sometimes as the only site in a patient otherwise in remission. Since the central nervous system has been a "sanctuary" shielded from the killing effects of systemic chemotherapy, it has been hypothesized that PCI could improve cure rate or at least delay central nervous system treatment failure. Superior quality of life would be derived by prolonging survival free of central nervous system disability. Most trials of PCI have found decreases in brain metastases but no survival improvement. Furthermore, with longer follow-up, the combination of PCI with chemotherapy seems to result in central nervous system dysfunction in about 45% of long-term survivors. Memory loss and decreased coordination and motor skills have sometimes been devastating.[157, 161–164]

Most studies reporting neurotoxicity with PCI have involved early, concurrent administration with chemotherapy. It may be that PCI damages the blood-brain barrier such that subsequent chemotherapy penetrates with greater concentration. A prospective Eastern Cooperative Oncology Group study is in progress testing whether administering PCI only after completion of chemotherapy will improve survival and decrease central nervous system relapse. Neurotoxicity will be another end point in this study. By administering no PCI until all chemotherapy is completed and allowing no chemotherapy after completion of PCI, it is hoped that disabling neurotoxicity will be avoided.[157]

Chemotherapy

Single-Agent Chemotherapy

In 1995, multiagent therapy is standard, but etoposide has proven useful as a single agent. In one study, etoposide administered every 3 weeks for a 5-day course resulted in a 10-month median survival. The drug may be administered orally. A trial of oral etoposide in an elderly population resulted in a 71% response rate, with median survivals of 16 months (LD) and 9 months (ED). Because etoposide is easily tolerated, some authorities consider it the best therapeutic choice for the frail, the elderly, and patients with comorbidities precluding toxic multidrug treatment.

Multiagent therapy has been shown to be superior in providing rapid cytoreduction and long-term survival. When treating LD with curative intent, multidrug treatment must be used. This is also the case in situations demanding rapid cytoreduction in order to preserve vital structures or their function, such as superior vena caval syndrome and airway obstruction. The best combinations of two to four drugs have been as effective as more complex combinations used in the past. Generally, combinations are administered in doses selected to avoid intolerable toxicity to specific organs. Some treatment plans alternate combinations of two to four drugs each. Originally this was done for two reasons: (1) to expose the tumor to as many active agents as possible within a short period of time and (2) to delay the emergence of drug resistance.

The issue of aggressiveness of treatment has been examined in published randomized trials for both LD and ED. No general dependence of therapeutic effect on dose was found within the usual clinical range of doses. Attempts to provide extremely high doses of chemotherapy have resulted in severe toxicity without survival advantage. Prolongation of the duration of treatment, a "maintenance" chemotherapy, is not supported by the literature. Treatment extended beyond 3 to 8 months has increased the duration of remission but has not improved survival. Salvage chemotherapy is more likely to promote response among patients who have relapsed if the duration of induction therapy was brief than if it had been relatively prolonged. However, the median survival resulting from salvage chemotherapy is poor (median survival from relapse, 8 to 12 weeks.)[157, 165–167]

Modern combination chemotherapy produces partial or complete responses in greater than 80% of patients in all stages of SCLC. A complete response is expected for at least 50% to 60% of patients with LD, with median survival of 12 to 16 months and 2-year survival rate approaching 20%. For ED patients, complete response rates up to 30% are achievable, with median survival of 7 to 12 months, but very few 2-year survivals are expected.[157, 168–170]

Cyclophosphamide in combination with doxorubicin (Adriamycin) and vincristine (CAV) is a common regimen. The combination of cisplatin (Platinol) with etoposide (PE) has the advantage of not having cardiac, esophageal, or pulmonary toxicities. Studies alternating CAV with PE show slight improvement of median survival compared with CAV alone. It is too early to conclude that this sequence itself is superior, since the improvement could be explained by a superiority of PE to CAV. Studies in progress should clarify whether PE can achieve, on its own, results superior to those with CAV.[170–173]

Surgery

For the most part, even localized SCLC presents as bulky unresectable disease. Infrequently, SCLC presents as a solitary nodule (T1-2, N0, M0), and the diagnosis is obtained only following resection. Retrospective studies of these patients has verified that much better survival is expected among patients who have been surgically resected: up to 60% 5-year survival for T1, N0, M0 tumors. However, long-term survival with surgery alone remains a curiosity. The advantage of surgery is immediate cytoreduction, but this advantage is generally lost if not followed by several cycles of chemotherapy for this almost invariably systemic disease.[157, 174, 175]

Combination Therapy

For LD, combination chemotherapy alone has been as successful as chemotherapy followed by radiotherapy. The primary site is a frequent site of first recurrence, however, justifying protocols continuing the irradiation of primary sites in localized disease. As previously mentioned, some chemotherapy combinations (e.g., CAV) are radiosensitizers, explaining improved local control but frequently at the expense of toxicity to bone marrow, heart, and esophagus.[157–160]

Long-term data are available from at least one trial administering PE concurrently with radiotherapy to a dose of 4500 cGy over 3 weeks. Responders were continued on six cycles of PE alternating with CAV. The combination of PE with radiotherapy can be given with few side effects. CAV following radiotherapy is less toxic than when it precedes radiotherapy (except as has already been mentioned, for the brain). Median survival has been 2 years, and 30% of patients have survived 5 years. Only larger trials comparing this regimen with standard ones in a prospective manner will confirm whether PE, with or without radiotherapy, with or without CAV, is superior treatment.

The role of surgery in extensive SCLC is limited to diagnostic and palliative procedures.

Shepherd and colleagues[176] at the University of Toronto have reviewed the role of surgery in combined-modality treatment of limited SCLC. There is almost universal agreement that even in the case of stage I resected disease, chemotherapy should be a part of the treatment in the postoperative period; 5-year survival rates of up to 60% have been described under these circumstances. The University of Toronto experience includes 119 patients who had had resection for limited disease: 79 prior to chemotherapy and radiotherapy and 40 with induction chemotherapy followed by resection and chemotherapy, most with CAV but frequently with PE in recent years. Postoperative radiotherapy was administered to the tumor bed and mediastinum (average, 3000 cGy) following resection and chemotherapy. Prophylactic cranial irradiation (2000 cGy) was administered. A complete response occurred in 45% of these patients and a partial response in 50%. The postoperative pathologic stages were: stage I, 35 patients; stage II, 36 patients; stage III, 48 patients. Overall 5-year survival rate was projected at 39%; 28% for stage III tumors. Shepherd and colleagues recommend initial treatment with induction chemotherapy followed by surgical resection in patients who respond.

Some groups have been able to convert stages II, IIIa, and IIIB SCLC to resectable disease with brief courses of well-tolerated chemotherapy,[177–179] but results seem to be similar whether surgery precedes or follows chemotherapy for stage I SCLC.[180, 181]

Prospective trials are being conducted to test multidisciplinary approaches. It is essential to ascertain that the unusual occurrence of early-stage SCLC truly is SCLC rather than a localized carcinoid tumor, which can appear very similar to SCLC under light microscopy.

References

1. Wynder EL, Graham EA: Tobacco smoking as a possible etiologic factor in bronchiogenic carcinoma. JAMA 143:329–336, 1950.
2. Doll R, Hill AB: Smoking and carcinoma of the lung. Br Med J 2:740–748, 1950.
3. Wingo PA, Tong T, Bolden S: Cancer statistics. CA 45:8–30, 1995.
4. Garfinkel L, Silverberg E: Lung cancer and smoking trends in the United States over the past 25 years. CA 41:137–145, 1991.
5. Meyer JA: Hugh Morriston Davis: And lobectomy for cancer, 1912. Ann Thorac Surg 46:472–474, 1988.
6. Davies HM: Recent advances in the surgery of the lung and pleura. Br J Surg 1:228, 1913.
7. Kittle CF: History of thoracic surgical oncology. In Beattie EJ, Bloom ND, Harvey JC (eds): Thoracic Surgical Oncology. New York: Churchill Livingstone, 1992, pp 1–18.
8. Graham EA, Singer JJ: Successful removal of an entire lung for carcinoma of the bronchus. JAMA 101:137–141, 1933.
9. Ochsner A, DeBakey M: Carcinoma of the lung. Arch Surg 42:209–258, 1941.
10. Doll R: Journal interview: Conversation with Sir Richard Doll. Br J Addict 86:365–377, 1991.
11. Doll R, Hill AB: A study of the aetiology of carcinoma of the lung. Br Med J 2:1271–1286, 1952.
12. White C: Research on smoking and lung cancer: A landmark in the

history of chronic disease epidemiology. Yale J Biol Med 63:29–46, 1990.
13. Doll R, Hill AB: The mortality of doctors in relation to their smoking habits. Br Med J 1:1451–1455, 1954.
14. Fisher R: Cigarettes, cancer and statistics. Centennial Rev 2:151–166, 1958.
15. Stolley PD: When genius errs: RA Fisher and the lung cancer controversy. Am J Epidemiol 133:416–425, 1991.
16. Fraumeni JF, Blot WJ: Lung and pleura. In Schottenfeld D, Fraumeni JF (eds): Cancer Epidemiology and Prevention. Philadelphia: WB Saunders, 1982, pp 564–582.
17. Morabia A, Wynder EL: Cigarette smoking and lung cancer cell types. Cancer 68:2074–2078, 1991.
18. Kabat GC: Recent developments in the epidemiology of lung cancer. Semin Surg Oncol 9:73–79, 1993.
19. Stockwell HG, Armstrong AW, Leverton RE: Histopathology of lung cancers among smokers and non-smokers in Florida. Int J Epidemiol 19(Suppl 1):s48–s52, 1990.
20. National Academy of Sciences: Environmental Tobacco Smoke: Measuring Exposure and Assessing Health Effects. Washington, DC: National Academy Press, 1986.
21. Hill AB: The environment and disease: Association or causation? Proc World Soc Med 58:295–300, 1965.
22. Wynder EL, Kabat GC: Environmental tobacco smoke and lung cancer: A critical assessment. In Kasuga H (ed): Indoor Air Quality. Berlin: Springer-Verlag, 1990, pp 5–15.
23. Hammond EC, Selikoff IS, Seidman H: Asbestos exposure, cigarette smoking, and death rates. Am NY Acad Sci 330:473–496, 1979.
24. Doll R, Peto R: The causes of cancer. Quantitative Estimates of Avoidable Risks of Cancer in the United States Today. Oxford: Oxford University Press, 1981.
25. Tomatis L, Aitio A, Wilbourn J, Shuker L: Human carcinogens so far identified. Jpn J Cancer Res 80:795–807, 1989.
26. Peto R, Schneiderman M: Quantification of Occupational Cancer. Banbury Report No. 9. Cold Spring Harbor, NY: Cold Spring Harbor Laboratory, 1981.
27. Parkin DM: Trends in lung cancer incidence worldwide. Chest 96:5S–8S, 1989.
28. Colditz, GA, Stampfer MJ, Willett WC: Diet and lung cancer: A review of the epidemiologic evidence in humans. Arch Intern Med 147:157–160, 1987.
29. LeMarchand L, Yoshizawa CN, Kolonel LN, et al: Vegetable consumption and lung cancer risk: A population-based case-control study in Hawaii. J Natl Cancer Inst 81:1158–1164, 1989.
30. Jain M, Burch JD, Howe GR, Miller AB: Dietary factors and risk of lung cancer: Results from a case-control study, Toronto, 1981–1985. Int J Cancer 45:549–553, 1990.
31. Packer JE, Mahood JS, Mora-Arellano VO, et al: Free radicals and singlet oxygen scavengers. Biochem Biophys Res Commun 98:901–906, 1981.
32. Malone WF: Studies evaluating antioxidants and beta-carotene as chemopreventives. Am J Clin Nutr 53:305S–313S, 1991.
33. Carmelli D, Swan GE, Robinette D, Fabsetz R: Genetic influence on smoking—a study of male twins. N Engl J Med 327:829–833, 1992.
34. Benowitz NL: The genetics of drug dependence: Tobacco addiction. N Engl J Med 327:881–883, 1992.
35. Doyle LA, Aisner J: Clinical presentation of lung cancer. In Roth JA, Ruckdeschel JC, Weisenberger TH (eds): Thoracic Oncology. Philadelphia: WB Saunders, 1989, pp 52–76.
36. Beattie EJ, Harvey JC, Pisch J: Atlas of thoracic surgery. In Beattie EJ, Bloom ND, Harvey JC (eds): Thoracic Surgical Oncology. New York: Churchill Livingstone, 1992, pp 65–184.
37. Corrin B (ed): The Lungs. New York: Churchill Livingstone, 1990.
38. World Health Organization: Histological Typing of Lung Cancer, 2nd ed. Geneva: World Health Organization, 1981.
39. Johnson BE, Kelly MJ: Overview of genetic and molecular events in the pathogenesis of lung cancer. Chest 103(Suppl 1):1S–3S, 1993.
40. Larismont D, Kiss R, DeLaunoit Y, Melamed MR: Characterization of the morpho-nuclear features and DNA ploidy of typical and atypical carcinoids and small cell carcinoma of the lung. Am J Clin Pathol 94:378–382, 1990.
41. Arrigoni MG, Woolner LB, Bernatz PE: Atypical carcinoid tumors of the lung. J Thorac Cardiovasc Surg 64:413–421, 1972.
42. Todd TR, Cooper JD, Weissberg D, et al: Bronchial carcinoid tumors: Twenty years experience. J Thorac Cardiovasc Surg 79:532–536, 1980.
43. Hause DR, Harvey JC: Endobronchial carcinoid and mucoepidermoid carcinomas in children. J Surg Oncol 46:270–272, 1991.
44. Harvey JC, Pisch J, Rubin E, Beattie EJ: Choice of procedure for surgical treatment of non–small cell lung cancer. Semin Surg Oncol 9:92–98, 1993.
45. 1989 Survey of physicians' attitudes and practices in early cancer detection. Cancer 40:77–101, 1990.
46. Boucot KR, Weiss W: Is curable lung cancer detected by semiannual screening? JAMA 224:1361–1365, 1973.
47. Early lung cancer detection: Summary and conclusions. Am Rev Respir Dis 130:565–570, 1984.
48. Tockman MS: Survival and mortality from lung cancer in a screened population. The Johns Hopkins study. Chest 89(Suppl):324S, 1984.
49. Melamed MR, Flehinger BJ, Zaman MD, Heelan RT, Perchick WA, Martini N: Screening for early lung cancer. Results of the Memorial Sloan-Kettering study in New York. Chest 86:44–53, 1984.
50. Sanderson DR: Lung cancer screening. The Mayo study. Chest 89(Suppl):324S, 1986.
51. Flehinger BJ, Melamed MR: Current status of screening for lung cancer. Chest Surg Clin North Am 4:1–16, 1994.
52. Mulshine JL, Tockman MS, Smart CR: Commentaries. Considerations in the development of lung cancer screening tools. J Natl Cancer Inst 81:900–905, 1990.
53. Naruke T, Kuroishi T, Suzuki T, Ikeda S, Japanese Lung Cancer Screening Research Group: Comparative study of survival of screen-detected compared with symptom-detected lung cancer cases. Semin Surg Oncol 9:80–84, 1993.
54. Beahrs OH, Henson DE, Hutter RVP, Kennedy BJ (eds): Manual for Staging of Cancer, 4th ed. Philadelphia: JB Lippincott, 1992, pp 115–119.
55. Ferguson MK: Synchronous primary lung cancers. Chest (Suppl)103:399S–400S, 1993.
56. Rubin E, Sanders C, Harvey JC, Beattie EJ: Diagnostic imaging and staging of primary lung cancer. Semin Surg Oncol 9:85–91, 1993.
57. Patterson GA, Ginsberg RJ, Poon PY, et al: A prospective evaluation of magnetic resonance imaging, computed tomography and mediastinoscopy in the preoperative assessment of mediastinal node status in bronchogenic carcinoma. J Thorac Cardiovasc Surg 94:649–684, 1987.
58. Pass HI, Progrebniak HW, Steinberg SM, et al: Randomized trial of neoadjuvant therapy for lung cancer: Interim analysis. Ann Thorac Surg 53:992–998, 1992.
59. Ginsberg RJ, Rubenstein L, Lung Cancer Study Group: A randomized trial of lobectomy versus limited resection for T1, N0 non-small cell lung cancer. Presented at the Sixth World Congress on Lung Cancer, Melbourne, Australia, November 10, 1991.
60. Crabbe MM, Patrissi GA, Fontinelli LJ: Minimal resection for bronchogenic carcinoma. Chest 95:968–971, 1989.
61. Miller JI, Hatcher CR: Limited resection of bronchogenic carcinoma in the patient with marked impairment of pulmonary function. Ann Thorac Surg 44:340–343, 1987.
62. Jensik RJ, Faber LP, Kittle CF: Segmental resection for bronchogenic carcinoma. Ann Thorac Surg 28:475–483, 1979.
63. Nagasaki F, Flehinger BJ, Martini N: Complications of surgery in the treatment of carcinoma of the lung. Chest 82:25–29, 1982.
64. Ginsberg RJ, Hill LD, Eagan RT, et al: Modern thirty day operative mortality for surgical resection in lung cancer. J Thorac Cardiovasc Surg 86:654–658, 1983.
65. Bechard DE: Pulmonary function testing. Chest Surg Clin North Am 2:565–586, 1992.
66. Warner MA, Divirtie MB, Tinker JH: Preoperative cessation of smoking and pulmonary complications in coronary bypass patients. Anesthesiology 60:380–383, 1984.
67. Jackson CV: Preoperative pulmonary evaluation. Arch Int Med 146:2120–2127, 1988.
68. Gass GD, Olsen GN: Preoperative pulmonary function testing to predict postoperative morbidity and mortality. Chest 89:127–135, 1986.
69. Goldman L, Caldera DL, Nussbaum SR, et al: Multifactorial index of risk in non-cardiac surgical procedures. N Engl J Med 297:845–857, 1977.
70. Goldman L: Cardiac risk and complications of non-cardiac surgery. Ann Intern Med 98:504–513, 1983.

71. Topkins MJ, Artusio JF: Myocardial infarction and surgery. A five year study. Anesth Analg 43:716–720, 1964.
72. DelGuercio LR, Cohn JD: Monitoring operative risk in the elderly. JAMA 243:1350–1354, 1980.
73. Foster ED, Davis KB, Carpenter J, et al: Risk of non-cardiac operations in patients with defined coronary artery disease. The Coronary Artery Surgery Study (CASS) Registry experience. Ann Thorac Surg 41:42–50, 1986.
74. Cooperman M, Pflug B, Martin EW, et al: Cardiovascular risk factors in patients with peripheral vascular disease. Surgery 84:505–509, 1978.
75. Delarue ND: Lung cancer in historical perspective: Lessons from the past, implications of present experience, challenges for the future. Can J Surg 23:549–555, 1980.
76. Pearson FG: Lung cancer: The past twenty five years. Chest 89:200s–205s, 1986.
77. Bains MS: Surgical treatment of lung cancer. Chest 100:826–837, 1991.
78. Naruke T, Goya T, Tsuchiya R, et al: Prognosis and survival in resected lung carcinoma based on the new international staging system. J Thorac Cardiovasc Surg 96:440–447, 1988.
79. Martini N, Burt ME, Bains MS, et al: Survival after resection of stage II non–small cell lung cancer. Ann Thorac Surg 54:460–466, 1992.
80. Mountain CF: Expanded possibilities for surgical treatment of lung cancer: Survival in stage IIIa disease. Chest 97:1045–1052, 1990.
81. Churchill ED, Belsey R: Segmental pneumonectomy in bronchiectasis. The lingula segment of the left upper lobe. Ann Thorac Surg 109:481–499, 1939.
82. McCormack PM, Martini N: Primary lung cancer: Results with conservative resection in treatment. NY State J Med 80:612–616, 1980.
83. Ginsberg RJ, Lung Cancer Study Group: Limited resection for peripheral T_1N_0 tumors. Lung Cancer Suppl 4:A80, 1988.
84. Landreneau RJ, Mack MJ, Hazelrigg SR, et al: Video-assisted thoracic surgery: Basic technical concepts and intercostal approach strategies. Ann Thorac Surg 54:800–807, 1992.
85. Coleman FP: Primary carcinoma of the lung with invasion of the ribs. Pneumonectomy and simultaneous block resection of the chest wall. Ann Surg 126:156–168, 1947.
86. Piehler JM, Pairolero PC, Weiland LH, et al: Bronchogenic carcinoma with chest wall invasion. Factors affecting survival following en bloc resection. Ann Thorac Surg 34:684–691, 1982.
87. McCaughan BC, Martini N, Bains MS, McCormack PM: Chest wall invasion in carcinoma of the lung. Therapeutic and prognostic implications. J Thorac Cardiovasc Surg 89:834–841, 1985.
88. Trastek VF, Pairolero PC, Piehler JM, et al: En bloc (non–chest wall) resection for bronchogenic carcinoma with parietal fixation: Factors affecting survival. J Thorac Cardiovasc Surg 87:352–358, 1984.
89. Pairolero PC, Trastek VF, Payne SP: Treatment of bronchogenic carcinoma with chest wall invasion. Surg Clin North Am 67:959–964, 1987.
90. McCormack PM, Bains MS, Beattie E, Martini N: New trends in skeletal reconstruction after resection of chest wall tumors. Ann Thorac Surg 31:45–52, 1981.
91. Choi NC: Curative radiation therapy for unresectable non–small cell carcinoma of the lung. Indications, techniques, results. In Grillo HC (ed): Thoracic Oncology. New York: Raven Press, 1983, pp 163–199.
92. Pisch J, Villamena P, Harvey J, et al: High dose rate endobronchial irradiation in malignant airway obstruction. Chest 104:721–725, 1993.
93. Shapshay SM, Dumon J-F, Beamis JF: Endoscopic treatment of tracheobronchial malignancy: Experience with the Nd:YAG and CO_2 lasers in 506 operations. Arch Otolaryngol Head Neck Surg 93:205–210, 1985.
94. Mair EA, Parsons DS, Lally K: Treatment of severe bronchomalacia with expanding endobronchial stints. Arch Otolaryngol Head Neck Surg 116:1087–1090, 1990.
95. Varila A, Mayner M, Irving D, et al: Use of Gianturco self-expanding stents in the tracheobronchial tree. Ann Thorac Surg 49:806–809, 1990.
96. Bloom N: Trachea. In Beattie EJ, Bloom N, Harvey JC (eds): Thoracic Surgical Oncology. New York: Churchill Livingstone, 1992, pp 273–281.
97. Grillo HC, Mathiesen DJ: Primary tracheal tumors: Treatments and results. Ann Thorac Surg 49:69–75, 1990.
98. Pearson FG, Todd TJ, Cooper JD: Experiences with primary neoplasms after trachea and carina. J Thorac Cardiovasc Surg 88:511–516, 1984.
99. Jensik RJ, Faber LP, Brown CM, Kittle CF: Bronchoplastic and conservative resectional procedures for bronchial adenoma. J Thorac Cardiovasc Surg 16:554–565, 1974.
100. Weisel RD, Cooper JD, Delarue NC, et al: Sleeve lobectomy for carcinoma of the lung. J Thorac Cardiovasc Surg 78:839, 1979.
101. DesLauriers J, Gaulin P, Beaulieu M, et al: Long term clinical and functional results of sleeve lobectomy for primary lung cancer. J Thorac Cardiovasc Surg 92:871–879, 1986.
102. Vogt-Moykopf I, Fritz T, Meyer G, et al: Bronchoplastic and angioplastic operation in bronchial carcinoma. Int Surg 71:211–220, 1986.
103. Goldberg M, Burkes R: Induction chemotherapy for Stage IIIA unresectable non–small cell lung cancer: The Toronto experience and an overview. Semin Surg Oncol 9:108–113, 1993.
104. Walter J, Miller H, Bomford CK: The Production of X- and Gamma Ray Beams. A Short Textbook of Radio-Therapy, 4th ed. Churchill Livingstone, Edinburgh: pp 17–33, 1979.
105. Hellman S: Cancer. Principles and Practice of Oncology, vol 1, 4th ed. Philadelphia: JB Lippincott, 1993, pp 248–249.
106. Hall EJ: New Radiation Modalities. Radiobiology for the Radiologist, 3rd ed. Philadelphia: JB Lippincott, 1988, pp 262–289.
107. Griffin TW: Particle-beam radiation therapy. In Perez LA, Brady LW (eds): Principles and Practice of Radiation Oncology, 2nd ed. Philadelphia. JB Lippincott, 1992, pp 376–379.
108. Hall EJ: Cell survival curves. In Hall EJ (ed): Radiology for the Radiologist, 3rd ed. Philadelphia: JB Lippincott, 1988, pp 24–26.
109. Cox JD, Azarnia N, Byhardt RW, et al: A randomized phase I/II trial of hyperfractionated radiation therapy with total doses of 60.0 Gy to 79.2 Gy: Possible survival benefit with >69.6 Gy in favorable patients with Stage III radiation therapy oncology group non-small-cell lung carcinoma: Report of Radiation Therapy Oncology Group 83-11. J Clin Oncol 8:1543–1555, 1990.
110. Cox JD, Azarnia N, Byhardt RW, et al: N2 (clinical) non–small cell carcinoma of the lung: Prospective trials of radiation therapy with total doses of 60 Gy by the Radiation Therapy Oncology Group. Int J Radiat Oncol Biol Phys 20:7–12, 1991.
111. Ball D, Matthews J, Worotniuk V, et al: Longer survival with higher doses of thoracic radiotherapy in patients with limited non–small cell lung cancer. Int J Radiat Oncol Biol Phys 25:599–704, 1993.
112. Wagner H Jr: Rational integration of radiation and chemotherapy in patients with unresectable stage IIIA or IIIB NSCLC. Results from the Lung Cancer Study Group, Eastern Cooperative Oncology Group, and Radiation Therapy Oncology Group. Chest 103:35s–42s, 1993.
113. Armstrong JG, Burman C, Leibel S, et al: Three dimensional conformal radiation therapy may improve the therapeutic ratio of high dose radiation therapy for lung cancer. Int J Radiat Oncol Biol Phys 26:685–689, 1993.
114. Henschke UK: Interstitial implantation in the treatment of primary bronchogenic carcinoma. Am J Roentgenol Radium Ther Nucl Med 79:6–13, 1958.
115. Hilaris BS, Gomez J, Nori D, et al: Combined surgery, intraoperative brachytherapy and postoperative external radiation in Stage III non–small cell lung cancer. Cancer 55:1226–1231, 1985.
116. Greenblatt DR, Nori D, Tankenbaum A, et al: New brachytherapy techniques using Iodine-125 seeds for tumor bed implants. Endocuriether Hyperthermia Oncol 3:73–80, 1987.
117. Fleischman ED, Kagan AR, Streeter OE, et al: Iodine interstitial brachytherapy in the treatment of carcinoma of the lung. J Surg Oncol 49:25–28, 1992.
118. Pisch J, Harvey JC, Alfieri A, et al: Utilization of absorbable mesh for afterloading HDR and LDR catheter placement in planar implant. Endocuriether Hyperthermia Oncol 9:127–132, 1993.
119. Pisch J, Berson AM, Harvey JC, et al: Absorbable mesh in placement of temporary implants. Int J Radiat Oncol Biol Phys 28:719–722, 1994.
120. Weisenberger TH, Lung Cancer Study Group: Effects of postopera-

tive mediastinal radiation on completely resected stage II and stage III epidermoid carcinoma of the lung. N Engl J Med 315:1377–1381, 1986.
121. Shields TW, Higgins GA, Lawton R, et al: Preoperative x-ray therapy as an adjuvant in the treatment of bronchogenic carcinoma. J Thorac Cardiovasc Surg 59:49–61, 1975.
122. Warram J: Preoperative irradiation of cancer of the lung: Final report of a therapeutic trial. Cancer 36:914–925, 1975.
123. Pancoast HK: Superior sulcus tumor. JAMA 99:1391–1396, 1932.
124. Shaw RR, Paulson DL, Kee JL: Treatment of the superior sulcus tumor by irradiation followed by resection. Ann Surg 154:29–40, 1961.
125. Darteville PG, Chapelier AR, Macchiarini P, et al: The anterior trans-cervical approach for radical resection of lung tumors invading the thoracic inlet. J Thorac Cardiovasc Surg 105:1025–1035, 1993.
126. Paulson DL: The importance of defining and staging of superior sulcus tumors. Ann Thorac Surg 15:549–551, 1973.
127. Paulson DL: Carcinoma of the superior sulcus. J Thorac Cardiovasc Surg 70:1095–1104, 1975.
128. Komaki R, Rok J, Cox JD, et al: Superior sulcus tumor. Results of irradiation of 36 patients. Cancer 48:1563–1568, 1981.
129. Hilaris BS, Luomenen RK, Beattie EJ: Integrated irradiation and surgery in the treatment of apical lung cancer. Cancer 27:1369–1378, 1971.
130. Martini N, Kris MG, Gralla RJ, et al: The side effects of pre-operative chemotherapy on the resectability of non–small cell lung carcinoma with mediastinal lymph node metastases (N2, M0). Ann Thorac Surg 45:370–379, 1988.
131. Gralla RJ, Kris MG, Martini N, et al: A neo-adjuvant trial in Stage IIIA non–small cell lung cancer in patients with clinically apparent mediastinal node involvement with MVP chemotherapy (mitomycin + *Vinca* alkaloid + cisplatin). Lung Cancer 4s:8–25, 1988 (abstract).
132. Pisters KMW, Kris MG, Gralla RJ, et al: Pre-operative chemotherapy in Stage IIIA non–small cell lung cancer: An analysis of a trial in patients with clinically apparent mediastinal node involvement. In Salmon SE (ed): Adjuvant Therapy of Cancer VI. Philadelphia: WB Saunders, 1988, pp 133–137.
133. Shepherd FA: Induction chemotherapy for locally advanced non–small cell lung cancer. Ann Thorac Surg 55:1585–1592, 1993.
134. Pisch J, Malamud S, Harvey J, Beattie EJ: Simultaneous chemo-radiation in advanced non-small-cell lung cancer. Semin Surg Oncol 9:120–126, 1993.
135. Bonomi P, Trybula M, Sandler S, et al: Comparison of neo-adjuvant chemotherapy alone to simultaneous chemotherapy-radiotherapy in locally advanced squamous cell bronchogenic carcinoma. Colloq INSERM 13:507–517, 1986.
136. Farley P, Giri J, Ronquillo A: Treatment of non–small cell lung cancer with simultaneous chemotherapy and radiation therapy. Proc ASCO 3:211, 1984 (abstract).
137. Johnson DH, Einhorn LH, Bartolucci A: Thoracic radiotherapy does not prolong survival in patients with locally advanced, unresectable non–small cell lung cancer. Ann Intern Med 113:33–38, 1990.
138. Taylor SG, Trybula M, Bonomi PD, et al: Simultaneous cisplatin fluorouracil infusion and radiation followed by surgical resection in regionally localized stage III, non–small cell lung cancer. Ann Thorac Surg 43:87–91, 1987.
139. Strauss G, Sherman D, Schwartz J, et al: Combined modality treatment for regionally advanced stage III non–small cell carcinoma of the lung (NSCLC) employing neo-adjuvant chemotherapy (CT), radiotherapy (RT), and surgery (S). Proc ASCO 5:172, 1986 (abstract).
140. Le Chevalier T, Arrigada R, Quoix E, et al: Radiotherapy alone versus combined chemotherapy and radiotherapy in non-resectable non-small-cell lung cancer: First analysis of a randomized trial in 53 patients. J Natl Cancer Inst 83:417–423, 1991.
141. Rosell R, Gomez-Codina J, Campo C, et al: A randomized trial comparing preoperative chemotherapy plus surgery with surgery alone in patients with non–small cell lung cancer. N Engl J Med 339:153–158, 1994.
142. Burt M, Wronski M, Arbit E, et al: Resection of brain metastases from NSCLC. J Thorac Cardiovasc Surg 103:399–411, 1992.
143. Speiser B, Spratling L: High-dose rate remote afterloading brachytherapy in the control of endobronchial carcinoma. Activity Suppl 1:7–15, 1991.
144. Khanavkar B, Stem P, Alberti V, et al: Complications associated with brachytherapy alone or with laser in lung cancer. Chest 99:1062–1065, 1991.
145. Feld R, Wierzbicki R, Walde PL, et al: Phase I-II study of high dose epirubicin in advanced non–small cell lung cancer. J Clin Oncol 10:297–303, 1993.
146. Shepherd FA, Evans WK, Goss PE, et al: Ifosfamide, cisplatin, and etoposide (ICE) in the treatment of advanced non–small cell lung cancer. Semin Oncol 19:54–58(s), 1992.
147. Makysmiuk AW, Jett JR, Earle JD, et al: Sequencing and schedule effects of cisplatin plus etoposide in small-cell lung cancer: Results of a North Central Cancer Treatment Group randomized clinical trial. J Clin Oncol 12:70–76, 1994.
148. Jaakkimainen L, Goodwin PJ, Pater J, et al: Counting the costs of chemotherapy in a National Cancer Institute of Canada randomized clinical trial. J Clin Oncol 8:1301–1309, 1990.
149. Callejas MA, Rami R, Catalan M, et al: Mediastinoscopy as an emergency diagnostic procedure in superior vena cava syndrome. Scand J Thorac Cardiovasc Surg 25:137–139, 1991.
150. Gauden SJ: Superior vena cava syndrome induced by bronchogenic carcinoma: Is this an oncological emergency? Australas Radiol 37:363–366, 1993.
151. Eng J, Sabanthan S: Management of superior vena cava obstruction with self-expanding intraluminal stents. Two case reports. Scand J Thorac Cardiovasc Surg 27:53–55, 1993.
152. Edwards RD, Jackson JE: Case report: Superior vena caval obstruction treated by thrombolysis, thrombectomy and metallic stents. Clin Radiol 48:215–217, 1993.
153. Watkinson AF, Hansell DM: Expandable wall stent for the treatment of obstruction of the superior vena cava. Thorax 48:915–920, 1993.
154. Larsson S, Lepore V: Technical options in reconstruction of large mediastinal veins. Surgery 111:311–317, 1992.
155. Piccione W Jr, Faber LP, Warren WH: Superior vena caval reconstruction using autologous pericardium. Ann Thorac Surg 50:417–419, 1990.
156. Faber LP: Resection for second and third primary lung cancer. Semin Surg Oncol 9:135–141, 1993.
157. Wittes RE: Small cell lung cancer: An overview of issues in therapy. Semin Surg Oncol 9:127–134, 1993.
158. Bunn PA, Lichter AS, Makuch RW, et al: Chemotherapy alone or chemotherapy with chest radiation therapy in limited stage small cell lung cancer: A prospective randomized trial. Ann Intern Med 106:655–662, 1987.
159. Perry MC, Eaton WL, Propert KJ, et al: Chemotherapy with or without radiation therapy in limited small cell carcinoma of the lung. N Engl J Med 316:912–918, 1987.
160. Viallet J, Ihde DC: Small cell carcinoma of the lung: Clinical and biologic aspects. Crit Rev Oncol Hematol 11:109–135, 1991.
161. Hirsch FR, Hansen HH, Paulson OB, et al: Development of brain metastases in small cell anaplastic carcinoma of the lung. In Kay J, Whitehouse J (eds): CNS Complications of Malignant Disease. London: Macmillan, 1979, pp 175–184.
162. Cox JD, Petrovich Z, Paig C, et al: Prophylactic cranial irradiation in patients with inoperable carcinoma of the lung. Cancer 42:1135–1140, 1978.
163. Pederson AG, Kristjansen PEG, Hansen HH, et al: Prophylactic cranial irradiation and small cell lung cancer. Cancer Treat Rev 15:85, 1988.
164. Johnson BE, Patronas N, Hayes W, et al: Neurologic, computed cranial tomographic, and magnetic resonance imaging abnormalities in patients with small-cell lung cancer: Further follow-up of 6- to 13-year survivors. J Clin Oncol 8:48–56, 1990.
165. Smit EF, Carney DN, Harford P, et al: A phase II study of oral etoposide in elderly patients with small cell lung cancer. Thorax 44:631–633, 1989.
166. Blackstein M, Eisenhauer EA, Wierzbicki R, et al: Epirubicin in extensive small-cell lung cancer: A phase I study of previously untreated patients: A National Cancer Institute of Canada Clinical Trials Group study. J Clin Oncol 8:385–389, 1990.
167. Slevin MI, Clarj PJ, Joel SP, et al: A randomized trial to evaluate the effect of schedule on the activity of etoposide in small-cell lung cancer. J Clin Oncol 7:1333–1340, 1989.
168. Carney DN: Biology of small-cell lung cancer. Lancet 339:843–846, 1992.

169. Hansen HH: Management of small-cell cancer of the lung. Lancet 339:846–849, 1992.
170. Seifter EJ, Ihde DC: Therapy of small cell lung cancer: A perspective on two decades of clinical research. Semin Oncol 15:278–299, 1988.
171. Evans WK, Feld R, Murray N, et al: Superiority of alternating non–cross resistant chemotherapy in extensive small cell lung cancer. Ann Intern Med 107:451–458, 1987.
172. Johnson DH, Einhorn LH, Birch R, et al: A randomized comparison of high-dose versus conventional-dose cyclophosphamide, doxorubicin, and vincristine for extensive-stage small-cell lung cancer: A phase III trial of the Southeastern Cancer Study Group. J Clin Oncol 5:1731–1738, 1978.
173. Ihde DC, Mulshine JL, Kramer BS, et al: Randomized trial of high versus standard dose etoposide and cisplatin in extensive stage small cell lung cancer. Proc Am Soc Clin Oncol 10:240, 1991.
174. Shields TW, Higgins GA, Matthews MJ, et al: Surgical resection in the management of small-cell carcinoma of the lung. J Thorac Cardiovasc Surg 84:481–488, 1982.
175. Ichinose Y, Hara N, Ohta M, et al: Comparison between resected and irradiated small-cell lung cancer in patients in stages I through IIIa. Ann Thorac Surg 53:95–100, 1992.
176. Shepherd FA, Ginsberg RJ, Feld R, et al: Surgical treatment for limited small-cell lung cancer. The University of Toronto Lung Oncology Group experience. J Thorac Cardiovasc Surg 101:385–393, 1991.
177. Zatopek NK, Holoye PY, Ellerbroek NA, et al: Resectability of small-cell lung cancer following induction chemotherapy in patients with limited disease (stage II-IIIb). Am J Clin Oncol 14:427–432, 1991.
178. Mentzer SJ, Reilly JJ, Sugarbaker DJ: Surgical resection in the management of small-cell carcinoma of the lung. Chest 103:349–351S, 1993.
179. Kaiser D, Fritzsche A, Matthiesen W: Indication for surgery in small-cell carcinoma of the lung. Thorac Cardiovasc Surg 40:185–189, 1992.
180. Hara N, Ohta M, Inchiose, et al: Influence of surgical resection before and after chemotherapy on survival small-cell lung cancer. J Surg Oncol 47:53–61, 1991.
181. Theuer W, Selawry O, Karrer K: The impact of surgery on the multidisciplinary treatment of bronchogenic small-cell carcinoma (updated review including ongoing studies). Med Oncol Tumor Pharmacother 9:119–137, 1992.

Secondary Lung Tumors

James C. Harvey, M.D. • Kenneth Lee, M.D.
Christopher Erdman, B.A. • Edward J. Beattie, M.D.

The first report from the United States of a planned resection of a metastasis to the lung was that of Barney and Churchill in 1939.[1] Previous episodic reports of the resection of metastatic tumors in the European literature of the nineteenth and early twentieth centuries are cited by Vogt-Moykopf et al.,[2] but such aggressive treatment did not become frequent even by the middle of this century. Thomford and colleagues[3] reported their experience with 205 patients who had metastases, predominantly solitary, resected at the Mayo Clinic from 1941 to 1962 with a 30.3% 5-year survival rate. They found no difference in the survival of patients with solitary metastases from that of the few patients with multiple metastases, but they cautiously concluded that "simultaneous bilateral pulmonary metastases is a grave prognostic sign, and is probably best treated by modalities other than surgery." However, at that time, there were few, if any, nonsurgical options for the treatment of secondary pulmonary tumors, at least with any chance of yielding a 30% 5-year survival rate. Pulmonary metastases were frequent, sometimes the only site of disease, and the cause of death among patients with cancer was frequently pulmonary insufficiency.[4–6]

Marcove and coworkers' life-history study of children treated for osteogenic sarcoma of the extremities in the prechemotherapy era revealed that in 83% of patients with normal chest radiographs at the time of amputation, pulmonary metastases developed.[7] Ninety-five percent of these patients were dead within 3 years. Because of the known life history of osteogenic sarcoma and the absence of effective nonsurgical treatment in the 1960s, Beattie and colleagues[8] planned to attempt complete resection in children with multiple pulmonary metastases from osteogenic sarcoma of the extremities. Twenty-two of 28 patients were successfully rendered disease-free, and 6 of these were 10-year survivors after multiple thoracotomies.[9] These results (Table 7–5) verified that resection alone can prolong survival and probably cure some patients previously without hope. The fact that second primary tumors occurred in three of the 10-year survivors during the second decade of follow-up indicates that close multisystem surveillance is required for patients with childhood tumors, whether or not they have had chemotherapy.[8]

DIAGNOSIS

Signs and Symptoms

Metastases to the lung tend to be at the periphery of their segments and frequently asymptomatic. Dyspnea may result from tumor compression of pulmonary parenchyma or from extrinsic airway compression. Acute dyspnea may result from hemorrhage into a tumor (Figs. 7–28 to 7–30), a situation that mandates relatively urgent surgery in a patient otherwise a candidate for treatment.

Spontaneous pneumothorax occasionally results from erosion of subpleural tumor through lung surface.[10] This

TABLE 7–5
Results At Greater Than 20 Years Following Resection of Pulmonary Metastases

Sex/Age	Amputation, Year	No. of Thoracotomies	No. of Metastases	Current Status
M	Femur, 1966	2	3	NED at 10 yr, lost to follow-up
F/14	Femur, 1966	2	4	NED at 24 yr
F/15	Hemipelvectomy, 1966	4	11	NED at 22 yr; stage III breast cancer 6/88; died of breast cancer 6/90
F/15	Femur, 1966	1	1	Diffuse histiocytic lymphoma 9/82; treated with chemotherapy and autologous bone marrow transplantation 12/82; NED for both diseases 12/92
F/11	Midthigh, 1968	4	13	New osteogenic sarcoma opposite knee; knee replaced 1982; died of disease 9/84
F/11	Hemipelvectomy, 1969	9	18	NED 1972–86; died with disease 2/88

Adapted from Beattie EJ, et al: Results of multiple pulmonary resections for metastatic osteogenic sarcoma after two decades. J Surg Oncol 46:154, 1991.
NED, No evidence of disease.

has especially been observed following a good response to chemotherapy. Chest pain results when tumor grows through visceral pleura into the chest wall or with diffuse pleural metastases.

Endobronchial metastases may present with obstructive symptoms (cough, wheezing, dyspnea, fever) or with hemoptysis. Breast, colon, kidney, and melanoma metastases have been most commonly reported, but other primary tumors have also presented in this fashion.[11–13]

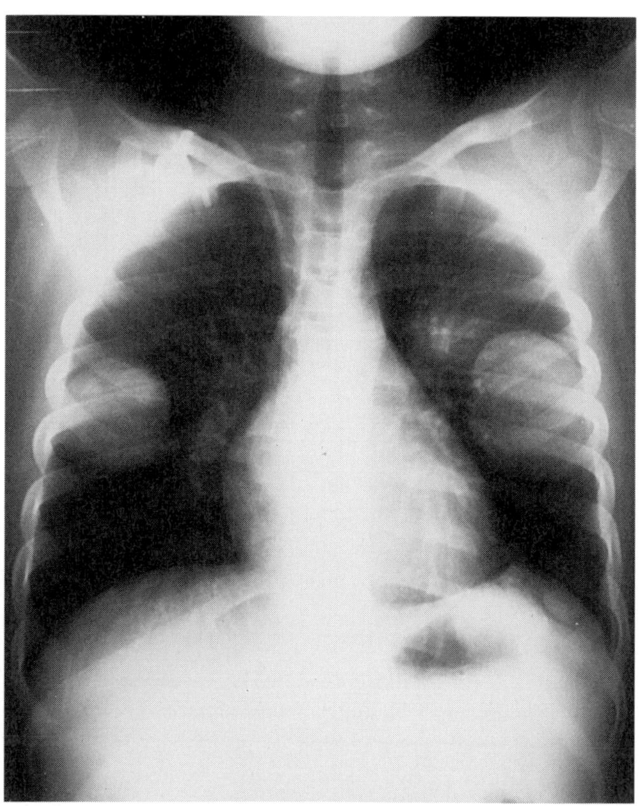

FIGURE 7–28. Preoperative chest radiograph of a 12-year-old boy who had had chemotherapy for metastatic osteogenic sarcoma. (From Harvey JC, et al: Utility of the neodymium:yttrium-aluminum-garnet [Nd:YAG] laser for extensive pulmonary metastasectomy. J Surg Oncol 54:175–179, 1993.)

Imaging Studies

Because the majority of secondary tumors of the lung are asymptomatic, the most frequent means of diagnosis are radiographic. For most tumor patients, chest roentgenograms are part of routine pretreatment staging and post-treatment surveillance. Computed tomography (CT) and magnetic resonance imaging (MRI) scans are more sensitive but less specific for tumor.[14, 15] No cost-benefit analyses are available to guide us in deciding on the additional expense involved in employing the more sensitive modalities, but baseline CT scans are recommended for patients with sarcomas, germ cell tumors, and other tumors with a strong propensity for pulmonary metastasis.

Solitary nodules at the threshold of CT scan detectability (3 mm) are malignant less than 50% of the time.[16] Therefore, we hesitate to recommend operations before an interval of observation unless other treatment planning (i.e., starting or discontinuing chemotherapy) depends on knowing. Most often, we request a repeated study in 2 months. Solitary nodules detected by chest roentgenography in patients with prior tumors elsewhere are more likely to be either a secondary tumor (64%) or a lung primary tumor (18%) than a benign mass.[17] Multiple nodules are usually related to the previous tumor (Fig. 7–31).

SURGERY

Selection of Surgical Candidates

We recommend excision of secondary tumors to the lung when the following conditions pertain[18]:

1. *The patient must be able to withstand the operation planned.* Complete assessment of the unique anatomic situation for each patient is carried out by studying the radiographs and bronchoscopic findings. Most tumors can be excised by wedge excisions, but a few require lobectomies, pneumonectomies, or bronchoplasty to accomplish complete resection. Whenever the original tumor was a carcinoma, a lobectomy is recommended for a solitary lung tumor because it

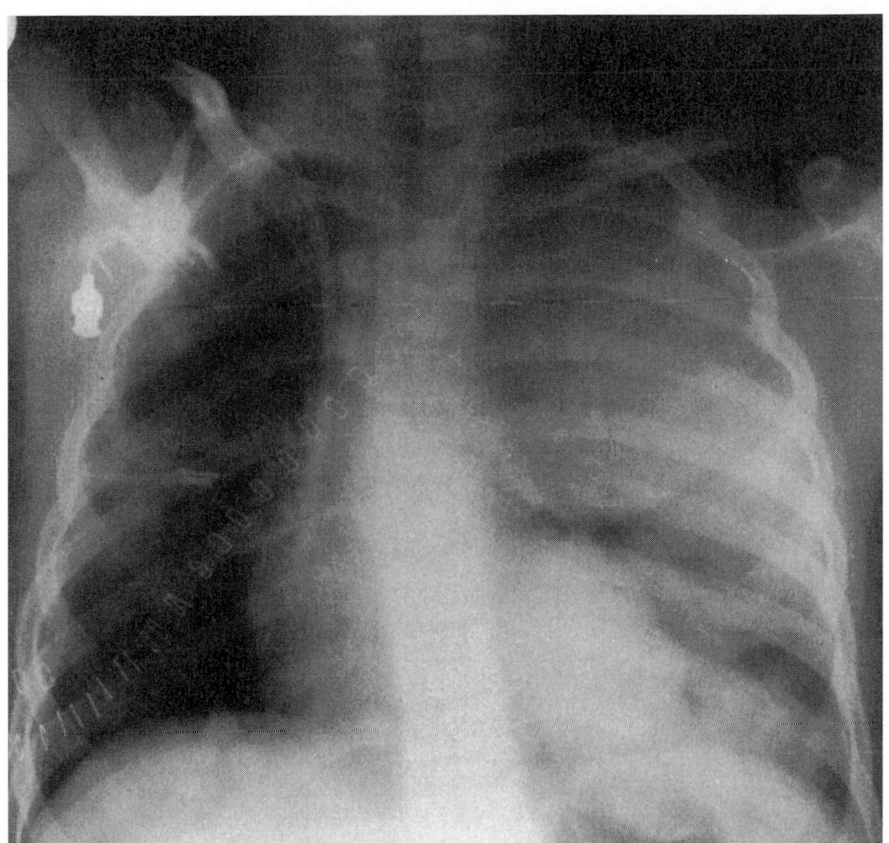

FIGURE 7–29. The patient in Figure 7–28 1 week after resection of metastatic masses in the right lung. Rapid growth of the mass had occurred in the interval. (From Harvey JC, et al: Utility of the neodymium:yttrium - aluminum - garnet [Nd:YAG] laser for extensive pulmonary metastasectomy. J Surg Oncol 54:175–179, 1993.)

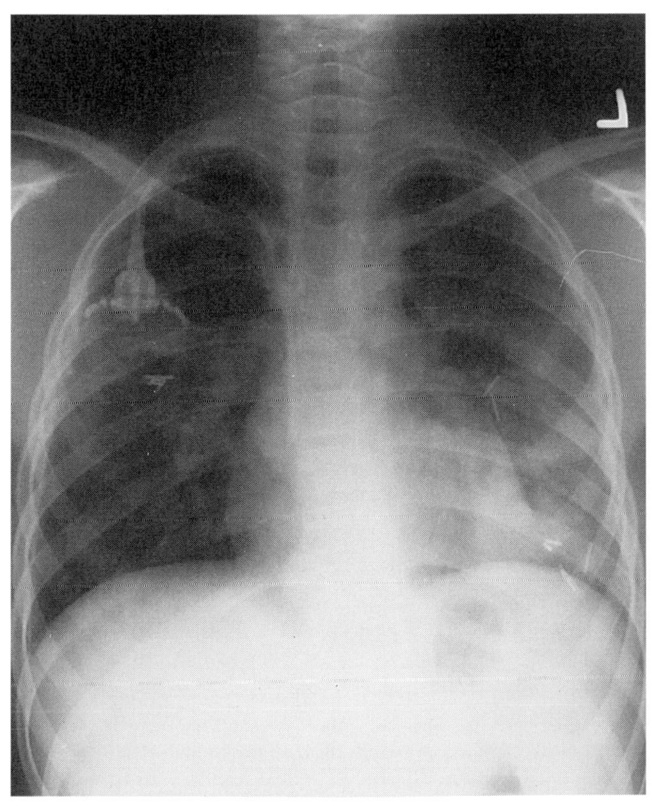

FIGURE 7–30. Postoperative radiograph after resection of left-lung masses in the patient in Figure 7–28. The rapid growth was due to hemorrhage into tumor. (From Harvey JC, et al: Utility of the neodymium:yttrium-aluminum-garnet [Nd:YAG] laser for extensive pulmonary metastasectomy. J Surg Oncol 54:175–179, 1993.)

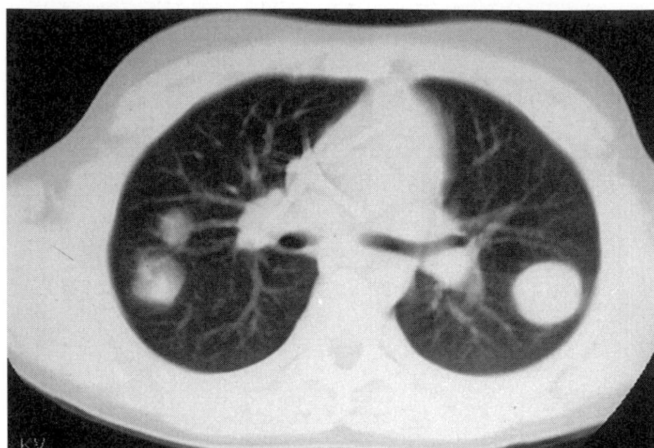

FIGURE 7–31. A preoperative CT scan showing typical rounded peripheral lesions due to metastatic osteogenic sarcoma. (From Harvey JC, et al: Utility of the neodymium:yttrium-aluminum-garnet [Nd:YAG] laser for extensive pulmonary metastasectomy. J Surg Oncol 54:175–179, 1993.)

is difficult to be certain that the lung tumor is not a primary lung cancer with frozen section analysis alone.

Pulmonary function tests, arterial blood gases, split-function lung scans, and diffusion studies are selectively employed to assist in the decision process. The same criteria as recommended for other pulmonary resections are employed in deciding the fitness of the patient to tolerate the proposed operation. Diffusion studies are sometimes necessary because of the frequent use of pulmonary toxic drugs in the treatment of primary tumors.

2. *It must be possible to remove all of the pulmonary metastases at operation.* The most important prognostic indicator for determining a successful outcome is the ability to render the patient disease-free.

A technical matter worth emphasizing is the fact that most metastatic tumors are located in the periphery of the involved segment. Even "central" tumors are frequently resectable with segmental dissection. Often on dissection of the segmental plane, the tumor is resectable while conserving most of the segment, allowing re-expansion of underlying compressed lung.

Two devices that have been found useful in achieving complete resection in patients with large numbers of nodules or masses in difficult locations are the Cavitron ultrasonic surgical aspirator (CUSA) and the Nd:YAG laser. Surgeons at Roswell Park Cancer Institute have described the CUSA as useful in patients who have centrally located metastatic tumors that would otherwise require lobectomy. The CUSA

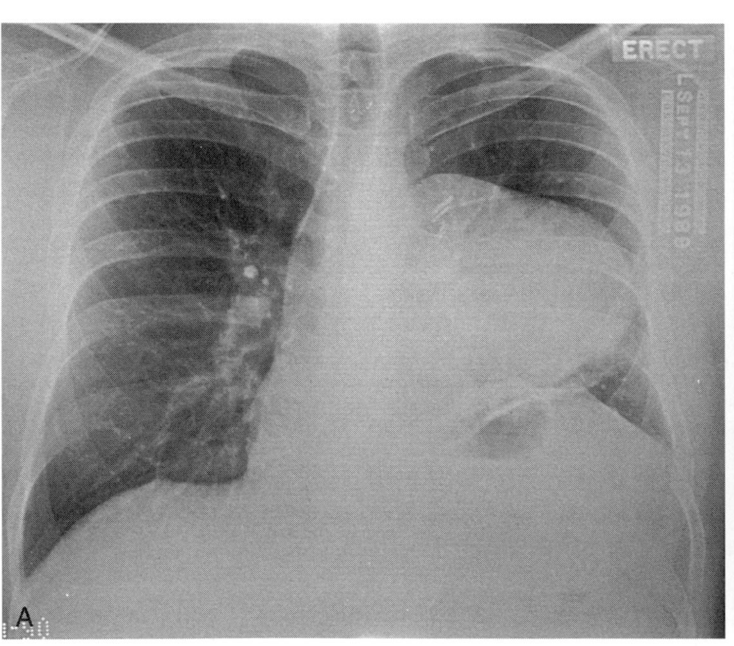

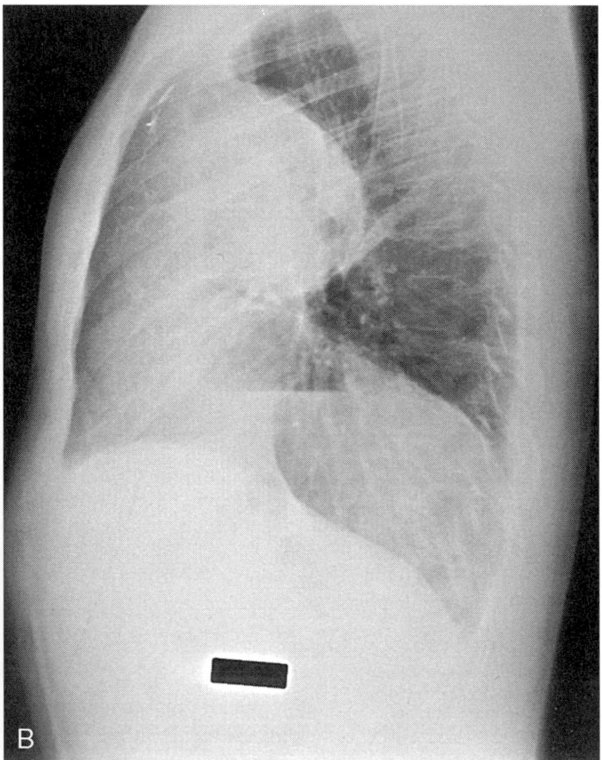

FIGURE 7–32. Posteroanterior *(A)* and lateral *(B)* views of a large residual germ cell mass invading phrenic nerve and obscuring hilar vessels. A complete resection preserving both lobes was accomplished using the Cavitron ultrasonic surgical aspirator. (From Harvey JC, et al: Resection of residual mediastinal germ cell masses with the Cavitron ultrasonic surgical aspirator. J Thorac Cardiovasc Surg 102:425–426, 1991.)

fragments and aspirates tumor at a selected margin from the tumor, preserving airways and vessels.[19] We have used the CUSA in resection of large masses of residual germ cell tumor following chemotherapy (Fig. 7–32). The device is inserted directly through the tumor pseudocapsule. Giant masses are fragmented, facilitating exposure of mediastinal vessels and nerves. The collapsed pseudocapsule is then excised, allowing underlying lung to expand normally.[20]

The Nd:YAG laser has been useful in accomplishing resection or vaporization of large numbers of tumors while preserving pulmonary parenchyma. Branscheid and colleagues[21] report that prior to employing this device, the mean number of metastases was 4 (range, 1 to 29); afterward, the mean number was 8 (range, 1 to 81). Ueda and coworkers[22] have reported resection or vaporization of 110 metastases in one patient alive and free of disease 51 months at the time of their report. We have resected 83 lesions in a patient with adenoid cystic tumor of the cheek. His chest roentgenogram remains unchanged 1 year following the second thoracotomy (Fig. 7–33).

3. *The tumor, including the primary site and extrapulmonary metastases, must be controlled or controllable.* We have gradually come to accept this position. Formerly, we required that the primary tumor be ''controlled or controllable'' and that no extrapulmonary metastases exist. Extrapulmonary metastases are recognized to increase the gravity of the situation but do not necessarily contradict resection. Highly selected patients with extrapulmonary disease (liver, brain, bowel, regional lymph nodes from the primary tumor, regional lymph nodes draining the lung secondary) are thought to have benefited from complete excision for sarcomas, carcinomas, and melanomas.[22–25] We have selectively been this aggressive but have treated only a small number of patients and with brief follow-up.
4. *There must be* ***no better treatment available*** *offering the same chance of cure or of superior palliation.* This condition has evolved over the years from the statement ''no other treatment available.'' In the current era of medical oncology, with the large selection of antitumor drug combinations and immunotherapies, there may no longer be situations in which ''no other treatment'' is available. It is presumed that treatments better than operations will continue to evolve. In patients with nonseminomatous germ cell tumors, chemotherapy combinations have been so successful that only a minority of tumors metastatic to the lung fail to disappear, and some of the residual masses lack viable tumor.[2, 26]

Patients with osteogenic sarcomas and other tumors have benefited from the development of chemotherapy over the past two decades, which has changed the life history of metastatic disease. In the early 1960s, children with osteogenic sarcoma metastatic to the lung, with rare exception, were doomed without surgical resection.[7] Currently, operation is no longer the only treatment available but remains an important part of the optimal treatment plan for residual lung masses after chemotherapy.[27, 28]

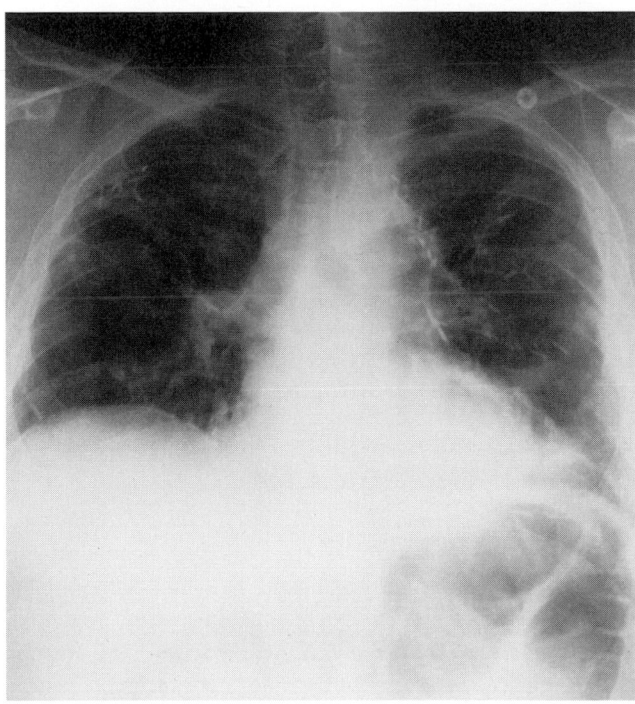

FIGURE 7–33. A postoperative chest radiograph after excision of 83 nodules secondary to metastatic adenoid cystic tumor. (From Harvey JC, et al: Utility of neodymium:yttrium-aluminum-garnet [Nd:YAG] laser for extensive pulmonary metastasectomy. J Surg Oncol 54:175–179, 1993.)

Incisions

The goal of pulmonary metastasectomy is complete excision. Many studies have verified that more tumors have been found at the time of operation than during preoperative imaging studies.[15, 21, 22, 28] Incisions such as median sternotomy[29] and bilateral transsternal thoracotomy,[21, 30] which permit bimanual palpation of both lungs, inflated and deflated, and have the potential of allowing complete excision with one operation, should be considered. Equally good results are obtained with bilateral staged thoracotomies.

We have no experience with bilateral transsternal thoracotomy, but very experienced surgeons are among its advocates. Median sternotomy, in our hands, provides access to most areas of both lungs but is not ideal for tumors of the left lower lobe, especially posterior ones in the region of the inferior pulmonary vein. We prefer conventional posterolateral thoracotomy for situations of difficult exposure, for sleeve resections, and for very large numbers of tumors.[31]

Video-Assisted Resections

A technique that we reserve only for special situations is video-assisted thoracic surgery (VATS). Frequently, it is not possible to find all of the tumors without the ability to palpate the lung bimanually, inflated and deflated. Furthermore, more parenchyma is conserved if resections are carried out with lung inflated. VATS may be useful for diagnosis before initiating chemotherapy and perhaps also for solitary tumors[32] but cannot be expected to produce complete resections of multiple tumors. Its misuse in the treatment of metastatic disease can only be regarded as a backward step.

PROGNOSTIC INDICATORS

Complete Resectability

The most important prognostic indicator is complete resectability. Disease in extrapulmonary sites, including intrathoracic sites (e.g., regional lymph nodes, pericardium, parietal pleura) is known to be a negative prognostic indicator. However, if all the tumors can be resected with minimal morbidity and the best possible conservation of pulmonary parenchyma, palliation and prolongation of survival can be accomplished,[27, 33] especially with judicious use of postoperative adjuvant treatments.[10, 34]

Number of Pulmonary Tumors

Completeness of resection is the most important prognostic indicator, but the surgeon's estimation of his or her own ability to accomplish this depends on an assessment of the number and location of nodules and of pulmonary reserve. However, when the number of nodules resected has been evaluated with respect to the impact on long-term survival, many investigators have found no certain threshold for a variety of sarcomas,[29, 35] carcinomas,[36, 37] and melanomas.[38] Our own experience[8] and that of others[21, 24, 32, 38] has verified that persistent reoperations prolong survival if complete resection can be accomplished.

Pogrebniak and coworkers[37] report similar mean survival after resection of metastatic renal tumors whether solitary (46 months) or multiple (47 months). Ueda and colleagues[22] found that a number of resected sarcoma nodules less than or equal to five versus greater than five did not affect survival; the 5-year survival rate was 25% among those completely resected versus no survivors among the cohort with incomplete resection. Branscheid and colleagues[21] reported 5-year survival rates of 19% for colorectal carcinoma, 53% for breast carcinoma, 38% for renal cell tumors, and 60% for testicular tumors. The number of nodules was found to be of prognostic significance in patients with breast cancer.[21] For patients with sarcomas, Branscheid et al. found a 5-year survival rate greater than 25%, with the number of resected nodules found to influence survival in patients with osteogenic sarcoma but not in those with soft tissue sarcomas. At the National Cancer Institute, no difference in the 5-year survival of patients with soft tissue sarcomas was detected when patients with less than four metastases were compared with those with greater than five.[29]

The presence of more than one metastasis was found to be a negative prognostic indicator for colorectal metastases in a study at the Mayo Clinic,[25] in which the 5-year survival rate was found to be 36.9% for patients undergoing resection of solitary metastasis, 19.3% for those with two metastases, and only 7.7% for those with more than two metastases. Another negative prognostic indicator was a greater than normal level of carcinoembryonic antigen. It was worthwhile, however, to resect extrapulmonary metastases and to perform a repeated resection.[25, 39]

Disease-Free Interval

The disease-free interval is defined as the interval from control of the primary tumor until recurrence. In general, it has been thought the longer the disease-free interval, the more likely the success of treatment of metastases, but this has not been uniformly verified. In fact, Putnam et al.[38] found no difference in the survival of patients whose lung secondary tumors were discovered synchronously with their primary sarcoma when compared with metachronous discovery. Other investigators have not found the disease-free interval to be of significance.[37] In circumstances in which chemotherapy has become important over the past two decades, prolonged survival is possible with synchronous disease. This is true for testicular tumors[7, 40, 41] and osteogenic sarcomas.[27, 28, 33, 42–46]

Tumor Doubling Time

Tumor kinetic studies have been performed in an attempt to determine the prognostic significance of rapid growth. Joseph and colleagues[43] report improved survival among patients with a tumor doubling time of greater than 40 days, and others have agreed.[47]

It is not our policy to observe for tumor doubling in patients with resectable tumors for whom operation is the best treatment. For tumors barely detectable on CT scans, we recommend repeated studies before making the decision to operate. Resection is recommended if an increase in the number or size of nodules is detected or if continuation of chemotherapy depends on knowing whether viable tumor exists in the nodules.

CONCLUSION

Aggressive surgical resection of metastatic tumors of the lung is of value in improving the life history of a variety of tumors as long as complete resection can be accomplished. No prognostic indicator more important than complete resection has been identified. Operation, with persistent reoperations, should be offered to all patients for whom there is no better alternative who can tolerate the proposed resection.[48] Use of the Nd:YAG laser will probably allow resection of larger numbers of metastatic tumors, preserving more lung parenchyma than past techniques, especially if dissection is performed along segmental planes.[21, 22, 31]

References

1. Barney JD, Churchill ED: Adenocarcinoma of the kidney with metastasis to the lung treated by pulmonary resection. J Urol 42:269, 1939.
2. Vogt-Mykopf I, Krysa S, Bülzebruck H, et al: Surgery for pulmonary metastases: The Heidelberg experience. Chest Surg Clin North Am 4:85–112, 1993.
3. Thomford NR, Woolner LB, Claggett OT: The surgical treatment of metastatic tumors in the lungs. J Thorac Cardiovasc Surg 49:357–363, 1965.
4. Farrell JT: Pulmonary metastasis: A pathologic, clinical roentgenologic study based on 78 cases seen at necropsy. Radiology 24:444–451, 1938.
5. Viadana E, Irwin D, Bross J, et al: Cascade spread of blood-borne metastases in solid and non-solid cancers in humans. In Weiss L, Gilbert H (eds): Pulmonary Metastasis. Boston: GK Hall, 1978, pp 143–155.
6. Willis RA: Secondary tumors of the lung. In The Spread of Tumors in the Human Body. London: Butterworth's, 1973, pp 167–185.
7. Marcove RC, Mike V, Hajek JC, et al: Osteogenic sarcoma under the age of 21: A review of 145 operative cases. J Bone Joint Surg 52:411–423, 1970.
8. Beattie EJ, Harvey JC, Marcove RC, et al: Results of multiple pulmonary resections for metastatic osteogenic sarcoma after two decades. J Surg Oncol 46:154–156, 1991.
9. Martini N, Huvos AG, Mike V, et al: Multiple pulmonary resections in the treatment of osteogenic sarcoma. Ann Thorac Surg 12:271–280, 1971.
10. O'Leary C, el Soussi M, Cowie J: Spontaneous bilateral pneumothoraces from synovial cell carcinoma. Respir Med 85:533–534, 1991.
11. Cahan WG: Excision of melanoma metastasis to the lung: Problems in diagnosis and management. Ann Surg 178:703–711, 1973.
12. Sheperd M: Endobronchial metastatic disease. Thorax 37:362–367, 1982.
13. Spencer H: Pathology of the Lung, 2nd ed. London: Pergamon Press, 1968.
14. Davis SD: CT evaluation for pulmonary metastases in patients with extrathoracic malignancy. Radiology 180:1–12, 1991.
15. Pass HI, Dwyer A, Makuch R, et al: Detection of pulmonary metastases in patients with osteogenic and soft-tissue sarcoma: The superiority of CT scan compared with conventional linear tomograms using dynamic analyses. J Clin Oncol 3:1261–1265, 1985.
16. Chang AE, Schaner RG, Conkle DM, et al: Evaluation of computed tomography in the detection of pulmonary metastases. Cancer: 43:913–916, 1979.
17. Adkins PC, Wesselhoeft CW Jr, Newman W, et al: Thoracotomy on the patient with previous malignancy: Metastasis or new primary? J Thorac Cardiovasc Surg 56:351–361, 1968.
18. Harvey JC, Beattie EJ: Aggressive pulmonary metastasectomy facilitated by the use of median sternotomy and Nd:YAG laser. Cancer 72:1807–1808, 1993.
19. Verazin GT, Regal AM, Antowiak JG, et al: Ultrasonic surgical aspirator for lung resection. Ann Thorac Surg 52:787–790, 1991.
20. Harvey JC, Fleischman EH, Applebaum H: Resection of residual mediastinal germ cell metastases using the Cavitron ultrasonic surgical aspirator. J Thorac Cardiovasc Surg 102:425–426, 1991.
21. Branscheid D, Krysa S, Wollkopf H, et al: Does Nd:YAG laser extend the indication for resection of pulmonary metastases? Eur J Cardiothorac Surg 6:590–596, 1992.
22. Ueda T, Uchida A, Kodorno K, et al: Aggressive pulmonary metastasectomy for soft-tissue sarcomas. Cancer 72:1919–1925, 1993.
23. Balch CM, Soong SJ, Murad TM: A multifactorial analysis of melanoma. IV. Prognostic factors in 200 patients with distant metastases. J Clin Oncol 1:126–134, 1983.
24. Ishida T, Kaneko S, Yokoyama H, et al: Metastasectomy for soft-tissue sarcoma. J Thorac Cardiovasc Surg 77:173–177, 1992.
25. McAfee MK, Allen MS, Trastek VF, et al: Colorectal lung metastases: Results of surgical excision. Ann Thorac Surg 53:780–786, 1992.
26. Mandelbaum I, Yaw PB, Einhorn LH, et al: The importance of one-stage median sternotomy and retroperitoneal node dissection in disseminated testicular cancer. Ann Thorac Surg 26:524–528, 1983.
27. Goorin AM, Shuster JJ, Baker A, et al: Changing pattern of pulmonary metastases with adjuvant chemotherapy in patients with osteosarcoma: Results from the multi-institutional osteosarcoma study. J Clin Oncol 9:600–605, 1991.
28. Skinner KA, Eliber FR, Holmes EC, et al: Surgical treatment and chemotherapy for pulmonary metastases from osteosarcoma. Arch Surg 127:1065–1071, 1992.
29. Jablons D, Steinberg SM, Roth J, et al: Metastasectomy for soft-tissue sarcoma. J Thorac Cardiovasc Surg 97:695–705, 1989.
30. Shimizu N, Ando A, Matsutani T, et al: Trans-sternal thoracotomy for bilateral pulmonary metastasis. J Surg Oncol 50:105–109, 1981.
31. Harvey JC, Lee KA, Beattie EJ: Utility of the neodymium:yttrium-aluminum-garnet (Nd:YAG) laser for extensive pulmonary metastasectomy. J Surg Oncol 54:175–179, 1993.
32. Dowling RD, Ferson FF, Landreneau RJ: Thoracoscopic resection of pulmonary metastases. Chest 102:1450–1454, 1992.
33. Rosen G, Caparros B, Huvos AG, et al: Preoperative chemotherapy for osteogenic sarcoma: Selection of postoperative adjuvant chemotherapy based on the response of the primary tumor to preoperative chemotherapy. Cancer 49:1221–1230, 1982.
34. Chawla SP, Rosen G, Lowenbraun S, et al: Role of high-dose ifosfamide (HDI) in recurrent osteosarcoma. Proc ASCO 31:198, 1990.
35. Pastorino U, Valente M, Gasparini M: Median sternotomy and multiple lung resections for metastatic sarcomas. Eur J Cardiothorac Surg 4:477–481, 1990.
36. Lanza LA, Natarajan G, Roth JA, et al: Long-term survival after resection of pulmonary metastases from carcinoma of the breast. Ann Thorac Surg 54:244, 1992.
37. Pogrebniak HW, Haas G, Linehean WM: Renal cell carcinoma: Resection of solitary and multiple metastases. Ann Thorac Surg 54:33–38, 1992.
38. Putnam JB, Roth JA, Wesley NM, et al: Analysis of prognostic factors in patients undergoing resection of pulmonary metastasis from soft-tissue sarcomas. J Thorac Cardiovasc Surg 87:260–268, 1984.
39. Pogrebniak HW, Stovroff M, Roth JA, et al: Resection of pulmonary metastases from malignant melanoma: Results of a 16-year experience. Ann Thorac Surg 46:20–23, 1988.
40. Bosl GJ, Gluckman R, Geller NL, et al: VAB-6: An effective chemotherapy regimen for patients with germ cell tumors. J Clin Oncol 4:1493–1499, 1986.
41. Einhorn LH, Williams SD, Troner M, et al: The role of maintenance therapy in disseminated testicular cancer. N Engl J Med 305:727–731, 1987.
42. Huvos AG, Rosen G, Marcove RC: Primary osteogenic sarcoma: Pathologic aspects in 20 patients after treatment with chemotherapy, en bloc resection and prosthetic bone replacement. Arch Pathol Lab Med 101:14–18, 1977.
43. Joseph WL, Morton DL, Adkins PC: Prognostic significance of tumor doubling time in evaluating operability in pulmonary disease. J Thorac Cardiovasc Surg 61:23–32, 1971.
44. Mori M, Tomoda H, Ishida T, et al: Surgical resection of pulmonary metastases from colorectal carcinoma: Special reference to repeated pulmonary resections. Arch Surg 126:1297–1301, 1991.
45. Rosen G, Huvos AG, Mosende C, et al: Chemotherapy and thoracotomy for metastatic osteogenic sarcoma: A model for adjuvant chemotherapy and the rationale for the timing of thoracic surgery. Cancer 41:841–849, 1978.
46. Beattie EJ, Martini N, Rosen G: The management of pulmonary metastases in children with osteogenic sarcoma with surgical resection combined with chemotherapy. Cancer 35:618–621, 1975.
47. Takita H, Edgerton F, Karakousis C, et al: Surgical management of metastases to the lung. Surg Gynecol Obstet 152:191–194, 1981.
48. Pogrebniak HW, Pass HI: Initial and reoperative pulmonary metastasectomy: Indications, technique and results. Semin Surg Oncol 9:142–149, 1993.

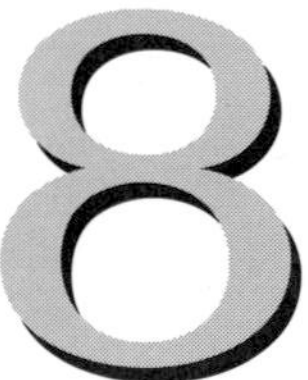

Melvyn Goldberg, M.D.
Ronald L. Burkes, M.D.

Tumors of the Mediastinum

Tumors situated in the mediastinum may be either primary or secondary in origin. In the majority of instances, secondary metastatic tumors are the result of lymphatic spread to mediastinal nodes from primary sites in the area, which include lung, laryngotracheobronchial tree, esophagus, thyroid, parathyroid, and proximal stomach.

Primary mediastinal tumors are relatively common and quite varied in origin. Specific tumors of the mediastinum usually occur in distinctive locations and age groups (Tables 8–1 and 8–2).

ANATOMIC COMPARTMENTS

The mediastinum is defined laterally by the two pleural cavities, superiorly by the bony structures of the thoracic inlet and inferiorly by the diaphragm (Fig. 8–1). Conventionally, the mediastinum has been divided into anterior, middle, and posterior compartments. This allows anatomic and diagnostic differentiation, since the tumors occur in specific locations.

Anterior Mediastinum

The anterior mediastinum is limited posteriorly by the heart and great vessels and the bodies of the first four thoracic vertebrae. It is bounded anteriorly by the sternum and laterally by the mediastinal pleura. The anterior mediastinum is divided into superior and inferior compartments. Most tumors of the anterior mediastinum occur in the superior compartment and include lymphoma, thymoma, and germ cell tumors. Thymoma and thyroid enlargements and neoplasms may also occur in the anteroinferior mediastinum.

Middle Mediastinum

This compartment is bounded posteriorly by the esophagus and anteriorly by the heart and great vessels. Circumferentially, it is contained by the pericardium and is limited laterally by the mediastinal pleura. The middle mediastinum is rich in lymphatics and is frequently involved by lymphoma and metastatic adenopathy from locally diseased structures. Rarely, it may also harbor thyroid enlargements and neoplasms.

Posterior Mediastinum

The posterior mediastinum lies between the pericardium anteriorly and the vertebral column and paravertebral gutters posteriorly. It includes the esophagus and the immediate surrounding structures. This region is almost exclusive for neurogenic tumors and enteric cysts of the esophagus. Esophageal tumors are excluded from this discussion.

DIAGNOSIS

Forty percent of mediastinal tumors are malignant and are usually associated with signs or symptoms. The remaining 60% are benign, and most are asymptomatic when initially identified.

TABLE 8–1
Incidence and Location of Primary Mediastinal Tumors in Adults

Type	Incidence (%)	Location
Neurogenic	21	Posterior
Cystic	20	All compartments
Thymoma	19	Anterior
Lymphoma	13	Anterior/middle
Germ cell	11	Anterior
Mesenchymal	7	All compartments
Endocrine	6	Anterior/middle

From Shields TW: General Thoracic Surgery, 3rd ed. Philadelphia: Lea & Febiger, 1989, pp 1096–1123.

TABLE 8–2
Relative Frequency of Various Mediastinal Tumors and Cysts in 1950 Adult Patients and 437 Children

	Adults		Children	
Type	*No.*	*%*	*No.*	*%*
Neurogenic	411	21	176	40
Thymoma	365	19	0	0
Lymphoma	246	13	80	18
Germ cell	207	11	47	11
Mesenchymal	138	7	38	9
Endocrine	125	6	0	0
Primary CA	57	3	16	4
Cyst	401	20	80	18
Total	1950	100	437	100

From Silverman NA, Sabiston DC Jr: Mediastinal mass. Surg Clin North Am 60:757, 1980.

The asymptomatic abnormalities are frequently identified and diagnosed with relative accuracy on routine chest films. Symptoms are commonly secondary to extrinsic compression on, or invasion of, adjacent structures, which include trachea and bronchi, esophagus, vena cava, chest wall, diaphragm, pleura, pericardium, spinal cord, recurrent laryngeal nerves, and stellate ganglia.

Imaging Techniques

Abnormalities are frequently displayed by routine chest films. Computed tomography (CT) scanning is essential to detail the size, contour, density, and location. When indicated, magnetic resonance imaging (MRI) may supply limited additional information in assessing bony structures, blood vessels, and the spinal column and cord.

Other ancillary procedures include angiography, radionuclide scanning techniques, and ultrasonography. Bronchoscopy and esophagogastroscopy may aid in the assessment of enlarged and abnormal contiguous structures.

Tissue Diagnosis

A fine-needle or core needle biopsy directed by fluoroscopic or CT control is exceedingly accurate in producing diagnostic material. Core biopsies of anterior mediastinal masses are safe and provide histologic specimens that can identify the architectural nature of lymphoma in order to direct appropriate therapy.

Cervical mediastinoscopy, limited anterior mediastinotomy, videothoracoscopy, and thoracotomy are more invasive procedures with indications for diagnosis or definitive therapy, or both.

Associated Criteria

Immunoassay for beta–human chorionic gonadotropin (βhCG) and alpha-fetoprotein (AFP) are of great value in the diagnosis and management of germ cell tumors.

Pheochromocytoma with hypertension is associated with elevated serum catecholamines. Thymoma may occur with myasthenia gravis and other biologic dysfunctions that result in elevated parameters. Parathyroid adenoma may produce hypercalcemia, and thyroid pathology may induce thyrotoxicosis.

MANAGEMENT

The management of mediastinal tumors ranges from observation only to radical extirpation. Intermediate treatments include aspiration, simple resection, radiotherapy, chemotherapy, and combination therapy.

This chapter updates the investigation and management of the common mediastinal tumors. Germ cell tumors and lymphoma are neoplasms primarily treated by nonsurgical means, but indications for surgical removal are discussed.

Diagnosis: Noninvasive Techniques

As discussed, the mediastinum is divided into anterior, middle, and posterior compartments. The anterior mediastinum contains the thymus gland or its remnants, branches of the internal mammary artery and vein, lymph nodes, and variable amounts of fat. The middle mediastinum con-

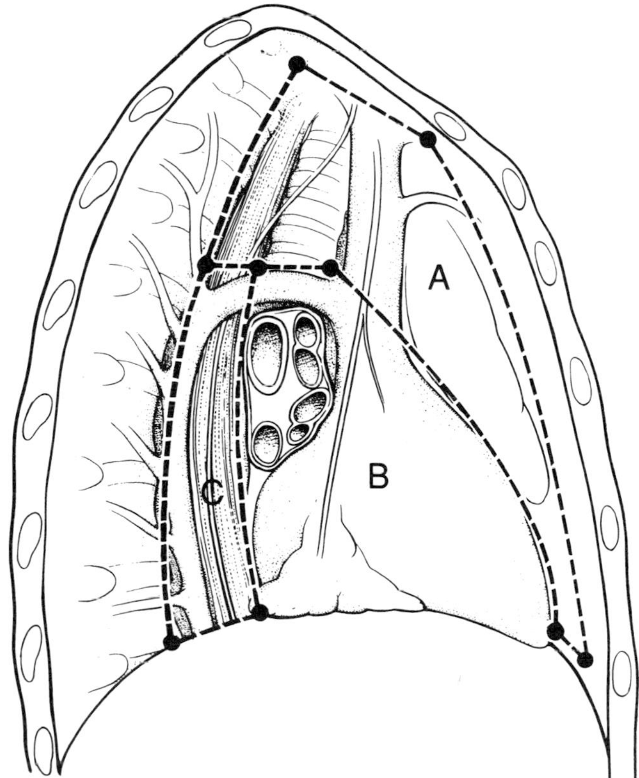

FIGURE 8–1. Lateral view of the chest dividing the mediastinum into the anterosuperior (A), middle (B), and posterior (C) mediastinum. (From Bloom ND: Tumors of the mediastinum. In Beattie EJ, et al [eds]: Thoracic Surgical Oncology. New York: Churchill Livingstone, 1992, p 238.)

tains the pericardium and its contents, ascending and transverse portions of the aorta, superior and inferior vena cava, brachiocephalic arteries and veins, phrenic nerves and upper portion of the vagus nerves, trachea and main bronchi, and contiguous lymph nodes and the pulmonary arteries and veins. The posterior mediastinal compartment contains the descending thoracic aorta, esophagus, thoracic duct, azygos and hemiazygos veins, nerves, fat, and lymph nodes.

Almost half of all patients with mediastinal masses are asymptomatic, with the abnormality being detected on a routine chest radiograph. Once a mediastinal abnormality is identified on chest film, the next procedure of choice is CT scanning of the mediastinum.[1] CT scan provides detail of size, contour, density, and anatomic relationships and can differentiate cystic from solid mediastinal masses. As well, CT scan can assess whether widening of the mediastinum is pathologic or simply an anatomic variation such as fat deposition (Fig. 8–2). Further, it may differentiate a solid mass from a vascular structure such as an aneurysm. The impact of MRI has yet to be established. The advantages include no ionizing radiation, no intravenous contrast, and multiplanar imaging of the mediastinum. Its ability to define bone, central nervous system, and vessel involvement is superb, and it may be able to differentiate radiation fibrosis from tumor mass with differing signal intensities. This may prove especially useful in patients with Hodgkin's disease and non-Hodgkin's lymphoma following chemotherapy or radiotherapy, or both.

Other noninvasive investigations include gallium scanning, which is important both in staging non-Hodgkin's lymphoma and, more importantly, in assessing a residual mass following chemotherapy or radiotherapy, or both, in order to help differentiate the presence of residual tumor versus fibrosis.[2]

Finally, tumor markers are especially valuable in patients with germ cell tumors of the mediastinum. Immunoassays for βhCG and AFP are important in both diagnosis and management of these tumors.[3]

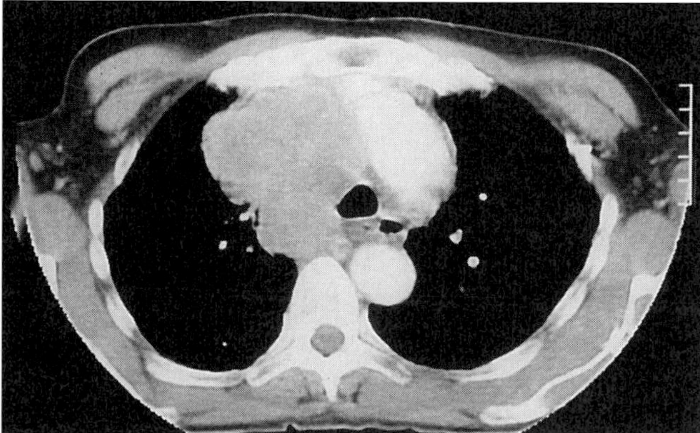

FIGURE 8–2. CT scan of the chest detailing a large anterosuperior mediastinal mass. This was a small cell carcinoma of the lung, which can on occasion mimic a primary mediastinal tumor.

Diagnosis: Invasive Techniques

Percutaneous Needle Biopsy

Percutaneous fine-needle aspiration biopsy is frequently used to diagnosis mediastinal pathology. An aspirate can be stained by the Papanicolaou technique and cytopathologically diagnosed. Needles with a larger diameter enable core biopsies to be performed; with these histologic specimens, not only can the type of malignancies be identified but, in the case of lymphoma, classification can also be determined. Many types of core biopsy needles are readily available.

The material can be assessed by light and electron microscopy using special staining techniques and immunohistochemical assays. Fine-needle biopsy should easily distinguish between benignity and malignancy. Tissue histology with core biopsy differentiates between types of lymphoma.

Needle biopsy should be performed by an experienced radiologist under fluoroscopic control and biplanar technique. In selected instances, CT guidance is required. There are very few contraindications for fine-needle aspiration of an anterior mediastinal mass.[4]

Anterior Mediastinoscopy

Anterior mediastinoscopy was originally described by McNeill and Chamberlain.[5] This procedure allows excellent access to the left or right precordium, usually through the second intercostal space parasternally. There is no need to remove a portion of intercostal cartilage, and, once access is gained into the mediastinum or medial pleural space, exploration can be performed initially with the finger and subsequently with either the mediastinoscope or the thoracoscope. Usually large anterior tumors can be directly visualized and sampled for biopsy. Adequate tumor volume should be removed to allow for the additional studies the pathologist may need to perform to make an absolute diagnosis.

The disadvantages of this incision is the increased incidence of wound infection and the disproportionate pain for an incision of this size. The infection may preclude a subsequent pneumonectomy or sternotomy until fully healed.

Cervical Mediastinoscopy

Cervical mediastinoscopy, as popularized by Pearson et al.,[6] affords easy access to the middle and upper part of the posterior mediastinum, where most involved mediastinal lymph nodes reside. Many anterior mediastinal masses may encroach on this space, allowing for easy biopsy and diagnosis. Right precordial tumors frequently descend inferiorly to the right because of the lack of the aortic arch to obstruct the descent. At times, both anterior mediastinotomy and cervical mediastinoscopy are combined to allow maximal access for adequate biopsy short of thoracotomy.

Thoracoscopy

Within the last few years, video-assisted thoracoscopic surgery (VATS) has developed as an adjunctive procedure in assessing and diagnosing intrathoracic disease.[7] The thoracoscope can be inserted through a selected intercostal space, allowing the operator to view and sample the mass through additional ports strategically positioned in other intercostal spaces. Special instruments have been devised for thoracoscopic use, but many general thoracic surgeons prefer to use conventional thoracotomy instruments through the interspace incisions.

The incisions are small and relatively painless postoperatively. The view of the pleural space is excellent, with access to all ipsilateral mediastinal structures. Direct biopsy under vision should preclude complications. Currently, VATS should be restricted to biopsy only, and excision should be performed through thoracotomy.

Thoracotomy

Thoracotomy, limited or full, may be used for incisional biopsy for diagnosis or for excisional biopsy and therapeutic cure. Either posterolateral thoracotomy or midline sternotomy is appropriate in the selected circumstance. In almost all instances with present radiographic localizing techniques for needle biopsy, a diagnosis can be made without thoracotomy. Resection of precordial lymphomas can be avoided by diagnosis with the lesser of invasive procedures.

One well-recognized characteristic of malignant thymoma is its ability to seed the pleural space or mediastinum after biopsy. The surgeon must be careful to transgress as few tissue planes as possible at subsequent resection and remove the area of biopsy en bloc with surrounding tissue.

THYMOMA

Thymoma is the most frequent neoplasm in the anterior precordial mediastinum. Fifteen percent of benign thymomas are associated with myasthenia gravis[8, 9] and considerably more with the malignant form. Other rare syndrome complexes may also be present. Because of local invasive features, the preoperative assessment and diagnosis may preclude biopsy.

Pathology

Thymomas are usually cytologically benign neoplasms with expression of malignancy by local invasion of adjacent structures. Rarely, the thymic tissue is cytologically malignant and described histologically as thymic carcinoma or thymic carcinoid tumor. Other rare benign tumors are also described infrequently (thymolipoma).

The benign neoplasms are usually encapsulated and easily removed. True invasion signifies malignancy. Even though thymomas are most frequent in the anterior mediastinum, they can occur in any portion of the mediastinum from the root of the neck to the posterior pleuropericardial recesses.

The histologic characteristics are lymphocytic, epithelioid, spindle cell (fusiform), or mixed.

Classification

Masaoka and colleagues[8] have classified thymoma on the basis of degree of invasion and have correlated this with prognosis (Table 8–3). Five-year survival rates of each clinical stage were 92.6% in stage I, 85.7% in stage II, 69.6% in stage III, and 50% in stage IV. The 5-year survival rate for the total resection group was 88.9% and for the nonradically treated group it was 44.4%.

The degree of invasion is determined intraoperatively by surgical assessment and multiple focal biopsies. Encapsulation and local adherence bode well, but invasion of surrounding structures does not, with increased local recurrence rates postoperatively.[8, 9]

Myasthenia Gravis

Myasthenia gravis is an autoimmune disorder of neuromuscular transmission. The causative agent is acetylcholine receptor antibody (AChRab), which blocks the muscle end-plate receptor and thereby interferes with neuromuscular transmission. With time, the receptors undergo atrophy and decrease in numbers. Most therapies act by attempts to decrease the levels of AChRab either chemically or surgically.

Symptoms may vary from minor complaints of ocular, facial, and pharyngopalatine weakness to severe generalized weakness and respiratory failure.

Edrophonium chloride (Tensilon) is diagnostic by reversing symptoms for several minutes to hours and may not always be positive. Single-fiber electromyography (SFEMG) is sensitive and specific for myasthenia gravis and should always be performed to document the diagnosis.

Thymectomy for myasthenia gravis (with or without

TABLE 8–3
Clinical Stages and Prognosis of Thymoma

Stage	Definition	5-Year Survival Rate (%)
Stage I	Completely encapsulated microscopically	92.6
Stage II	1. Macroscopic invasion into surrounding fatty tissue or mediastinal pleura or 2. Microscopic invasion into the capsule	85.7
Stage III	Macroscopic invasion into adjacent organs	69.6
Stage IVA	Diffuse pleural or pericardial involvement	50.0
IVB	Lymphatic or hematogenous metastasis	<50

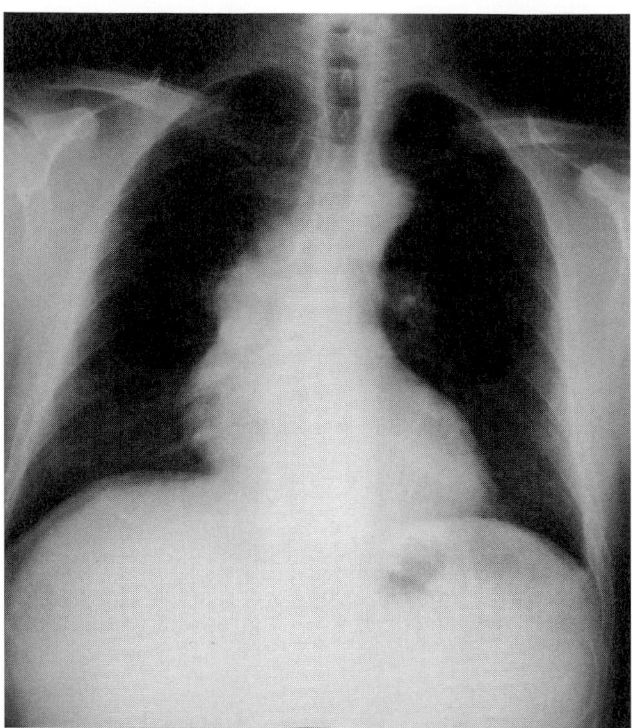

FIGURE 8–3. Chest radiograph identifying a well-encapsulated stage I thymoma as a large right suprahilar precordial mass.

thymoma) is now a relatively safe procedure as compared to earlier reports. With better anticholinesterase medications, plasmapheresis to remove AChRab preoperatively, and discrete use of immunosuppressive agents like corticosteroids and azathioprine, thymectomy is now usually an elective procedure with a routine postoperative recovery period. Patients should be conjointly cared for preoperatively and postoperatively by surgeon and neurologist.

Clinical Features

Most patients with mediastinal tumors present in the fifth or sixth decades,[10] and those with thymoma at an earlier age. The majority of patients present with stage I or II disease and no localizing symptoms, with initial detection on routine chest radiograph.

With extensive involvement of the mediastinum, patients may complain of the effects of superior vena cava obstruction, dysphagia due to esophageal compression, wheeze or severe central airway obstruction due to tracheal involvement or encasement, and chest pain due to involvement of mediastinal autonomic innervation.

Rarer symptom complexes include red cell aplasia, hypogammaglobulinemia, pancytopenia, rheumatoid arthritis, ulcerative colitis, sclerosing cholangitis, Hashimoto's thyroiditis, and lupus erythematosus.

Predictors of Outcome

With improvement in preoperative and postoperative managements, myasthenia gravis should no longer influence the outcome of surgical treatment.

The degree of invasion is the most reliable predictor of outcome and relates to the clinical staging of Masaoka (see Table 8–3).

Recent efforts have been made to determine whether cellular and molecular biologic techniques might predict outcome. DNA ploidy was identified as a predictor of prognosis, with aneuploid tumors being generally associated with greater degrees of invasion, myasthenia gravis, and increased incidence of recurrence.[11] Others have found no relationship between DNA content and prognosis.[12]

Diagnosis

Most tumors are detected by routine chest radiography followed by thoracic CT (Figs. 8–3 and 8–4). Anterior precordial mediastinal masses are usually thymic in origin. Patients with myasthenia gravis should routinely have thoracic CT scans.

Other anterior mediastinal masses that are not treated surgically must be excluded. Percutaneous fine-needle aspiration biopsy can usually differentiate between thymoma, germ cell tumor, and lymphoma or Hodgkin's disease. If lymphoma is suspected, usually a more substantial biopsy is required to better classify the tumor, and this can be accomplished by needle core biopsy, cervical mediastinoscopy, or anterior mediastinotomy. Percutaneous fine-needle aspiration biopsy was specific in 94% of cases and sensitive in 87% in a recent survey of 33 patients.[13] With light and electron microscopy, immunohistochemical techniques, and serum marker assays, this approach is highly reliable (Fig. 8–5).

Open biopsy is used if the diagnosis is still in doubt after simpler measures have been performed. If the tumor appears invasive by imaging, open assessment may confirm this impression and validate neoadjuvant treatment prior to total extirpation.

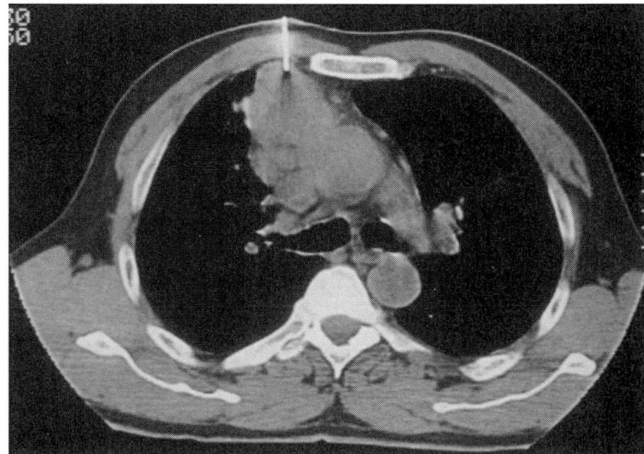

FIGURE 8–4. CT scan of the chest identifying a large precordial thymoma and its use in guiding a fine-needle aspiration biopsy.

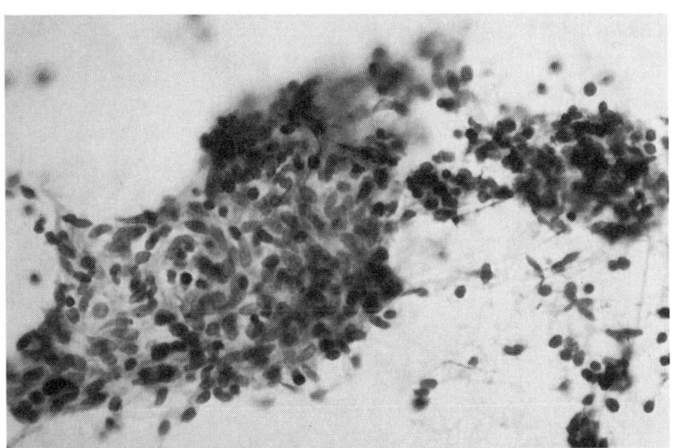

FIGURE 8–5. Cytopathologic specimen from an aspiration of a benign thymoma demonstrating a positive keratin stain.

Surgery

The optimal treatment for localized thymoma is wide total removal. Locally invaded tissue should be removed without disabling the patient severely postoperatively. Our technique at the Fox Chase Cancer Center entails a full sternotomy and complete removal of the tumor, including the remaining thymus from the root of the neck to the posterior pericardiophrenic recesses. This includes the entire precordial tissue to the phrenic nerves laterally.

On occasion when performing a transcervical thymectomy for myasthenia gravis, a small thymoma is unexpectedly discovered. The incision should be converted to a full sternotomy and the appropriate procedure then performed.

These tumors respond well to radiotherapy, which can be effectively delivered intraoperatively via external beam or, if residual tumor remains after surgery, via external beam, brachytherapy through afterloading catheters, or radiation seeds implanted at operation. Obviously, bilateral phrenic neurectomies are not tolerated, so at least one phrenic nerve must be preserved in invasive stage III disease by carefully filleting it out of the tumor mass. Vascular invasion with resection and reconstruction is advised by several groups, with extended survivals to 5 and 10 years postoperatively (100% and 94.7%, respectively) with the addition of postoperative radiation.[4, 14, 15]

Repeated resections for recurrent disease, including pleural deposits that are localized, are frequently encouraged and are combined with radiotherapy or chemotherapy, or both.

Radiotherapy

Although surgery remains the primary therapy for thymoma, recurrence of disease in patients undergoing complete resection is seen. The routine use of adjuvant radiotherapy for all postoperative patients remains controversial. Local intrathoracic recurrence and pleural dissemination are the major causes of initial treatment failure, and whether adjuvant mediastinal irradiation prevents recurrence has not yet been established. Urgosi et al.[16] have showed that postoperative radiotherapy is useful in selected patients with stage III disease. The risk of local recurrence was reduced and survival was prolonged in patients resected with locally advanced disease.

Haniuda and coworkers[17] suggest that better selection of patients for postoperative radiotherapy may be based on the pleural factor. They found that postoperative radiotherapy prevented recurrence in pleural stage II patients, whereas postoperative mediastinal radiation did not reduce the recurrence rate in late stage II and stage III patients. Further, patients with stage I or II disease and no pleural involvement had a good prognosis with or without adjuvant radiation. Macchiarini et al.[18] investigated the role of neoadjuvant chemotherapy with surgery followed by postoperative radiotherapy in seven patients with stage IIIA invasive thymoma. All but one patient is currently alive and disease-free, including three patients who underwent an incomplete resection. However, conclusions are difficult to make, as the numbers are small and the follow-up is short. Further, it is difficult to sort out the contribution of neoadjuvant chemotherapy as opposed to postoperative radiotherapy in this group of patients.

Chemotherapy

Although experience with systemic chemotherapy for patients with locally advanced or metastatic thymoma is limited, reports do suggest that thymoma is a chemosensitive tumor. Cisplatin, corticosteroids, and doxorubicin appear to produce the best objective response rates when used as single agents in patients with metastatic thymoma. Hu and Levine[19] classify the combination chemotherapy regimens as platinum- or nonplatinum-containing regimens. Among the nonplatinum-containing regimens, cyclophosphamide, vincristine (Oncovin), prednisone, and procarbazine (COPP) as well as cyclophosphamide, vincristine, and prednisone (CVP) or cyclophosphamide, doxorubicin, Oncovin, and prednisone (CHOP) achieved response rates of approximately 60%.[20, 21] Cisplatin-containing regimens appeared to improve these results, at least in phase II studies. Fornasiero and colleagues[22] reported their results in 37 patients with stage III or IV invasive thymoma treated with cisplatin (Adriamycin), doxorubicin, Oncovin (vincristine), and cyclophosphamide (ADOC).[22] The overall clinical response rate was 92%, with 43% being complete remissions. Seven of the 16 complete remissions were pathologically confirmed at subsequent thoracotomy. Loehrer et al.[23] reviewed 20 patients treated with cisplatin (Platinol), doxorubicin (Adriamycin), and cyclophosphamide (PAC) and found a 70% response rate with a median survival of 59 months.

The demonstration that systemic chemotherapy has shown efficacy both as first-line therapy and after surgery or radiotherapy stimulated investigation of neoadjuvant chemotherapy approaches. As mentioned, Macchiarini and coworkers[18] reported their results in seven patients treated with neoadjuvant cisplatin, epirubicin, and etoposide followed by postoperative radiotherapy. All patients showed a partial response, and four patients underwent a complete resection. Histologic analysis of the surgical specimens showed no evidence of disease in two patients. All but one patient is alive and disease-free. Although longer follow-up and a larger number of patients are needed to assess the impact of neoadjuvant chemotherapy on survival, this study demonstrates the feasibility of this approach.

MEDIASTINAL GERM CELL TUMORS

Primary mediastinal germ cell tumors are rare neoplasms, accounting for approximately 1% to 3% of germ cell tumors and about 10% of all mediastinal tumors. After the testis and the retroperitoneum, the mediastinum represents the third most frequent site of malignant germ cell tumors. Despite the common histologic and serologic features of testicular tumors and mediastinal germ cell tumors, the latter are recognized as clinically and biologically distinct entities.

Etiology

Initially thought to represent metastases from an occult testicular primary tumor, it is now generally accepted that mediastinal germ cell tumors arise by malignant transformation of residual germinal elements distributed to the mediastinum. Autopsy studies have not revealed any evidence of a small testicular primary tumor, nor has any fibrotic reaction been detected in the testis.[24] Further, testicular germ cell tumors rarely metastasize to the mediastinum. Finally, patients with germ cell tumors of the mediastinum have been cured, with testicular recurrences only rarely reported.

The distribution to the mediastinum may arise as a consequence of abnormal migration of germ cells during embryogenesis, or, alternatively, the mediastinum may represent one area of widespread distribution of germ cells as part of normal embryogenesis.[25]

Histopathology

Mediastinal germ cell tumors appear identical histologically to germ cell tumors arising in the testis. All histologic variants are found, the most common being benign teratoma, which constitutes approximately 70% of mediastinal germ cell tumors in childhood and 60% in adults.[26] The most common malignant tumor is seminoma, accounting for approximately one third of all cases. The remaining two thirds contain nonseminomatous elements, including teratoma with embryonal cell carcinoma (teratocarcinoma), while endodermal sinus tumor, choriocarcinoma, and embryonal cell carcinoma are much less frequent.

Clinical Presentation

Benign teratomas and dermoid tumors that may contain teeth are frequently discovered incidentally on chest radiograph. In contrast, malignant germ cell tumors are frequently associated with symptoms, including chest pain, dyspnea, cough, and signs and symptoms of superior vena cava syndrome.[27] Weight loss and fever may be present. Patients may present with symptoms of metastatic disease, most frequently to lung, liver, and bone. Physical examination is often normal, although signs of local complications such as superior vena cava syndrome or pericardial and pleural effusions may be present.

Roentgenographic Findings

In more than 95% of cases, the standard posteroanterior and lateral chest radiograph is abnormal within the anterior mediastinum (Fig. 8–6). Only 3% to 8% of mediastinal tumors arise within the posterior mediastinum. CT scan typically shows a large homogeneous mass without areas of necrosis or calcification in patients with seminoma (Fig. 8–7). In contrast, the radiologic features of nonseminomatous germ cell tumors often show a large heterogeneous mass with areas of hemorrhage and necrosis.[28]

Laboratory Findings

Serum markers are usually normal in patients with a pure seminoma, although this may be associated with a low elevation of hCG. Significant elevation of AFP indicates the presence of a nonseminomatous component.[29]

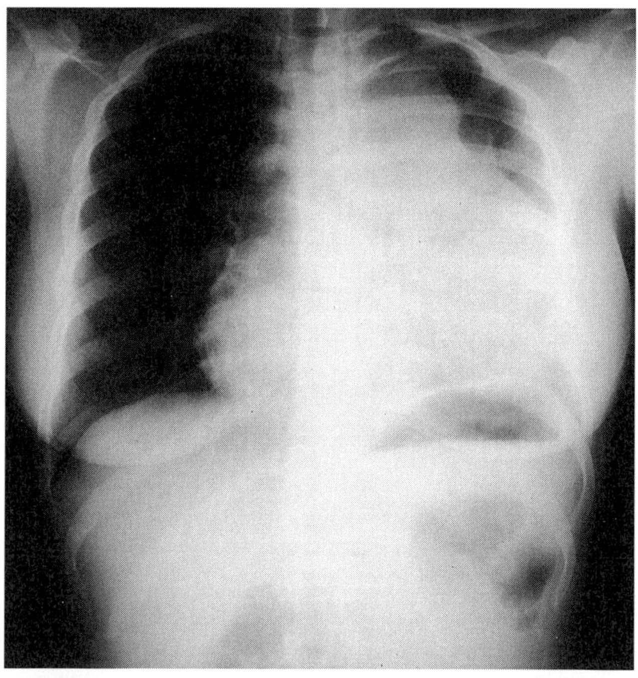

FIGURE 8–6. Chest radiograph demonstrating the left precordial and hilar position of a large primary germ cell tumor (yolk sac tumor) in a woman.

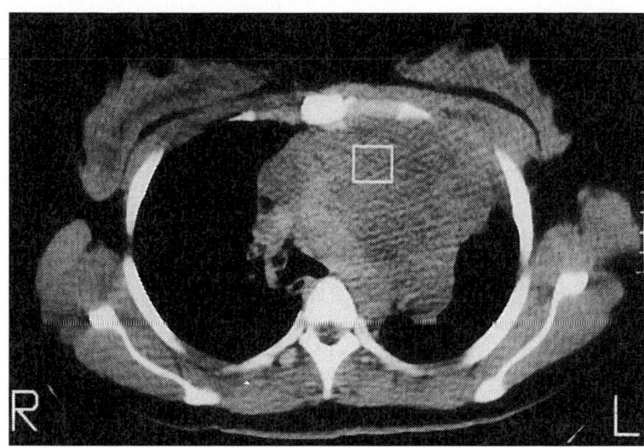

FIGURE 8–7. CT scan of the chest identifying the characteristics of the yolk sac tumor.

AFP is elevated in approximately 80% of patients, whereas hCG is elevated in only 30%. This differs somewhat from advanced testicular cancer, in which elevation of both hCG and AFP occurs with equal frequency.

Clinical Staging

In addition to chest radiograph and tumor markers, CT scan of the chest and abdomen should be obtained to determine the extent of disease. Careful physical examination of the testis should be carried out, and patients with significant retroperitoneal adenopathy on CT scan should undergo a testicular ultrasound. Further investigations should depend on symptoms. There is no role for blind orchidectomy in patients with a normal testicular examination and ultrasound.

Management

Benign Teratoma

Resection is the treatment of choice for benign teratoma, resulting in near-universal cure rates. There is no role for radiotherapy or chemotherapy. As these tumors may be densely adherent to adjacent structures, more extensive surgery may be required. Lewis et al.[30] from the Mayo Clinic reviewed their data on 86 patients with benign teratoma. Of 69 patients for whom follow-up information was available, 64 were healthy with no evidence of recurrent disease with an average follow-up of 10 years. Of the five patients who died, four died of intraoperative complications and one of unknown causes 6 months postoperatively.

Pure Seminoma

Mediastinal and testicular seminomas are both very sensitive to radiotherapy, resulting in a 60% to 80% long-term survival. Surgical resection alone may also be curative in patients with small tumors, although postoperative radiotherapy is usually recommended. In recent years, certain prognostic factors as well as experience with chemotherapy has led to a reassessment of the role of radiotherapy. An age greater than 35 years and the presence of superior vena cava syndrome, with adenopathy and hilar disease on chest film, worsen the prognosis.[26] These tumors can be very bulky at presentation, with invasion into adjacent intrathoracic structures and extension to hilar parenchyma, thus necessitating large radiotherapy ports, which risk damage to normal mediastinal structures and the lung.[31] One third of patients fail at distant sites.

Currently, cisplatin-based chemotherapy is recommended as primary treatment for patients with mediastinal seminoma. Lemarie and coworkers[32] treated 13 patients with pure seminoma, resulting in 12 complete responses, with only 2 patients relapsing after achieving a complete response.

Jain et al.[31] from the Memorial Sloan-Kettering Cancer Center retrospectively reviewed 21 patients with extragonadal seminoma treated either with surgery followed by postoperative radiotherapy (10 patients) or with cisplatin-based chemotherapy followed by radiotherapy or surgery (11 patients). Five of the 10 patients not receiving chemotherapy experienced recurrent disease, with 4 eventually dying; whereas only 1 of 11 patients receiving chemotherapy died of metastatic disease, the remaining patients being free of disease at 19 to 46 months following therapy.

In summary, with optimal therapy most patients with seminoma will be cured. Patients with small tumors may undergo thoracotomy and complete resection followed by postoperative radiotherapy. Clearly, all patients with distant metastases at diagnosis should receive cisplatin-based combination chemotherapy. For patients with locally advanced disease, induction chemotherapy with cisplatin-based chemotherapy is curative in instances. Residual masses after conventional therapy may require surgical extirpation to define and totally remove residual disease: benign, malignant, or residual fibrous tissue.

Nonseminomatous Germ Cell Tumors

Unlike in mediastinal seminoma, for which the treatment options remain controversial, the primary therapy in mediastinal nonseminomatous tumors is preferentially cisplatin-based chemotherapy.[33–35] Local treatment modalities, including surgery and radiotherapy, as primary treatment have little role in this disease. Although initially thought to carry a poor prognosis relative to their testicular counterparts, recent data suggest that the therapeutic outcome for nonseminomatous germ cell tumors is improving with modern treatment.

Bleomycin, etoposide, and cisplatin (Platinol) (BEP)[36] appear to constitute the optimum therapy. Patients with normal tumor markers and CT scan following four courses of chemotherapy should receive no further treatment. For patients in whom the tumor markers have normalized but residual tumor remains, debulking surgery of the residual mass is performed. If residual tumor is found, patients should receive further chemotherapy with a salvage regimen. The best results to date having been with combination etoposide (or vinblastine), ifosfamide, and Platinol (VIP).[37] Patients with markers that do not normalize should also undergo salvage chemotherapy.

In summary, treatment strategy for nonseminomatous mediastinal germ cell tumors requires cooperation between medical oncologists and thoracic surgeons. Although there has been a marked improvement in the prognosis of these patients with cisplatin-based chemotherapy, only approximately 50% of patients are long-term survivors, justifying future improvements in therapy.

Biologic Associations with Mediastinal Germ Cell Tumors

The association between mediastinal germ cell tumors and hematologic malignancies was identified in 1985. The hematologic malignancies that occur in this setting appear to be primary rather than secondary leukemias related to cisplatin-based chemotherapy. Unlike secondary leukemias, which rarely develop before 2 years after treatment, 70% of leukemias associated with mediastinal germ cell tumors present within 12 months of treatment and may even precede the diagnosis. The subtypes of leukemia are primarily megakaryocytic leukemia, erythroleukemia, and malignant histiocystosis. The most common cytogenetic abnormality is an isochrome of the short arm of chromosome 12 (i[12p]). The abnormality has been noted in both the bone marrow and the mediastinal germ cell tumor. This syndrome has been found only in patients with mediastinal nonseminomatous germ cell tumors and is associated with a very short survival.[38–40]

In addition to these hematologic neoplasms, mediastinal germ cell tumors have been associated with thrombocytopenia, malignant histiocytosis, essential thrombocythemia, and the hemophagocytic syndrome.[41] Mediastinal nonseminomatous germ cell tumors have been associated with Klinefelter's syndrome. At Indiana University, 4 of 22 patients had the karyotype 47,XXY. Other reports in the literature suggest an incidence of 20%.[42]

Role of Surgery

Mediastinal germ cell tumors are neoplasms that are primarily treated by radiotherapy, chemotherapy, or a combination owing to their extreme sensitivities to these modalities of therapy.[43, 44] Over the past decade, a specific role for surgery of these diseases has slowly evolved.

In many instances, surgery may play an important role in the diagnosis and treatment of these neoplasms. There may be a role for surgery in the treatment of residual mediastinal seminomatous lesions. In nonseminomatous neoplasms, treated primarily by cisplatin-based therapy, adjuvant surgical resection is frequently necessary to identify the nature of residual disease in order to plan appropriate additional therapy if necessary.[45–47]

Benign teratomas produce local symptoms due to encroachment on adjacent structures. To prevent or relieve symptoms, teratomas are removed surgically, occasionally with the adjacent involved structure.[30, 40]

Primary Nonseminomatous Germ Cell Tumors

Surgery is useful as a diagnostic tool and may also be a therapeutic procedure. If a diagnosis remains uncertain after assay of serum tumor markers and fine-needle aspiration biopsy, an anterior mediastinotomy may be necessary to establish the diagnosis. Germ cell tumors seldom involve the superior mediastinum, and cervical mediastinoscopy is seldom fruitful in diagnosing this disease.

After induction chemotherapy, residual tumor may be present on imaging studies with normalized serum tumor markers (Fig. 8–8). In order to plan continued therapy, the residual disease is removed surgically to determine its nature: fibrosis, benign teratoma, or active malignancy. All areas of previous involvement should be explored[33] by the appropriate incision. All vestiges of disease must be completely excised, with preservation of vital structures such as vagi, phrenic nerves, and vessels of the mediastinum. Usually only fibrosis is found adjacent to vital structures, and the residuum can be cleanly shaved off the structure with no underlying damage. Frozen section results dictate the degree of the resection.

Frequently, the surgeon removes residual disease when serum markers are elevated. Removal of all viable malignancy followed by high-dose chemotherapy and bone mar-

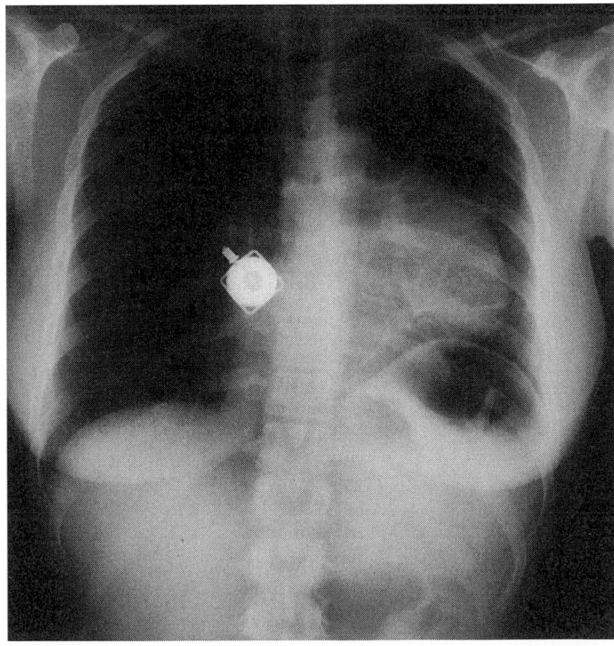

FIGURE 8–8. Chest radiograph after chemotherapy identifying a major reduction in the size of the yolk sac tumor. The resected specimen contained benign teratoma only.

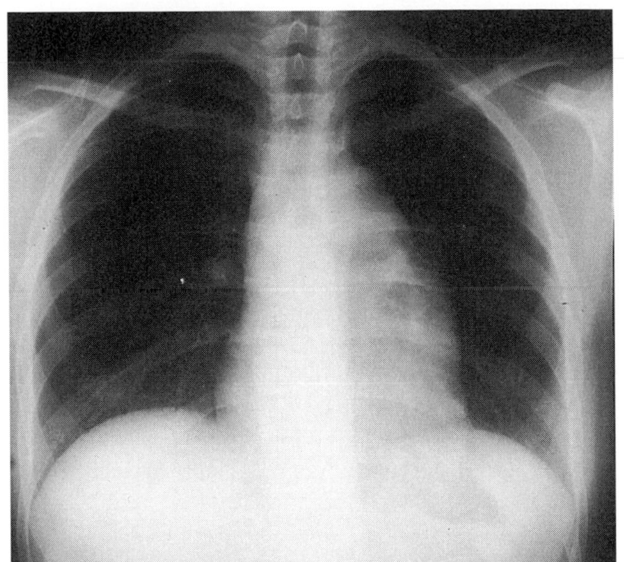

FIGURE 8–9. Chest radiograph identifying a large left precordial mass with obliteration of the aortopulmonary window secondary to Hodgkin's lymphoma.

row transplantation occasionally yields beneficial results. With no radiographic residual disease and negative serum markers, no surgery should be performed.

Metastatic Nonseminomatous Germ Cell Tumors

Nonseminomatous germ cell tumors frequently metastasize to lung, mediastinal nodes, and retroperitoneal nodes. After induction chemotherapy, excision of residual disease is performed to define and remove the residua. The surgical approach depends on the site of involvement and may necessitate sternotomy, laparotomy, thoracotomy, or thoracoabdominal approaches.

Active localized or metastatic germ cell tumor patients can often do well after conventional nonsurgical treatment, with prolonged 5-year survival after salvage extirpative surgery. Nonseminomatous germ cell tumors may require an aggressive multidisciplinary approach and further research into better treatment.

PRIMARY MEDIASTINAL MALIGNANT LYMPHOMA

Mediastinal involvement occurs in 60% to 90% of patients presenting with Hodgkin's disease and in 18% to 46% of patients with non-Hodgkin's lymphoma. The presentation of lymphoma primary to the mediastinum is uncommon.[48–50] Primary mediastinal lymphoma may be defined as lymphoma presenting clinically and radiologically as an intrathoracic neoplasm arising from the mediastinum in the absence of peripheral adenopathy or readily detectable or accessible disease beyond the thorax. The vast majority of these neoplasms include Hodgkin's disease, large cell lymphoma, and lymphoblastic lymphoma. Significant differences exist with respect to presentation, natural history, approach to therapy, and prognosis. Therefore, a definitive diagnosis is of critical importance in determining subsequent management.

Presentation

The majority of patients with primary mediastinal lymphoma present with symptoms due to an enlarging intrathoracic mass: chest pain, nonproductive cough, dyspnea, dysphagia, hoarseness, or signs and symptoms of superior vena cava obstruction.[48] Patients may also present with symptoms directly related to the lymphoma—that is, fever, night sweats, and weight loss (B symptoms). Physical examination may reveal physical signs related to involvement of the anterior or middle mediastinum. Peripheral adenopathy and splenomegaly are usually not present with primary mediastinal disease.

Radiologic Features

Evaluation of the mediastinum is critical in patients with Hodgkin's and non-Hodgkin's lymphoma. Because the mediastinum is so commonly involved, both treatment planning and disease staging are influenced by the anatomic extent of disease at the time of initial diagnosis or at the time of relapse.

CT has replaced conventional tomography in assessing the mediastinum (Figs. 8–9 and 8–10). Radiologic involvement of the mediastinum may occur in a variety of ways, including a permeating continuum, discrete lymphadenopathy, or parietal involvement. Enlargement of a single node or nodal group is more common in non-Hodgkin's lymphoma than in Hodgkin's disease. In permeating continuum, contiguous mass involvement in lymph nodes is pres-

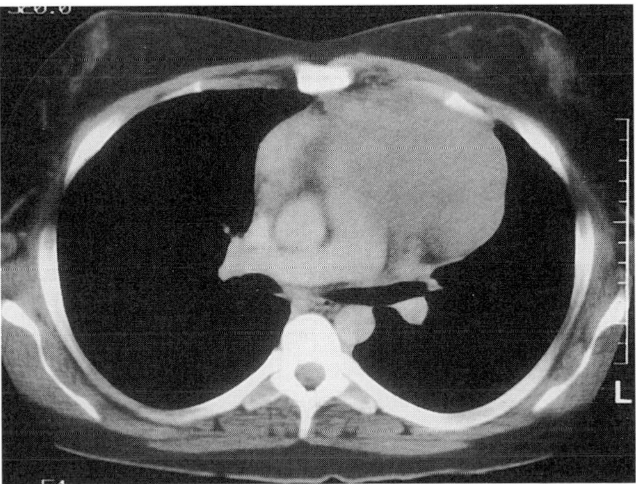

FIGURE 8–10. CT scan of the chest identifying the proximity of the lymphoma to the anterior chest wall and the relative ease and safety of performing a core needle biopsy for diagnosis and typing of lymphoma.

ent, possibly arising from the thymus, and may blend with the cardiac silhouette. With parietal involvement, the nodes in the internal mammary chain, paravertebral chains, or epicardiac and diaphragmatic nodes are involved and may extend to involve sternum or chest wall.[49]

Histologic Categories

Hodgkin's disease, diffuse large cell lymphoma, and lymphoblastic lymphoma constitute more than 90% of primary mediastinal lymphomas. Although Hodgkin's disease is known to have a bimodal age-incidence pattern, patients with primary mediastinal involvement tend to have an early age peak, from late teens to early thirties, with the nodular sclerosing subtype being the most common histologic pattern.

Lymphoblastic lymphoma is classified as a high-grade malignant lymphoma in the working formulation, presenting primarily in adolescent males. Histologically, this neoplasm is primarily of an immature T-cell phenotype, although occasionally a tumor of B-cell origin has been seen, and characteristically contains high levels of terminal deoxynucleotidyl transferase (TdT) activity.[51] Untreated, this disease is rapidly fatal, with early involvement of the central nervous system and bone marrow progressing to a leukemic phase.[52]

Diffuse large cell non-Hodgkin's lymphoma of the mediastinum is the most common primary non-Hodgkin's lymphoma of the mediastinum in adults. Various series show a predilection for young women, with a median age of 24 to 34 years, although older men may also be affected.[53] The mediastinal mass is usually large and may invade adjacent structures such as lung, pleura, pericardium, or chest wall. This disease may be quite heterogeneous histologically. The most common types are diffuse large cell lymphoma with morphologic features of follicular center cells, most often of large noncleaved cells. These tumors are of B-cell phenotype and are frequently accompanied by sclerosis. Other histologic appearances include B-cell immunoblastic sarcoma as well as T-cell immunoblastic sarcoma.[54]

Treatment

The prognosis for Hodgkin's disease is excellent. Although radiotherapy may be used as primary therapy, radiocurability is based on the bulk of disease and evidence of disease extension beyond the mediastinum.[55, 56]

Various chemotherapeutic regimens exist for the management of Hodgkin's disease. The traditional regimen is the MOPP program, consisting of mechlorethamine, Oncovin, procarbazine, and prednisone.[57] More recently, there has been a move toward an alternative regimen, consisting of Adriamycin, bleomycin, vinblastine, and dacarbazine (ABVD), which appears to be more efficacious than MOPP but with substantially less long-term toxicity with respect to second malignancy and gonadal dysfunction.[58] Other regimens include the alternating sequence of MOPP and ABVD or the MOPP/ABV hybrid.[59, 60]

Combination chemotherapy is the treatment of choice for patients with primary mediastinal non-Hodgkin's lymphoma. Owing to the intermediate or high-grade nature of this disease as well as to the frequent presence of bulky disease and rapid dissemination, radiotherapy alone is not considered curative, supporting the role for combination chemotherapy. Doxorubicin-based regimens are the most effective chemotherapy programs for the large cell lymphomas.[61–63] Lymphoblastic lymphoma, because of its high-grade nature and propensity for central nervous system and marrow involvement, must be treated much more aggressively, including prophylaxis of the central nervous system employing intrathecal chemotherapy with or without cranial irradiation.[64]

Although heterogeneity of outcome for patients with primary mediastinal lymphoma is reported in the literature, a cure rate in excess of 50% should be achieved with an intensive, combined-modality approach.[65, 66] For patients who fail primary therapy, the long-term survival is poor, with the median survival measured in months. The ability to achieve a complete remission is of great importance for long-term survival. Patients who relapse after primary chemotherapy or fail to achieve a complete remission should proceed to salvage therapy such as high-dose chemotherapy followed by autologous bone marrow transplantation.[67]

Role of Surgery

Pretreatment Procedure

Sufficient material must be obtained to secure a diagnosis of malignancy, to determine that the neoplasm is a lymphoma, and to allow the appropriate histopathologic procedures to type the lymphoma. Histologic material can be obtained by supraclavicular nodal biopsy, cervical mediastinoscopy, anterior parasternal mediastinotomy, and, on occasion, thoracotomy.[68, 69]

The portion of the tissue must be adequate (at least 1 cc), removed cleanly to avoid crush artifact, and given directly to the surgical pathologist, who can then direct appropriate preservation techniques to aid in ancillary histoimmunochemical assay. Exploration of the neoplasm's extent and its fixation to adjacent tissue is valuable information in determining future treatment modalities.

Post-treatment Procedure

Intrathoracic relapse rate with bulky mediastinal diseases is more likely to occur in those treated with chemotherapy alone.[70–72] Occasionally, the distinction between residual mediastinal disease and a complete remission must be made. Imaging techniques may be used to attempt to differentiate viable persistent tumor from fibrosis, but in many instances this can be determined only by open biopsy.

Treatment-related complications may require surgical

resolution. Combination chemoradiotherapy to the mediastinum can produce pericardial effusion requiring pericardiocentesis, constrictive pericarditis requiring pericardectomy, esophageal stricture requiring repeated dilatations, and premature coronary artery disease requiring possible corrective surgery.

Treatment

Any type of lymphoma may occur in the thymus as a solitary neoplasm. At times, it may be impossible to differentiate a lymphocytic-predominant thymoma from a true lymphoma. If the disease is localized to the thymus, it should be removed completely by surgical extirpation, should be diagnosed with accuracy, and should receive postoperative therapy either by local radiotherapy to the surgical bed or by systemic chemotherapy, depending on the type of lymphoma.

METASTATIC TUMORS

Metastatic involvement of the mediastinum occurs by direct invasion from adjacent compartments or by lymphangitic spread resulting in lymphadenopathy. Indications for resection must be individualized and are based on the need for diagnosis, palliation, or cure. Diagnostic techniques have been described previously in the chapter. Palliative resection may be necessary with tumor encroachment on airway, esophagus, or vena cava, or with pericardial involvement with effusion and tamponade.[73] Curative resection most frequently involves thyroid carcinoma invading the mediastinum by direct extension or by local involvement of mediastinal lymph nodes, with the pretracheal and paratracheal lymph nodes most commonly involved.[74, 75]

Currently, the indications for radical lymphadenectomy of the anterior mediastinum have been established.[76, 77] This radical approach can provide meaningful cures in the majority of instances.[78] Superior mediastinal nodes are involved in 10% of differentiated thyroid carcinomas and, if not removed, produce local compression problems in 60% of the cases. Removal increases the therapeutic effectiveness of radioiodine and radiotherapy. Poorly differentiated thyroid carcinoma is almost uniformly fatal and rarely warrants extensive surgical extirpation.

Other rare indications for resection of metastatic disease include secondary melanoma, carcinoma of unknown origin,[79] pheochromocytoma,[80] pericardial metastases,[81] and laryngectomy with mediastinal tracheostomy.[82, 83]

Neurogenic Tumors

This group of tumors is most commonly situated in the posterior mediastinum. Neurogenic tumors comprise three groups: nerve sheath tumors (neurolemmoma, neurofibroma, neurosarcoma), mostly in adults; tumors of the autonomic nervous system (ganglioneuroma, ganglioneuroblastoma, neuroblastoma), mainly in children; and tumors of the paraganglionic system (chemodectoma, pheochromocytoma), which are uncommon.

In children, the majority are malignant, whereas only 1% to 4% are malignant in adults.[84, 85] Symptoms are rare in adults and are the result of local mechanical or compressive effects of the tumor. Occasionally, neuroblastomas and pheochromocytomas produce catecholamines and hypertension.

Roentgenography demonstrates a smooth homogeneous mass in the posterior mediastinum adjacent to the vertebral body in the paravertebral sulcus. Chronic pressure atrophy of ribs or vertebral bodies does not signify malignancy. CT scanning and, more recently, MRI demonstrate extension of the mass into the intervertebral foramen and its approximation with the spinal cord (Fig. 8–11). Pressure atrophy may produce bone resorption in the foramen and lead to its widening. Dumbbell conformation, with portions of the tumor extraforaminal and intraspinal, connected by a waist in the foramen, is infrequent (10%), and 40% of these cases are symptomatic.[86]

Fine-needle aspiration biopsy is usually successful in establishing a diagnosis even though the tumors are relatively acellular. Treatment in children is surgical, with combination chemotherapy in the more malignant varieties. Treatment in adults is expectant, with surgery advised only for patients with very large lesions (> 5 cm), those with impending symptoms, those producing symptoms, or those with intraspinal extension.

Endocrine Tumors

Thyroid tumors and more commonly benign goiters may occasionally descend into the anterior mediastinum.[87–90] The middle and posterior mediastinum are less frequently involved.[91] Usually patients are euthyroid (85%) and

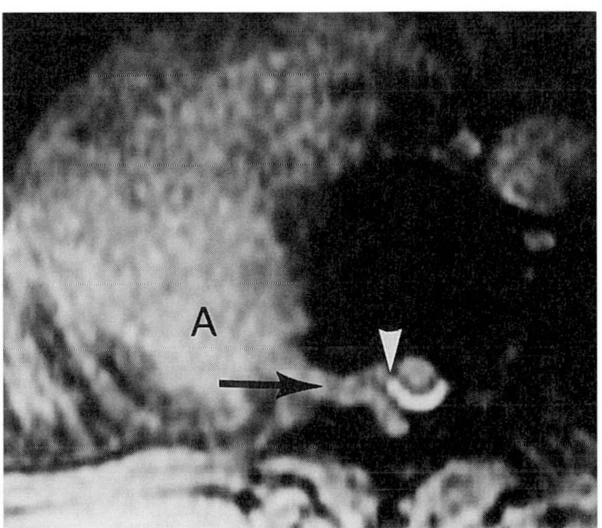

FIGURE 8–11. MRI scan detailing a large benign schwannoma (A) involving the intervertebral foramen (black arrow) and the ipsilateral one half of the spinal column with cord approximation (white arrow).

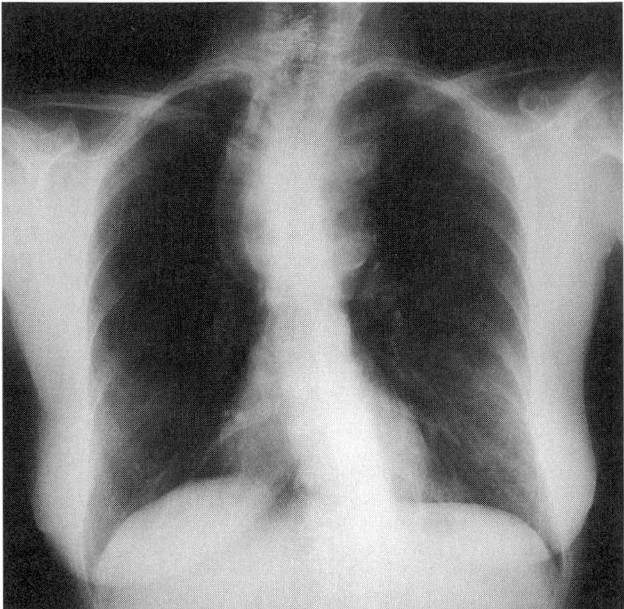

FIGURE 8–12. Posteroanterior chest radiograph identifying a large retrosternal goiter with displacement of the trachea to the right and extension below the aortic arch. This patient presented with stridor and hoarseness.

asymptomatic but, on occasion, may demonstrate symptoms of thyroid dysfunction and local compressive effects: dyspnea, dysphagia, impairment of venous return, and hoarseness (Figs. 8–12 and 8–13). Effective treatment for intrathoracic goiter is aimed primarily at reducing the size of the goiter, since the majority of symptoms are secondary to compression. Early removal of an enlarged thyroid electively can preclude emergency acute compression and compromise of the airway. Rarely does medical treatment, consisting of either radioiodine or hormone replacement, produce a satisfactory response. For these reasons, plus the fact that a goiter may contain an occult carcinoma, medical therapy should be reserved for patients that are unwilling or medically unfit to have surgery.

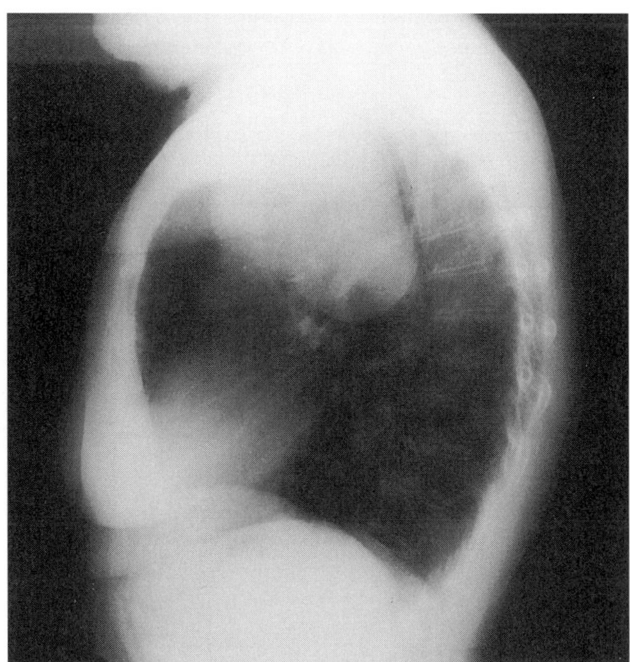

FIGURE 8–13. Lateral chest radiograph of a patient with a retrosternal goiter.

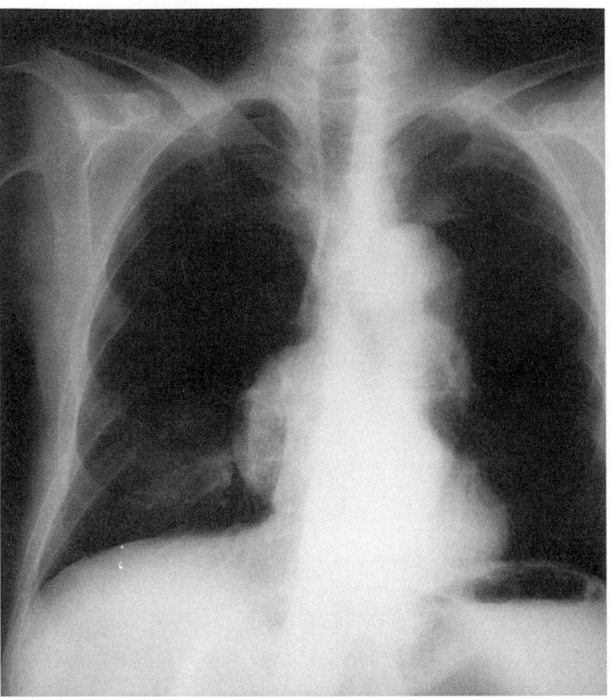

FIGURE 8–14. Chest radiograph of a patient with a liposarcoma of the posterior mediastinum seen as a large mass in the right parapericardial region.

Twenty percent of patients with hyperparathyroidism have parathyroid adenomas or hyperplastic parathyroid glands in the mediastinum, and 80% are associated with the thymus gland.[92] Most of these benign conditions are found in the mediastinum after unsuccessful neck exploration. Most can be identified and resected through the same collar incision, and only the rare intrathymic tumors require sternotomy.[93] If hypercalcemia persists after a complete neck exploration, the mediastinum should be explored after initial investigations with high-resolution CT scanning, ultrasonography, and technetium-thallium subtraction imaging.[94]

Mesenchymal Tumors

A variety of mesenchymal tumors are seen infrequently in the mediastinum, and 50% are malignant.[95] Lipomas are the most common soft tissue tumor, usually located in the anteroinferior mediastinum and often confused with the omental fat in a Morgagni hernia and thymolipoma. Liposarcoma is rare, highly malignant, and presents clinically quite late (Fig. 8–14).[96]

Endothelial tumors, cystic hygromas, and hemangiomas

are also rare. The majority of cystic hygromas (lymphangiomas) are cervical, with 10% extending into the mediastinum. Less than 10% are primary mediastinal.[97] Mediastinal hemangiomas are usually benign, asymptomatic, and, when removed, seldom recur.[98] Mediastinal fibroma (benign fibrous mesothelioma) may be associated with hypoglycemia and may transform into fibrosarcoma.[88] Each of these rarities dictates its own approach to treatment. With enlargement or symptoms, or both, most are removed surgically.

References

1. Baron RL, Levitt RG, Sagel SS, et al: Computed tomography in the evaluation of mediastinal widening. Radiology 138:107–113, 1981.
2. Front D, Ben-Haim S, Israel O, et al: Lymphoma: Predictive value of Ga-67 scintigraphy after treatment. Radiology 182:359–363, 1992.
3. Nichols CR: Mediastinal germ cell tumors: Clinical features and biologic correlates. Chest 99:472–479, 1991.
4. Weisbrod GL: Percutaneous fine needle biopsy of the mediastinum. Clin Chest Med 8:27–41, 1987.
5. McNeill TM, Chamberlain JM: Diagnostic anterior mediastinotomy. Ann Thorac Surg 2:532–540, 1966.
6. Pearson FG, Nelems JM, Henderson RD, et al: The role of mediastinoscopy in the selection of treatment for bronchial carcinoma with involvement of superior mediastinal lymph nodes. J Thorac Cardiovasc Surg 64:382–390, 1972.
7. Lewis RJ, Caccavale RJ, Sisler GE: Special report: Video endoscopic thoracic surgery. N Engl J Med 88:473–475, 1991.
8. Masaoka A, Monden Y, Nakahara K, et al: Follow-up study of thymomas with special reference to their clinical stages. Cancer 48:2485–2492, 1981.
9. Wilkins EW, Grillo HC, Scannell JG, et al: Role of staging in prognosis and management of thymoma. Ann Thorac Surg 51:888–892, 1991.
10. Percarmona E, Rendina EA, Venuta F, et al: Analysis of prognostic factors and clinicopathologic staging of thymoma. Ann Thorac Surg 55:534–538, 1990.
11. Davis SE, McCartney JC, Camplejohn RS, et al: DNA flow cytometry of thymomas. Histopathology 15:77–83, 1989.
12. Asamura H, Nakajima T, Mukai K, et al: Degree of malignancy of thymic epithelial tumors in terms of nuclear DNA content and nuclear area: An analysis of 39 cases. Am J Pathol 133:615–622, 1988.
13. Herman SJ, Holub RV, Weisbrod GL, et al: Anterior mediastinal masses: Utility of transthoracic needle biopsy. Radiology 180:167–170, 1991.
14. Nakahara K, Ohno K, Hashimoto J, et al: Thymoma: Results with complete resection and adjuvant postoperative irradiation in 141 consecutive patients. J Thorac Cardiovasc Surg 95:1041–1047, 1988.
15. Masuda H, Ogata T, Kikuchi K, et al: Total replacement of superior vena cava because of invasive thymoma: Seven year's survival. J Thorac Cardiovasc Surg 95:1083–1085, 1988.
16. Urgosi A, Monetti U, Rossi G, et al: Role of radiation therapy in locally advanced thymoma. Radiother Oncol 19:273–280, 1990.
17. Haniuda M, Morimoto M, Nishimura H, et al: Adjuvant radiotherapy after complete resection of thymoma. Ann Thorac Surg 54:311–315, 1992.
18. Macchiarini P, Chella A, Ducci F, et al: Neoadjuvant chemotherapy, surgery, and postoperative radiation therapy for invasive thymoma. Cancer 68:706–713, 1991.
19. Hu E, Levine J: Chemotherapy of malignant thymoma: Case report and review of the literature. Cancer 57:1101–1104, 1986.
20. Evans WK, Thompson DM, Simpson WJ, et al: Combination chemotherapy in invasive thymoma: Role of COPP. Cancer 46:1523–1527, 1980.
21. Goldel N, Boning L, Fredrik A, et al: Chemotherapy of invasive thymoma: A retrospective study of 22 cases. Cancer 63:1493–1500, 1989.
22. Fornasiero A, Daniele O, Ghiotto C, et al: Chemotherapy for invasive thymoma: A thirteen year experience. Cancer 68:30–33, 1991.
23. Loehrer PJ, Perez CA, Roth IM, et al: Chemotherapy for advanced thymoma: Preliminary results of an intergroup study. Ann Intern Med 113:520–524, 1990.
24. Luna MA, Johnson DE: Postmortem findings in testicular tumors. In Johnson DE (ed): Testicular Tumors. New York: Medical Examination Publishing, 1975.
25. Willis RA: Borderland of Embryology and Pathology, 2nd ed. Washington, DC: Butterworth's, 1962, p 442.
26. Knapp RH, Hurt RD, Payne WS, et al: Malignant germ cell tumors of the mediastinum. J Thorac Cardiovasc Surg 89:82–89, 1985.
27. Dehner LP: Germ cell tumors of the mediastinum. Semin Diagn Pathol 7:266–284, 1990.
28. Lee KS, Im JG, Han CH, et al: Malignant primary germ cell tumors of the mediastinum: CT features. AJR 153:947–951, 1989.
29. Nichols CR, Saxman S, Williams SD, et al: Primary mediastinal non-seminomatous germ cell tumors—a modern single institution experience. Cancer 65:1641–1646, 1990.
30. Lewis BD, Hurt RD, Payne WS, et al: Benign teratomas of the mediastinum. J Thorac Cardiovasc Surg 86:727–731, 1983.
31. Jain KK, Bosl GJ, Bains MS, et al: The treatment of extragonadal seminoma. J Clin Oncol 2:820–827, 1984.
32. Lemarie E, Assouline PS, Diot P, et al: Primary mediastinal germ cell tumors: Results of a French retrospective study. Chest 102:1477–1483, 1992.
33. Wright CD, Kesler KA, Nichols CR, et al: Primary mediastinal nonseminomatous germ cell tumors: Results of a multimodality approach. J Thorac Cardiovasc Surg 99:210–217, 1990.
34. Kay PH, Wells FC, Goldstraw P: A multidisciplinary approach to primary nonseminomatous germ cell tumors of the mediastinum. Ann Thorac Surg 44:578–582, 1987.
35. Saxman S, Nichols CR, Williams SD, Loehrer PJ, Einhorn LH: Mediastinal yolk sac tumor, the Indiana University experience, 1976–1988. J Thorac Cardiovasc Surg 102:913–916, 1991.
36. Williams SD, Birch R, Einhorn LH, et al: Treatment of disseminated germ cell tumors with cisplatin, bleomycin, and either vinblastine or etoposide. N Engl J Med 316:1435–1440, 1987.
37. Loehrer P, Einhorn L, Williams S: VP-16 plus ifosfamide and cisplatin as salvage therapy in refractory germ cell cancer. J Clin Oncol 4:528–536, 1986.
38. Nichols CR, Roth BJ, Heerema N, et al: Haematologic neoplasia associated with primary mediastinal germ cell tumors. N Engl J Med 322:1425–1429, 1990.
39. DeMent SH: Association between mediastinal germ cell tumors and haematologic malignancies. Hum Pathol 21:699–703, 1990.
40. Ladanyi M, Samaniego F, Reuter VE, et al: Cytogenetic and immunohistochemical evidence for the germ cell origin of a subset of acute leukemias associated with mediastinal germ cell tumors. J Natl Cancer Inst 82:221–227, 1990.
41. Myers TJ, Kessimian N, Schwartz S: Mediastinal germ cell tumor associated with the hemophagocytic syndrome. Ann Intern Med 15:504–505, 1988.
42. Nichols CR, Heerema NA, Palmer C, et al: Klinefelter's syndrome associated with mediastinal germ cell neoplasms. J Clin Oncol 5:1290–1294, 1987.
43. Hurt RD, Bruckman JE, Farrow GM, et al: Primary anterior mediastinal seminoma. Cancer 49:1658–1663, 1982.
44. Lee YM, Jackson SM: Primary seminoma of the mediastinum: Cancer Control Agency of British Columbia experience. Cancer 55:450–452, 1985.
45. Einhorn LH: Treatment of testicular cancer: A new and improved protocol. J Clin Oncol 8:1777–1781, 1990.
46. Vogelzang NJ, Raghavan D, Anderson RW, et al: Mediastinal nonseminomatous germ cell tumors: The role of combined modality therapy. Ann Thorac Surg 33:333–339, 1982.
47. Lack EE, Weinstein HJ, Welch KJ: Mediastinal germ cell tumors in childhood: A clinical and pathological study of 21 cases. J Thorac Cardiovasc Surg 89:826–835, 1985.
48. Lichtenstein AK, Levine A, Taylor CR, et al: Primary mediastinal lymphoma in adults. Am J Med 68:509–514, 1980.
49. Blank N, Castellino RA: The mediastinum in Hodgkin's and non-Hodgkin's lymphomas. J Thorac Imaging 2:66–71, 1987.
50. Jones SE, Fuks Z, Bull M, et al: Non-Hodgkin's lymphomas. IV. Clinicopathologic correlation in 405 cases. Cancer 31:806–823, 1973.
51. Murphy S, Jaffe ES: Terminal transferase activity and lymphoblastic neoplasms. N Engl J Med 311:1373–1374, 1984.

52. Rosen PJ, Feinstein DI, Pattengale PK, et al: Convoluted lymphocytic lymphoma in adults: A clinicopathologic entity. Ann Intern Med 89:319–324, 1978.
53. Lamarre L, Jacobson JO, Aisenberg AC, et al: Primary large cell lymphoma of the mediastinum: A histologic and immunophenotypic study of 29 cases. Am J Surg Pathol 13:730–739, 1989.
54. Sutcliffe SB: Primary mediastinal malignant lymphoma. Semin Thorac Cardiovasc Surg 4:55–67, 1992.
55. Lee CK, Blumfield CD, Goldman AI, et al: Prognostic significance of mediastinal involvement in Hodgkin's disease treated with curative radiotherapy. Cancer 46:2403–2409, 1980.
56. Hoppe RT: The management of bulky mediastinal Hodgkin's disease. Hematol Oncol Clin North Am 3:265–276, 1989.
57. DeVita VT Jr, Serpick AA, Carbone PP: Combination chemotherapy in the treatment of advanced Hodgkin's disease. Ann Intern Med 73:881–895, 1970.
58. Bonadonna G, Zucali R, Monfardini S, et al: Combination chemotherapy of Hodgkin's disease with Adriamycin, bleomycin and vinblastine and imidazole carboxamide versus MOPP. Cancer 36:252–259, 1975.
59. Klimo P, Connors JM: An update on the Vancouver experience in the management of advanced Hodgkin's disease treated with the MOPP/ABV hybrid program. Semin Hematol 25(Suppl 2):34–40, 1988.
60. Canellos GP, Anderson JR, Propert KJ, et al: Chemotherapy of advanced Hodgkin's disease with MOPP, ABVD, or MOPP alternating with ABVD. N Engl J Med 327:1478–1484, 1992.
61. Yi PI, Coleman M, Saltz L, et al: Chemotherapy for large cell lymphoma: A status update. Semin Oncol 17:60–73, 1990.
62. Fisher RI, Gaynor ER, Dahlberg S, et al: Comparison of a standard regimen (CHOP) with three intensive chemotherapy regimens for advanced non-Hodgkin's lymphoma. N Engl J Med 328:1002–1006, 1993.
63. Armitage JO: Treatment of non-Hodgkin's lymphoma. N Engl J Med 328:1023–1030, 1993.
64. Bertino JR: Long-term remissions in lymphoblastic lymphoma. J Clin Oncol 1:515, 1983.
65. Todeschini G, Ambrosetti A, Meneghini V, et al: Mediastinal large B-cell lymphoma with sclerosis: A clinical study of 21 patients. J Clin Oncol 8:804–808, 1990.
66. Jacobson JO, Aisenberg AC, Lamarre L, et al: Mediastinal large cell lymphoma: An uncommon subset of adult lymphoma curable with combined modality therapy. Cancer 62:1893–1898, 1988.
67. Canellos GP, Nadler L, Takvorian T: Autologous bone marrow transplantation in the treatment of malignant lymphoma and Hodgkin's disease. Semin Hematol 25(Suppl 2):58–65, 1988.
68. Yellin A, Pak HY, Burke JS, et al: Surgical management of lymphoma involving the chest. Ann Thorac Surg 44:363–369, 1987.
69. Ricci C, Rendina EA, Venuta F, et al: Surgical approach to isolated mediastinal lymphoma. J Thorac Cardiovasc Surg 99:691–695, 1990.
70. Jochelson M, Mauch P, Balikian J, et al: The significance of the residual mediastinal mass in treated Hodgkin's disease. J Clin Oncol 3:637–640, 1985.
71. Radford JA, Cowan RA, Flanagan M: The significance of residual mediastinal abnormality of the chest radiograph following treatment for Hodgkin's disease. J Clin Oncol 6:940–946, 1988.
72. Orlandi E, Lazzarino M, Brusamolino E, et al: Residual mediastinum widening following therapy in Hodgkin's disease. Hematol Oncol 8:125–131, 1990.
73. Goldberg M: Metastatic tumors to the mediastinum. Semin Thorac Cardiovasc Surg 4:68–69, 1992.
74. Crile G Jr: The fallacy of the conventional radical neck dissection for papillary carcinoma of the thyroid. Ann Surg 145:317–320, 1957.
75. Gordon PR, Huvos AG, Strong EW: Medullary carcinoma of the thyroid gland. Cancer 31:915–924, 1973.
76. Thompson NW, Nishiyama RH, Harness JK: Thyroid carcinoma: Current controversies. Curr Probl Surg 15:33, 1978.
77. Lynn J, Gamoros OI, Taylor S: Medullary thyroid cancer. World J Surg 5:27–32, 1981.
78. Niederle B, Roka R, Fritsch A: Transsternal operations in thyroid cancer. Surgery 98:1154–1161, 1985.
79. Greco FA, Vaughn WK, Hainsworth JD: Advanced poorly differentiated carcinoma of unknown primary site; recognition of a treatable syndrome. Ann Intern Med 104:547–553, 1986.
80. Thompson NW, All MD, Shapiro B, et al: Extraadrenal and metastatic pheochromocytoma: The role of I meta-iodobengyl-guanadine (^{131}I-MIBG) in localization and management. World J Surg 8:605–611, 1984.
81. Hankins JR, Satterfield JR, Aisner J, et al: Pericardial window for malignant pericardial effusion. Ann Thorac Surg 30:465–471, 1980.
82. Grillo HC: Terminal or mural tracheostomy in the anterior mediastinum. J Thorac Cardiovasc Surg 51:422–427, 1966.
83. Orringer MB, Sloan H: Anterior mediastinal tracheotomy. J Thorac Cardiovasc Surg 78:850–859, 1979.
84. Gale AW, Jelihovsky T, Grant AF, et al: Neurogenic tumors of the mediastinum. Ann Thorac Surg 17:434–443, 1974.
85. Reed J, Hallet KK, Feigen DS: Neural tumors of the thorax: Subject view from the AFIP. Radiology 126:9–17, 1978.
86. Akwari OE, Payne WS, Onofrio BM, et al: Dumbbell neurogenic tumors of the mediastinum. Mayo Clinic Proc 53:353–358, 1978.
87. Katlic RM, Grillo HC, Wang CA: Substernal goiter: Analysis of eighty Massachusetts General Hospital cases. Am J Surg 149:283–287, 1985.
88. Wychulis AR, Payne WS, Clagett OT, et al: Surgical treatment of mediastinal tumors: A 40 year experience. J Thorac Cardiovasc Surg 62:379–385, 1971.
89. Michel LA, Bradpiece HA: Surgical management of substernal goiter. Br J Surg 75:565–569, 1988.
90. Wakeley CPG, Mulvaney JH: Intrathoracic goiter. Surg Gynecol Obstet 70:702–710, 1940.
91. Sweet RH: Intrathoracic goiter located in the posterior mediastinum. Surg Gynecol Obstet 89:57–66, 1949.
92. Nathaniels EK, Nathaniels AM, Wang C: Mediastinal parathyroid tumors. Ann Surg 171:165–170, 1970.
93. Russell CF, Edis AJ, Scholz DA, et al: Mediastinal parathyroid tumors: Experience with 38 tumors requiring mediastinotomy for removal. Ann Surg 193:805–809, 1981.
94. Stark DD, Gooding GA, Clark OH: Noninvasive parathyroid imaging. Semin Ultrasound CT MR 6:310–320, 1985.
95. Davis RD, Oldham HN, Sabiston DC: Primary cysts and neoplasms of the mediastinum: Recent changes in clinical presentation, methods of diagnosis, management, and results. Ann Thorac Surg 44:229–237, 1987.
96. Schweitzer DL, Aguam AS: Primary liposarcoma of the mediastinum. Report of a case and review of the literature. J Thorac Cardiovasc Surg 74:83–97, 1977.
97. Rice TW: Benign neoplasms and cysts of the mediastinum. Semin Thorac Cardiovasc Surg 4:25–33, 1992.
98. Cohen AJ, Sbashing RJ, Hochholzer L: Mediastinal hemangiomas. Ann Thorac Surg 43:656–659, 1987.

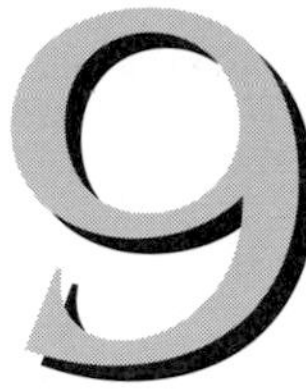

Tumors of the Chest Wall and Malignancies of the Pleura

Chest Wall Tumors

Kushagra Katariya, M.D. • Norman D. Bloom, M.D.
James C. Harvey, M.D. • Julianna Pisch, M.D.
Edward J. Beattie, M.D.

Chest wall tumors, whether primary or secondary, encompass a wide variety of bone and soft tissue disease. Most present as painful enlarging masses. Tumors may have recurred or persisted following previous resection or irradiation. All are diagnostic and therapeutic challenges. Surgical extirpation is often the best treatment. A team approach is required in diagnosis, excision, and reconstruction of chest wall defects.[1]

Primary neoplasms are uncommon. Those of the bony chest comprise 7% to 8% of all intrinsic bone tumors.[2, 3] Neoplasms of the ribs are far more common than those of the sternum.[2–5] Primary tumors of the ribs are as frequently benign as they are malignant, but benign tumors of the sternum are uncommon.

The surgical treatment and results depend on the tumor.[2–9] The prognosis of patients with benign tumors is excellent after excision, whereas the 10-year survival rate of patients with primary malignant chest wall tumors is only 13.3%.[10] A familiarity with the natural history of these tumors is fundamental for early recognition and proper treatment.

Chest wall tumors are twice as common in males as in females. Age may suggest the diagnosis.[11] The average age for the presentation of benign tumors is 26 years. Eosinophilic granulomas, aneurysmal bone cysts, and osteochondromas occur in younger populations; fibrous dysplasias and bone islands occur in older individuals. The average age for presentation with malignant lesions is 40 years. The incidence of Ewing's sarcoma peaks in adolescence. Osteogenic sarcoma, lymphoma, chondrosarcoma, and plasmacytoma occur more frequently among adults. Metastatic lesions to the thoracic skeleton are the most common lesions, and the average age of these patients is in the fifth and sixth decades of life (Table 9–1).

CLINICAL FEATURES

Pain and presence of a mass are the most frequent presenting complaints. Most patients experience both. Up to 20% of patients are asymptomatic, and their tumor is detected on routine radiographic examination.[1, 12] Other clinical features include muscle weakness, pleural effusion, and atrophy in an upper extremity in cases of brachial plexus compression by a tumor of the first or second rib.[12]

Laboratory examinations are of little value. The erythrocyte sedimentation rate (ESR) may be elevated in Ewing's sarcoma, and the alkaline phosphatase level may be elevated in osteogenic sarcoma. Electrophoresis may reveal

TABLE 9–1
Average Age of Patients with Benign or Malignant Chest Wall Tumors

Type of Tumor	Age (yr)
Benign	
Eosinophilic granuloma	10
Osteochondroma	15
Chondroma	25
Fibrous dysplasia	40
Malignant	
Ewing's sarcoma	10
Osteogenic sarcoma	15
Chondrosarcoma	30
Plasmacytoma	50

proteins specific for myeloma, although the Bence Jones protein has only rarely been identified in solitary plasmacytomas.

Radiographic examination of the chest wall is helpful in making the diagnosis and determining the extent of the disease. A local abnormality is almost always visible. Rib lesions, although visualized on posterior and lateral radiographs, are often better defined on oblique views. Computed tomography (CT) scanning is superior in defining the tumor and the extent of its local involvement. Sharp delineation and intact cortical margins as seen in radiographs are characteristic of benign tumors, whereas malignant tumors are usually poorly defined and commonly show cortical disruption. Occasionally, old rib fractures, calcified prominent costal cartilages, myositis ossificans, prominent or bifid xiphoids, and osteomyelitis of bony structures in the chest can give misleading pictures that suggest tumor. Because of this, an accurate histologic diagnosis is essential for the treatment of all chest wall tumors. Suspected primary neoplasms (benign or malignant) should be diagnosed by excisional biopsy unless larger than 2 cm, in which setting an incisional biopsy is recommended.[1] Necrotic tumors should be diagnosed by excision. However, if there is a known history of a primary neoplasm elsewhere and the chest wall mass is a suspected metastasis, needle or incisional biopsy may establish the diagnosis.[1]

Small tumors (<2 cm) should be excised, a procedure that is curative in most cases. For larger tumors, a carefully planned open biopsy is recommended to obtain adequate tissue. The incision should be made so as not to compromise a future definitive resection.[11] Opinions differ regarding "adequate" resection, method for reconstruction of the bony thorax, and manner of soft tissue reconstruction. A margin of resection grossly free of tumor by several centimeters is considered wide resection by most surgeons. This is adequate for chest wall metastases, benign tumors, and certain low-grade primary malignant bone tumors such as chondrosarcoma. More aggressive tumors, such as osteosarcoma, have the potential to spread within the marrow cavity, along the periosteum, or along the parietal pleura, and, consequently, an en bloc resection is necessary.[1] Surgical resection of advanced tumors is often incomplete, leaving microscopic margins. Such surgery is usually followed by radiotherapy.

Radiotherapy may be given by external irradiation alone or in combination with brachytherapy. Doses in the range of 60 to 65 Gy over a period of 6 to 7 weeks achieve local-regional control rates of about 85% to 90%.[13] If brachytherapy is used, the tumor bed may be implanted with afterloading catheters about 1 cm away from each other, taken through the skin. Usually, 2 to 3 days later, iridium 192 seeds in nylon ribbons are inserted into the catheters, and 20 to 30 Gy is given over the next 48 or 72 hours. To ensure even spacing of the catheters, an absorbable Vicryl mesh may be used to secure them over areas of scant tissue (Figs. 9–1 to 9–3). High total doses of radiation may be delivered when external beam irradiation is combined with brachytherapy because the rapid dose falloff outside the implanted region avoids high doses to the surrounding normal tissue.[13]

TYPES OF CHEST WALL TUMORS

The reported distribution of benign and malignant chest wall tumors in several large series is summarized in Tables 9–2 and 9–3.[11] The most common benign lesions are fibrous dysplasias, enchondromas, osteochondromas, and eosinophilic granulomas. The most common malignant lesions are chondrosarcomas, Ewing's sarcoma, plasmacytomas, and osteogenic sarcomas.

Benign Tumors

Fibrous Dysplasia

Fibrous dysplasias are usually asymptomatic and are discovered on routine radiographic examination of the chest. The characteristic lesion is a central, fusiform, lytic lesion with a homogeneous ground-glass appearance and a sharply defined edge. Throughout the mass there may be trabeculae of bone, but calcification is not prominent.[12] Pathologically, the major feature is proliferation of fibroblasts, which produces a dense, collagenous matrix. These lesions typically show extreme uptake on bone scans, presumably due to diffuse microscopic ossification.

Treatment is wide excision. Recurrences are extremely rare.[12]

Enchondroma

Enchondromas are typically located at costochondral junctions of patients in the second and third decades of life. Clinically, they are usually a painless mass on the anterior chest wall. Radiographically, the typical enchondroma is a well-defined oval or slightly lobulated area of rarefaction in the medulla, which may be situated centrally or eccentrically, with or without expansion of the cortex.[12]

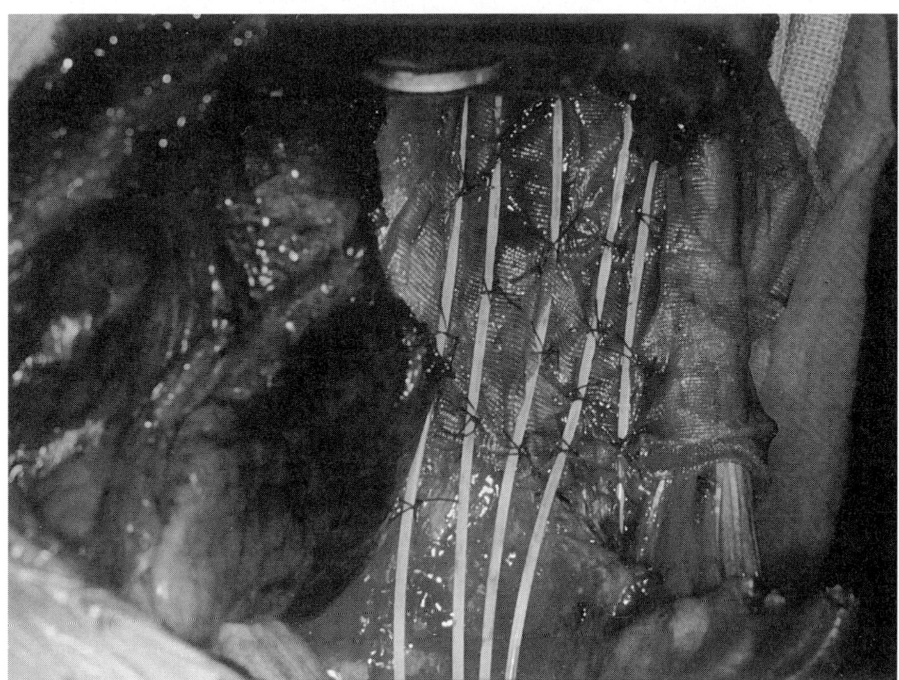

FIGURE 9–1. Plastic catheters sutured to absorbable mesh after resection of tumor. Catheter margination is reduced by using a two-layer "sandwich" of the mesh.

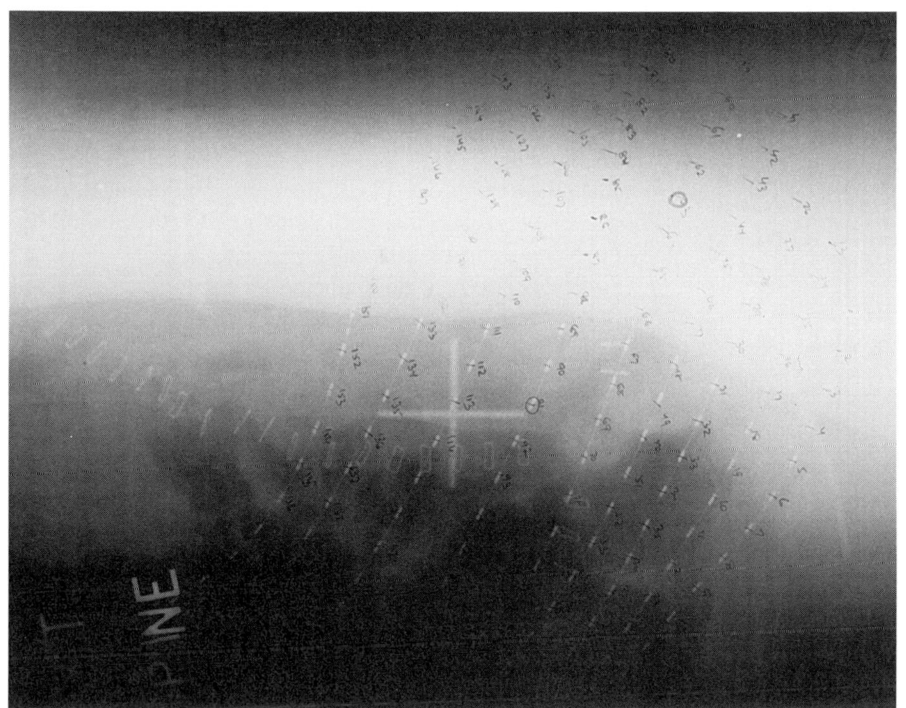

FIGURE 9–2. Radiograph with dummy sources for dose calculation in a patient with a large recurrent chest wall sarcoma. The even parallel spacing needed for good dose distribution is evident.

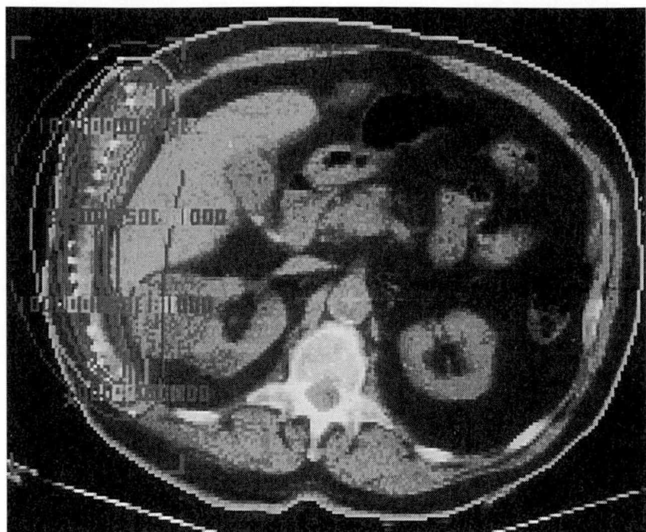

FIGURE 9–3. CT scan with superimposed isodose curves showing that the tumor bed is adequately covered for the planned radiation dose.

Calcification may be either diffuse, giving a dense, radiopaque appearance, or focal, resulting in stippling (Fig. 9–4).

Grossly, enchondromas are composed of bluish hyaline material, with foci of calcification presenting a well-defined lobular lesion located in the medullary cavity. Histology shows cartilage of varying cellularity. Untreated tumors can grow very large, sometimes exceeding 4 cm, which some pathologists believe is the upper limit for benign tumors.[14]

Excision of the involved costal cartilage along with a short segment of the accompanying rib is curative.

Osteochondromas

Osteochondromas are usually seen in the first two decades of life. There is no sex predilection. Ordinarily, the only finding is a palpable mass. Radiographically, the characteristic appearance is a projection of cortical bone with a cartilaginous cap. Irregular calcifications may be present in this cap (Fig. 9–5). Grossly, the tumor cortex and its peripheral covering are continuous with underlying bone, with which it often merges. Microscopically, a benign cartilaginous cap with overlying bony trabeculae formed by orderly enchondral ossification is seen.[12]

TABLE 9–2
Histologic Classification of Benign Chest Wall Tumors Reported in the Literature[2,3,10,12,34]

Type of Tumor	No. of Patients	Percentage
Fibrous dysplasia	32	29.6
Enchondroma	22	20.3
Osteochondroma	21	19.4
Eosinophilic granuloma	8	7.4
Aneurysmal bone cyst	6	5.5
Osteoblastoma	4	3.7
Bone islands	3	2.7
Hemangioma	2	1.8
Xanthoma	2	1.8
Fibroma	2	1.8
Fibroxanthoma	1	0.9
Giant cell tumor	1	0.9
Lipoma	1	0.9
Osteoid osteoma	1	0.9
Angiomatosis	1	0.9
Chondroblastoma	1	0.9
Total	108	100

TABLE 9–3
Histologic Classification of Malignant Chest Wall Tumors Reported in the Literature[2,3,10,12,34]

Type of Tumor	No. of Patients	Percentage
Chondrosarcoma	42	37.1
Myeloma	37	32.7
Ewing's sarcoma	17	15.0
Osteogenic sarcoma	10	8.8
Lymphoma	7	6.2
Total	113	

Surgical excision is necessary only in patients with pain, abnormal increase in tumor size, or atypical radiographic features. Excision of the tumor along with the entire cartilaginous cap is performed to avoid recurrence. For a tumor located on a rib, en bloc resection is often necessary.

Eosinophilic Granuloma

Most patients with eosinophilic granuloma present in the first two decades of life. Peak incidence is between 5 and 10 years of age. Radiographically, these are lytic lesions with well defined margins, with or without a reactive sclerotic rim. Grossly, the lesions contain well-demarcated areas showing focal hemorrhage. Histology reveals the characteristic infiltrate of various cells, predominantly histiocytes and eosinophils, with some giant cells, fibroblasts, lymphocytes, and plasma cells.

Some lesions heal spontaneously, but most are treated by local excision. Curettage, steroid injections, and radiotherapy have also been used.

Malignant Tumors

Chondrosarcoma

Chondrosarcomas are the most common primary malignant tumors of the chest wall. As with their benign counterpart (chondroma), the costochondral junction is the most frequent location, although the tumors may occur anywhere along the rib.

Radiography often reveals a large, lobulated tumor destroying cortical bone, calcified in a mottled manner. Grossly, the tumors show a firm, lobulated, smooth, bluish surface. Although apparently well demarcated, they cause destruction of the cortex and surrounding soft tissues. Foci of hemorrhage, calcification, and necrosis along with myxoid material are commonly present. The classic histologic

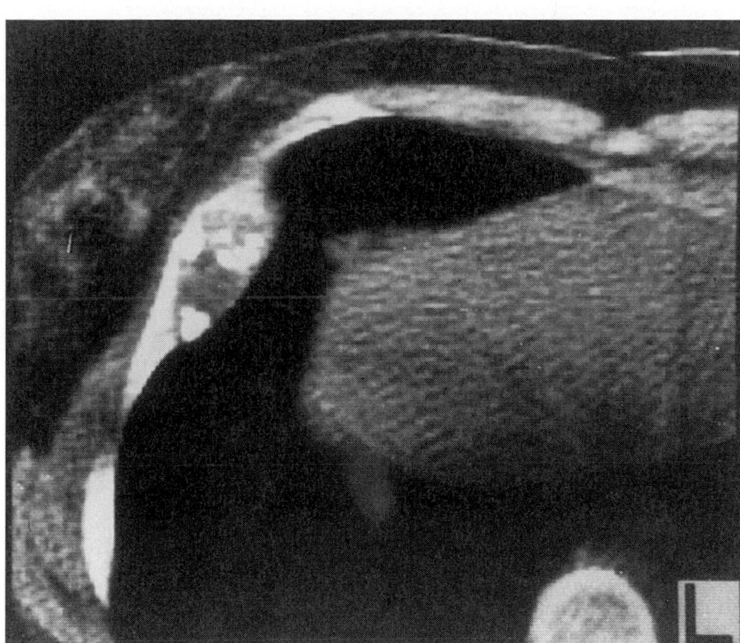

FIGURE 9–4. CT scan demonstrating an enchondroma of the fifth rib in a 17 year old.

picture shows the presence of many cells with plump nuclei and giant cartilaginous cells with large single or multiple nuclei or clumps of chromatin. There is a wide range of features, from a poorly differentiated spindle cell sarcoma showing only microscopic areas of chondroid differentiation to extremely well differentiated lesions that are indistinguishable from a benign cartilaginous tumor. Grading systems of chondrosarcomas emphasize mitotic rate and cellularity.[15–17]

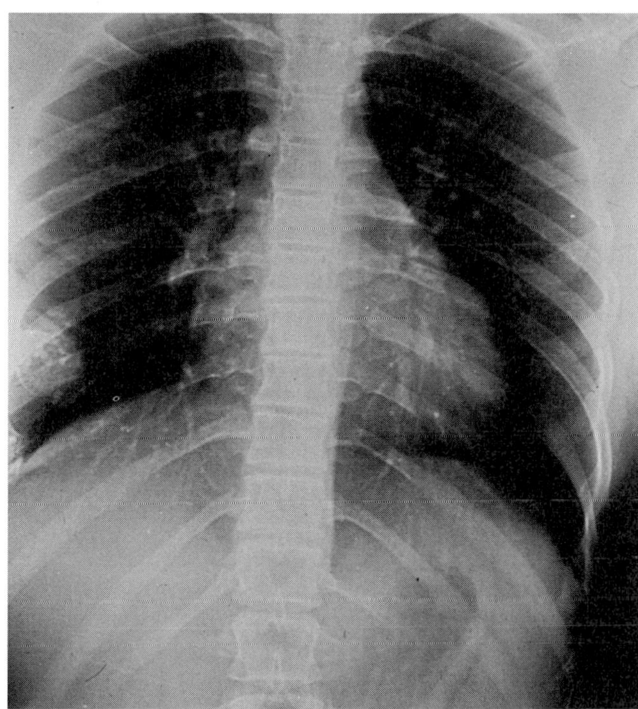

FIGURE 9–5. Osteochondromas arising in the seventh and ninth ribs found on a routine chest radiograph.

Grade I chondrosarcoma has a 5% rate of metastasis, a 92% 5-year survival rate, and an 85% 10-year survival rate; a grade II lesion has a 20% rate of metastasis, a 70% 5-year survival rate, and a 50% 10-year survival rate; a grade III lesion has a 55% rate of metastasis, a 44% 5-year survival rate, and a 28% 10-year survival rate.[11]

Definitive surgical resection is the treatment of choice, with prosthetic reconstruction whenever necessary to close the chest wall defect.[11] Opinions differ regarding what constitutes a wide resection. We advocate a surgical margin of 2 cm with a wider margin (4 cm) for higher-grade lesions. Chemotherapy and radiotherapy have no proven efficacy in the management of these tumors.

Ewing's Sarcoma Tumors

Ewing's sarcoma, a primary bone malignancy, is more often seen in younger patients, with peak incidence between 10 and 20 years of age. Patients usually present with pain, gradually increasing in severity over several months. Other clinical features include a mass, tenderness, and local erythema with or without systemic manifestations, including malaise, low-grade fever, leukocytosis, anemia, and an elevated ESR.[11]

The only consistent radiographic finding is destruction or lysis of bone, in itself a nonspecific finding,[12] with a laminated periosteal reaction (Fig. 9–6). In some instances there is widening of the medulla with sclerosis of the widened cortex and multiple layers of periosteal new bone formation, thereby producing the characteristic onion-peel appearance. Although the tumor is usually confined to a single rib, it is not uncommon for it to involve more than one. There is frequently an associated extraosseous soft tissue mass. Incisional biopsy is the initial management. Grossly, these tumors are firm, fibrous, and sometimes

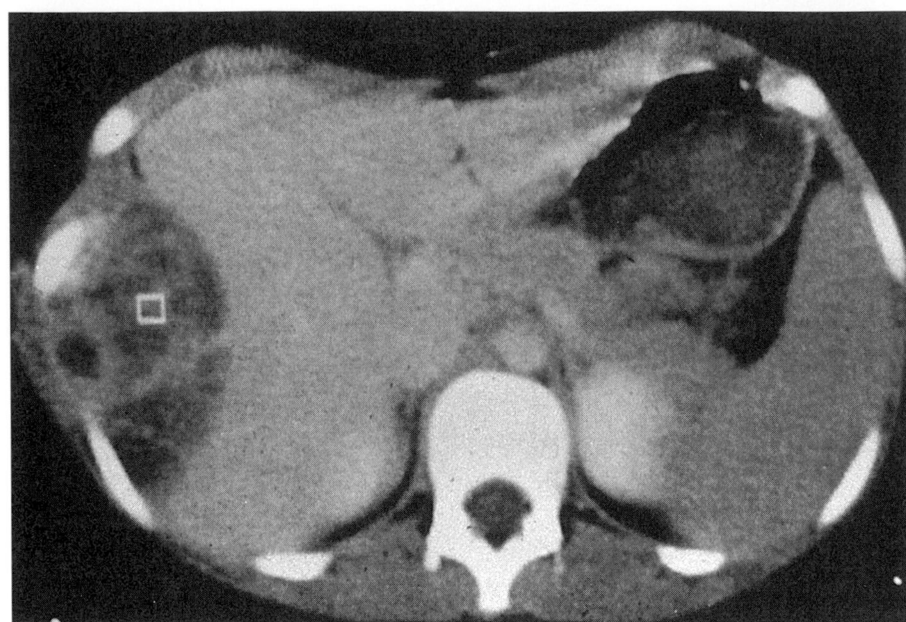

FIGURE 9–6. Ewing's sarcoma in a 12-year-old girl involving the diaphragm and compressing the right lobe of the liver.

gelatinous, with variable amounts of hemorrhage, necrosis, and cyst formation. Microscopy shows sheets of uniform, closely packed cells larger than lymphocytes with scanty cytoplasm. Tumor cells aggregate around blood vessels, thus forming perivascular rosettes.

Treatment involves a combined-modality approach with multiagent chemotherapy and radical excision. Survival rates up to 52% at 5 years have been reported.[18–20]

Plasmacytoma

Solitary plasmacytomas of bone are uncommon, occurring in 3% to 7% of patients with plasma cell myeloma.[21, 22] Approximately 30% of primary malignant tumors of the chest wall are plasmacytomas. Ribs are the third most common site after the spine and the pelvis (Fig. 9–7). Radiographically, these are well-defined punched-out, lytic lesions in the ribs. In the sternum, cortex is usually destroyed in several places and tumor invades soft tissue.[12] Solitary plasmacytomas are grossly and microscopically indistinguishable from multiple myeloma deposits. If radiographic examination of the entire skeleton and bone scans reveal no additional lesions, tissue should be obtained by needle biopsy initially. If the location of the tumor precludes a safe approach for a needle biopsy, an open surgical biopsy may be accomplished. Grossly, myeloma tissue is soft reddish gray and friable. Microscopically, it is composed of sheets of plasma cells varying in maturity, with nuclear polymorphism and prominent nucleoli noted in the poorly differentiated lesions.

Local control of a solitary plasmacytoma can be achieved with radiotherapy.[23] Radical surgery is reserved for those who fail radiotherapy and have symptomatic localized disease. Systemic chemotherapy is reserved for patients with manifestation of disease progression and dissemination. Overall, patients with plasmacytomas have an indolent course, although progression to disseminated disease eventually occurs. The median survival time is 47 months, and the 5-year survival rate is 32% after disease progression. The 5-year survival rate is 75%, 10-year survival is 52%, and 20-year survival is 37%.[11]

Osteogenic Sarcoma

Osteogenic sarcomas are the second most common primary tumors of bony origin after myelomas. In the ribs, however, they are the fourth most common and were re-

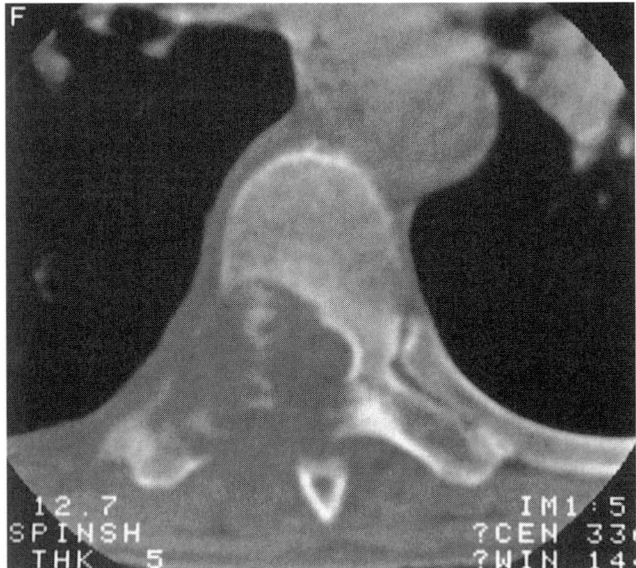

FIGURE 9–7. A solitary plasmacytoma arising from the articulation of the seventh rib with the transverse process of the thoracic vertebral body. Partial destruction of the vertebral body is noted, as well as extension into the canal with spinal cord compression.

sponsible for only 10% of the tumors reported in a collected series.[24] There is a male predilection. Peak incidence is in the second decade of life. Clinically, the tumor usually presents as a painful, rapidly expanding mass (Fig. 9–8). The duration of symptoms varies from a few weeks to many months. Radiographically, the typical sunburst appearance due to reactive periosteal new bone formation is often present; in about one half of osteosarcomas the diagnosis can be made on the radiographic appearance.

Treatment includes induction and postoperative chemotherapy with multiple drugs, including cisplatin, doxorubicin (Adriamycin), and high-dose methotrexate. Preoperative chemotherapy is used to shrink the tumor size prior to en bloc resection. Various studies, including those of Rosen et al.,[25] the Children's Cancer Study Group,[26] and the German-Austrian osteosarcoma study group,[27–29] have focused on preoperative chemotherapy, with 2-year disease-free survival rates ranging from 4% in poor responders to 91% in good responders. Additional regimens have involved intra-arterial therapy preoperatively,[30] with a disease-free survival rate of more than 80% in good responders versus only 34% in patients who had a poor or no response.

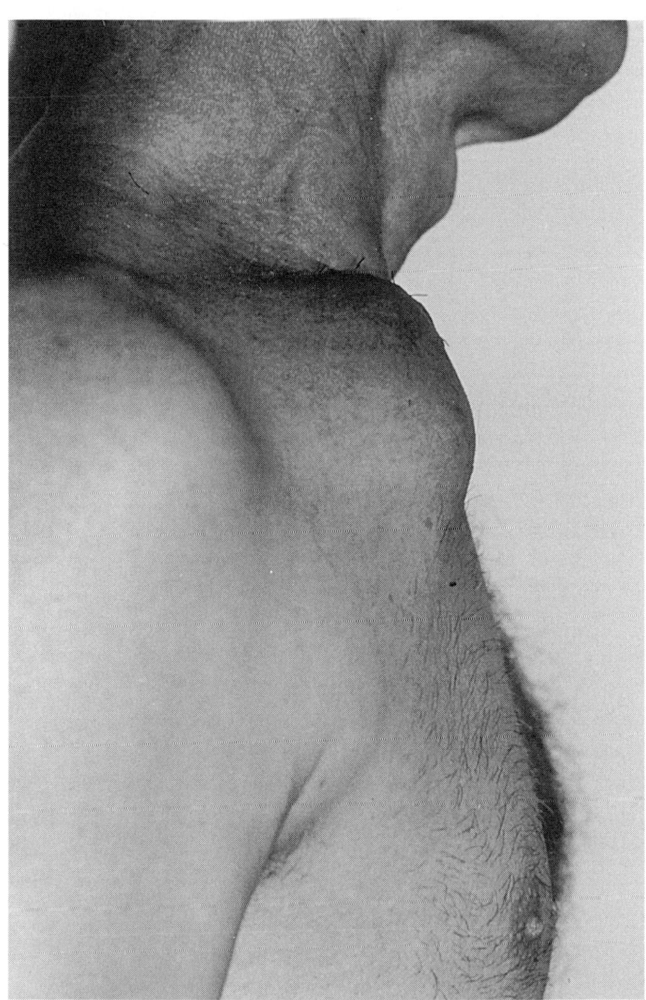

FIGURE 9–8. Radiation-induced osteogenic sarcoma of the clavicle with involvement of the first and second ribs.

Soft Tissue Sarcomas

The most common type of soft tissue sarcomas arising in the thoracic skeleton are fibrous in origin, predominantly malignant fibrous histiocytomas.[11] Others, including dermatofibrosarcoma protuberans, liposarcomas, fibrosarcomas, angiosarcomas, and primitive neuroectodermal tumors, have been reported.[31–35] Neuroectodermal tumors are a rare, highly malignant, small cell neoplasm that most often arises from the chest wall or paravertebral region.[36] Askin's tumors, originally described in children, may be a subset of this small cell neuroectodermal group. Predisposing factors to the development of sarcomas include a history of irradiation or one of the various hereditary syndromes, such as von Recklinghausen's neurofibromatosis, Werner's syndrome, or Gardner's syndrome.[32]

Wide excision is the mainstay of therapy. Prognosis depends on the histologic grade of the tumor. Fibrosarcomas have a 5-year survival rate of 55%.[33] Other sarcomas with similar prognosis include liposarcomas and dermatofibrosarcomas.[34] Angiosarcomas and neuroectodermal tumors have the worst prognosis.[35] Past surgical reports have not stressed the need for an aggressive approach in treating Askin's tumors. The importance of complete excision when possible cannot be overemphasized. This may be followed by aggressive combinations of chemotherapy.[37]

CHEST WALL RECONSTRUCTION

There has been considerable discussion in the literature regarding how the thorax should be reconstructed.[38–40] Whether or not to reconstruct depends on the size and location of the defect, the presence of wound infection, and whether the tumor has been previously irradiated.[39] With large resections, reconstruction may be necessary to obtain sufficient chest wall fixation for vital respiratory effort and function.

Various prosthetic meshes[1, 41, 42] have been used to stabilize the bony thorax (Fig. 9–9*A* and *B*). Prolene has a double-stitch knit and is therefore rigid in all directions, while Marlex has a single-stitch knit and is rigid in only one direction.[11] Gore-Tex has the advantage of being impermeable to the flow of air and water across the chest wall.[11] Rigid mesh sandwiches of methyl methacrylate have also been used.[1] Other materials used to repair defects include periosteum, rib grafts, titanium mesh, and fiberglass, but these have not gained wide acceptance.[11] Muscle transposition alone may provide adequate chest wall stability.

Soft tissue reconstruction is best accomplished by muscle transposition.[43–46] All chest wall muscles can be elevated and rotated a significant distance with or without the overlying skin (Fig. 9–10*A* to *D*). Campbell[47] first reported the use of a latissimus dorsi muscle flap in 1950. The transverse rectus abdominis myocutaneous (TRAM) flap is useful for chest wall defects as well (Fig. 9–11*A* and *B*). Large omental flaps and microvascular flaps are also used

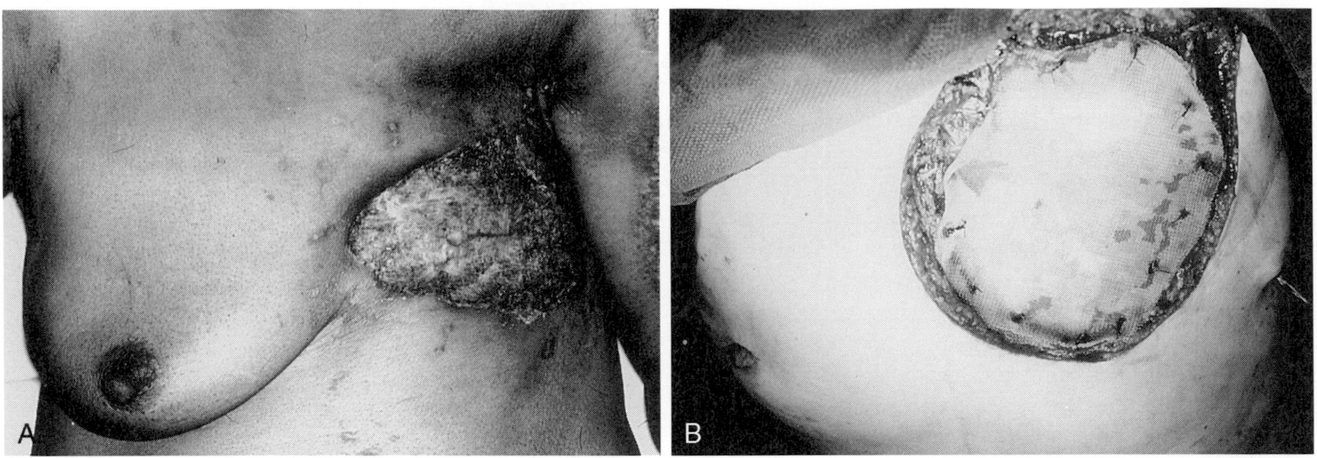

FIGURE 9–9. *A,* Ulcerative recurrent breast carcinoma after mastectomy and radiotherapy. *B,* Chest wall resection and prosthetic mesh reconstruction of the defect.

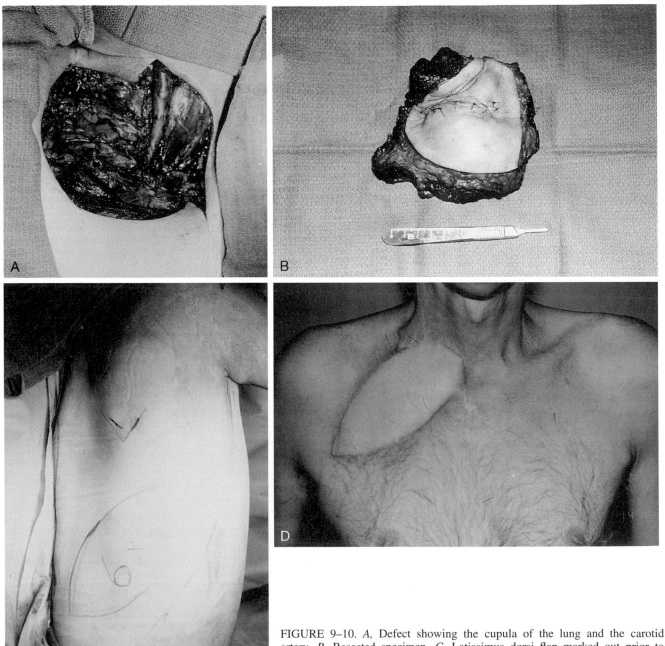

FIGURE 9–10. *A,* Defect showing the cupula of the lung and the carotid artery. *B,* Resected specimen. *C,* Latissimus dorsi flap marked out prior to elevation and rotation. *D,* Flap in position 1 month after resection.

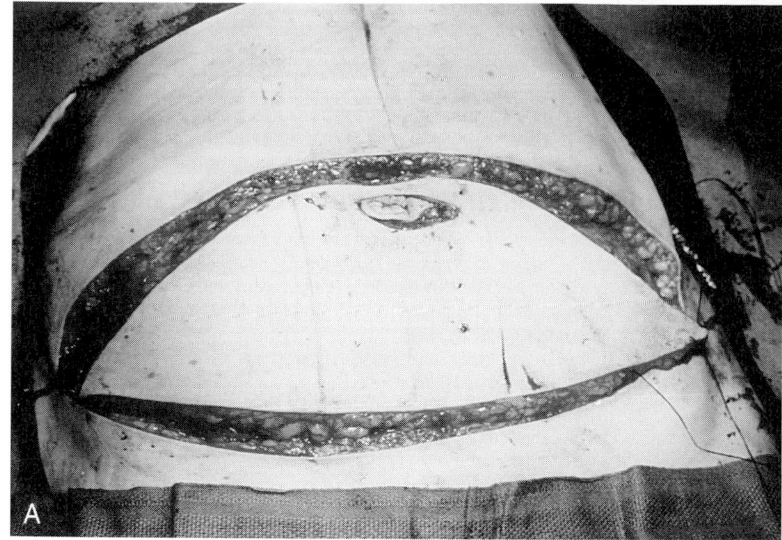

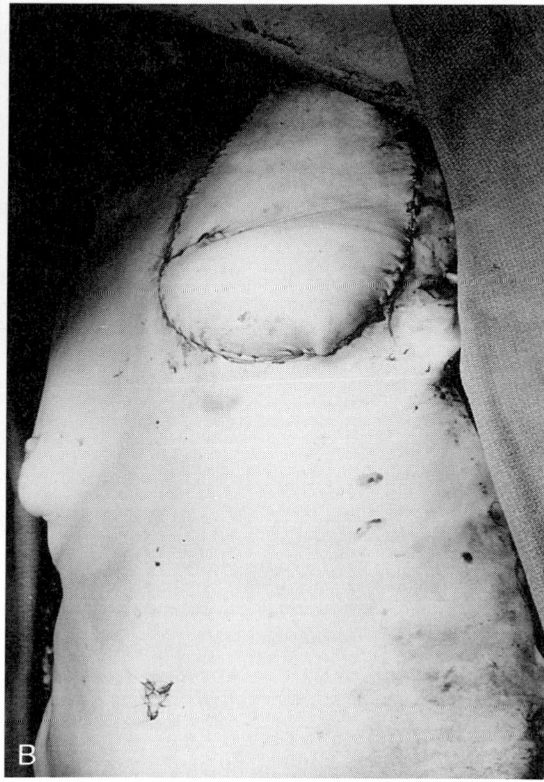

FIGURE 9–11. *A,* TRAM flap being elevated. *B,* Flap in position with a reconstructed umbilicus.

to close large chest wall defects.[48–51] The latter technique is particularly useful if local flaps have previously failed of if the area had been irradiated.

References

1. Pairolero PC, Phillip GA: Chest wall tumors. J Thorac Cardiovasc Surg 90:367–372, 1985.
2. Pascuzzi CA, Dahlin DC, Clagett OT: Primary tumors of the ribs and sternum. Surg Gynecol Obstet 104:390–406, 1957.
3. Teitelbaum SL: Twenty years' experience with tumors of the bony thorax at a large institution. J Thorac Cardiovasc Surg 66:776–782, 1972.
4. Ochsner A, Lucas GL, McFarland GB: Tumors of the thoracic skeleton: Review of 134 cases. J Thorac Cardiovasc Surg 52:311–319, 1966.
5. Hochberg LA, Crastnopol P: Tumors of the ribs. Dis Chest 28:406–414, 1955.
6. Hedblom CA: Tumors of the bony chest wall. Arch Surg 3:56–63, 1921.
7. Martini N, Huvos AG, Smith J, Beattie EJ: Primary malignant tumors of the sternum. Surg Gynecol Obstet 138:391–397, 1974.
8. Hochberg LA: Primary tumors of the ribs: Review of the literature and presentation of eleven cases not reported previously. Arch Surg 67:566–576, 1953.
9. Sommer GNJ, Major RC: Neoplasms of the bony thoracic wall. Ann Surg 115:51–59, 1942.
10. Threlkel JB, Adkins RB Jr: Primary chest wall tumors. Ann Thorac Surg 11:450–459, 1971.
11. Bloom ND: Chest wall, pleura and sternum. In Beattie EJ, Bloom ND, Harvey JC (eds): Thoracic Surgical Oncology. New York: Churchill Livingstone, 1992 pp 251–272.
12. Sabanathan S, Salama FD, Morgan WE, Harvey JA: Primary chest wall tumors. Ann Thorac Surg 39:4–15, 1985.
13. Pisch J, Berson AM, Harvey JC, et al: Absorbable mesh in the placement of temporary implants. Int J Radiat Oncol Biol Phys 28:719–722, 1994.
14. Jaffe HL: Tumors and Tumorous Conditions of the Bones and Joints. Philadelphia: Lea & Febiger, 1958.
15. Evans HL, Ayala AG, Romsdahl MM: Prognostic factors in chondrosarcoma of bone. Cancer 40:818–831, 1971.
16. Marcove R, Huvos A: Cartilaginous tumors of the ribs. Cancer 27:794–808, 1971.
17. Gitelis S, Bertoni F, Picci P, et al: Chondrosarcoma of bone. J Bone Joint Surg 63A:1248–1257, 1981.
18. Fernandez CH, Lindbergh RD, Sautow WW, et al: Localized Ewing's sarcoma: Treatment and results. Cancer 34:143–148, 1974.
19. Hustu OH, Pinkel D, Pratt CB: Treatment of clinically localized Ewing's sarcoma with radiotherapy and combination chemotherapy. Cancer 30:1522–1527, 1972.
20. Pomeray TC, Johnson RE: Combined modality therapy of Ewing's sarcoma. Cancer 35:36–47, 1975.
21. Chak L, Coix RS, Bostwick DC, et al: Solitary plasmacytoma of bone: Treatment progression and survival. J Clin Oncol 5:1811–1815, 1987.
22. Knowling MA, Harwood AR, Bergsagel DE: Comparison of extramedullary plasmacytomas with solitary and multiple plasma cell tumors of the bone. J Clin Oncol 1:255–262, 1983.
23. Mill WB, Griffith R: The role of radiation therapy in the management of plasma cell tumors. Cancer 45:647–652, 1980.
24. Lichtenstein L: Bone Tumors. St. Louis: CV Mosby, 1977.
25. Rosen G, Marcove R, Caparros B, et al: Primary osteogenic sarcoma. The rationale for preoperative chemotherapy and delayed surgery. Cancer 43:2163–2169, 1979.
26. Krailo M, Ertel I, Makley J, et al: A randomized study comparing high dose methotrexate with moderate dose methotrexate as components of adjuvant chemotherapy in childhood nonmetastatic osteosarcoma: A report from the Children's Cancer Study Group. Med Pediatr Oncol 15:69–76, 1987.
27. Winkler K, Beron G, Kotz R: Neoadjuvant chemotherapy for osteogenic sarcoma: Results of a cooperative German/Austrian study. J Clin Oncol 2:617–621, 1984.
28. Winkler K, Beron G, Kotz R: Adjuvant and neoadjuvant chemotherapy of osteosarcoma: Experience of the German-Austrian cooperative osteosarcoma studies (COSS). In Van Oosteram AT, Van Unnik JAM (eds): Management of Soft Tissue and Bone Sarcomas. New York: Raven Press, 1986, p 275.

29. Jaffe N, Prudich J, Knappo J: Treatment of primary osteosarcoma with intraarterial and intravenous high dose methotrexate. J Clin Oncol 1:428–433, 1983.
30. Jaffe N, Raymond K, Ayala A: Effect of cumulative courses of intra-arterial *cis*-diaminedichloroplatin-II on the primary tumor in osteosarcoma. Cancer 63:63–67, 1989.
31. Mindell ER, Shah NK, Webster JH: Postradiation sarcoma of the bone and soft tissue. Orthop Clin North Am 8:821–826, 1977.
32. Lynch HT, Krush AS, Harlan WL, et al: Association of soft tissue sarcoma, leukemia and brain tumors in families affected with breast cancer. Am Surg 39:194–199, 1973.
33. Graeger JA, Patel MK, Briele HA, et al: Soft tissue sarcoma of the adult thoracic wall. Cancer 59:370–377, 1987.
34. Graeber GM, Snyder RJ, Fleming AW, et al: Initial and long term results in the management of primary chest wall neoplasms. Ann Thorac Surg 34:664–674, 1982.
35. Stefanko J, Turnbul AD, Helson LA, et al: Primitive neuroectodermal tumors of the chest wall. J Surg Oncol 37:33–38, 1982.
36. Askin FB, Rosa J, Siobley RK, et al: Malignant small cell tumor of the thoracopulmonary region in childhood. Cancer 43:2438–2451, 1979.
37. Harvey JC, Bergland R, Pisch J, et al: Superior results with complete resection of Askin's tumor. Semin Surg Oncol 9:156–159, 1993.
38. McCraw JB, Penix JO, Baker JW: Repair of the major defects of the chest wall and spine with the latissimus dorsi myocutaneous flap. Plast Reconstr Surg 62:197–206, 1978.
39. Larson DL, McMurtrey MJ: Musculocutaneous flap reconstruction of chest wall defects. An experience with 50 patients. Plast Reconstr Surg 73:734–740, 1984.
40. Arnold PG, Pairolero PC: Chest wall reconstruction. An experience with 100 consecutive patients. Ann Surg 199:725–732, 1984.
41. Graham J, Usher FC, Perry SL: Marlex mesh as a prosthesis in the repair of chest wall defects. Ann Surg 151:469–478, 1960.
42. Arnold PG, Pairolero PC: Chest wall reconstruction. Ann Thorac Surg 31:45–52, 1981.
43. Arnold PG, Pairolero PC: Use of pectoralis major muscle flap to repair defects of the anterior chest wall. Plast Reconstr Surg 63:205–213, 1979.
44. Bostwick J III, Nahai F, Wallace JG, Vasconez LO: Sixty latissimus dorsi flaps. Plast Reconstr Surg 63:31–41, 1979.
45. Hodgkinson DJ, Arnold PG: Chest wall reconstruction using the external oblique muscle. Br J Plast Surg 33:216–220, 1980.
46. Arnold PG, Pairolero PC, Waldorf JC: The serratus anterior muscle: Intrathoracic and extrathoracic utilization. Plast Reconstr Surg 73:240–246, 1984.
47. Campbell DA: Reconstruction of the anterior thoracic wall. J Thorac Cardiovasc Surg 19:456–468, 1950.
48. Carberry DM, Ballantyne LW: Omental pedicle graft in the closure of large anterior chest wall defects. NY State J Med 75:1705–1709, 1975.
49. Jacobs EW, Hoffman S, Kirschner P, et al: Reconstruction of large chest wall defects using greater omentum. Arch Surg 113:886–893, 1978.
50. Jurkiewicz MJ, Arnold PG: The omentum: An account of its use in the reconstruction of the chest wall. Ann Surg 185:548–554, 1977.
51. Arnold PG, Witzke DJ, Irons GB, et al: Use of omental transposition flaps for soft tissue reconstruction. Ann Plast Surg 11:508–512, 1983.

Diffuse Malignant Pleural Mesothelioma

James C. Harvey, M.D. • Christopher Erdman, B.A.
Julianna Pisch, M.D. • Edward J. Beattie, M.D.

Prior to Wagner and colleagues' report of a cluster of cases of diffuse malignant pleural mesothelioma (DMPM) among residents of the Asbestos Hills of the northwestern Cape Province of South Africa,[1] reports of primary tumors of the pleura were only sporadic and their very existence was in question by some pathologists. Although asbestos had been in use since ancient times because of its properties of superior insulation and durability, widespread industrial use was delayed until the discovery of large deposits in Canada and South Africa in the nineteenth century.

The pathogenicity of asbestos dust in the workplace was suspected by the turn of the century, when serious pulmonary disease, including pulmonary fibrosis and tuberculosis, was reported to be of high incidence among exposed workers. The term "asbestosis" was not used until 1924, when Cooke mentioned the presence of mineral particles in the lungs that he later termed "asbestos bodies."[2]

Industrial use of asbestos proliferated in the early twentieth century, with products such as asbestos cement, brake linings, clutch facings, and insulation. A great surge in demand occurred during World War II, when asbestos was used for protective clothing, gas masks, and sprayed insulation in ships. It was also used as a filter for wines and as a component of cement pipes, plastics, paints, and asphalt. Environmental controls introduced in the 1930s reduced the death rates associated with heavy exposures (asbestosis). These controls allowed epidemiologists to recognize the long-term potential for slowly developing malignancies associated with much lower dose exposures and much longer latency intervals.[2]

EPIDEMIOLOGY

The incidence rate of DMPM is not precisely known, but it is estimated that approximately 2200 new cases arise annually in the United States, afflicting at least three times as many men as women.[3, 4] Asbestos is the most important risk factor. Smoking is unrelated.[5]

Clinical studies fail to reveal a history of asbestos exposure in about 30% of cases,[5, 6] but intensive, repeated interviews of patients who fail to recall exposures to asbes-

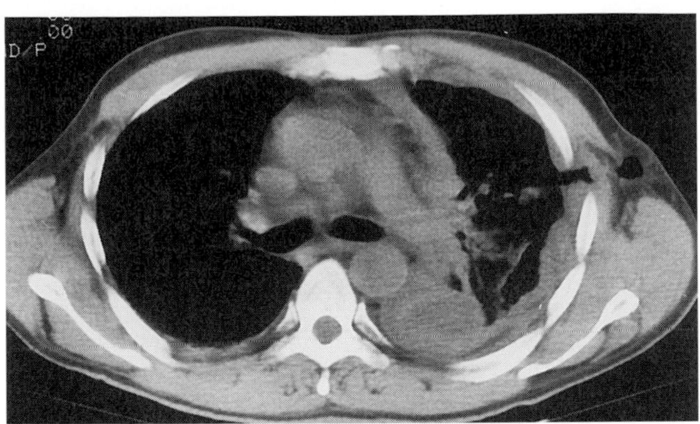

FIGURE 9–12. Computed tomogram at level of carina showing large pleural mass in left posterior thorax with nodular thickening of pleura laterally.

tos sometimes reveal an exposure rate of close to 100%. Cochrane and Webster[7] reinterviewed 70 patients in South Africa who had not initially given a history of asbestos exposure and found that 69 had had exposures to visible airborne asbestos dust, had had prolonged room contact with loose asbestos fibers, or had resided in areas of known asbestos pollution. The incidence of DMPM peaks 35 years after exposure to asbestos.[8] Peto and colleagues[9] have constructed a model predicting death rates due to pleural and peritoneal mesothelioma to be proportional to the third or fourth power of time interval from first exposure. Age itself is not a risk factor.[9] There may be no safe threshold dose, since tumors have been reported after only 1 day of exposure.[10]

There are differing degrees of carcinogenicity for the four major types of asbestos fibers. Crocidolite (the type prevalent in the Asbestos Hills area of South Africa) is the most carcinogenic, followed by amosite, anthophyllite, and chrysotile (the type found in North American deposits).[11] Occupational exposure in North America was mostly to native chrysotile until the 1930s, when amosite was used in small quantities. Amosite use increased during and subsequent to World War II.[2] Imported crocidolite used in the manufacturing of gas masks in Canada during World War II resulted in an increasing death rate due to mesothelioma as compared to that of chrysotile-exposed miners and millers in Canada.[10] A fifth type of fiber, zeolite, has been postulated to be related to DMPM in an Anatolian village,[11] but this was not verified in a North American study.[12]

LIFE HISTORY

The usual patient with pleural mesothelioma is a man with a remote history of occupational asbestos exposure.[10] The exposure need be of only brief duration. Families of workers may have a history of exposure to contaminated clothing from the workplace.[13] Children have had the disease, and it has been hypothesized that in utero exposure may be implicated.[14]

Symptoms are dyspnea and nonpleuritic chest pain.[15] Death is due to pulmonary insufficiency, usually within 12.5 months from first symptom or 8.4 months from diagnosis.[16] Favorable prognostic indications include relative youth (age <65 years),[17] good performance status,[18] disease confined to one pleural cavity without nodal involvement,[19] absence of chest pain,[20, 21] and epithelial cell type.[20, 22, 23]

LOCAL-REGIONAL ANATOMY

The pleura is composed of a single layer of mesothelial cells lining the thoracic cavity. Its blood supply is provided by intercostal, internal mammary, superior phrenic, and anterior mediastinal arteries. Lymphatics lie in connective tissue beneath mesothelial cells and drain into regional nodes, including intercostal, phrenic, and mediastinal nodes.

PATHOLOGY

Mesotheliomas arise from cells lining the pleura. Histologic characteristics may be sarcomatous with spindle cells, epithelial, or a combination of the two cell types.[24] The majority of tumors have an epithelial element; pure sarcomatous tumors account for only about 20% of tumors.[24] The epithelial element is responsible for pleural effusions and also for the frequent difficulty in histologically distinguishing the tumors from metastatic carcinomas.[4] In contrast, sarcomatous tumors tend to produce pleural thickening rather than effusions and tend to be bulkier and localized at presentation.[4, 25]

The tumor tends to grow in sheets, and the parietal pleura may become centimeters thick (Fig. 9–12).[25] Tumor on visceral pleura invades lung earlier, leading to encasement and fixation. Eventually, tumor invades through chest wall (Fig. 9–13) and also into mediastinal structures. As the tumor advances, it may penetrate the diaphragm,

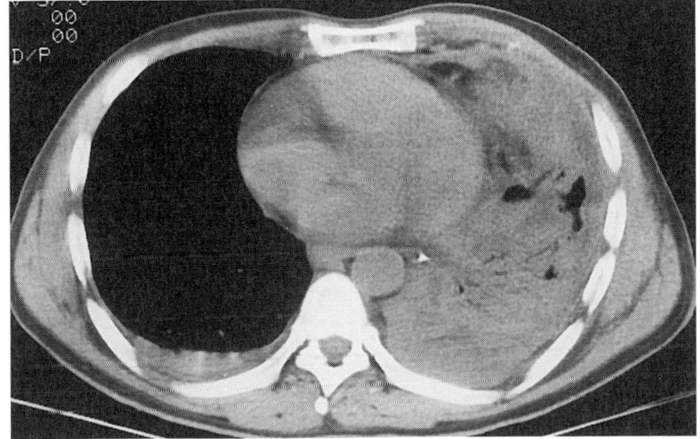

FIGURE 9–13. Computed tomogram through lower lungs showing pleural tumor occupying most of the left hemithorax. Tumor extends through left chest.

invade the lymph nodes, and ultimately become bloodborne, reaching the opposite lung, brain, kidney, and other organs.

DIAGNOSIS, SCREENING, AND EARLY DETECTION

The clinical diagnosis of mesothelioma should be entertained in any case of pleural effusion or chest wall tumor of an asbestos-exposed patient, but it is not excluded by the patient's not recalling such exposure. Confirmation depends on a generous tissue sample because special studies, including immunohistochemistries and electron microscopy, are often required to distinguish mesothelioma from carcinomas (in the case of epithelial tumors) and from other sarcomas in the case of sarcomatous and mixed tumors. Other sarcomas with epithelial components are more often localized than diffuse, originating either in the chest wall or in the lung.[25]

Malignant mesothelioma remains difficult to detect. Even among trade-union members being followed for asbestos-related pathology, diagnosis is usually made when symptoms of chest pain or dyspnea arise. Only a minority of patients with DMPM have roentgenographic signs of asbestos exposure such as pleural plaques, interstitial fibrosis, or low diaphragms.[3]

STAGING

There has been no uniformly accepted staging method for malignant pleural mesothelioma. The Butchart classification (Table 9–4)[26] has most often been used in the rare circumstances of any attempt at staging.

The American Joint Committee on Cancer has proposed a TNM staging system (Table 9–5).[27]

Clinical staging is dependent on computed tomography (CT) scans to investigate

- Confinement to "one capsule of parietal pleura" (stage I in Butchart staging)
- Invasion of ipsilateral lung, endothoracic fascia, diaphragm, or pericardium (T2 in TNM staging)
- Invasion of chest wall or mediastinal organs (T3 in TNM or stage II in Butchart)
- Extension to contralateral pleura, lung, peritoneum, intra-abdominal organs, or cervical tissues (T4 in TNM)

CT is also useful in assessing nodal status, but with the same limitations that apply for lung cancer. Because treatment planning depends on accurate staging, mediastinoscopy is recommended.

TABLE 9–4
Butchart Staging System

Stage	Definition
I	Within the capsule of the parietal pleura: ipsilateral pleura, lung, pericardium, diaphragm
II	Invading chest wall or mediastinum: esophagus, heart, opposite pleura Positive lymph nodes within the chest
III	Through diaphragm to peritoneum: opposite pleura Positive lymph nodes outside the chest
IV	Distant bloodborne metastases

From Butchart EG, et al: Pleuropneumonectomy in the management of diffuse malignant mesothelioma of the pleura: Experience with 29 patients. Thorax 31:15, 1976.

TABLE 9–5
AJCC TNM Staging System

Primary Tumor (T)	
TX	Primary tumor cannot be assessed
T0	No evidence of primary tumor
T1	Tumor limited to ipsilateral parietal and/or visceral pleura
T2	Tumor invades any of the following: ipsilateral lung, endothoracic fascia, diaphragm, or pericardium
T3	Tumor invades any of the following: ipsilateral chest wall muscle, ribs, or mediastinal organs or tissues
T4	Tumor directly extends to any of the following: contralateral pleura, lung, peritoneum, intra-abdominal organs, or cervical tissues
Regional Lymph Nodes (N)	
NX	Regional lymph nodes cannot be assessed
N0	No regional lymph node metastasis
N1	Metastasis in ipsilateral peribronchial and/or ipsilateral hilar lymph nodes, including direct extension
N2	Metastasis in ipsilateral mediastinal and/or subcarinal lymph node(s)
N3	Metastasis in contralateral mediastinal, contralateral hilar, ipsilateral or contralateral scalene, or supraclavicular lymph node(s)
Distant Metastasis (M)	
MX	Distant metastasis cannot be assessed
M0	No evidence of distant metastasis
M1	Distant metastasis

AJCC, American Joint Committee on Cancer.

TREATMENT

Surgical treatment options include

1. No surgery ("supportive care").
2. Parietal pleurectomy with decortication.
3. Extrapleural pneumonectomy (EPP).

Chemotherapy, irradiation, and photodynamic therapy have been used as adjuvants or as part of investigative protocols, but their value is not established.[28]

No Surgery

At the Southern California Permanente Medical Group, the majority (76 of 94) of patients treated had supportive care only. Surgical diagnosis, pleurocenteses, and attempts at sclerotherapy were performed. Thirty-three patients had some form of treatment, including chemotherapy in a variety of doses, combinations, and schedules and a variety of doses of external beam irradiation.

TABLE 9–6
Supportive Care

Study	No.	1-Year Survival	2-Year Survival	Median Survival (mo)
Harvey et al.[6]	76	NS	NS	7.7
Hulks et al.[21]	68	NS	NS	7
Ruffie et al.[18]	176	NS	NS	6.8
Rusch et al.[32]	37	NS	18.5%	NS

NS, Not stated.

Median survival in this group was 231 days, but four patients survived more than 2 years.[6] Similar median survivals of 6 to 7 months have been reported by a number of others, leading some to advocate this option over others (Table 9–6).[18, 21, 29]

Parietal Pleurectomy with Decortication

Nine patients were treated with parietal pleurectomy with decortication at the Southern California Permanente Medical Group. One of these patients also had a pericardiectomy, four also received chemotherapy, and one also received external beam irradiation.

There was no operative mortality. None of these patients survived 2 years, but the median survival was 360 days. Many have reported mortalities close to zero, with survivals in the range of 9 to 20 months.[7, 30, 31] It is our choice and that of others (Table 9–7)[30] that the treatment for most patients is parietal pleurectomy with decortication and internal irradiation (Figs. 9–14 and 9–15).

Principal morbidity is prolonged air leak.[28] Martini and coworkers[25] observed that pleurectomy is not feasible in about 20% of explored patients because of obliteration of the pleural space; in this situation it must be decided whether the patient is better served by either terminating the operation or performing EPP (see Table 9–7).[28]

Extrapleural Pneumonectomy

EPP involves a circumferential extrapleural mobilization of the lung, often through two intercostal spaces (but only one skin incision). The specimen includes lung in its pleural envelope, pericardium, and diaphragm (Figs. 9–16 to 9–22).

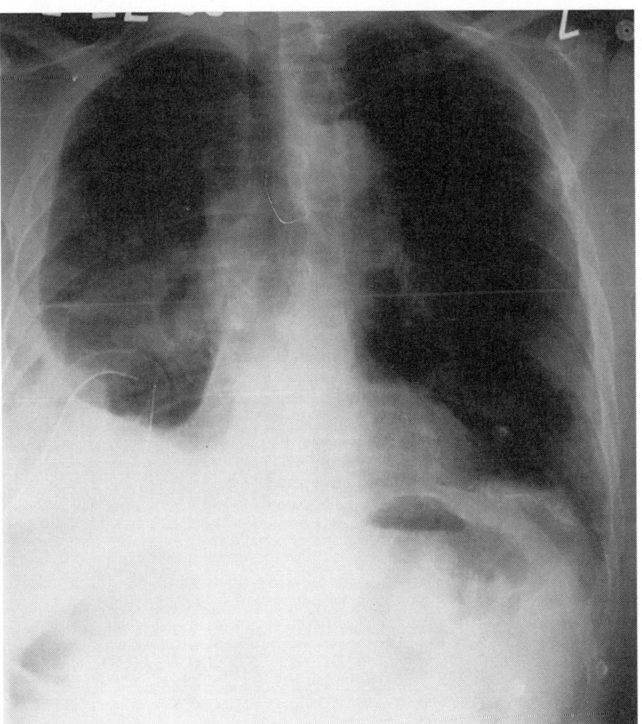

FIGURE 9–14. Preoperative chest radiograph showing a right chest tube in place with pleural thickening. A full-thickness pleural biopsy confirmed pleural mesothelioma, epithelial type.

At the Southern California Permanente Medical Group, seven such procedures were performed with one operative mortality. The median survival was less than 6 months, but there were two 5-year survivors.[6] It is noteworthy that in most series, median survival for EPP is no longer than that achieved by pleurectomy with decortication,[28] and the procedure is accompanied by an operative mortality rate of approximately 15%.[6, 18, 32] However, there are long-term survivors among selected patients treated with EPP (Table 9–8), and some experienced groups have performed the operation with a mortality rate less than 10%.[12, 28, 31] Local control is superior, so initial recurrence is at distant sites.[28]

Text continued on page 290

TABLE 9–7
Pleurectomy with Decortication

Study	No.	Morbidity (%)	Mortality (%)	1-Year Survival (%)	2-Year Survival (%)	Median Survival (mo)
Allen et al.[28]	56	26.8	5.4	30.4	8.9	9
Brancatisano et al.[33]	45	16	2.2	58	21	16
Chahinian et al.[17]	30	NS	0	57	27	13
McCormack et al.[30]	64	25	1.5	49	NS	NS
Mychalsak et al.[34]	105	NS	NS	52	23	12.6
Rusch et al.[32]	26	1.8	NS	NS	20	NS

NS, Not stated.

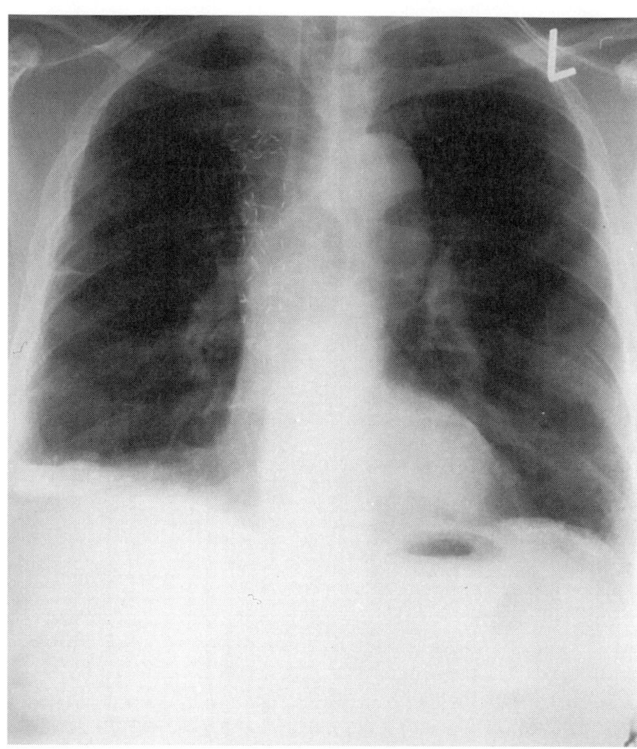

FIGURE 9–15. Postoperative chest radiograph after parietal pleurectomy and decortication. Iodine 125 seeds are seen implanted in residual mass in the paravertebral area.

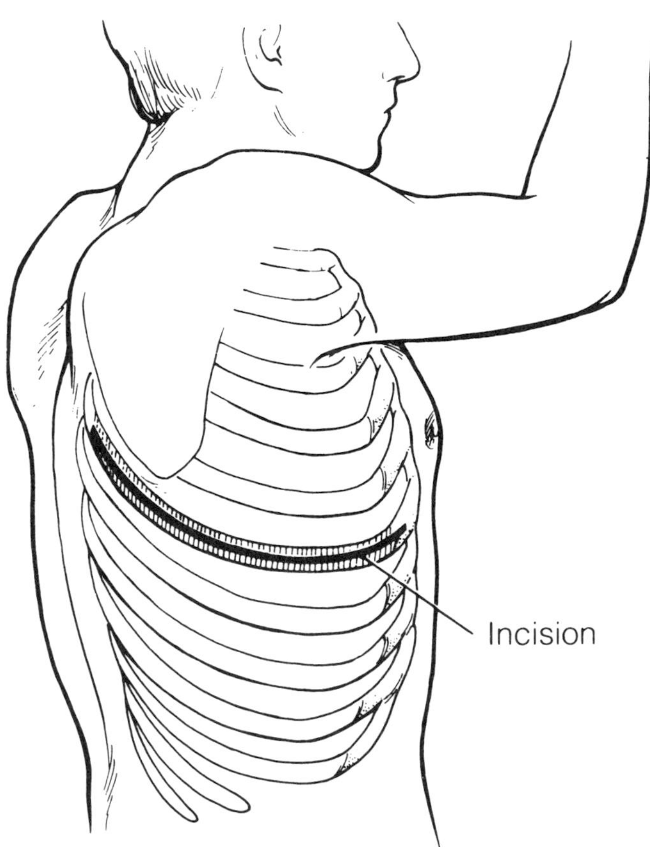

FIGURE 9–16. An extended thoracotomy incision is required to safely perform the procedure. The sixth rib is resected to facilitate exposure. If necessary, an additional lower incision may also be performed through the same skin incision. (From Sugarbaker DJ, Mentzer SJ, Strauss G: Extrapleural pneumonectomy in treatment of malignant pleural mesothelioma. Ann Thorac Surg 54:941–946, 1992.)

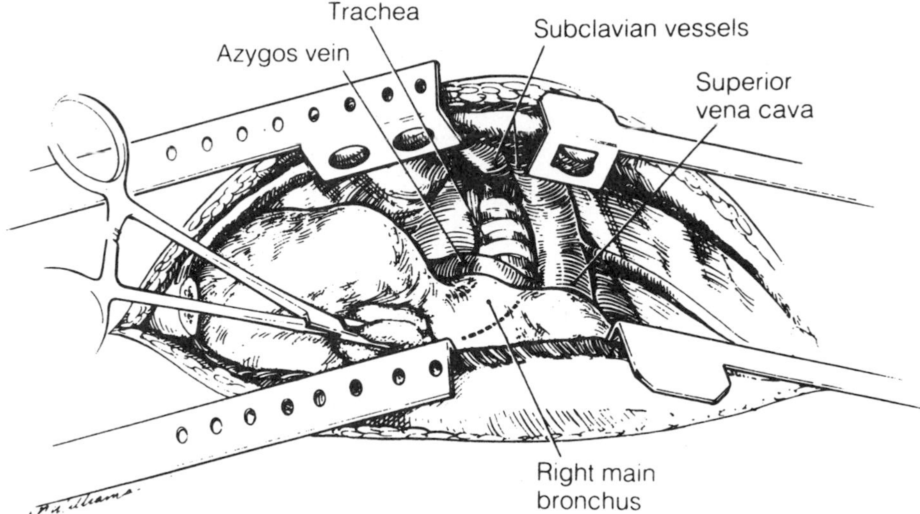

FIGURE 9–17. Wide exposure is achieved with two retractors into the incision. Extrapleural dissection of the lung has been performed, revealing important landmarks. (From Sugarbaker DJ, Mentzer SJ, Strauss G: Extrapleural pneumonectomy in treatment of malignant pleural mesothelioma. Ann Thorac Surg 54:941–946, 1992.)

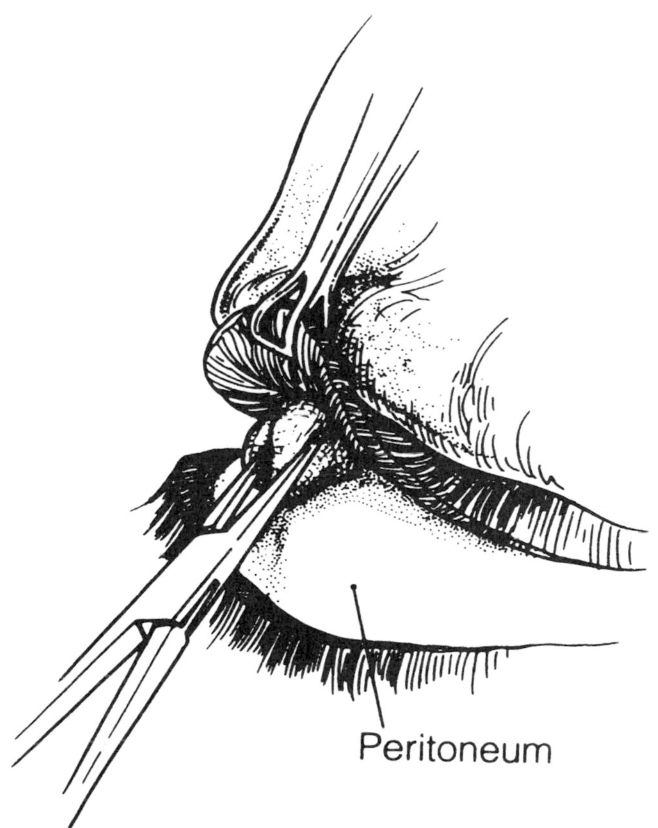

FIGURE 9–18. Dissection of diaphragm from underlying peritoneum. It is not necessary to incise the peritoneal surfaces of diaphragm. Care is taken to keep the pleural envelope intact during this dissection. (From Sugarbaker DJ, Mentzer SJ, Strauss G: Extrapleural pneumonectomy in treatment of malignant pleural mesothelioma. Ann Thorac Surg 54:941–946, 1992.)

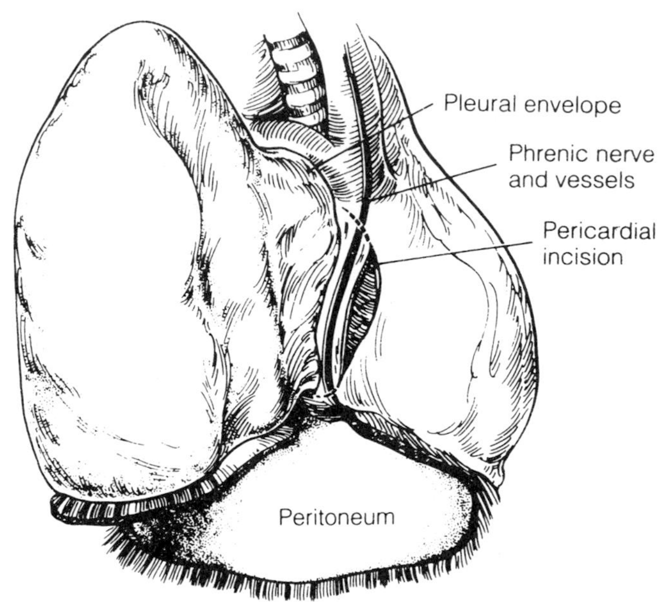

FIGURE 9–19. The pericardium is incised anterior to the phrenic nerve and hilar vessels, again taking care to keep the parietal envelopes intact. (From Sugarbaker DJ, Mentzer SJ, Strauss G: Extrapleural pneumonectomy in treatment of malignant pleural mesothelioma. Ann Thorac Surg 54:941–946, 1992.)

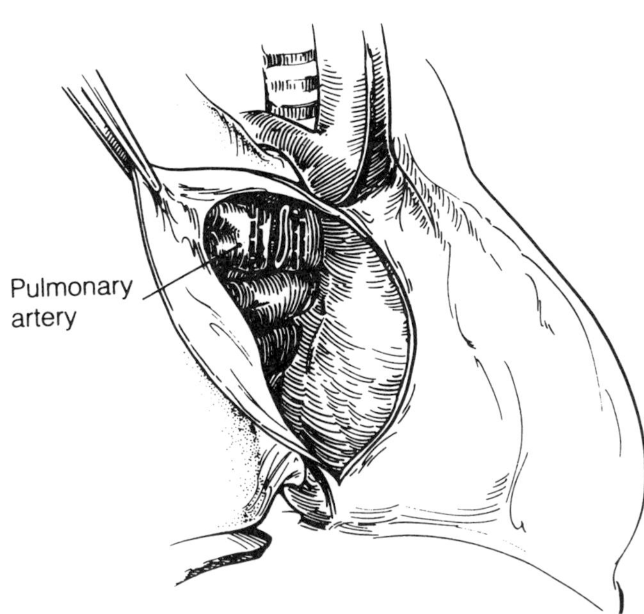

FIGURE 9–20. Reflecting the pericardium posteriorly, hilar vessels may be stapled and ligated. (From Sugarbaker DJ, Mentzer SJ, Strauss G: Extrapleural pneumonectomy in treatment of malignant pleural mesothelioma. Ann Thorac Surg 54:941–946, 1992.)

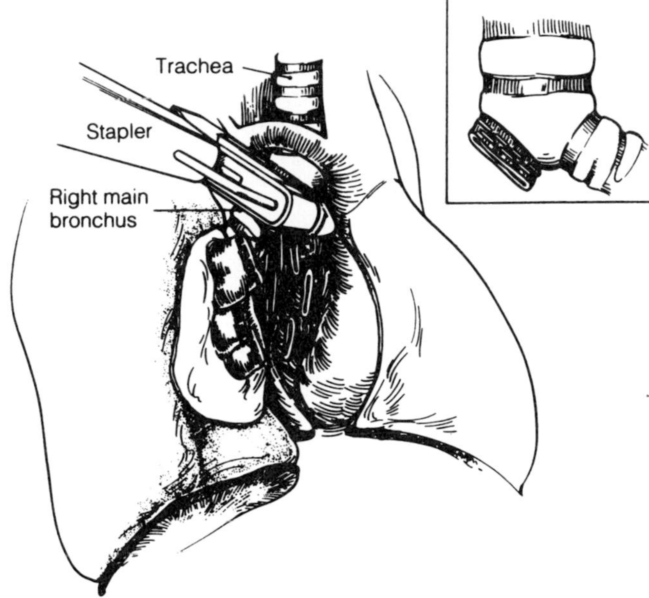

FIGURE 9–21. After ligation of the hilar vessels, it is easy to perform a high stapling of the bronchus.

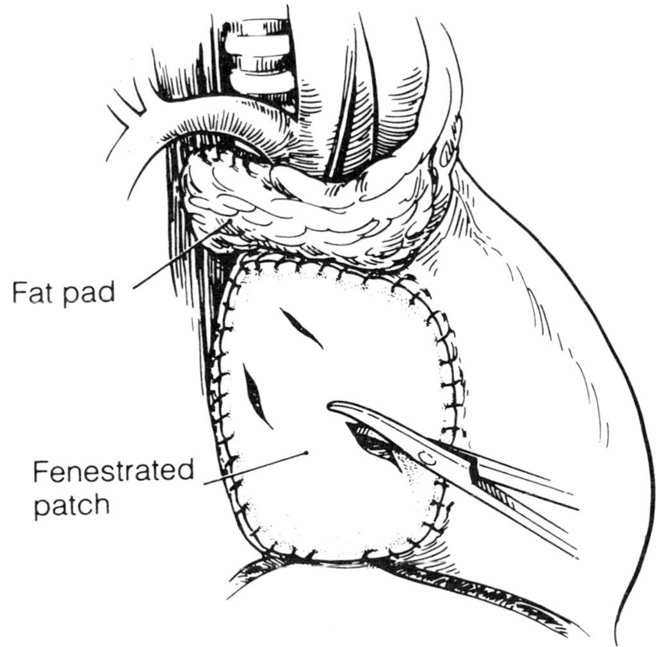

FIGURE 9–22. Protective covering of the bronchial stump using pericardial fat pad. Other appropriate tissue, such as chest wall muscle or omentum, may be selected. The large pericardial defect is repaired with a patch and fenestrated to minimize the risk of tamponade. We use bovine pericardium for our replacement patch.

TABLE 9–8
Extrapleural Pneumonectomy

Study	No.	Mortality (%)	Morbidity (%)	1-Year Survival (%)	2-Year Survival (%)	5-Year Survival (%)	Median Survival (mo)
Allen et al.[28]	40	7.5	30	52.5	22.5	10.0	13.3
Butchart et al.[26]	29	31.0	43	NS	10.0	3.5	NS
DeValle et al.[35]	33	9.1	24	NS	24	6	NS
Harvey et al.[6]	7	14	NS	28.5	28.5	28.5	<6
Ruffie et al.[18]	23	14	24	NS	17.0	NS	9.3
Rusch et al.[32]	20	15	40	NS	33	NS	10.0
Sugarbaker et al.[36]	31	6	19	70	48	NS	NS

NS, Not stated.

The procedure should be considered in situations in which complete resection can be accomplished with low operative mortality.

References

1. Wagner JC, Sleggs CA, Marchand P: Diffuse pleural mesothelioma and asbestos exposure in the North Western Cape Province. Br J Ind Med 17:260–227, 1960.
2. Lee DHK, Selikoff IJ: Historical background to the asbestos problem. Environ Res 18:300–314, 1979.
3. Antman KH: Natural history and epidemiology of malignant mesothelioma. Chest 103:373S–376S, 1993.
4. Wanebo HJ, Martini N, Melamed MR, Hilaris B, Beattie EJ Jr: Pleural mesothelioma. Cancer 38:2481–2488, 1976.
5. Hammond EC, Selikoff IJ, Seidman H: Asbestos exposure, cigarette smoking and death rates. Ann NY Acad Sci 330:473, 1979.
6. Harvey JC, Fleischman EH, Kagan AR, Streeter OE: Malignant pleural mesothelioma: A survival study. J Surg Oncol 45:40–42, 1990.
7. Cochrane JC, Webster I: Mesothelioma in relation to asbestos fibre exposure. S Afr Med J 54:279–281, 1978.
8. Selikoff IJ: Mortality experience of insulation workers in the United States and Canada, 1943–1976. Ann NY Acad Sci 330:91–116, 1977.
9. Peto J, Seidman H, Selikoff IJ: Mesothelioma mortality in asbestos workers: Implications for models of carcinogenesis and risk assessment. Br J Cancer 45:124–135, 1982.
10. Lemen RA, Dement JM, Wagoner JK: Epidemiology of asbestos-related diseases. Environ Health Perspect 34:1–11, 1980.
11. Artvinli M, Baris YI: Environmental fiber-induced pleuro-pulmonary diseases in an Anatolian village: An epidemiologic study. Arch Environ Health 37:177–181, 1982.
12. McDonald AD, McDonald JC: Malignant mesothelioma in North America. Cancer 46:1650–1656, 1980.
13. Anderson HA, Lilis R, Daum SM, et al: Household-contact asbestos neoplastic risk. Ann NY Acad Sci 271:311, 1976.
14. Grundy GW, Miller RW: Malignant mesothelioma in childhood. Report of 13 cases. Cancer 30:1216–1218, 1972.
15. Sridhar KS, Doria R, Raub WA, et al: New strategies are needed in diffuse malignant pleural mesothelioma. Cancer 70:2969–2979, 1992.
16. Ribak J, Selikoff IJ: Survival of asbestos insulation workers with mesothelioma. Br J Ind Med 49:732–735, 1992.
17. Chahinian AP, Pajak TF, Holland JF, et al: Diffuse malignant mesothelioma: Prospective evaluation of 69 patients. Ann Intern Med 96:746–755, 1982.
18. Ruffie P, Feld R, Minkin S, et al: Diffuse malignant mesothelioma of the pleura in Ontario and Quebec: A retrospective study of 332 patients. J Clin Oncol 7:1157–1168, 1989.
19. Sugarbaker DJ, Strauss GM, Lynch TJ, et al: Node status has prognostic significance in multimodality therapy of diffuse, malignant mesothelioma. J Clin Oncol 11:1172–1178, 1993.
20. Antman K, Shemin R, Ryan L, et al: Malignant mesothelioma: Prognostic variables in a registry of 108 patients, the Dana-Farber Cancer Institute and Brigham and Women's Hospital experience over two decades, 1965–1985. J Clin Oncol 6:147–153, 1988.
21. Hulks G, Thomas JS, Waclawski E: Malignant pleural mesothelioma in Western Glasgow 1980–1986. Thorax 44:496–500, 1989.
22. Schildge J, Kaiser D, Henss H, et al: Prognostiche faktoren bein diffusen malignen mesotheliom der pleura. Pneumologie 43:660–664, 1989.
23. Sugarbaker DJ, Strauss GM, Lynch TJ, et al: Node status has prognostic significance in the multimodality therapy of diffuse, malignant mesothelioma. J Clin Oncol 11:1172–1178, 1993.
24. Qua JC, Rao UNM, Takita H: Malignant pleural mesothelioma: A clinicopathologic study. J Surg Oncol 54:47–50, 1993.
25. Martini N, McCormack PM, Bains MS, et al: Pleural mesothelioma. Ann Thorac Surg 43:113–120, 1987.
26. Butchart EG, Ashcroft T, Barnsley WC, et al: Pleuropneumonectomy in the managment of diffuse malignant mesothelioma of the pleura: Experience with 29 patients. Thorax 31:15–24, 1976.
27. American Joint Committee on Cancer: TNM Staging Manual. Beahrs OH, Henson DE, Hutter RVP, Kennedy BJ. Philadelphia: JB Lippincott, 1993, pp 123–125.
28. Allen KB, Faber P, Warren WH: Malignant pleural mesothelioma: Extrapleural pneumonectomy and pleurectomy. Chest Surg Clin North Am 4:113–126, 1994.
29. Law MR, Gregor A, Hodson ME, et al: Malignant mesothelioma of the pleura: A study of 52 treated and 64 untreated patients. Thorax 39:255–259, 1984.
30. McCormack PM, Nagasaki F, Hilaris BS: Surgical treatment of pleural mesothelioma. J Thorac Cardiovasc Surg 84:843–842, 1982.
31. Hilaris BS, Dattatreyudu N, Kwong E, et al: Pleurectomy and intraoperative brachytherapy and postoperative radiation in the treatment of malignant pleural mesothelioma. Int J Radiat Oncol Biol Phys 10:325–331, 1984.
32. Rusch VW, Piantadosi S, Holmes EC: The role of extrapleural pneumonectomy in malignant pleural mesothelioma. J Thorac Cardiovasc Surg 102:1–9, 1991.
33. Brancatisano RP, Joseph MG, McCaughan BC: Pleurectomy for mesothelioma. Med J Aust 154:455, 1991.
34. Mychalsak BR, Nori D, Armstrong JG, et al: Results of treatment of malignant pleural mesothelioma with surgery, brachytherapy and external beam irradiation. Endocuriether Hypertherm Oncol 5:245–250, 1989.
35. DeValle MJ, Faber LP, Kittle CF, et al: Extrapleural pneumonectomy for diffuse malignant mesothelioma. Ann Thorac Surg 42:612–618, 1986.
36. Sugarbaker DJ, Mentzer SJ, DeCamp M, et al: Extrapleural pneumonectomy in the setting of a multimodality approach to malignant mesothelioma. Chest 103:377s–381s, 1993.

Malignant Pleural Effusions

Edward M. Pina, M.D. • James C. Harvey, M.D.
Kushagra Katariya, M.D. • Edward J. Beattie, M.D.

Malignant pleural effusion (MPE) is a sign of advanced metastatic tumor. The clinician is required to verify the diagnosis, since not all effusions in the cancer patient are malignant. Treatment is required even though life expectancy is brief because symptoms may be so disabling.

We present a brief discussion of MPE, emphasizing recent developments in surgical treatment.[1, 2]

EPIDEMIOLOGY

Of newly diagnosed pleural effusions, 28% to 60% are reported to be malignant. About 75% of cases are due to lung cancer and breast cancer.[3]

Lung carcinoma, especially adenocarcinoma, is the leading cause of MPE. At initial evaluation of patients with lung carcinoma, about 15% have a pleural effusion and at least 50% have one during the course of their disease.

Metastatic breast carcinoma is the second leading cause of MPE. In a review of 265 breast cancer patients who died from disseminated disease, 46% had pleural effusions on autopsy, of which 56% were ipsilateral to the primary carcinoma, 26% contralateral, and 16% bilateral.[4]

LIFE HISTORY

In general, the majority of patients with MPE die within 6 months because of progression of tumor. Lung cancer patients have a median survival considerably less than that of patients with solid tumors having more treatment options (breast, ovary).

In a review of 96 patients with MPE, 44 (46%) did not have a prior history of carcinoma.[5] Martini et al.[6] reported that 64% of 106 patients reviewed had a pleural effusion at the initial presentation of disease. Most MPEs are symptomatic; the most common complaints are dyspnea, nonproductive cough, and pleuritic chest pain. However, 25% of patients have minimal or absent symptoms at the time of diagnosis. Clinical findings of patients with a pleural effusion reveal a reduced air entry on the involved side, dullness to percussion, and decreased breath sounds. Suspicion that a pleural effusion is malignant should be high in case of previous cancer, but the diagnosis must be confirmed.

PATHOPHYSIOLOGY

The blood supply to the parietal pleura is provided by the intercostal arteries. The visceral pleura's blood supply is predominantly from the pulmonary artery and veins with systemic contributions from bronchial vessels being only a minor contribution.

The pleural cavity, under normal circumstances, contains approximately 15 ml of fluid. However, the daily fluid exchanged through this space is up to several liters. Pleural fluid is a filtrate from the parietal pleura that enters the pleural space, where it is absorbed by the pleural lymphatics and visceral pleural capillaries. Between 10% and 20% of the pleural fluid is absorbed by the lymphatics, including proteins of large molecular weight. The formation of pleural fluid is determined by Starling's law, relating the interaction of interstitial hydrostatic pressure, plasma oncotic pressure, and interstitial protein oncotic pressure. Any imbalances between these factors disturb the normal equilibrium and lead to an increase of fluid within the pleural cavity. These changes may occur in several ways when malignancy is present. The most common mechanism is lymphatic obstruction, due to either parietal pleural deposits, leading to an increase in capillary permeability, or visceral pleural deposits, reducing capillary absorption, or both. Other mechanisms include obstruction of the pulmonary veins by tumor increasing the capillary hydrostatic pressure and increased intrapleural colloid osmotic pressure due to the shedding of necrotic material, which decreases the pleural fluid reabsorption capacity of the visceral pleura.[7, 8]

DIAGNOSIS

The diagnosis of effusion is usually revealed by chest roentgenogram obtained either routinely or for investigation of symptoms. Specific diagnosis may be suggested by associated findings of pulmonary nodules, rib lucencies, or pleural thickening. Computed tomography (CT) is more sensitive in revealing pleural fluid and detail (Fig. 9–23).

Diagnostic thoracentesis confirms the presence of pleural fluid and provides material for analysis and cytology. Ultrasound may be useful in localizing effusions in patients whose effusions are small or in those who have loculated fluid collection.

Pleural fluid is grossly bloody in more than half the cases of MPE, but not all bloody effusions are malignant. Usually MPE fluid is exudative, with a ratio of pleural protein to serum protein greater than 0.5, but some may be transudates. Cytology reveals a diagnosis in most cases as long as at least 250 ml of fluid is submitted in 95%

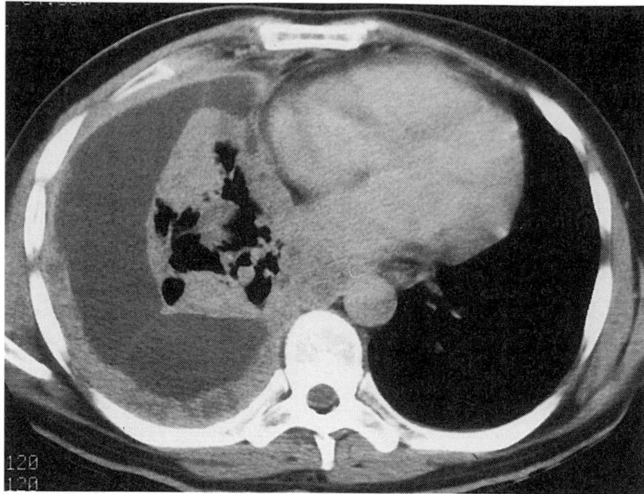

FIGURE 9–23. A 32-year-old man with malignant disease. Pleural biopsy confirmed adenocarcinoma. The right lower lung is encased by a rind of pleural tumor. Nodular excrescence extends into the azygoesophageal recess and involves the right posterior pericardium.

alcohol for cell block. Diagnosis rates may be improved by cytogenic analysis, with correct diagnosis achieved in more than 80% of the cases in which cytologic and chromosomal analyses were combined.[9]

Closed pleural biopsy alone has a lower diagnostic yield than fluid cytology, but, in combination with cytology, the diagnosis is achieved in greater than 80% of cases.[10] The biopsy should be performed with a Cope or Abrams needle prior to thoracentesis to avoid lung injury, the pleural fluid protecting the lung during the procedure.

In cases of uncertainty following closed pleural biopsy and thoracentesis, more invasive measures are required. Open pleural biopsies under local anesthesia may improve the yield. Thoracoscopy, under local anesthesia, allows inspection of the pleura with a diagnostic yield of close to 100%. Videothoracoscopic techniques may also be employed (Fig. 9–24), allowing generous biopsies.

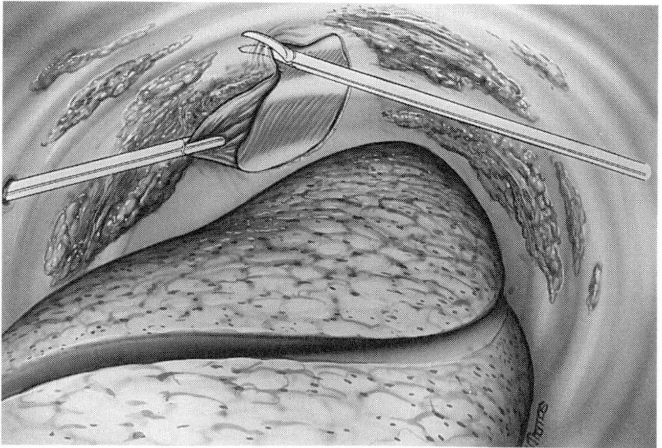

FIGURE 9–24. Drawing of a videothoracoscopic biopsy of a pleural tumor.

TREATMENT

Initial treatment of MPE should be tube thoracostomy, since thoracentesis alone results in almost inevitable recurrence within a month.[11] Systemic therapy is given, depending on cell type and the patient's overall performance status. Lymphomas are the only tumors with significant response to external beam irradiation.

Sclerotherapy

If, and only if, complete expansion of the lung is achieved, the pleural space may be obliterated by sclerotherapy. Any of a number of irritating agents, including antibiotics (e.g., tetracycline), antineoplastic agents (e.g., nitrogen mustard, bleomycin), and talc, have been infused. These agents are thought to work by means of promoting pleural fibrosis rather than any direct antineoplastic activity. Consistently good results have not been achieved, except in the case of talc, which has achieved control of MPE through the patient's life span in 90% of cases.[12] It may be administered in aerosol form via thoracoscope or instilled in a suspension into a chest tube.

Table 9–9 demonstrates different sclerosing agents with response rates.

Pleurectomy

In our experience, parietal pleurectomy has been the most effective means of controlling MPE.[6] However, the morbidity of a major thoracotomy precludes all but highly selected patients from the conventional (open) procedure. Recently, we have been able to perform parietal pleurectomy by means of a video-assisted (thoracoscopic) technique.[16] Early experience indicates that we are accomplishing an operation equivalent to that formerly performed by "open" technique, which had a success rate of close to 100%.[6]

The videothoracoscopic procedure is performed under general anesthesia with a double-lumen endotracheal tube and with the patient in a lateral decubitus position. With a

TABLE 9–9
Sclerosing Agents for the Management of Malignant Pleural Effusion

Agent/Study	No.	Reponse (%)	Days
Bleomycin			
Maiche et al.[13]	9	64	30
Hartman et al.[14]	28	64	30
Gupta et al.[15]	12	54	60
Tetracycline			
Hartman et al.[14]	27	33	30
Gupta et al.[15]	12	58	30
Mitoxantrone		67	30
Maiche et al.[13]	11		
Talc (VATS)			
Hartman et al.[14]	33	97	30

VATS, Video-assisted thoracic surgery.

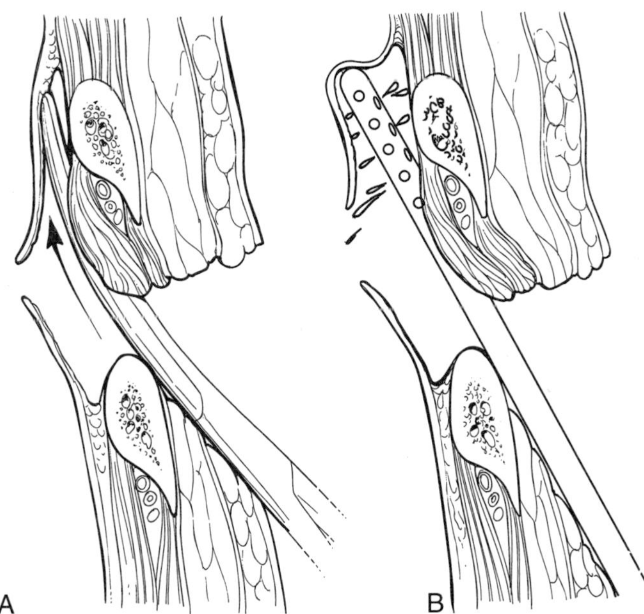

FIGURE 9–25. *A,* A curved clamp dissecting an extrapleural plane through a thoracostomy port incision. *B,* Insertion of an irrigation device into the extrapleural space.

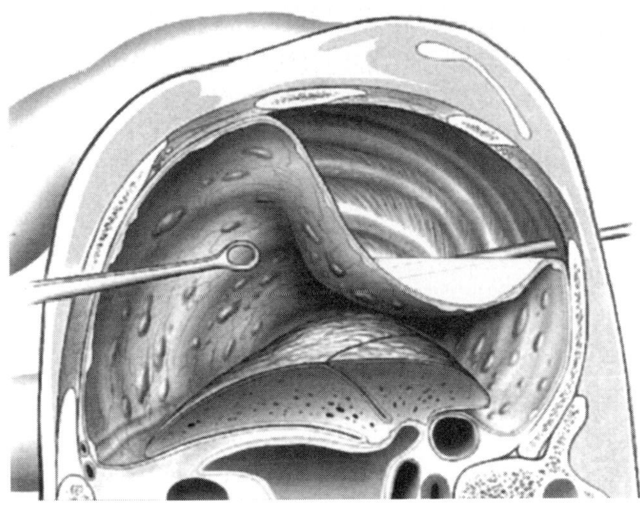

FIGURE 9–27. Videothoracoscopic view of "tent" of pleura detached from chest wall with combined irrigation and sweeping motion.

thoracoscope inserted through a 12-mm trochar in the seventh intercostal space, the thoracic cavity is inspected. The second and third ports are directly placed in the fourth anterior interspace and fifth posterior interspace. Subpleural planes are developed with a curved clamp and a disposable high-pressure irrigation device inserted into the plane (Fig. 9–25). The simultaneous maneuver of sweeping and irrigation dissects the pleura free from the chest wall (Fig. 9–26). The maneuver is repeated through the opposite port. It is possible to detach a "tent" of pleura from the chest wall (Fig. 9–27), which may be grasped to provide countertraction while the pleura is cut free and withdrawn through one of the ports (Fig. 9–28).

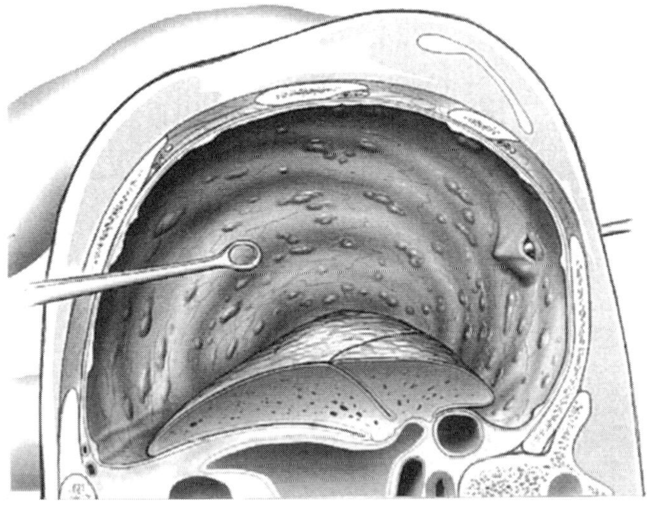

FIGURE 9–26. Cross section of the seventh thoracic vertebra demonstrating a "tent" of pleura dissected from chest wall with a combined irrigation and sweeping motion.

During the past 1½ years, we have performed 10 such procedures. The patients required chest drainage tubes for a median of 4 days (range, 2 to 13 days), at which time they were ready for discharge. There was one perioperative death, a patient with multiple metastases from an unknown primary tumor who developed adult respiratory distress syndrome and had treatment withdrawn at his and his family's request. One patient (the one whose drainage tubes were required for 13 days) needed bronchoscopy for retained secretions, after which his lung expanded, the drainage diminished, and the chest tubes were able to be withdrawn. Only one patient needed transfusion. She was anemic and had had previous systemic chemotherapy and an anteropleural sclerotherapy that failed. She required a more than usual dissection to take down adhesions and free loculated fluid and had an air leak until the fifth postoperative day. No others needed transfusion, nor did they have air leak beyond postoperative day 4. None have required further treatment to relieve their symptoms of pleural effusion.

Pleuroperitoneal Shunt

The pleuroperitoneal shunt, introduced in 1982, has increasingly become recognized as an attractive alternative in the management of MPE.[17] It is especially useful in cases of incomplete pulmonary expansion, a situation not satisfactorily treated by any means other than decortication—not an attractive option for sick patients with a short life expectancy. It is also an alternative for patients who prefer not to have tube thoracostomy.

We have reported our initial experience with the shunt.[18] Insertion of the shunt is performed in the operating room, under local anesthesia with intravenous sedation for most

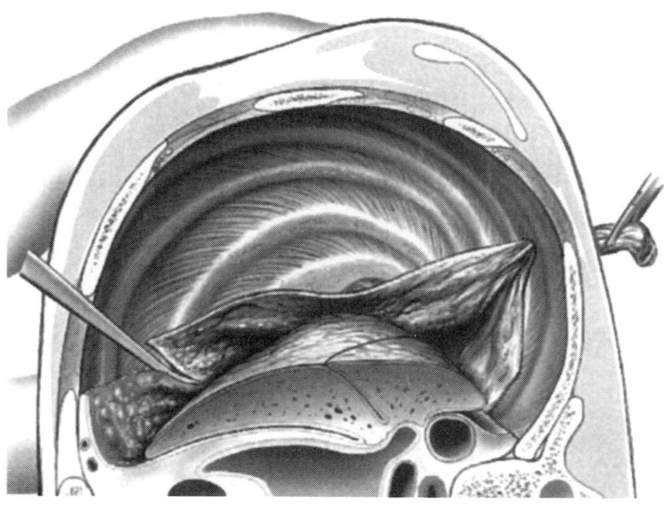

FIGURE 9–28. The diseased pleura being incised through the anterior port and withdrawn through the posterior port.

patients, but 40% receive general anesthesia. An incision is made over the anterior chest wall (usually in the inframammary crease), such that a subcutaneous pocket can be created (Fig. 9–29). The pumping chamber is positioned over the costal margin. A second incision is made over the upper abdomen. A double pursestring suture is placed in the peritoneum, and the device is passed through a subcutaneous tunnel (Fig. 9–30). The Seldinger technique is employed to introduce the pleural catheter into the hemithorax via a 16 French peel-away catheter (Figs. 9–31 and 9–32). The distal limb is then placed into the peritoneal cavity through a muscle-splitting stab wound into the peritoneum. The pursestrings are then secured. The chamber is fixed in its position with sutures, and the skin is closed with a running subcuticular suture. The patient and nursing staff are instructed to pump the chamber for 10 minutes every hour while the patient is awake for the first 2 days, and then for 10-minute intervals four times a day.

All of the patients have been satisfied with the performance of the shunt and were relieved of their shortness of breath. One patient had been in a hospice, unable to be discharged due to recurrent effusions and shortness of

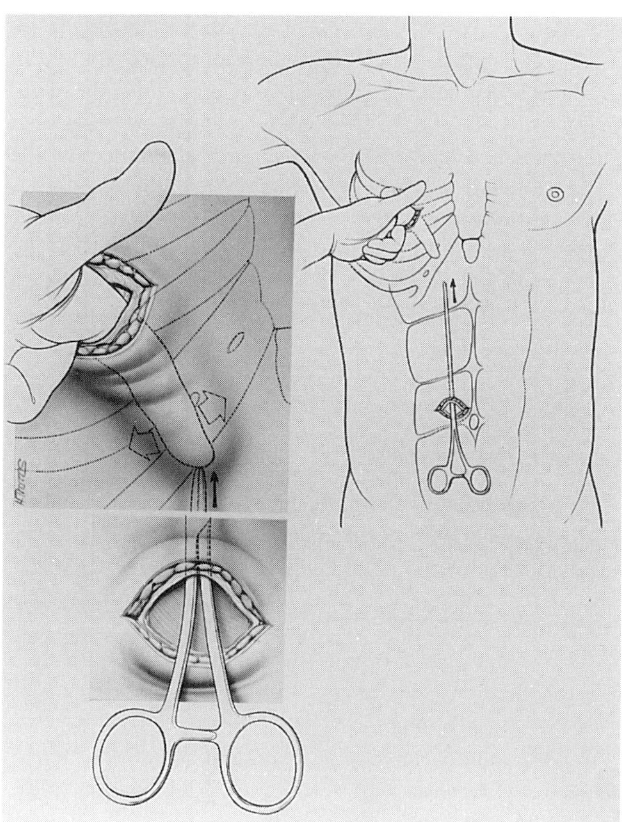

FIGURE 9–29. A subcutaneous pocket is created in the inframammary region and connected to a subcutaneous tunnel leading to an abdominal insertion site.

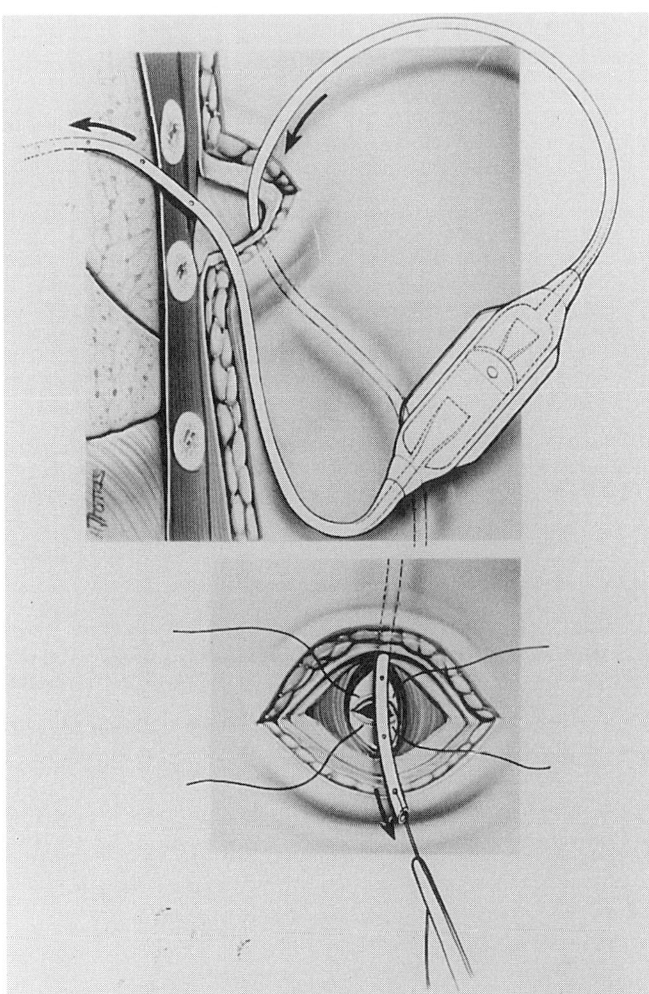

FIGURE 9–30. The distal limb device is tunneled down to the peritoneal insertion site, where it may be inserted through pursestring sutures. The pumping chamber is positioned over the costal margin.

breath. She underwent an uneventful shunt insertion and was released 4 days later. She died less than 1 month after surgery breathing comfortably at home.

The average length of patency of the shunts (either until clotting or the patient's demise) was 2.5 months (range, 6 days to 8 months).

DISCUSSION

In the past, the standard of care for recurrent MPEs included repeated thoracentesis followed by tube thoracostomy and instillation of sclerosing agents. This often required prolonged stays in the hospital, painful sclerotherapy, and a failure rate of at least 20% to 30%.[2] This also depleted the patients of valuable fluid and proteins. We have recently been investigating options that either would increase the success rate or would allow the patient with an MPE to ambulate, undergo a relatively painless procedure, and for the end-stage cancer patient, gain control over his or her care.

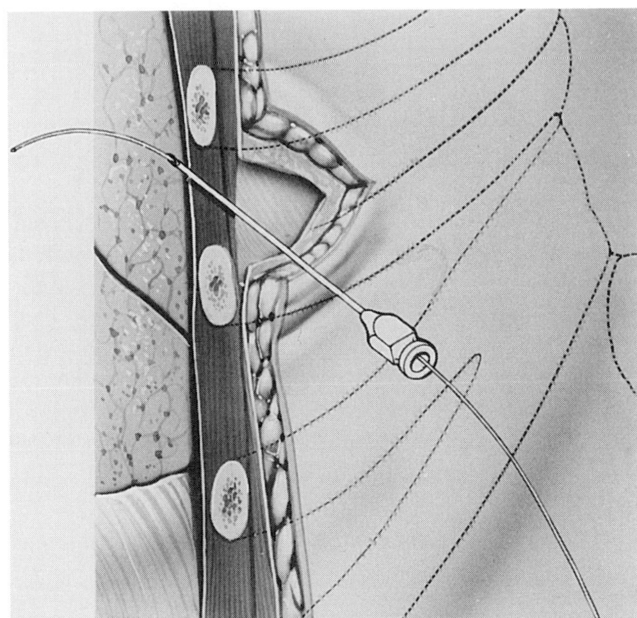

FIGURE 9–31. The guide wire is inserted through a needle into the pleural cavity.

Parietal pleurectomy is the most effective means of controlling MPE. Others have found talc, either aerosolized or in a suspension, and pleural abrasion satisfactory. We have no experience with talc, but the limited experience with videothoracoscopic pleural abrasion, in our hands, resulted in unsatisfactory control of the effusion. When we turned our attention to videothoracoscopic pleurectomies, hydrodissection was found to be technically easy, permitting a pleurectomy equivalent to that achieved by open thoracot-

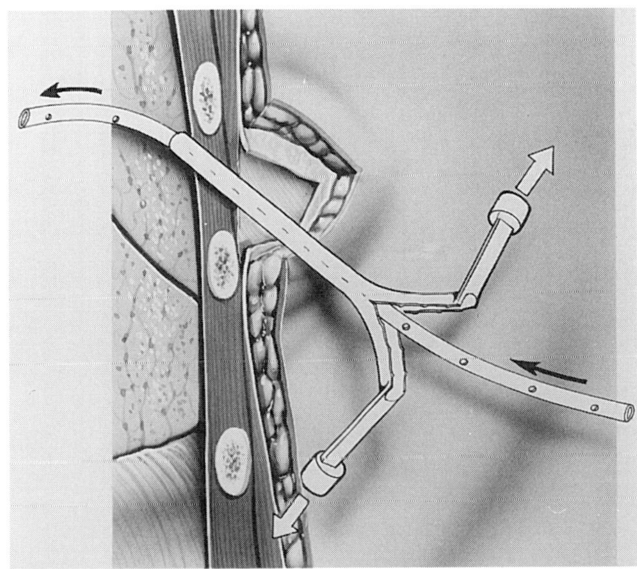

FIGURE 9–32. The proximal limb of the pleuroperitoneal shunt introduced through a peel-away catheter.

omy. If the same results as open procedures are verified with long-term follow-up, fewer recurrences will be seen with this technique than with alternative ones. This minimally invasive surgical technique may allow the benefits of pleurectomy to be provided to patients formerly excluded from the open procedure.

The pleuroperitoneal shunt remains an important alternative for MPE among patients too sick for general anesthesia or those with incomplete expansion of the lung. It is useful even for patients with a limited life expectancy when compared to the discomfort of repeated thoracenteses. A shunt does require that the patient be oriented and not too debilitated to press the device as required. An occasional obese patient has found it difficult to find the shunt placed deep in the subcutaneous tissues. We have had a very high level of satisfaction from patients selected for the procedure, and a shunt life exceeds the life expectancy of most patients who require it.

References

1. Light RW, Macgregor MI, Luchsinger PC, et al: Pleural effusions, the diagnostic separation of transudates and exudates. Ann Intern Med 77:507–513, 1972.
2. Hausheer FH, Yarlo JW: Diagnosis and treatment of malignant pleural effusion. Semin Oncol 12:54–75, 1985.
3. Cohen S, Hossain SA: Primary carcinoma of the lung: A review of 417 histologically proved cases. Dis Chest 49:67–74, 1966.
4. Goldsmith HS, Bailey HD, Callahan EL, et al: Pulmonary lymphangitic metastases from breast carcinoma. Arch Surg 94:483–488, 1967.
5. Chernow B, Shan SA: Carcinomatous involvement of the pleura. Am J Med 63:695–702, 1977.
6. Martini N, Bains MS, Beattie EJ Jr: Indications for pleurectomy in malignant pleural effusion. Cancer 35:734–738, 1975.
7. Light RW: Pleural effusions. Med Clin North Am 61:1339–1352, 1977.
8. Miles DW, Knight R: Diagnosis and management of malignant pleural effusion. Cancer Treat Rev 19:151–168, 1993.
9. Giazza G, Cosimi MF, Lanero M, et al: Cytologic diagnosis and chromosome analysis: Sensitivity, specificity, accuracy and predictive value in malignant and benign pleural effusions. Pathologica 82:33–40, 1990.
10. Shan SA: The pleura. Am Rev Respir Dis 138:184–234, 1988.
11. Ruckdeschel JC: Management of malignant pleural effusion: An overview. Semin Oncol 15:24–28, 1988.
12. Fentiman IS, Rubens RD, Hayward JL: A comparison of intracavitary talc and tetracycline for the control of pleural effusions secondary to breast cancer. Eur J Cancer Clin Oncol 22:1079–1081, 1986.
13. Maiche AG, Virkkunen P, Kontkanen T, et al: Bleomycin and mitoxantrone in the treatment of malignant pleural effusions. Am J Clin Oncol 16:50–53, 1993.
14. Hartman DL, Gaither JM, Kesler KA, et al: Comparison of insufflated talc under thoracoscopic guidance with standard tetracycline and bleomycin pleurodesis for control of malignant pleural effusions. J Thorac Cardiovasc Surg 105:743–748, 1993.
15. Gupta N, Opfell RW, Padova J, et al: Intrapleural bleomycin vs. tetracycline for control of malignant pleural effusions: A randomized study. Proc Am Soc Clin Oncol 189:366, 1980.
16. Harvey JC, Beattie EJ: Videothoracoscopic hydrodissection pleurectomy for malignant pleural effusions. J Surg Oncol 56:165–166, 1994.
17. Weere JL, Schouter JT: Pleural peritoneal shunts for the treatment of malignant pleural effusions. Surg Gynecol Obstet 154:391–392, 1982.
18. Reich H, Beattie EJ, Harvey JC: Pleuroperitoneal shunt of malignant pleural effusions: A one year experience. Semin Surg Oncol 9:160–162, 1993.

10

Soft Tissue Sarcomas

Soft Tissue Sarcomas of the Extremities

Daniel B. Frost, M.D. • *A. Robert Kagan, M.D.*

This subchapter covers soft tissue sarcomas of the extremities. Bone primary lesions, along with tumors of the head and neck and retroperitoneal sites, are not covered here. The surgical, radiotherapeutic, and combined-modality approaches to soft tissue sarcomas of the extremities, both for primary treatment and for salvage, are discussed. The respective advantages and limitations of these approaches are examined. Adjuvant therapy trials and approaches to, and results of, treatment of locally recurrent and metastatic disease are also considered.

EPIDEMIOLOGY

Incidence

The incidence of soft tissue sarcoma in the United States was estimated to be 6000 new cases in 1994.[1] Over half of all soft tissue sarcomas are located in extremity sites. Incidence in males generally outnumbers that in females. Incidence increases with advancing age, rising from less than 1 in 100,000 population per year for patients less than 25 years old to 8 in 100,000 population for patients over 80 years old.[2]

Causes

A history of trauma to the site is very common. However, the trauma is almost invariably recent and, therefore, served to cause the tumor to be found, but it cannot be implicated in its etiology. Several, but not all, epidemiologic studies have suggested a link between pesticide exposure and soft tissue sarcoma.[3–5] The implicated compounds are trichlorophenols and phenoxyacetic acids. The assessment of risk is complicated by the presence of contaminants such as the dioxin TCDD (2,3,7,8-tetrachlorodibenzo-para-dioxin, a known tumor promotor) in the phenoxyacetic acid 2,4,5-T. The latency period is long, with a median of 21 years in one study.[2] The soft tissue sarcomas are all of visceral origin, in contrast to the distribution in the general population (Fig. 10–1).

Other studies have linked the use of tobacco with soft tissue sarcoma.[6, 7] The association between smokeless tobacco use and excess rates of squamous cell carcinomas of the upper aerodigestive tract is well established. A similar association was found for soft tissue sarcomas.[6] However, an analysis of the 248,046-member prospective veterans' cohort of Harold Dorn failed to confirm the finding of an excess risk from smokeless tobacco use but did find an association with cigarette use.[7] The relative risks in all studies are on the order of 1.5 to 2.2. The site of increased risk is the upper aerodigestive tract.

To date, there are no known epidemiologic associations for extremity soft tissue sarcomas.

Radiotherapy-Induced Sarcoma

While irradiation-induced sarcoma is an accepted entity, the actual risk is very difficult to determine, as most reported series have a vague idea of the number of patients in the denominator. Given these uncertainties, the incidence

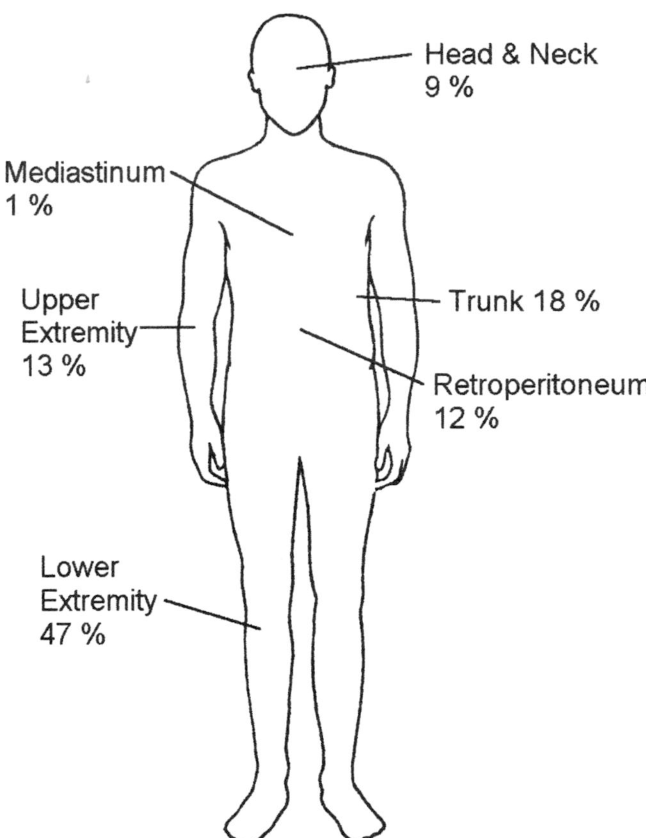

FIGURE 10–1. Distribution of soft tissue sarcomas by site. (Data from Lawrence W, Jr, et al: Ann Surg 205:349–359, 1987 [ACS Patterns of Care Study, 4550 patients].)

is estimated to be about 0.5% of patients receiving irradiation. Most secondary sarcomas are osteosarcomas.[8] Survivors of childhood cancer are at increased risk for many types of cancer. The Late Effects Study Group estimated the relative risk to be 133 for osteosarcoma and 41 for soft tissue sarcomas.[8] The cumulative risk for development of a secondary cancer was 12% at 25 years. In a series of patients treated for Ewing's sarcoma, the calculated risk for development of a secondary sarcoma was 9% at 11¼ years and 44% at 19 years.[9] Only three patients were at risk at 19 years. This makes it statistically precarious to accept an increasing cumulative risk with time as proven. The median time interval, or latent period, for development of a secondary sarcoma is 10 to 15 years.[9–12] The prognosis appears to be worse than for spontaneously occurring sarcomas.[12, 13]

Foreign-Body Induced Sarcoma

Reports of soft tissue sarcomas arising next to or around chronic foreign bodies are anecdotal, and these tumors usually have a latent period of several decades.[14]

Syndromes That Include Sarcomas

Li-Fraumeni Syndrome

In 1969, Li and Fraumeni published a review of the 280 records and 418 death certificates of childhood rhabdomyosarcoma patients and identified five families with a cluster of cancers. These associated cancers were most often soft tissue sarcomas and breast cancers.[15, 16] The addition of more families added osteosarcomas, brain tumors, adrenocortical cancers, and leukemias to the list.[17] In Li-Fraumeni syndrome, as in most hereditary cancers, the tumors tend to develop in childhood or young adulthood.[18] Multiple primary tumors are common, as are multiple histologic types (e.g., leiomyosarcoma followed by an osteosarcoma or a liposarcoma or an epithelial tumor).

Tumor suppressor genes are the class of genes most often associated with familial cancer syndromes. The best known of these are the WT1 and RB1 genes, which are associated with Wilms' tumor and retinoblastoma, respectively. The p53 tumor suppressor gene has recently been identified as the probable etiology of the Li-Fraumeni syndrome. The p53 gene, which is about 20 kb long and is located on chromosome 17[19] encodes a 53-kd protein.[20] This protein, which was first identified in SV40-transformed cells, probably acts as a negative regulator of cell growth. Wild-type p53 may be involved in programmed cell death (apoptosis).[21] Cells that lack a normal p53 gene do not exhibit the normal G1 arrest in the cell cycle.[22]

Lane[23] recently proposed a model to account for what is known of p53 function; in normal cell division, p53 is unnecessary. When DNA is damaged, p53 levels rise, resulting in cell-cycle arrest at the G1 stage. This allows for repair of the DNA strand damage or sets up the cell for apoptosis. In cells lacking normal p53, the damaged DNA is replicated, resulting in mutation. This mutation, in turn, may lead to mitotic failure and cell death or to a malignant cell clone. With the ability to repair sublethal damage thus impaired, soft tissue sarcomas in patients with this syndrome might be more radiosensitive than nonsyndrome soft tissue sarcomas. There is no convincing evidence that soft tissue sarcomas in patients with Li-Fraumeni syndrome respond to irradiation differently than soft tissue sarcomas occurring in the general population. Patients with Li-Fraumeni syndrome are, however, at greater risk for development of second primary cancers.

Von Recklinghausen's Neurofibromatosis

Von Recklinghausen's disease (neurofibromatosis type 1), an autosomal dominant trait, occurs in about 1 in 3000 persons.[24] Patients with von Recklinghausen's neurofibromatosis have an increased risk for development of soft tissue sarcoma, Wilms' tumor, nonlymphocytic leukemias, and brain tumors. In a review by Blatt et al.,[25] 3 of 121 patients with von Recklinghausen's neurofibromatosis who were under 18 years of age had or went on to have a neurofibrosarcoma or fibrosarcoma, while 3 others had or went on to have malignant astrocytomas.[25] The incidence in adult-patient series is similar.[24] There are anecdotal reports and small series of patients that have implied that patients with von Recklinghausen's neurofibromatosis may be more susceptible to irradiation-induced cancers.[25] It is therefore significant that there are 12 children who underwent irradiation with doses from 41 to 60 Gy and had no evidence of recurrence or new tumor in the irradiation fields after a median follow-up of 6 years.[25]

These and other data[26] suggest that adjuvant irradiation should be safe to use in patients with von Recklinghausen's neurofibromatosis.

Distribution

Liposarcomas, leiomyosarcomas, and malignant fibrous histiocytomas predominate in most large series.[27, 28] Liposarcomas predominate in the lower extremity. Extremity sites account for 60% of all soft tissue sarcomas (Table 10–1; see Fig. 10–1).

EVALUATION

Biopsy Technique

While some surgical oncologists advocate an extensive work-up (computed tomography [CT] scans, radiographs) before biopsy of any soft tissue mass, we agree with those who prefer to do a limited incisional biopsy first. There is less anxiety for the patient because a diagnosis is made more quickly. We also believe this avoids unnecessary tests and, therefore, costs. If a sarcoma is diagnosed, appropriate studies can be scheduled. If the mass is benign, complete excision can be done when convenient. There has been excellent acceptance of this approach by our patients when the reason for a two-stage procedure is explained to them.

The biopsy should be done with a possible definitive resection in mind. This usually requires a vertical or longitudinal rather than a transverse incision so that the biopsy scar can easily be excised en bloc with the tumor at the time of the definitive resection. For any tumor but the smallest and obviously subcutaneous, an incisional biopsy should be done before excision. A limited incisional biopsy is preferable so that there is as little disturbance of the site and hematoma formation as possible. Both of these factors can theoretically disseminate tumor cells beyond the wound in an unpredictable pattern. There is also less chance of infection. This type of biopsy can almost always be done under local anesthesia in the office or ambulatory surgery suite. Fine-needle aspirates for cytologic examination can also be done if a cytopathologist with soft tissue sarcoma experience is available.[29] Of course, a negative, or nondiagnostic, aspirate should be followed by an incisional biopsy.

Another option is a core needle biopsy (Tru-Cut, Travenol Laboratories, Deerfield, IL). In a study of 37 patients, Barth et al.[30] showed that core needle biopsy correctly diagnosed 16 of 16 sarcomas and 10 of 11 benign tumors. In the same study, fine-needle aspiration biopsy was equally good at diagnosing malignant tumors as core needle biopsy but less capable of identifying benign tumors, largely because of the difficulty of getting a good smear.

If chemotherapy or radiotherapy, or both, is to be given preoperatively, an incisional biopsy should be done first, as chemotherapy or irradiation can cause maturation or extensive necrosis, either of which can make accurate histologic diagnosis and grading difficult or impossible.

TABLE 10–1
Distribution of Soft Tissue Sarcomas by Histology

Histologic Type	Percent
Malignant fibrous histiocytoma	25.9
Liposarcoma	17.7
Leiomyosarcoma	14.8
Miscellaneous sarcomas	12.8
Fibrosarcoma	6.6
Sarcoma, NOS	5.4
Malignant nerve sheath tumor	4.0
Rhabdomyosarcoma	3.6
Synovial sarcoma	3.6
Angiosarcoma	2.9
Extraskeletal chondrosarcoma	1.2
Malignant mesenchymoma	1.0
Alveolar soft part sarcoma	0.6
Extraskeletal osteosarcoma	0.6
Total*	100.70

Data from Lawrence W, et al: Adult soft tissue sarcomas. Ann Surg 205:349–359, 1987 (ACS Patterns of Care Study, 4550 patients).

NOS, Not otherwise specified.

*Some patients had more than one histologic type.

Imaging

Preoperative imaging studies begin with a chest radiograph or chest CT scan. The decision as to which is more appropriate is perhaps more philosophic than scientific. CT is more sensitive than plain radiographs for detecting small nodules, especially in the lung apex, posterior sulcus, or subpleural areas. The increased sensitivity of CT makes it less useful in the setting of either a low probability of pulmonary metastasis (e.g., grade 1 sarcoma) or a high incidence of benign nodules (e.g., coccidioidomycosis granulomas). Both of these situations, particularly in adults, increase the frequency of false-positive findings. In our opinion, unless a therapeutic decision such as amputation versus limb-sparing surgery will be based on the result, plain radiographs of the chest are preferable to CT.

Imaging of the primary tumor is best done by magnetic resonance imaging (MRI).[31] The advantages of MRI over CT are enhanced contrast of the soft tissues and the ability of the software to generate sagittal, coronal, and axial images. The result is increased anatomic detail. A side effect has been the virtual elimination of the need for arteriograms.

The detection of local recurrence is clinical. When there is suspicion of recurrence, confirmation can be obtained with CT, MRI, or ultrasonography. Ultrasonography was compared with MRI for the detection of local recurrence in a study by Fornage.[32] Specificity and sensitivity were equal. Ultrasonography had the advantage of being able to guide a biopsy needle and was less costly. Ultrasonography

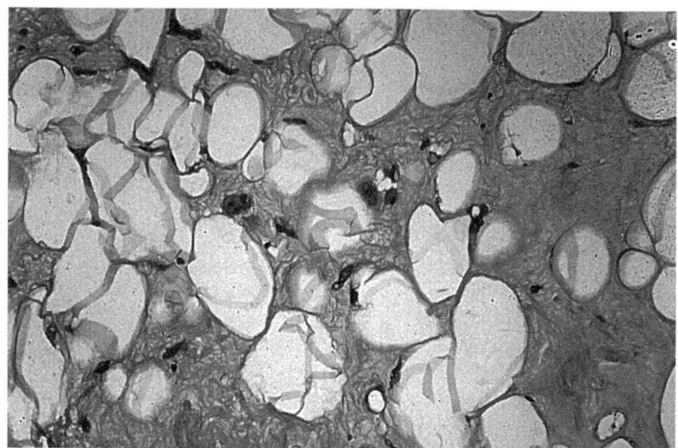

Figure 10–2. Grade 1 liposarcoma showing scattered atypical cells with hyperchromatic nuclei (hematoxylin-eosin, original magnification × 180).

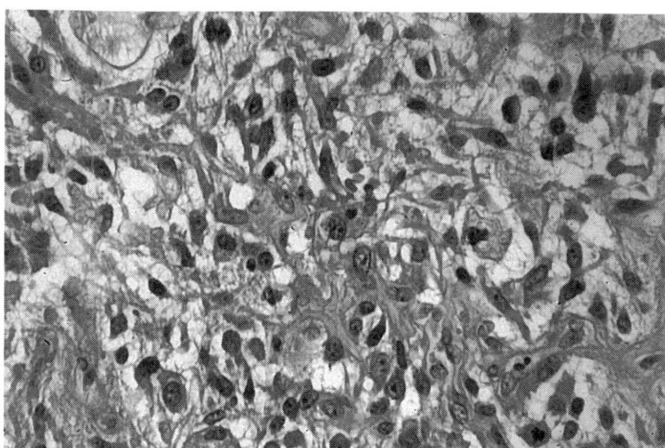

FIGURE 10–3. Grade 2 liposarcoma with moderate variation in size and shape of lipoblasts (hematoxylin-eosin, original magnification × 180).

is very operator-dependent, and these results would not apply to every hospital.

The evaluation of pulmonary metastases for possible pulmonary metastasectomy is best done by CT. Whether 1-cm or 0.5-cm cuts are required is controversial.

Staging

The latest American Joint Committee on Cancer staging manual was released in 1992. The current staging of localized soft tissue sarcomas is based on grade and tumor size. Nodal metastasis is unusual, and patients with positive lymph nodes are classified as metastatic. Distant metastasis is handled in the usual fashion. This staging system was developed before multimodal treatment was widely used, and local recurrence rates were higher; it probably needs revision.

T Staging

Stage T1 comprises soft tissue sarcomas less than 5 cm in diameter. Stage T2 soft tissue sarcomas are 5 cm or greater in size. Prior to the last revision, there was a stage T3, which comprised those tumors that invaded bone, major vessel, or nerve. The reason for the choice of 5 cm as the division point is not clear. The original TNM staging system of the American Joint Committee Task Force on Soft Tissue Sarcoma uses this size without comment on its origin.[33]

G Staging

While tumor grading has remained the principal factor in soft tissue sarcoma staging, it is notoriously subjective. In a report from the Scandinavian Sarcoma Group, when the pathology was reviewed by a committee the grade was changed in 40% of cases.[34] While four grades are advocated by some,[34] in virtually all American series three grades are recognized (Figs. 10–2 to 10–4). An exception is the Memorial Sloan-Kettering Cancer Center, which distinguishes only between high grade and low grade. Several distinct histologic patterns may exist in one tumor; therefore, it is essential that the entire specimen be sampled.

N Staging

If the regional lymph nodes are involved, the patient is staged N1. The incidence of nodal metastasis is low for all histologic types (Table 10–2).

M Staging

If distant metastasis is present, the patient is staged M1.

Stage Groupings

It may be possible to simplify this cumbersome system (Table 10–3) on the basis of a recent review from the Memorial Sloan-Kettering group. In this study, 174 adult patients (10% of the entire adult extremity soft tissue sarcoma cohort) with extremity soft tissue sarcomas 5 cm

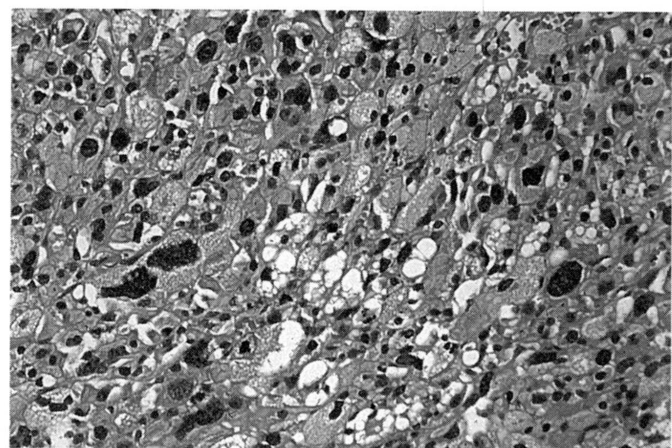

FIGURE 10–4. Grade 3 liposarcoma with extreme cellular pleomorphism (hematoxylin-eosin, original magnification × 180).

TABLE 10–2
Incidence of Nodal Metastasis

Histologic Type	No. with Involved Nodes*	Total No. with Histology	Percent
Angiosarcoma	8	151	5.3
Synovial sarcoma	10	214	4.7
Rhabdomyosarcoma	12	293	4.1
Malignant fibrous histiocytoma	44	1246	3.5
Alveolar soft part sarcoma	1	30	3.3
Leiomyosarcoma	24	837	2.9
Liposarcoma	26	1158	2.2
Fibrosarcoma	9	489	1.8
Malignant nerve sheath	2	214	1.4
Malignant mesenchymoma	0	66	0
Other	42	1289	4.0
Total	178	5987	2.97

Data from Lawrence W, et al: Adult soft tissue sarcomas. Ann Surg 205:349–359, 1987 (ACS Patterns of Care Study, 4550 patients).
*Clinically suspicious or involved.

or less in size and treated after mid-1982 were evaluated. Survival (and local recurrence rate) was not affected by grade.[35] Other series have reported low local recurrence rates for sarcomas 5 cm or less in size regardless of grade, and low local recurrence for grade 1 tumors regardless of size.[36] Others have described low local recurrence rates for grade 1 tumors regardless of size but an increasing local recurrence rate for increasing grade for T1 tumors.[110]

Despite, or perhaps because of, these conflicting results, the most important prognostic variable may be the type and quality of treatment used.[37] The stage groupings could probably be simplified, as in Table 10–4. Other modifications have been proposed.[38]

TABLE 10–3
AJCC Stage Groupings

Stage	*Grade*	*Tumor*	*Node*	*Distant Metastasis*
1992				
IA	G1	T1	N0	M0
IB	G1	T2	N0	M0
IIA	G2	T1	N0	M0
IIB	G2	T2	N0	M0
IIIA	G3, G4	T1	N0	M0
IIIB	G3, G4	T2	N0	M0
IVA	Any G	Any T	N1	M0
IVA	Any G	Any T	Any N	M1
1983 and 1988				
IA	G1	T1	N0	M0
IB	G1	T2	N0	M0
IIA	G2	T1	N0	M0
IIB	G2	T2	N0	M0
IIIA	G3, G4	T1	N0	M0
IIIB	G3, G4	T2	N0	M0
IIIC	Any G	T1, T2	N1	M0
IVA	Any G	T3	Any N	M0
IVA	Any G	Any T	Any N	M1

AJCC, American Joint Committee on Cancer.

TABLE 10–4
Proposed Revised Stage Groupings

Stage	Grade	Tumor	Node	Distant Metastasis
IA	G1	Any T	N0	M0
IB	Any G	T1	N0	M0
II	G2	T2	N0	M0
III	G3, G4	T2	N0	M0
IVA	Any G	Any T	N1	M0
IVB	Any G	Any T	Any N	M1

Prognostic Factors

Prognostic Variables

Prognostic variables for primary, locally recurrent, and metastatic soft tissue sarcomas are summarized in Figure 10–5.

Histologic Subtype

There is no evidence that the various histologic types of sarcoma behave differently enough to warrant separating them out.[89] It is possible that, with a large enough number of patients, statistically significant differences in overall survival or local recurrence might be seen. Liposarcomas may have a better prognosis and rhabdomyosarcomas a worse prognosis than the "average" sarcoma.

TREATMENT

Surgical

Definitions of Surgical Margins

Enneking's definitions of surgical margins are used so often that it is worthwhile to review them.[39] There are four categories, the first of which is *intralesional.* This is defined as leaving gross tumor behind, essentially a cut-through. The second category, a *marginal* resection, is one in which the tumor pseudocapsule is the plane of resection, implying residual microscopic disease. The third category is the *wide* margin, in which a margin (thickness not specified) of normal tissue is taken on the entire periphery of the tumor. This may leave microscopic disease. The fourth category is the *radical* margin, which is taken to be a "compartmental" resection. Since sarcomas often extend beyond the boundaries of any one compartment, the definition is sometimes difficult to determine. As with the wide margin, there is potentially microscopic disease, although theoretically it should occur less frequently.

Technique

Approach to Resection

The approach to the resection of soft tissue sarcomas has changed greatly over the last 15 years, with the recognition that limb preservation is feasible in most patients.

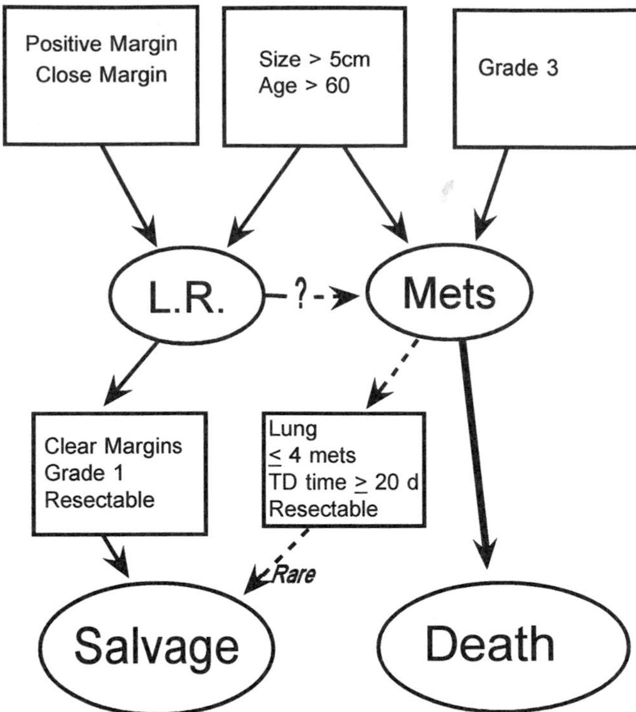

FIGURE 10–5. Prognostic factors for soft tissue sarcomas. L.R., Local recurrence; Mets, metastases; TD time, tumor doubling time.

The success of the combined-modality approach is responsible for this change in attitude on the part of surgical oncologists. What has not changed is the need to place cure as the absolute first priority in planning and executing the resection. In the usual case, concerns about function are subjugated to the achievement of clear margins, even if this means amputation. Certain exceptions can be made in specific circumstances, as discussed in the next section.

Technique of Resection

There will always be patients for whom amputation is required. These patients have large tumors in anatomically unfavorable sites, surrounding the major neurovascular bundles, making total excision impossible without sacrificing a major vessel. In the occasional patient, a vascular reconstruction may be possible. Most patients will have received or will be scheduled to receive irradiation and chemotherapy, which may make reconstruction too hazardous. Major nerves, however, can be resected with good functional results. The surgeon must weigh the level of function of the amputated extremity with prosthesis against that achieved with the limb intact but the palsy due to the specific nerve cut.

The usual soft tissue sarcoma resection does not involve these major neurovascular structures. Resection in this situation requires obtaining adequate margins. Careful preparation of the skin is essential, and plastic orthopedic extremity drapes are desirable. Prophylactic antibiotics are used if the biopsy incision is not well healed. If the tumor is located posteriorly in the lower extremity, the patient should be placed in a lateral or semiprone position.

If an excisional biopsy (sometimes referred to as an "oops") was done, there is the problem of determining where the tumor was located. Re-excision is essential, as there is at least a 49% incidence of macroscopic residual disease.[40] The only recourse is to try to reconstruct the tumor volume and location. It is important to remember that the incision may not have been centered on the tumor. The location of the seroma or hematoma is one guide. Initial (if available) and postbiopsy scans should also be used to determine the anatomic location and extent of the resection.

The biopsy scar should always be excised en bloc with the tumor; however, a wide ellipse of skin is required only for sarcomas involving the skin. If the biopsy scar is oriented incorrectly (e.g., transversely), it should be excised en bloc by means of a curvilinear (S) incision. For a subcutaneous tumor (Fig. 10–6*A*), a simple excision with a margin of fat and, if located deep, the underlying muscular fascia is all that is required. An intramuscular tumor (Fig. 10–6*B*) requires resection of the involved muscle or muscle group around the tumor. After the skin and subcutaneous tissue have been incised, flaps are raised in the plane of the muscular fascia. When an adequate margin of muscle is obtained, the muscular fascia is incised and the muscle fibers divided. A margin of a few centimeters of normal muscle is maintained. A true origin to insertion type of resection is rarely needed. The ideal is an even margin of normal tissue around the tumor. Tumors located on or near the bone (Fig. 10–6*C*) are resected in similar fashion to intramuscular tumors, with the addition that the periosteum underlying the tumor is incised and stripped off the bone for the appropriate distance. If the tumor abuts a nerve but does not encase it (Fig. 10–6*D*), the perineurium should be incised and stripped off the underlying nerve.

If there is an area of the resection margin that cannot be safely resected farther that may have pathologic tumor

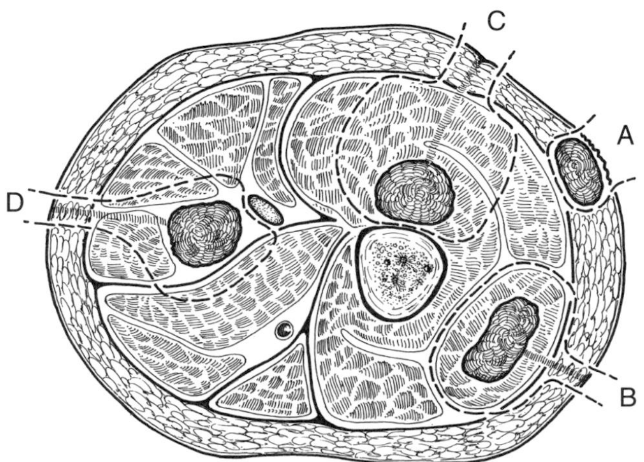

FIGURE 10–6. *A* to *D*, Types of tumor resections.

involvement, small clips should be placed in that area. This will facilitate accurate planning of the postoperative irradiation fields.

Closed suction drains are commonly used and are left in place for 3 to 5 days. If the plan is to leave them in longer, prophylactic antibiotics should be given beginning the day of surgery. In our experience, drains are not necessary, and healing occurs normally without them. Theoretically, at least, there should be less chance of infection if drains are omitted. Soft tissues are approximated as well as possible using absorbable suture. Skin sutures are left in for 3 to 6 weeks if the patient received irradiation or chemotherapy preoperatively.

The specimen's major regions should be marked with sutures to orient the pathologist. Ideally, the surgeon and the pathologist should go over the specimen together. All surfaces should be inked prior to fixation so that, microscopically, the status of the margin can be clearly determined.

Specific procedures and operative details are well covered in soft tissue tumor surgical atlases.[41, 42]

Management of Specific Situations

When Wide Margins Are Impossible to Achieve

The Relationship Between Local Recurrence and Metastasis

Controversy exists over whether local recurrence increases the risk for distant metastasis. Several studies have looked at this issue because of its importance in choosing primary treatment in borderline cases. It has been suggested that local recurrence results in higher rates of distant metastasis[43] and that improved local control would translate into improved survival.[44] While intuitively appealing, it is not clear that there is a significant association. If there is no such association, a close or questionable margin could be accepted if, for example, amputation was the only means of obtaining a better margin. A subsequent local recurrence could be treated without fear that cure had been compromised by the initial procedure. The real issue is whether local recurrence is in itself a cause of distant metastasis or is a marker of a biologically aggressive tumor.

Stotter and colleagues[37, 45] argue that local recurrence should be treated as a time-dependent variable. In their study of 175 patients with extremity soft tissue sarcoma, local recurrence, when treated as time-dependent in the multivariate analysis, emerged as an independent risk factor for distant metastasis. If local recurrence was treated as a conventional prognostic factor (e.g., local recurrence versus no local recurrence), no association was seen. Only 23 of 55 patients (42%) who experienced metastases had a prior local recurrence. A second study that treated local recurrence as a time-dependent variable for multivariate analysis also found local recurrence to be an independent predictor of distant metastasis.[46]

In a later study from the same group, 49% of patients with soft tissue sarcoma in whom metastases developed had a prior local recurrence.[47] The time from treatment to the diagnosis of the distant metastases was identical for those with and without local recurrence. When the highest-grade tumors were examined separately, the same pattern was seen.[48] These authors argue that if distant metastases originate from the recurrence, a time lag should have been seen in the group with distant metastasis after local recurrence, given normal tumor kinetics.

The local recurrence rate in all these studies is high, ranging from 30% to 50% for the grade 4 tumors; thus, there are adequate numbers of patients in both groups for analysis. A recent report comparing amputation and limb-sparing surgery failed to find any impact of local recurrence on survival.[84]

While multivariate analysis may be statistically valid, it does not prove a causal relationship. The same factors that predict local recurrence (e.g., high grade) predict metastasis. It is likely that the same patient and tumor characteristics that result in local recurrence promote or allow distant metastasis. Another argument against local recurrence as a risk factor for distant metastasis is the lack of a significant drop in distant metastasis in series in which local recurrence rate has been reduced to less than 5%.[36, 108, 133]

All of these studies suffer from unequal distribution of prognostic variables. There are, however, two randomized studies in which two groups are stratified for the major prognostic variables.[49, 50] Despite local recurrence rates varying from 0% to 33%, there was no significant difference in overall survival (Table 10–5).

Management. There is enough doubt about the relationship between local recurrence and the development of distant metastasis that accepting a small increased risk of local recurrence for a major functional gain is reasonable. As a case in point, it is National Cancer Institute (NCI) policy that if the tumor abuts a major nerve or vessel, as good a surgical margin as possible should be obtained and postoperative radiotherapy given.[51]

TABLE 10–5
Results of Two Randomized Trials: Local Recurrence and Survival Rates

Study (Institution)	Treatment	Local Recurence Rate (%)	Overall Survival Rate (%)
Rosenberg et al., 1982[50]	Amputation	0	88
(NCI)	LSS + Postoperative RT	15	83
Harrison et al., 1993[49]	LSS + BRT	18	76
(MSKCC)	LSS	33	76

NCI*, National Cancer Institute; LSS, limb-sparing surgery; RT, radiotherapy; MSKCC, Memorial Sloan-Kettering Cancer Center; BRT, brachytherapy.
*Disease-free survival.

When Tumor Is in the Popliteal or Antecubital Fossa

Extremity soft tissue sarcomas located in the antecubital or popliteal fossa present a challenge, as these are virtually always extracompartmental, and wide margins are impossible. Surgical resection alone was successful in only two of seven patients treated at the Memorial Sloan-Kettering Cancer Center.[52] The same report includes 10 patients who were treated with resection and iridium 192 brachytherapy (median dose, 45 Gy*, estimated BED† = 55 Gy). Local control was 100%. Three patients had major complications; one required an amputation. Function was judged to be good in all of the nine patients who retained their limb.

When Tumor Is in the Hand or Foot

Soft tissue sarcomas arising in the hand or foot also pose a problem because of the confined space within which the surgeon must work. It is impossible to preserve function and obtain clear surgical margins in many patients. In contrast to the overall distribution, synovial sarcomas are the most common histologic type, accounting for 38% to 64% of all soft tissue sarcomas found in hand or foot sites.[53–55] Liposarcomas are rare.

In a series of patients with sarcomas of the hand or foot treated surgically between 1949 and 1973, 74% underwent a major amputation, with no local recurrences.[53] Only 13% had a local excision; the remainder had a minor amputation. These last two groups, with a median follow-up of 13 years, had a combined local recurrence rate of 32%.

Okunieff and coworkers[54] reported a group of 15 patients with hand or wrist soft tissue sarcomas treated by excision and postoperative external beam radiotherapy to a median dose of 68 Gy. Eight had intralesional, five had marginal, and two had wide excisions. Median follow-up is only 33 months. Local recurrence was seen in two (13%). A nonfunctional hand was noted in only one patient. Selch et al.[55] reviewed the University of California, Los Angeles (UCLA) experience with 20 patients with soft tissue sarcomas of the foot: 16 were treated under a neoadjuvant protocol and 4 received postoperative irradiation. Of the 20 patients, 7 had a microscopic positive final margin, 1 had a cut-through, and 1 underwent primary amputation. None of the neoadjuvant protocol patients received postoperative radiotherapy, despite positive margins. The local recurrence rate was 10%. Both of these patients had positive margins. The median follow-up was 36 months. Three acute and four late complications occurred, and all salvaged feet were said to be functional.

Both of the last two series used a conservative surgical approach, accepting close or positive margins to preserve function. The use of adjuvant irradiation appears to give acceptable local recurrence rates; however, follow-up is limited, and the true local recurrence rate may be higher.

Brachytherapy, using a system that delivered full dose to the skin, was used to treat five foot soft tissue sarcomas.[98] Severe flap necrosis occurred in all patients. The use of brachytherapy in the hand or foot should be considered investigational.

*One gray (Gy) = 100 cGy (centigray) = 100 rad (radiation absorbed dose).

†For definition of $BED_{2\ Gy}$, see later section on radiotherapy. (BED, Biologically equivalent irradiation dose.)

When Tumor Invades Major Blood Vessel, Bone, or Nerve

Major Vessels

As discussed elsewhere in this subchapter, tumor involvement of a major vessel, nerve, or bone is not an absolute indication for amputation. The profunda femoris artery, for example, can be ligated. Either the radial or the ulnar artery can be ligated in most patients. Major veins, if involved, are usually occluded, and collaterals already exist. Ligation can therefore be undertaken with an acceptable risk of venous insufficiency. The use of vascular grafts (e.g., reversed saphenous vein) in irradiated fields is controversial. Few vascular surgeons would willingly place a vascular graft in an irradiated area unless tissue reaction was minimal.

The preoperative use of chemotherapy and radiotherapy carries an increased risk of wound dehiscence, which in the presence of a graft could result in loss of limb. While one could argue that the limb was going to be lost anyway, it is clear that use of a graft should be limited. The use of a vascular graft in an area that will be irradiated postoperatively is being done, but the risk of vascular blow-out alone and the long-term incidence of occlusion and pseudoaneurysm formation are unreported. In a series of 13 patients who had carotid artery reconstruction after radical cancer surgery and large-fraction intraoperative irradiation, three strokes were observed and there was one vascular blowout.[56] Three patients with major arterial resection (who may or may not have been irradiated) are included in a series from the Memorial Sloan-Kettering Cancer Center, with 3- ,6- and greater than 10-year survivals respectively.[117] Another report includes nine patients who had resection and prosthetic reconstruction of the femoral or iliac arteries[57]; no details or results are given. Two vascular reconstructions (type not specified), which were apparently successfully performed, are included in a series of 60 patients who received preoperative doxorubicin and irradiation.[58] If a graft is used, it should be covered by muscle or a myocutaneous flap to protect it in case of wound breakdown.

Bone

In the usual case, the tumor abuts the bone, and an adequate margin is achieved by simple stripping of a section of the underlying periosteum. If the bone is involved beyond the periosteum (a rare occurrence), bone can be removed with an osteotome. If there is extensive involve-

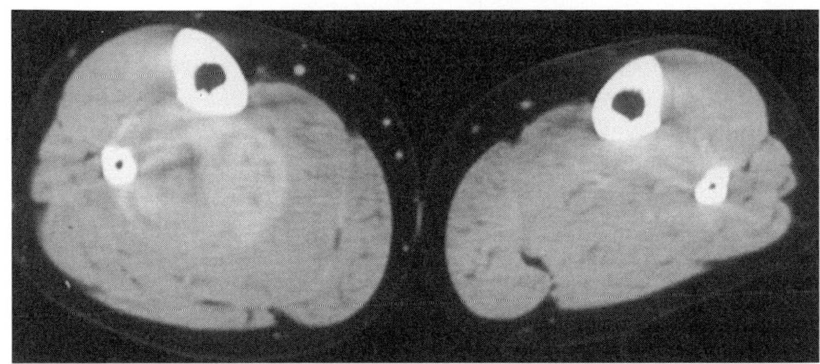

FIGURE 10–7. CT scan of a sarcoma in the calf involving the sciatic nerve and popliteal artery. Resection included the nerve, but the tumor was shaved off the vessel. Postoperative irradiation was given. There was local recurrence within 12 months.

ment and the bone is weight bearing, the involved bone segment can be resected and an endoprosthesis inserted. This, obviously, must be planned preoperatively.

Nerve

Major nerves can be resected if required. Tumors involving the femoral nerve can be resected intact, including the nerve, as the tensor fascia lata is innervated separately and will provide stability of the knee (see later section on function). If the flexors and extenders of the hip are intact, it is possible to walk well on level ground, although stair climbing is impaired. The peroneal nerve can be cut to avoid above-knee amputation and the ankle braced. The sciatic nerve can be divided to avoid hip disarticulation or hemipelvectomy, again using a brace to compensate for the resulting paralysis (Figs. 10–7 and 10–8).

Survival after extended resections as described above parallels that for conventional resections.[117]

When Tumor Violation Occurs

Cut-Through or Exposure of the Pseudocapsule

Even the most careful surgeon can inadvertently cut through tumor and thereby contaminate the wound with tumor cells. The best management of this situation, or its impact on local recurrence, is unclear. There are, not surprisingly, few institutions willing to report such data. In one report of 28 patients, 7 of whom had soft tissue sarcomas, a policy of re-excision and closure of the capsule with copious saline lavage was followed.[59] Three patients had cut-through and four had violation of the capsule. Three received adjuvant postoperative irradiation. There was one local recurrence within a minimum follow-up time of 24 months. In this patient, the policy of re-excision was not followed.

A recent study reports 40 similar patients, 24 of whom had soft tissue sarcomas.[60] In 12 of the 24 patients, the pseudocapsule was exposed. Local recurrence occurred in three of the five patients in whom no additional excision was done and in none of the seven patients in whom additional re-excisions were done. In the other 12 patients, the tumor was cut through. Three of the five local recurrences occurred in patients with no additional re-excision. The use of adjuvant irradiation did not make a difference; however, while the average dose was 56 Gy, some patients received as little as 30 Gy.

On the basis of these findings, we recommend that if the tumor is violated, the defect should be sutured closed and that area re-excised. Copious lavage with saline solution may be useful. The role of adjuvant irradiation after re-excision is unclear.

Positive Margin

If a pathologic positive or close (< 1 mm) margin is found, and the specimen was well identified, it is possible

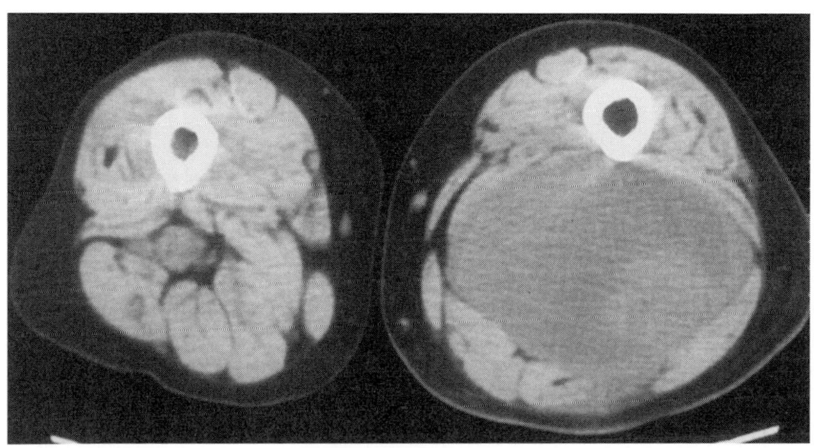

FIGURE 10–8. CT scan of a neurofibrosarcoma in the posterior thigh involving the sciatic nerve. The nerve was resected along with the tumor. Postoperative radiotherapy was given. There has been no local recurrence, and the patient walks with the aid of a cane and brace.

to take the patient back to the operating room and reresect the area. Although no data exist, local recurrence rate should be similar to that if clear margins were obtained at the primary surgery. If the patient was not treated with irradiation preoperatively, postoperative radiotherapy can be given. If the area was marked with clips, the volume to be treated can be defined with greatly enhanced accuracy.

If the patient received irradiation preoperatively and if re-excision is not feasible, reirradiation is an option. Eleven patients treated with preoperative chemotherapy and large-fraction irradiation were found to have pathologic tumor involving the margins.[113] These patients, who received 17.5 or 28 Gy preoperatively, were given 30 to 60 Gy postoperatively (median total split-course dose, 73 Gy; median interval, 1 month). There were three (27%) local recurrences, four patients experienced severe edema, and six had impaired function.

Another option, of course, is to amputate the extremity if this will achieve a wide margin.

The final option is simply to observe the patient, and in certain circumstances this may be the only option, as amputation either has already been done or will not provide better margins.

Several recent studies have looked at the effect that very close or positive margins have on local recurrence rates (Table 10–6). The results are remarkably consistent, with the exception of the group with negative margins treated by resection alone, in which the local recurrence rate is noticeably greater than in the combined-modality studies. Positive margins are associated with a high risk of local recurrence, but the recurrence rate is still only one of three in the surgery-only group. The data for positive margins in Table 10–6 cast doubt on the efficacy of irradiation to sterilize microscopic residual disease. However, the same data support a policy of observation in many cases in which the final pathologic margin is microscopically positive. This is all the more true given the small, if any, effect that local recurrence has on overall survival.

The next issue is what width of tissue margin is required to minimize the local recurrence rate. Sadoski et al.[61] looked at the effect of surgical margins on local recurrence rates in 132 patients. Following preoperative irradiation and resection, a boost was given to 100 patients, most often by means of external beam radiotherapy to a volume defined by clips placed at the edges of the tumor bed. The authors state that the boost was given without regard for the surgical margins. No residual tumor was found in 22 instances. A margin that was negative, even if less than 1 mm, yielded, in their study, as low a local recurrence rate as did a wider margin. Another recently published series of 74 patients stratified the surgical margins at 5 mm.[92] An advantage was reported for margins of greater than 5 mm. Because of the small numbers of patients in each group in both studies, no definite conclusions about the minimal surgical margins necessary can be made. The data do suggest that the necessary margin is very small.

When Lymph Nodes Are Positive

The low incidence of nodal metastasis (see Table 10–2) makes prophylactic regional lymph node dissection unwarranted. Clinically suspicious nodes can be confirmed by fine-needle aspiration cytology. A standard node dissection should be performed. There are reports of the successful use of radiotherapy to treat involved lymph nodes; however, only two patients were treated.[62]

When Tumor Is Inoperable

Patients with inoperable tumors can be (1) technically unresectable or (2) medically unable to withstand surgery. Medically inoperable patients are candidates for palliative treatment or primary radiotherapy.

TABLE 10–6
Margin Status and Local Recurrence

Study (Institution)	Treatment	No. of Patients	Margin	LR Rate (%)	Notes
Sadoski et al., 1993[61] (MGH)	Preoperative 50 Gy	28	Positive	18	Boost given without regard to margin in 71% of patients
	Resection	46	≤1 mm	6	
	± 14–18 Gy boost	36	>1 mm	3	
Herbert et al., 1993[92] (Fox Chase)	Resection	19	Positive	32	1 of 2 patients with grossly positive margins recurred;
	Postoperative 40–71 Gy	10	≤5 mm	10	
		45	>5 mm	0	7% preoperative XRT
Harrison et al., 1993[49] (MSKCC)	Group 1: Resection	11	Positive	36	
		59	Negative	30	Randomized study
	Group 2: Resection	11	Positive	27	
	Brachytherapy	44	Negative	15	
Abbatucci et al., 1986[98] (Baclesse)	Preoperative 27 Gy*				50% received preoperative actinomycin D
	Resection	23	Positive	44	
	Postoperative 23–43 Gy	54	Negative	2	

LR, Local recurrence; MGH, Massachusetts General Hospital; XRT, radiotherapy; MSKCC, Memorial Sloan-Kettering Cancer Center.
*$dBED_{2\,Gy}$. Actual 2 fractions of 6.5 Gy each.

Technically inoperable tumors are difficult to define. To some degree, it is dependent on the experience of the surgeon. There are tumors that are in fact not safely resectable, usually because of size and location or fixation to major vascular structures and prior high-dose irradiation to the area. In this situation, after discussion of the consequences and risks of surgical intervention, the patient may decline to be operated on. For this patient, there is a role for definitive radiotherapy.

There are series with small to modest numbers of patients who received irradiation with curative intent for inoperable soft tissue sarcomas.[63–65, 108] In all these series, which are retrospective, the criteria for inoperability are vague, irradiation techniques are heterogeneous, and doses vary considerably. A third problem is that two of the larger series include patients treated from 1935 and after in one and from 1954 and after in the other. In one series of 36 patients treated from 1971 to 1982, who received 64 Gy or its equivalent, 25 tumors were less than 10 cm.[63] In this group of 25 patients, there was a 47% local recurrence rate; 43% of patients were alive 5 years following treatment. For patients with tumors larger than 10 cm, the local recurrence rate was approximately 70%, and none were cured. These results are representative of other reported series.

Another approach is preoperative (or neoadjuvant) chemotherapy. A group of 46 patients with large, high-grade soft tissue sarcomas were given a preoperative regimen of Cy(V)ADIC (cyclophosphamide, [some patients also received vincristine], doxorubicin [Adriamycin], and dacarbazine [DIC]). Although the tumors were not technically inoperable, their mean size was 10.6 cm, and 87% were grade 3.[66] There was an 11% complete response and a "major" partial response in another 13%. Severe side effects, including a mean of 2.3 hospitalizations, occurred in 80%. Although not reported as a neoadjuvant regimen for soft tissue sarcomas, in our experience the combination of mesna, Adriamycin, ifosfamide, and dacarbazine (MAID) also gives good results.

Radiotherapy

Comparing Radiotherapy Doses

Oncologic surgeons have a good understanding of the biologic implications of 50 to 60 Gy given in 2-Gy fractions. The sections that follow contain references to irradiation doses more and less than 50 Gy, some given in very different fractions than the standard 2 Gy. It is important to understand how different irradiation doses and fractionation schedules are compared.

Dosages can be calculated as the given dose or as the tumor dose (the amount of radiation calculated to reach the tumor center). It is, unfortunately, not often specified which system is used. The tumor dose will be equal to or less than the given dose depending on the depth of the tumor in relationship to the depth at which the radiation reaches its maximum effect, which in turn depends on its energy. A "standard" course of preoperative or postoperative radiotherapy is given using a fraction of 2 Gy/day, 5 days a week. Other fractionation schemes must be converted to the "standard" of an equivalent of 10 Gy/week in five fractions of 2 Gy before comparisons may be made. Currently, it is thought that the best conversion is based on a mathematical model termed the linear-quadratic equation. Before calculation, however, it must be decided whether we are interested in acute effects (e.g., mucositis, tumor kill) or late effects (e.g., fibrosis, myelitis), as there is a term in the equation, known as the α/β ratio, that is different for the two types of effect. The α/β ratio is a number that is a measure of tissue-specific radiosensitivity factors. This number has been estimated for most tissues. For acute effects, the α/β ratio is around 8 to 20 Gy, and 10 is a commonly used figure. For late effects, the α/β ratio is in the range of 1 to 6 Gy, and 2 is a commonly used value.

$$\frac{BED_{2\,Gy} = D(\alpha/\beta + d)}{\alpha/\beta + 2}$$

where $BED_{2\,Gy}$ is the 2-GY equivalent dose
D is the dose, and
d is the fraction dose.

As an example, the initial UCLA protocol called for 35 Gy given in 10 fractions. What is this dosage equal to in terms of a "standard" radiotherapy course in its effect on the patient and the tumor? Using the equation (which equates to our standard of 2-Gy fractions), for early effects ($\alpha/\beta = 10$) the $BED_{2\,Gy}$ is approximately 40 Gy, while for late effects ($\alpha/\beta = 2$) the $BED_{2\,Gy}$ is approximately 48 Gy. This illustrates an important point: with larger fractions, late effects will be increased over early effects for a given effect on the tumor.

The above refers only to external beam radiotherapy given as a single course. In some situations, the irradiation course is divided, or split, with the segments separated by weeks or years. The linear-quadratic equation has no time factor; thus, the BED of split-course irradiation cannot be accurately determined, only approximated. There are animal data suggesting that, with delays ranging from months to years, late damage can be repaired to some degree. Thus, in reirradiation for local recurrence, which usually involves a long interval between the radiotherapy courses, the BED of the two irradiation doses can only be guessed at, but it would be less than a simple sum of the two doses. The effects of irradiation, independent of fraction size, may be altered by the field size and the accompanying use of chemotherapy.

With brachytherapy, the dosimetry is very subjective and dependent on the alignment, spacing, and loading of the sources. In the United States, there are no generally accepted guidelines or dose definitions. Computerized planning produces isodose curves of different dose rates, which allows the physician to individualize the tumor dose. With brachytherapy, a distance of only 0.5 cm will change the dose rate by more than 10%. Common dose rates are usually in the range of 0.4 to 0.6 Gy/hour and are higher in the center of the implanted volume. Unless two institutions use exactly the same system (placement, spacing, loading, and interpretation), it is impossible to equate dosages. Identical stated implant doses may, in reality, vary by a factor of three.[67]

Radiation Tolerance

Much has been written about the advantages and disadvantages of preoperative or postoperative irradiation; either way, the surgical oncologist should be familiar with the basic facts underlying postirradiation morbidity. The functional disability depends not only on the amount of normal tissue irradiated but also on the anatomic site. For example, an 8 × 8 cm volume of postirradiation indurated stiff tissue in the thigh may cause only a minor functional disability; that same unyielding tissue in the wrist, elbow, or knee may cause significant loss of range of movement. That same irradiated tissue in the supraclavicular or inguinal regions may cause neurovascular damage and pain.

The irradiation tolerance of connective tissue and muscle without chemotherapy is equivalent to 76 Gy in 38 fractions of 2 Gy/day, 10 Gy/week. In a series reporting results of brachytherapy for soft tissue sarcoma, four patients receiving a total estimated dose to a major peripheral nerve of 91 to 148 Gy experienced a radiation-induced nerve injury.[68] No patients whose total dose was less than 90 Gy had neurotoxicity. Because of the uncertainties of brachytherapy dosimetry, the 90-Gy threshold should be considered provisional. The irradiation tolerance of peripheral arteries or veins is poorly documented. Radiotherapy injury to an artery (e.g., axillary) appears to take 8 to 10 years to become symptomatic.[69] Tolerance depends on the total dose as well as on the daily dose and, ultimately, the weekly dose rate. For example, wound dehiscence is almost guaranteed after preoperative 30 Gy in three fractions of 10 Gy; however, normal healing would be expected with 30 Gy in 15 fractions of 2 Gy given preoperatively.

The use of irradiation doses such as 50 Gy for subclinical disease, 65 Gy for positive microscopic margins, and 75 Gy for gross disease has its support in soft clinical data. The choice of postirradiation volume, larger for grade 3 or intramuscular sarcomas, and the blocking of a minimum 1-cm strip of skin and subcutaneous tissue to prevent edema are guidelines based on recommendation rather than on precise studies.

External Beam Radiotherapy

In most centers in the United States, external beam radiotherapy for extremity soft tissue sarcoma is delivered using a linear accelerator rated at 4 to 6 MeV. Cobalt 60 teletherapy is also used. Radiation is generally given as photons (x-rays or gamma rays), although on occasion an electron beam may be used for part of the treatment. The field size used depends on whether the irradiation is being given pre- or postoperatively. A preoperative field may range from 5 to 15 cm, depending on the tumor size. The margin is increased for high-grade tumors. A postoperative field must include the entire surgical wound plus a margin and, in most instances, will be larger than the preoperative field for the same size tumor. Anteroposterior-posteroanterior parallel opposed fields are commonly used. In certain patients, oblique fields may be advantageous. The limb is immobilized in a fixture so that its position and orientation are reproduced for each treatment. Normally, a strip of skin and subcutaneous tissue is left out of the irradiation field to decrease the risk of distal edema. If possible, one half of the bone diameter is excluded. If the tumor is large in relation to the extremity, it may be necessary to include the whole bone or even the whole limb circumference (Fig. 10–9).

Brachytherapy

Placement of brachytherapy sources can be done percutaneously under local anesthesia or as part of a surgical procedure. Whenever possible in order to minimize irradiation exposure to the medical personnel, afterloading catheters (polyethylene tubing) are used. With afterloading technique, the catheters when placed do not contain the radioactive source. Typically, the source, iridium 192, is prepared as small "seeds" spaced at 1-cm intervals along a wire. The wires are passed into the catheters at the bedside.

Extremity tumors are well suited for afterloading techniques. After the surgeon and the radiotherapist decide on the size of the tumor bed, the target volume or area is then defined by adding margins of 2 cm.[49] The catheters are passed percutaneously into the wound, laid in position about 1 cm apart and as parallel as possible, and loosely secured with an absorbable suture. The wound is then closed, and, since collapse of the postresection cavity (dead space) is essential to obtaining adequate irradiation doses to the resection margins, good drains are essential. Proper placement of the catheters is crucial if a good dose distribution is to be had. A plan for loading the catheters is completed with the aid of a computer to deliver a dose of 42 to 45 Gy over 4 to 6 days (30 to 45 cGy/hour) to a point 0.5 cm from the plane of the sources, near the corner of the implant. The catheters are loaded 6 days postoperatively. This interval, which was originally 3 to 4 days, has been steadily increased in an attempt to decrease the number of patients with wound-healing problems. While iridium 192 has been the source used, iodine 125 may have some advantage in tumor sites close to vital organs.[70] Modifications are used by other centers.[71, 72]

A problem with this general technique is that if the catheters do not lie in a flat plane, the dosimetry becomes complex and therefore uncertain. Such a flat plane is difficult to obtain in a large wound. The potential benefit

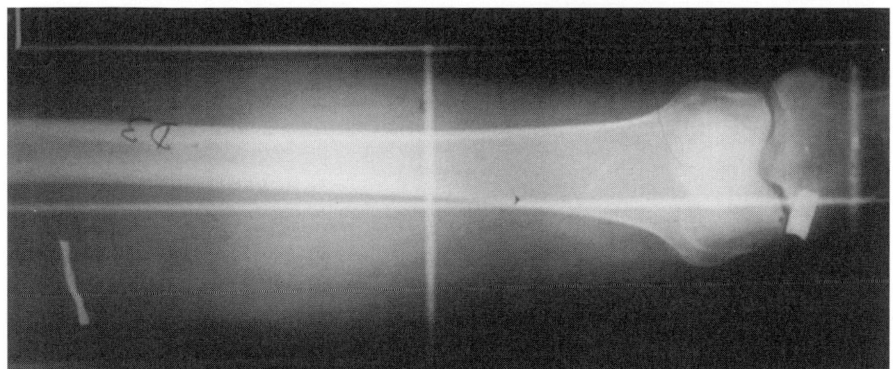

FIGURE 10–9. Simulation film for patient in Figure 10–7. The radiotherapy portal encompasses the tumor, the biopsy site, and, in this case, the entire limb as well.

compared with external beam radiotherapy is a shorter time to deliver the radiotherapy (6 days vs. 5 to 6 weeks for the conventional 50 to 60 Gy). The need for several days of hospitalization offsets any cost advantage. Hypofractionation protocols (e.g., 28 Gy in 8 days) also negate this advantage. Any dosimetric advantage is theoretic at this juncture.

Multimodality Therapy

Intra-arterial Catheters

Multimodality therapy protocols that use chemotherapy require an access to the vascular system. Intra-arterial delivery necessitates that an arterial catheter be placed, normally percutaneously using the Seldinger technique. The catheter can be placed retrograde and inserted in the opposite side for proximally located tumors, or antegrade and ipsilaterally inserted for distal tumors. The position of the catheter is confirmed by injection of fluorescein dye viewed under ultraviolet light (Wood's lamp). This should be done while the patient is still in the angiography suite. The presence of a "hot spot," or area of excessive perfusion, can be detected and the catheter repositioned. The distribution of the dye should cover the tumor bed with a wide margin. If necessary, the catheter can be withdrawn slightly to provide more proximal perfusion.

The position of the catheter is checked every morning at the patient's bedside by injecting fluorescein dye and examining the limb under the Wood's lamp. The distribution of the dye should match that seen in the radiology suite. Occasionally, a patient will need to be returned to the angiography room for adjustment. Catheter placement for 72 hours is well tolerated; longer time intervals are accompanied by a significant catheter-related morbidity.[73] Intra-arterial catheters may be unnecessary, at least for doxorubicin, as equal results have been obtained with intravenous infusion.[74]

Complications

Complications following resection of soft tissue sarcomas are generally minimal, with primary healing of the wound the rule. Major complications (e.g., those requiring reoperation for correction) occur in less than 5% of cases, moderate complications (e.g., seroma, wound dehiscence) occur in 11% to 25%, and minor complications (e.g., small seroma, small dehiscence) occur in 20% to 25%.[75–78] The complication rate increases when preoperative irradiation or combined chemotherapy and radiotherapy are used. The range of possible morbidity and sequelae are shown in Table 10–7.

Bujko and colleagues[75] analyzed the outcome of 202

TABLE 10–7
Complications and Sequelae of Preoperative Irradiation

	Complication	Morbidity Grade	Morbidity	Outcome
Early	Dermatitis	Minor	Dry desquamation	Early healing
		Moderate	Moist desquamation	Healing
	Wound healing	Moderate	Dehiscence	Late healing
		Major	Necrosis	Late healing
				Amputation
Late	Fibrosis	Minor	Induration	None/edema
		Moderate	Decreased motion	Mild loss of function
		Major	Contracture	Major loss of function
	Radionecrosis	Moderate	Bone loss	Resection, reconstruction
		Major	Fracture	Amputation
	Neuritis	Moderate	Sensory loss	Numbness
		Major	Motor loss	Loss of function
	Vascular	Moderate	Occlusion	Angioplasty, reconstruction
		Major	Blow-out	Reconstruction, amputation

patients who received preoperative irradiation at an average dose of 47.5 Gy (range, 16 to 70 Gy) (Table 10–8). They found that wound-healing problems occurred significantly more often when the sarcoma was grade 3 and located in the leg, when estimated blood loss exceeded 1000 cc, and when the patient's age was over 40 years. An increased risk was also associated with hyperfractionated radiotherapy, which would be expected. Surprisingly, patients with diabetes mellitus or hypertension displayed no increased delay in healing.

Function

When performing limb-sparing surgery, there may be concern that the extent of the resection required may impair function to such a degree that an amputation might be preferable. A few studies have examined function following limb-sparing surgery and give some guidelines. Markhede and Stener,[79] in a careful study of 46 patients undergoing resection of a soft tissue tumor from the hip or thigh, or both, found that postoperative impairment could be predicted from the type of resection. Muscles that could be resected without causing impairment to any degree were the iliopsoas, the gluteus maximus, a single hamstring muscle, and one to two of the quadriceps muscles. Muscles that when resected caused a moderate degree of impairment were the tensor fascia latae, all three of the major adductors (longus, brevis, magnus), and all of the hamstrings. They also noted that while no patient complained spontaneously of impaired function, almost all experienced a feeling of unsteadiness and reduced running ability. All but 1 of the 46 patients was able to return to his occupation.

Stinson and colleagues[80] from the NCI studied acute toxicity and long-term function after resection and "definitive" adjuvant external beam radiotherapy. Postoperative radiotherapy was given to a total dose of 63 to 70 Gy. "Long term" was defined as persisting for greater than 1 year after treatment. Contracture occurred in 27 (20%) patients but persisted in only 1 patient. Contracture was positively correlated with irradiation to a joint and with a total dose of 70 Gy. While 7% of patients required a cane or other walking aid, one half of these were eventually able to walk without any aids. Irradiation doses greater than 63 Gy (1.8-Gy fractions) were associated with chronic pain (requiring narcotics), moderate to severe edema, moderate to severe decreased strength, and moderate to severe decrease in range of motion. Radiotherapy fields larger than 35 cm in length were associated with edema and decreased muscle strength. Robinson et al.[81] has reported similar results.

The NCI reported a study of quality of life after limb-sparing surgery versus amputation.[82] No difference was found. The evaluations were self-assessed, however, and, as noted by Markhede and Stener,[79] patients learn to cope and adapt. The NCI study should not be taken to mean that patients accept amputation, as almost all patients elect limb-sparing surgery over amputation, but rather that patients who need amputation will adjust and have a good quality of life.

TABLE 10–8
Risk Factors for Delayed Healing After Preoperative Radiotherapy

	Risk Factor	*P* Value	Odds Ratio	Not Associated with Increased Risk
Patient	Lower extremity site	0.001	3.8 1.0	Diabetes mellitus
	Increasing age	0.034	—	Hypertension
	Increasing grade	0.020		Tumor size
Treatment	Estimated blood loss >1000 cc	0.010	2.9	Preoperative irradiation dose
	Hyperfractionated irradiation	0.026	1.8	Adjuvant chemotherapy

Adapted from Bujko K, et al: Wound healing after preoperative radiation for sarcoma of soft tissues. Surg Gynecol Obstet 176:124–134, 1993. By permission of Surgery, Gynecology, and Obstetrics, now known as the Journal of the American College of Surgeons.

Treatment Summary

Grade 1 Tumors

Grade 1 tumors can be treated by simple excision if clear margins can be obtained (see earlier discussion of technique). Neoadjuvant protocols are not normally used for grade 1 soft tissue sarcomas, as the consensus is that this is overtreatment. While many series report grade 1 tumors in the overall group receiving adjuvant radiotherapy, they were probably either large with positive or questionable margins or histology was borderline. It is appropriate to give radiotherapy in this subgroup. It does not appear to matter much whether the irradiation is given pre- or postoperatively (see later discussion of surgery and radiotherapy under Results). There are tradeoffs: preoperative irradiation may shrink the tumor, making the resection easier, but may also predispose the site to healing problems (see earlier discussion of complications).

Grade 2 and 3 Tumors

Grade 2 and 3 (and 4 in some series) soft tissue sarcomas should be treated by a multimodality limb-preserving approach. Ideally, the surgeon and the radiotherapist (and, perhaps, the medical oncologist) plan treatment together. The proven options are pre- or postoperative radiotherapy or a UCLA-type neoadjuvant approach (see earlier discussion of multimodality therapy). We favor the latter. Even very large soft tissue sarcomas are candidates for limb salvage if located in the thigh (see earlier discussion of function). Neoadjuvant protocols are not a substitute for adequate surgery. Every effort must be made to get clear margins (see earlier discussion of technique). The minimum margin needed is apparently very small, on the order of 1 mm (see earlier discussion of positive margin). A grossly positive margin should be re-excised (see earlier discussion of when tumor violation occurs), being as aggressive as needed (see discussions of function, and when tumor invades major blood vessel, nerve, or bone). A close margin should be observed (see discussion of when wide margins are impossible to achieve).

Regional Nodal Involvement

Positive regional nodes should be excised using standard lymphadenectomy techniques (see earlier discussion of when lymph nodes are positive). While successful irradiation of positive lymph nodes has been reported, the standard remains surgical resection.

Local Recurrence

The treatment of locally recurrent soft tissue sarcoma depends entirely on the initial treatment used. If excision was the primary modality, the options are the same as for a previously untreated sarcoma. An aggressive approach should be used, with the expectation of a significant rate of salvage (see later discussion of treatment of local recurrence).

Metastatic Disease

Metastatic soft tissue sarcoma can be approached surgically in selected patients (see later discussion of treatment of distant metastasis).

RESULTS

Surgery

Amputation

Surgical resection is the backbone of the treatment of soft tissue sarcoma. The amount of resection has been the source of considerable controversy. Most surgical series contain patients treated by local excision (equivalent to marginal resection), wide excision, and amputation.[83–86, 108, 109] The reasons for choosing the particular type of operation are individualized and doubtless based on tumor size and location, with amputation generally reserved for tumors with the worst prognosis.

The results after amputation are fairly consistent (Table 10–9), as few marginal amputations are done for cure. The number of patients alive 5 years following treatment is consistent with the inclusion of generally poorer prognosis tumors in this treatment category.[84]

While once considered the standard approach to the treatment of soft tissue sarcomas, fewer amputations are currently being done as the primary surgical procedure, as there is no evidence that amputation improves survival.[83, 84] Willard and colleagues[84] attempted to compare the results of amputation and limb-sparing surgery for similar tumors and found no advantage for amputation. This result applied to all tumor sizes and grades. This series is somewhat difficult to interpret, as 16 of the 92 patients undergoing amputation had distant metastasis at presentation and 8 had amputation of a digit only. The number of patients with distant metastasis in the limb-sparing surgery group is not given. The limb-sparing surgery group includes patients who received adjuvant irradiation. Local control was better in the amputation group, but the efficacy of salvage treatment eliminated any survival advantage. The question remains, what patients are best served by amputation? The answer appears to be only those patients in whom limb-sparing surgery would leave a useless limb.

Limb-Sparing Surgery

Virtually all centers now report combined-modality results, or reserve purely surgical treatment for small, superficial and grade 1 tumors. There are exceptions.[85, 86, 109] Earlier series give local recurrence rates of 12% to 70% after wide excision (Table 10–10). The large discrepancies in the local recurrence rates probably reflect more the definition of "wide" that was used than the surgical technique employed. The success of salvage is reflected in the percentage of patients alive 5 years following treatment. Of great interest is a randomized series evaluating brachytherapy that contains a surgery-only arm.[49] While 11 patients in this group had positive margins, only 4 had local recurrence.

TABLE 10–9
Results After Amputation

Study (Institution)	No. of Patients	Grade 2–4 (%)	LR Rate (%)	% Alive 5 yrs After Treatment	Notes
Berli et al., 1990[109] (Gothenburg)	35	87	3	~43	
Rosenberg et al., 1982[50] (NCI)	16		13	55	81% were T2 or T3 Part of a randomized study
Shiu et al., 1975[117] (MSKCC)	106	N/A	7	45	
Gerner et al., 1975[111] (RPCI)	38		8 0	43	

LR, Local recurrence; NCI, National Cancer Institute; MSKCC, Memorial Sloan-Kettering Cancer Center; N/A, Not available; RPCI, Roswell Park Cancer Institute.

TABLE 10–10
Results After Limb-Sparing Surgery

Study (Institution)	No. of Patients	Grade 2 or 3 (%)	Surgical Margin No. of Patients	LR Rate (%)	% Alive 5 yr After Treatment	Notes (No. of Patients in Group)
Harrison et al., 1993[49] (MSKCC)	70	74	Pos. 16% Neg. 84%	33	76 DFS	Part of a randomized study Only 4/11 (36%) patients with positive margins failed locally
Karakousis et al., 1991[57] (RPCI)	80	?	>2 cm	7	(71%)*	For whole group, not just surgery-only patients*
Rydholm et al., 1991[85] (Lund)	70 49	83 89	Wide (56) Wide (14)	7 29	91%* 79%*	Site: SC (40) or IM (30); F/U 4.5 yr Site: Extramuscular
Berli et al., 1990[109] (Gothenburg)	37	87	Wide (26) Mgl (9)	19 56	Mgl ~45	Site: SC (26) IM (11)
	60		Wide (44) Mgl (16)	9 69	Wide ~70	Site: Extramuscular or deep; F/U 6 yr
Leibel et al., 1982[108] (UCSF)	31	50	Wide Comp	70 18	74 82	
Shiu et al., 1975[117] (MSKCC)	178	N/A	Wide (178)	12	63	
Gerner et al., 1975[111] (RPMI)	102	N/A	Mgl (58) Wide (44)	93 71	50	

LR, Local recurrence; MSKCC, Memorial Sloan-Kettering Cancer; DFS, disease free survival; RPCI, Roswell Park Cancer Institute; SC, subcutaneous; IM, intramuscular; F/U, follow-up; Mgl, marginal resection; UCSF, University of California, San Francisco; Comp, compartmental resection; N/A, not available.

*Absolute cancer-specific 4½ year survival.

Two recently reported series have tried to define the best results obtainable by surgery alone. The University of Göteborg, Sweden, reported 97 patients; 84% of the tumors were greater than 5 cm, and 87% were grade 3 or 4.[109] Local recurrence data were reported by type of resection and by location of the tumor. Wide resections resulted in an overall local recurrence rate of 13%, while the local recurrence rate after marginal resections was 64%. Another Swedish group has reported an overall local recurrence rate after wide excision of 16% (7% and 29%, depending on location of the tumor).[85] Again, there was a high proportion of high-grade and T2 tumors. Most patients with marginal resections received irradiation postoperatively, and thus there are no data for marginal resection. Both series used strict criteria for defining resection margins, and in one,[85] even patients with open biopsies were excluded.

The Roswell Park Cancer Institute recently updated their results.[57] Minimum follow-up is probably 4 years or so, and about one third of tumors were grade 1. Eighty patients in whom margins of at least 2 cm were obtained were not given adjuvant irradiation. Local recurrence was observed in only 7% of the 80 patients.

These three series probably represent the best results obtainable by surgery alone.

TABLE 10–11
Possible Advantages and Disadvantages of Preoperative Radiotherapy

Possible Advantages	Possible Disadvantages
Decreased irradiation volume	Impaired wound healing
Decreased tumor size at surgery	Altered specimen for pathology
Sterilization of tumor capsule	
Sterilization of disturbed biopsy site	

It is evident that patients who have had a marginal resection require further treatment, either surgical (e.g., re-excision of the involved margin) or an effective second modality for what is really salvage, not adjuvant, therapy. It is less clear that patients who have had a successful wide excision require adjuvant treatment.

Surgery and Radiotherapy

Preoperative Radiotherapy

Relatively few reports of preoperative irradiation exist that do not include preoperative chemotherapy as well. In these series, some or all patients presented with initially inoperable tumors.[87] The definition of "inoperable" is obviously subjective. There are theoretic benefits, and risks, from preoperative irradiation (Table 10–11). For tumors that are considered inoperable because of the bulk, preoperative irradiation may shrink the sarcoma to a size that is amenable to resection or decrease operative blood loss and morbidity. Sterilization of the pseudocapsule is a theoretic concept at present. There are no reports of using preoperative radiotherapy specifically for disturbed (e.g., hematoma) wounds. Wound healing is impaired after moderate-to high-dose irradiation (60 to 70 Gy), but careful wound closure and the judicious use of flaps and grafts can obviate these problems. An adequate biopsy specimen can reduce the chance of sampling error in tumors that may be inhomogeneous with respect to histologic grade.

Tepper and Suit[88] reported a series of 60 patients treated at the Massachusetts General Hospital with preoperative irradiation with a postoperative small boost intended to keep wound complications down while still delivering 62 to 64 Gy (Table 10–12). Seventeen tumors were larger than 15 cm, and 24 were considered initially inoperable.

TABLE 10–12
Results of Preoperative Adjunctive Radiotherapy

Study (Institution)	No. of Patients	Grade 2 or 3 (%)	Surgical Margin (No. of Patients)	Dose (Gy)	LR Rate (%)	% Alive 5 yr After Treatment	Notes
Robinson et al., 1992[87] (RMH)	70	79	Mgl (40) Wide (30)	50	11	62	21 patients got <50 Gy 6 patients got 70–80 Gy
Barkley et al., 1988[89] (MDACC)	110	90	Mgl	50	10	56 DFS	8 patients received mixed beam with photon and neutrons
Sadoski et al., 1993[61] (MGH)	132	92	Positive (28) Negative (104)	50	6	?	14–18 Gy postoperative boost in 100 patients

LR, local recurrence; RMH, Royal Marsden Hospital; MDACC, M.D. Anderson Cancer Center; DFS, disease free survival; MGH, Massachusetts General Hospital.

Compared with their postoperative patients, almost twice as many preoperatively treated patients had high-grade tumors. The authors believed that there was a 17% advantage in local control for preoperative over postoperative irradiation for tumors larger than 15 cm. There were only nine patients with tumors of this size in their postoperative group; thus, this difference is not significant. Sadoski et al.[61] recently updated the Massachusetts General Hospital results. Of 132 patients treated preoperatively with 50 Gy, 22 had no residual tumor. One-hundred patients received a postoperative boost of 14 to 18 Gy, apparently without regard for the surgical margin. The actuarial local recurrence rate was 6%. Overall survival is not given.

Barkley et al.[89] reported the M.D. Anderson Cancer Center experience with preoperative radiotherapy (see Table 10–12). They treated 90 patients who had intact primary tumors with 50 Gy followed by a conservative resection. Minimum follow-up was less than 12 months; mean follow-up, however, was 52 months. Local control in the subset of 90 patients who presented with intact primary tumors and who were able to complete the protocol was 91%. Twelve patients had disturbed biopsy wounds (defined as piecemeal excision or excision without margins) and had no "deleterious consequences" from a conservative surgical resection. Complications occurred in 14% and in all eight who received neutrons. Amputation was necessary in two patients. No effect of histologic type on outcome was seen, while histologic grade correlated well.

Another recent series is from the Royal Marsden Hospital, London (see Table 10–12).[87] All patients were thought to be inoperable. Radiotherapy fractionation schemes included 50 patients treated daily, 13 treated twice daily, and 3 treated once a week. Total dose ranged from 20 to 80 Gy. Four patients received preoperative intra-arterial doxorubicin. This was early in the series and was abandoned because of marked late toxicity. A response (defined as a ≥50% decrease in tumor size) was seen in 42 cases (60%), and four had a complete histologic response. A dose-response relationship was noted; 80% of patients receiving 60 Gy or more responded, compared with 50% of patients whose dose was less than 60 Gy. Nine patients (13%) experienced major complications; two needed amputation. There was an increased incidence of complications in patients older than 60 years.

The Royal Marsden Hospital has also reported the use of a hyperfractionated (more than one fraction per day) protocol using 1.25 Gy twice daily (6-hour interval) to a total irradiation dose of 62.5 to 75 Gy.[90] Median follow-up for these 29 patients is less than 2 years. Despite the theoretic ability of hyperfractionation to increase the tumor response ratio, and despite the short follow-up, an increase in both early and late toxicity was seen. They are now using both a lower total dose (60 Gy) and dose per fraction (1.2 Gy).

Postoperative Radiotherapy

Postoperative irradiation is the most widely used form of adjuvant therapy for soft tissue sarcomas. Most series include patients who received chemotherapy. These patients are usually those who had grade 3 sarcomas or had signs considered to be bad prognostic features. The exception is the NCI randomized study, one arm of which falls into this group. Since the consensus is that adjuvant chemotherapy has little, if any, effect on the outcome, it is ignored in the following analysis (Table 10–13).

The M.D. Anderson Cancer Center reported 300 patients, 200 of whom had extremity sarcomas.[110] Their surgical philosophy was to perform a conservative resection, preserving as much function as possible. Resection margins varied from wide to marginal, and some patients probably had microscopically positive margins. This study spans a 14-year period. A shrinking-field technique was employed. For the first 8 years, the irradiation dose was carried to 75 Gy to the tumor volume and 50 Gy to the larger field. For the last 6 years, the tumor volume dose was 65 Gy, with 60 Gy to the wider field. Local recurrence occurred in 20%, and 69% of patients were alive 5 years following treatment. No analysis of local recurrence rate in relation to margin status was done. Major complications were seen in 7%, and 1.5% had poor range of movement.

Rosenberg and colleagues[50] reported on the NCI trial of limb-sparing surgery plus irradiation versus amputation. All tumors were high grade. The irradiation dose was 60 to 70 Gy. Compared with the amputation arm, there was

TABLE 10–13
Results of Postoperative Radiotherapy

Study (Institution or Group)	No. of Patients	Grade 2 or 3	Surgical Margin (%)	Dose (Gy)	LR Rate (%)	% Alive 5 yr After Treatment	Notes
Herbert et al., 1993[92] (Fox Chase)	74	76%	Positive 26% Mgl 14% Wide 50%	63	11	70	Preoperative irradiation in 6 patients LR 45% if positive margin LR 20% if close margin (P = .003)
Wiklund et al., 1993[91] (SSG)	26	100%	Mgl or microscopically positive	62	18	?	
Karakousis et al., 1991[57] (RPCI)	64	?	<2 cm	60	8	?	
Tepper and Suit, 1985[88] (MGH)	110	?	?	64	16	73	LR 39% for T >15 cm
Rosenberg et al., 1982[50] (NCI)	27	100%	?	60–70	15	83	One arm of a randomized trial
Lindberg et al., 1981[110] (MIDACC)	200	75%	Mgl	60 (mean)	20	69	30% of LRs were out of field

LR, Local recurrence; SSG, Scandinavian Sarcoma Group; RPCI, Roswell Park Cancer Institute; MGH, Massachusetts General Hospital; NCI, National Cancer Institute; MDACC, M.D. Anderson Cancer Center.

no difference in local recurrence, disease-free survival, or overall survival. The authors mention that the local recurrence rate was increased in those patients who had positive margins, but no numbers are given. Another series was reported in the same year that did look at the influence of margin status.[108] Forty-seven patients who had resection only and 29 patients who had irradiation (55 to 70 Gy) postoperatively are included. Seventeen patients had wide resections, six were irradiated. There were three local failures, none of which were in the postoperative radiotherapy group. Forty-three patients had a limited or marginal resection, 23 were irradiated. Local recurrence occurred in 70% of surgical patients and 13% of postoperatively irradiated patients. Ultimate local control of approximately 90% was obtained by salvage surgery and radiotherapy. Given the limited statistical capability of such a small series, postoperative irradiation appeared to reduce the local recurrence rate after marginal resection.

The analysis of Tepper and Suit included 110 patients who received postoperative irradiation in a series that includes preoperative irradiation and radiotherapy-alone groups.[88] Local recurrence was recorded in 13 of 110 patients, while the actuarial local failure rate was 16%. They state that for patients with stage IIB, IIIB, and IVA tumors, local recurrence increased from 17% to 42% for complete resection compared with incomplete resection. Overall survival was similar. Function was felt to be good; complications are not listed.

A series of 144 patients treated at Roswell Park Memorial Institute contains 64 patients whose surgical margins were less than 2 cm and who were referred for radiotherapy. The minimum margin is not given. The irradiation dose was 60 Gy. The local recurrence rate was low at 8%.

The Scandinavian Sarcoma Group recently published their results with marginal surgery and postoperative irradiation.[91] These 26 patients, 22 of whom had extremity tumors, were extracted from a database of 240 patients enrolled in their protocols. All patients' margins were close or microscopically positive, or tumor violation occurred during surgery. Median follow-up was 62 months. Hypofractionated irradiation using 3-Gy fractions to a total dose of 51 Gy ($BED_{2\ Gy}$ = 63.75 Gy) was used in most; however, some patients received approximately 54 Gy in conventional fractions. The local recurrence rate was 18%. There were nine major complications, including three amputations. Seven of these patients had daily fractions of greater than 2.7 Gy.

Herbert et al.[92] reported 74 patients, 19 (26%) of whom had microscopically positive margins, 10 (14%) had close margins, and 2 (3%) had grossly positive margins. Six patients were irradiated preoperatively. Brachytherapy was used as part of the radiotherapy in 14 patients. The dose used was 50 Gy given by external beam plus 16 Gy given as brachytherapy. Median follow-up was 48 months. The actuarial local recurrence rate was 45% for patients with positive margins, 20% for patients with close margins, and 0% for patients with wide margins. This was statistically significant (P = .003). No effect on survival was seen.

Brachytherapy

The use of brachytherapy (interstitial implants) has never been as popular as that of external beam radiotherapy (Table 10–14). In the United States, the use of brachytherapy for soft tissue sarcomas has been championed by the group at the Memorial Sloan-Kettering Cancer Center. They have reported its use for locally advanced tumors and as a postoperative adjuvant therapy in a randomized trial.[49, 68] This trial entered, over a 5-year period, 126 patients who were previously untreated or who had recurrent sarcoma but had not received radiotherapy or chemotherapy. All patients underwent "grossly complete" resections; 18% had positive margins. Minimum follow-up, while not stated, is probably 4 to 5 years. There was a

TABLE 10–14
Results of Brachytherapy

Study (Institution)	No. of Patients	Grade 2 or 3 (%)	Surgical Margin	Dose (Gy)	LR Rate (%)	% Alive 5 yr After Treatment	Notes
Harrison et al., 1993[49] (MSKCC)	55	80	Positive 20%	4 2–45	18	76 DFS	One arm of a randomized study All patients had "grossly complete" resection
Shiu et al., 1991[68] (MSKCC)	33	70	Mgl	40 (25–60)	12	?	Locally advanced tumors, 16 were recurrent
	45	68	Mgl or positive 69%	44 (25–54) 13 got EBRT	30	66 DFS	All were abutting or invading a major neurofascular bundle
Habrand et al., 1991[72] (IGR)	48	85	22 < 2 cm 26 ?	60 (25–72) 4 got EBRT	33	58	30% got 2 or 3 plane implants, 7 are H&N sites
Schray et al., 1990[71] (Mayo)	63	75	Mgl	15–20 61 got EBRT	8	?	EBRT 45–50 Gy Median follow-up only 22 mo

LR, Local recurrence; MSKCC, Memorial Sloan-Kettering Cancer Center; DFS, disease free survival; Mgl, marginal resection; EBRT, external beam radiotherapy; IGR, Institut Gustave Roussy; H&N, head and neck.

decrease in the local recurrence rate in the brachytherapy arm. Subset analysis showed that this effect was limited to those patients with high-grade tumors. The actuarial recurrence rates for the other three subsets (high grade no brachytherapy, low grade with brachytherapy, low grade no brachytherapy) were the same. Brachytherapy had no effect on reducing local recurrence when margins were positive. There were 11 patients with positive margins in each arm; the local recurrence rate was 36% (4 of 11) and 27% (3 of 11) for the no brachytherapy and brachytherapy arms, respectively. Cancer-specific survival was the same for all groups. Reported complications are limited to wound healing. A major or moderate wound healing complication occurred in 48%; patients treated after 1985 experienced a 14% incidence. Most of this improvement is probably due to delaying loading of the catheters to 5 and then 6 days postoperatively.

The use of brachytherapy in the treatment of locally advanced soft tissue sarcomas was reported by Shiu and coworkers.[68] Two groups are presented. The first, a group of 33 patients with locally advanced tumors, 16 recurrent, were treated with resection (probably marginal) and brachytherapy. The local recurrence rate was 12%. Complications were seen in 39%; this was probably due to early (postoperative day 3) loading of the catheters. The second group consisted of 45 patients whose tumor abutted or invaded a major neurovascular bundle. Resections were marginal or margins were positive in 69%. Invasion of the adjacent structure was documented in 28%. High dosages were used, with one patient receiving an estimated total dose of 148 Gy. The observed local recurrence rate was 30%. Four peripheral nerve injuries occurred, all in patients who received an estimated total dosage of more than 90 Gy (three of these patients had prior irradiation).

Habrand et al.,[72] from the Institut Gustave Roussy, treated a group of 48 patients, including 32 with extremity tumors. Twenty-two patients were treated because the surgical margins were less than 2 to 3 cm. The other 26 patients were treated for recurrence. Some of these patients had positive or close surgical margins; however, details are not given. In seven patients, the tumor was located in the head or neck. Median follow-up is 82 months, but the minimum follow-up is only 16 months. Local recurrence occurred in 16 patients (33%); only two recurrences were believed to be within the irradiated volume. The margin status was not predictive of local recurrence. Complications were significant. The probable explanation is that, unlike the Memorial Sloan-Kettering group, full dosage (45 to 50 Gy) was delivered to the scar. Radiation necrosis was seen in 35%, one as late as 9½ years after treatment. All 5 of 5 patients with foot sarcomas experienced necrosis.

The Mayo Clinic combined low-dose brachytherapy and external beam radiotherapy in treating 63 patients.[71] There was good local control, but the follow-up is too short to draw any conclusions.

Surgery, Chemotherapy, and Radiotherapy

Multimodality Therapy

In the 1970s, (1) the arrival of a chemotherapeutic agent, doxorubicin (Adriamycin), effective against soft tissue sarcoma; (2) the established effectiveness of radiotherapy; (3) and the room for improvement left by then-current treatments led to initiation of combined-therapy (multimodality) protocols. The sequential trials undertaken by Eilber and colleagues[93] at UCLA are unique for using a consistent therapeutic approach and for a systematic evaluation of irradiation dose-time relationships. To date, 416 patients with grade 2 or 3 extremity soft tissue sarcomas have been treated under neoadjuvant protocols. Overall survival for the group is 95% for grade 2 and 65% for grade 3 soft tissue sarcomas. The first trial used doxorubicin given intra-arterially to the affected extremity followed by radiotherapy. The original dose was 35 Gy given over 2 weeks, 3.5 Gy per fraction ($BED_{2\,Gy}$ = 48 Gy). This was followed within 5 to 14 days by resection. At surgery, a wide resection was done, with the goal of achieving clear margins. In this initial study of 77 patients (group 1), while a low local recurrence rate was obtained (Table 10–15), there was a 16% major complication rate, including one amputation. In an effort to reduce the rate of complications, the irradiation dose was decreased to 17.5 Gy given in 1 week, 3.5 Gy per fraction ($BED_{2\ Gy}$ = 23 Gy) for the next 137 patients (group 2). The number of major complications did decrease, but so did local control. Attempting to find a balance, the irradiation dose was then increased to 28 Gy given in eight fractions ($BED_{2\ Gy}$ = 38 Gy). At the same time, 96 patients (group 3) were randomized to intra-arterial versus intravenous delivery of the doxorubicin.[74] In this group of 112 patients, the local recurrence rate returned to under 10% and the complication rate remained stable. Two newer trials examine the addition of cisplatin and ifosfamide to the preoperative treatment. Follow-up is too short to formulate any conclusions.

In our own practice, we have used Eilber and colleagues' initial protocol (35 Gy in 10 fractions) for grade 2 or 3 soft tissue sarcomas since 1979. Forty-two patients have been followed for a minimum of 5 years. We have detected a local recurrence in 10%, and the overall survival rate is 62%. Our major complication rate is less than 10%.

Several other trials have been based on the UCLA model.[73, 94–96] In some hospitals, the UCLA protocol was abandoned after a few patients had been treated because of a perceived excessive rate of complications.[97] In most, the treatment program was modified.[94, 95] Wanebo et al.[95] reported the combined results of three institutions: Brown University, the University of Cincinnati, and the University of Calgary. The radiotherapy dose varied by 25% between centers (Table 10–15). The institution giving 35 Gy reduced the dose to 30 Gy ($BED_{2\ Gy}$ = 37 Gy) during the study because of a large number of wound complications. They state that this reduction halved the number of wound complications, which parallels the UCLA results for a similar dose reduction. In this trial, two patients underwent pulmonary metastasectomy during treatment. Overall survival was related to grade and patient age. For grade 1 or 2, compared with grade 3, overall survival was 90% and 38%, respectively. Patients over age 60 had an overall survival of 25%, while overall survival for younger patients was 69%. None of nine patients with a tumor larger than 15 cm was cured. Major complications were seen in 8%.

The University of California, Davis, studied 25 patients, 17 of whom had soft tissue sarcomas. The irradiation dose was decreased to 40 Gy midstudy owing to a number of wound-healing problems. The dose reduction did not make

TABLE 10–15
Results of Multimodality Therapy

Study (Institution)	No. of Patients	F/U (yr)	Grade 2 or 3 (%)	Surgical Margin	Dose* (Gy)	Chemotherapy	LR Rate (%)	% Alive 5 yr After Treatment	Complications
Eilber et al., 1993[93] (UCLA)	77	11	100	Mgl	Pre 48	Adria 90 mg IA	9	58 (10 yr)	16% major, 1 ampt
	137	8	100	Mgl	Pre 23	Adria 90 mg IA	15	72	
	112	5	100	Mgl	Pre 39	Adria 90 mg IA or IV	9	74	
	46	1½	100	Mgl	Pre 39	Adria 90 mg CDDP 120 mg/m²	11	70	
	44	1½	100	Mgl	Pre 23	Ifosfamide 2 g/m² × 12 IV	2	86	
Levine et al., 1993[73] (Univ. of Illinois)	28	7½	87	Wide	Pre 28	Adria 100 mg/m² IA 10 days	25	69	7%, 4 catheter-related
	27			Mgl	Pre 28 Post 32		4		
Moseley, 1992[96] (GSH)	18		100	Mgl	Post 60	Adria 90 mg	0	61	17% major, 1 ampt
	20					CDDP perfusion	5		10% major, 1 neuritis
Wanebo et al., 1990[95] (Tricenter)	60 (7 bone)	4½	97	Ampt 5% Wide 83% Mgl 12%	38–46 Gy	Adria 90 mg IA	2	58	8% major, 2 ampt Poor ROM 5%
Pezzi et al., 1990[66] (MDACC)	46		All > T1	Ampt 14%	55	Cy(V)ADIC Adria 90 mg/m²	24	38	N/A
Abbatucci et al., 1986[90] (Baclesse)	89		60 >T1	Wide 61% Mgl 26% ? 13%	Pre 27 Post	Act D in 44%	14	75	
Goodnight et al., 1985[94] (UCD)	25 (8 bone)	2½	76	?	48/40	Adria 90 mg iA	0	N/A	16% major

F/U, Follow-up; LR, local recurrence; UCLA, University of California, Los Angeles; Mgl, marginal resection; Pre, preoperative; Adria, Adriamycin (doxorubicin); IA, intra-arterially; IV, intravenously; CDDP, cisplatin; Post, postoperative; GSH, Good Samaritan Hospital, Portland, OR; Tricenter, Brown University, the University of Cincinnati, the University of Calgary; Ampt, amputation; ROM, range of motion; MDACC, M.D. Anderson Cancer Center; Cy(V)ADIC, cyclophosphamide, vincristine, Adriamycin, dacarbazine; N/A, not available; Act D, actinomycin D; UCD, University of California, Davis.

*Irradiation doses expressed as $BED_{2\ Gy}$ calculated with α/β = 2 Gy.

†Different radiotherapy doses were used in each center.

a difference. Follow-up is too short to determine overall survival, and the local recurrence rate has undoubtedly increased over time.

Some trials have incorporated notable modifications. Levine and coworkers[73] reported on 55 patients treated with intra-arterial doxorubicin delivered over 10 days followed by irradiation to a dose of 25 Gy in 10 fractions ($BED_{2\ Gy}$ = 28 Gy). Approximately one half were irradiated postoperatively with an additional mean dose of 32 Gy because of close margins. These 55 patients accounted for 10% of all extremity soft tissue sarcomas seen at that center, and therefore were highly selected. A majority of the tumors were grade 3 and larger than 5 cm. The local recurrence rate was 15%, which is comparable to the UCLA group 2, which received approximately the same irradiation dose ($BED_{2\ Gy}$ = 23 Gy). Confirming the inadequacy of the preoperative irradiation dose, there was a reduction in the local recurrence rate from 25% to 4% in the group that received postoperative radiotherapy, even though this was the group with the problematic margins. The increased doxorubicin dose did not improve the overall survival or the local recurrence rate. The prolonged infusion did create a new set of complications related to the arterial puncture site, which resulted in an amputation in one patient.

Moseley,[96] from Good Samaritan Hospital in Portland, Oregon, reported a comparison of intra-arterial doxorubicin versus hyperthermic perfusion with cisplatin, either followed by postoperative irradiation to a dose of 60 Gy. The overall survival rate and local recurrence rate are similar. Because different agents were used, the added benefit, if any, of hyperthermic perfusion is unknown. Given these results and the expense of the procedure, hyperthermic perfusion hardly seems justified.

Surprisingly few reports of alternative preoperative programs exist. Pezzi et al.[66] reported on 46 patients treated at the M.D. Anderson Cancer Center with preoperative Cy(V)ADIC, of whom 16 received preoperative irradiation and 7 received postoperative irradiation. The mean irradiation dose was 55 Gy (range, 50 to 66 Gy). The average tumor size was greater than 10 cm, and all were high grade. The local recurrence rate of those 23 patients receiving radiotherapy is not reported, and complications are not given. Results from the Centre Regional Françqis Baclesse have been reported by Abbatucci and colleagues.[98] In this study of 113 patients, 58 had extremity sites and 60% were larger than 5 cm; 50% received preoperative actinomycin D. All patients were treated with preoperative and postoperative radiotherapy. The preoperative dose was two fractions of 6.5 Gy ($BED_{2\ Gy}$ = 27 Gy). If the excision was considered to be adequate, a postoperative dose was given to bring the total to the equivalent of 50 Gy given in conventional fractions. If the excision was thought to be inadequate, the total dose was brought to 60 Gy. For some patients, 70 Gy was given to an area of residual tumor marked with clips by the surgeon. The results for the extremity sites are not listed separately. Overall survival for the 89 patients treated for cure was 75% at 5 years and 70% at 10 years of follow-up. An increase in the local recurrence rate (2% vs. 44%) and a decrease in overall survival rate (88% vs. 35%) was demonstrated for patients who had resections with microscopically positive margins. Good or acceptable functional results were achieved in 91% of 44 patients evaluable at 2 years following treatment. There were three amputations.

Radiotherapy

Primary Radiotherapy

Radiotherapy by itself (Table 10–16) has a very limited role in the management of soft tissue sarcomas. In 1975, Gilbert and coworkers,[99] in a review of the literature, could not find evidence for a dose-response effect in 197 patients but reported a local control rate just above 50%, similar to that reported by Lindberg and colleagues,[134] allowing leeway for differences in tumor size and grade.

Slater et al.,[100] in a series of 72 patients with unresectable soft tissue sarcoma, all of whom were irradiated for cure, were able to show an acceptable level of local control only in patients with desmoids, dermatofibrosarcoma protuberans, and well-differentiated liposarcomas. No dose-response correlation was noted. There was no change in the local recurrence rate depending on the tumor size. The major complication rate was dose-dependent: for doses less

TABLE 10–16
Results of Radiotherapy Alone

Study (Institution)	No. of Patients	Grade 2 or 3	Dose (Gy)	LR Rate (%)	% Alive 5 yr After Treatment
Slater et al., 1986[100] (MDACC)	57	?	T <5 cm 61 T 5–8 cm 64 T >8 cm 65	72*	48 DFS
	15	?	60–80†	68*	?
Tepper and Suit, 1985[101] (MGH)	36	?	64	44	28

LR, Local recurrence; MDACC, M.D. Anderson Cancer Center; DFS, disease free survival; MGH, Massachusetts General Hospital.

*Actuarial local recurrence rate.

†Calculated (relative biologic effectiveness 3.1 for neutrons) total dose. Actual 30–43 Gy photons plus 9 to 22 Gy neutrons. Three patients received neutrons alone, calculated photon equivalent dose 60–70 Gy.

than 70 Gy there was a 2% incidence, and for doses greater than 70 Gy there was a 28% incidence.

Tepper and Suit[101] reported 36 patients treated only by radiation; the overall actuarial survival at 5 years was 28%, with a 44% local recurrence rate. In contrast to Slater and colleagues' study, they thought that there was an improved local control with decreasing tumor size; the local recurrence rate was 13% and 70% for T1 tumors and tumors larger than 10 cm, respectively. The restricted success of radiotherapy can be further understood by a review of 36 patients with synovial cell sarcoma. Little benefit could be shown in recurrent disease, poorly differentiated tumors, or those tumors that grossly invaded bone, major blood vessel, or nerve.

Systemic Adjuvant Chemotherapy

At least 11 trials of systemic adjuvant chemotherapy for soft tissue sarcoma have been published. While several show a trend toward a better survival, in only two trials was overall survival improved enough to reach statistical significance.[102, 103] A problem with most trials is that accrual is slow and the number of patients small, which limits their ability to detect a modest improvement in survival. The four largest trials are shown in Table 10–17. The Dana-Farber Cancer Institute, the Massachusetts General Hospital, the Eastern Cooperative Oncology Group, and the Intergroup Sarcoma Study Group pooled data from three similar trials.[104] Eligible patients had stage IIB to IVA soft tissue sarcomas. Visceral sites were excluded. Single-agent doxorubicin was used. While there were trends toward improved disease-free and overall survival, at a median follow-up of 54 months there was no statistically significant difference.

The European Organization for Research and Treatment of Cancer trial was inclusive of all stages (except IVB) and sites. Forty percent were grade 3. Of 374 eligible patients, 233 had extremity sarcomas.[105] The multiagent chemotherapy program, Cy(V)ADIC, was compared with observation. At a median follow-up of 44 months, there is no statistically significant difference between the two groups.

The Scandinavian Sarcoma Group compared single-agent doxorubicin with observation in 181 evaluable patients, 155 of which were located in an extremity.[106] All were high grade. At 40 months median follow-up, there was no significant benefit from chemotherapy. Results are reported for two local modalities (wide resection or marginal resection with postoperative irradiation), giving four groups. The results listed in Table 10–17 are an average of the two groups in the observation arm and the treatment arm, respectively. The overall and disease-free survivals are stated to be not statistically different; however *P* values are not given.

The fourth study, done at UCLA, again compared single-agent doxorubicin with observation in 119 patients with grade 3 extremity soft tissue sarcomas treated under a standardized protocol.[107] At 28 months' median follow-up, there was no statistically significant difference in overall or disease-free survival reported. *P* values are not given.

Summary of Treatment Results

Results of the various treatment modalities are summarized in Table 10–18. Because of the disparities in follow-up, inconsistent patient selection, variations within treatment groups, and variable end points, any attempt at meta-analysis would be meaningless. The "typical" results listed in the table are, rather, estimates based on the results presented in Tables 10–9, 10–10, and 10–12 to 10–16. The "best" columns list the best results reported (that have reasonable median follow-up times) for each treatment group. It is clear that with the exception of radiotherapy alone, all methods are capable of giving good results. For limb-sparing surgery alone to be effective, however, careful patient selection is essential. The same is probably true for adjuvant brachytherapy. We think that, given the large number of patients treated and the inclusion of poor-prognosis tumors, the results with multimodality neoadjuvant treatment are the current standard for comparison, at least

TABLE 10–17
Results of Four Clinical Trials of Systemic Adjuvant Chemotherapy

Study (Institution or Group)	No. of Patients	Grade	Agent(s)	Overall Survival Rate (%)		*P* Value	Cardiac Toxicity (%)
				Control Group	*Treated Group*		
Antman et al., 1990[104] (Tricenter)	101	2–3	Doxorubicin	67	79	0.31 (NS)	6.25
Alvegärd et al., 1989[106] (SSG)	240	3	Doxorubicin	72	72	NS*	1.7 (3 died)
Bramwell et al., 1988[105] (EORTC)	233	1–3	CyVADIC	68	74	0.26 (NS)	
Eilber et al., 1988[107] (UCLA)	119	3	Doxorubicin	80	84	NS*	None clinical

Tricenter, Dana-Farber Cancer Institute, Massachusetts General Hospital, Eastern Cooperative Oncology Group, Intergroup Sarcoma Study Group; NS, not significant; SSG, Scandinavian Sarcoma Group; EORTC, European Organization for the Research and Treatment of Cancer; CyVADIC, cyclophosphamide, vincristine, Adriamycin, dacarbazine; UCLA, University of California, Los Angeles.

TABLE 10–18
Summary of Treatment Results

Treatment	Typical LR Rate (%)	Typical OS Rate (%)	Best LR Rate (%)	Best OS Rate (%)
Amputation	5	50	0	88
Limb-sparing surgery	25	70	7	90
Preoperative RT*	10	60	6	62
Postoperative RT*	15	70	8	83
Brachytherapy*	20	70	12	76
Multimodality therapy*	8	70	2	86
RT	60	30	44	48

LR, Local recurrence; OS, overall survival; RT, radiotherapy.
*As an adjuvant to resection.

as practiced at a few centers. Not all institutions that have adopted this program have had good results, and most have felt the need to modify it, especially the irradiation dose. Some have abandoned it. This has been due to a perceived high rate of wound-healing problems. In our experience with our neoadjuvant program, primary healing is the rule, and those few wounds with dehiscence eventually healed, with good functional results.

The results for radiotherapy alone are skewed by the preponderance of inoperable tumors referred for treatment, and thus the true efficacy of irradiation as a primary modality is unknown.

There is no evidence that single-agent doxorubicin or doxorubicin-based adjuvant chemotherapy is effective in increasing overall survival or even disease-free survival. The reported trials are small, and it is therefore possible that a small benefit was not detectable. Trials using newer combinations, notably doxorubicin and ifosfamide, are being prepared or are under way. It remains to be seen whether these will be effective.

FOLLOW-UP

Patterns of Recurrence

Pulmonary metastasis and, to a much lesser extent, local recurrence are the predominant sites of failure for high-grade (grade 2-3, 4) soft tissue sarcomas. Isolated lung metastasis occurs in 50% to 66% of all patients with recurrent disease.[115, 133] Pulmonary metastasis in combination with other sites occurs in 67% to 90% of patients who experience distant metastasis.[108, 133] This pattern holds for patients with second to fourth recurrences. Local recurrence can occur in any patient; however, the incidence varies tremendously. Regional nodal metastasis occurs in 2% to 3% of recurrent sarcomas. Other sites, such as liver, bone, or brain, are rare.

Sixty percent to 70% of local recurrences occur within 2 years after treatment, up to 15% may recur after 5 years, and recurrence after 10 years has been reported.[109–111]

Recommended Schedule

Low-Grade Tumor

Low-grade (grade 1) soft tissue sarcomas are unlikely to recur locally or metastasize to the lungs. Thrice-yearly examinations for the first few years, then yearly, are sufficient. Chest radiographs are ordered as clinically indicated.

High-Grade Tumor

Patients with high-grade (grade 2-3, 4) soft tissue sarcomas are at significant risk for pulmonary metastasis. Other metastatic sites are uncommon until the patient is being treated for second recurrence. Examination every 2 months for the first 2 or 3 years, with a chest radiograph at each visit, is commonly recommended. No other laboratory tests are needed.

TREATMENT OF RECURRENT DISEASE

Treatment of Local Recurrence

Indications

The incidence of local recurrence has decreased with the advent of multimodality treatment protocols. Nevertheless, local recurrences still occur in 5% to 10% of patients. Salvage surgery is indicated whenever the local recurrence is resectable and the patient has no evidence of metastatic disease or a major interval illness. Occasionally, resection in the presence of metastasis is indicated in order to prevent limb loss or loss of limb function. In rarer circumstances, debulking may be justified for relief of pain from nerve compression or stretching.

Management

The traditional treatment of locally recurrent soft tissue sarcoma of the extremity has been amputation. There is still a role for amputation when there is multifocal recurrence or when there is an infield recurrence after radiotherapy was used in the primary treatment and clear margins cannot be obtained because the tumor involves a major neurovascular bundle or bone. In selected cases, resection and arterial reconstruction may be feasible. Involvement of a major nerve is less of a reason to amputate, as the loss of motor function (e.g., an ankle drop) can be compensated for with a brace. When the recurrence is in the proximal thigh, this usually results in a more functional extremity than can be obtained with a hip disarticulation or hemipelvectomy and prosthesis. The sensory loss can be accommodated for by good skin care on the patient's part.

In the unirradiated patient, resection alone, radical or not, is seldom advisable; therefore, planning with adjuvant radiotherapy in mind is essential. The multimodality neoadjuvant protocols can also be used.

Results

Amputation for local recurrence yields second recurrence rates of 10%, with 40% of patients alive 5 years following treatment. Wide resections result in local recurrence rates of 44%, with 58% of patients alive 5 years following treatment.[117]

A few institutions have looked at alternatives to amputation (Table 10–19). The UCLA group applied their preoperative intra-arterial doxorubicin plus irradiation protocol to recurrent soft tissue sarcomas. At the time of their initial report, they were using 35 Gy given in 10 fractions.[112] Sixteen patients, most of whom probably had wide excisions and no irradiation, were treated. There were no local recurrences, and 87% were projected to be alive at 5 years. Complications are not reported but presumably were on a par with those of patients treated primarily. A more recent report includes patients whose primary treatment included irradiation.[113]

Retreatment included excision and either preoperative intra-arterial doxorubicin plus 28 Gy in eight fractions or "conventional" irradiation to 50 Gy, depending on the treatment of the primary soft tissue sarcoma. Only the group (seven patients; median follow-up, 59 months) treated initially by excision and irradiation (median, 60 Gy) and whose local recurrence was treated with the preoperative multimodality protocol (doxorubicin + 28 Gy) had good results. Because the intervals between the courses of radiotherapy are not consistent, the total BED can only be estimated. In this group, the local recurrence rate was 14%, and it was projected that 86% would be alive at 5 years. Complications included a 33% incidence of severe edema and a 14% severe loss of range of motion. Considering that these patients received a $BED_{2\,Gy}$ of approximately 80 Gy, plus the effect of the doxorubicin, the complication rate is unexpectedly low.

A series of 40 reirradiated patients was recently reported from Memorial Sloan-Kettering.[114] For 32 of the patients, primary treatment consisted of excision plus external beam radiotherapy, dose unknown. Retreatment consisted of excision plus brachytherapy using an afterloading technique with iridium 192 (median dose calculated to be equivalent to 45 Gy). At a median follow-up of 40 months, the local recurrence rate was 18%, with a projected 85% of the patients alive at 5 years, if the local recurrence being treated was the first or second. The local recurrence rate increased to 53%, and the projected 5-year survival rate fell to 55%, for those patients being treated for their third or more local recurrence. These results are all the more remarkable because the authors state that more than 50% of the resections had microscopically or grossly positive margins. Unfortunately, no breakdown of the local recurrence rate by status of the margins is given, making analysis of this very important variable impossible. Four severe skin ulcerations, requiring surgical intervention, and one femoral fracture occurred.

Patients with multiple sites of recurrence have a very poor prognosis, with less than 10% surviving 24 months.[115]

A study of the use of hyperthermia for the treatment of locally recurrent tumors, including five soft tissue sarcomas, demonstrated no response in any of the five sarcoma patients.[116]

The choice of the optimal treatment for a local recurrence of a soft tissue sarcoma remains a test of the surgeon's judgment. Putting together the results of the above reports, and the current approach to primary treatment, we can make a few recommendations. Patients who recur after excision only should have re-excision and adjuvant irradiation or pre-reoperative irradiation plus intravenous doxorubicin or cisplatin. Because most patients are now treated with adjuvant irradiation, the results of the two reirradiation series suggest that amputation need not be the only option for local recurrence in these patients.

TABLE 10–19
Reirradiation for Locally Recurrent Soft Tissue Sarcomas*

Study	Group	No. of Patients	Initial Treatment	Interval (mo)	Treatment	Total Dose (Gy)	LRR Rate (%)	% Alive 5 yr After Treatment	Complications
Essner et al, 1991[113]	1	7 MFU 59 mo	Excision/60 Gy	28	Protocol† 28 Gy	98.5	14	86	Edema 33% ROM 86% 1 amputation
	2	10 MFU 46 mo	Protocol 28 Gy	22	Excision/50 Gy	88.5	60	50	Edema 64% fx 10% ROM 50%
	3	4	Excision/50 Gy	37	Excision/50 Gy	100	100	0	Severe 100%
Nori et al., 1991[114]	1	40‡ MFU 36 mo	32 Excision/EBRT 5 Excision/EBRT/CT 3 misc.	Not given	Excision/brachytherapy 45 Gy§	? + 45	18 2 LR + DM	85 if 1st or 2nd LR	12.5% 1 fx and 4 ulcers

LRR, Local re-recurrence; MFU, median follow-up; ROM, range of motion; fx, fracture; EBRT, external beam radiotherapy; CT, chemotherapy; DM, distant metastasis.
*Extremity sites, others excluded.
†Protocol, intra-arterial Adriamycin, 90 mg in 72 hours, followed by irradiation with 350-cGy fractions.
‡50% positive margins at excision of local recurrence; patients are lumped together and cannot be separated out.
§Estimated dose.

Reirradiation fields should be planned so that amputation, if necessary, can be done at the same level as would have been possible prior to reirradiation. Although not proven, the preservation of an unirradiated strip of skin and subcutaneous tissue is probably important in regard to function. Until there is longer follow-up to determine the late effects, reirradiation should be undertaken with caution.

Treatment of Regional Lymph Node Recurrence

Isolated regional lymph node recurrence is seen in 2% to 3% of patients. The treatment is a standard lymph node dissection. The few published results of survival after therapeutic lymphadenectomy each contain a small number of patients. The best estimate is that about 20% to 40% are alive 5 years following lymphadenectomy.[53, 110, 117]

Treatment of Distant Metastasis

Pulmonary Metastasis

Indications

The unquestioned first prerequisite for pulmonary metastasectomy is that the primary site be controlled and that there be no evidence of other metastatic disease. The second is that the patient be able to withstand the proposed operation. The third is that it be feasible to remove all of the pulmonary metastases, by way of either a sternotomy or staged thoracotomies. Other factors, such as the number of nodules, the disease-free interval, or the tumor doubling time, are controversial.

Results

Because more than one half of patients whose tumor recurs have pulmonary metastases as the only site of recurrence,[133] pulmonary metastasectomy has been recommended as being potentially curative. The recent literature contains several articles advocating "aggressive" pulmonary metastasectomy, with as many as 110 nodules excised or vaporized at one operation.[118–120] Other authors have suggested that the only limiting factor is the amount of residual lung that must be left "to provide a satisfactory physiological outcome."[121] Still others have advocated extended resections.[132]

No prospective or randomized studies have been published. The usual "control" group comprises those patients with unresectable metastasis.[122–124] The usual median survivals are 9 to 12 months and 14 to 20 months for the unresected and resected groups, respectively. Median follow-ups are almost always less than 5 years and occasionally less than 3 years. The 5-year survival rates range from 15% to 35% for first-time pulmonary metastasectomy and from 12% to 52% for reoperative pulmonary metastasectomy. The median value is 25%, the often-quoted 5-year survival figure after pulmonary metastasectomy for soft tissue sarcoma.

In those studies in which data beyond 5 years of follow-up are given, although there are patients alive at 5 years, the survival curve still has a steep slope and few patients are alive by 7 years. Standard error values are never given. In an attempt to evaluate the true efficacy of pulmonary metastasectomy, one study identified a group of 12 patients with pulmonary metastasis (2 from soft tissue sarcoma) that on retrospective clinical and radiologic grounds were candidates for resection but did not undergo surgery.[125] When compared with 70 operated patients (9 with soft tissue sarcoma), there was no survival difference. While this investigation has obvious flaws, it is the only study to attempt a valid comparison.

When the results of pulmonary metastasectomy for soft tissue sarcomas are analyzed, some trends appear (Tables 10–20 and 10–21). The only patients surviving beyond 5 years either had a solitary pulmonary metastasis[126] or less than four nodules.[121, 127, 128] In one study, the two patients surviving beyond 5 years both had alveolar soft part sarcomas.[118] In a recent review of a large number of patients with alveolar soft part sarcoma, of those patients with metastatic alveolar soft part sarcoma at diagnosis, approximately 40% were alive at 5 years.[129] It is difficult in this case to separate the effect of the pulmonary metastasectomy from the biology of the tumor on outcome. In another series, there is a reported 33% 5-year survival rate for patients with metastatic soft tissue sarcoma; however, no long-term results are given and the survival curve lumps osteosarcomas and soft tissue sarcomas together, so the trend for soft tissue sarcomas is impossible to determine.[120] In this study, the number of nodules did not predict survival, although there is a trend toward lower recurrence rates with decreasing numbers of nodules. Another factor in this series, which includes patients treated since 1947, is that 7% of the unresected patients were alive at 5 years, which is in contrast to the other cited series, in which the unresected patients all died within 3 years. In a series that reported the results of a preoperative chemotherapy protocol, while 22% were alive at 5 years, all were dead by 78 months.[130] In the other reported series, when the number at risk at 5 years can be determined, only two or three patients per series are alive at 5 years following pulmonary metastasectomy.[118, 126, 131] These small numbers of patients at risk make the actuarial projections of survival questionable.

A recent report has focused on extended resection for pulmonary metastasis and includes patients undergoing pneumonectomy (1 patient with soft sarcoma) or composite resection (12 patients with soft tissue sarcoma).[132] Of these 13 patients, 2 are surviving at 17 and 25 months' follow-up, respectively. The longest survival after resection was 40 months. There was a postoperative death in the pneumonectomy group.

It would appear that for soft tissue sarcomas, pulmonary metastasectomy may benefit only a subset of patients: those with one to three nodules, or longer tumor doubling times,

TABLE 10–20
Results of Primary Pulmonary Metastasectomy for Soft Tissue Sarcomas

Study (Institution)	No. of Patients	Mortality Rate (%)	No. of Nodules	5 Year Survival Rate (%)	10 Year Survival Rate (%)
Roth et al., 1985[127] (NCI)	67	?	1–?	15	?
Roth et al., 1986[122] (NCI)	65	0	1–61 (9.5)	18	?
Jablons et al., 1989[121] (NCI)	74	0		27	21 at 8 yr (2 patients)
Mountain et al., 1984[120] (MDACC)	49	?	1–?	33	?
Casson et al., 1991[126] (MDACC)	24*	2.6†	NA	22	0 at 78 mo
Pastorino et al., 1989[123] National Cancer Institute (Milan)	28	?	NA	35	18
Liénard et al., 1989[124] Institute Jules Bordet (Brussels)	8	0	?	25	0
Ueda et al., 1993[118] Osaka University	23	0	1–110	25	?

NCI, National Cancer Institute; MDACC, M.D. Anderson Cancer Center; NA, not available.
*All patients received chemotherapy preoperatively.
†One patient who underwent a composite resection.

or low-grade tumors. While a proportion of these selected patients are alive at 5 years or more following resection, it is impossible at this time to know what the impact of the surgical procedure might be over and above the biology (natural history) of the tumor. Since it is clear that there is no benefit from incomplete resection, every effort should be made to determine the extent and resectability of all metastases preoperatively. Exploratory thoracotomy is rarely, if ever, justified.

Other Metastatic Sites

Indications

Metastasectomy for sites other than lung must be evaluated on a case-by-case basis. Only well-documented solitary lesions should be attempted. Patients rendered disease-free for sites such as liver, brain, or multiple sites are anecdotal. An exception may be subcutaneous sites. A report on recurrence patterns from the NCI reported that six of eight (75%) patients with subcutaneous metastasis were made disease-free by salvage excision.[133] No long-term results were reported.

Technique

Technique of salvage resection for these sites is tailored to the site. Resection should not be undertaken unless there is a reasonable certainty that clear margins can be obtained. Certain situations may justify partial excision for palliation (e.g., tumor causing pain by either nerve compression or stretching).

FUTURE PROSPECTS

With the use of multimodality protocols, local control of grade 3 soft tissue sarcomas is probably as good as can be expected. Randomized trials are planned to test the need for radiotherapy in grade 1 soft tissue sarcomas and to evaluate the role of irradiation and chemotherapy for grade 2 and 3 sarcomas.

TABLE 10–21
Results of Repeated Pulmonary Metastasectomy for Soft Tissue Sarcoma

Study (Institution)	No. of Patients	Mortality Rate %	No. of Nodules	5-Year Survival Rate %	10-Year Survival Rate %
Rizzoni et al., 1986[128] (NCI)	29	0	?	22	22 at 8 yr (2 patients)
Pogrebniak et al., 1991[131] (NCI)	43	0	?	12	12
Casson et al., 1991[126] (MDACC)	39	0	?	19 if n > 1 52 if n = 1	0 if n >1 33 at 7 yr if n = 1

NCI, National Cancer Institute; MDACC, M.D. Anderson Cancer Center.

Adjuvant chemotherapy trials using the MAID combination have been initiated.

References

1. Wingo PA, Tong T, Bolden S: Cancer statistics, 1995. CA 45:8–30, 1995.
2. Brennan MF: The James Ewing Lecture. Arch Surg 127:1290–1293, 1992.
3. Hardell L, Eriksson M: The association between soft tissue sarcomas and exposure to phenoxyacetic acids. Cancer 62:652–656, 1988.
4. Hardell L, Sandstrom A: Case control study: Soft tissue sarcomas and exposure to phenoxyacetic acids or chlorphenols. Br J Cancer 39:711–717, 1979.
5. Moses M, Selikof IJ: Soft tissue sarcomas, phenoxy herbicides, and chlorinated phenols. Lancet 1:1370, 1981.
6. Zahm SH, Heineman EF, Vaught JB: Soft tissue sarcoma and tobacco use: Data from a prospective cohort study of United States veterans. Cancer Causes Control 3:371–376, 1992.
7. Zahm SH, Blair A, Holmes FF, et al: A case control study of soft tissue sarcoma. Am J Epidemiol 130:665–674, 1989.
8. Tucker MA, Meadows AT, Boice JD, et al: Cancer risk following treatment of childhood cancer. Prog Cancer Res Ther 26:211–224, 1984.
9. Plager C, Lamoheir PC, et al: The risk of secondary sarcomas after radiation therapy for Ewing's sarcoma. Proc Annu Meet Am Soc Clin Oncol 8:PA1233, 1989, (meeting abstract).
10. Wethersby RP, Dahlin DC, Ivins JC: Postradiation sarcoma of bone: Review of 78 Mayo Clinic cases. Mayo Clin Proc 56:294–306, 1981.
11. Amendola BE, Amendola MA, McSlatchey KD, Miller CH Jr: Radiation-associated sarcoma: A review of 23 patients with postradiation sarcoma over a 50 year period. Am J Clin Oncol 12:411–415, 1989.
12. Laskin WB, Silverman TA, Enzinger FM: Postradiation sarcomas. An analysis of 53 cases. Cancer 62:2330–2340, 1988.
13. Davidson T, Westbury G, Harmer CL: Radiation induced soft tissue sarcoma. Br J Surg 73:308–309, 1986.
14. Lindeman G, McKay MJ, Taubman KL, et al: Malignant fibrous histiocytoma developing in bone 44 years after shrapnel trauma. Cancer 66:2229–2232, 1990.
15. Li FP, Fraumeni JF: Soft tissue sarcomas, breast cancer and other neoplasms: A familial syndrome? Ann Intern Med 71:741–745, 1969.
16. Li FP, Fraumeni JF: Rhabdomyosarcoma in children: Epidemiologic study and identification of a familial cancer syndrome. J Natl Cancer Inst 43:1365–1370, 1969.
17. Li FP, Fraumeni JF: Prospective study of a family cancer syndrome. JAMA 247:2692–2694, 1982.
18. Strong LC, Stine M, Norsted TL: Cancer in survivors of childhood soft tissue sarcoma and their relatives. J Natl Cancer Inst 79:1213–1216, 1987.
19. McBride OW, Merry D, Givol D: The gene for human p53 cellular tumor antigen is located on chromosome 17 short arm (17p13). Proc Natl Acad Sci 83:130, 1986.
20. Lamb P, Crawford L: Characterization of the human p53 gene. Mol Cell Biol 6:1379–1380, 1986.
21. Yonish-Rouach E, Resnitsky D, et al: Wild-type p53 induces apoptosis of myeloid leukemic cells that is inhibited by interleukin 6. Nature 352:345–347, 1992.
22. Martinez J, Georgoff I, et al: Cellular localization and cell cycle regulation by a temperature sensitive p53 protein. Genes Dev 5:151–153, 1919.
23. Lane DP: p53, Guardian of the genome. Nature 358:15, 1992.
24. Riccardi VM: Von Recklinghausen's neurofibromatosis. N Engl J Med 305:1617–1627, 1981.
25. Blatt J, Jaffe R, Deutsh M, et al: Neurofibromatosis and childhood tumors. Cancer 57:1225–1229, 1986.
26. Raney RB, Littman P, et al: Results of multimodal therapy in children with neurogenic sarcoma. Med Pediatr Oncol 7:229–236, 1979.
27. Lawrence W, Donegan WL, Natarajan N, et al: Adult soft tissue sarcomas. Ann Surg 205:349–359, 1987.
28. Rydholm A: Management of patients with soft tissue tumors managed at a regional oncology center. Acta Orthop Scand Suppl 203:13–77, 1983.
29. Layfield LJ, Anders KH, Glasgow BJ, Mirra JM: Fine needle aspiration of primary soft tissue tumors. Arch Pathol Lab Med 110:420–424, 1986.
30. Barth RJ, Merino MJ, Solomon D, et al: A prospective study of the value of core needle biopsy and fine needle aspiration in the diagnosis of soft tissue masses. Surgery 112:536–543, 1992.
31. Kransdorf MJ, Jelinek JS, Moser RP: Imaging of soft tissue tumors. Radiol Clin North Am 31:359–372, 1993.
32. Fornage BD: Recurrent soft tissue sarcoma: A comparison between ultrasonography and magnetic resonance imaging. Thirty-Sixth Annual Clinical Conference and Twenty-Fifth Annual Special Pathology Program: Patterns and Mechanisms of Failure After Cancer Treatment, Houston, TX, 1992, pp 51–53, (meeting abstract).
33. Russell WO, Cohen J, Enzinger F, et al: A clinical and pathological staging system for soft tissue sarcomas. Cancer 40:1562–1570, 1977.
34. Alvëgard TA, Berg NO: Histopathology peer review of high-grade soft tissue sarcoma: The Scandinavian Sarcoma Group experience. J Clin Oncol 7:1845–1852, 1989.
35. Geer RJ, Woodruff J, Casper ES, Brennan MF: Management of small soft tissue sarcoma of the extremity in adults. Arch Surg 127:1285–1289, 1992.
36. Eilber FR, Giuliano AE, Huth J, et al: Limb salvage for high-grade soft tissue sarcomas of the extremity: Experience at the University of California, Los Angeles. Cancer Treat Symp 3:49–57, 1985.
37. Stotter AT, A'Hern RP, Fisher C, et al: The influence of local recurrence of extremity soft tissue sarcoma on metastasis and survival. Cancer 65:1119–1129, 1990.
38. Watkins KT, Souba WW, Bland KI: Staging of soft tissue sarcomas of the extremity. Surg Oncol Clin North Am 2:537–546, 1993.
39. Enneking WF, Spanier SS, Malawer MM: The effect of the anatomic setting on the results of surgical procedures for soft parts sarcoma of the thigh. Cancer 47:1005–1022, 1981.
40. Giuliano AE, Eilber FR: The rationale for planned reoperation after unplanned total excision of soft tissue sarcomas. J Clin Oncol 3:1344–1348, 1985.
41. Sugarbaker PH, Nicholson TH: Atlas of Extremity Sarcoma Surgery. Philadelphia: JB Lippincott, 1984.
42. Lawrence W, Neifeld JP, Terz JJ: Manual of Soft-Tissue Tumor Surgery. New York: Springer-Verlag, 1983.
43. Cantin J, McNeer GP, Chu FC, Booher RJ: The problem of local recurrence after treatment of soft tissue sarcoma. Ann Surg 168:47–53, 1968.
44. Suit HD, Tepper JE: Impact of improved local control on survival in patients with soft tissue sarcoma. Int J Radiat Oncol Biol Phys 12:699–700, 1986.
45. Barr LC, Stotter AT, A'Hern RP: Influence of local recurrence on survival: A controversy reviewed from the perspective of soft tissue sarcoma. Br J Surg 78:648–650, 1991.
46. Rööser B, Attewell R, Berg NO, Rydholm A: Survival in soft tissue sarcoma: Prognostic variables identified by multivariate analysis. Acta Orthop Scand 58:516–522, 1987.
47. Gustafson P, Rööser B, Rydholm A: Is local recurrence of minor importance for metastases in soft tissue sarcoma? Cancer 67:2083–2086, 1991.
48. Rööser B, Gustafson P, Rydholm A: Is there no influence of local control on the rate of metastasis in high grade soft tissue sarcoma? Cancer 65:1727–1729, 1990.
49. Harrison LB, Franzese F, Gaynor JJ, Brennan MF: Longterm results of a prospective randomized trial of adjuvant brachytherapy in the management of completely resected soft tissue sarcomas of the extremity and superficial trunk. Int J Radiat Oncol Biol Phys 27:259–265, 1993.
50. Rosenberg SA, Tepper J, Glatstein E, et al: The treatment of soft tissue sarcomas of the extremities—prospective randomized evaluations of (1) limb sparing surgery plus radiation therapy compared with amputation and (2) the role of adjuvant chemotherapy. Ann Surg 196:305–315, 1982.
51. Stinson SF, DeLaney TF, Greenberg J, et al: Acute and long-term effects on limb function of combined modality limb sparing therapy for extremity soft tissue sarcoma. Int J Radiat Oncol Biol Phys 21:1493–1499, 1991.
52. Shiu MH, Collin C, Hilaris BS, et al: Limb preservation and tumor

control in the treatment of popliteal and antecubital soft tissue sarcomas. Cancer 57:1632–1639, 1986.
53. Owens JC, Shiu MH, Smith R, Hajdu SI: Soft tissue sarcomas of the hand or foot. Cancer 55:2010–2018, 1985.
54. Okuneiff P, Suit HD, Proppe KH: Extremity preservation by combined modality treatment of sarcomas of the hand and wrist. Int J Radiat Oncol Biol Phys 12:1923–1929, 1986.
55. Selch MT, Kopald KH, Ferreiro GA, et al: Limb sparing therapy for soft tissue sarcomas of the foot. Int J Radiat Oncol Biol Phys 19:41–48, 1990.
56. McCready RA, Miller SK, Hamaker RC, et al: What is the role of carotid arterial resection in the management of advanced cervical cancer? J Vasc Surg 10:274–280, 1989.
57. Karakousis CP, Emrich LJ, Rao U, Khalil M: Limb salvage in soft tissue sarcomas with selective combination of modalities. Eur J Surg Oncol 17:71–80, 1991.
58. Wanebo HJ, Temple MD, Popp MB, et al: Combination regional therapy for extremity sarcoma. Arch Surg 125:355–359, 1990.
59. Enneking WF, Maale GE: The effect of inadvertent tumor contamination of wounds during the surgical resection of musculoskeletal neoplasms. Cancer 62:1251–1256, 1988.
60. Ogihara Y, Sudo A, Fujinami S: Inadvertent tumor violation during musculoskeletal sarcoma surgery and risk of recurrence. Jpn J Clin Oncol 22:264–269, 1992.
61. Sadoski C, Suit HD, Rosenberg A, et al: Preoperative radiation, surgical margins, and local control of extremity sarcomas of soft tissues. J Surg Oncol 52:223–230, 1993.
62. Robinson M, Barr L, Fisher C, et al: Treatment of extremity soft tissue sarcomas with surgery and radiation therapy. Radiother Oncol 18:221–233, 1990.
63. Tepper JE, Suit HD: Radiation therapy alone for sarcoma of soft tissue. Cancer 56:475–479, 1985.
64. Slater JD, McNeese MD, Peters LJ: Radiation therapy of unresectable soft tissue sarcomas. Int J Radiat Oncol Biol Phys 12:1724–1729, 1986.
65. McNeer GP, Cantin J, Chu F, Nickson JJ: Effectiveness of radiation therapy in the management of sarcoma of the soft somatic tissues. Cancer 22:391–397, 1968.
66. Pezzi CM, Pollock RE, Evans HL, et al: Preoperative chemotherapy for soft tissue sarcomas of the extremities. Ann Surg 211:476–481, 1990.
67. Olch AJ, Kagan AR, Wollin M, et al: Multi-institutional survey of techniques in volume iridium implants. Endocuriether Hypertherm Oncol 2:193–197, 1986.
68. Shiu MH, Hilaris BS, Harrison LB, Brennan MF: Brachytherapy and function-saving resection of soft tissue sarcoma arising in the limb. Int J Radiat Oncol Biol Phys 21:1485–1492, 1991.
69. Granmayeh M, Libschitz HI: Vascular system. In Libshitz HI (ed): Diagnostic Roentgenology of radiotherapy Change. Baltimore: Williams & Wilkins, 1979, pp 195–201.
70. Genest P, Hilaris BS, Nori D, et al: Iodine-125 as a substitute for iridium-192 in temporary interstitial implants. Endocuriether Hypertherm Oncol 1:223–228, 1985.
71. Schray MF, Gunderson LL, Sim FH, et al: Soft tissue sarcoma. Integration of brachytherapy, resection and external irradiation. Cancer 66:451–456, 1990.
72. Habrand JL, Gerbaulet A, Pejovic MH, et al: Twenty years experience of interstitial iridium brachytherapy in the management of soft tissue sarcomas. Int J Radiat Oncol Biol Phys 20:405–411, 1991.
73. Levine EA, Trippon M, Das Gupta TK: Preoperative multimodality treatment for soft tissue sarcomas. Cancer 71:3685–3689, 1993.
74. Eilber FR, Giuliano AE, Huth JF, et al: Intravenous (IV) vs. intraarterial (IA) Adriamycin, 2800 r radiation and surgical excision for extremity soft tissue sarcomas: A randomized prospective trial. Proc ASCO 9:304, 1990 (abstract).
75. Bujko K, Suit HD, Springfield DS, Convery K: Wound healing after preoperative radiation for sarcoma of soft tissues. Surg Gynecol Obstet 176:124–134, 1993.
76. Arbeit JM, Hilaris BS, Brennan MF: Wound complications in the multimodality treatment of extremity and superficial truncal sarcomas. J Clin Oncol 3:480–488, 1987.
77. Ormsby MV, Hilaris BS, Nori D, Brennan MF: Wound complications of adjuvant radiation therapy in patients with soft tissue sarcomas. Ann Surg 210:93–99, 1989.
78. Saddegh MK, Bauer HC: Wound complication in surgery of soft tissue sarcoma: Analysis of 103 consecutive patients managed without adjuvant therapy. Clin Orthop 289:247–253, 1993.
79. Markhede G, Stener B: Function after removal of various hip and thigh muscles for extirpation of tumors. Acta Orthop Scand 52:373–395, 1981.
80. Stinson SF, DeLaney TF, Greenberg J, et al: Acute and long-term effects on limb function of combined modality limb sparing therapy for extremity soft tissue sarcoma. Int J Radiat Oncol Biol Phys 21:1493–1499, 1991.
81. Robinson MH, Spruce L, Eeles R, et al: Limb function following conservation treatment of adult soft tissue sarcoma. Eur J Cancer 12:1567–1574, 1991.
82. Sugarbaker PH, Barofsky I, Rosenberg SA, et al: Quality of life assessment of patients in extremity sarcoma trials. Surgery 91:17–21, 1982.
83. Collin C, Godbold J, Hajdu SI, Brennan MF: Localized extremity soft tissue sarcoma: An analysis of factors affecting survival. J Clin Oncol 5:601–612, 1987.
84. Willard WC, Hajdu SI, Casper ES, Brennan MF: Comparison of amputation with limb-sparing operations for adult soft tissue sarcoma of the extremity. Ann Surg 215:269–275, 1992.
85. Rydholm A, Gustafson P, Rööser B, et al: Limb-sparing surgery without radiotherapy based on anatomic location of soft tissue sarcoma. J Clin Oncol 9:1757–1765, 1991.
86. Markhede G, Angerval L, Stener B: A multivariate analysis of the prognosis after surgical treatment of malignant soft tissue tumors. Cancer 49:1721–1733, 1982.
87. Robinson MH, Ball ABS, Schofield J, et al: Preoperative radiation therapy for initially inoperable extremity soft tissue sarcomas. Clin Oncol 4:36–43, 1992.
88. Tepper JE, Suit HD: Radiation therapy of soft tissue sarcomas. Cancer 55:2273–2277, 1985.
89. Barkley HT, Martin RG, Romsdahl MM, et al: Treatment of soft tissue sarcomas by preoperative irradiation and conservative surgical resection. Int J Radiat Oncol Biol Phys 14:693–699, 1988.
90. Robinson M, Cassoni A, Harmer C, et al: High dose hyperfractionated radiation therapy in the treatment of extremity soft tissue sarcomas. Radiother Oncol 22:118–125, 1992.
91. Wiklund TA, Alvëgard TA, Mourisdon HT, et al: Marginal surgery and postoperative radiation therapy in soft tissue sarcomas. Eur J Cancer 29:306–309, 1993.
92. Herbert SH, Corn BW, Solin LJ, et al: Limb-preserving treatment for soft tissue sarcomas of the extremity. Cancer 72:1230–1238, 1993.
93. Eilber FR, Eckhardt JJ, Rosen G, et al: Neoadjuvant chemotherapy and radiation therapy in the multidisciplinary management of soft tissue sarcomas of the extremity. Surg Oncol Clin North Am 2:611–620, 1993.
94. Goodnight JE, Bargar WL, Voegeli T, Blaisdell FW: Limb sparing surgery for extremity sarcomas after preoperative intraarterial doxorubicin and radiation therapy. Am J Surg 150:109–113, 1985.
95. Wanebo HJ, Temple WJ, Popp MB, et al: Combination regional therapy for extremity sarcoma. Arch Surg 125:355–359, 1990.
96. Moseley HS: An evaluation of two methods of limb salvage in extremity soft tissue sarcomas. Arch Surg 127:1169–1174, 1992.
97. Mason M, Harmer CL, Westbury G: Late normal tissue damage following intra-arterial Adriamycin plus radiation therapy and conservation surgery for soft tissue sarcomas. Br J Cancer 56:878, 1987, (abstract).
98. Abbatucci JS, Boulier MD, de Ranieri J, et al: Local control and survival in soft tissue sarcomas of the limbs, trunk walls and head and neck: A study of 113 cases. Int J Radiat Oncol Biol Phys 12:579–586, 1986.
99. Gilbert HA, Kagan AR, Winkley J: Soft tissue sarcomas of the extremities: Their natural history, treatment, and radiation sensitivity. J Surg Oncol 7:303–317, 1975.
100. Slater JD, McNeese MD, Peters LJ: Radiation therapy for unresectable soft tissue sarcomas. Int J Radiat Oncol Biol Phys 12:1729–1734, 1986.
101. Tepper JE, Suit HD: Radiation therapy alone for sarcoma of soft tissue. Cancer 56:475–479, 1985.
102. Picci P, Bacci G, Gherlinzoni R, et al: Results of a randomized trial for the treatment of localized soft tissue tumors in adult patients. In Ryan JR, Baker LH (eds): Recent Concepts in Sarcoma Treatment. Dordrecht: Kluwer, 1988, p 144.

103. Ravaud A, Binh BN, Coindre JM: Adjuvant chemotherapy with CYVADIC in high risk soft tissue sarcoma: A randomized prospective trial. In Salmon SE (ed): Adjuvant Treatment of Cancer VI. Philadelphia: WB Saunders, 1990, pp 556–562.
104. Antman K, Ryan L, Borden E, et al: Pooled results from three randomized adjuvant studies of doxorubicin versus observation in soft tissue sarcoma: 10 year results and review of the literature. In Salmon SE (ed): Adjuvant Treatment of Cancer VI. Philadelphia: WB Saunders, 1990, pp 529–533.
105. Bramwell V, Rouesse J, Steward W, et al: Reduced rate of local recurrence following CYVADIC chemotherapy in localized soft tissue sarcoma: An EORTC randomized trial. Proc Annu Meet Am Soc Clin Oncol A1243, 1989, (meeting abstract).
106. Alvëgard TA, Sigurdsson H, Mouridsen H, et al: Adjuvant chemotherapy with doxorubicin in high-grade soft tissue sarcoma: A randomized trial of the Scandinavian Sarcoma Group. J Clin Oncol 7:1504–1513, 1989.
107. Eilber FR, Giuliano AE, Huth JF, Morton DL: A randomized prospective trial using postoperative adjuvant chemotherapy (Adriamycin) in high-grade extremity soft tissue sarcoma. Am J Clin Oncol 11:39–45, 1988.
108. Leibel SA, Tranbaugh RT, Wara WM, et al: Soft tissue sarcomas of the extremities. Cancer 50:1076–1083, 1982.
109. Berli Ö, Stener B, Angervall L, et al: Surgery for soft tissue sarcoma in the extremity. Acta Orthop Scand 61:475–486, 1990.
110. Lindberg RD, Martin RG, Romsdahl MM, Barkley HT: Conservative surgery and postoperative radiotherapy in 300 adults with soft tissue sarcomas. Cancer 47:2391–2397, 1981.
111. Gerner RE, Moore GE, Pickren JW: Soft tissue sarcomas. Ann Surg 181:803–808, 1975.
112. Giuliano AE, Eilber FR, Morton DL: The management of locally recurrent soft tissue sarcoma. Ann Surg 196:87–91, 1982.
113. Essner R, Selch M, Eilber FR: Reirradiation for extremity soft tissue sarcomas. Cancer 67:2813–2817, 1991.
114. Nori D, Shupak K, Shiu MH, Brennan MF: Role of brachytherapy in recurrent extremity sarcoma in patients treated with prior surgery and irradiation. Int J Radiat Oncol Biol Phys 20:1229–1233, 1991.
115. Huth J, Eilber FR: Patterns of metastatic spread following resection of extremity soft tissue sarcomas and strategies for treatment. Semin Surg Oncol 4:20–26, 1988.
116. Gabriele P, Orecchia R, Ragona R, et al: Hyperthermia alone in the treatment of recurrences of malignant tumors. Experience with 60 lesions. Cancer 66:1691–1695, 1990.
117. Shiu MH, Castro EB, Hajdu SI, Fortner JG: Surgical treatment of 297 soft tissue sarcomas of the lower extremity. Ann Surg 182:597–602, 1975.
118. Ueda T, Uchida A, Kodama K, Doi O, et al: Aggressive pulmonary metastasectomy for soft tissue sarcomas. Cancer 72:1919–1925, 1993.
119. Beattie EJ: Surgical treatment of pulmonary metastases. Cancer 54:2729–2731, 1984.
120. Mountain CF, McMurtrey MJ, Hermes KE: Surgery for pulmonary metastasis: A 20-year experience. Ann Thorac Surg 38:323–329, 1984.
121. Jablons D, Steinberg SM, Roth J, et al: Metastasectomy for soft tissue sarcoma. J Thorac Cardiovasc Surg 97:695–705, 1989.
122. Roth JA, Pass HI, Wesley MN, et al: Comparison of median sternotomy and thoracotomy for resection of pulmonary metastasis in patients with adult soft tissue sarcomas. Ann Thorac Surg 42:134–138, 1986.
123. Pastorino U, Maurizio V, Gasparini M, et al: Lung resection for metastatic sarcomas: Total survival from primary treatment. J Surg Oncol 40:275–280, 1989.
124. Liénard D, Rocmans P, Lejeune FJ: Resection of lung metastasis from sarcomas. Eur J Surg Oncol 15:530–534, 1989.
125. Åberg T, Malmberg KÅ, Nilsson B, Nõu E: The effect of metastasectomy: Fact or fiction? Ann Thorac Surg 30:378–384, 1980.
126. Casson AG, Putnam JB, Natarajan G, et al: Efficacy of pulmonary metastasectomy for recurrent soft tissue sarcoma. J Surg Oncol 47:1–4, 1991.
127. Roth JA, Putnam JB, Wesley MN, Rosenberg SA: Differing determinates of prognosis following resection of pulmonary metastasis from osteosarcomas and soft tissue sarcoma patients. Cancer 55:1361–1366, 1985.
128. Rizzoni WE, Pass HI, Wesley MN, et al: Resection of recurrent pulmonary metastasis in patients with soft tissue sarcomas. Arch Surg 121:1248–1252, 1986.
129. Lieberman PH, Brennan MF, Kimmel M, et al: Alveolar soft part sarcoma. Cancer 63:1 13, 1989.
130. Lanza LA, Putnam JB, Benjamin RS, Roth JA: Response to chemotherapy does not predict survival after resection of sarcomatous pulmonary metastasis. Ann Thorac Surg 51:219–224, 1991.
131. Pogrebniak HW, Roth JA, Steinberg SM, et al: Reoperative pulmonary resection in patients with metastatic soft tissue sarcoma. Ann Thorac Surg 52:197–203, 1991.
132. Putnam JB, Suell DM, Natarajan MS, Roth JA: Extended resection of pulmonary metastasis: Is the risk justified? Ann Thorac Surg 55:1440–1446, 1993.
133. Potter DA, Glenn JG, Kinsella T, et al: Patterns of recurrence in patients with high-grade soft tissue sarcomas. J Clin Oncol 3:353–366, 1985.
134. Benjamin RS, Lindberg RD, Martin RG, et al: Limb salvage for patients with sarcomas of soft tissue and bone. Cancer Bull 35:11–15, 1983.

Soft Tissue Sarcomas of the Retroperitoneum

Norman D. Bloom, M.D.

Soft tissue sarcomas account for 1% of all solid tumors, with an incidence of approximately 2 in 100,000, or about 6000 new cases in the United States per year. Of these, 12% or 750 cases occur in the retroperitoneum.

DIAGNOSIS

Up to 90% of patients are asymptomatic and present with an abdominal mass only. Mild symptoms such as abdominal discomfort or pain can be elicited from approximately half of all patients on detailed inquiry. Less then 20% have gastrointestinal, urologic, or peripheral neurologic deficits secondary to more invasive disease at the time of presentation.[1]

The most definitive radiographic study is abdominal computed tomography (CT). CT scan establishes the retroperitoneal origin of the large "abdominal" mass and the presence or absence of necrosis and liver metastases (Fig. 10–10). An abdominal magnetic resonance imaging (MRI)

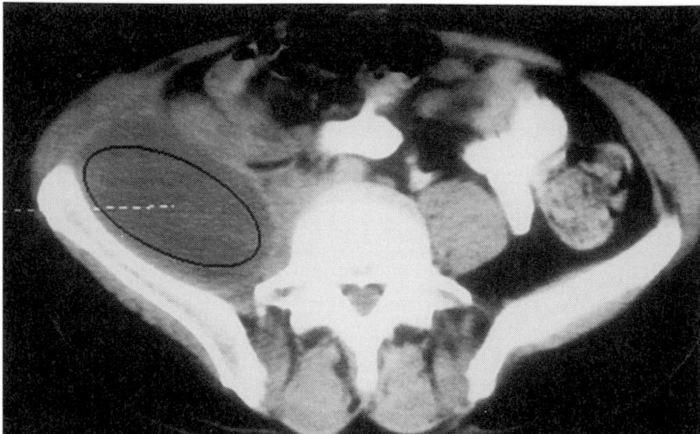

FIGURE 10–10. Malignant fibrous histiocytoma arising in the iliac muscle with extensive central necrosis.

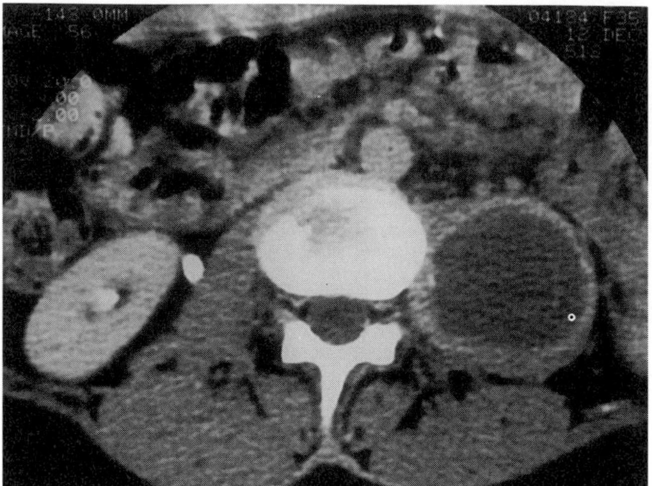

FIGURE 10–12. Benign neurofibroma arising from the L-1 nerve root with involvement of the psoas muscle and central necrosis.

scan may better delineate the nature and extent of the neoplasm. Coronal sections may show the location and patency of the vena cava. The T1-weighted images better define the relationship of the tumor to other solid organs (e.g., liver spleen, kidney). T2-weighted MR images can better define the extent of the tumor within the psoas (Fig. 10–11) or quadratus muscles, as well as any extension into the spinal canal through the spinal foramina.

An aortogram is beneficial prior to surgical therapy. Displacement, encasement, or invasion of normal vessels can be delineated, and bilateral renal function evaluated. Feeding vessels supplying the tumor can be clearly defined as well.

A venacavogram is indicated if there is evidence of peripheral edema or suggestion of vena caval obstruction on CT or MRI. This is not performed routinely.

To complete the preoperative evaluation, CT scan of the chest is performed. Pulmonary metastasis from retroperitoneal sarcomas is less common than for extremity sarcomas (occurring in only 15% of cases), but CT scans are a prerequisite before major abdominal surgery.

The differential diagnosis of tumors arising in the retroperitoneum includes benign tumors (neurofibromas, atypical lipoma) (Figs. 10–12 and 10–13), lymphomas (Fig. 10–14), urogenital malignancies presenting as a large retroperitoneal mass (Fig. 10–15), or primary retroperitoneal sarcomas. Benign lesions are suspected on the basis of lack of invasiveness associated with these lesions. Lymphomas often manifest with multinodular involvement. Urogenital tumors tend to be more homogeneous than sarcomas. Serology for the germ cell tumor markers (human chorionic gonadotropin, alpha fetoprotein, lactate dehydrogenase) or testicular ultrasound may preclude laparotomy in the latter cases.

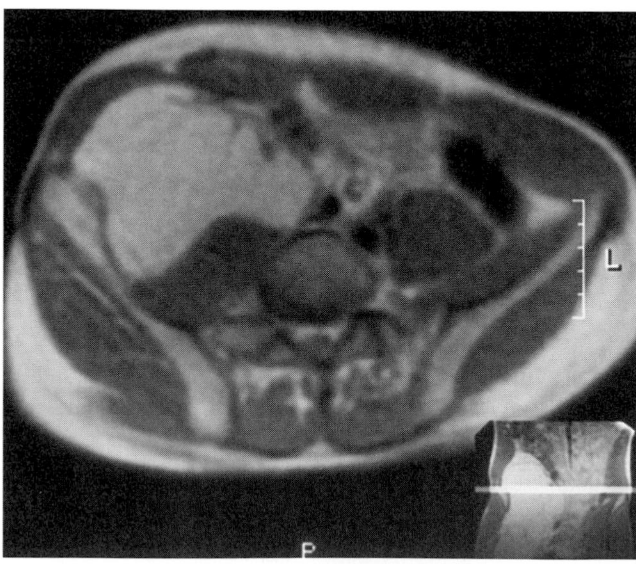

FIGURE 10–11. MRI scan of a large mass arising in the psoas muscle with a displaced but fully patent vena cava.

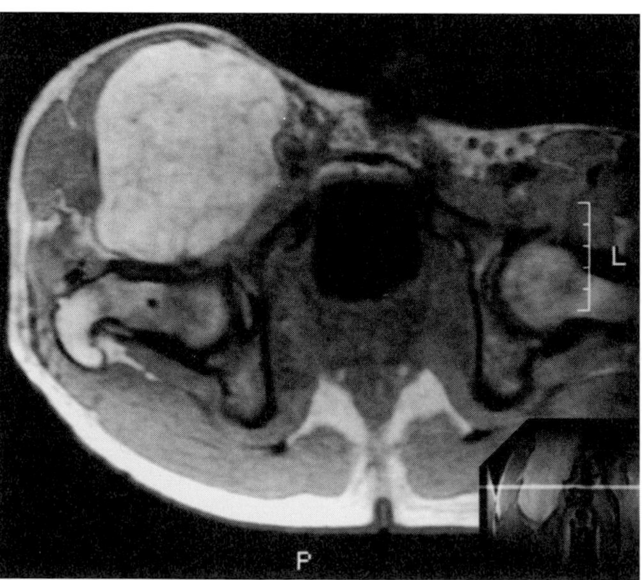

FIGURE 10–13. Large atypical lipoma arising in the retroperitoneum and extending below the inguinal ligament into the thigh.

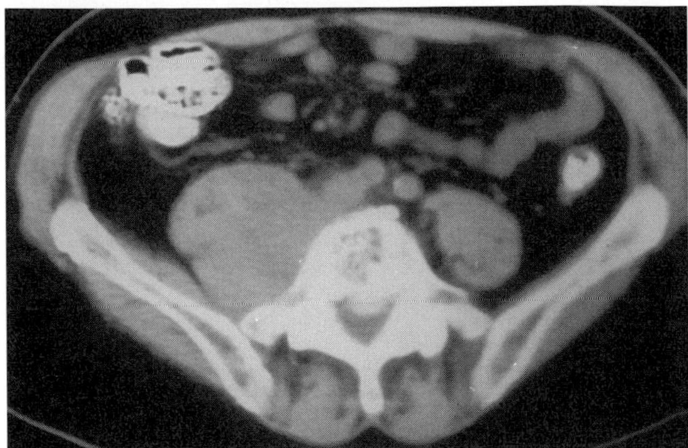

FIGURE 10–14. A 67-year-old man presenting with a B-cell lymphoma arising in right common iliac nodes.

To establish a definitive diagnosis, biopsy of the mass is indicated. Ultrasound or CT-guided fine-needle biopsies or core needle biopsies often do not provide sufficient tissue to establish a definitive diagnosis. An open biopsy with frozen section analysis is often sufficient to establish the diagnosis and allow for a definitive procedure at the same setting. Care should be taken in performing the biopsy to prevent spillage of the tumor, and it should be performed through a limited incision initially.

RESULTS

There are no prospective, randomized studies of treatment results for retroperitoneal sarcomas. The end results of several retrospectively reviewed series over the last 20 years reveals numerous consistent findings.[3–9] On the basis of a cumulative series of 606 patients, the most common retroperitoneal sarcomas are, in descending order of frequency, liposarcomas, leiomyosarcomas, malignant fibrous histiocytomas, and fibrosarcomas (Table 10–22). As with the extremity sarcomas, the grade of the tumors is the most important factor defining the stage of the disease (Table 10–23).

TABLE 10–22
Common Histologies of Retroperitoneal Sarcomas

Histology	No.	%
Liposarcomas	203	33.5
Leiomyosarcomas	172	28.4
Malignant fibrous histiocytoma	48	7.9
Fibrosarcoma	40	6.6
Neurogenic	38	6.3
Embryonal rhabdomyosarcoma	22	3.6
Spindle cell	12	2.0
Other	71	11.7
Total	606	100

In analyzing these series for end results, resectability of the tumor is of primary importance. Of the 606 patients, only 285 (47%) were resectable. Resectability rates range from 30% to 61% (Table 10–24). Overall survival rates for the total series of patients was 35% at 5 years and approximately 15% at 10 years (Table 10–25). However, in those patients in whom the tumor was completely resected, the 5-year survival rate was 65% to 70%, with a 10-year survival rate of 40% to 45%.[5, 7, 8] A 5-year survival rate of 8% occurred in those patients who underwent partial resection or biopsy only.[5] The most common reasons for unresectability in 46 of 114 cases analyzed by Jacques et al.[7] were vascular involvement, peritoneal implants, distant metastasis, root of mesentery involvement, spinal cord involvement, or extensive disease (Table 10–26). In this series of patients, half were operated on for recurrent disease, which would account for the higher incidence of peritoneal implants.

SURGICAL TECHNIQUES

It is important to assess appropriately the resectability of all retroperitoneal sarcomas intraoperatively. These lesions occupy the right or left side of the abdomen or pelvis. For lesions above the pelvic brim, the vena cava or aorta forms the medial line of the resection. Initial dissection along these major vessels is the first step in determining resectability as well as in controlling blood supply. If the vena cava is involved, resection without reconstruction is often feasible. Those portions of the large and small intestines, kidney, spleen, or distal pancreas that may be included in the resection are assessed at this time. Posteriorly, the

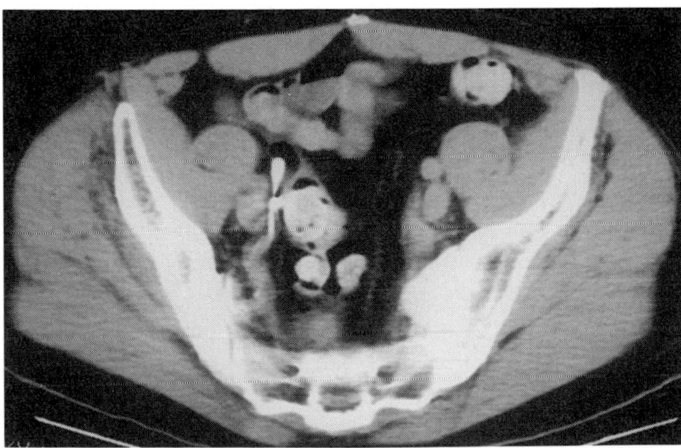

FIGURE 10–15. Germ cell tumor with bilateral iliac nodal disease.

TABLE 10–23
Sarcoma Staging

Designation	Grade	Stage
G1	Low	I
G2	Intermediate	II
G3	High	III

TABLE 10–24
Resectability Rates for Retroperitoneal Sarcomas

Study	Total No. of Patients	Resectable	Percent
Storm et al.[3]	54	33	61
Cody et al.[4]	158	47	30
McGrath et al.[5]	47	18	38
Zornig et al.[6]	51	30	59
Jacques et al.[7]	114	67	59
Karakousis et al.[8]	68	27	40
Dalton et al.[9]	116	63	54
	606	285	47

paraspinal musculature to the midline is exposed. If there is extension of the tumor into the spinal canal via spinal foramina, an en bloc resection can be performed (Fig. 10–16*A* to *E*).

For tumors arising in the pelvis, one can partially or completely resect the bony pelvis. Simple reconstructive techniques can be employed following resection of the iliac wing or pubic rami (Fig. 10–17*A* to *C*). Bowel and bladder resection may necessitate construction of a colostomy or urinary conduit.

For extremity sarcomas adequately resected, the local control rate can approach 90%. The biologic behavior of the retroperitoneal tumors is different in that recurrences are predominantly local. Storm and colleagues[3] reported an 85% local recurrence rate and a 15% distant failure rate in 27 of 33 resected patients, with a median time to recurrence of 20 months. In the series reported by Jacques et al.[7] 75% of all tumors recurred locally while 50% recurred locally among tumors completely resected. Among patients completely resected for primary disease (n = 41), there was a 40% recurrence rate, and 65% of the recurrences were local only. Among patients resected for recurrent disease (n = 39), 62% recurred, and 90% of the recurrences were local only.

In spite of an "adequate" surgical excision, the local control rate for these tumors has been unsatisfactory.

ADJUNCTIVE THERAPIES

Because of the high incidence of local failure, the role of radiotherapy as an adjunctive or primary treatment modality has been evaluated.

TABLE 10–25
Survival Rates of Patients with Retroperitoneal Sarcomas

Study	No. Patients	5 Years (%)	10 Years (%)
Storm et al.[3]	54	35	10
Cody et al.[4]	158	40	
McGrath et al.[5]	47	33	10
Zornig et al.[6]	51	35	15
Jacques et al.[7]	154	35	20
Karakousis et al.[8]	68	34	
Dalton et al.[9]	116	40	22

TABLE 10–26
Common Reasons for Unresectability

Reason	%
Vascular involvement	43
Peritoneal implants	28
Distant metastasis	19
Root of mesentery involvement	8
Spinal cord involvement	6
Extensive disease	17

As a primary treatment modality, the results obtained by radiotherapy have been dismal. In the Yale experience, only 4 of 10 patients survived for 1 year, and there was only 1 3-year survival.[12] The patient ultimately recurred at 4 years and died at 8 years. This result and similar results reported by Kinne and coworkers[13] and Braasch and Mona[14] indicate that only rarely will radiotherapy alone induce long-term disease-free survival and local control. In these rare instances, the tumors were all well-differentiated liposarcomas or fibrosarcomas.

In most of the series reviewed, previously adjunctive radiotherapy was utilized in a variety of uncontrolled ways. Tepper et al.[15] in evaluating the role of adjunctive radiotherapy following surgical excision, noted that complete resection was associated with better survival but that the radiation dose level was also important. Local failure was seen in 67% of patients who received less than 5000 cGy and in only 17% of those who received greater than 6000 cGy. However, the ability to deliver 6000 cGy to the retroperitoneum after resection is severely limited owing to gastrointestinal toxicities if only external beam radiotherapy is employed.

In order to evaluate an alternative method of delivering radiotherapy to the surgical bed, a prospective, randomized trial comparing 20 cGy of intraoperative radiotherapy in combination with postoperative low-dose (35 to 40 cGy) versus postoperative high-dose (50 to 55 cGy) external beam radiotherapy was performed. Fifteen patients who received intraoperative radiotherapy and 20 control patients were followed for a minimum of 5 years. Median survival times were similar for both groups. The number of local-regional recurrences were significantly lower among the patients who received intraoperative radiotherapy (6 of 15) than among the control patients (16 of 20). Patients who received intraoperative radiotherapy had fewer complications of disabling radiation-related enteritis (2 of 15) than did control patients (10 of 20), but radiation-related peripheral neuropathy was more frequent among those who received intraoperative radiotherapy (9 of 15) than among control patients (1 of 15). The neuropathy resolved or improved in two thirds of the patients, but three had a permanent significant disability.[16]

Brachytherapy is an alternative for radiotherapy to the tumor bed, but there are no data to substantiate the superior effectiveness of this technique.

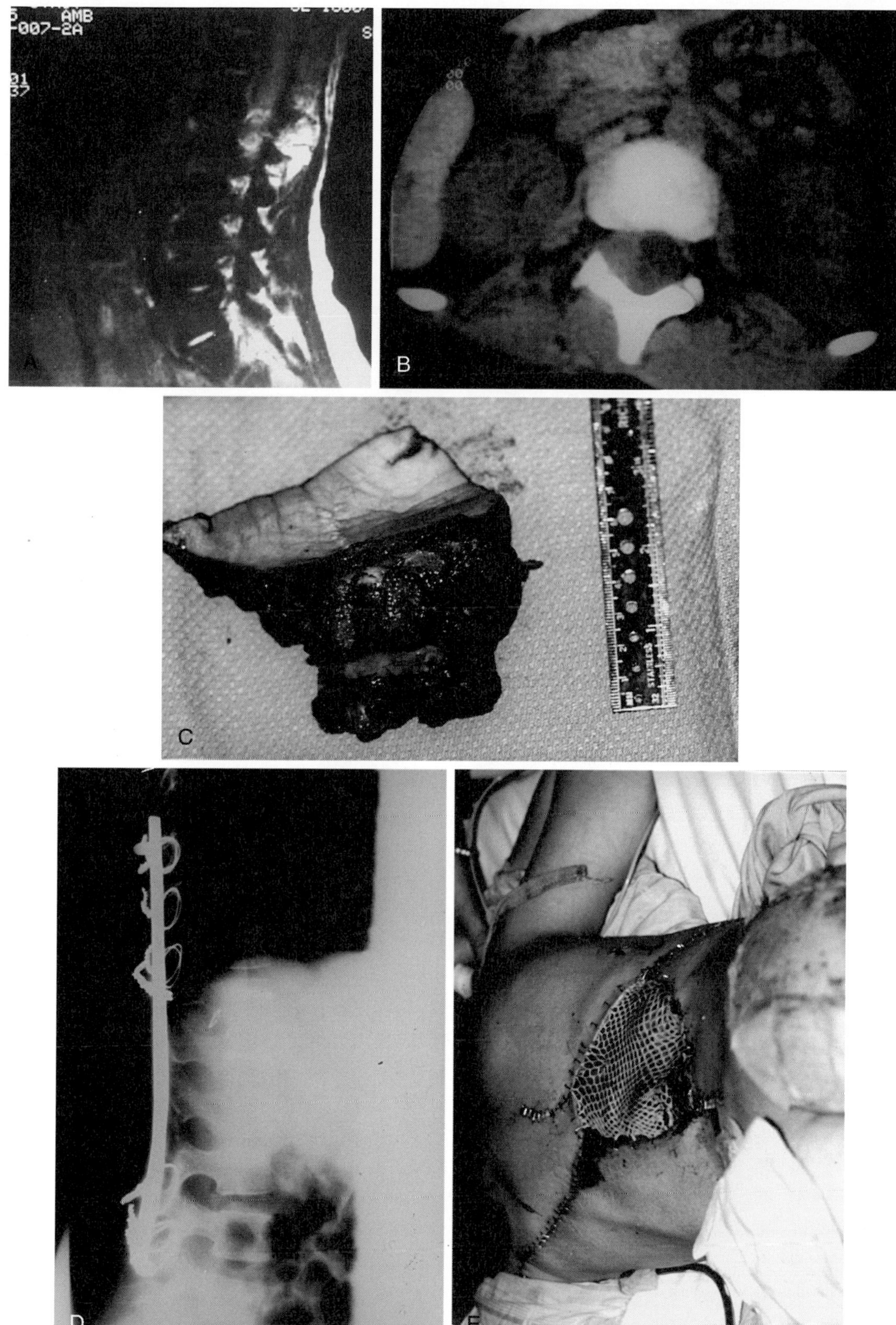

FIGURE 10–16. *A,* MRI scan demonstrating a paraspinal recurrence of an extraosseous Ewing's sarcoma with extension into the spinal canal. *B,* Coronal CT scan clearly demonstrating the intraspinal extension of the tumor. *C,* Resected tumor containing three hemivertebrae and dura. *D,* Stabilization of the spine with Cotrel-Dubousset rods. *E,* Rotated latissimus flap with a skin graft to fill the full-thickness defect and cover the spinal instrumentation.

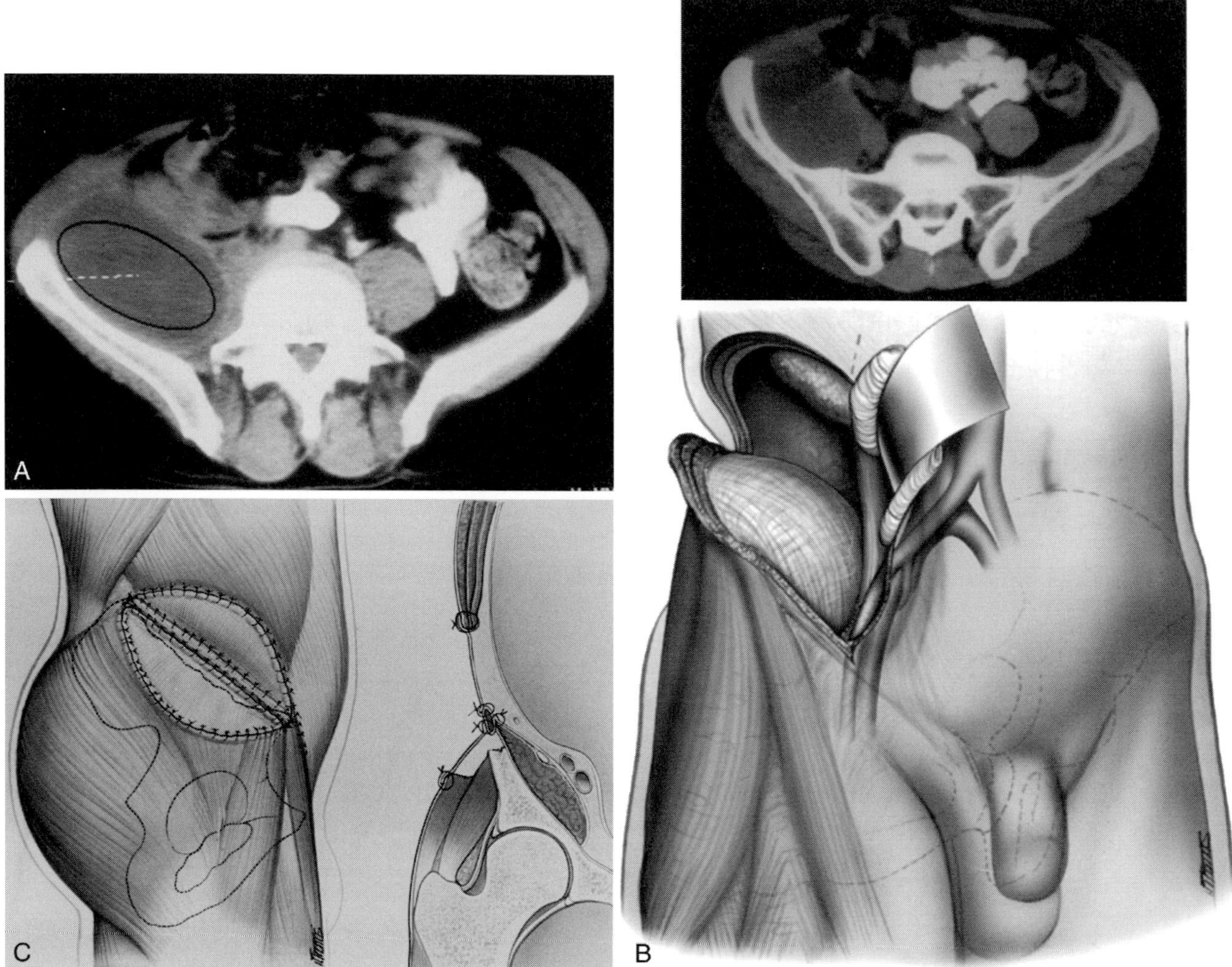

FIGURE 10–17. *A,* Soft tissue sarcoma arising in the iliac muscle and involving the iliac wing. *B,* Resection of tumor and iliac wing. *C,* Marlex mesh reconstruction of the surgical defect.

The role of adjunctive radiotherapy for retroperitoneal sarcomas is still not defined. High morbidity associated with higher radiation dosages precludes its use. The role of intraoperative radiotherapy is still unclear.

Adjunctive chemotherapy with doxorubicin hydrochloride, cyclophosphamide, and methotrexate was shown to improve disease-free survival in one National Cancer Institute study of sarcomas of the extremities[17]; another study showed that chemotherapy did not benefit patients with retroperitoneal sarcomas.[18]

References

1. Storm KF, Mahoi DM: Diagnosis and management of retroperitoneal soft tissue sarcomas. Ann Surg 214:1–15, 1991.
2. Niefeld JP, Walsh JW, Lawrence W Jr: Computerized tomography in the management of soft tissue tumors. Surg Gynecol Obstet 155:535–540, 1982.
3. Storm FK, Eilber FR, Mirra J, et al: Retroperitoneal sarcomas: A reappraisal of treatment. J Surg Oncol 17:1–17, 1981.
4. Cody HS, Turnbull AD, Forter JG, et al: The continuing challenge of retroperitoneal sarcomas. Cancer 47:2147–2152, 1981.
5. McGrath P, Niefield JP, Lawrence W: Improved survival following complete excision of retroperitoneal sarcomas. Ann Surg 200:200–204, 1984.
6. Zornig C, Welter HS, Krull A, et al: Retroperitoneal sarcoma in a series of 51 adults. Eur J Surg Oncol 18:475–480, 1992.
7. Jacques DP, Coit DG, Hajd S, et al: Management of primary and recurrent soft tissue sarcomas of the retroperitoneum. Ann Surg 212:51–59, 1990.
8. Karakousis C, Velez AF, Emrich L: Management of retroperitoneal sarcomas and patient survival. Am J Surg 150:376–380, 1985.
9. Dalton R, Donohue J, Mucha P, et al: Management of retroperitoneal sarcomas. Surgery 106:725–733, 1989.
10. Costa J, Wesley RA, Glatstein E: The grading of soft tissue sarcomas. The results of a clinicohistopathologic correlation in a series of 163 cases. Cancer 53:530–541, 1984.
11. Russell WO, Cohen J, Enzince F, et al: A clinical and pathologic staging system for soft tissue sarcomas. Cancer 40:1562–1570, 1977.
12. Harrison LB, Gutierrez E, Fischer J: Retroperitoneal sarcomas: The Yale experience and a review of the literature. J Surg Oncol 32:159–164, 1986.
13. Kinne D, Chu F, Huvos A, et al: Treatment of primary and recurrent retroperitoneal liposarcoma. Cancer 31:53–64, 1973.
14. Braasch J, Mon A: Primary retroperitoneal tumors. Surg Clin North Am 47:663–670, 1967.
15. Tepper J, Suit H, Wood W, et al: Radiation therapy of retroperitoneal soft tissue sarcomas. Int J Radiat Oncol Biol Phys 10:825–830, 1984.
16. Sindelar W, Kinsella TJ, Chen PW, et al: Intraoperative radiotherapy in retroperitoneal sarcomas. Final results of a prospective, randomized, clinical trial. Arch Surg 128:402–410, 1993.
17. Chang AE, Kinsella T, Glatstein E, et al: Adjunctive chemotherapy for patients with high grade soft-tissue sarcomas of the extremity. J Clin Oncol 6:1491–1500, 1988.
18. Glenn J, Sindelar WF, Kinsella T, et al: Results of multimodality therapy of resectable soft-tissue sarcomas of the retroperitoneum. Surgery 97:316–324, 1985.

11

Michael Gross, M.D.

Skeletal Tumors of the Extremities

EPIDEMIOLOGY

Musculoskeletal tumors arise from mesenchymally derived tissues, and the overall incidence of such tumors is low. This is especially true in comparison with the vast number of cancers arising from epithelial and endothelial tissue origins. Of all cancers, musculoskeletal tumors constitute less than 1%. Although the absence of a national tumor registry makes the figure imprecise and difficult to validate, the incidence of malignant bone tumors in North America is around 8.5 cases per million per year.

Most musculoskeletal sarcomas arise in the second decade of life, usually during the period of maximal growth velocity. The age of the patient, particularly with respect to epiphyseal closure, is a major determinant of the likelihood of a particular cancer occurring. The variation in the incidence of cancers with respect to age is demonstrated stylistically in Figure 11–1. The peaks of tumor incidence are not meant to be relative to one another but to demonstrate that among certain age groups, a particular histologic type is more likely to occur than any other type. For instance, it is very unusual to see chondrosarcomas in children, and it is very unusual to see giant cell tumors in patients whose epiphyses have not yet closed.[1]

No specific risk factors have been identified for musculoskeletal tumors as a whole. Soft tissue and bone sarcomas arising from bones with total joint arthroplasty in situ have been reported, but the incidence is low, and the tumor occurs some years after implantation.[2, 3] Risk factors and prognostic factors are discussed separately for each tumor.

DIAGNOSIS

Musculoskeletal tumors present with pain, a lump, or both. Patients often associate the pain with a recent injury, particularly active adolescents. However, the pain usually does not settle, and patients' requirements for analgesics increase. Patients then complain of pain with activity, which is not modified by rest. When the pain persists through the night and prevents sleep, an opinion is usually sought. This classic escalation of pain should make the treating physician suspicious of a malignant neoplasm.

In the case of tumors in the vicinity of joints, such as the knee or elbow, it is usually possible to palpate a mass. There is increased warmth associated with the swelling. The mass is usually firm in consistency. The patient may demonstrate signs of increased vascular activity around the mass, such as an increase in venous markings, and there is occasionally a thrill in a tumor such as a telangiectatic osteosarcoma. Masses around the hip are more difficult to diagnose, but the patient walks with an antalgic gait and often a trunk shift and exhibits a restricted range of motion; all are indicative of proximal femoral or hip pathology, or both.

Patients presenting with tumors involving the pelvis are often diagnosed at a later stage, because it is difficult to palpate much of the skeletal pelvis, apart from the iliac wings. Tumors involving the acetabular area and the ischial area are usually diagnosed late because the patient is treated for ischial bursitis, trochanter bursitis, or other such diagnoses. The diagnosis of tumor is usually made when the patient continues to suffer pain and a radiograph demonstrates abnormalities in the pelvic osseous architecture.

With an adequate history, appropriate physical examination, and plain radiographs, the diagnosis is apparent in 90% of patients. An enormous amount of information is gleaned from a plain radiograph, which is cheap, easy to perform, and easy to transmit to an experienced oncologist for an opinion. In general, there are three questions to be answered when looking at a plain radiograph of a lesion:

1. Where is the lesion in relation to the anatomy of the bone involved?
2. What is the bone's response to the lesion?

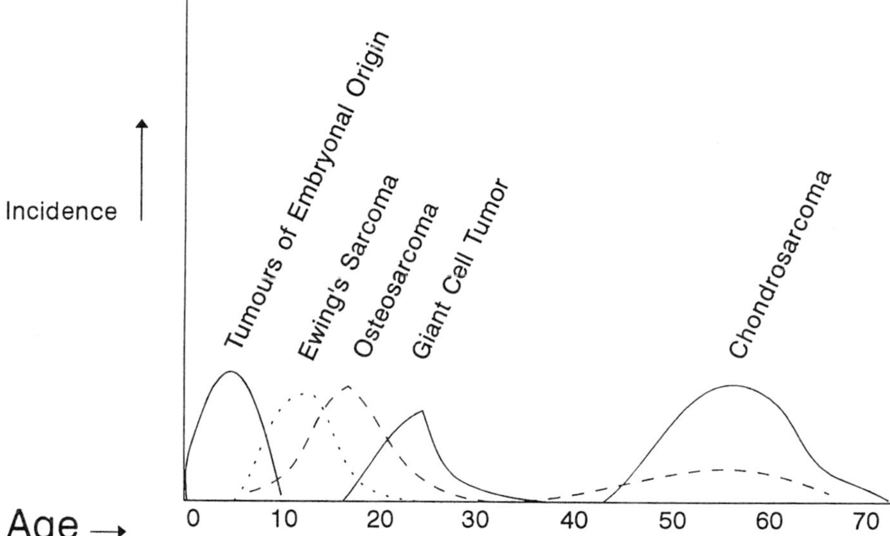

FIGURE 11–1. Variation in incidence of different cancers with respect to age.

3. What are the radiographic characteristics of the lesion itself?

Where Is the Lesion? Certain bone tumors have a predilection for a particular area of a bone. For example, osteosarcoma often occurs in the metaphysis, and Ewing's sarcoma often appears in the diaphysis. Giant cell tumors are more likely to appear in the epiphysis and metaphysis if the epiphyseal plate is closed,[4] whereas an epiphyseal tumor that occurs with the growth plate open is most likely a chondroblastoma.

What Is the Bone Doing to the Lesion? This question is crucial in determining the biology of the tumor. If the tumor is growing extremely quickly, the bone may not be able to respond to it at all. Codman was the first to describe the elevation of the periosteum and its subsequent ossification, which takes place when the tumor expands through the cortex, lifting the periosteum off the bone. A lesion that is completely surrounded by periosteal bone indicates a fairly slow rate of growth, and a lesion with no periosteal response indicates a rapid rate of growth.[5]

What Is the Radiographic Appearance of the Lesion? The lesion itself may produce either tumor osteoid, which shows up as ossification, or areas of calcification described as flocculant or circular ring forms. Intralesional calcification is more common in chondrosarcoma. Intralesional ossification is characteristic of osteosarcoma, which can produce the classic sun-ray spicules as the tumor cells grow out from the bone.

When an abnormality in the bone is suggestive of a malignant tumor, the patient should be referred to a musculoskeletal oncology group.[5] Figure 11–2 schematically suggests an appropriate decision sequence. This group consists of a surgeon, chemotherapists, radiation oncologists, diagnostic radiologists, and pathologists who are appropriately trained and experienced in the diagnosis and treatment of musculoskeletal tumors. Close association with palliative care and social work services within the institution is highly desirable.

Good-quality radiographs are acquired. A computed tomography (CT) scan defines changes in osseous structures. Tumor osteoid or intralesional calcification is better seen with a CT scan than with other imaging modalities.

A bone scan is important to confirm that the disease is localized. Multiple hot spots in the bone scan should alert

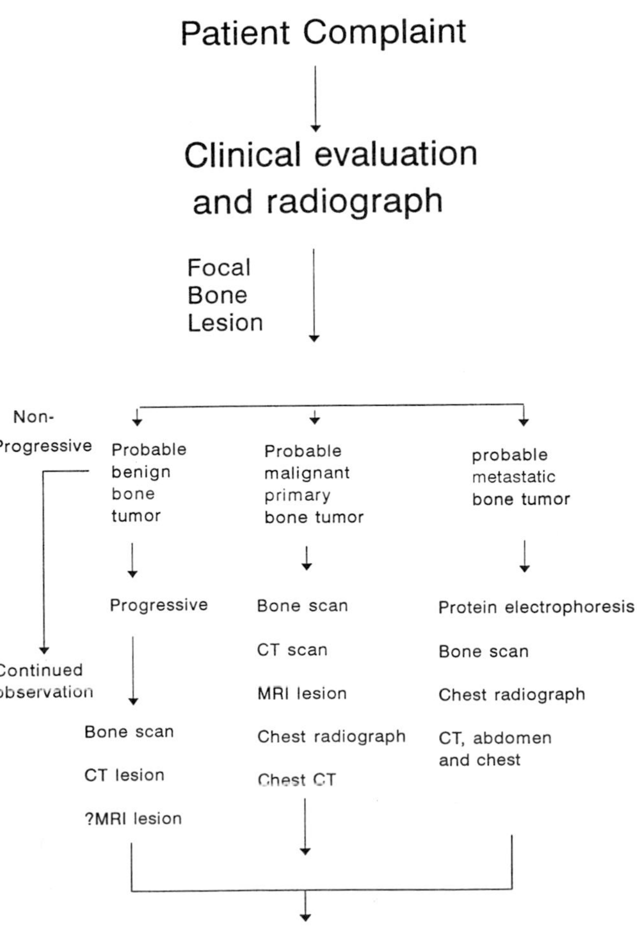

FIGURE 11–2. Decision sequence for diagnosis of bone tumors.

one to the possibility of a metastatic tumor or a primary osteosarcoma with skip lesions.[6] A bone scan is a sensitive but nonspecific tool for the diagnosis of bone tumors; a pattern of increased activity indicates only that there is increased bone formation at a particular area. It does not always correspond to tumor activity, and certain tumors, such as multiple myeloma and histiocytosis, have little association with "hot" bone scans.

Magnetic resonance imaging (MRI) defines soft tissue involvement and intramedullary involvement better than a CT scan.[7] Soft tissue involvement is usually outlined by the presence of increased inflammation around the tumor and a concomitant increase in edema within that inflammatory zone. This shows up well on T2-weighted MR images. The intramedullary extent of the tumor is best seen on an MRI scan, as demonstrated in Figures 11–3 and 11–4.

A chest radiograph and CT scan of the chest are important to rule out the presence of metastases. Cuts finer than 1 cm have an increasing sensitivity and a decreasing specificity. If a solitary lesion of less than 1 cm in the peripheral lung field is seen, excisional biopsy should be performed to determine the patient's stage of disease. If metastases are present at the time of the examination, this may affect the chemotherapist's choice of a chemotherapy regimen.

Appropriate blood work includes a complete blood count, erythrocyte sedimentation rate, and tests for levels of calcium and alkaline phosphatase. Alkaline phosphatase is often elevated in adolescents and therefore does not serve as a prognostic marker in patients with osteosarcoma, but in older patients, elevated alkaline phosphatase is unusual. It is also unusual to see massive changes in serum calcium in a patient presenting with a primary musculoskeletal tumor. Abnormalities in serum calcium should therefore alert the treating physician to the possibility of metastasis or a giant cell tumor secondary to hyperparathyroidism.

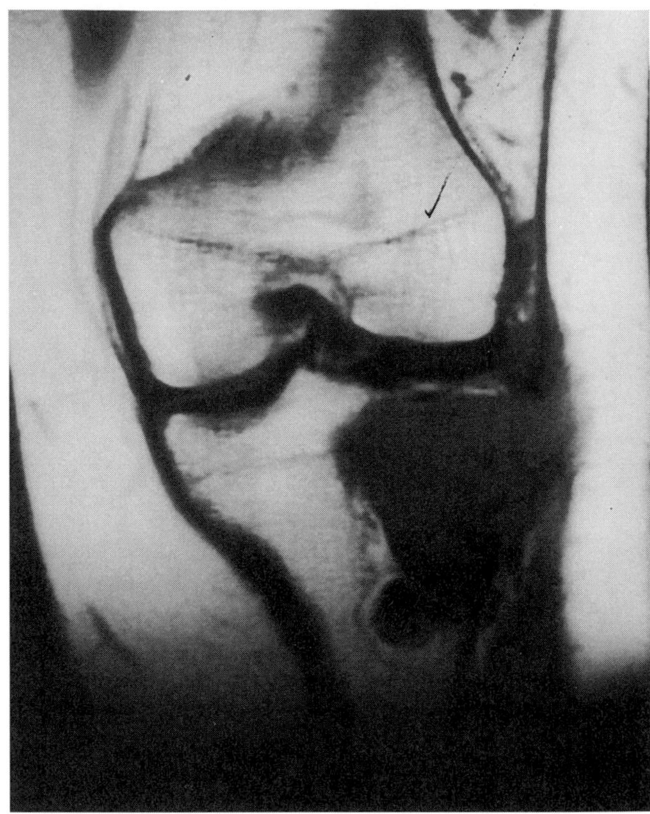

FIGURE 11–4. Coronal-slice MRI scan of a lesion in a 22-year-old woman. MRI clearly delineates the extent of the tumor within the bone and demonstrates that the tumor has grown outside the osseous compartment into the soft tissues. The tumor was found to be an osteosarcoma on biopsy.

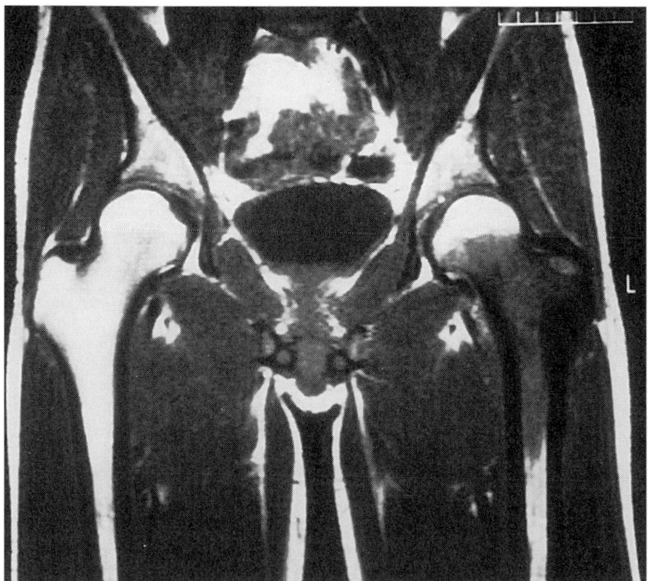

FIGURE 11–3. MRI scan of pelvis and proximal femur in an 18 year old presenting with a tumor of the proximal left femur. MRI clearly delineates the extent of the tumor infiltration in the bone marrow. The tumor was found to be a Ewing's sarcoma on biopsy.

STAGING

Any staging system must be designed to allow for an accurate estimate of the presenting patient's tumor burden, an evaluation of the treatment plan, and a prediction of the outcome of the patient's treatment based on historical data from similar patients.

Musculoskeletal tumors are now staged according to the Musculoskeletal Tumor Society recommendations, which were based on Enneking's initial classification system.[8, 9] Lesions are defined in relation to anatomic compartments, which have a distinct barrier between them. For example, cortical bone, including periosteum, is one compartment; the extensor compartment of the thigh bounded by fascial barriers is another. A lesion is extracompartmental if it has crossed the barrier between one compartment and another.

The staging system also depends on an assessment of the biology or grade of the tumor. Pathologists determine

TABLE 11–1
Surgical Stages

Stage	Grade	Site
IA	Low (G1)	Intracompartmental (T1)
IB	Low (G1)	Intracompartmental (T2)
IIA	High (G2)	Intracompartmental (T1)
IIB	High (G2)	Extracompartmental (T2)
III	Any (G) Regional or distant metastasis	Any (T)

from the histology whether the tumor is high grade or low grade in terms of its histologic appearance (Table 11–1). This staging system contrasts with the TNM method (whose components are primary tumor [T], regional nodes [N], and metastasis [M]). Because few musculoskeletal tumors metastasize to lymph nodes, the TNM methodology is not favored by musculoskeletal oncologists. With the staging system given in Table 11–1, there is more of a correlation between the extent of tumor spread and long-term survival.

THE SURGICAL MARGINS

The surgical margins of tumor resection are determined by pathologists, who examine the resected specimen, biopsy samples from the resected tumor bed, or both. The resected specimen is dissected by a pathologist, who determines the tumor's anatomic extent—specifically, the involved compartment or compartments. Suspicious areas are prepared to allow for the identification of the surgical margin; white paper correction fluid is used, which defines the surgical excision line on histologic examination.

Margins are defined as intralesional, marginal, wide, or radical (Table 11–2). An intralesional resection involves direct entry into the tumor and incomplete resection. It is often the result of curettage of a lesion that subsequently turns out to be malignant on review of the histology.

A marginal excision involves dissecting through the zone surrounding a tumor. This zone consists of inflammatory cells, neovascular tissues, and edema. It is sometimes erroneously described as a pseudocapsule around the tumor. The danger of a marginal excision is that the tumor often extends microscopically beyond its obvious gross margins.

TABLE 11–2
Surgical Procedures*

Margin	Local Procedure	Amputation
Intralesional	Curettage or debulking	Debulking amputation
Marginal	Marginal excision	Marginal amputation
Wide	Wide local excision	Wide through-bone amputation
Radical	Radical local resection	Radical disarticulation

*Classified by the type of margin they achieve and whether it is obtained by a local or ablative procedure.

A wide excision involves a resection of the tumor with a cuff of normal tissue surrounding it. This is the preferred surgical margin to achieve. Thick, fibrous membrane, such as fascia lata, is an effective barrier to tumor spread. Muscle, however, is an extremely poor barrier to tumor spread, and a more generous margin of 3 to 5 cm is often suggested. The difficulty with most resections comes from tumors extending into a compartment that has no normal anatomic barriers, such as a popliteal space. An osteosarcoma of the distal femur may grow down toward a popliteal artery and vein and be separated only by fat. By the time the tumor has become fixed, decalcified, and sectioned, the margins appear to be critically measured in millimeters. This kind of resection is classified as a contaminated wide margin if there is any sign that the tumor has extended absolutely to the margin of the resected specimen. Further treatment consisting of either surgical excision or brachytherapy may be advisable in this situation.

A radical resection is one in which the whole compartment is resected. A historical example is the use of hip disarticulation for distal femoral osteosarcoma, as a means of removing all the bone involved. Radical resections are rarely performed and are not considered necessary.

Amputation is reserved for those patients whose neurovascular bundles are involved by tumor and in whom a wide en bloc excision would have inadequate margins. Limb-sparing surgery is widely accepted as the treatment of choice, with an expected recurrence rate of less than 5%.[10–12]

With certain tumors, further adjuncts to staging are suggested. Patients with malignant fibrous histiocytomas and synovial cell sarcomas involving bones of the lower limb should have CT scans of the abdomen to rule out lymph node involvement. Certain tumors, such as telangiectatic osteosarcoma, are highly vascular, and an arteriogram may be indicated. Pelvic tumors often displace the major vessels, and angiography demonstrates the extent (Fig. 11–5).

THE BIOPSY

The biopsy should be performed by the treating surgeon. North American and English experiences support the impression that problems occur 3 to 10 times more commonly when the biopsy is performed prior to referral to a tumor treatment center.[13–15] The periphery of a lesion is most likely to yield viable tumor tissue, and the pathologist should be informed as to which part of the tumor the specimen came from.

The biopsy is performed through a longitudinal incision chosen so that the site can be excised as part of the definitive surgical procedure to follow. Sharp dissection of the tumor prevents the seeding of soft tissues around the biopsy site. The frozen section of soft tissue parts confirms the presence of viable tumor tissue. The histologic material may require many immunologic tests to determine the

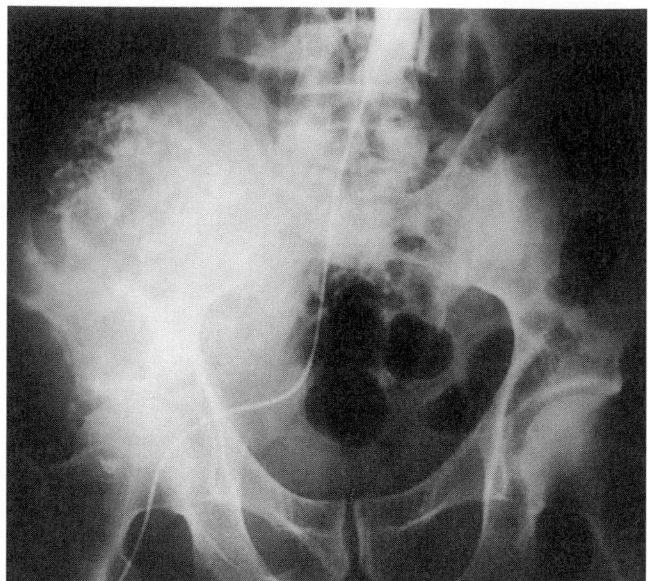

FIGURE 11–5. Radiograph of pelvis in a 55-year-old man presenting with a large pelvic mass. The intra-arterial catheter is clearly seen being displaced by the tumor, which was found to be a chondrosarcoma on biopsy.

true diagnosis. Tumor tissue may be quick-frozen for later examination by electron microscopy and possible genetic examination.[16]

If the cortex of a bone is breached during the biopsy process, polymethylmethacrylate bone cement may be used to plug the hole and prevent bleeding out of the intramedullary cavity into the soft tissues. In theory, hemorrhage from the bone tumor will result in contamination of tissue planes and possible seeding of tumor cells. These areas should be excised en bloc with the resected specimen.

Up to 20% of primary musculoskeletal tumors are not easily diagnosed by experienced bone pathologists.[17] It is not uncommon to refer specimens to other institutions when difficult diagnostic conundrums are encountered. A close dialogue must be maintained among the surgeon, the pathologist, and the radiologist, as there are classic traps for the unwary. An osteosarcoma presenting with a predominant fibrous component may be diagnosed as either fibrosarcoma or malignant fibrous histiocytoma. If the biopsy is not conducted in a way that provides adequate sampling of all the tumor, it is possible to miss a small area where tumor osteoid is found. For this reason, the author prefers open biopsy rather than needle biopsy, as the sampling error is larger with needle biopsy.[13]

TREATMENT

The goal of treatment is to render patients disease-free 10 years after their treatment programs.[18]

The treatment of a primary malignant bone tumor is surgical. The goal of surgery is to resect the tumor without compromising surgical margins so that the patient's survival is not compromised. Surgical techniques have progressed to the point where limb-sparing surgery is commonly performed; the recurrence rate of a primary tumor is 5% or less, equivalent to historical recurrent rates for amputation as the initial treatment of choice.[11, 19, 20] Surgical reconstruction along with limb-sparing surgery has become the treatment of choice when possible. There are many different methodologies employed for reconstructing a limb, including prosthetic replacement, allograft with or without prosthesis, vascularized fibula grafts, and limb rotation–plasty. The failure rate of all modalities of reconstruction is approximately 40% at 5 to 10 years follow-up.[21] The patient population is young and highly active and puts stresses on materials that are not able to undergo spontaneous repair, as occurs in the living bone skeleton.[22]

Role of Chemotherapy

The role of chemotherapy is to eradicate micrometastatic disease that is present at the time of presentation of a musculoskeletal tumor. Current chemotherapy regimens used in the treatment of osteosarcoma involve the institution of chemotherapy before surgical resection. This allows the treating oncologist to assess the efficacy of the chemotherapy in terms of tumor necrosis at the primary site after surgical resection.

Jaffe[23] was the first to establish that osteogenic sarcoma responds to high doses of methotrexate with citrovorum factor rescue. Since then, more aggressive chemotherapy regimens have been developed and have been submitted to randomized controlled studies. The Pediatric Oncology Group organized a multicenter study randomizing patients to receive either Rosen's T7 chemotherapy protocol after surgery or no chemotherapy. After the first 36 patients were reviewed, this study was closed because there was a significantly poorer survival among patients who did not receive immediate chemotherapy.[24] This established a role for chemotherapy as an adjuvant therapy to decrease the incidence of metastasis, which is the major cause of death following successful surgery.

In North America, the role of chemotherapy has evolved as a result of work initially performed at the Memorial Sloan-Kettering Cancer Center by Rosen et al.[25] At that institution, patients were being treated surgically with en bloc excision and fabrication of a custom endoprosthetic reconstruction device. During the wait for fabrication of the device, patients were placed on chemotherapy.[26] It was noted that the patients on a pre–prosthetic implant chemotherapy protocol had a better survival rate than their counterparts on the protocol that included only postamputation chemotherapy. Subsequently, patients were given a T7 protocol preoperatively, and it was noted that resected tumors were more necrotic; those patients appeared to have a superior survival pattern, compared with patients in whom the tumor was largely viable.[27, 28] Spontaneous necrosis in osteosarcoma is minimal, so necrosis seen following chemotherapy may be attributed to the treatment.[29]

Neoadjuvant chemotherapy, given prior to definitive resection of the tumor, has become the standard treatment. It allows an early assessment of the tumor's response. A change in chemotherapy agents is possible if the response is not satisfactory, that is, if greater than 90% tissue necrosis is not achieved.

The role of chemotherapy in the treatment of osteosarcoma and Ewing's sarcoma is clearly established. The role of chemotherapy in other musculoskeletal tumors is more controversial and is the subject of ongoing randomized controlled studies. Treatment of fibrosarcoma and malignant fibrous histiocytoma with chemotherapy regimens similar to those used in treating osteosarcoma has not proved beneficial. Ongoing nonrandomized studies have failed to show any significant improvement with preoperative or postoperative chemotherapy regimens for these diagnoses. Chondrosarcoma is generally resistant to chemotherapy and radiotherapy. In highly dedifferentiated chondrosarcoma—the most aggressive type—chemotherapy and radiotherapy may be indicated, usually for palliation.

Role of Radiotherapy

Radiotherapy is not used in the isolated treatment of bone tumors.[30] Use of radiotherapy in a skeletally immature child results in premature closure of epiphyseal plates and secondary limb deformities due to failure of growth. There is an increased pathologic fracture rate later in life in children who have received radiotherapy for Ewing's sarcoma.[31] The role of surgery and radiotherapy in this disease is being more closely examined in children; in adults, it remains controversial whether radiotherapy should be used alone or in combination with surgery, or whether surgery alone is sufficient.

OSTEOSARCOMA

Osteosarcoma constitutes about 20% of all primary malignant bone tumors, and the incidence of conventional osteosarcoma in North America is approximately two cases per million per year. The disease most often affects adolescents in the second decade of life, during the period of maximal growth activity. The male to female ratio is approximately 1.6:1.

The tumor has a predilection for the metaphysis of tubular long bones, especially the distal femur, proximal tibia, and proximal humerus. Approximately 50% of cases occur around the knee.

Osteosarcoma is a rapidly growing tumor. It is often associated with swelling and definite radiographic abnormalities. The most classic radiographic abnormality relates to the formation of new bone or tumor osteoid, which can grow out at right angles to the bone and form the so-called sun-ray spicules (Fig. 11–6).

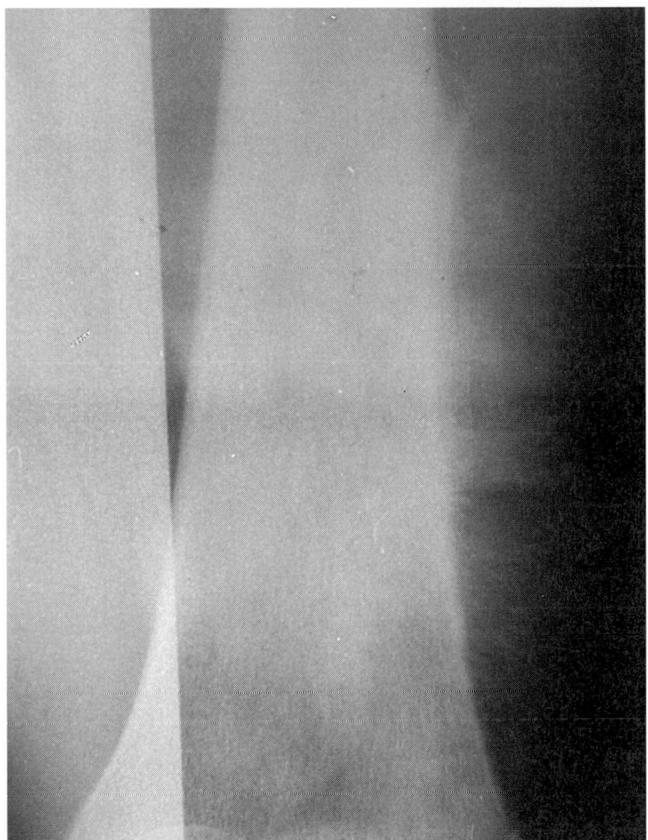

FIGURE 11–6. Osteosarcoma of the distal femur displaying the characteristic sun-ray spicules of bone as the periosteum is elevated.

The pathologic diagnostic marker is the presence of tumor osteoid.[11] Some osteosarcomas form only small amounts of tumor osteoid, but any lesion that produces tumor osteoid is usually classified as an osteosarcoma, even though great areas of the tumor may look like fibrous histiocytoma or fibrosarcoma. Prognostic variables for osteosarcoma are not easily determined. DNA analysis has been performed on osteosarcoma and other benign tumors, demonstrating that the vast majority of high-grade osteosarcomas are hyperploid.[16] However, with the identification of a retinoblastoma gene using molecular cloning techniques,[32] 30% to 40% of patients were noted to have a heritable predisposition to tumor as well as to other cancers, including osteosarcoma. It may be possible in the future to identify which genetic locus predisposes individuals to development of osteosarcoma.

Subclassifications of osteosarcoma are related to the anatomic location on the bone and the histologic appearance. The variants of osteosarcoma are shown in Table 11–3. Variations in the histologic presentation of osteosarcoma correlate with outcome.

Telangiectatic sarcoma is an unusual variant. It may mimic aneurysmal bone cysts radiologically, as it consists of large blood-filled spaces that look like cysts. However, these spaces are lined with tumor cells that produce malig-

TABLE 11–3
Classification of Osteosarcoma

Primary	Anatomic Variance
Conventional	Parosteal
Small cell	Periosteal
Fibrohistiocytic	Endosteal
Telangiectatic	
Multicentric	
Secondary	
Paget's disease	
Radiation-induced	

nant osteoid, as compared with the more benign cells appearing in aneurysmal bone cysts. Telangiectatic sarcoma has a predilection for heavy blood loss at biopsy. The prognosis is poor compared with that of classic osteosarcoma.

Small cell osteosarcoma is similar to Ewing's sarcoma histologically, but immunohistochemical staining can be diagnostic, as can chromosome analysis for translocation at chromosome 22, which is classic for Ewing's sarcoma. This variant has a worse prognosis than does classic osteosarcoma.

Secondary osteosarcomas are defined as those sarcomas occurring in pre-existing lesions of bone. They usually occur in patients aged 50 to 70. Most commonly, osteosarcoma arises in Paget's disease of the bone, although the sarcomatous degeneration can also yield malignant fibrous histiocytoma and fibrosarcoma. Osteosarcoma can also arise in a radiated bone 10 to 25 years after radiation treatment. The prognosis for these two types of osteosarcoma is usually poor, and they are not as responsive to chemotherapy as are osteosarcomas arising in younger age groups.

Another diagnostic conundrum relates to the surface osteosarcomas, that is, parosteal and periosteal osteosarcomas. A parosteal osteosarcoma is a low-grade osteosarcoma that arises in close apposition to the periosteum. It is usually separated from the underlying bone by a distinct margin.[33] This tumor is often mistaken for an exostosis but has a tendency to recur 2 to 5 years after a marginal or intralesional excision. The diagnosis is usually made on its characteristic radiographic appearance rather than on the histologic appearance.

A periosteal osteosarcoma is a high-grade osteosarcoma that occurs on the surface of the bone and usually extends into the soft tissue surrounding the bone.

Surgical Reconstruction Techniques

Limb-sparing surgery has not decreased the overall survival of patients with osteosarcoma.[34] There are many different ways of performing limb salvage. Allografts are a logical method of reconstruction in cases of large bone defects.[35] Gebhardt and coworkers[36] reported a 70% satisfactory outcome in patients at 2 or more years of follow-up. Allografts incorporated by the host may offer improved longevity of the reconstruction compared with metallic implants. However, fractures are a significant long-term complication of allografts. In young individuals, it remains to be seen whether allografts will become fully incorporated into the actual skeleton and behave like normal living bone. In a series of 16 massive retrieved human allografts, only 20% had become involved in a repair process by 5 years. This internal repair process took place very slowly and was confined to the superficial surface and ends of the graft.[37] The deep unrepaired portions of the graft retained their architecture, and the most rapid area of incorporation was the cancellous junctions, where internal cancellous tissue had advanced from the host to the allograft.[37] Power and associates[38] reported the results of revision of osteoarticular allografts in weight-bearing joints. In a series of 16 patients who required further allografting for failure of their primary allografts, 50% had graft survival at an average follow-up of 4 years (Fig. 11–7).

The use of vascularized bone transfer from the iliac crest

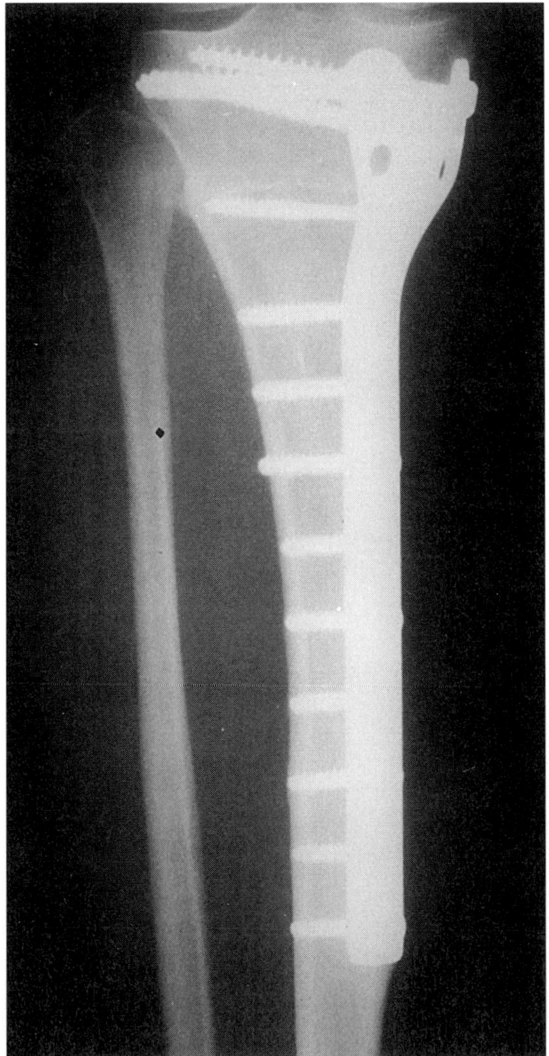

FIGURE 11–7. Four-year follow-up on an intercalary allograft demonstrating its complete union. Radiographically it is difficult to tell where the allograft ends and the patient's tibia starts.

or fibula to reconstruct defects following bone resection has become popular. At the Mayo Clinic between 1979 and 1989, 69 patients were treated with vascularized bone transfers after resection of tumors.[39] Sixty-seven percent had union after the primary procedure, and an additional 10 patients (14%) had union after a secondary procedure, for an overall union rate of 81%. The most favorable rate of union was among patients who had stable internal fixation with or without additional bone grafting.[39] The author prefers a vascularized fibular graft in conjunction with an allograft for areas that are going to undergo increased physiologic stress, such as hip or knee fusions and long intercalary grafts of the femur (Figs. 11–8 and 11–9).

Custom-designed arthroplasty can be performed for patients whose tumors involved joints that had to be resected. Any prosthetic device has to take into account the problems associated with wide resections of large tumors: loss of bone, loss of soft tissues, and instability of joints (particularly of the lower limb).[40] Long-term follow-up of many different devices demonstrated a consistent pattern of complications involving infections, aseptic loosening of the stems, and mechanical failures of the components.[41, 42] Reactions to metallic debris generated by loosening of the prosthesis have also been reported.[43, 44]

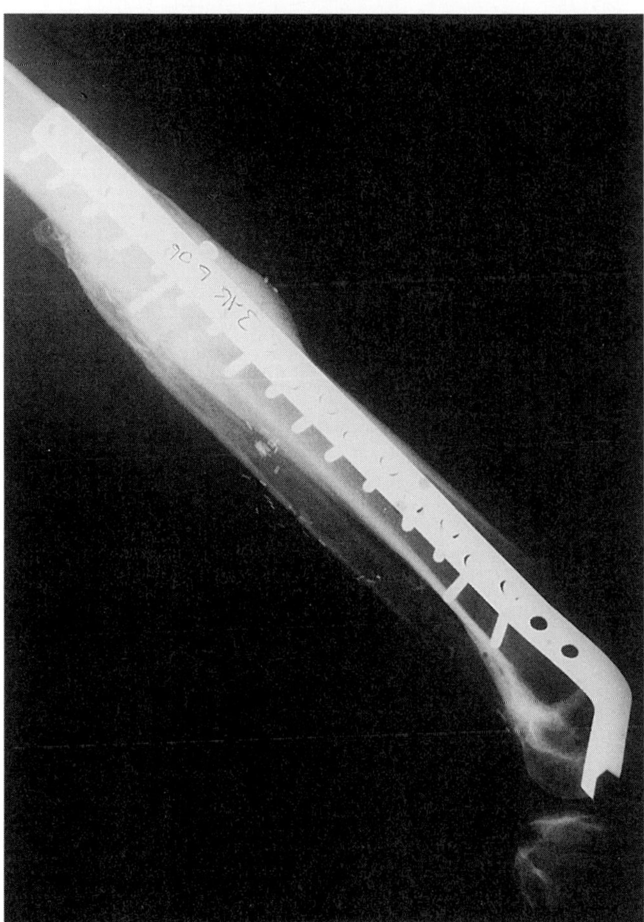

FIGURE 11–9. Lateral radiograph of the same patient in Figure 11–8 demonstrating a 3-year follow-up of an intercalary distal femoral allograft with a posteriorly placed vascularized fibular autograft. There has been complete union of both the allograft and the fibula to the distal femur and the proximal femoral shaft of the patient.

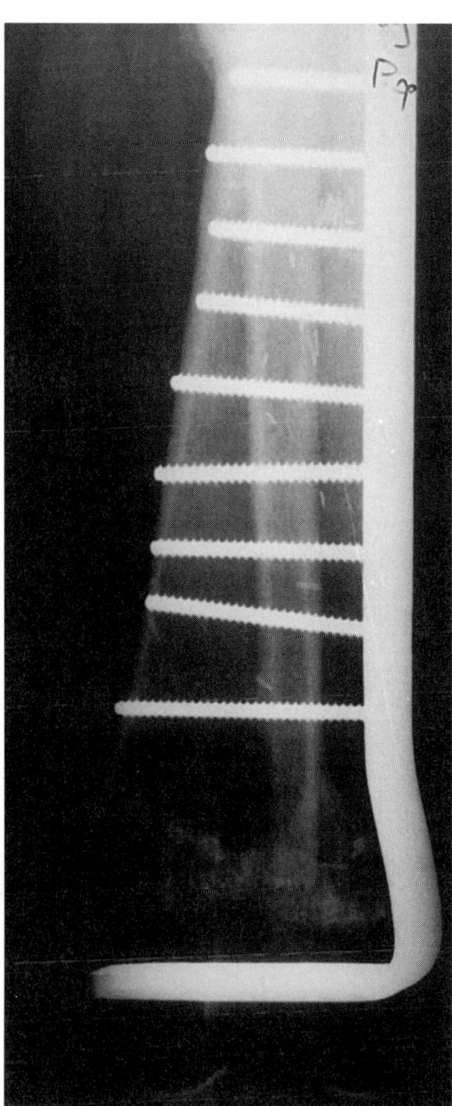

FIGURE 11–8. Anteroposterior radiograph demonstrating a 3-year follow-up on an intercalary allograft of the distal femur with a posteriorly placed vascularized fibular graft.

The use of expandable metallic prostheses has been explored in treating bone and joint defects in children. Such a prosthesis would expand as the child grew and allow for restoration of normal limb length and later reconstruction once complete growth was attained. In series other than from the originators, however, these prostheses have had a high incidence of complications and are now infrequently used.[43, 45]

Creative amputation is another method for treating tumors of the distal femur and proximal tibia. The modified van Ness rotation–plasty has been popularized in the treatment of such tumors, originally for the treatment of femoral dysplasia in congenitally short limbs.[46] After resection, the remaining distal limb is rotated 180° on its longitudinal axis and fixed to the proximal femur with plates and screws. The ankle joint becomes the knee joint, and it can be constructed so that at the end of maturity, both knee joints are at the same level. The functional results of this amputation—when it is successful—have been good, with electromyographic analysis demonstrating that there is more symmetry in gait with this procedure than with an above-knee amputation.[47, 48]

The Role of Chemotherapy

The use of chemotherapy is now well established in osteosarcoma.[34] Results in North America indicate that a disease-free survival of up to 80% of patients at 5 years, and 60% at 10 years, can be expected using modern chemotherapeutic regimens.[49]

The European literature, however, varies in long-term survival figures. Data from a cancer registry in England indicates that up to 1984, chemotherapy had not significantly improved the long-term survival of younger patients, and the overall survival was approximately 30% at 5 years.[50] The German experience is of a 5-year survival rate of approximately 64% in a group of children under the age of 15.[51] The results from Denmark up to 1984 indicate a survival rate of approximately 30% at 10 years.[10] This study addressed prognostic factors in osteosarcoma by performing a regression analysis on a number of clinical and pathologic variables. Tumors localized to the trunk, pelvis, or femur and symptom duration of less than 6 months were poor prognostic factors. Tumors dominated by fibroblastic cells in patients aged 25 to 30 were associated with an especially good prognosis. These researchers also noted that cancer deaths continued 10 years after the initial treatment and that the estimated hazard rate was four times greater than that of a group of healthy age- and sex-matched individuals.[10]

EWING'S SARCOMA

Ewing's sarcoma arises from nonmesenchymal elements of bone marrow.[52] Ewing's tumor constitutes approximately 6% of malignant bone tumors and tends to affect children more commonly than adults. Ninety percent of patients are younger than 30 years old at clinical presentation. Males are more commonly affected than females. Although there is no pattern of hereditary transmission, whites are affected more often than blacks. A chromosomal translocation described in Ewing's sarcoma cells suggests that a particular oncogene participates in its development.[52]

Most often the pelvis and lower limbs are the sites of Ewing's sarcoma. Metastases are often present at the time of presentation, leading some to believe that this is a systemic disease.[53] Pain and swelling are the most common symptoms, both tending to be progressive. A certain number of patients have symptoms for many months before diagnosis. Some are mistakenly treated for infection. An elevated erythrocyte sedimentation rate is frequent, along with leukocytosis or anemia or both. Often a low-grade fever supports the misdiagnosis of infection.

Ewing's tumor can have a characteristic radiographic appearance, involving the diaphysis of a long bone.[52] The intramedullary canal may demonstrate a loss of bone, having a moth-eaten appearance. If the tumor has eroded through the cortex, there may be reactive onion skinning of periosteal new bone (Fig. 11–10).

Biopsy results from the tumor are often similar to those of infection, with the tumor appearing as a semiliquid, resembling pus.[54] It is essential that appropriate biopsy specimens are taken. Histologically, the tumor consists of sheets of small cells that are uniform and quite characteristic. The tissue contains considerable glycogen and is positive on specific stains, such as periodic acid–Schiff.

The prognosis of Ewing's sarcoma has consistently improved with the use of aggressive multiagent chemotherapy, from 10% to approximately 50% survival at 5 years.[55, 56] Long-term follow-up of Ewing's sarcoma indicates that there are prognostic indicators for survival: age above 25 years, high serum lactate dehydrogenase, and central primary tumors are associated with a poor long-term prognosis.[57]

Metastatic disease used to be the principal cause of treatment failure, but control of local disease has become increasingly critical to long-term survival. Late recurrence of local disease following radiotherapy and chemotherapy has been reported when Ewing's sarcoma patients are

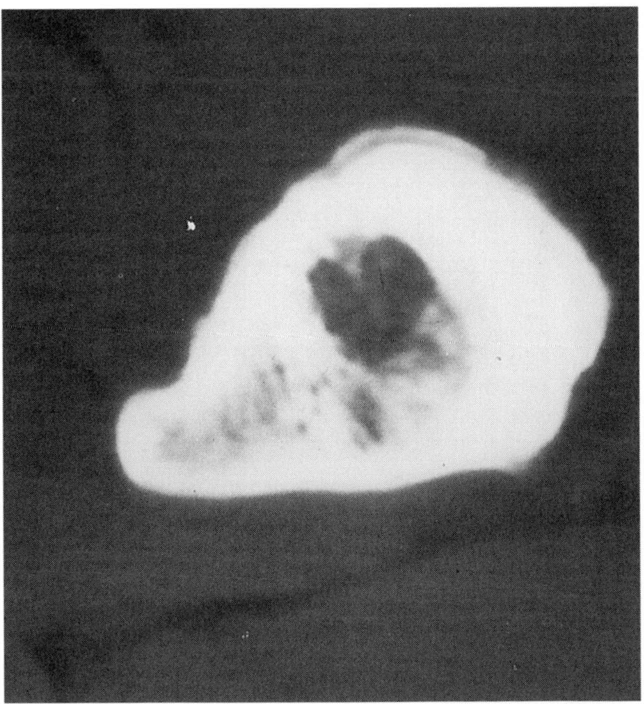

FIGURE 11–10. CT transaxial radiograph of a proximal femur demonstrating an anterior periosteal response in Ewing's sarcoma.

subjected to careful long-term clinical follow-up. It had been thought that chemotherapy and radiotherapy for local disease were adequate treatment. More recently, however, surgical excision of the primary lesion has been advocated. An increased survival (74% at 5 years) has been obtained by adding complete surgical excision of the primary lesion, compared with those treated without surgery.[58] In the Mayo Clinic experience with Ewing's sarcoma of the pelvis, local failure was 44% in the group treated with chemotherapy and radiotherapy alone, compared with 13% in patients that had resection.[59] At present, recommendations for surgery include excision of the primary lesion when feasible.[56]

Osteosarcoma can develop as a secondary malignant neoplasm in children who have received radiotherapy for previous tumors, including Ewing's sarcoma. Osteosarcoma arises an average of 10 years (range, 5 to 21 years) following treatment. The prognosis of this type of osteosarcoma is poor.[53] Ewing's sarcoma is also associated with the development of secondary cancers in long-term irradiated survivors. The actuarial risk was calculated as 8% at 5 years for development of a second cancer, and 4% for development of a bone sarcoma.[60] The Pediatric Oncology Group reported on the prognostic features of Ewing's sarcoma. In that study, which compared pretreatment and post-treatment CT scans, medullary involvement was associated with the worst chance of survival.[61]

POST-TREATMENT CARE

It must be recognized that musculoskeletal surgery carries a high complication rate. A high anxiety level and high expectations from the patient and relatives, coupled with a diagnosis of bone cancer, exacerbates any latent or submerged psychological problems in the patient and family.

The musculoskeletal oncology team must be prepared for many varied complications relating to the extent of the surgical resection, the method of reconstruction, and complications of adjacent therapy, such as radiotherapy-induced delayed wound healing or postchemotherapy neutropenia and increased risk of infection.[22]

In the immediate postoperative period, the patient should be closely assessed for common complications such as deep venous thrombosis, pneumonia, wound-healing problems, dislocations of prosthetic devices, and loss of position of internal fixation apparatus. A pre-emptive approach to the diagnosis of complications allows for early intervention and possible salvage of potentially disastrous outcomes. Early evacuation of wound hematomas and correction of bleeding points or bleeding disorders are essential. Early recognition of a declining white blood cell count could result in the early administration of a granulocyte colony–stimulating factor.

Major extremity surgery is associated with a marked increase in postoperative pain, and all attempts must be made to prevent the patient from suffering excessively. Continuous postoperative infusion with regional analgesia has become an accepted modality of treating such patients, as major nerves are often accessible following wide surgical excisions, and it is easy to place an epidural catheter in the nerve sheath.[62] The author has had considerable experience with this treatment and has found that patients progress more quickly and have a markedly lower incidence of phantom limb pain following amputation.

Once the patient is discharged from the hospital, therapy must continue. Each team member must be aware of the implications of his or her own treatments on colleagues' areas of treatment. For example, chemotherapy is often aggressive and toxic and can result in the development of an opportunistic infection. The patient must therefore be seen in follow-up in the oncology clinic by the surgeon during the period of chemotherapy to assess and prevent any infectious seeding of a prosthetic replacement caused by an opportunistic infection associated with a low white count and cell activity.

A regular surveillance program is essential. A full clinical examination, chest radiograph, and appropriate radiographs of the surgical reconstruction are recommended every 3 months for the first 2 years following surgery. No specific tumor markers are available. The chest radiograph allows for the early identification of metastasis in the lung. Since most metastases are asymptomatic, such a program of surveillance is mandatory. Chemotherapy has been observed to delay the presentation of metastasis, so a 5-year follow-up is essential, and a 10-year follow-up program is advantageous. Success of treatment cannot be determined until 5 to 10 years have passed, to ascertain the success of both the tumor treatment and the surgical reconstruction.

References

1. Kransdorf MJ, Sweet DE, Buetow PC, Giudici MAI, Moser RP: Giant cell tumor in skeletally immature patients. Radiology 184:233–237, 1992.
2. Brien WW, Salvati EA, Healey JH, Bansal M, Ghelman B, Betts F: Osteogenic sarcoma arising in the area of a total hip replacement. J Bone Joint Surg [Am] 72:1097–1099, 1990.
3. Martin A, Bauer TW, Manley MT, Marks KE: Osteosarcoma at the site of total replacement. J Bone Joint Surg [Am] 70:1561–1567, 1988.
4. McDonald DJ, Sim FH, McLeod RA, Dahlin DC: Giant-cell tumor of bone. J Bone Joint Surg [Am] 68:235–242, 1986.
5. Simon MA, Finn HA: Diagnostic strategy for bone and soft-tissue tumors. J Bone Joint Surg [Am] 75:622–631, 1993.
6. Enneking WF, Kagan A: "Skip" metastases in osteosarcoma. Cancer 36:2192–2205, 1975.
7. Berquist TH: Magnetic resonance imaging of primary skeletal neoplasms. Radiol Clin North Am 31:411–424, 1993.
8. Enneking WF, Spanier SS, Goodman M: A system for the surgical staging of musculoskeletal sarcoma. Clin Orthop 153:106–120, 1980.
9. Enneking WF: Limb Salvage in Musculoskeletal Oncology. New York: Churchill Livingstone, 1987.
10. Bentzen SM, Poulsen HS, Kaae S, et al: Prognostic factors in osteosarcomas; a regression analysis. Cancer 62:194–202, 1988.
11. Klein MJ, Kenan S, Lewis MM: Osteosarcoma; clinical and pathological considerations. Orthop Clin North Am 20:327–345, 1989.
12. Simon MA, Aschlman MA, Thomas N, Mankin HJ: Limb-salvage

treatment versus amputation for osteosarcoma of the distal end of the femur. J Bone Joint Surg [Am] 68:1331–1337, 1986.
13. Enneking WF: The issue of the biopsy [editorial]. J Bone Joint Surg [Am] 64:1119–1120, 1982.
14. Grimer RJ, Davies AM, Evans N: Editorial: Fatigue fractures of the proximal tibia simulating malignancy. Br J Radiol 730:903–908, 1988.
15. Mankin HJ, Lange TA, Spanier SS: The hazards of biopsy in patients with malignant primary bone and soft-tissue tumors. J Bone Joint Surg [Am] 64:1121–1127, 1982.
16. Bauer HC, Kreicbergs A, Silfversward C, Tribukait B: DNA analysis in the differential diagnosis of osteosarcoma. Cancer 61:2532–2540, 1988.
17. Schojowicz F, McGuire MH: Diagnostic difficulties in skeletal pathology. Clin Orthop 240:281–310, 1989.
18. Sweetnam R: Malignant bone tumor management; 30 years of achievement. Clin Orthop 247:67–73, 1989.
19. Campanacci M: Local recurrence after amputation for osteosarcoma. J Bone Joint Surg [Br] 62:201–207, 1980.
20. Grimer RJ, Sneath RS: Diagnosing malignant bone tumors. J Bone Joint Surg [Br] 72:754–756, 1990.
21. Brown KLB: Complications of Limb Salvage: Prevention, Management and Outcome. Montreal: ISOLS, 1991.
22. Quill G, Gitelis S, Morton T, Piasecki P: Complications associated with limb salvage for extremity sarcomas and their management. Clin Orthop 264:242–250, 1990.
23. Jaffe N: Chemotherapy for malignant bone tumors. Orthop Clin North Am 20:487–505, 1989.
24. Link MP, Goorin AM, Miser AW, et al: The effect of adjuvant chemotherapy on relapse-free survival in patients with osteosarcoma of the extremity. N Engl J Med 314:1600–1606, 1986.
25. Rosen G, Murphy ML, Huvos AG, Gutierrex M, Marcove RC: Chemotherapy, en bloc resection, and prosthetic bone replacement in the treatment of osteogenic sarcoma. Cancer 37:1–11, 1976.
26. Rosen G, Marcove RC, Caparros B, Nireberg A, Kosloff C, Huvos AG: Primary osteogenic sarcoma; the rationale for preoperative chemotherapy and delayed surgery. Cancer 43:2163–2177, 1979.
27. Rosen G, Caparros B, Huvos AG, et al: Preoperative chemotherapy of osteogenic sarcoma; selection of postoperative adjuvant chemotherapy based on the response of the primary tumor to preoperative chemotherapy. Cancer 49:1221–1230, 1982.
28. Rosen G, Nirenberg A: Neoadjuvant chemotherapy for osteogenic sarcoma; a five year follow-up (T-10) and preliminary report of new studies (T-12). Prog Clin Biol Res 201:39–51, 1985.
29. Springfield DS, Schakei ME, Spanier SS: Spontaneous necrosis in osteosarcoma. Clin Orthop 263:233–237, 1991.
30. Kalnicki S: Radiation therapy in the treatment of bone and soft tissue sarcomas. Orthop Clin North Am 20:505–512, 1989.
31. Springfield DS, Pagliarulo C: Fractures of long bones previously treated for Ewing's sarcoma. J Bone Joint Surg [Am] 67:477–481, 1985.
32. Wiggs J, Nordenskjold M, Yandell D, et al: Prediction of the risk of hereditary retinoblastoma, using DNA polymorphisms within the retinoblastoma gene. N Engl J Med 318:151–157, 1988.
33. Enneking WF, Springfield D, Gross M: The surgical treatment of parosteal osteosarcoma in long bones. J Bone Joint Surg [Am] 67:125–135, 1985.
34. Yasko AW, Lane JM: Chemotherapy for bone and soft tissue sarcomas of the extremities. J Bone Joint Surg [Am] 73:1263–1271, 1991.
35. Mnaymeneh W, Malinin T: Massive allografts in surgery of bone tumors. Orthop Clin North Am 20:455–467, 1989.
36. Gebhardt C, Flugstad DI, Springfield DS, Mankin HJ: The use of bone allografts for limb salvage in high-grade extremity osteosarcoma. Clin Orthop 270:181–196, 1991.
37. Enneking WF, Mindell ER: Observations on massive retrieved human allografts. J Bone Joint Surg [Am] 73:1123–1142, 1991.
38. Power RA, Wood DJ, Tomford WW, Mankin HJ: Revision osteoarticular allograft transplantation in weight-bearing joints. J Bone Joint Surg [Br] 73:595–599, 1991.
39. Han C, Wood MB, Bishop AT, Cooney WP: Vascularized bone transfer. J Bone Joint Surg [Am] 74:1441–1449, 1992.
40. Horowitz SM, Lane JM, Healey JH: Soft-tissue management with prosthetic replacement for sarcomas around the knee. Clin Orthop 275:226–231, 1992.
41. Horowitz SM, Lane JM, Otis JC, Healey JH: Prosthetic arthroplasty of the knee after resection of a sarcoma in the proximal end of the tibia. J Bone Joint Surg [Am] 73:286–293, 1991.
42. Ward WG, Johnston KS, Dorey FJ, Eckardt JJ: Extramedullary porous coating to prevent diaphyseal osteolysis and radiolucent lines around proximal tibial replacements. J Bone Joint Surg [Am] 75:976–987, 1993.
43. Lavy CBD, Briggs TWR: Failure of growing endoprosthetic replacement of the humerus. J Bone Joint Surg [Br] 74:626, 1992.
44. Shinto Y, Uchida A, Yoshikawa H, Araki N, Kato T: Inguinal lymphadenopathy due to metal release from a prosthesis. J Bone Joint Surg [Br] 75:266–269, 1993.
45. Safran MR, Eckardt JJ, Kabo JM, Oppenheim WL: Continued growth of the proximal part of the tibia after prosthetic reconstruction of the skeletally immature knee. J Bone Joint Surg [Am] 74:1172–1179, 1992.
46. Merkel KD, Gebhart M, Springfield DS: Rotationplasty as a reconstructive operation after tumor resection. Clin Orthop 270:231–236, 1991.
47. Capanna R, Ruggieri P, Biagini R, et al: The effect of quadriceps excision on functional results after distal femoral resection and prosthetic replacement of bone tumors. Clin Orthop 267:186–196, 1991.
48. Steenoff JR, Daanen HAM, Taminiau AHM: Functional analysis of patients who have had a modified van Ness rotationplasty. J Bone Joint Surg [Am] 75:1451–1456, 1993.
49. Glasser DB, Lane JM: Stage IIB osteogenic sarcoma. Clin Orthop 270:29–39, 1991.
50. Gill M, Murrells T, McCarthy M, Silcocks P: Chemotherapy for the primary treatment of osteosarcoma: Population effectiveness over 20 years. Lancet 1:689–691, 1988.
51. Michaelis J: Osteosarcoma. Lancet 1:1174, 1988.
52. Eggli KD, Quiogue T, Moser RP: Ewing's sarcoma. Radiol Clin North Am 31:325–337, 1993.
53. Beehler JR, Robertson WW, Meadows AT, Womer RB: Osteosarcoma as a second malignant neoplasm in children. J Bone Joint Surg [Am] 74:1079–1083, 1992.
54. Pritchard DJ: Small round cell tumors. Orthop Clin North Am 20:367–375, 1989.
55. Nesbit ME, Gehan EA, Burgert EO, et al: Multimodal therapy for the management of primary, nonmetastatic Ewing's sarcoma of bone: A long term follow-up of the first intergroup study. J Clin Oncol 8:1664–1674, 1990.
56. O'Connor MI, Pritchard DJ: Ewing's sarcoma; prognostic factors, disease control and the reemerging role of surgical treatment. Clin Orthop 262:78–87, 1991.
57. Kinsella TJ, Miser JS, Waller B, et al: Long term follow-up of Ewing's sarcoma of bone treated with combined modality therapy. Int J Radiat Oncol Biol Phys 20:389–395, 1991.
58. Wilkins RM, Pritchard DJ, Burgert EO, Unni KK: Ewing's sarcoma of bone; experience with 140 patients. Cancer 58:2551–2555, 1986.
59. Frassica FJ, Frassica DA, Pritchard DJ, Schomberg PJ, Wold LE, Sim FH: Ewing sarcoma of the pelvis. J Bone Joint Surg [Am] 75:1457–1465, 1993.
60. Smith LM, Cox RS, Donaldson SS: Second cancers in long term survivors of Ewing's sarcoma. Clin Orthop 274:275–281, 1992.
61. Reinus WR, Gilula LA, Donaldson S, Shuster J, Glicksman A, Vietti TJ: Prognostic features of Ewing's sarcoma on plain radiograph and computed tomography scan after initial treatment: A pediatric oncology group study (8346). Cancer 72:2503–2510, 1993.
62. Malawer MM, Buch R, Khurana JS, Garvey T, Rice L: Postoperative infusional continuous regional analgesia; a technique for relief of postoperative pain following major extremity surgery. Clin Orthop 266:227–237, 1991.

Norman D. Bloom, M.D.

12

Amputations of the Shoulder and Pelvis

HEMIPELVECTOMY

Hemipelvectomy has been employed successfully for the treatment of bone and soft tissue sarcomas of the upper thigh, hip, or pelvis;[1] unremitting osteomyelitis of the pelvis; and trauma.[2] In most of the latter instances, the amputation was traumatic, and the surgeon's role was limited to débridement and wound management. However, situations arise in which uncontrollable pelvic bleeding necessitates a hemipelvectomy. Occasionally, patients with recurrent squamous cell cancers of the cervix and penis extending to the pelvic sidewall benefit from hemipelvectomy as well.[3]

The first successful hemipelvectomy was performed by Girard in 1895, although Billroth performed a resection 6 years earlier. Prohibitive blood loss usually resulted in a high operative morbidity rate. Pringle reported a 75% morbidity rate among patients operated on before 1909; this was reduced to 58% in the years between 1909 and 1945.

Gordon-Taylor[4] described the operation as "a simple surgical exercise, well suited for an elderly surgeon with a modicum of anatomy and the physical ability to stand by an operating table for a mere 50 to 60 minutes." The need for speed was emphasized in order to adequately control the hemorrhage.

Between 1925 and 1952, Gordon-Taylor became the most experienced surgeon in the performance of this operation. In 1935, he reported an operative mortality rate of 51% in 79 patients.[5] By 1952, this rate had been reduced to 22%.[6] This reduction was attributed to a constant refinement of operative technique and the control of intraoperative hemorrhage. Improvements in blood transfusion and anesthetic techniques after World War II had a significant impact on operative mortality.

In 1966, Higinbotham and associates[7] reported a surgical mortality rate of 7% in 100 patients, in 5 due directly to uncontrollable hemorrhage. The average blood loss in this series of patients was 12 units. A later series of patients reported by Miller[8] had an average blood loss of only 8 units. In some more recent series, blood loss has been further reduced.[9]

In Higinbotham and colleagues' series, 75% of patients experienced hematoma, seroma, infection, or skin necrosis. The latter occurred in 26 of the 100 patients, and gross infections occurred in 22. In Miller's series of 50 patients, skin flap necrosis occurred in 80% of the patients; débridement in the operating room was required in 50%.

The classic incision utilized for a hemipelvectomy relies on a posterior flap consisting of skin and some gluteal vessels that arise from the internal iliac (Fig. 12–1). With a high ligation of the common iliac vessels, the blood supply to the flap becomes more tenuous, relying on collaterals from the lumbar branches (Fig. 12–2). The anterior flap is more generously supplied via the superior epigastrics. The loss of the inferior epigastric supply is of less significance. The compromised blood supply to the large posterior flap contributes significantly to the wound complication rate.

Bowden and Booher[10] initially described the anterior flap in conjunction with a hemipelvectomy to cover a large posterior defect caused by a tumor arising in the buttock. Sugarbaker and Chretian[11] designed a myocutaneous flap consisting of the quadriceps musculature supplied by the superficial femoral system. The use of this myocutaneous

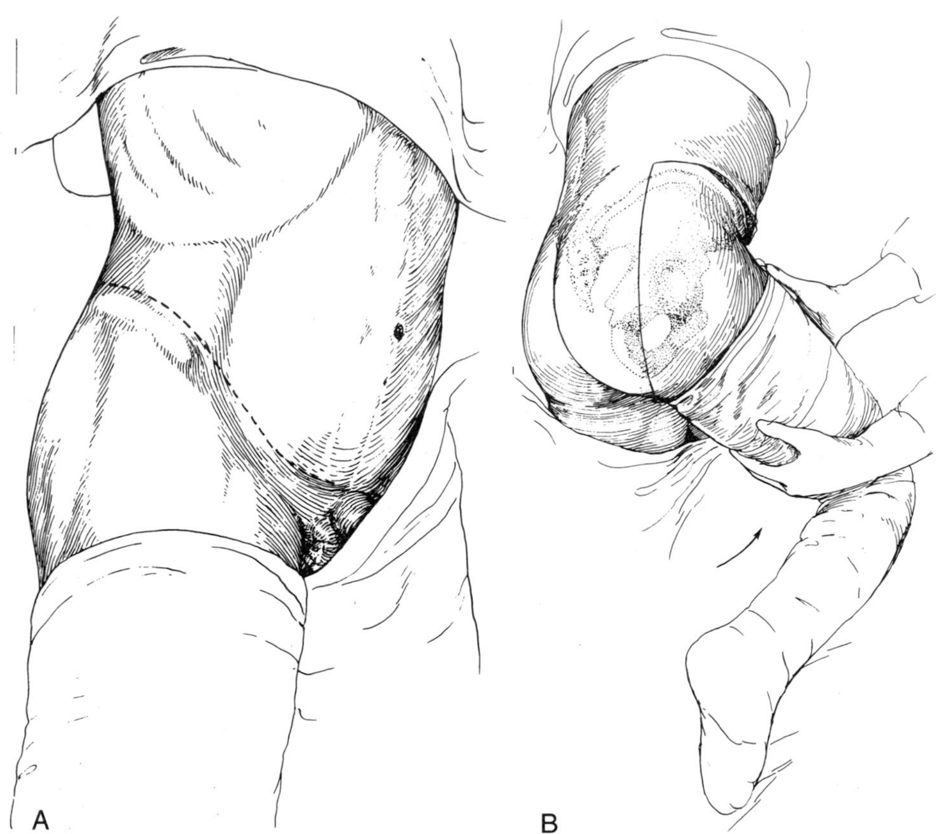

FIGURE 12–1. *A,* The anterior incision employed for a classic hemipelvectomy. *B,* The posterior skin incision following the line of the gluteus maximus. (From Nora P: Textbook of Operative Surgery, 3rd ed. Philadelphia: WB Saunders, 1990, p 1275.)

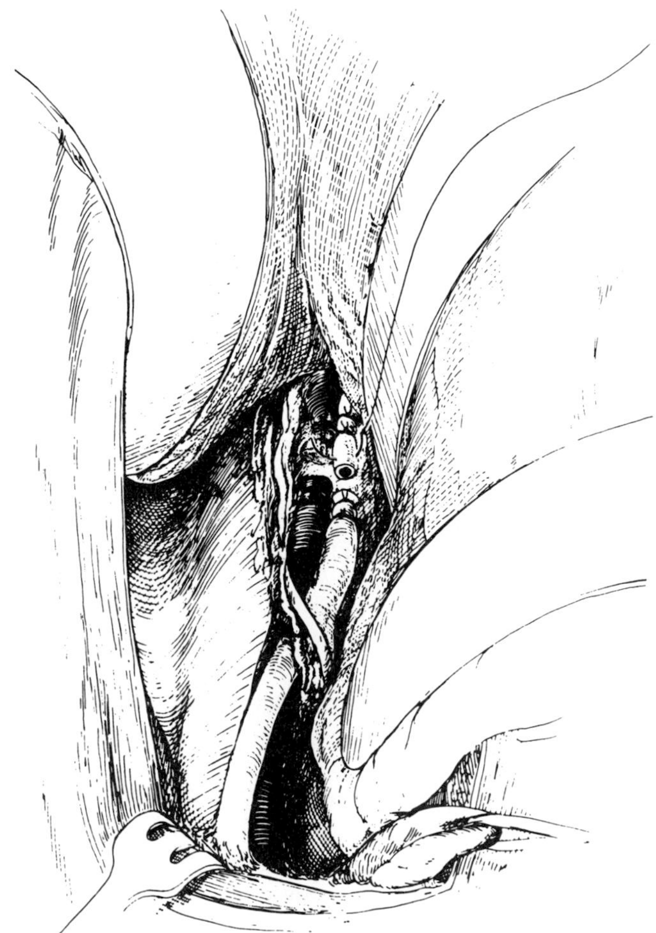

FIGURE 12–2. High ligation of the common iliac artery and vein in the retroperitoneal space. (From Nora P: Textbook of Operative Surgery, 3rd ed. Philadelphia: WB Saunders, 1990, p 1275.)

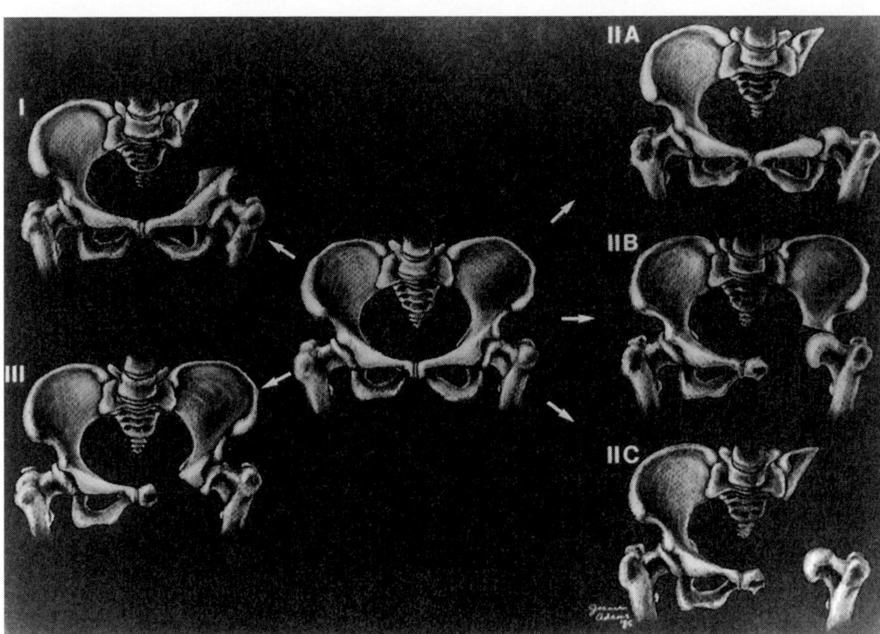

FIGURE 12–3. Subclassifications of the internal hemipelvectomy. (From Enneking WF: Limb Salvage in Musculoskeletal Oncology. New York: Churchill Livingstone, 1987, p 174.)

flap wherever possible has reduced the wound complication rate by allowing for a well-vascularized skin flap.

INTERNAL HEMIPELVECTOMY

Over the past decade, various surgical techniques have been employed to resect the hemipelvis and preserve the lower extremity. Prior to 1978, there were only a handful of reported cases.[12, 13] In 1978, Enneking and colleagues[14] published results of limb salvage in 32 patients with primary neoplasms involving the innominate bone. Each resection could be classified into one of three patterns: type 1, resection of the ilium; type II, resection of the periacetabular region with sacrifice of the hip joint; and type III, resection of the pubic rami (Fig. 12–3). The type II resection is subclassified according to whether the iliac wing or symphysis is included with the hip joint.

Type I Hemipelvectomy

The type I hemipelvectomy is technically the easiest and yields excellent functional and oncologic results. Campanacci and Capanna[15] reported on 34 patients undergoing type I resection; the overall complication rate was 58%. The most frequent complication was infection, followed by neurologic damage, injury to the iliac vessels, and abdominal wall hernia. Healey and coworkers[16] reported similar complication rates in their series of patients.

For type I resections, functional results have been variable. Eilber et al.,[17] reporting on 10 patients, had two excellent results, three good results, four fair results, and one poor result. In Campanacci and Capanna's series of 34 patients, 15 were assessed for functional results. Excellent results were obtained in 10 patients, with good results in 4 and fair results in 1. In these patients, there were 10 infectious complications, 5 hernias, and 5 cases of nerve damage.

In a recent series of 12 patients, Marlex mesh was used to reconstruct the surgical defect.[18] There were no infections or hernias, but two patients required resection of a major nerve. The functional results were excellent in nine patients, good in two, and fair in one. Marlex mesh reduces the dead space, stabilizes the abdominal wall, and allows earlier ambulation (Fig. 12–4*A* and *B*).

Type II Hemipelvectomy

Type II or periacetabular resection is the most difficult to perform and reconstruct. In a symposium, several investigators reported on the end results achieved in 127 cases with a follow-up time of 20 months to 20 years.[19–26] The most common tumors resected were chondrosarcoma (61%), osteosarcoma (19%), Ewing's sarcoma (5%), and malignant fibrous histiocytoma (5.5%) (Table 12–1). Surgical margins were obtained in two thirds of cases. The resection was limited to the acetabulum (type II) in 21

TABLE 12–1
Histology in 127 Cases of Periacetabular Resection

Histology	No.	%
Chondrosarcoma	77	61.0
Osteosarcoma	24	19.0
Ewing's sarcoma	6	5.0
Malignant fibrous histiocytoma	7	5.5
Lymphoma	1	0.8
Plasmacytoma	1	0.8
Benign lesions	7	5.5
Other	4	3.0

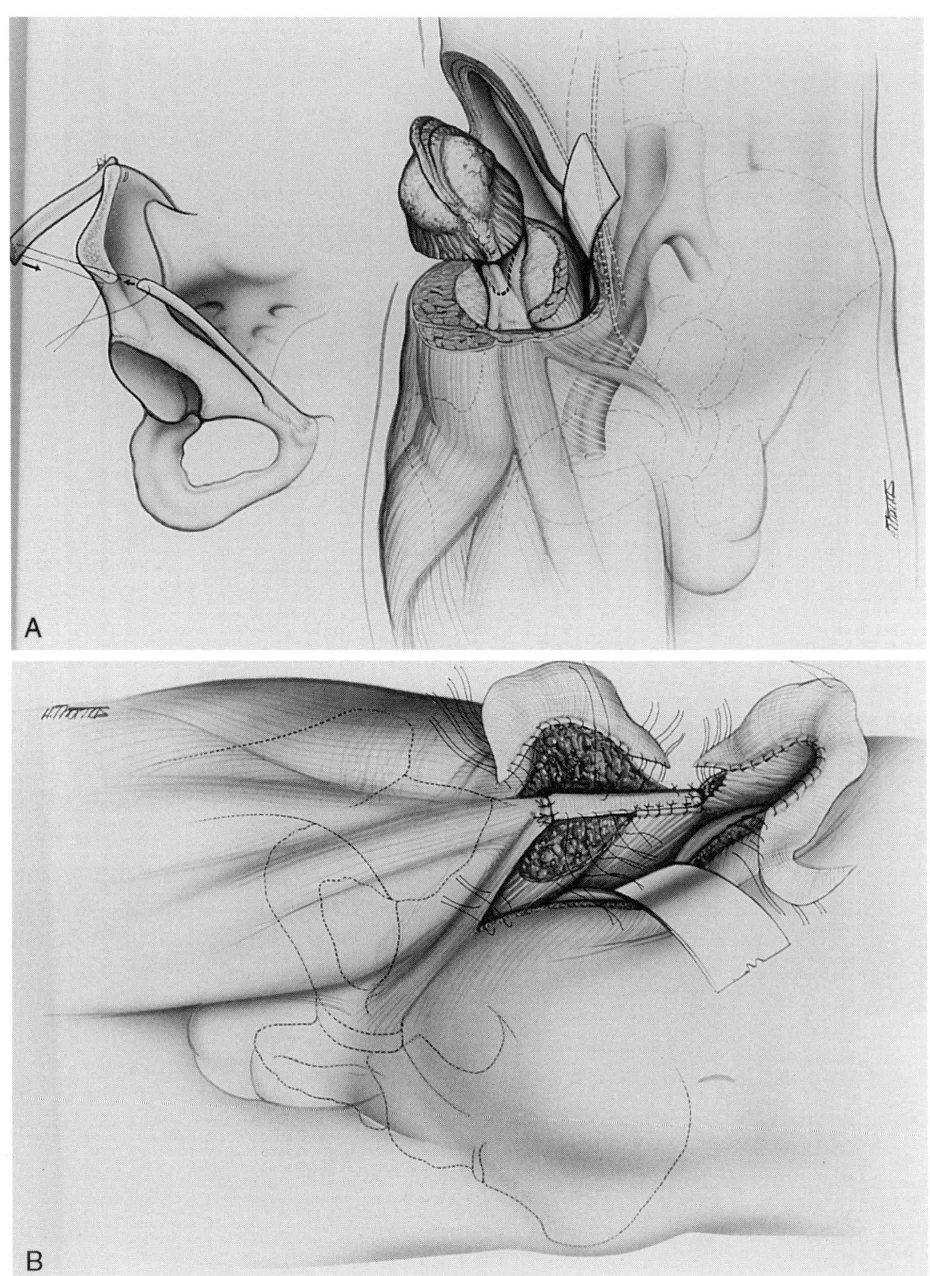

FIGURE 12–4. *A,* Type I resection of the iliac wing. *B,* Marlex mesh reconstruction of the resulting deficit.

cases; it included the acetabulum and part or all of the ilium (types I and II) in 22 cases, the acetabulum and pubis (types II and III) in 46 cases, and almost the entire pelvis (types I, II, and III) in 38 cases.

A variety of reconstructive techniques were utilized. No reconstruction of the skeleton (with the goal of spontaneous pseudarthrosis or a flail hip) was performed in 48 cases. Twenty-one cases had iliofemoral or ischiofemoral synthesis using metal wires, with the goal of pseudarthrosis or arthrodesis (Fig. 12–5). Iliofemoral or ischiofemoral synthesis using screws or plates, with or without bone grafts, was employed in 34 cases (Fig. 12–6). In the remaining patients, reconstruction was attempted by a combination of bone grafts and a femoral prosthesis (7 cases), by a pelvic prosthesis (10 cases) (Fig. 12–7), or by pelvic allograft (7 cases) (Table 12–2).

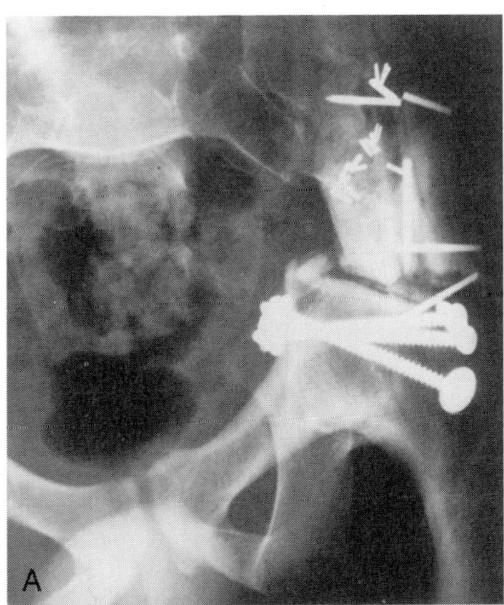

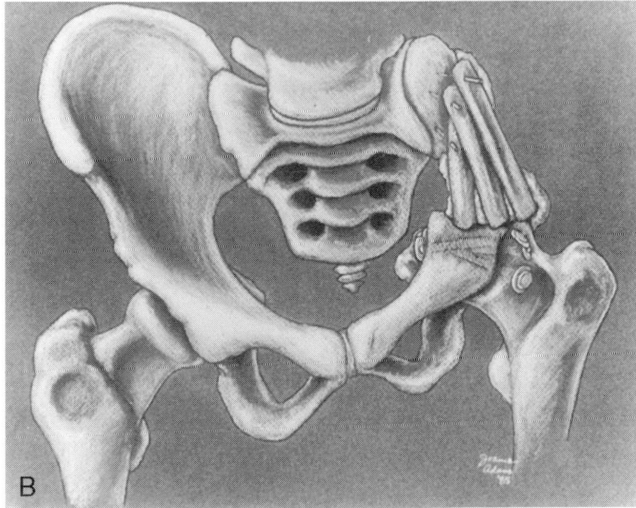

FIGURE 12–5. Postoperative radiograph *(A)* and illustration *(B)* of a type I and II resection of a pelvic lesion. Reconstruction was accomplished by arthrodesis of the hip, fibular autografts, and methyl methacrylate. (From Enneking WF: Limb Salvage in Musculoskeletal Oncology. New York: Churchill Livingstone, 1987, p 176.)

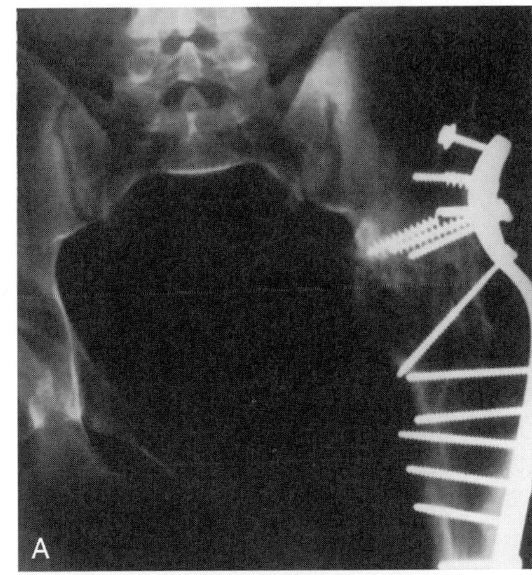

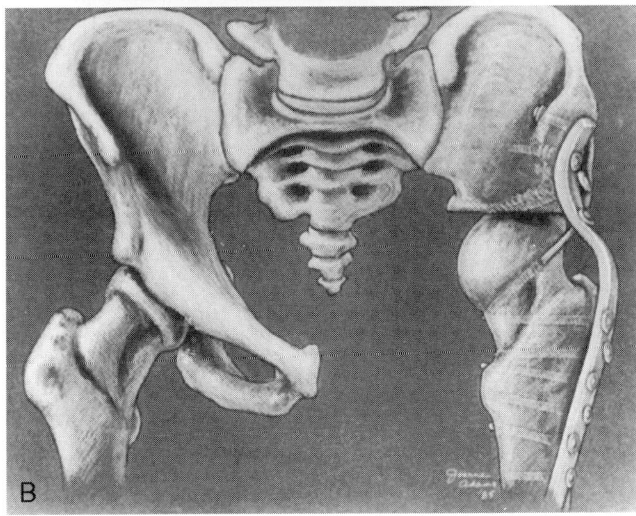

FIGURE 12–6. Postoperative radiograph *(A)* and illustration *(B)* of a type II and III resection and reconstruction by iliofemoral arthrodesis. (From Enneking WF: Limb Salvage in Musculoskeletal Oncology. New York: Churchill Livingstone, 1987, p 178.)

Only two patients died in the perioperative period, but more than one third of the patients had major complications; one quarter required supplementary surgery. The most frequent complication was infection, with or without flap necrosis (14%), followed by flap necrosis (5%), nerve

TABLE 12–2
Types of Reconstruction Used in
127 Cases of Periacetabular Resection

Type of Reconstruction	No.	%
No reconstruction	48	38.0
Iliofemoral or ischiofemoral wiring	21	16.5
Iliofemoral or ischiofemoral synthesis ± bone grafts	34	27.0
Bone grafts and femoral prosthesis	7	5.5
Pelvic prosthesis or allograft	17	13.0

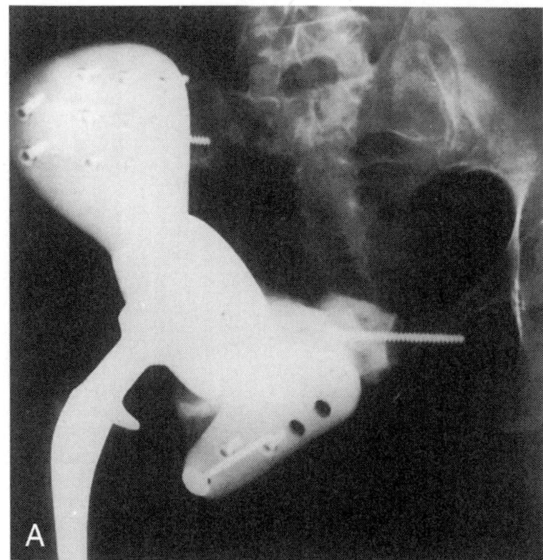

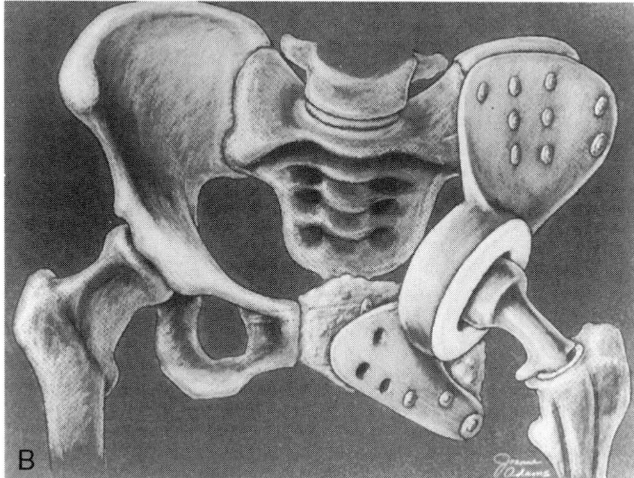

FIGURE 12–7. Postoperative radiograph *(A)* and illustration *(B)* of a custom-made hemipelvis reconstruction for a type I, II, and III resection. (From Enneking WF: Limb Salvage in Musculoskeletal Oncology. New York: Churchill Livingstone, 1987, p 179.)

damage (4%), and vascular damage (2%). Seven patients subsequently underwent amputation. Infections were twice as common in those patients undergoing more complex reconstructions.

The overall results obtained in this combined series were 5% excellent, 31% good, 38% fair, and 26% poor. Patients who had no reconstruction had the worst functional results, but complications increased among reconstructed patients (Table 12–3).

In a recent report by Harrington,[27] 14 patients underwent either an autoclaved autograft replacement (4 patients) or allograft replacement (10 patients). Five patients had excellent results and seven had good results. Follow-up on these patients ranged from 5 to 11 years. Fatigue fractures of the grafts occurred in three patients at 5, 6, and 8.5 years, at which time previous excellent functional results became fair or poor.

Type III Hemipelvectomy

Type III hemipelvectomy is the least common type of internal hemipelvectomy. Results are excellent or good in the majority of cases (Fig. 12–8). Technical considerations include full mobilization of the iliac vessels, bladder, and urethra. Reconstruction of the resected pelvis with Marlex mesh eliminates the hernias that have been reported after this procedure.

INTERSCAPULOTHORACIC AMPUTATION

Interscapulothoracic amputation consists of an en bloc resection of the entire clavicle, scapula, shoulder, and upper extremity. Ralph Cumming, surgeon at the Naval Hospital in Antigua, is credited with performing the first elective forequarter amputation for a gunshot wound in 1808.[28] Berger introduced the term interscapulothoracic amputation in 1887 and described the anterior approach.[29] Littlewood first witnessed the posterior approach in 1882; his description of it was published posthumously in 1922.[30] The current approach utilizes a combination of both these classic incisions (Figs. 12–9 to 12–13).

In 1958, Pack[31] reported results obtained in 88 amputations performed from 1926 to 1953. More than half (53%) of the operations were for primary soft tissue sarcomas. The remainder were for primary bone lesions, skin cancers, extensive axillary nodal disease of various etiologies, or

TABLE 12–3
Functional Results According to Enneking's System in 97 Cases of Periacetabular Resection with Follow-Up of 20 Months to 20 Years

Technique	No.	Excellent (%)	Good (%)	Fair (%)	Poor (%)
Flail hip	21	1 (5)	4 (19)	8 (38)	8 (38)
Iliofemoral pseudarthrosis	28	2 (7)	9 (32)	14 (50)	3 (11)
Iliofemoral arthrodesis	15	1 (7)	5 (33)	5 (33)	4 (27)
Ischiofemoral pseudarthrosis	7	—	1 (14)	3 (43)	3 (43)
Ischiofemoral arthrodesis	7	1 (14)	3 (43)	1 (14)	2 (29)
Bone graft and femoral prosthesis	6	—	4 (67)	1 (17)	1 (17)
Pelvic prosthesis	9	—	3 (33)	3 (33)	3 (33)
Pelvic allograft	4	—	1 (25)	2 (50)	1 (25)
Total		5 (5)	30 (31)	37 (38)	25 (26)

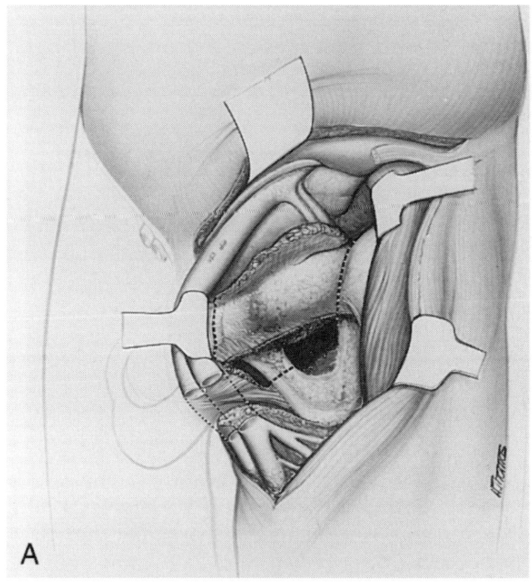

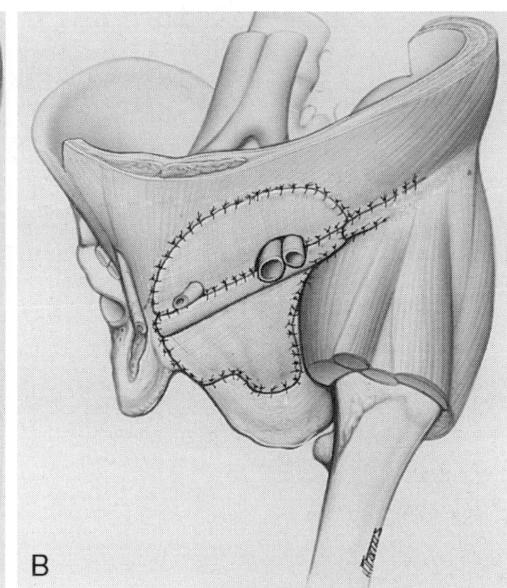

FIGURE 12–8. *A,* Type III resection of the pelvis for a lesion of the superior pubic ramus. *B,* Marlex mesh reconstruction of the defect.

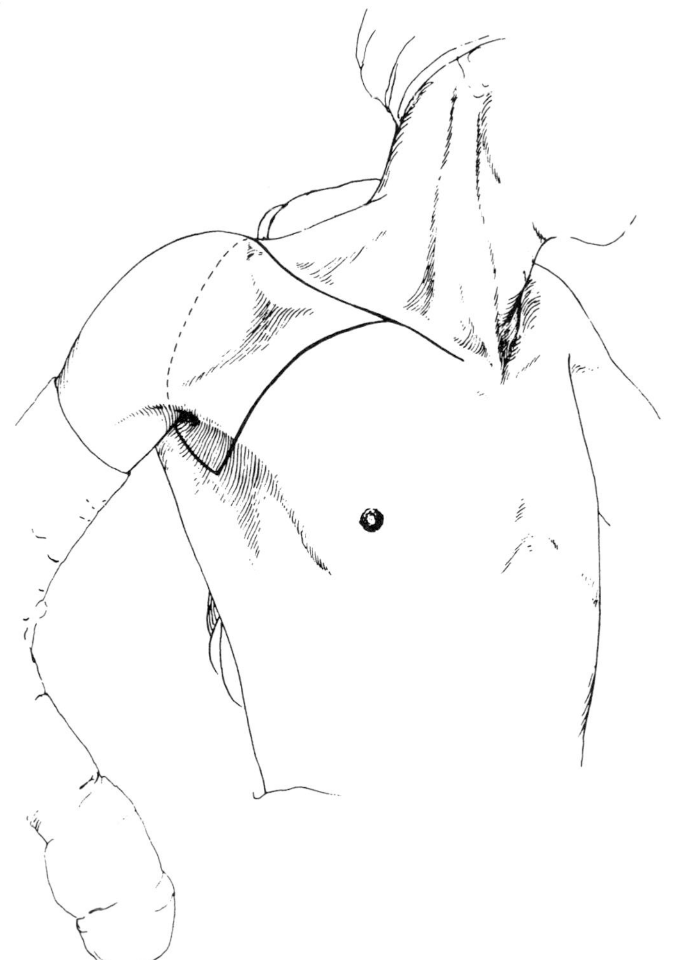

FIGURE 12–9. Anterior skin incision for a forequarter amputation. (From Nora P: Textbook of Operative Surgery, 3rd ed. Philadelphia: WB Saunders, 1990, p 1269.)

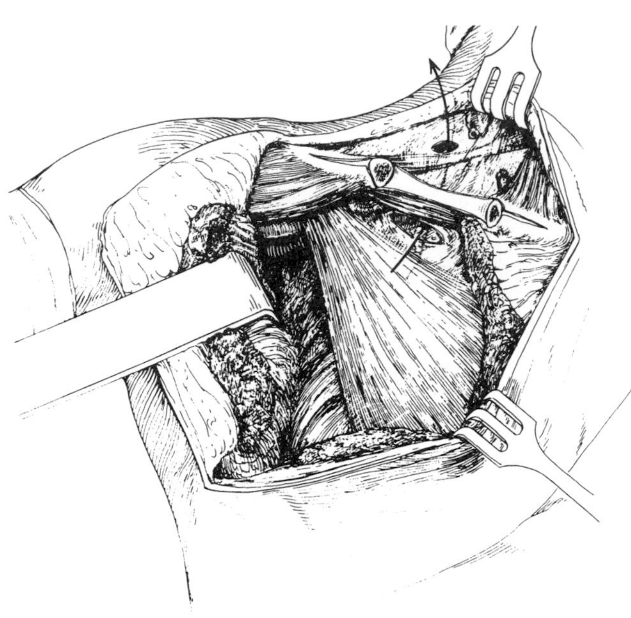

FIGURE 12–10. The pectoralis major muscle is divided to expose the pectoralis minor muscle, clavipectoral fascia, and clavicle. (From Nora P: Textbook of Operative Surgery, 3rd ed. Philadelphia: WB Saunders, 1990, p 1269.)

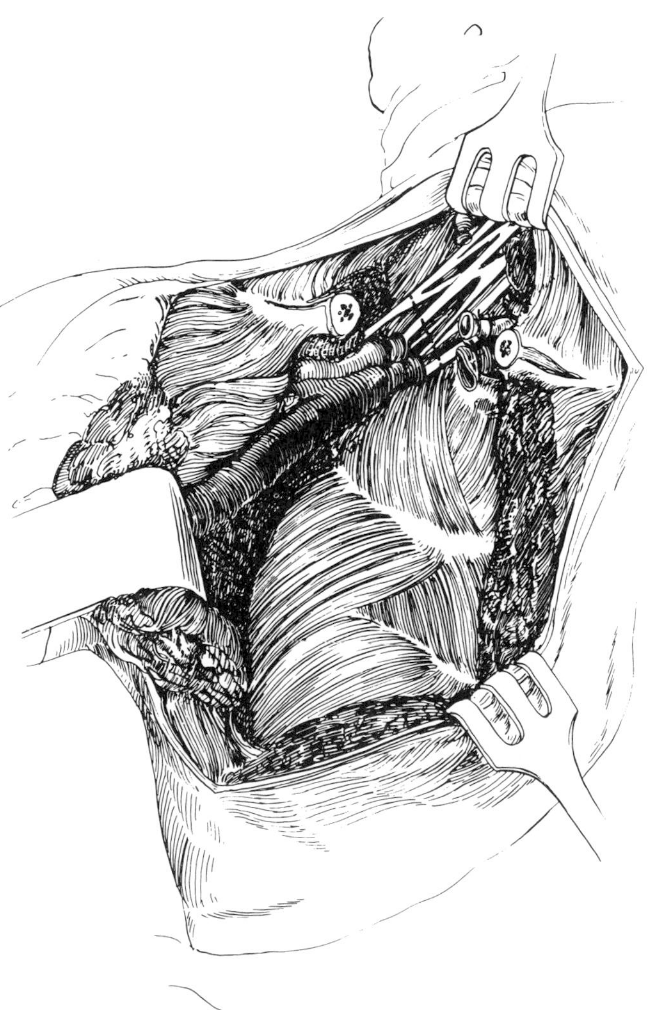

FIGURE 12–11. After the division of the pectoralis minor muscle and clavicle, the subclavian vessels are divided and the line of resection on the brachial plexus is defined. (From Nora P: Textbook of Operative Surgery, 3rd ed. Philadelphia: WB Saunders, 1990, p 1230.)

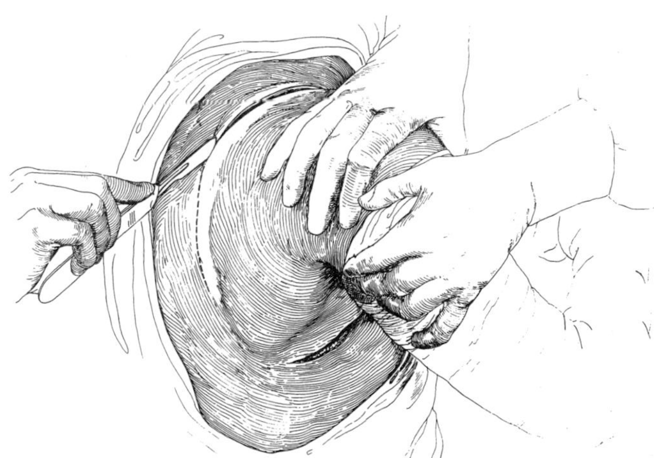

FIGURE 12–12. The posterior skin incision is made paralleling the medial border of the scapula. (From Nora P: Textbook of Operative Surgery, 3rd ed. Philadelphia: WB Saunders, 1990, p 1271.)

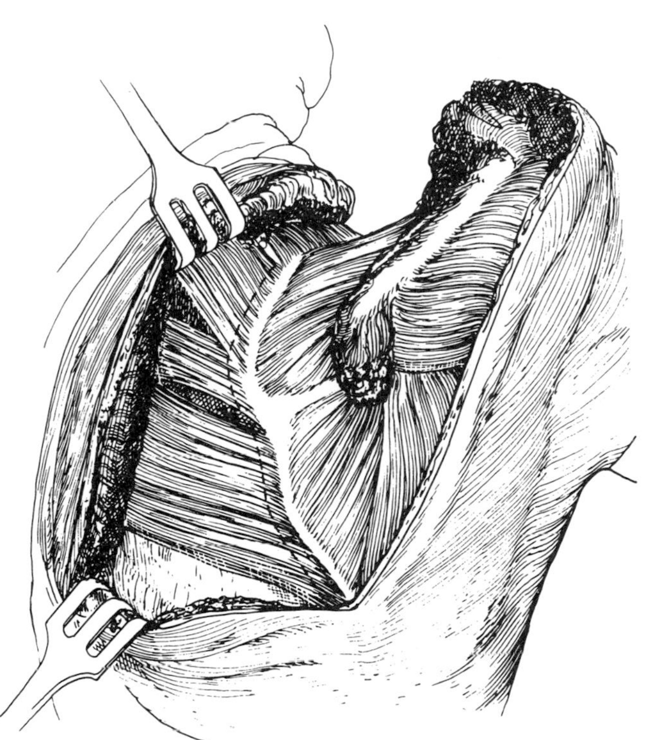

FIGURE 12–13. All the parascapular musculature is incised. (From Nora P: Textbook of Operative Surgery, 3rd ed. Philadelphia: WB Saunders, 1990, p 1271.)

TABLE 12–4
Survival in 86 Patients Undergoing Forequarter Amputation for Primary Bone Tumors

Histology	No.	5-YearSurvival	%
Osteogenic sarcoma	56	17	30
Chondrosarcoma	19	9	47
Ewing's sarcoma	3	1	33
Fibrosarcoma	6	2	33
Reticulum cell sarcoma	2	0	0

metastatic lesions. Of the 39 determinant cases in this series, the 5-year survival rate was 30% for soft tissue sarcoma patients. In the majority of these patients, the operation was for palliation. Pack's paper defined the indications for this procedure.

Sim et al.[32] reviewed the Mayo Clinic experience in 1977. One-hundred and seventy-three forequarter amputations were performed between 1942 and 1977. Eighty-six were for primary tumors arising in the bone, and 87 were for primary soft tissue tumors. The majority of the primary bone tumors (70) arose in the humerus, and the majority of these patients had osteosarcomas. Other primary lesions included chondrosarcoma (19), fibrosarcoma (6), Ewing's sarcoma (3), and reticulum cell sarcoma (2). Approximately one third of these patients survived 5 years (Table 12–4). Of the 87 soft tissue sarcoma patients, fibrosarcomas were the most common histologic type, and the 5-year survival was similar to that obtained in patients with primary bone tumors (Table 12–5). During this period, there were no operative deaths among these patients, and the average blood replacement was 1500 mL. Only 10 patients suffered wound complications.

TIKHOFF-LINDBERG PROCEDURE

Although the results achieved with interscapulothoracic amputation are acceptable with regard to mortality, morbidity, and cure rates, the current emphasis is on performing more conservative operations with limb preservation.

The first report of an upper extremity limb salvage operation appeared in the Russian literature in 1914. Bauman alluded to a 1908 report by Pranishkov of the removal of the scapula and surrounding soft tissue, with resection

TABLE 12–5
Survival in 87 Patients Undergoing Forequarter Amputation for Primary Soft Tissue Sarcomas

Histology	No.	5-Year Survival	%
Liposarcoma	11	4	36
Fibrosarcoma	20	10	50
Synovial sarcoma	5	2	40
Rhabdomyosarcoma	10	3	30
Lymphangiosarcoma	13	2	15
Miscellaneous	28	7	25

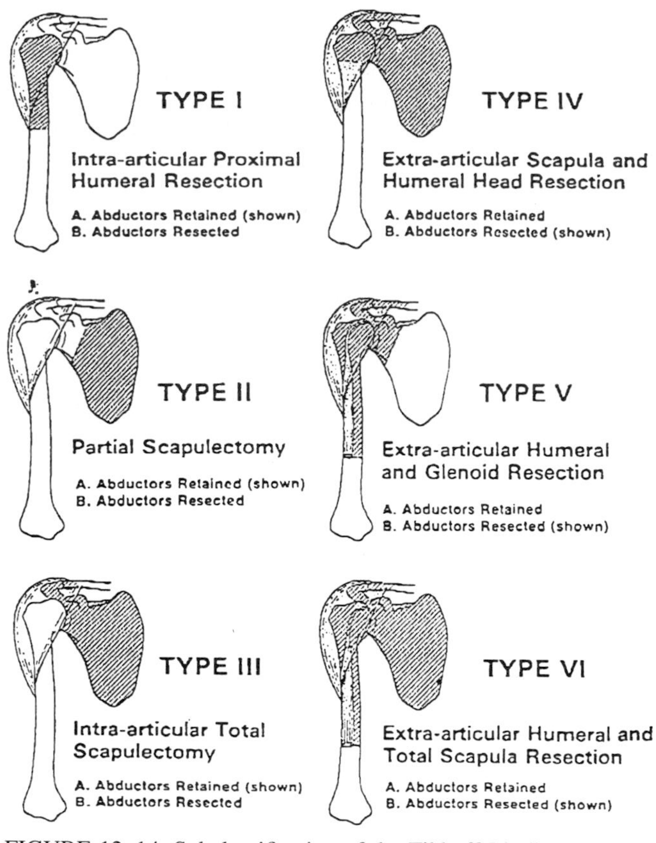

FIGURE 12–14. Subclassification of the Tikhoff-Lindberg operation as proposed by Malawer.

of the head of the humerus and outer third of the clavicle. Tikhoff and Bauman performed three additional operations, and the results were published in Russian in 1914.[33] In 1927, Lindberg read a paper before the Nineteenth All Russian Congress of Surgeons in Leningrad in which he reported on three interscapulothoracic resections for malignant tumors around the shoulder joint and credited Professor Tikhoff of Tomsk University for first performing this

TABLE 12–6
Histologic Type of Tumors in 60 Patients Undergoing Shoulder Girdle Resection with Limb Salvage

Histology	No.
Osteogenic sarcoma	11
Chondrosarcoma	10
Malignant fibrous histiocytoma	7
Ewing's sarcoma	6
Fibrosarcoma	3
Alveolar cell sarcoma	1
Lymphoma	1
Malignant schwannoma	1
Fibromatosis	1
Hemangioendotheliosarcoma	1
Rhabdomyosarcoma	1
Chondroblastoma	1
Giant cell tumor	6
Metastatic tumors	10

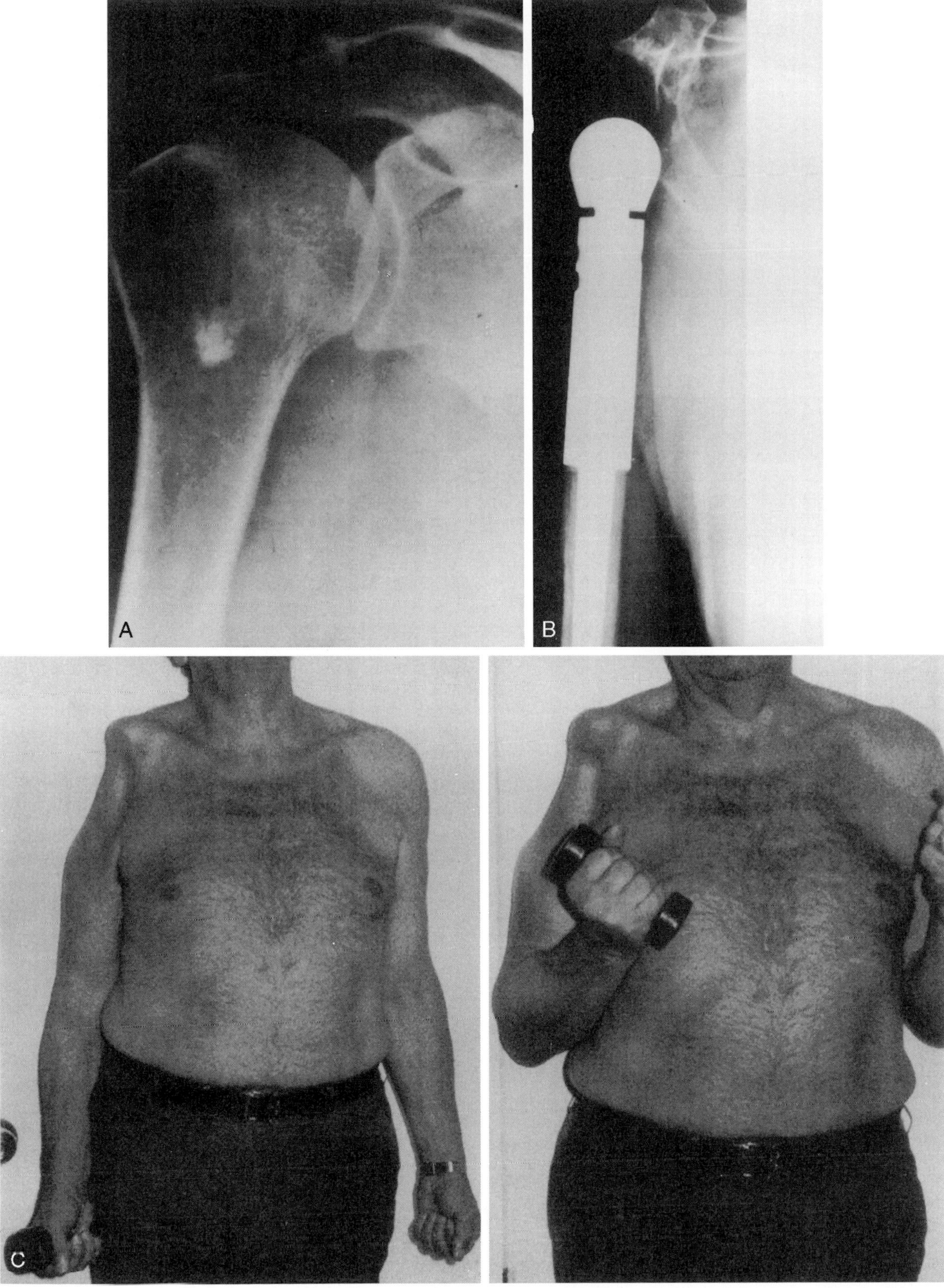

FIGURE 12–15. *A,* Radiograph of a 65-year-old man with a chondrosarcoma involving the proximal humerus. *B,* A proximal humerus prosthesis was employed after an en bloc resection. *C,* The functional result obtained.

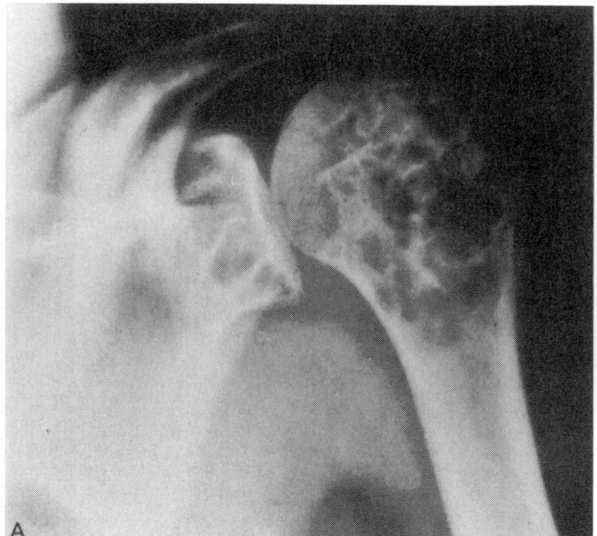

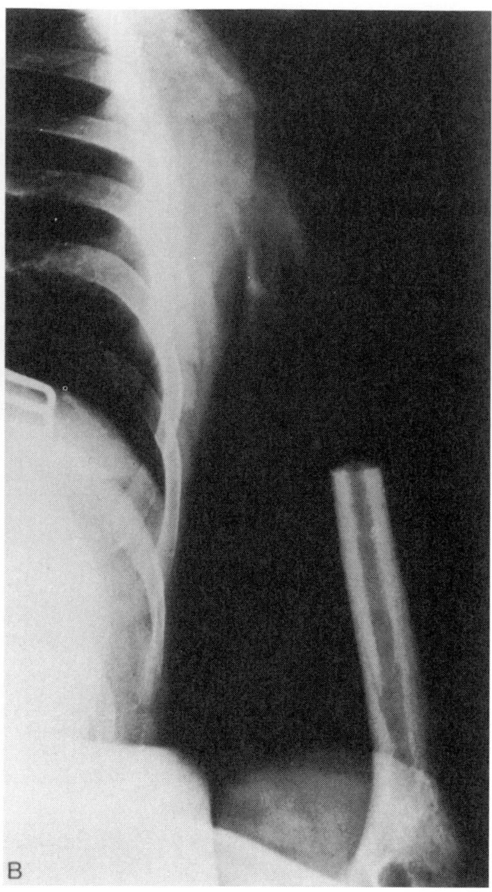

FIGURE 12–16. *A,* Radiograph of a 60-year-old patient with a dedifferentiated chondrosarcoma. *B,* The result after a type VI Tikhoff-Lindberg resection.

operation.[34] Up until 1976, there were only six additional cases reported in the English literature.[35] In 1977, Marcove and associates[36] reported 17 cases, and in 1985, Malawer and colleagues[37] reported another 10 cases.

The limiting factor in determining resectability is the ability to dissect the neurovascular bundle. If this can be accomplished, the results of this procedure will be comparable to those achieved by forequarter amputation.

The majority of tumor resections of the shoulder girdle in the past decade have been performed for tumors arising in the proximal humerus. Resections of these lesions can be performed with preservation of the scapula. This led Malawer to propose that the Tikhoff-Lindberg operations be divided into six subgroups (Fig. 12–14). This system is based on the anatomic and functional structures removed during surgery. Type I involves an intra-articular proximal humeral resection. Type II entails a partial scapular resection, with preservation of the glenohumeral joint. Type III involves a total scapulectomy. Type IV involves an extra-articular total scapulectomy and humeral head resection. Type V involves resection of the humeral head and glenoid of the scapula. Type VI is a classic Tikhoff-Lindberg resection.

In a personal series of patients operated on from 1978 to 1988, 60 patients underwent resections for tumors arising around the shoulder girdle. The age of the patients ranged from 3 to 82 years. There were 31 males and 29 females in this series.

The histologic types are presented in Table 12–6. Ten patients who underwent type I proximal humeral resection had metastatic disease. The most common histologic type of the metastatic lesions was hypernephroma, which has a predilection for solitary metastasis to the proximal humerus.

A majority of patients underwent type I resection (Table 12–7, Fig. 12–15). Malawer[38] reported a similar distribution in 50 patients undergoing resections. The local recurrence rate was low in this series (three patients).

A variety of reconstruction options exist for those patients undergoing this type of procedure. Endoprosthetic

TABLE 12–7
Distribution of Modified Tikhoff-Lindberg Procedures in 110 Patients

Type	No.	%
I	49	57
II	6	2
III	11	12
IV	10	3
V	20	5
VI	14	21

replacement with either a metal or a ceramic prosthesis is widely used for type I and type V resections. Cadaveric allografts or vascularized bone transfers have been reported.[39–42] Cheng and Gebhardt[43] recently reported on an endoprosthetic replacement following a classic Tikhoff-Lindberg (type VI) resection (Fig. 12–16).

On the basis of the results obtained with these limb salvage procedures, it is the rare individual who requires a forequarter amputation as an initial procedure for tumors arising in the shoulder girdle. The amputative procedure can be reserved for local recurrences and advanced primary lesions.

References

1. Speed-Kellog H: Hemipelvectomy. Ann Surg 95:167–178, 1932.
2. Meester GL, Myerley WH: Traumatic hemipelvectomy: A case report and review of the literature. J Trauma 15:541–542, 1975.
3. Pringle JH: The interpelvic-abdominal amputation: Notes on two cases. Br J Surg 4:283–292, 1932.
4. Gordon-Taylor G: On malignant disease in the region of the hip joint. J R Coll Surg Edinb 5:1–6, 1959.
5. Gordon-Taylor G, Wiles P: Interabdominal (hindquarter) amputation. Br J Surg 22:671–678, 1935.
6. Gordon-Taylor G: The technique and management of the hindquarter amputation. Br J Surg 39.536–547, 1952.
7. Higinbotham NL, Marcove RC, Casson P: Hemipelvectomy: A clinical study of 100 cases with 5 year follow up on 60 patients. Surgery 59:706–718, 1966.
8. Miller TR: Hemipelvectomy in lower extremity tumors. Orthop Clin North Am 8:903–908, 1977.
9. Frey C, Matthews LS, Benjamin H, et al: A new technique for hemipelvectomy. Surg Gynecol Obstet 143:753–758, 1986.
10. Bowden L, Booher RH: Surgical considerations in the treatment of sarcoma of the buttock. Cancer 6:89–93, 1953.
11. Sugarbaker PH, Chretian PH: Hemipelvectomy for buttock tumors utilizing an anterior myocutaneous flap quadriceps femoris muscle. Ann Surg 197:106–116, 1983.
12. Milch H: Partial resection of the ischium. J Bone Joint Surg 17:166–174, 1935.
13. Radley RJ, Liebig CA, Brown JR: Resection of the pelvic bones, the superior and inferior pubiramus, and the ischial tuberosity: A surgical approach. J Bone Joint Surg [Am] 36:855–874, 1959.
14. Enneking WF, Dunham WK: Resection and reconstruction for primary neoplasms involving the innominate bone. J Bone Joint Surg [Am] 60:731–746, 1978.
15. Campanacci M, Capanna R: Pelvic resections: The Rizzoli Institute experience. Orthop Clin North Am 22:65–86, 1991.
16. Healey JH, Lane JM, Marcove RL, et al: Resection and reconstruction of periacetabular malignant and aggressive tumors. In Yamamuro T (ed): New Developments for Limb Salvage in Musculoskeletal Tumors. Tokyo: Springer Verlag, 1989, pp 443–450.
17. Eilber FR, Eckhardt JJ, Grant T: Resection of malignant bone tumors of the pelvis: Evaluation of local recurrence, survival and function. In Enneking WF (ed): Limb Salvage in Musculoskeletal Oncology. New York: Churchill Livingstone, 1987, pp 136–140.
18. Bloom ND: Marlex mesh reconstruction of the pelvis following partial resection of the innominate bone with limb salvage. Am J Surg (in press).
19. Salzer M, Knohr K, Sehera J, et al: Resection and treatment of malignant pelvic bone tumors. In Enneking WF (ed): Limb Salvage in Musculoskeletal Oncology. New York: Churchill Livingstone, 1987, pp 104–111.
20. Shiver JC, Sim FH, Prichard D, et al: Limb salvage for tumors about the pelvic girdle. In Enneking WF (ed): Limb Salvage in Musculoskeletal Oncology. New York: Churchill Livingstone, 1987, pp 112–117.
21. Enneking WF, Menendez LR: Functional evaluation of various reconstructions after periacetabular resection of iliac lesions. In Enneking WF (ed): Limb Salvage in Musculoskeletal Oncology. New York: Churchill Livingstone, 1987, pp 117–138.
22. Capanna R, Guernelli N, Ruggieiri P, et al: Periacetabular pelvic resections. In Enneking WF (ed): Limb Salvage in Musculoskeletal Oncology. New York: Churchill Livingstone, 1987, pp 141–146.
23. Tumeno B, Languepin A, Gerber C: Local resection with limb salvage for the treatment of periacetabular bone tumors: Functional results in nine cases. In Enneking WF (ed): Limb Salvage in Musculoskeletal Oncology. New York: Churchill Livingstone, 1987, pp 147–156.
24. Mutschler N, Bruri C, Kiefer H: Functional results after pelvic resection with endoprosthetic replacement. In Enneking WF (ed): Limb Salvage in Musculoskeletal Oncology. New York: Churchill Livingstone, 1987, pp 156–166.
25. Lune JM, Duone K, Glosser DB, et al: Periacetabular resection for malignant sarcomas. In Enneking WF (ed): Limb Salvage in Musculoskeletal Oncology. New York: Churchill Livingstone, 1987, pp 166–170.
26. Dunham N: Acetabular resections for sarcoma. In Enneking WF (ed): Limb Salvage in Musculoskeletal Oncology. New York: Churchill Livingstone, 1987, pp 170–188.
27. Harrington KD: The use of hemipelvic allografts or autoclaved grafts for reconstruction after wide resections of malignant tumors of the pelvis. J Bone Joint Surg [Am] 74:331–341, 1992.
28. Keevil HF: Ralph Cumming and the interscapulothoracic amputation in 1808. J Bone Joint Surg [Am] 31:318–589, 1949.
29. Berger P: L'Amputation du Member Superieur dans la Contiguite du Trone C (Amputation Interscapulo Thoracique). Paris: Masson, 1887.
30. Littlewood H: Amputations at the shoulder and at the hip. Br Med J 1:381–383, 1922.
31. Pack GT: Major extra articulations for malignant neoplasms of the extremities: Interscapulothoracic amputation, hip joint disarticulation, and interilioabdominal amputation: A report of end results in 228 cases. J Bone Joint Surg [Am] 38:249–262, 1958.
32. Sim FH, Prichard DS, Ivins JC: Forequarter amputation. Orthop Clin North Am 8:921–931, 1977.
33. Bauman PK: Resection of the upper extremity in the region of the shoulder joint. Khirurg Arkg Velyaminoua 30:145–149, 1914.
34. Lindberg BE: Interscapulothoracic resection for malignant tumors of the shoulder joint. J Bone Joint Surg [Am] 10:344–349, 1928.
35. Francis KC, Worcester JN: Radical resection for tumors of the shoulder with preservation of the functional extremity. J Bone Joint Surg [Am] 44:1423–1429, 1962.
36. Marcove RC, Lewis MM, Huvos AG: En bloc upper humeral interscapulothoracic resection: The Tikhoff-Lindberg procedure. Clin Orthop 124:219–228, 1977.
37. Malawer MM, Sugarbaker PH, Zambart M, et al: Tikhoff-Lindberg procedure report of 10 patients and presentation of a modified technique for tumors of the proximal humerus. Surgery 97:518–528, 1985.
38. Malawer MM: Tumors of the shoulder girdle. Orthop Clin North Am 22:7–35, 1991.
39. Bos G, Sim F, Pritchard D, et al: Prosthetic replacement of the proximal humerus. Clin Orthop 224:178–185, 1987.
40. Ross AC, Wilson UN, Scales JF: Endoprosthetic replacement of the proximal humerus. J Bone Joint Surg [Br] 69:656–668, 1983.
41. Sekera J, Ramach W, Pongracz N, et al: Experience with ceramic and metal implants for the proximal humerus in cases of malignant bone tumors. In Enneking WF (ed): Limb Salvage in Musculoskeletal Oncology. New York: Churchill Livingstone, 1987, pp 211–215.
42. Mankin HS, Gebhardt MC: The use of frozen cadaveric allografts in the management of patients with bone tumors of the extremities. Orthop Clin North Am 18:275–291, 1987.
43. Cheng EY, Gebhardt MC: Allograft reconstructions of the shoulder after bone tumor resections. Orthop Clin North Am 22:37–48, 1991.

13

Narayan Sundaresan, M.D. • George Krol, M.D.
James E. O. Hughes, M.D. • Laura Hough, R.N.

Tumors of the Spine

The last decade has witnessed dramatic changes in the approach to tumors of the spine, brought about by several factors. Improvements in surgical approaches to the entire vertebral column have now made it technically feasible to resect tumors involving the spine at all levels, and a clearer understanding of spinal biomechanics has led to the development of a vast array of instrumentation systems that allow reconstruction of the spine following tumor surgery.[1–10] In addition, the widespread availability of magnetic resonance imaging (MRI) and computed tomography (CT) has improved the radiologic diagnosis of spinal tumors and greatly enhanced the surgeon's ability to visualize the tumor in its entirety, plan the proper approach, and assess the results of therapy. Unfortunately, there is a prevailing pessimistic attitude toward the treatment of spinal tumors, in part due to the results obtained with limited decompressive procedures. Although the goal of complete tumor resection is widely accepted as the treatment of choice for benign tumors, it is less accepted that the extent of tumor resection is of major importance in the long-term results for malignant tumors. The concept that surgery serves only to provide tissue diagnosis or palliative neural decompression should be abandoned. More appropriate goals are cancer therapy and spinal stabilization.[11, 12] However, these goals are not tenable in patients with widespread cancer in whom only limited palliation is possible. In patients with primary malignancies of the spine or with solitary metastases from biologically indolent tumors, the goal of surgery should be complete resection.[13–15] Frequently, when a tumor involves more than one element of the spine, combined anterior-posterior approaches or staged procedures are necessary.[16–18] In addition, adjuvant treatment (local irradiation) or systemic therapy to eradicate metastases may be recommended.[19–21] The integration of these approaches requires the collaboration of several disciplines. Close collaboration among the involved specialists will do much to reduce morbidity from therapy.

INCIDENCE

Primary tumors of the spine are extremely rare.[22–25] According to the American Cancer Society, approximately 2000 new cases of bone cancer and 6000 cases of soft part sarcomas are diagnosed each year.[26] Of these, approximately 5% involve the spine. Some bone tumors have a special predilection for the vertebral column (e.g., osteoblastoma); others (chordoma) occur exclusively in the spine.

Although primary tumors are relatively uncommon, metastases to the spine are a common feature of many solid tumors.[27–38] Approximately 1.1 million new cases of cancer are diagnosed annually in the United States, and 40% to 50% of those patients die of uncontrolled metastatic disease. Autopsy studies show that 5% to 30% of all cancer patients have metastases to the spine, 20% of which are symptomatic.[35, 39, 40–44] In most series, four primary sites account for more than two thirds of all metastases to the spine: breast, lung, hematopoietic system, and prostate.[29, 31, 32, 45–49] The propensity for some tumors to metastasize preferentially to the spine and skeletal system is called osteotropism. A clear understanding of this phenomenon may one day allow us to prevent the development of bone metastases.

PATHOGENESIS

In patients with cancer, involvement of the spine results from several different mechanisms.[50–53] In the majority, the tumor is disseminated by the vascular system to the vertebral body. Progressive replacement of the red marrow results in the spread of tumor toward the epidural space. Although, radiologically, the pedicle represents the initial site of involvement, experimental data suggest that tumor emboli spread to the vertebral body through the basivertebral plexus.[54, 55]

In addition, the spine may be directly invaded by the spread of malignancies arising in the paraspinal region. The retroperitoneum and posterior mediastinum are frequent sites of origin of tumors that encroach on the spine by destruction of the vertebral column, as seen in sarcomas. Tumors may also spread through the intervertebral foramina without bone destruction, a feature commonly seen with dumbbell neurogenic tumors and lymphomas. Finally, a tumor may extend along the perineurium of the intervertebral nerves directly through the dura to invade the spinal cord.

Several animal models of experimental neoplastic cord compression have been developed.[53, 54, 56–59] These studies indicate that the primary process may be one of compression of the venous plexus, resulting in progressive vasogenic edema, hemorrhage, loss of myelin, and ischemia.[60] Unfortunately, there is little direct correlation between the extent of neural injury and the histologic findings. The vasogenic edema is accompanied by an increase in the synthesis of prostaglandin E_2, and in at least one animal model, the effects of vasogenic edema could be reversed by nonsteroidal anti-inflammatory agents such as indomethacin.[43, 61]

Compression of the spinal cord may arise from a variety of mechanisms: expansion of the periosteum or cortex, with resulting pain; pathologic compression fractures; instability of the spine; and compression or invasion of the nerve roots and dural sac. In addition, neurologic symptoms and pain may result from indirectly mediated tumoral factors such as hypercalcemia.[62]

CLINICAL PRESENTATION

Pain is the most common initial complaint of patients presenting with a suspected spinal tumor.[34, 63–67] Unfortunately, pain symptoms in the initial stages are relatively nonspecific and cannot easily be differentiated from disc disease. By careful questioning, it is sometimes possible to differentiate mechanical causes such as disc disease and spondyloarthritis from tumor-related pain. Mechanical pain is generally intensified by activity and relieved by bed rest, whereas nonmechanical pain is constant and unremitting; it is not relieved by rest and is intensified at night. Spinal column tumors may present with constant focal, radicular, or referred pain. Focal pain is due to local tumor growth, which causes expansion of the vertebral body cortex and distortion of the overlying periosteum. This may progress to vertebral collapse, invasion of paravertebral soft tissues, spinal instability, or cord compression, all of which may result in intensification of local pain. Specific segment pain may be reproduced by pressure or percussion over the involved region. Radicular pain results from irritation or compression of the dural sac or nerve roots, indicating extrinsic compression from a tumor mass with paravertebral extension or edema. Radicular pain is common in lesions of the cervical or lumbar segments; in the thoracic region, radicular pain presents as a circumferential girdle of bandlike dysesthesia and paresthesia. Finally, spinal deformity resulting from collapse or kyphoscoliosis may result in paraspinal muscular spasms and pain.

A careful review of the patient's medical history and a thorough neurologic examination often reveal the anatomic level of spinal involvement. Patients with compressive lesions of the spinal cord generally present with paraparesis; spasticity; early bowel and bladder dysfunction; abnormal reflexes, including hyperreflexia; a sensory level to pain and temperature; and abnormal plantar responses. Conus medullaris tumors are associated with urinary urgency, hesitancy, constipation, and impotence. Autonomic dysfunction is a late manifestation of compression of the spinal cord. If the correct diagnosis is not made at this stage, the clinical syndrome may evolve into complete paralysis, which is often irreversible.

In young patients, torticollis is a common presenting feature of cervical spine tumors. Painful scoliosis resulting from nerve root irritation and muscle spasm may result from an osteoid osteoma or osteoblastoma of the spine.[68–70] In such cases, the tumor generally lies within the concavity of the scoliotic curve. A kyphotic disfigurement (gibbus) may be the result of a vertebral collapse. Outward cutaneous manifestations (café-au-lait spots) associated with intraspinal neoplasms may indicate a neurofibroma. Birthmarks or nevi suggest spinal dysraphism. The physical examination should include a rectal examination to rule out a presacral tumor or a malignancy involving the prostate.

Anemia, an elevated sedimentation rate, and abnormalities of bone or liver enzymes should be noted. In all patients presenting with pathologic compression fractures of the spine, serum protein electrophoresis (SPE) and immunoelectrophoresis (IEP) should be requested to rule out myeloma. Urine electrophoresis may be the only abnormality seen in 20% of patients with multiple myeloma. Prostate-specific antigen (PSA), carcinoembryonic antigen (CEA), serum lactate dehydrogenase (LDH), and CA 125 antigen levels are tumor markers for various malignancies. Vanillic acid derivatives are often seen in the urine of children with neuroblastoma.

Two clinical features are considered in evaluating the potential malignancy of a lesion in the spine: age and location. More than 75% of lesions located in the vertebral body are malignant, whereas only one third of lesions in the posterior elements are malignant. More than two thirds of all lesions seen in children under 18 are benign; this figure is reversed in adults.

RADIOLOGY

The majority of patients with spinal tumors are evaluated because of an evolving neurologic deficit. Accurate assessment of the spinal segments involved, including staging studies to determine the extent of systemic metastases, are required. Over the past 5 years, there has been extraordinary progress in the imaging of the spine. It is now necessary to integrate information from a variety of studies, including plain radiographs, radiographic and radionuclide imaging, CT, myelography, and MRI.

In the radiographic evaluation, several questions are relevant. What kind of abnormality is present? If initial radiographic evaluation is negative or nonspecific, what additional studies should be performed? What is the differential diagnosis? What is the extent of local and systemic involvement?

Radiographic evaluation requires technically adequate images. Most tumors of the spine arise from the medullary spaces of the bone, and subtle changes in bone density are difficult to detect. The vertebral body is composed of approximately 95% trabecular bone and 5% cortical bone, whereas the posterior elements are largely cortical. Experimental studies have shown that 30% to 50% of the medullary space must be destroyed before radiographic changes are visible. In osteopenic patients, even greater trabecular destruction may be necessary. Signs of tumor involvement include focal lytic destruction or osteopenia, vertebral collapse, destruction of the pedicle ("winking owl" sign), and malalignment of the spine. Certain tumors, such as lymphoma and Ewing's sarcoma, are difficult to detect on plain radiography because the pattern of bone destruction is "permeative" rather than lytic. In such patients, alteration of the trabecular pattern may be the only visible sign.

Attention should also be given to the margin between the bone and the tumor. A slowly growing benign lesion usually produces a well-demarcated rim of marginal sclerosis, enlargement of a neural foramen, or scalloping of the posterior edge of the body. In lesions with a faster growth rate, the margin may be discrete, without any reaction ("punched out"). In more rapidly growing, high-grade tumors, numerous areas of bone rarefaction with intervening residual bone may be seen, or innumerable minuscule slitlike areas of bone destruction with no margin may be encountered.

Location in the spinal axis is an important consideration in the differential diagnosis. For example, the sacrum is the most common site for chordoma and other tumors such as giant cell tumors and Ewing's sarcoma. The portion of the vertebra from which the lesion arises is also important: osteoblastoma, osteoid osteoma, and aneurysmal bone cysts predominate in the posterior elements, whereas metastatic lesions frequently involve the pedicle or the junction of the pedicle and the vertebral body. Conversely, the majority of malignant primary tumors, such as osteosarcoma, giant cell tumors, and lymphoma, originate within the vertebral body.

In patients presenting with pain and nondiagnostic plain films, radionuclide bone scanning with technetium-labeled phosphate analogues provides a significant improvement in sensitivity over plain radiographs.[71] Exceptions to this include multiple myeloma, chordoma, and histiocytosis X, as well as rapidly growing anaplastic tumors. In addition, radionuclide bone scans may help in the differential diagnosis, since the majority of metastatic lesions are multifocal. Technetium scans are sensitive to increases in osteoid formation and may detect lesions as small as 2 mm. However, they are nonspecific, since increased uptake is seen in patients with fractures, infection, or soft tissue inflammation.[72] In patients in whom a malignancy is only suspected, the bone scan may suggest an accessible site for biopsy. In patients with solitary abnormalities, false-positive bone scans are seen in up to one third of cases.[73]

The introduction of MRI has revolutionized the imaging of bone tumors.[74–78] The major advantages of MRI are its unsurpassed contrast resolution and its ability to image directly in any plane. MR images use a reflection of hydrogen density and the response of mobile hydrogen protons to various sequences of radiofrequency stimulation. The response varies with tissue density, depending on the biophysical environment of the protons and the relaxation time constants T1 and T2. Signal intensities depend not only on hydrogen density but also on the pulse sequence used. Cortical bone, ligaments, tendons, and fibrocartilage have very little signal (black); soft tissue, fat, and marrow have a strong signal intensity. MRI of spinal tumors should include T1- and T2-weighted sequences. Most tumors have a low signal in the T1-weighted image, and these provide the best contrast with the high signal of marrow and fat. T2-weighted images provide the best contrast between the high signal of tumor and the low signal of cortical bone, muscle, and fibrous structures. Several studies have suggested that MRI may be superior to CT. CT technology has stabilized, but MR technology continues to improve.

Gadolinium has been used to provide vascular-enhanced MR images but has not improved the detection of spinal tumors. It has been suggested that contrast MRI is a reliable indicator of tumor response to therapy.

CT is indicated to determine bony architecture and soft tissue extension in the paraspinal tissues and the epidural space. The major advantages of CT are its wide availability and relative low cost in comparison with MRI. Adequate imaging requires image manipulation using appropriate window width and levels. CT scans are more reliable than MRI in demonstrating the cortical outlines of bone and calcification. CT allows accurate assessment of needle placement during biopsies. In patients with soft tissue components, intravenous contrast may be needed to define tumor extension, distinguish tumor from residual fibrosis, and delineate major blood vessels.

Evaluation of the preoperative CT images with bone windows allows assessment of pedicle width, vertebral body diameters, and other measurements, resulting in proper selection of spinal implants. In patients who have undergone instrumentation, periodic re-evaluation for tumor recurrence may require CT myelography. To minimize the artifacts resulting from instrumentation, the use of CT- and MRI-compatible implants (titanium) is recommended.

Myelography, especially in conjunction with CT, has been the gold standard for evaluation of the subarachnoid space in patients with spinal tumors, but it has largely been supplanted by MRI. In centers where "emergency" MRI studies are not available, myelography is often used to evaluate the entire spinal axis in patients with suspected cord compression. It is not uncommon for patients to deteriorate after lumbar puncture; therefore, all patients with epidural tumors should be treated with an intravenous bolus of dexamethasone (Decadron, 20 to 100 mg) after the myelographic procedure.

In patients with hypervascular tumors, spinal angiography is indicated to demonstrate the location of critical arteries, such as the artery of Adamkiewicz. A variety of therapeutic agents are currently used for preoperative embolization. The most popular is polyvinyl alcohol foam (Ivalon) in particles ranging in size from 150 to 500 μm in diameter. For effective embolization, the smallest-sized particle should be used. Absolute alcohol can also be used as a sclerosing agent for permanent tumor necrosis before surgery. Patients with metastases from kidney, thyroid, and sarcoma should be embolized preoperatively. Reducing intraoperative blood loss has a major impact not only on morbidity but also on the extent of tumor resection that is feasible. Of the primary spinal tumors, notoriously vascular lesions include giant cell tumors, hemangiomas, and aneurysmal bone cysts; these should be embolized as well.

BIOPSY

In patients with malignant bone tumors, it is common to perform a needle biopsy prior to radical surgery. The hazards of biopsy in musculoskeletal tumors must be carefully considered, since poorly planned biopsies increase the local risk of recurrence by tumor dissemination along fascial planes and the biopsy tract.[79] Biopsies are divided into three different categories: needle biopsy, open incisional biopsy, and excisional biopsy.[9, 80, 81] For tumors limited to the posterior elements, such as osteoblastoma or aneurysmal bone cysts, an excisional biopsy is both diagnostic and therapeutic.

The most common indication for biopsy is the confirmation of suspected metastatic disease. It is particularly useful in establishing the diagnosis of round cell tumors (such as Ewing's sarcoma or lymphoma), for which the initial treatment is nonsurgical. In other primary malignant tumors, such as osteosarcoma, for which delayed definitive surgery is indicated, needle biopsy may provide the diagnosis. Finally, biopsy is indicated to document recurrence.

Most needle biopsies are performed under fluoroscopic or CT control. Fluoroscopy is faster and easier to perform than CT-guided biopsy. For smaller, more difficult lesions in the thoracic spine, CT guidance offers greater safety. Review of all available studies, including CT scans and radionuclide scans, is indicated to determine the site of the lesion, choice of needle, and route of approach. Most biopsies are performed under local anesthesia, usually using a localizing 22-gauge needle followed by a larger needle once the target is reached. A careful history to rule out bleeding tendency or ingestion of nonsteroidal anti-inflammatory drugs is obtained, and clotting parameters are checked prior to biopsy.

The choice of the needle depends on the type of lesion (osteoblastic, osteolytic, or mixed), the location (bony or soft tissue), and the amount of tissue needed for diagnosis. A trephine-type needle may be required if an intact cortex is to be perforated. Sufficient tissue should be obtained to provide the pathologist material for cultures, immunoperoxidase studies, and electron microscopy. Close cooperation among the radiologist, clinician, and pathologist is necessary to confirm the adequacy of the tissue and to perform smear preparations of aspirates.

Complications include pain, bleeding, and pneumothorax. However, the most frequent adverse outcome is a nondiagnostic biopsy. This is particularly true of densely blastic lesions, necrotic tumors, or vascular lesions, which may yield insufficient tissue for diagnosis. In experienced hands, the accuracy rate ranges from 80% to 90%. However, in our experience, needle biopsy of the spine fails to provide the correct diagnosis in 25% of patients.

If an open incisional biopsy is performed, the incision must be planned so that it can be excised at a definitive operation. Meticulous surgical techniques and homeostasis are essential. Postoperative hematomas carry the potential to disseminate tumor cells along fascial planes. Bone windows should be small and planned so that pathologic fractures do not result; they are packed with Gelfoam and bone wax.

PRIMARY TUMORS

Primary tumors are generally classified based on the cell of origin; in this section, the most common tumors arising in the spine are considered.

Osteoid Osteoma and Osteoblastoma

The most common tumors of osteoblastic origin are osteoid osteoma and osteoblastoma (Fig. 13–1). These benign lesions have a special propensity for the spine and are differentiated mainly by size.[69] Twenty-five percent of osteoid osteomas and 40% of osteoblastomas occur in the spine, where they tend to involve the posterior elements such as the facet or pedicle. Patients present predominantly with pain, which may be noticeable at night. Traditionally, the pain has been thought to be responsive to aspirin; although this is considered a pathognomonic feature, exceptions are relatively common. Plain radiography may miss the tumor, but the radionuclide bone scan provides the correct diagnosis because of the intensity of uptake and can also be used to localize the tumor during surgery.

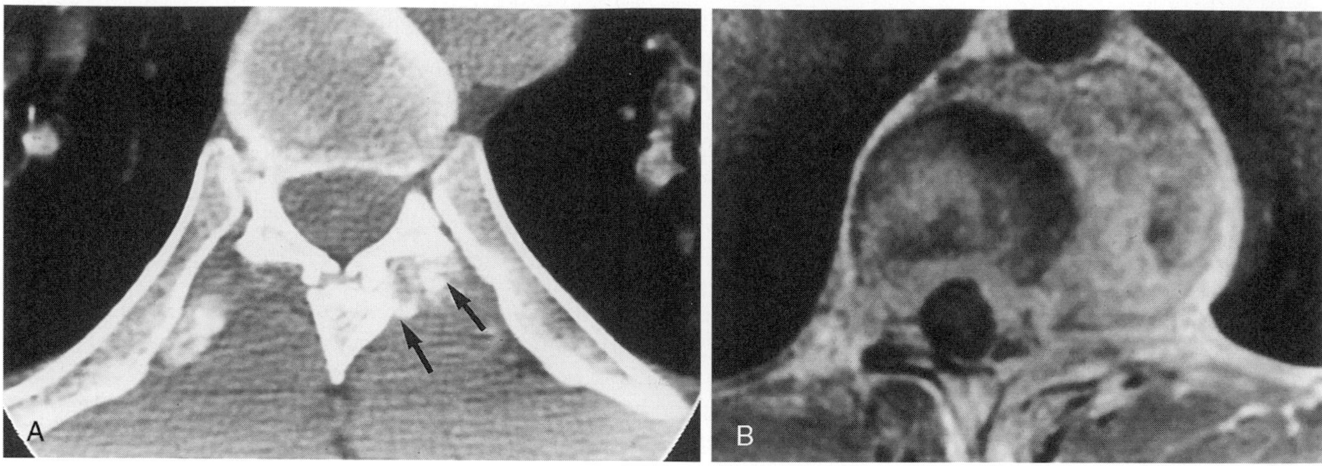

FIGURE 13–1. Osteoblastoma. *A,* A 33-year-old man with progressive back pain. There is sclerotic change of the lamina (arrows), characteristic of this neoplasm. *B,* Malignant osteoblastoma. There is a large paravertebral soft tissue component with intracanal extension.

Osteoblastomas are larger, are apparent on plain radiographs, and frequently have soft tissue extension or cross apophyseal joints. Approximately half of patients present with painful scoliosis, which resolves when the tumor is removed.[68, 70]

Complete surgical excision is the treatment of choice. In benign lesions, this may be achieved by curettage and packing the resected area with bone. A small number of osteoblastomas, especially those that are larger or locally invasive, may behave aggressively like low-grade sarcomas. Thus, careful evaluation of the specimen by an experienced bone pathologist is mandatory, and the resection should be extensive enough to involve normal bone.

A rare form of tumor may present as an enostosis (osteochondroma). These may show calcification and be a component of the syndrome of multiple osteocartilaginous enostosis. In patients with multiple exostoses, the major complication—apart from cord compression—is the development of malignant transformation.[82, 83] This generally involves the cartilaginous component, which becomes chondrosarcoma in 5% to 25% of patients.

Vascular Tumors

The most common vascular tumor is a hemangioma, which may be seen on plain radiography. The classic vertical striations produced by abnormally thickened trabeculae of bone should pose no diagnostic difficulty. On occasion, patients present with pain, which may be site specific or diffuse and poorly localized. Exceptionally, patients present with neurologic deficits. Neurologic deficits can result from bone expansion, soft tissue or epidural extension of the tumor, or pathologic compression fractures (Fig. 13–2).

In the past, vascular tumors were treated by decompressive laminectomy and postoperative irradiation because their profuse vascularity often precluded curative resection. Currently, however, with the widespread availability of angiography and presurgical embolization, complete removal of the tumor can be safely accomplished. Although the decision to perform surgery on symptomatic patients is relatively easy, it is difficult to determine whether patients with only vague pain will benefit from operation. In a recent review from the Mayo Clinic, vertebral hemangiomas were discovered incidentally in 35 patients; pain was the presenting complaint in 13 patients, and 11 were treated for neurologic deficits.[84] Progression to neurologic symptoms was found in only two cases. No recurrence was noted among patients who had subtotal excision plus radiotherapy of 2600 to 4500 cGy. The authors recommend annual radiologic and neurologic examination for patients with hemangiomas associated with pain, especially young females with thoracic lesions. They recommend radiotherapy or embolization as an effective therapeutic alternative for patients with medically refractory pain.

A similar vascular lesion is the aneurysmal bone cyst; this is defined as a tumorlike lesion of bone consisting of an arteriovenous fistula that creates, via hemodynamic forces, a reactive bone lesion.[22] Approximately 80% of aneurysmal bone cysts occur in patients under the age of 20. These tumors constitute 6% of all bone lesions and predominate in the axial skeleton and spinal column. The major radiographic feature is that of an expanding lesion without sclerotic borders. Aneurysmal bone cysts predominate in the posterior elements and generally expand the contour of the vertebra. CT may show multiple fluid levels resulting from hemorrhage, and MRI may reveal a vascular lesion of the spine (Fig. 13–3).

Histologically, it is important to recognize that secondary aneurysmal bone cysts may be seen in conjunction with other tumors, such as osteoblastoma, giant cell tumor, chondroblastoma, or fibrous dysplasia.[85] Typically, aneurysmal bone cysts exhibit numerous cavernous spaces that usually lack an endothelial lining. The walls of these spaces consist of fibrous connective tissue mixed with immature

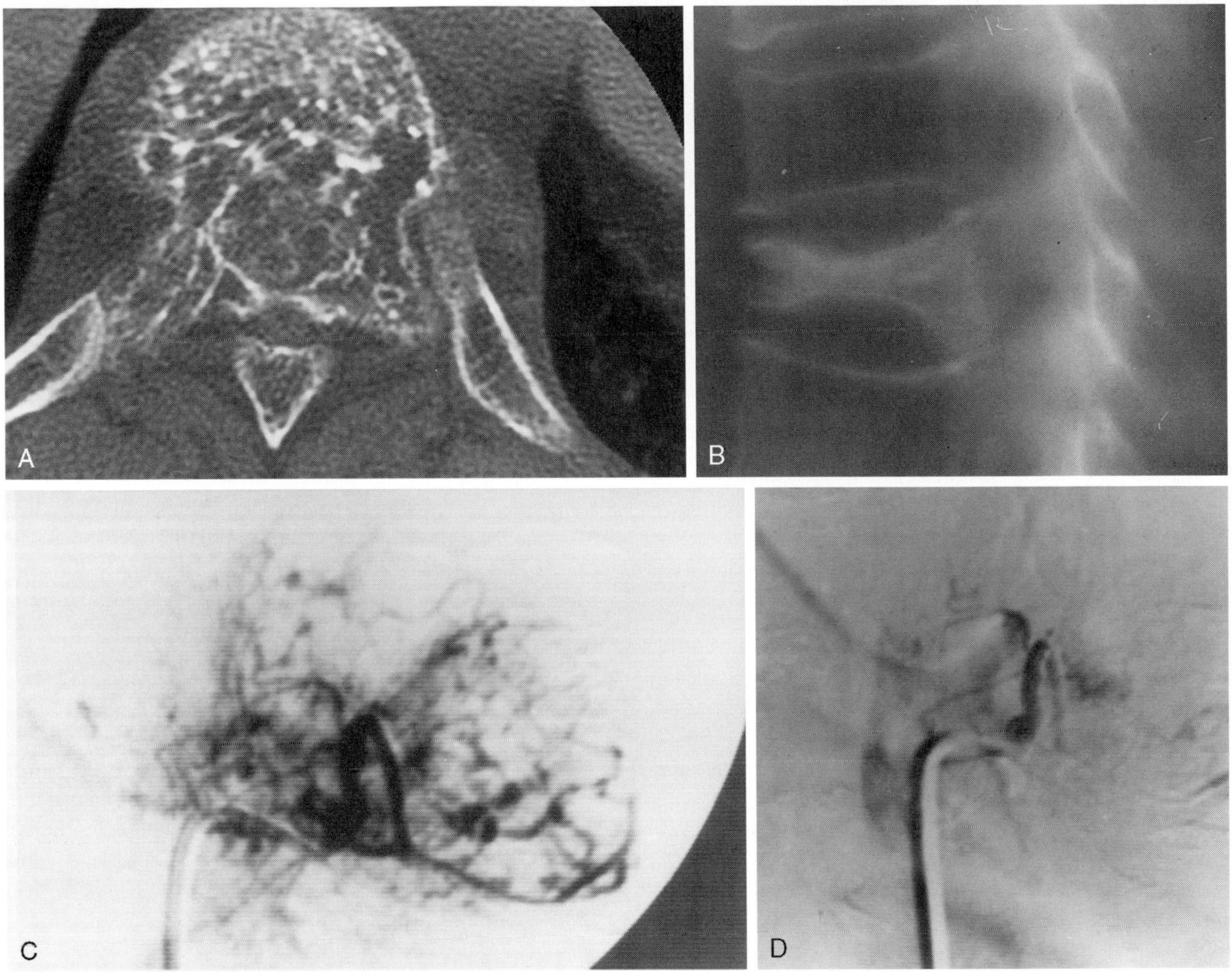

FIGURE 13–2. Lower thoracic hemangioma. *A,* CT scan showing coarsened trabecular pattern. *B,* Conventional tomogram in the lateral plane revealing almost total collapse and patchy sclerosis of vertebral body. Although uncomplicated hemangioma may show characteristic vertical striations on radiographs, a reliable differentiation from malignant tumor in case of collapse is not possible. *C,* Preoperative spinal angiogram demonstrating prominent vascularity of the tumor. *D,* There is significant decrease in perfusion after particular embolization of the tumor.

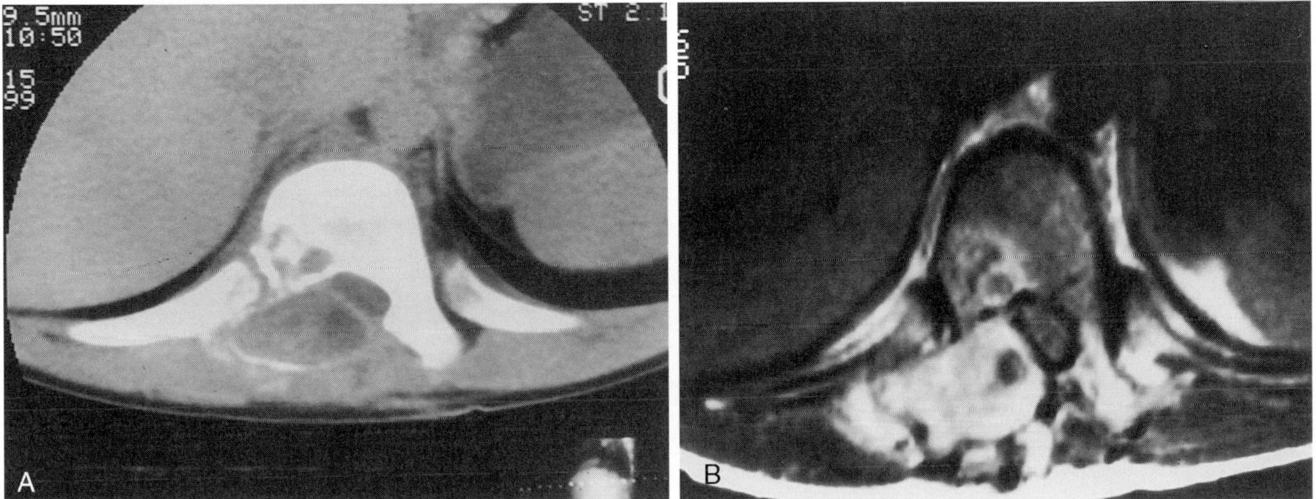

FIGURE 13–3. Aneurysmal bone cyst in a 10-year-old girl. *A,* Axial CT section through lower thoracic spine. There is extensive destruction of T-12 vertebra associated with soft tissue mass. Expansion of the bone with preservation of fragments is characteristic of these lesions. *B,* Corresponding axial MR image showing intracanal extension of the mass with compression of the spinal cord.

bone. The lesion itself is characterized by a rich, honeycombed network of small or large, distended, thin-walled, blood-containing spaces, with hemosiderin-laden macrophages and multinucleate giant cells in the septa lining the blood channels. Occasionally, a solid variant of aneurysmal bone cyst with predominant spindle cell proliferation and mitotic figures may be seen; it is important to distinguish this from other spindle cell neoplasms.

A combination of curettage and bone grafting may be successful in eradicating the lesion. However, with incomplete resections, recurrences in the range of 20% to 30% may be expected. The high incidence of local recurrence following curettage indicates unsuccessful treatment at the time of surgery. These lesions can be successfully eradicated by presurgical embolization followed by resection.

Giant Cell Tumors

Giant cell tumors constitute 5% of all primary bone tumors and are histologically characterized by a vascular spindle cell stroma in addition to numerous multinucleated giant cells. The majority occur in skeletally mature patients. Although more than three quarters of giant cell tumors occur in the articular end of a long bone, they are occasionally seen in the vertebrae. In the vertebrae, giant cells involve the body, in contrast to aneurysmal bone cysts, which predominate in the posterior elements.[86, 87]

Radiographically, giant cell tumors are characterized by a lytic, eccentric bone destruction exhibiting a "soap-bubble" effect (Fig. 13–4). Unfortunately, the radiographic features of giant cells are completely consistent with those of other malignant tumors. The majority of these tumors are highly vascular, and preoperative angiography with

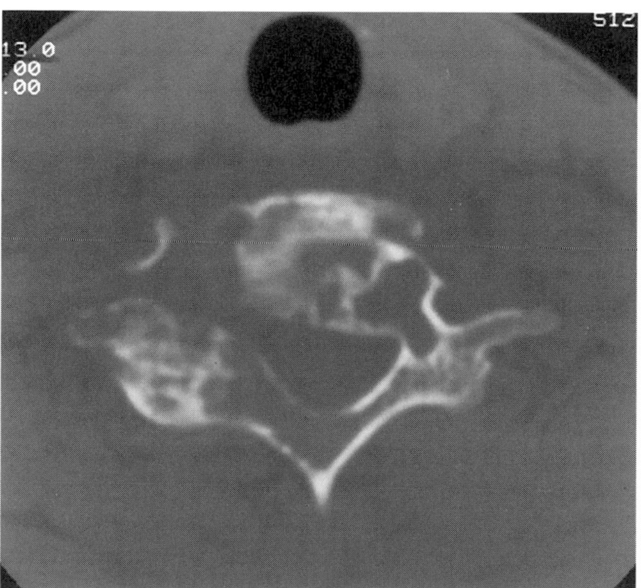

FIGURE 13–4. Destructive lesion of C-6, subsequently diagnosed as a giant cell tumor. Although a "soap-bubble" appearance is suggestive of this neoplasm, differentiation from other malignancies is not possible.

embolization is indicated. Histologically, these tumors are classified into three different grades, which indicate their malignant potential; unfortunately, making a distinction between intermediate- and high-grade tumors may be difficult. In general, as the proliferative potential of a giant cell tumor increases, the actual number of giant cells in the specimen diminishes.

The ideal treatment for giant cell tumors of the spine is initial complete removal. Although cryosurgery, using liquid nitrogen, is useful in minimizing the risk of local recurrence in extraspinal lesions, its use is contraindicated in spinal tumors because of the possibility of neural injury. Because many of these tumors are locally invasive, it was customary to recommend postoperative radiotherapy following incomplete resection; however, this has been associated with a high incidence of malignant transformation.[88] The natural history of giant cell tumors in the spine suggests that vertebral lesions have a more favorable prognosis than tumors arising from the appendicular skeleton. Thus, we do not favor the use of radiation following incomplete resection.

Eosinophilic Granuloma

Eosinophilic granuloma is a benign, self-limited condition that produces focal destruction of bone.[89] Solitary eosinophilic granuloma is a disease of children and young adults. Typically, the findings consist of a radiolucent oval area of bone destruction that is well demarcated, without peripheral sclerosis. In the spine, the classic sign in children and young adults is one of vertebral collapse, producing the classic "vertebra plana" (Fig. 13–5).[90, 91] If a wedged vertebral collapse is noted in a child or adolescent, a skeletal survey is indicated to discover the presence of multifocal lesions. Spinal cord compression may result from vertebral collapse and segmental kyphosis. This disease is part of the generalized syndrome complex termed "histiocytosis X," or Langerhans cell granulomatosis. The diagnosis is generally established by biopsy. Histologic evaluation often reveals hemorrhagic and cystic tissue with clusters of mononuclear histiocytes, although the basic proliferating cell is the Langerhans cell. Ultrastructural studies reveal rodlike or tennis racket–shaped cytoplasmic inclusions called Langerhans' or Birbeck granules, which are normally absent in histiocytes.[22]

The clinical syndrome of eosinophilic granuloma fluctuates considerably and is characterized by both spontaneous regression and occasional reactivation. Partial intralesional curettage, chemotherapy, and low-dose radiation have been suggested for lesions involving the spine. For multifocal lesions, systemic chemotherapy with methotrexate and vinblastine has been recommended.

Multiple Myeloma and Plasmacytoma

Multiple myeloma is the major malignancy of plasma cells. Osteolytic bone destruction or diffuse osteoporosis

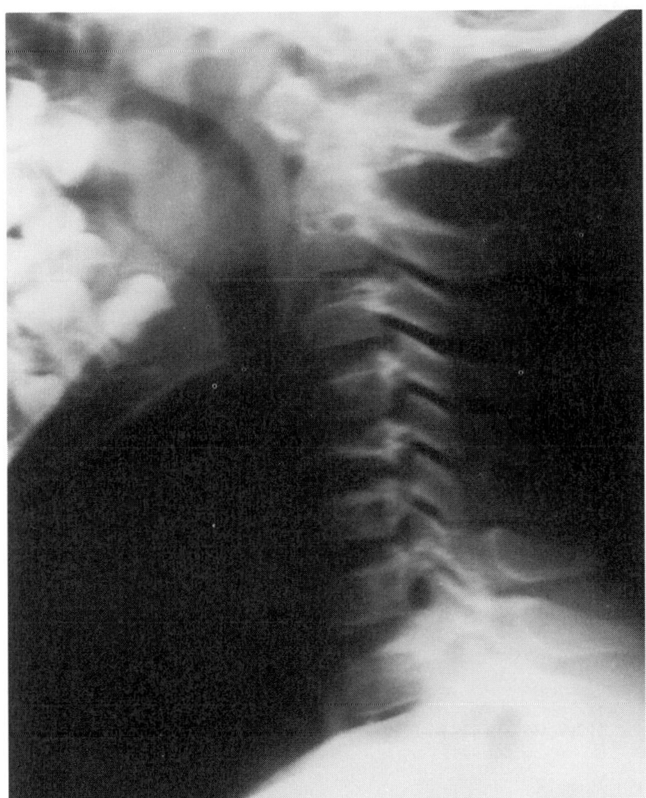

FIGURE 13–5. Eosinophilic granuloma in a 5-year-old boy with a history of neck pain. There is almost complete collapse of the C-5 vertebral body. The child was treated successfully with irradiation after the diagnosis was made. (Courtesy of Dr. R. Marcove, Department of Orthopedic Surgery, Memorial Sloan-Kettering Cancer Center, New York, New York.)

with or without fractures distinguishes myeloma from related lymphoid malignancies. Multiple myeloma has an annual incidence of 2 to 3 in 100,000 in the general population, and patients present with a variable spectrum of symptoms and at different stages of disease development. Clinically, the disease is characterized by malignant plasma cells in the bone marrow and monoclonal immunoglobulins in the serum or urine or both in 99% of patients. In approximately 5% of patients, the disease manifests as a solitary plasmacytoma of bone, a frequent site of which is the vertebral column.[92–95]

Although most plasmacytomas represent a forme fruste of myeloma, in some cases the disease may remain truly localized, with patients achieving long-term disease-free survival from local radiation alone.[96] In general, patients with solitary plasmacytoma are younger and have greater male predominance, and only two thirds show evidence of a secreting paraprotein. The median survival in patients with multiple myeloma is 28 months, whereas the median survival of patients with solitary plasmacytoma is greater than 60 months. In addition, if a paraprotein is secreted, the quantitative levels are generally lower and disappear after local treatment. Bone marrow aspirates show less than 5% of plasma cells, and the majority of patients generally have uninvolved immunoglobulins.

Solitary plasmacytoma or myeloma frequently presents with spinal cord compression (Fig. 13–6). Serum protein electrophoresis and immunoelectrophoresis should be performed in all cases of pathologic compression fractures of the spine in which an obvious primary malignancy is not evident. Decompression of the spinal cord is frequently required. If possible, complete tumor resection should be attempted and the spine stabilized. Since patients with solitary plasmacytoma have an expected median survival of more than 5 years, bone grafts may be used to reconstruct the spine instead of methyl methacrylate. Following surgery, most oncologists prefer to use postoperative radiotherapy for local control. However, if bone grafts have been used for stabilization, early irradiation may result in nonunion. We recommend that radiotherapy be delayed for 3 to 6 months to allow a solid bony fusion.

A major rationale for surgery is the provision of stability.[82] A substantial proportion of patients with clinically obvious myeloma experience progressive pain and disability from segmental instability after irradiation. Careful serial radiographic evaluation should allow this diagnosis to be made so that spine stabilization can be performed. Prophylactic stabilization is indicated in patients with impending fractures as well. In our view, the role of stabilization in myeloma has been understated in the literature and deserves considerable emphasis.

In patients who achieve complete clinical remission, all paraproteins in the serum and urine should disappear. The persistence of myeloma protein after irradiation may identify patients who are at high risk for early progression. However, even in the presence of persistent myeloma protein, 15% of patients remain free of disease for more than 10 years. Thus, it may be prudent to withhold systemic therapy in younger patients who achieve complete remission with radiation alone. However, elderly patients presenting with pathologic fractures, as well as those discovered to have disseminated disease, may require more vigorous therapy.

At present, the current standard treatment for myeloma is palliation. Most drug combination therapies consist of melphalan and prednisone but are unable to achieve complete remissions. However, since 1989, new insights have been gained into the biology of myeloma. These have raised hopes for the potential curability of this disease with high-dose chemotherapy and bone marrow transplantation.[97–99]

Chordoma

Chordomas are rare primary tumors of bone that are thought to arise from the notochord. They constitute between 1% and 4% of bone tumors and are traditionally considered slow-growing, locally invasive neoplasms with little tendency to metastasize.[100–102] The actual incidence of these tumors, calculated from demographic data in two

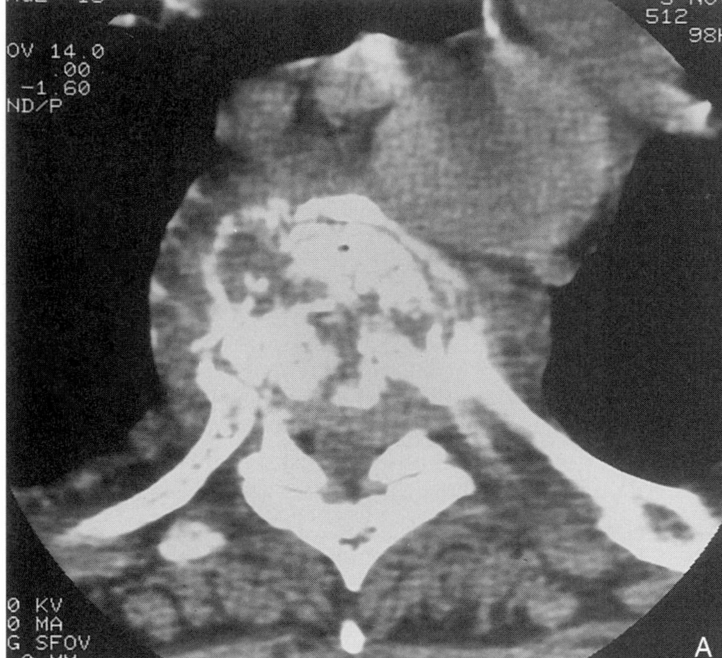

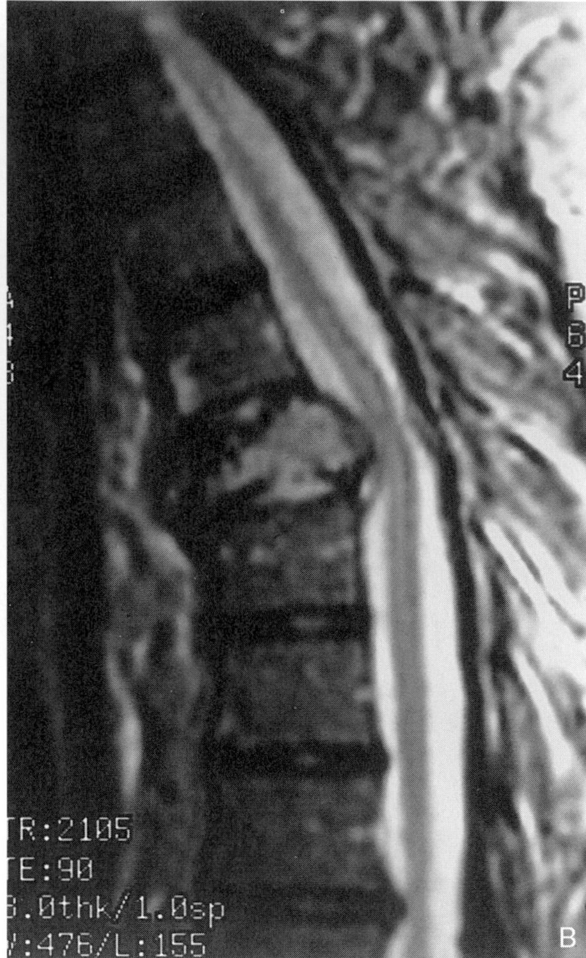

FIGURE 13–6. Axial CT section through T-5 level demonstrates extensive destruction of vertebral body and paraspinal extension *(A)*. There is posterior displacement and angulation of the spinal cord at the level of collapse as shown on sagittal MR image *(B)*.

Scandinavian studies, is approximately 0.5 to 1 case per million population. Thus, this tumor should be included in the differential diagnosis of all tumors of the spinal axis, from the clivus to the sacrum. Approximately 50% arise in the sacrococcygeal region, 35% in the spheno-occipital region, and 15% in the true vertebrae.[22, 25]

Although reported in infancy and childhood, chordoma occurs predominantly in the older population. More than half the cases occur from the fifth through seventh decades of life. In our experience, patients with vertebral lesions are generally younger than those with sacral tumors. Furthermore, although the biologic activity of chordomas varies considerably, more aggressive behavior and "malignant" chordomas are seen only in the younger age groups.

Symptoms are generally of short duration in patients with tumors involving the true vertebrae. Almost all patients present with neck or back pain, often with a radicular component. More than two thirds present with weakness or neurologic deficit; a minority may be symptomatic from the anterolateral soft tissue mass.

Historically, the most consistent feature on plain radiography was the finding of destruction of the vertebra with an associated soft tissue mass. In a 1987 review, Smith and coworkers[103] noted the presence of bone destruction in only 78% of patients; of those showing evidence of bone destruction, approximately half had sclerotic margins and half had ill-defined margins. Although calcification is considered a hallmark of chordomas, this is seen in less than half the cases on plain films. In the true vertebra, the combination of destruction and reactive sclerosis should suggest the possibility of this tumor. In more recent cases, following the advent of MRI, we have been impressed by the relative paucity of plain radiographic findings.

Not surprisingly, CT scans demonstrate both the bony and the soft tissue components of the tumor with ease. More than 90% of sacral tumors have both large presacral and posterior extensions of tumor. These soft tissue extensions are generally located in the midline and involve the lower segments. The soft tissue mass generally has a uniform density, but in 35% of cases, there may be irregular lucencies, indicating necrosis. Although the term "calcification" is frequently used to describe the mottled densities seen in the sacrum, it would be more appropriate to use the term "calcific debris."

Since the spinal theca is close to the epidural space, it was axiomatic in the pre-MRI era to use myelography with water-soluble media to define the epidural extension of tumor. Although the thecal sac ends at the S1-2 level, we routinely used myelography to define the soft tissue extent of the tumor. With the current availability of MRI, however, myelography is rarely indicated. Radionuclide scans show reduced uptake in the majority of patients; on occasion, a specific pattern may be seen that is helpful in the differential diagnosis of sacral tumors. The main portion of the tumor tends to be cold or photopenic, and its peripheral margin is surrounded by a halo of increased activity.

Although experience with MRI is still evolving, it is currently the best tool for evaluating spinal tumors (Fig. 13–7), but it has to be interpreted in conjunction with CT scans. A major advantage of MRI is the ability to display tumor extension in axial, sagittal, and coronal planes. Several authors have suggested that MRI is superior to CT because of the prolonged T1 and T2 times of the tumors. Soft tissue tumor extension is shown especially well with long TR (repetition time) and TE (echo time) (T2-weighted) images, and the presence or absence of a tissue plane between the tumor and the rectum is easily seen. There is a characteristic tendency for the tumor to invade the perineurium of spinal nerves and for recurrences to present as high signal intensities on the T2-weighted images. MR scanning is thus the examination of choice in evaluating for tumor recurrences.

Grossly, chordomas are lobulated, gray, partially translucent, glistening, cystic or solid masses that resemble cartilage tumors or, occasionally, a mucin-producing carcinoma. The consistency varies from firm and focally ossified or calcified tissue to extremely soft, myxoid, gelatinous, or even semifluid material. These tumors appear to be well circumscribed, owing to a pseudocapsule formation within soft tissue. In all sacral tumors, the intact and elevated periosteum anteriorly forms the pseudocapsule of the tumor. In the bone itself, the tumor appears to be multifocal, invading between trabeculae without a clear margin of reactive bone. Microscopically, the tumors are characterized by a distinct, lobular architecture that is formed by the physaliphorous ("soap bubble") cells, with ample vacuolated cytoplasm, as well as by the "signet-ring"–type cells; in between the cells, there are fibrous septa, which are incomplete and densely infiltrated by lymphocytes.

Although the typical chordoma is easy to recognize, this tumor may show a wide range in its histologic appearance and pattern. In addition to the areas showing physaliphorous cells, an occasional tumor may show a typical spindle cell sarcomatous arrangement or a round cell pattern; others may show an epithelial arrangement. Following treatment with radiotherapy, areas of spindle cell sarcoma formation may be seen. On occasion, the chordoma may be transformed into a malignant fibrous histiocytoma. This frequently results after radiotherapy but may also be seen de novo. In difficult cases, immunoperoxidase studies may be helpful in distinguishing chordoma from adenocarcinoma and cartilage tumors. Chordomas are usually positive for keratin and S-100 protein, whereas cartilage tumors are keratin negative and adenocarcinomas are S-100 protein negative.

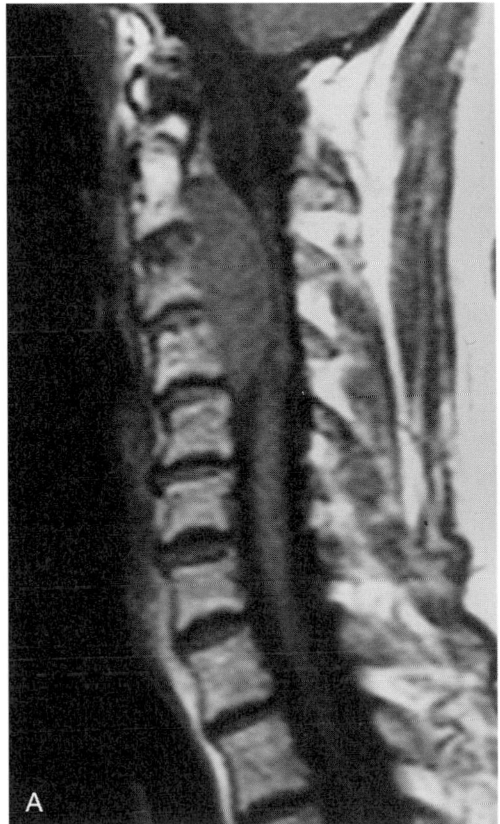

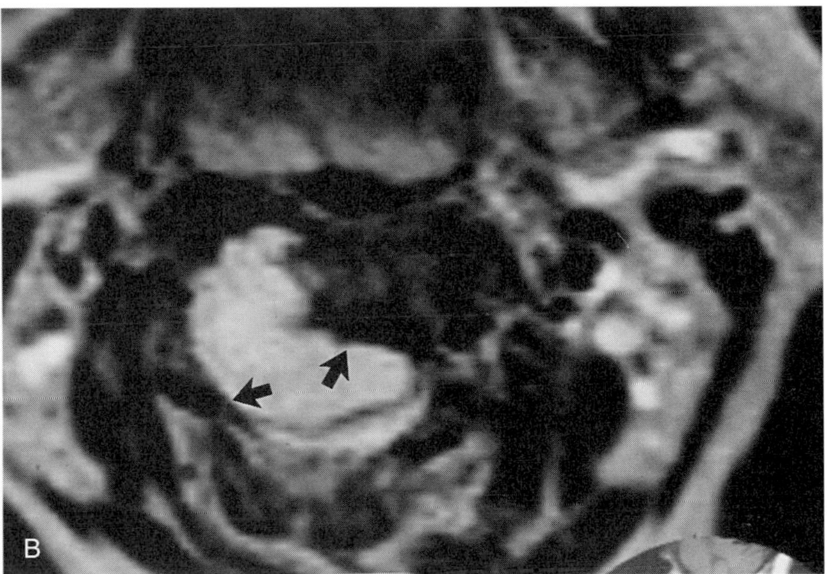

FIGURE 13–7. Cervical chordoma with predominant epidural component in 61-year-old woman. *A,* Sagittal T1-weighted MR image showing fusiform, homogeneous mass in the anterior compartment of the spinal canal with posterior displacement and compression of the spinal cord. *B,* Axial T2-weighted MR image. The tumor is predominantly right-sided, and there is involvement of the vertebral body.

While the tendency of chordomas to recur locally is well known, the propensity for these tumors to metastasize may not be. Between 10% and 30% of chordomas show evidence of distant metastases, predominantly to soft tissues, lymph nodes, lung, bone, liver, and other intra-abdominal viscera.[101–104] Occasionally, widely disseminated metastases to organs, including the heart, pleura, and brain, have been found. In our more recent experience, 30% of patients experienced metastases.[105] Metastatic lesions in chordoma have little impact on overall survival, because death frequently results from complications of local recurrence.

There is general agreement that complete surgical resection is the treatment of choice in chordomas, but this type of surgery may not always be technically feasible in elderly patients with comorbid illnesses.

For chordomas arising in the vertebral body, the true bony and anterolateral soft tissue extent should be defined; generally, the anterolateral soft tissue component is significantly larger than the vertebral component. In the past, laminectomy and tumor resection from a posterior approach were useful in relieving cord compression and reducing pain, but recurrences occurred within the first 2 years in all those who had such limited resections.[102] Although long-term survival has been reported in isolated cases following limited surgery, complete resection frequently requires an anterior approach. With involvement of anterior and posterior elements, complete resection requires removal of the entire vertebra—a procedure called spondylectomy.[13] Reconstruction of the spine with anterior and posterior instrumentation as well as bone grafts may be required. A variety of techniques allow complete excision of the vertebra, including its lateral elements (subtotal spondylectomy), using an anterior approach. Although en bloc tumor removal cannot be achieved, complete resection of all gross disease, including the involved soft tissues and muscles, should be attempted at the initial operation. Our current data suggest that with such aggressive surgery, more than two thirds of patients are disease-free at 5 years.[105]

The value of radiotherapy is controversial. Postoperative radiotherapy is used following biopsy or subtotal resection, but its role following complete resection is not established. In an extensive review of the literature, Cummings and associates[106] found no difference in survival between those who had undergone prior biopsy only and those who had had subtotal resection prior to radiotherapy. Since the growth rate of chordoma tissue is slow, the actual response of the tumor mass to radiation may be difficult to measure. There may be a role for this modality as palliative treatment for subjective control of pain and neurologic deficit.

It has been suggested that chordoma is sensitive to higher doses of radiation than that conventionally available by external photon beam therapy. Suit and colleagues[107] suggested that an increased response might be seen by combining both photon and high-energy proton beam therapy, thus delivering doses comparable to 7000 to 8000 cGy.[107] This combination improves the dose distribution compared with more conventional external beam therapy. High doses can therefore be delivered to critical areas such as the base of the skull and the cervical spine, with reduced risk of necrosis of the central nervous system. Current data on charged particle beam therapy with either proton beams or helium-neon suggest that local control can be achieved in more than two thirds of prior untreated patients. This treatment is worthy of consideration in skull base and cervical chordomas following surgery.

Chordomas are resistant to chemotherapy. The majority of patients are referred for chemotherapy only after maximum radiotherapy has been given or for treatment of metastatic disease. Reports in the literature suggest occasional subjective and objective responses to chemotherapy. In our recent series, seven patients were treated with combination chemotherapy using the most effective doxorubicin (Adriamycin)-containing sarcoma regimens. No major response was noted. In patients with sarcomatous elements, it may be worthwhile using doxorubicin-cisplatin or ifosfamide-doxorubicin-cisplatin combinations, such as that used for high-grade spindle cell sarcomas.

Primary Lymphoma

Malignant lymphomas account for 10% of all cancers in patients under the age of 15 years.[108] Approximately 60% of lymphomas in children are non-Hodgkin's lymphoma, and occasionally lymphoma arises primarily in bone (Fig. 13–8).[109–112] Spinal cord compression may result from soft tissue tumor within the epidural space without apparent bone involvement: so-called epidural lymphoma.[113] The majority of these patients are in the fifth or sixth decade of life. Between 5% and 25% of non-Hodgkin's lymphomas arise at extranodal sites; thus, primary lymphoma of bone constitutes 5% of all bone tumors.

Originally called reticulum cell sarcoma or lymphosarcoma, the term non-Hodgkin's lymphoma is preferred to describe this tumor, with morphologic subtypes corresponding to various stages of lymphocytic differentiation.[107] To allow correlation between several histologic classifications, a working formulation was developed. The spinal cord may be compressed by two separate mechanisms: tumors may appear to originate in the vertebra or from retroperitoneal nodes and secondarily involve the epidural space.

In those patients presenting with spinal cord compression, urgent decompression may be necessary. If the diagnosis of lymphoma is suspected, fresh tissue should be sent for marker studies, immunoperoxidase testing, and electron microscopy. Proper clinical staging includes the performance of bone scans, CT evaluation of the chest and abdomen, and bone marrow biopsy. For many years, the most popular staging system was the Ann Arbor system; thus, tumors arising from a vertebra would be stage IE (denoting a single extranodal site) or stage IV if other sites

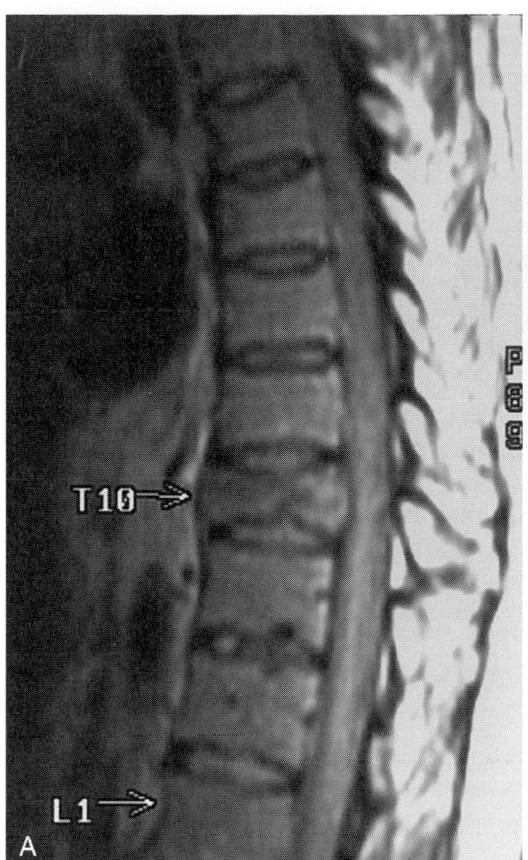

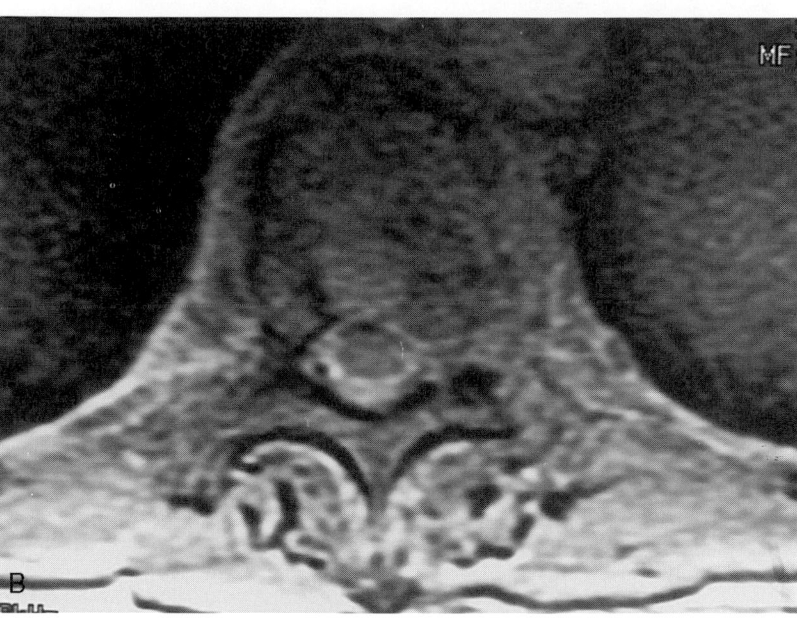

FIGURE 13–8. Lymphoma of thoracic spine. Axial *(A)* and sagittal *(B)* T2-weighted MR images demonstrate partial collapse of vertebral body and diffuse paraspinal mass with epidural extension.

of involvement were noted. The staging also took into account the presence or absence of constitutional symptoms such as fever, night sweats, or weight loss (designated A or B). Recently, other important factors have been found to be of prognostic value, including maximal diameter of tumor, specific site of extranodal origin, performance status, and serum lactate dehydrogenase levels. Thus, patients with diffuse large cell or immunoblastic non-Hodgkin's lymphoma that involves the epidural space require central nervous system prophylaxis.

If the spinal cord has been satisfactorily decompressed by laminectomy, we currently recommend the use of systemic chemotherapy prior to radiotherapy, since the majority of patients have occult stage IV disease. Truly localized lymphoma in the epidural space is extremely rare. Chemotherapy regimens incorporating CHOP are most appropriate. Local radiotherapy should be deferred until several cycles of chemotherapy have been completed.

Osteosarcoma and Malignant Spindle Cell Tumors

Osteosarcoma is the most common primary malignancy of bone, and its incidence ranges from one to two cases per million in the United States and most Western countries.[22, 23, 25] It originates predominantly in long bones, and less than 5% arise in the spine.[114] Although osteosarcomas may occur at any age, the incidence peaks in the second decade of life. Osteosarcomas may also result from malignant transformation in a variety of pathologic conditions: in Paget's disease, following radiotherapy, in fibrous dysplasia, and in some benign bone tumors.[115] In general, older patients with osteosarcoma often have secondary tumors.

Therapeutic ionizing radiation is associated with an increased risk of secondary bone and soft tissue tumors, of which osteosarcoma is clearly the most common histologic type. Long-term survivors of bilateral retinoblastoma have a risk 2000 times greater than the rest of the population, and the gene for malignant transformation in these tumors has been identified in the long arm of chromosome 13 within band 13q14.

Primary osteosarcomas involving the spine present complex therapeutic problems unlike those seen in extremity lesions. In the two largest institutional series reported, fewer than 30 cases per institution were encountered over a 40-year period.[116, 117] The majority of patients present with pain and neurologic deficit related to tumor extension into the spinal cord. Plain radiographic findings may be variable. In the spine, a combination of osteolytic, sclerotic, or mixed patterns may be seen. Pathologic fractures may also occur, and in 90% of cases, the vertebral body is predominantly involved. Both CT and MRI are recommended to demonstrate the extent of bone and soft tissue invasion (Fig. 13–9). The MR image appearance depends

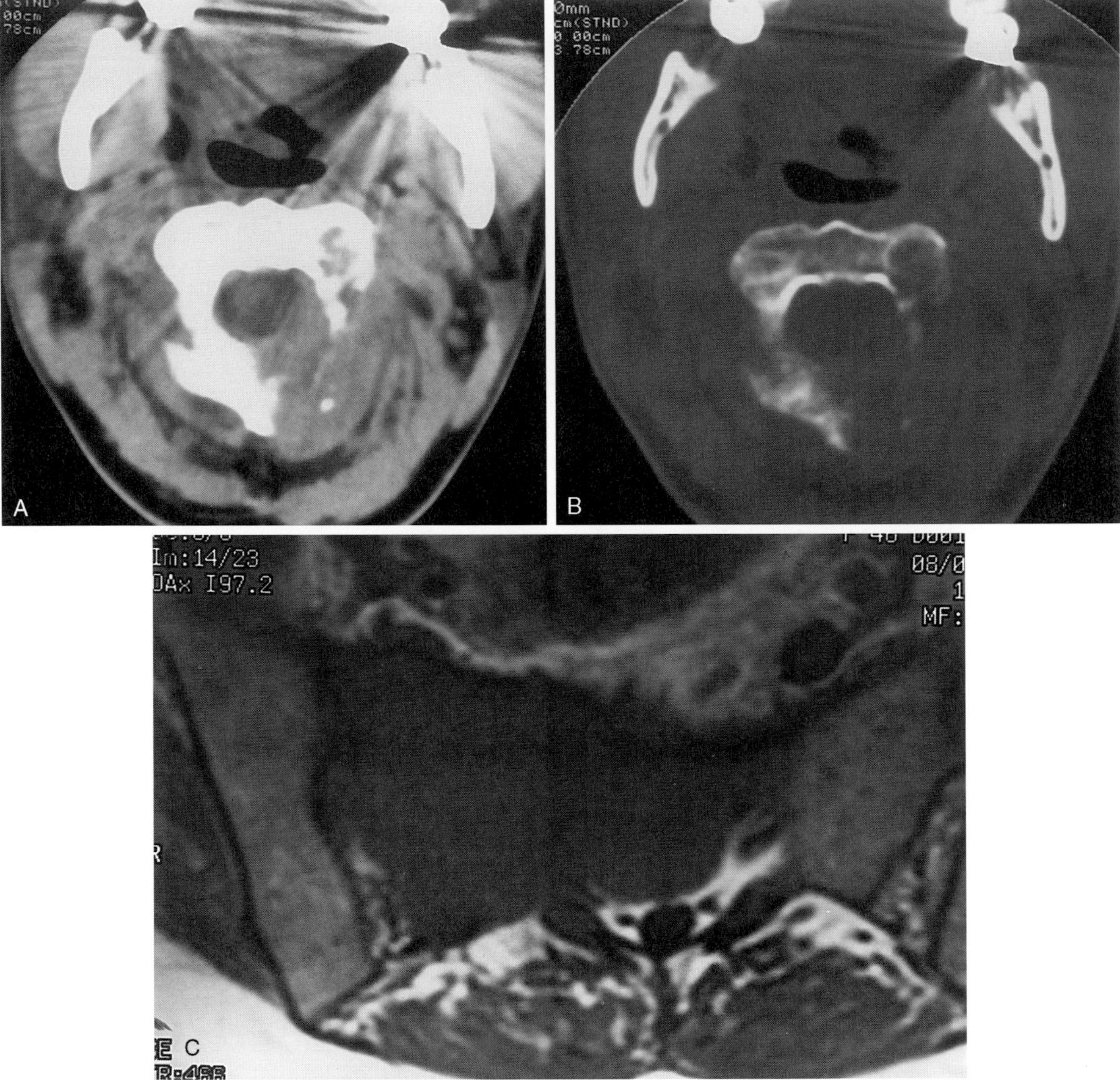

FIGURE 13–9. Osteogenic sarcoma. *A* and *B,* CT scans of the cervical spine in a young woman. There is destruction and considerable new bone production involving posterior elements of C-2 and C-3 vertebrae. *C,* MR image of the pelvis of a 44-year-old woman. There is extensive infiltration of the sacrum with extension into the epidural space of the distal canal on the right side.

heavily on the extent of mineralization: nonmineralized tumor has a relatively low signal intensity on T1-weighted images and a bright signal on T2-weighted images. Mineralized tumors may appear dark on all sequences. Radioisotopes using technetium and thallium are particularly helpful in demonstrating either skip or satellite lesions. In the spine, especially in those who have undergone chemotherapy or surgery, serial scans are useful in determining local and systemic relapses.

When the diagnosis of osteosarcoma is suspected, confirmation by biopsy is indicated before definitive surgery is undertaken. In extremity lesions, such biopsies can be performed using a Tru-Cut needle, but open biopsies may be required in spinal lesions. In such cases, the surgical approach should be carefully planned and meticulous hemostasis achieved so that postoperative hemorrhage does not result in tracking of the tumor along tissue planes. If the pathologist can confirm the diagnosis, it may be appropriate to perform a subtotal spondylectomy at this stage. Frequently, however, the diagnosis of osteosarcoma can be established only by permanent sections.

Grossly, the tumor has a reddish, gritty, granular quality

because of bone production. All osteosarcomas, regardless of subtype, have as a common feature: the production of bone (osteoid) by neoplastic osteoblasts. For simplicity, four divisions can be used to describe the predominant cell type: osteogenic, chondroblastic, fibroblastic, and secondary osteosarcoma.[9] Histologically, all osteosarcomas have disorganized, haphazardly arranged spicules or masses of woven bone in a rich vascular stroma. The malignant osteoblasts spring from the background stroma; there is no prominent osteoblastic palisading about the bone spicules. Foci of hemorrhage or necrosis are common features. In all spindle cell and cartilage-producing or giant cell malignancies, a diligent search should be made for foci of bone production. If bone production is not evident in a spindle cell malignancy, the tumor may be designated a malignant fibrous histiocytoma or fibrosarcoma based on its overall morphology.

The treatment of osteosarcoma of the extremities has been greatly improved by the introduction of multiagent chemotherapy. If the diagnosis of osteogenic sarcoma is established by biopsy, staging studies are indicated to determine the presence of metastases. In many centers, definitive surgery is often delayed so that early systemic (neoadjuvant) chemotherapy can be instituted. The rationale for early chemotherapy is based on three premises: First, since there is a high likelihood of systemic micrometastases, chemotherapy is used to eradicate these micrometastases when the tumor burden is relatively small and responsive, prior to the emergence of resistant clones. Second, regression of the primary tumor allows more effective and less mutilating surgery and, in the case of spinal lesions, allows intralesional surgery to be performed with less risk of systemic dissemination. Third, the histologic effects of chemotherapy can be observed in the resected primary specimen, which allows appropriate planning of future chemotherapy.

In patients with vertebral column tumors who have had the diagnosis established by decompressive laminectomy, we favor the initial use of systemic chemotherapy if the patient is neurologically stable. If the patient has persistent compression and neurologic deficits or has an unstable spine, tumor resection and stabilization may need to be completed prior to chemotherapy. Currently, the only effective treatment for osteosarcoma is total spondylectomy, which implies total removal of the entire vertebra or vertebrae involved by tumor. This can be accomplished either in a single procedure or by staged approaches. In our view, external radiotherapy should not be used, since these tumors are highly resistant to standard doses of external photon beam radiation. In addition, the use of irradiation may increase the incidence of local wound complications following surgery.

Chondrosarcoma

Chondrosarcoma is a malignant tumor in which the basic neoplastic tissue is fully developed cartilage without tumor osteoid being directly formed by a sarcomatous stroma. Myxoid changes, calcification, or ossification may be present. These tumors constitute 10% of bone tumors but are exceedingly rare in the spine.[118] Chondrosarcoma may arise de novo in previously normal bone or result from sarcomatous transformation from a pre-existing benign cartilage tumor. Repeated surgical excisions following recurrences often precede malignant transformation. As with other primary tumors of bone, males are at higher risk than females. The mean age of presentation is approximately 40 years, with patients' ages ranging from the first to the ninth decades of life.

Histologically, tumors may be divided into three grades of increasing malignancy. Since histologic analysis may not always suffice to predict biologic activity, DNA analysis of individual tumor cells using flow cytometry has been recommended to provide additional prognostic information.

The most common presenting feature is pain, associated with neurologic deficit. In the spine, tumors can present as a destructive lesion within the spine or, more commonly, as a paraspinal mass with calcification. In evaluating the biopsy specimen, the pathologist should use additional information available from the radiographs and CT scan. Large lesions greater than 8 to 10 cm in diameter and bone destruction are features that support the diagnosis of malignancy (Fig. 13–10). In at least 10% of tumors there is a progression toward more anaplasia with local recurrence. Variants of chondrosarcoma include dedifferentiated chondrosarcoma of the spine, which behaves like a high-grade spindle cell sarcoma, as well as mesenchymal chondrosarcoma; both of these tumors are moderately responsive to chemotherapy.

In all patients, treatment should be complete surgical excision.[15] Cryosurgery has also been used to prevent local recurrence of chondrosarcomas. This technique requires careful protection of the dura and nerves, with liquid nitrogen being applied in a controlled manner with a probe or funnel. Three complete freeze-thaw cycles are recommended.

Ewing's Sarcoma

Ewing's sarcoma is the prototype of the small, round cell neoplasm of childhood and represents approximately 30% of primary bone tumors in this age group.[20] Before the development of systemic chemotherapy, less than 20% of all patients with Ewing's sarcoma survived. Currently, with aggressive multimodality treatment, approximately 50% to 60% of patients with localized tumors achieve long-term, relapse-free survival.[19, 119–125]

Approximately 80% of reported cases occur within the first two decades of life. The majority of patients present with pain, swelling, and systemic symptoms including fever; this may mistakenly suggest a diagnosis of infection. In spinal lesions, early onset of neurologic symptoms with cord compression is common.[126, 127] The sacrum is a com-

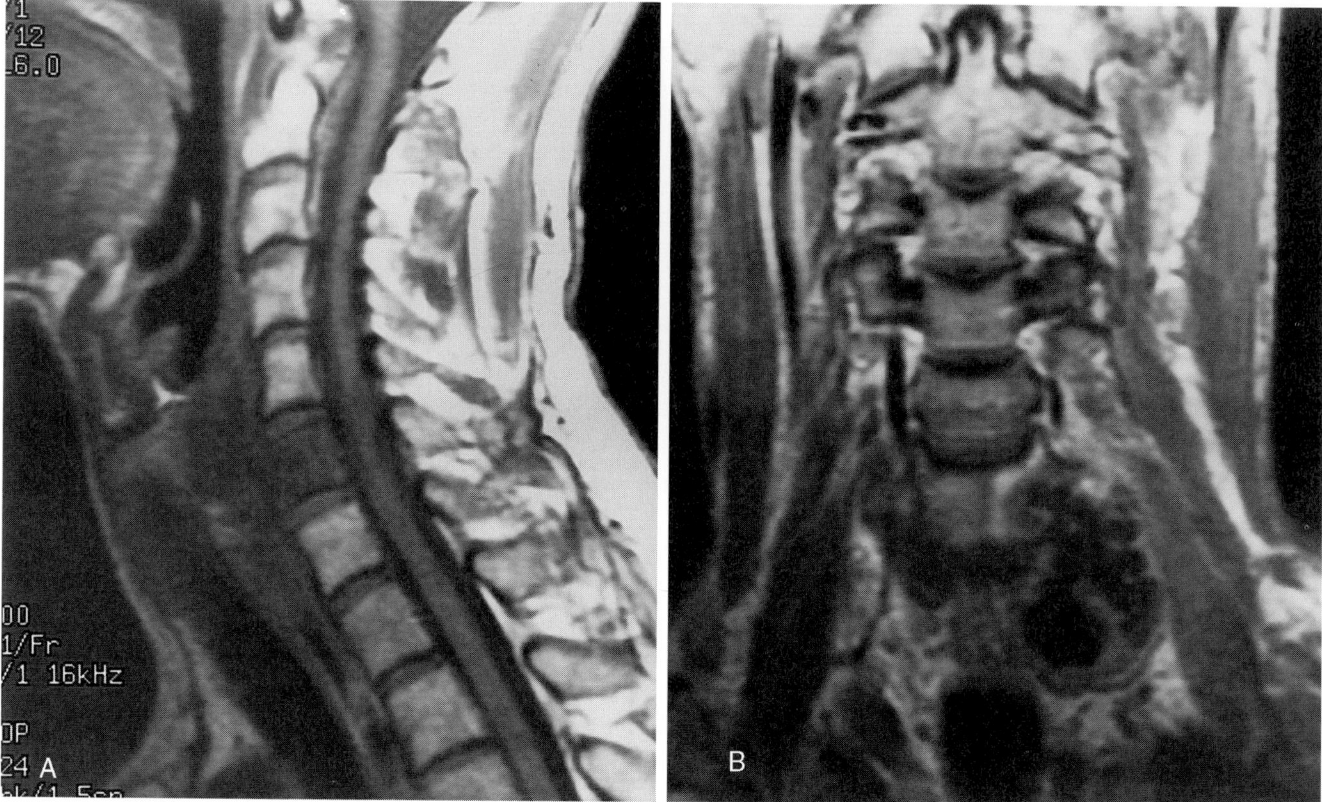

FIGURE 13–10. Chondrosarcoma of the lower cervical spine in a 47-year-old woman. Sagittal *(A)* and coronal *(B)* MR images show abnormal intensity of C-6 vertebral body and lobulated soft tissue mass arising from its lateral elements on the left side. There is no canal compromise or cord compression.

mon site for axial tumors, which may grow to a large size prior to the onset of pain. In young patients, pelvic lesions may present as a neurogenic bladder. The only reliable blood marker is serum lactate dehydrogenase, which should be monitored closely as an indicator of tumor burden. The radiographic features include a mottled, moth-eaten appearance of irregular bone destruction with poorly defined margins (Fig. 13–11). In the sacrum, the destroyed bone may be replaced with a ground-glass appearance resembling cracked ice. Both CT and MRI should be performed to evaluate the true extent of soft tissue and bone marrow abnormalities. However, MRI is exquisitely sensitive to change in normal tissue, such as edema or denervation of muscle, and it is important not to overestimate local tumor extent.

Approximately 20% of patients present with gross metastatic disease, but the incidence of micrometastases is very high. Evaluation for metastatic disease should include chest CT, bone scan, and bone marrow aspiration and biopsy. If the bone scan reveals suspicious lesions, attempts should be made to obtain histologic verification. Because chemotherapy has the potential for cardiac, renal, and hepatic toxicity, assessment of these organs should be included in the pretreatment evaluation.

Ewing's sarcoma encompasses a group of small, round cell malignancies of childhood that include peripheral neuroectodermal tumor (PNET) of bone and Askin's tumor, as well as other round cell tumors. Results of electron microscopy study and immunoperoxidase staining have led to the belief that Ewing's sarcoma and PNET share a common

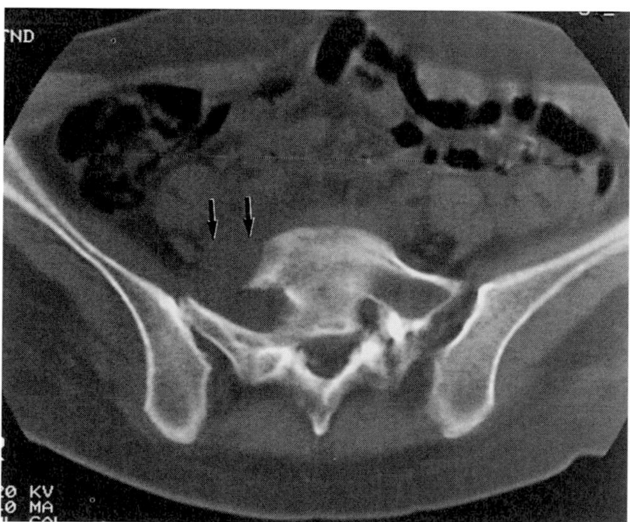

FIGURE 13–11. Ewing's sarcoma. CT scan of the pelvis demonstrates destructive process involving the upper sacrum on the right side associated with soft tissue mass.

origin from a precusor neural cell that may arise interchangeably in bone or soft tissue. Cytogenetic studies have shown that Ewing's sarcoma and PNET share a specific abnormality, a reciprocal translocation (11;22). In addition, these tumors share a consistent pattern of proto-oncogene expression, that is, high levels of c-*myc,* c-*myb,* and c-*mil*/c-*raf* RNA and a lack of N-*myc* amplification. These tumors also produce a high level of acetylcholinesterase, as seen in parasympathetic nerve endings. The differential diagnosis of round cell tumors includes small cell osteosarcoma, rhabdomyosarcoma, mesenchymal chondrosarcoma, lymphoma, and neuroblastoma. Since these round cell tumors cannot always be distinguished at the light microscope level, electron microscopy and immunocytochemistry along with cytogenetic and molecular genetic studies should be part of the initial biopsy evaluation.

The treatment of Ewing's sarcoma should be based on the concept of early systemic chemotherapy. At present, with multimodality treatment, more than half the patients with localized tumors can be cured.[20, 128] At present, there is considerable debate over the methods used for local control, that is, surgery versus radiation.[122, 129–131]

Local control rates with radiotherapy as the primary modality have varied from 55% to 90%. Factors that influence local control include size greater than 8 to 10 cm as well as pelvic or axial location. Classic radiation dose recommendations are 4000 to 4500 cGy to the whole field or involved bone, followed by a booster dose using a coned-down field to deliver 5000 to 6000 cGy to the tumor. Several studies have demonstrated superior results for patients who have had resection as part of local therapy following induction chemotherapy. In some situations, surgery is clearly the primary local control modality. These include small tumors of expendable bone, such as the clavicle or fibula, and of other weight-bearing bones when radiation would include the major growth sites. In our view, surgery should be used to eradicate local spinal disease after induction chemotherapy.

Several studies for Ewing's sarcoma have shown that systemic therapy with VAC-doxorubicin produces the best response. Recently, 214 patients with Ewing's sarcoma were entered in a study that tested high-dose intermittent chemotherapy versus moderate-dose continuous chemotherapy with VAC-doxorubicin. This study showed a significant disease-free and overall survival advantage for the high-dose therapy group.[128] A more recent follow-up study of 107 patients treated at the National Cancer Institute showed a 37% 5-year, 35% 10-year, and 33% 15-year actuarial disease-free survival rate for those presenting with localized tumors; there was a 2% 5-year survival rate for those with clinically evident metastatic disease at diagnosis.[19]

New chemotherapy regimens include the incorporation of ifosfamide plus etoposide (IE) into the standard VAC-doxorubicin regimen. Early data suggest that IE chemotherapy is as effective as VAC-doxorubicin.[121]

METASTATIC TUMORS

The management of spinal metastases causing neurologic deficits continues to be the focus of intense debate.[29–31] In the past decade, the pendulum swung from a philosophy of emergency decompressive laminectomy in all patients to a conservative approach of steroids and radiation.[34, 132] Thus radiotherapy was recommended in all patients without consideration of the clinical status, the nature of compression within the canal, or the presence or absence of associated instability. Although some attempt has been made to compare various modalities, the absence of well-controlled prospective studies is responsible for the lack of clear guidelines.

Although metastases to the spine frequently represent a manifestation of advanced cancer, the clinical syndrome is so variable that it is difficult to apply generalizations regarding treatment. Approximately 10% of patients in most surgical series present with spinal metastases as their initial symptom of cancer; in more than half these patients, the primary focus is occult. Although virtually any neoplasm can metastasize to the spine, the most common primary sites are the breast, lung, prostate, and hematopoietic system.[32, 34, 46, 133–135]

In general, symptoms are back pain with or without a radicular component. At the time of diagnosis, neurologic deficits are common. Up to three quarters of patients have varying degrees of weakness, with associated bladder and bowel dysfunction in approximately half.[38, 49, 66, 67, 136–138] Approximately 10% of patients are severely paraparetic or paraplegic at the time of diagnosis, and 20% of ambulatory patients deteriorate while undergoing radiotherapy.[43, 47, 48] Since the results of treatment depend to a large extent on pretreatment neurologic status, it is critical to identify the subset of patients who might benefit from surgery early.

Several factors have been identified as important indicators of post-treatment outcome; of these, the most important are tumor biology, pretreatment neurologic status, progression of symptoms (tempo), location of tumor, and therapy used.[30, 38, 46, 66, 139–145]

Biologic aggressiveness of the primary tumor has an important bearing on post-treatment survival rate. Patients with relatively slow-growing tumors such as breast and prostate cancer, as well as lymphoma, have a more favorable prognosis. Patients with exclusively osseous metastases from kidney and thyroid cancer may live for many years, whereas the chance of survival of patients with metastatic bronchogenic carcinoma is generally poor.

There is little doubt that there is a clear correlation between pretreatment neurologic status and outcome. Several studies have shown that approximately 70% of patients who are ambulatory at the beginning of treatment remain so following treatment, by either radiation or laminectomy; only one third of paraparetic patients become ambulatory, and the response rate for severely paraparetic patients is less than 10%. These data emphasize the value of early diagnosis. More recent surgical series have shown much greater improvement rates if surgical approaches are tailored to the site of spinal cord compression.

The tempo of neurologic progression and initial response to steroid therapy are important prognostic factors. Approximately 10% to 20% of patients experience acute onset of cord compression (within 24 to 48 hours); in the absence of a response to high-dose steroid therapy, the outlook is poor. Siegal and Siegal[43, 146] noted that the site of tumor compression within the spinal canal has prognostic significance. In a prospective study, they noted that the success rate for ventrally located tumors was 80% when the tumor was decompressed through an anterior route and only 39% for posteriorly located tumors decompressed by laminectomy.[43, 146]

The most important treatment variable is the initial therapy used. Several retrospective studies have shown that the ambulatory rates obtained by either radiotherapy alone or laminectomy plus radiotherapy are approximately 50%. There are few data to support the use of laminectomy, even if the goal is neural decompression.

Therapeutic options available in the initial management of spinal metastases include chemotherapy, steroids plus radiotherapy, and surgery. There is general agreement that corticosteroids should be given initially to all patients with spinal metastases. The most common corticosteroid used is dexamethasone, but the dosage remains controversial.[147–149] Initially, there was enthusiasm for extremely high doses of dexamethasone (100 mg intravenously) followed by 24 mg given intravenously four times a day. However, there are few clinical data to support the use of such high doses, and a more accepted approach is to use 10 to 20 mg intravenously, followed by 4 mg four times a day. Although many clinicians continue to use high doses, serious side effects can arise, including hyperglycemia, gastrointestinal bleeding, perforation from stress ulcers, myopathy, steroid psychosis, and suppression of immune function.[149] For the surgeon, the most important side effects are failure of the surgical wound to heal and the development of sepsis and wound infections from immune suppression.[150]

If the tumor is highly sensitive to chemotherapy (round cell sarcoma, lymphoma, or germinoma), it may be possible to use systemic chemotherapy in place of local radiotherapy. Similarly, hormonal ablation by orchiectomy or drug therapy may produce dramatic relief of pain and partial reversal of neurologic deficits in patients with metastases from prostate cancer.

External radiotherapy is considered the mainstay of treatment in patients with spinal metastases who are not surgical candidates due to otherwise advanced disease or poor performance status. Approximately one third to one half of treated patients improve and are able to walk following treatment.[34, 49, 151] Pain relief is seen in half the patients treated, although the actual impact of radiation in controlling pain in patients who concomitantly receive steroids and narcotics is difficult to discern. The outcome is dependent largely on ambulatory status, since patients who are nonambulatory are less likely to show significant improvement. Patients with radiosensitive tumors (such as breast, prostate, and lymphoma) are more likely to show improvement. Most patients are generally treated at a dose rate of 200 cGy/day, for a total of 3000 cGy, using a single posterior port whose field encompasses two segments above and below the level of involvement. This dose approaches cord tolerance in the thoracic region, and retreatment is not an option. In patients with potentially curable disease in the lumbar segments (solitary metastases from breast cancer), more protracted courses using lower-dose fractions (150 cGy/day) to a total dose of 5000 cGy may be used.

The major limiting factor with regard to improving cure rates by external radiotherapy alone is the limited radiation tolerance of the spinal cord.[152, 153] Thus, treatment with conventional doses generally results in local relapses from tumor recurrence or instability within 3 to 6 months. To improve the response rates for spinal tumors, several different methods have been tried, including the use of radiosensitizers (such as mizonidazole), the concurrent use of chemotherapy such as 5-fluorouracil or cisplatin, and the use of brachytherapy with permanent or removable implants. In selected cases, the use of particle beams (proton or helium-neon) in conjunction with photon beam therapy has been recommended for potentially curable tumors. The advantages of such treatment include better dose distribution, sparing of neural tissue, and an enhanced radiobiologic effect for heavy particles such as helium.[21, 107] These treatment options are available in only a few centers and are time-consuming and expensive.

The two major problems of surgery on irradiated patients are related to wound healing and obtaining bone fusion following spinal reconstruction. Several studies have shown that the wound dehiscence rate following surgery in irradiated patients may approach 30%, especially if instrumentation is used.[154] In a study of surgery alone compared with surgery following irradiation, we noted a statistically significant increased rate of complications (36% vs. 16%) in patients who had undergone radiation.[155] We advocate avoiding incisions in the irradiated field if surgery is performed and recommend closures with myocutaneous flaps if instrumentation is used.

INDICATIONS FOR SURGERY

The scope and extent of surgery are individualized for each patient. Outcome depends on the site of the primary tumor, histology, the pretreatment neurologic deficit, and overall performance status.[145, 156] The major goal of treatment is palliation. Tumor resection and stabilization can be accomplished in the majority of patients, but it is important not to apply treatment indiscriminately. In our view, ambulatory patients are better candidates for surgical intervention; patients who are paraplegic or near-paraplegic benefit little from extensive surgery. Patients who develop rapid deficits within a 24-hour period have a poor outcome regardless of therapy. Patients with spinal instability, retropulsed bone fragments, or acute collapse of the vertebral body will not benefit from radiotherapy alone. Patients who have widespread disease or those who have failed prior treatment are much less likely to respond to surgery. We recommend radiotherapy plus steroids as the initial treatment of choice in the following conditions: patients with widespread metastases whose survival can be measured in weeks, patients with lymphoma or other round cell malignancies such as neuroblastoma and Ewing's sarcoma, and patients with breast or prostate cancer without spinal abnormalities. In all other patients with spinal metastases, neurosurgical evaluation should be sought. Because the objective of therapy varies for each patient, we have classified indications for surgical intervention into five major categories: cancer therapy, stabilization, neurologic salvage, tissue diagnosis, and pain relief.

Cancer Therapy

In patients with primary osseous neoplasms, localized paraspinal tumors with direct spine involvement, and solitary sites of relapse, local treatment has a major bearing on overall survival. Other patients with pathologic compression fractures and radioresistant tumors, such as kidney cancer, with limited systemic disease also fall into this category. In these patients, magnitude of epidural extension and the presence or absence of neurologic deficit have little bearing on the timing of surgery; rather, the goal of surgery should be maximal reduction of tumor bulk.

Stabilization

Another major objective of surgery is providing stability to the spine by either maintenance of the spinal alignment or correction of a deformity caused by tumor growth. Patients with fracture-dislocations, localized kyphosis, or collapsed vertebrae with retropulsion of a bone fragment may require operative decompression in conjunction with radiotherapy. In these patients, the radiosensitivity of the primary tumor has little bearing on the indication for therapy. A major subgroup of patients in this category have segmental instability of the spine. This is clinically manifest by pain aggravated by movement and is usually seen after radiotherapy. Plain radiographs may show progressive collapse of the vertebral bodies, or MRI may show retropulsion of bony elements with a local kyphosis. Surgical reduction of movement across this motion segment generally results in prompt relief of pain. This can be accomplished by anterior stabilization following vertebral body resection or by posterior stabilization with or without instrumentation.[2, 3, 5–8, 154, 157–161]

Neurologic Salvage

Surgery is indicated for neurologic palliation in patients who relapse after a course of radiotherapy and in others who deteriorate while undergoing radiotherapy. In such patients, the salvage rate is relatively poor, and the morbidity is high. There may be no discernible effect on survival; the major impact is on the quality of survival. Several different techniques have been advocated to measure improvement in the quality of life, and these should be used to measure the results of treatment.[162]

Tissue Diagnosis

Another major indication for surgical intervention is to distinguish between benign and malignant spinal cord compression. It is not uncommon to encounter benign causes of cord compression in cancer patients, such as that resulting from disc disease or osteoporosis.[163]

Pain Relief

Pain relief is generally achieved in most patients who undergo tumor resection; it may result from restoration of spinal stability, decompression of nerve roots, or direct removal of tumor compressing the brachial or sacral plexus.[164] In patients with incapacitating pain, relief of pain is a worthwhile goal even if motor deficits are permanent and irreversible. Pain-relieving procedures such as rhizotomy, cordotomy, and implantation of drug-delivering devices fall into this category.[165]

SURGICAL APPROACHES

The surgical approach must allow adequate access for tumor resection, neural decompression, and satisfactory exposure for stabilization with instrumentation (Figs. 13–12, 13–13, and 13–14).[18, 47, 48] Thus, spinal tumors may be operated on from posterior or lateral anterior approaches or combinations of these.[7, 16, 140, 160, 166–171]

A posterior decompressive laminectomy has been largely abandoned except in patients whose lesions are located strictly posterior to the dura. Laminectomy provides improvement in only one third of patients, and complications are numerous, including added instability, kyphosis, and neurologic deterioration from translation or angulation. In most studies, no additional palliation was seen in comparison with radiotherapy alone. In a meta-analysis, Findlay[172] noted that of the 1816 patients reviewed, 32% of those treated by laminectomy, 38% of those treated by laminectomy and radiotherapy, and 51% of those treated by radiotherapy were able to walk at the end of treatment. Approximately 20% of patients in each group experienced neurologic deterioration. In addition, 11% of patients undergoing operation experienced perioperative complications, with a mortality rate of 9%. Laminectomy is contraindicated when the tumor mass lies anterior to the cord, if the vertebral body is collapsed, or in the presence of a kyphotic deformity or subluxation of one vertebra over another.[173] The fact that it is technically easy to perform

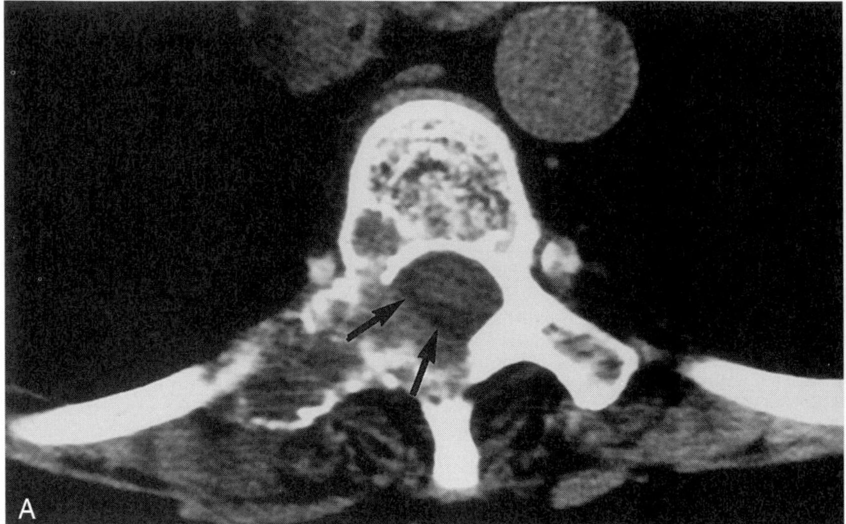

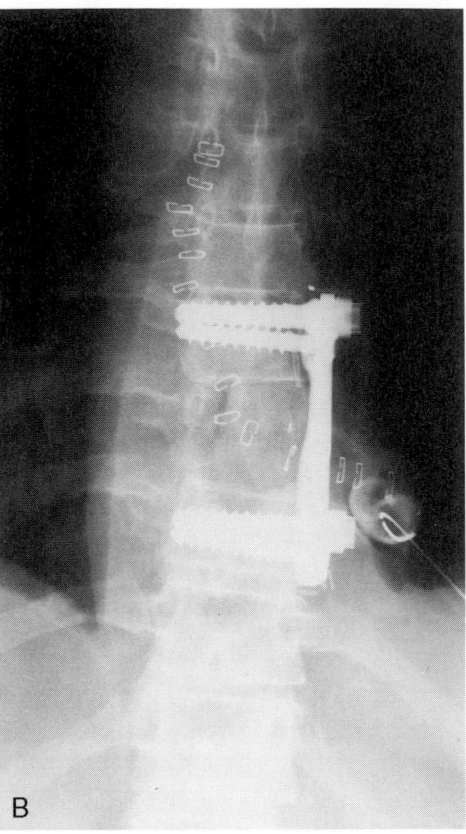

FIGURE 13–12. Breast carcinoma with metastases to the thoracic spine. CT scan *(A)* shows destruction of the T-10 vertebra. There is mild epidural extension (arrows). The lesion was resected and the spine stabilized with lateral plates and screws *(B)*.

and is well tolerated does not justify its use, except for tissue diagnosis.

Since laminectomy does not allow adequate access to the anterior aspect of the cord, a variety of extended posterolateral approaches have been reported that produce short-term improvement rates of 75%, especially in conjunction with instrumentation.[174] Major indications for posterolateral procedures include multisegment involvement, radiographic demonstration of a posterolateral tumor mass, three-column instability, and patient inability to tolerate thoracotomy.[157] Perrin and colleagues[154, 168] reported pain relief in 80%, a post-treatment ambulation rate of 65%, and a mortality rate of 8% in a series of 200 consecutive patients undergoing posterolateral approaches. Currently, posterior stabilization may be accomplished following decompression using a variety of instrumentation systems. In the cervical spine, a combination of Luque rods (L rods or rectangles) and sublaminar cables allows easy contouring of the instrumentation to the cervical curvature. Alternatively, lateral mass plates in conjunction with screws may be used. In the lumbar and thoracic regions, the instrumentation must resist a greater axial load. Thus, posterior rod systems in conjunction with hooks and screws into the pedicles are commonly used. These allow secure segmental fixation at multiple levels. In the past, the most common systems were the Harrington rod and Luque rod systems, but they have been largely replaced by more modular systems. In the United States, the Texas Scottish Rite Hospital (TSRH), Isola, and Cotrel-Dubousset systems are the major ones in use at present (Fig. 13–15).

Even if posterior stabilization is performed, there can be substantial motion anteriorly in response to physiologic compression and bending loads, especially in patients whose anterior and middle columns have been destroyed by tumor. For this reason, anterior stabilization using methyl methacrylate or a bone graft may be required.

Since the majority of tumors involve the vertebral body, it is logical that anterior vertebral body resection is most appropriate in the majority of patients. In our experience, the anterior approach fulfills all the requirements for adequate surgery: it allows adequate access for complete tumor resection and immediate stabilization. In patients with neoplasms, the importance of adequate internal fixation by rigid instrumentation stabilization cannot be overemphasized. Although autologous bone grafts are clearly indicated for spine reconstruction in patients with benign tumors or slow-growing malignancies, they should not be used in patients with limited life expectancy or others who require postoperative radiation to the surgical site. When postoperative radiotherapy is used to improve local control in slow-growing malignant tumors, we recommend that it be delayed for 12 weeks to allow adequate incorporation of the graft. If bone grafts are used for reconstruction of the spine, additional instrumentation is generally required. In the cervical spine, anterior plate fixation with Morscher or Caspar plates is recommended. In the thoracic and

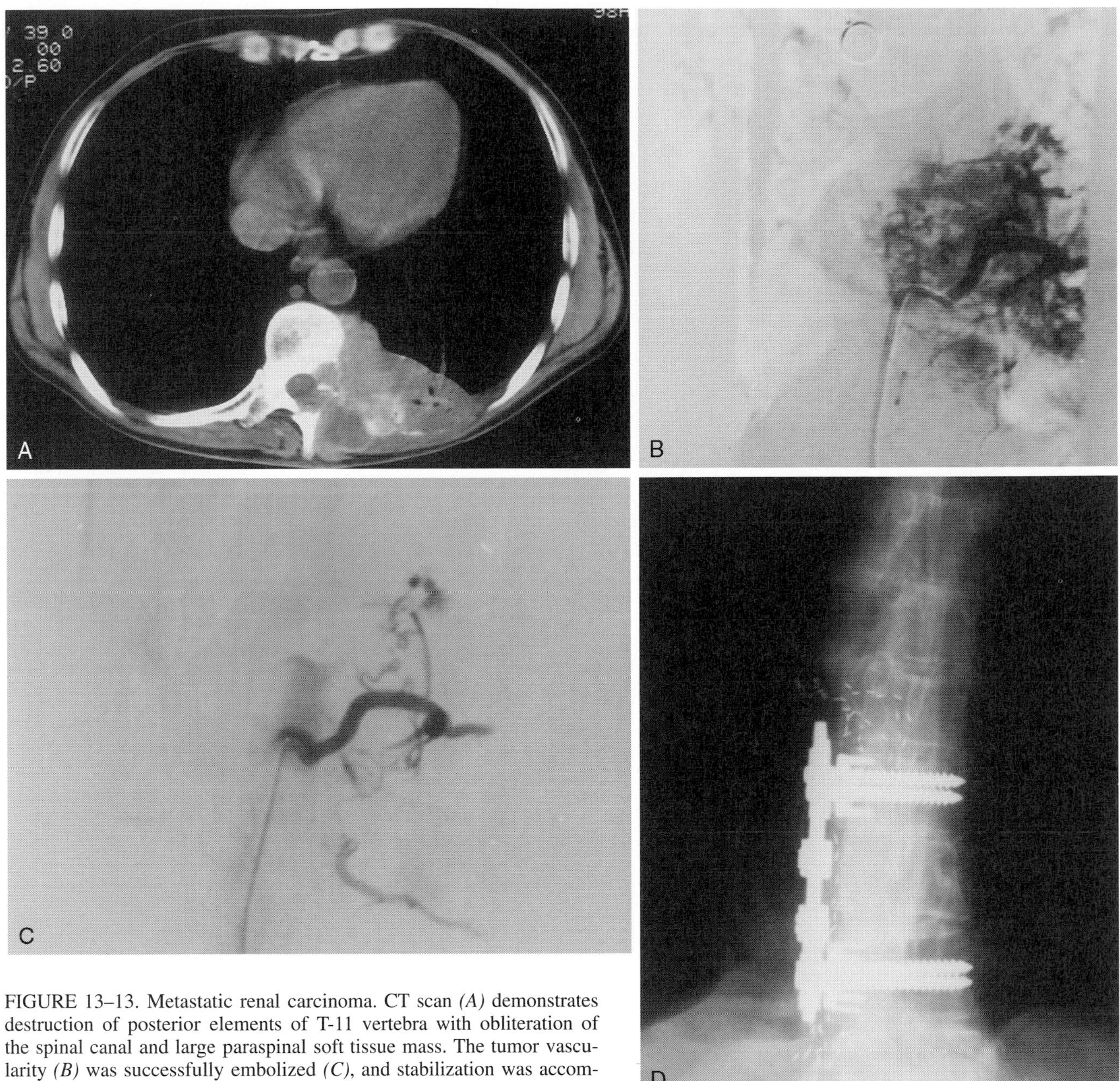

FIGURE 13–13. Metastatic renal carcinoma. CT scan *(A)* demonstrates destruction of posterior elements of T-11 vertebra with obliteration of the spinal canal and large paraspinal soft tissue mass. The tumor vascularity *(B)* was successfully embolized *(C)*, and stabilization was accomplished *(D)*.

lumbar regions, a variety of anterior instrumentation systems are available, although clinical experience is still limited. Biomechanically, the strongest anterior constructs are the TSRH anterior system, the Z-plate (both available from Danek, Memphis, TN), and the Kaneda device (Acromed, Cleveland, OH). We have found the Z-plate to be relatively easy and expeditious to use, and an additional feature is its compatibility for postoperative MRI studies.

At present, the optimal construct following anterior vertebrectomy is polymethyl methacrylate.[48, 158, 170, 175–177] Although there have been some doubts regarding its long-term stability, it is extremely strong in resisting compressive forces when used as an anterior construct. Fixation of the methyl methacrylate is achieved by the use of Steinmann pins driven into intact vertebrae above and below the level of resection.[48] Long-term studies of methyl methacrylate constructs have shown no clinical evidence of loosening, although there have been several fatigue fractures of the Steinmann pins. A major advantage of this technique is its simplicity and low cost in comparison with other instrumentation systems. In addition, a major consideration in all reconstructive procedures is the use of MRI-compatible titanium implants for follow-up evaluation.

Although the superiority of surgery over radiotherapy has not been established by prospective controlled studies, several retrospective studies have shown that the anterior approach provides improvement rates in the 80%

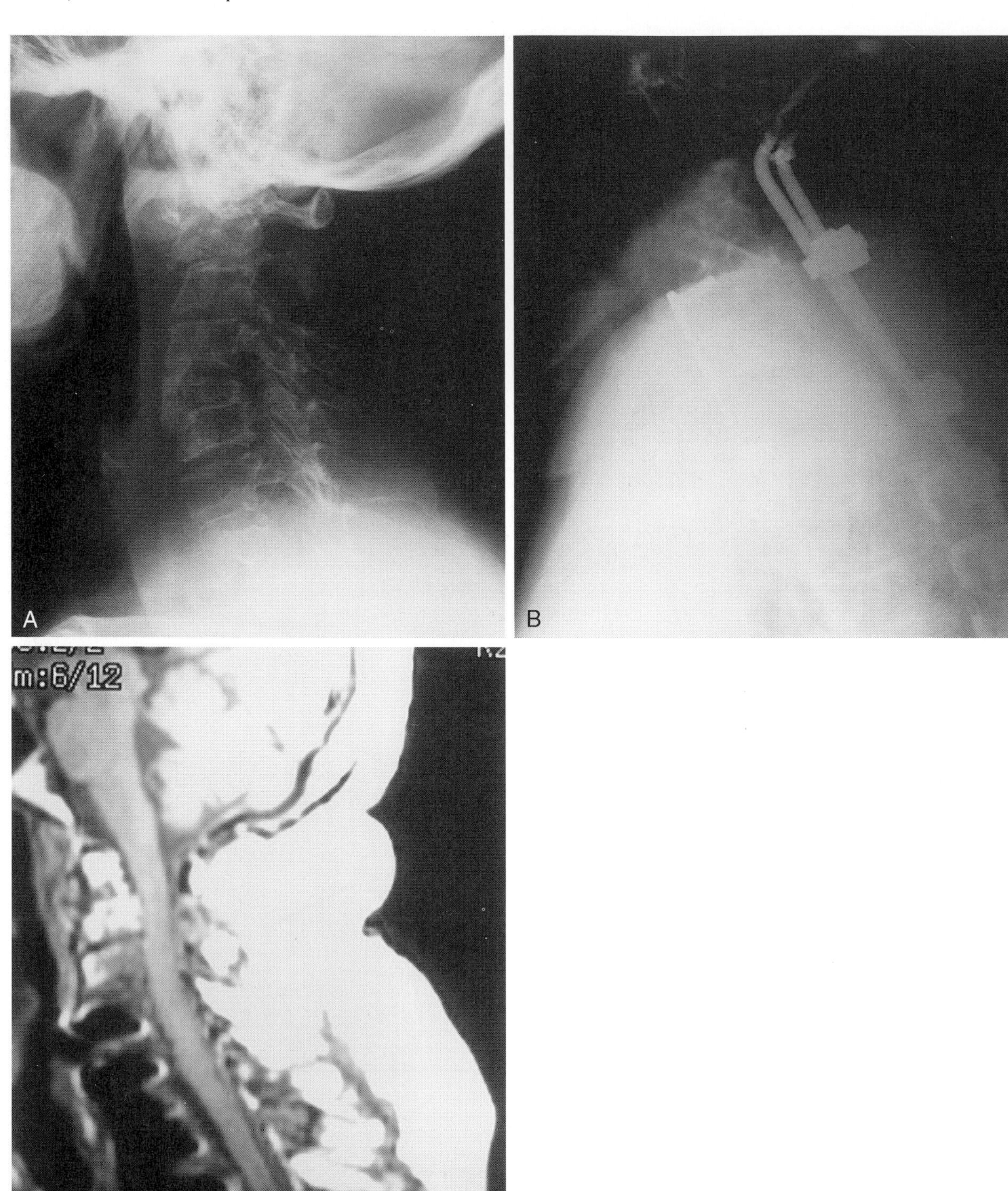

FIGURE 13–14. Supportive treatment of multilevel metastases from breast carcinoma. Lateral view of the cervical spine *(A)* reveals diffuse bone lesions with multilevel collapse and grade I C1–2 and C5–6 subluxation. Posterior stabilization provided by customized occipital-cervical-thoracic rods *(B)*. Postoperative MR image shows good alignment and no compromise of the spinal canal *(C)*.

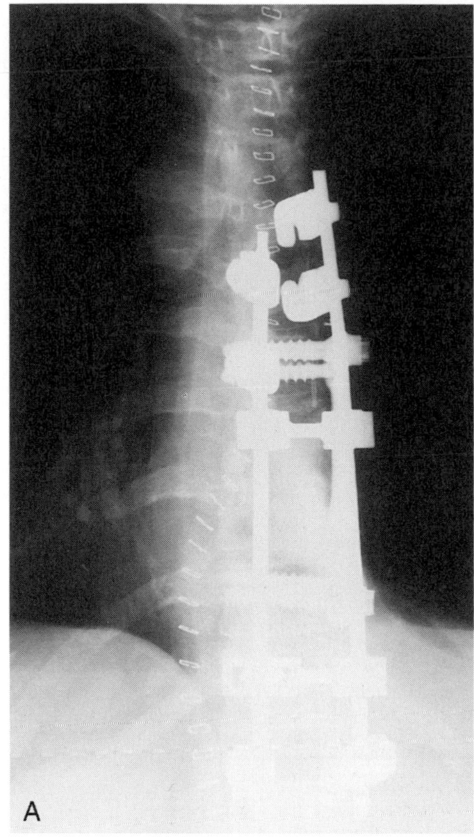

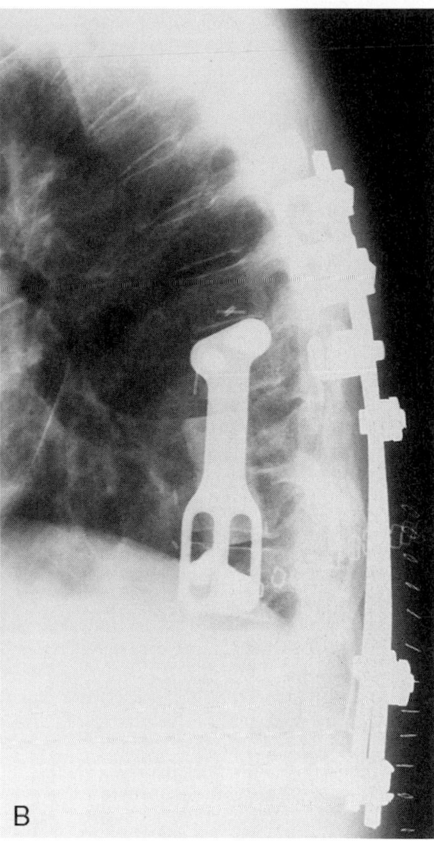

FIGURE 13–15. T-10 metastases, status post resection (the same patient as in Fig. 13–12). Stability maintained by combination of anterior and posterior plates, graft, rods, and screws. (Frontal *(A)* and lateral *(B)* radiographs of the thoracic spine.)

range—substantially better than that reported following radiotherapy alone.[17, 43] To determine the role of surgery in patients with spinal metastases, we recently reported a prospective study of 54 patients with radioresistant solid tumors.[178] Prior to surgery, 24 (44%) were nonambulatory. Following surgery, the ambulation rate was 100%, with three patients (6%) dying of various causes over a 30-day period. At 2 years, 23 of 25 patients remained ambulatory, although repeated operations for local recurrences were required in 25% of patients. The successful ambulation rate in our study reflects accurate and complete radiologic identification of the site of compression, careful preoperative management to minimize the incidence of complications, proper selection of the operative approach, the availability of ancillary support, and the use of newly developed spinal instrumentation. Because multidisciplinary team approaches are required, early neurosurgical consultation is recommended for optimal results. We believe that early aggressive surgical management of spinal metastases will have a major impact on survival in the subset of patients with limited disease, as well as in others with biologically slow-growing tumors. In such patients, the goal of operation is complete resection of the tumor, which often requires staged or simultaneous anterior-posterior approaches to the spine.

References

1. Cotrel Y, Dubousset J, Guillaumat M: New universal instrumentation in spinal surgery. Clin Orthop 227:10–23, 1988.
2. Cusick J, Larson S, Walsh P, Steiner R: Distraction stabilization in the treatment of metastatic carcinoma. J Neurosurg 59:861–866, 1983.
3. Cybulski G, Von Roenn K, D'Angelo C, DeWald R: Luque rod stabilization for metastatic disease of the spine. Surg Neurol 28:277–283, 1987.
4. Denis F: Spinal instability as defined by the three column spine concept in acute spinal trauma. Clin Orthop 189:65–76, 1984.
5. DeWald R, Bridwell K, Prodromas C, Rodts M: Reconstructive spinal surgery as palliation for metastatic malignancies of the spine. Spine 10:21–62, 1985.
6. Sundaresan N, Schmidek HH, Schiller AL, Rosenthal A: Tumors of the Spine: Diagnosis and Management. Philadelphia: WB Saunders, 1990.
7. Kaneda K: Anterior approach and Kaneda instrumentation for lesions of the thoracic and lumbar spine. In Bridwell KH, DeWald RL (eds): The Textbook of Spinal Surgery. Philadelphia: JB Lippincott, 1991, pp 959–990.
8. Kostuik J, Errico T, Gleason T, Errico C: Spinal stabilization of vertebral column tumors. Spine 13:250–256, 1988.
10. Sundaresan N, Krol G, Hughes J: Treatment of malignant tumors of the spine. In Youmans J (ed): Neurological Surgery, 3rd ed. Philadelphia: WB Saunders, 1990, pp 249–274.
11. Sundaresan N, Galicich J, Lane J, Scher H: Stabilization of the spine involved by cancer. In Dunsker S, Schmidek H, Frymoyer J, III (eds): The Unstable Spine. Orlando, FL, Grune & Stratton, 1986.
12. Sundaresan N, DiGiacinto G, Hughes J: Surgical approaches to primary and metastatic tumors of the spine. In Schmidek H, Sweet W (eds): Operative Neurosurgical Techniques: Indications, Methods, Results, vol 2. Orlando, FL: Grune & Stratton, 1988.
13. Sundaresan N, DiGiacinto G, Krol G, Hughes J. Spondylectomy for malignant tumors of the spine. J Clin Oncol 7:1485–1491, 1989.
14. Stener B, Johnsen O: Complete removal of three vertebrae for giant cell tumor. J Bone Joint Surg [Br] 53:278–287, 1971.
15. Stener B: Total spondylectomy in chondrosarcoma arising from the seventh thoracic vertebra. J Bone Joint Surg [Br] 23:288–295, 1971.
16. Weinstein J: Surgical approach to spine tumors. Orthopaedics 12:897–905, 1989.

17. Weinstein J: In Frymoyer J (ed): The Adult Spine: Principles and Practice. New York: Raven Press, 1991. Differential diagnosis and surgical treatment of benign and malignant neoplasms, pp 829–860.
18. Cooper P, Errico T, Martin R, Crawford B, DiBartolo T: A systematic approach to spinal reconstruction after anterior decompression for neoplastic disease of the thoracic and lumbar spine. Neurosurgery 32:1–8, 1993.
19. Kinsella T, Miser J, Waller B, et al: Long-term follow-up of Ewing's sarcoma of bone treated with combined modality therapy. Int J Radiat Oncol Biol Phys 20:389–395, 1991.
20. Horowitz M: Ewing's sarcoma: Current status of diagnosis and treatment. Oncology 3:101–106, 1989.
21. Suit H: The problem of primary tumor control. Cancer 61:2148–2152, 1988.
22. Huvos A: Bone Tumors: Diagnosis and Prognosis. Philadelphia: WB Saunders, 1991.
23. Mirra J, Picci P, Gold R: Bone Tumors. Clinical Radiologic, and Pathologic Correlations. Philadelphia: Lea & Febiger, 1989.
24. Weinstein J, McLain R: Primary tumors of the spine. Spine 12:843–851, 1987.
25. Dahlin D, Unni K: Bone Tumors: General Aspects and Data on 8,542 Cases. Springfield, IL: Charles C Thomas, 1986.
26. American Cancer Society: Cancer statistics, 1993. CA 43:1–63, 1993.
27. Bach F, Larsen B, Rohde K, et al: Metastatic spinal cord compression. Occurrence, symptoms, clinical presentations and prognosis in 398 patients with spinal cord compression. Acta Neurochir 107:37–43, 1990.
28. Black P: Spinal metastases: Current status and recommended guidelines for management. Neurosurgery 5:726–746, 1979.
29. Boland P, Lane J, Sundaresan N: Metastatic disease of the spine. Clin Orthop 169:95–102, 1982.
30. Byrne T, Desorges J: Spinal cord compression from epidural mestastases. N Engl J Med 327:614–619, 1992.
31. Delaney T, Oldfield E: Spinal cord compression. In Devita V, Hellman S, Rosenberg S (eds): Cancer: Principles and Practice of Oncology. Philadelphia: JB Lippincott, 4th ed, 1993, pp 2118–2126.
32. Constans J, et al: Spinal metastases with neurological manifestations: Review of 600 cases. J Neurosurg 59:111–118, 1983.
33. Chein L, Kalwinsky D, Peterson G, et al: Metastatic epidural tumors in children. Med Pediatr Oncol 10:455–462, 1977.
34. Gilbert R, Kim J, Posner J: Epidural spinal cord compression from metastatic tumor: Diagnosis and treatment. Ann Neurol 3:40–51, 1978.
35. Lewis D, Packer R, Raney B, et al: Incidence, presentation, and outcome of spinal cord disease in children with systemic cancer. Pediatrics 78:438–443, 1986.
36. Rodriguez M, Dinapoli R: Spinal cord compression: With special reference to metastatic epidural tumors. Mayo Clin Proc 55:442–448, 1980.
37. Shaw M, Rose J, Paterson A: Metastatic extradural malignancy of the spine. Acta Neurochir 52:113–120, 1980.
38. Sorensen P, Borgesen S, Rohde K, et al: Metastatic epidural spinal cord compression: Results of treatment and survival. Cancer 65:1502–1508, 1990.
39. Barron K, Hisano A, Araki S, Terry R: Experiences with metastatic neoplasms involving the spinal cord. Neurology 9:91–106, 1959.
40. Fornasier V, Horne J: Metastases to the vertebral column. Cancer 36:590–594, 1975.
41. Galasko C: Skeletal Metastases. London: Butterworth's, 1986.
42. Leeson M, Makley J, Carter J: Metastatic skeletal disease in the pediatric population. J Pediatr Orthop 5:261–267, 1985.
43. Siegal T, Siegal T: Current considerations in the management of neoplastic spinal cord compression. Spine 14:223–228, 1989.
44. Torma T: Malignant tumors of the spine and the spinal epidural space: A study based on 250 histologically verified cases. Acta Chir Scand 225:1–138, 1957.
45. Bruckman J, Bloomer W: Management of spinal cord compression. Semin Oncol 5:135–140, 1978.
46. Harrington K: Metastatic disease of the spine. J Bone Joint Surg [Am] 68:1110–1115, 1986.
47. Sundaresan N, Galicich J, Bains M, Martini N, Beattie E Jr: Vertebral body resection in the treatment of cancer involving the spine. Cancer 53:1393–1396, 1984.
48. Sundaresan N, Galicich J, Lane J, Bains M, McCormack P: Treatment of neoplastic epidural spinal cord compression by vertebral body resection and stabilization. J Neurosurg 63:676–684, 1985.
49. Sundaresan N, DiGiacinto G, Hughes J: Surgical treatment of spinal metastases. Clin Neurosurg 33:503–522, 1986.
50. Berrettoni B, Carter J: Mechanisms of cancer metastasis to bone. J Bone Joint Surg [Am] 68:308–312, 1986.
51. Cramer S, Fried L, Carter K: The cellular basis of metastatic bone disease in patients with lung cancer. Cancer 48:2649–2660, 1981.
52. Galasko C, Bennett A: Relationship of bone destruction in skeletal metastases to osteoclast activation and prostaglandins. Nature 263:508–510, 1976.
53. Aoki J, Yamamoto I, Hino M, et al: Osteoclast mediated osteolysis in bone metastases from renal cell carcinoma. Cancer 62:98–104, 1988.
54. Arguello F, Boggs R, Duerst R, et al: Pathogenesis of vertebral metastasis and epidural spinal cord compression. Cancer 65:98–106, 1990.
55. Batson O: The role of the vertebral veins in metastatic processes. Ann Intern Med 16:38–45, 1942.
56. Delattre J, Arbit E, Thaler H, Rosenblum M, Posner J: A dose-response study of dexamethasone in a model of spinal cord compression caused by epidural tumor. J Neurosurg 70:920–925, 1989.
57. Ikeda H, Ushio Y, Hayakawa T: Edema and circulatory disturbances in the spinal cord compressed by epidural neoplasm in rabbits. J Neurosurg 52:203–209, 1980.
58. Manabe S, Tanaka H, Higo Y, et al: Experimental analysis of the spinal cord compressed by spinal metastasis. Spine 14:1308–1315, 1989.
59. Ushio Y, Posner R, Posner J, Shapiro W: Experimental spinal cord compression by epidural neoplasm. Neurology 27:422–429, 1977.
60. Hashizume Y, Iljima S, Kishimoto H, Hirano A: Pencil-shaped softening of the spinal cord: Pathologic study in 12 autopsy cases. Acta Neuropathol (Berl) 61:219–224, 1983.
61. Siegal T, Siegal T: Participation of serotonergic mechanisms in the pathophysiology of experimental neoplastic spinal cord compression. Neurology 41:574–580, 1991.
62. Bockman R: Hypercalcemia in malignancy. Clin Endocrinol Metab 9:317–333, 1980.
63. Graus F, Krol G, Foley K: Early diagnosis of spinal epidural metastasis: Correlation with clinical and radiologic findings (abstract). Proc Am Soc Clin Oncol 98:269, 1985.
64. Jaeckle K, Young D, Foley K: The natural history of lumbosacral plexopathy in cancer. Neurology 35:8–15, 1985.
65. Kori S, Foley K, Posner J: Brachial plexus lesions in patients with cancer. Neurology 31:45–50, 1981.
66. Redmond J III, Friede K, Cornett P, et al: Clinical usefulness of an algorithm for the early diagnosis of spinal metastatic disease. J Clin Oncol 6:154–157, 1988.
67. Rodichok L, Harper G, Ruckdeschel J, et al: Early diagnosis of spinal epidural metastases. Am J Med 70:1181–1188, 1981.
68. Akbarnia B, Rooholamini S: Scoliosis caused by benign osteoblastoma of the thoracic or lumbar spine. J Bone Joint Surg [Am] 63:1146–1155, 1981.
69. Marsh B, Bonfiglio M, Brady L, Enneking W: Benign osteoblastoma: Range of manifestations. J Bone Joint Surg [Am] 57:1–9, 1975.
70. Ransford A, Pozo J, Hutton P, Kirwan E: The behavior pattern of the scoliosis associated with osteoid osteoma or osteoblastoma of the spine. J Bone Joint Surg [Br] 66:16–20, 1984.
71. Galasko C: The significance of occult skeletal metastases, detected by skeletal scintigraphy, in patients with otherwise apparent "early" mammary carcinoma. Br J Surg 67:694–696, 1975.
72. Harbin W: Metastatic disease and the nonspecific bone scan: Value of spinal computed tomography. Radiology 145:105–107, 1982.
73. Corcoran R, Thrail J, Kyle R, et al: Solitary abnormalities in bone scans of patients with extra-osseous malignancies. Radiology 121:663–666, 1976.
74. Godersky J, Smoker W, Knutzon R: Use of magnetic resonance imaging in the evaluation of metastatic spinal disease. Neurosurgery 21:676–680, 1987.
75. Smoker W, Godersky J, Knutzon R, et al: The role of MR imaging in evaluating metastatic spinal disease. AJR Am J Roentgenol 149:1241–1248, 1987.
76. Sze G, Abramson A, Krol F, et al: Gadolinium-DTPA in the evalua-

tion of intradural extramedullary spinal disease. AJNR 9:153–163, 1988.
77. Li K, Poon P: Sensitivity and specificity of MRI in detecting malignant spinal cord compression and distinguishing malignant from benign compression fractures of vertebrae. Magn Reson Imaging 6:547–556, 1988.
78. Zimmerman R, Bilaniuk L: Imaging of tumors of the spinal canal and cord. Radiol Clin North Am 26:965–1007, 1988.
79. Mankin H, Lange T, Spanier S: The hazards of biopsy in patients with malignant primary bone or soft tissue tumors. J Bone Joint Surg [Am] 64:1121, 1982.
80. Fyfe I, Henry A, Mulholland R: Closed vertebral biopsy. J Bone Joint Surg [Br] 65:140–143, 1983.
81. Ghelman B, Lospinuso M, Levine D, O'Leary P, Burke S: Percutaneous computed tomography–guided biopsy of the thoracic and lumbar spine. Spine 16:736–739, 1991.
82. Loftus C, Michelsen C, Rapoport F, Antunes J: Management of plasmacytomas of the spine. Neurosurgery 13:30–36, 1983.
83. Malat J, Virapongse C, Levine A: Solitary osteochondroma of the spine. Spine 11:625–628, 1986.
84. Fox M, Onofrio B: The natural history and management of symptomatic and asymptomatic vertebral hemangiomas. J Neurosurg 78:36–45, 1993.
85. Vergel De Dios A, Bond J, Shives T, McLeod R, Unni K: Aneurysmal bone cyst. Cancer 69:2921–2931, 1992.
86. Di Lorenzo N, Spallone A, Nolletti A, Nardi P: Giant-cell tumors of the spine: A clinical study of six cases, with emphasis on the radiological features, treatment, and follow-up. Neurosurgery 6:29–34, 1980.
87. Savini R, Gherlinzoni F, Morandi M, et al: Surgical treatment of giant-cell tumor of the spine. J Bone Joint Surg [Am] 65:1283–1289, 1983.
88. Dahlin D: Giant-cell tumor of vertebrae above the sacrum. Cancer 39:1350–1356, 1977.
89. Green N, Robertson W, Kilroy A: Eosinophilic granuloma of the spine with associated neural deficit. J Bone Joint Surg [Am] 62:1198–1202, 1980.
90. Ippolito E, Farsetti P, Tudisco C: Vertebra plana. J Bone Joint Surg [Am] 66:1364–1368, 1984.
91. Sherk H, Nicholson J, Nixon J: Vertebra plana and eosinophilic granuloma of the cervical spine in children. Spine 3:116–121, 1978.
92. Corwin J, Lindberg R: Solitary plasmacytoma of bone vs. extramedullary plasmacytoma and their relationship to multiple myeloma. Cancer 43:1007–1013, 1979.
93. Knowling M, Harwood A, Bergasagel D: A comparison of extramedullary plasmacytoma with multiple and solitary plasma cell tumors of bone. J Clin Oncol 1:255–262, 1983.
94. McLain R, Weinstein J: Solitary plasmacytomas of the spine: A review of 84 cases. J Spine Disorders 2:69–74, 1989.
95. Valderrama J, Bullough P: Solitary myeloma of the spine. J Bone Joint Surg [Br] 50:82–90, 1988.
96. Dimopoulos M, Goldstein J, Fuller L, Delasalle K, Alexanian R: Curability of solitary bone plasmacytoma. J Clin Oncol 10:587–590, 1992.
97. Attal M, Huguet F, Schlaifer D, Payen C, Laroche M: Intensive combined therapy for previously untreated aggressive myeloma. Blood 79:1130–1136, 1992.
98. Barlogie B, Epstein J, Selvanayagam P, Alexanian R: Plasma cell myeloma—new biological insights and advances in therapy. Blood 73:865–879, 1989.
99. Gosta G, Sante T, Ljunman P, et al: Allogeneic bone marrow transplantation in multiple myeloma. N Engl J Med 325:1267–1273, 1991.
100. Kaiser T, Pritchard D, Unni K: Clinicopathologic study of sacrococcygeal chordoma. Cancer 54:2574–2578, 1984.
101. Rich T, Schiller A, Suit H, Mankin H: Clinical and pathological review of 48 cases of chordoma. Cancer 56:182–187, 1985.
102. Sundaresan N, Galicich J, Chu F, Huvos A: Spinal chordomas. J Neurosurg 50:312–319, 1979.
103. Smith J, Ludwig R, Marcove R: Sacrococcygeal chordoma. A clinicoradiologic study of 60 patients. Skeletal Radiol 16:37–44, 1987.
104. Sundaresan N: Spinal chordomas. Clin Orthop 204:135–142, 1986.
105. Sundaresan N, Huvos A, Krol G, Lane J, Brennan M: Surgical treatment of spinal chordomas. Arch Surg 122:1479–1481, 1987.
106. Cummings B, Stephen E, Harwood A: The treatment of chordomas. Cancer Treat Rev 9:299–311, 1982.
107. Suit H, Goiten M, Munzenreder J, et al: Definitive radiation therapy for chordoma and chondrosarcoma of base of skull and cervical spine. J Neurosurg 56:377–385, 1982.
108. Furman W, Fitch S, Hustu O, Callihan T, Murphy S: Primary lymphoma of bone in children. J Clin Oncol 7:1275–1280, 1989.
109. Clayton F, Butler J, Ayala A, Jae Y, Zornoza J: Non-Hodgkin's lymphoma in bone: Pathologic and radiologic features with clinical correlates. Cancer 60:2494–2501, 1987.
110. Loeffler J, Tarbell M, Kozalewich J, et al: Primary lymphoma of bone in children: Analysis of treatment results with adriamycin, prednisone, onloxin and local radiation therapy. J Clin Oncol 4:496–501, 1986.
111. Mendendenhall N, Jones J, Kramer B, et al: The management of primary lymphoma of bone. Radiother Oncol 9:137–145, 1987.
112. Ostrowski M, Unni K, Banks P, et al: Malignant lymphoma of bone. Cancer 58:2646–2655, 1986.
113. Perry J, Deodhare S, Bilbao J, Murry D, Muller P: The significance of spinal cord compression as the initial manifestation of lymphoma. Neurosurgery 32:157–162, 1993.
114. Barwick K, Huvos A, Smith J: Primary osteogenic sarcoma of the vertebral column. Cancer 46:595–604, 1980.
115. Huvos A, Woodward H, Cahan W, Higinbotham N: Postirradiation osteogenic sarcoma of bone and soft tissue: A clinicopathologic study of 66 patients. Cancer 56:1244, 1985.
116. Shives T, Dahlin D, Sim F, et al: Osteosarcoma of the spine. J Bone Joint Surg [Am] 68:660–668, 1986.
117. Sundaresan N, Rosen G, Huvos A, Krol G: Combined treatment of osteosarcoma of the spine. Neurosurgery 23:714–719, 1988.
118. Shives T, McLeod R, Unni K, Schray M: Chondrosarcoma of the spine. J Bone Joint Surg [Am] 71:1158–1165, 1989.
119. Hayes F, Thompson E, Hustu H, et al: The response of Ewing's sarcoma to sequential cyclophosphamide and adriamycin induction therapy. J Clin Oncol 1:45–51, 1983.
120. Jergens H, Gadner H, Gobel U, et al: Update of the cooperative Ewing's sarcoma studies (CESS) of the German society of pediatric oncology (GPO). Med Pediatr Oncol 17:284, 1989.
121. Meyer W, Kyn L, Marina N, et al: Ifosfamide plus etoposide in newly diagnosed Ewing's sarcoma of bone. J Clin Oncol 10:1737–1742, 1992.
122. Nesbit M Jr, Gehan E, Burgert E Jr, et al: Multimodal therapy for the management of primary, nonmetastatic Ewing's sarcoma of bone: A long-term follow-up of the first intergroup study. J Clin Oncol 8:1664–1674, 1990.
123. Rosen G, Caparros B, Nirenberg A, et al: Ewing's sarcoma: Ten-year experience with adjuvant chemotherapy. Cancer 47:2204–2213, 1981.
124. Vetti J, Gehan E, Nesbit M Jr, et al: Multimodal therapy in metastatic Ewing's sarcoma: An intergroup study. J Natl Cancer Inst 56:279–284, 1981.
125. Wilkins R, Douglas P, Burgert E Jr, Krishnan U: Ewing's sarcoma of bone. Cancer 58:2551–2555, 1986.
126. Pilepich M, Vetti T, Nesbit M, et al: Ewing's sarcoma of the vertebral column. Int J Radiat Oncol Biol Phys 7:27–31, 1981.
127. Kornberg M: Primary Ewing's sarcoma of the spine. Spine 11:54–57, 1986.
128. Burgert N Jr, Nesbit M, Garnsey L, et al: Multimodal therapy for the management of nonpelvic, localized Ewing's sarcoma of bone: Intergroup study IESS-II. J Clin Oncol 8:1514–1524, 1990.
129. Horowitz M, Neff J, Kun L: Radiotherapy versus surgery for local control. Pediatr Clin North Am 38:365–380, 1991.
130. Kinsella T, Lichter A, Miser J, et al: Local treatment of Ewing's sarcoma: Radiation versus surgery. Cancer Treat Rep 68:695–701, 1984.
131. Neff J: Nonmetastatic Ewing's sarcoma of bone: The role of surgical therapy. Clin Orthop 204:111–118, 1986.
132. Greenberg H, Kim J, Posner J: Epidural cord compression from metastatic tumor: Results with a new treatment protocol. Ann Neurol 8:361–366, 1980.
133. Dunn R, Kelly W, Whons R, Howe J: Spinal epidural neoplasia. A 15 year review of the results of surgical therapy. J Neurosurg 52:47–51, 1980.
134. Fer M, Greco F, Oldham R: Poorly Differentiated Neoplasms and Tumors of Unknown Origin. Orlando, FL: Grune & Stratton, 1987.

135. Fontana M, Pompili A, Cattani F, Mastrostefano R: Metastatic spinal cord compression. Follow-up study. J Neurosurg Sci 24:141–146, 1980.
136. Rodichok L, Ruckdeschel J, Harper G, et al: Early detection and treatment of spinal epidural metastases: The role of myelography. Neurology 20:696–702, 1986.
137. Ruff R, Lanska D: Epidural metastases in prospectively evaluated veterans with cancer and back pain. Cancer 63:2243–2241, 1989.
138. Stark R, Henson R, Evans S: Spinal metastases: A retrospective survey from a general hospital. Brain 105:189–213, 1982.
139. Harper G, Rodichuk L, Prevosti L, et al: Early diagnosis of spinal metastases leads to improved treatment outcome. Proc Am Soc Clin Oncol 1:6, 1982 (abstract).
140. Harrington K: Anterior decompression and stabilization of the spine as a treatment for vertebral body collapse and spinal cord compression from metastatic malignancy. Clin Orthop 233:177–197, 1988.
141. Kim R, Spencer S, Meredith R, et al: Extradural spinal cord compression: Analysis of factors determining functional prognosis—prospective study. Radiology 176:279–282, 1990.
142. Klein S, Sanford R, Muhlbauer M: Pediatric spinal epidural metastases. J Neurosurg 74:5–70, 1991.
143. Livingston K, Perrin R: The neurosurgical management of spinal metastases causing cord and cauda equina compression. J Neurosurg 53:839–843, 1978.
144. Manabe S, Tateishi A, Abe M, Ohno T: Surgical treatment of metastatic tumors of the spine. Spine 14:41–47, 1989.
145. Tokuhashi Y, Matsuzaki H, Sadayoshi T, Kawano H, Ohsaka S: Scoring system for the preoperative evaluation of metastatic spine tumor prognosis. Spine 15:1110–1113, 1990.
146. Siegal T, Siegal T: Surgical decompression of anterior and posterior malignant epidural tumors compressing the spinal cord: A prospective study. Neurosurgery 17:424–432, 1985.
147. Delattre J, Arbit E, Rosenblum M, et al: High dose versus low dose dexamethasone in experimental epidural spinal cord compression. Neurosurgery 22:1005–1007, 1988.
148. Vecht C, Haaxma-Reiche H, Van Putten W, et al: Initial bolus of conventional versus high-dose dexamethasone in metastatic spinal cord compression. Neurology 39:1255–1257, 1989.
149. Weisman D: Glucocorticoid treatment for brain metastases and epidural spinal cord compression: A review. J Clin Oncol 6:543–551, 1988.
150. Falcone A, Nappi J: Chemotherapy and wound healing. Surg Clin North Am 64:779–794, 1984.
151. Calkins A, Olson M, Ellis J: Impact of myelography on the radiotherapeutic management of malignant spinal cord compression. Neurosurgery 19:614–616, 1986.
152. Dorfman L, Donaldson S, Gupta P, Bosley T: Electrophysiologic evidence of subclinical injury to the posterior columns of the spinal cord after therapeutic radiation. Cancer 50:2815–2819, 1982.
153. Goodwin-Austin R, Howell D, Worthing B: Observations on radiation myelopathy. Brain 98:557–568, 1975.
154. Heller M, McBroom R, MacNab T, Perrin R: Treatment of metastatic disease of the spine with postero-lateral decompression and Luque instrumentation. Neuroorthopedics 2:70–74, 1986.
155. Macedo N, Sundaresn N, Galicich J: Decompressive laminectomy for metastatic cancer: What are the current indications? Proc Am Soc Clin Oncol 4:278, 1985.
156. Barcena A, Lobato R, Rivas J, et al: Spinal metastatic disease: Analysis of factors determining functional prognosis and choice of treatment. Neurosurgery 15:820–827, 1984.
157. Bridwell K, Jenny A, Saul T, et al: Posterior segmental spinal instrumentation (PSSI) with posterolateral decompression and debulking for metastatic thoracic and lumbar spine disease: Limitations of the technique. Spine 13:1383–1394, 1988.
158. Fidler M: Anterior decompression and stabilization of metastatic spinal fractures. J Bone Joint Surg [Br] 68:83–90, 1986.
159. Flatley T, Anderson M, Anast G: Spinal instability due to metastatic disease: Treatment by segmental spinal stabilization. J Bone Joint Surg [Am] 66:47–52, 1984.
160. Kostuik J: Anterior spinal cord decompression for lesions of the thoracic and lumbar spine: Techniques, new methods of internal fixation, results. Spine 8:512–531, 1983.
161. O'Neil J, Gardner V, Armstrong G: Treatment of tumors of the thoracic and lumbar spinal column. Clin Orthop 227:103–112, 1988.
162. Cella D, Tulsky D, Gray G, et al: The functional assessment of cancer therapy scale: Development and validation of the general measure. J Clin Oncol 11:570–579, 1993.
163. Carr B, Goodkin R: Breast cancer with osseous metastasis and herniated lumbar disc: A cautionary tale. Cancer 56:1701–1703, 1985.
164. Sundresan N, DiGiacinto G: Antitumor and anti-nociceptive approaches to cancer pain. Med Clin North Am 71:329–348, 1987.
165. Foley K: The treatment of cancer pain. N Engl J Med 31:84–95, 1985.
166. Harrington K: Anterior cord compression and spinal stabilization for patients with metastatic lesions of the spine. J Neurosurg 61:107–117, 1984.
167. Overby M, Rothman A: Anterolateral decompression for metastatic epidural spinal cord tumors. Neurosurgery 62:344–348, 1985.
168. Perrin R, McBroom R: Anterior vs. posterior decompression for symptomatic spinal metastasis. J Can Sci Neurol 14:75–80, 1987.
169. Sherman R, Waddell J: Laminectomy for metastatic epidural spinal cord tumors. Clin Orthop 207:55–63, 1986.
170. Siegal T, Tiqva P, Siegal T: Vertebral body resection for epidural compression by malignant tumors. J Bone Joint Surg [Am] 67:375–382, 1985.
171. Watkins R: Surgical Approaches to the Spine. New York: Springer-Verlag, 1983.
172. Findlay G: Adverse effects of the management of malignant spinal cord compression. J Neurol Neurosurg Psychiatry 47:761–768, 1984.
173. Findlay G: The role of vertebral body collapse in the management of malignant cord compression. J Neurol Neurosurg Psychiatry 50:151–154, 1987.
174. Fessler R, Dietle D, MacMillan M, Peace D: Lateral parascapular extrapleural approach to the upper thoracic spine. J Neurosurg 75:349–355, 1991.
175. Clark C, Keggi K, Panjabi M: Methyl methacrylate stabilization of the cervical spine. J Bone Joint Surg [Am] 66:40–46, 1984.
176. Fidler M: Pathological fractures of the cervical spine. Palliative surgical treatment. J Bone Joint Surg [Br] 67:83–90, 1985.
177. Harrington K: The use of methylmethacrylate for vertebral body replacement and anterior stabilization of pathologic fracture dislocations of the spine due to metastatic malignant disease. J Bone Joint Surg [Am] 63:36–46, 1981.
178. Sundaresan N, DiGiacinto G, Hughes J, Cafferty M, Vallejo A: Treatment of neoplastic spinal cord compression: Results of a prospective study. Neurosurgery 29:645–650, 1991.

14

Gynecologic Malignancies

Introduction and Anatomy

Allan J. Jacobs, M.D.

Gynecologic malignancies include tumors of the vulva, vagina, cervix, uterus, fallopian tube, and ovaries, as well as gestational trophoblastic neoplasms. Numerous tumors of different histology arise from each site; these may differ markedly from one another in their epidemiology, natural history, and response to treatment. The etiology and, in some cases, the molecular biology of these tumors are relatively well understood. This has led to the widespread employment of measures that have reduced the incidence and mortality of some of these diseases through prevention and early detection.

The adoption of worldwide staging systems for all these malignancies by the International Federation of Gynecology and Obstetrics (FIGO) has standardized the analysis of clinical trials. This has contributed greatly to the control of gynecologic neoplasms in all sites. It can be said of carcinomas of any site in the female reproductive tract that at least 75% of patients whose stage I lesions (i.e., lesions confined to the primary organ) are appropriately treated will survive for 5 years; this is virtually tantamount to cure. At least half of patients with stage II disease (limited regional disease) should survive 5 years, irrespective of site. The 5-year survival rate in women with primary ovarian and endometrial stage III carcinomas (those with extensive regional involvement) approaches 25% and exceeds this figure with primary cervical carcinoma.

Staging of these tumors is based on a detailed and sophisticated understanding of their patterns of spread. Gynecologic neoplasms may spread in four ways:

1. Direct extension to adjacent organs.
2. Lymphatic metastasis.
3. Hematogenous metastasis. Veins draining the vagina and the uterine corpus and cervix may carry metastases to the spine as well as to the lung because of anastomoses with the paravertebral veins.
4. Transperitoneal spread, except for vulvar cancer.

The predilection of cancers to preferentially follow each of these potential metastatic pathways varies according to the primary site, histologic type, and grade of each tumor.

Gynecologic oncologists were quick to recognize the utility of multimodality treatment. Operation plays a significant part in the treatment of most gynecologic neoplasms, but the majority of patients with gynecologic cancer are best treated using more than one modality. This chapter describes how surgery is integrated with the complementary modalities of chemotherapy and radiotherapy in the treatment of these lesions.

The operative aspects of management of gynecologic malignancies frequently require extensive pelvic dissection involving both intraperitoneal and retroperitoneal planes. Furthermore, these surgical procedures often require resection of bowel, bladder, or ureter, with subsequent repair or anastomosis. Gynecologic cancer surgeons must therefore be familiar with these techniques and with the surgical anatomy of the entire pelvis.

PELVIC SIDEWALL

It seems reasonable to begin the discussion with a description of the structures of the pelvic sidewall, since this is where pelvic surgical dissection begins in oncologic procedures.

Pelvic Sidewall Peritoneum

The peritoneum lateral to the uterus, fallopian tubes, and ovary on either side, together with its underlying areolar tissue, is known as the broad ligament (Fig. 14–1). This structure reflects anteriorly lateral to the uterus, allowing the peritoneum to envelop the round ligament. The bilateral round ligaments are structures homologous with the spermatic cord. They originate in the uterine cornua anterior to the fallopian tube, pass through the ipsilateral inguinal canal, and insert in the labium majus. The artery of the round ligament (Sampson's artery) originates from the inferior epigastric artery and runs medially near the posterior aspect of the round ligament to supply the uterus. The areolar tissue posterior to the round ligament is somewhat thicker and more vascular than other pelvic retroperitoneal areolar tissue. The pelvic peritoneum also reflects over the ovarian vessels superolaterally to the ovaries to form the infundibulopelvic ligament.

Transection of the round ligament is ordinarily the safest place to enter the retroperitoneum, but in some cases, this structure is obscured by tumor. In that circumstance, it is best to incise the peritoneum anterolaterally to the uterus and ovary. The infundibulopelvic ligament lies fairly close to the ureter, and it is best not to transect it until the ureter has been identified.

Psoas and Great Vessels

The largest pelvic retroperitoneal structure is the psoas muscle. This muscle is constant in location unless major axial malformations are present. Because it is an easily identified landmark that is difficult to injure, it serves as a good starting point for retroperitoneal dissection. The surgeon may identify it by dividing the round ligament or incising the broad ligament peritoneum anterolateral to the ovarian vessels; blunt lysis of the underlying areolar tissue exposes the muscle. The psoas is oriented in a superoinferior direction, arising from the anterior and lateral thoracic spine and inserting into the lesser trochanter of the ipsilateral femur. It is highlighted by a tendinous "racing stripe" that runs along its length. The femoral nerve runs through the body of the psoas, so prolonged retraction may cause injury. The psoas muscle serves to orient the surgeon to the location of the common iliac and external iliac arteries, which, in turn, serve as landmarks for the other great vessels of the pelvis.

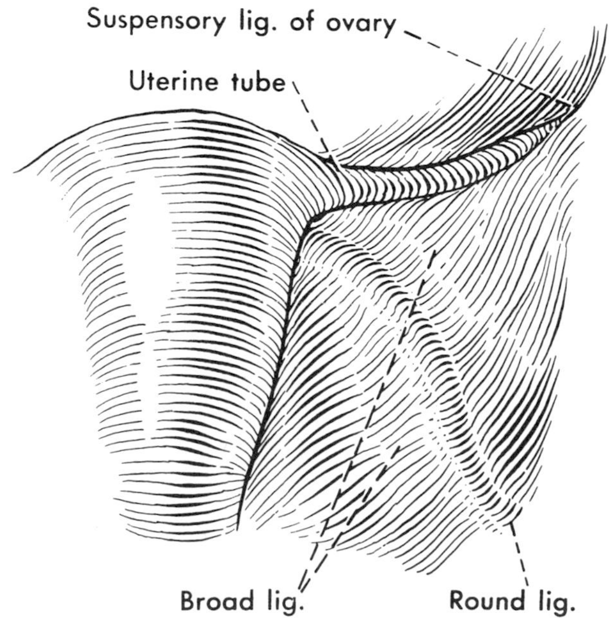

FIGURE 14–1. The broad ligament envelops the suspensory ligament of the ovary (infundibulopelvic ligament) and the round ligament. (From Hollinshead WH: Anatomy for Surgeons, vol 2, The Thorax, Abdomen and Pelvis, 2nd ed. Philadelphia: Harper & Row, 1971, p 794.)

The aorta bifurcates into the left and right common iliac arteries just anterior to the fifth lumbar vertebra, lying directly posterior to the umbilicus (Fig. 14–2). Each common iliac artery runs along the anteromedial edge of the psoas with important branches. It bifurcates at the pelvic brim into the external iliac and internal iliac arteries. The external iliac artery continues along the anteromedial aspect of the psoas, to which it contributes branches in 10% of people. It gives off the deep iliac circumflex and the inferior epigastric arteries as it reaches the inguinal ligament.

The internal iliac arteries course in a posteroinferior direction, giving off a posterior division with numerous somatic branches, and terminating deep in the pelvis in the uterine, obturator, and superior vesical arteries (Fig. 14–3). The obturator artery passes inferolaterally through the obturator fossa and the obturator foramen. The uterine artery travels medially through the cardinal ligament to supply the uterus and upper vagina. The superior vesical artery courses anteriorly to reach the bladder near the lateral aspect of the dome. Anomalies of the internal iliac arterial system are frequent.

The left common and external iliac veins are posteromedial to their respective arteries, as is the right external iliac vein. The right common iliac vein starts lateral to the artery and passes behind it to arrive at a posteromedial location at its bifurcation. The only major tributary is the circumflex iliac vein, which enters the external iliac vein anteriorly and passes anteriorly over the external iliac artery just anterior to the inguinal ligament and proximal to the origin of the deep circumflex iliac and inferior epigastric arteries.

Each internal iliac vein is situated posterolaterally to the respective artery. Traced caudally, it ramifies into a venous plexus that lies at the base of the obturator fossa and pararectal space.

Pelvic Lymph Nodes and Obturator Fossa

The pelvic nodes consist of the external iliac, internal iliac, and obturator node groups, all of which drain the

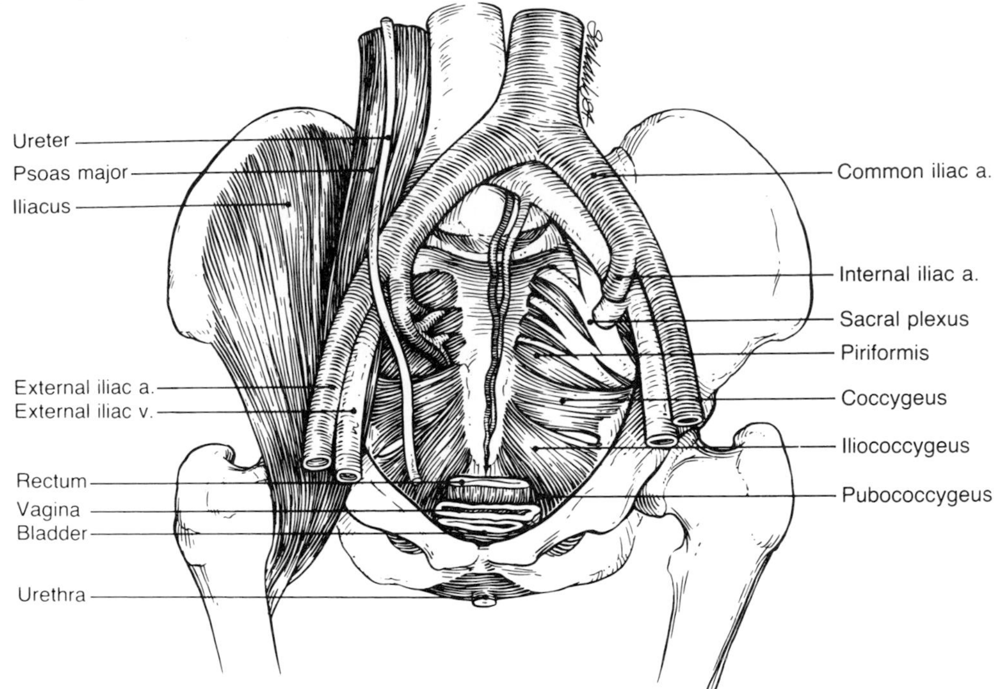

FIGURE 14–2. The aorta bifurcates at about the level of the fourth lumbar vertebra, and the vena cava bifurcates slightly caudal to the aortic bifurcation. The ureter passes from lateral to medial anterior to the bifurcation of the common iliac artery, crossing the great vessels at that point. (From Gould SF: Anatomy. In Gabbe SG, et al [eds]: Obstetrics: Normal and Problem Pregnancies, 2nd ed. New York: Churchill Livingstone, 1991, p 24.)

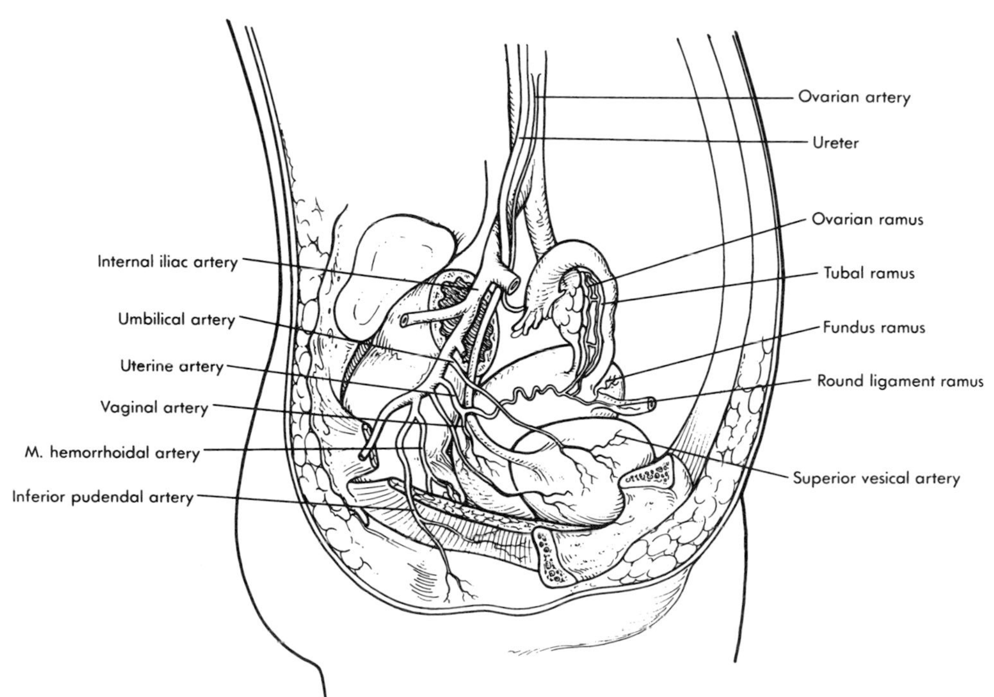

FIGURE 14–3. The branches of the internal iliac artery. In general, the branches of the anterior division of the internal iliac supply visceral structures, while the posterior division ramifies to nourish skeletal structures. (From Reiffenstuhl G: Practical pelvic anatomy for the gynecologic surgeon. In Nichols DH [ed]: Gynecologic and Obstetric Surgery. St. Louis: Mosby, 1993, p 30.)

pelvic viscera and must be removed in surgical staging or treated when pelvic lymph node metastasis is likely. These nodes drain into the ipsilateral common iliac nodes, which drain into the aortic nodes on both sides.

The external iliac and common iliac lymph nodes lie embedded in a strip of adipose tissue sitting on the anterior surface of their associated arteries. The genitofemoral nerve, a sensory nerve, runs within or lateral to the node bundle. The internal iliac nodes (a misnomer) lie on the medial surface of the external iliac vein, from which they are easily separated (Fig. 14–4). They are often adherent to the retrocelomic surface of the broad ligament peritoneum near the ureter. They join the common iliac node chain near the bifurcation of the common iliac vessels.

The obturator nodes are located in the obturator fossa. The obturator fossa is bounded anteriorly by the psoas; medially by the internal iliac artery; and posteriorly, inferiorly, and laterally by the pelvic wall musculature. The obturator nerve courses through it in a superoinferior direction, passing through the obturator foramen to innervate the abductors of the thigh and to provide sensation to the medial thigh and knee. Numerous blood vessels pass through the fossa, mostly posterior to the obturator nerve. The remainder of the fossa is filled with the obturator nodes and the fat that envelops them. The node bundle narrows superiorly, just inferior to the bifurcation of the common iliac vein, before joining the common iliac trunk. This facilitates ligation. Distally, the obturator node bundle narrows as it joins the internal iliac bundle posterior to the internal iliac vein near the inguinal ligament.

Presacral nodes are often seen medial to the distal common iliac vein. They may be involved in advanced uterine and cervical malignancies when obstruction of primary lymph node drainage opens anastomoses through lymphatics in the uterosacral ligaments.

Ureters and Ovarian Vessels

The ureters and ovarian vessels are considered together because they lie close together through most of their course. In addition, the ureters pass close to structures that require division in most gynecologic ablative surgery. The ureters are variable in size, and their location is easily distorted by pelvic disease. They are close to several other tubular structures that also run in a superoinferior direction, including the ovarian vessels, the iliac vessels, vessels of the sigmoid mesentery, and even the common iliac node bundle. Ureteral injury is one of the most frequent serious consequences of gynecologic operations. When not markedly dilated or attenuated, a ureter may be recognized by its peristalsis and its consistency, which resembles that of a rubber band. Aspiration of blood or urine from a vascular structure using a 25-gauge needle attached to a syringe helps identify vascular pelvic structures. Arteries usually pulsate, but they may not do so in a woman with marked atherosclerosis or calcification. When these maneuvers do

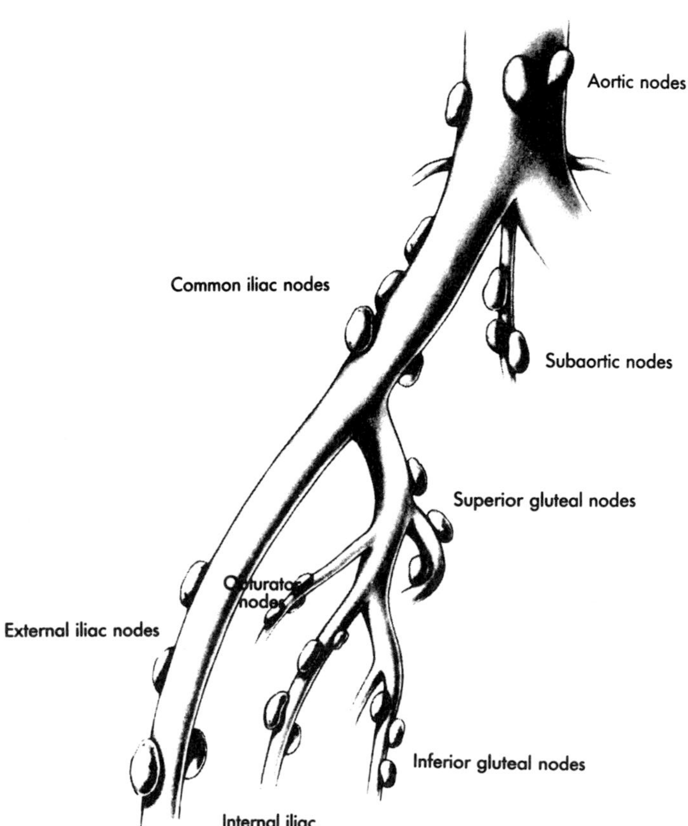

FIGURE 14–4. Location of the major pelvic node groups. (From Droegemueller W: Anatomy. In Herbst AL, et al [eds]: Comprehensive Gynecology, 2nd ed. St. Louis: Mosby Year Book, 1992, p 62; Plentl AA: Lymphatic System of the Female Genitalia. Philadelphia: WB Saunders, 1971, p 13.)

not help, it may be necessary to trace a tubular structure superiorly to the renal pelvis or inferiorly to the cardinal ligament to identify it as a ureter.

The ureter arises from the renal pelvis and travels inferiorly. It may be just lateral to, or even overlying, the vena cava or aorta (Fig. 14–5). Usually, however, the abdominal portion of the ureter sits near the anteromedial or anterior aspect of the psoas. It lies anterior to the great vessels and posterior to the ovarian vessels. At the pelvic brim, the ureter passes over the bifurcation of the common iliac artery and travels posteromedially (Fig. 14–6). It courses just lateral to the posterior peritoneum of the broad ligament in an inferior direction parallel to the infundibulopelvic ligament and ovary, but 1 to 6 cm posterior to them. The ureter enters the cardinal ligament 1 to 2 cm lateral to the cervix or upper vagina, passing posterior to the uterine artery. It curves posteromedially to enter the base of the bladder anterior to the upper third of the vagina. The ureters derive their blood supply from adjacent vessels. The renal and ovarian vessels supply the abdominal ureters, and the internal iliac, uterine, and inferior vesical vessels supply the pelvic ureter.

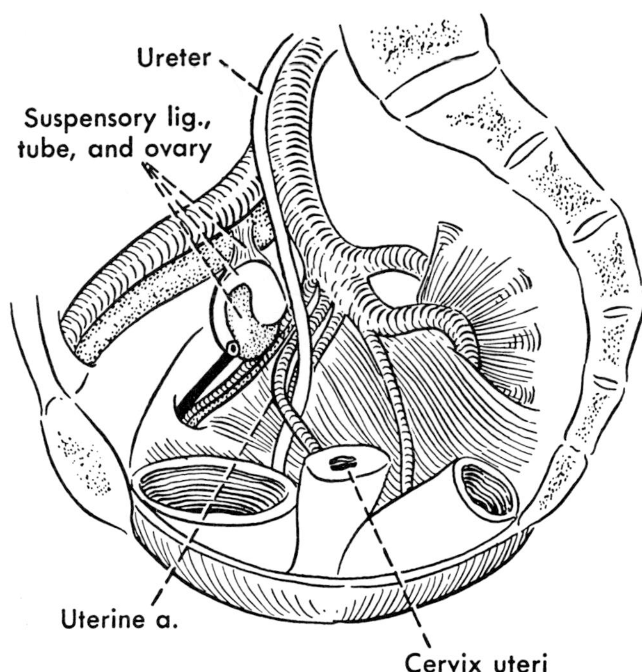

FIGURE 14–6. The ureter passes medially, and anterior to the great vessels, at the pelvic brim. (From Hollinshead WH: Anatomy for Surgeons, vol 2, The Thorax, Abdomen and Pelvis, 2nd ed. Philadelphia: Harper & Row, 1971, p 723.)

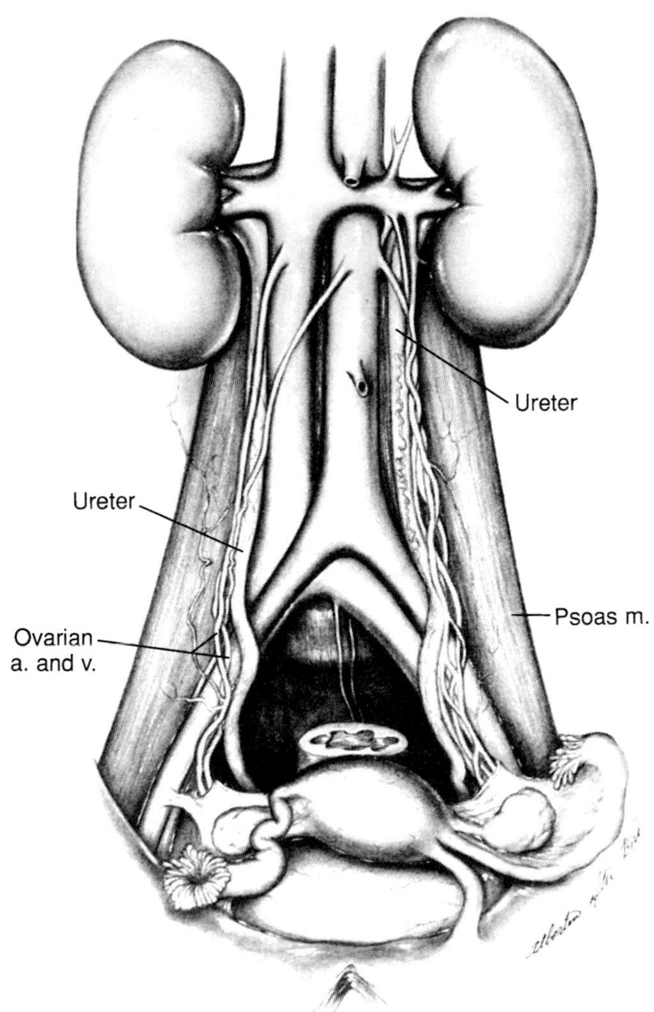

FIGURE 14–5. Relation of the abdominal ureters to the psoas muscle, the vena cava, the aorta, and the ovarian vessels. (From Hollinshead WH: Anatomy for Surgeons, vol 2, The Thorax, Abdomen and Pelvis, 2nd ed. Philadelphia: Harper & Row, 1971, p 537.)

The ovarian vessels lie close to, and in a fixed relationship to, the ureters. Both ovarian arteries arise from the abdominal aorta 3 to 5 cm distal to the renal vessels. They course inferiorly, parallel and anterior to the ureters, to which they may give off branches. The position of both the arteries and the ureters becomes more lateral and anterior as they course distally, and they cross the bifurcation of the common iliac artery anteriorly at the pelvic brim. At this point, the ovarian arteries approach the peritoneum, where they are enveloped in a fold of broad ligament known as the infundibulopelvic ligament. Each ovarian artery approaches its ovary from a lateral direction, passing dorsal to the ovary through the mesovarium, giving off ovarian branches, and finally anastomosing with the uterine artery anterior to the utero-ovarian ligament. The ovarian veins run immediately adjacent to the ovarian arteries. The right ovarian vein enters the inferior vena cava, and the left ovarian vein contributes to the left renal vein.

PELVIC VISCERA

Uterus and Cervix

The uterus sits in the center of the pelvis, where its posterior surface and the anterior surface of the fundus are invested by peritoneum. The upper, muscular portion is the

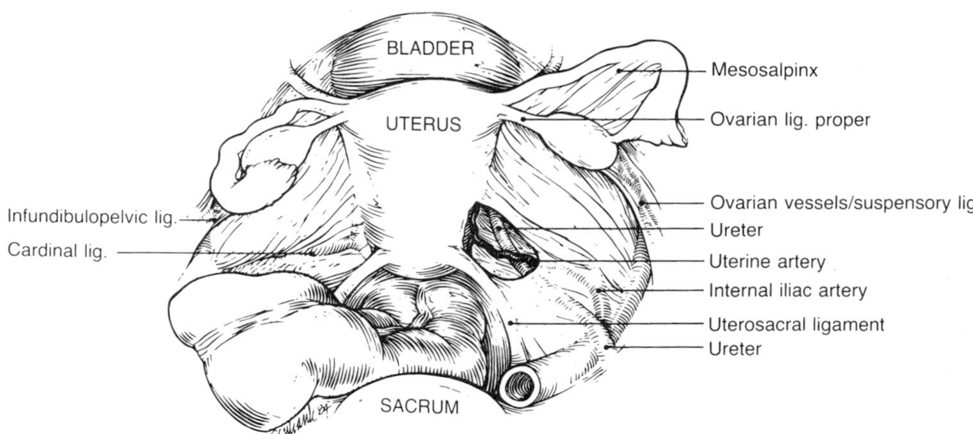

FIGURE 14–7. The uterine ligaments, seen from a posterior view. (From Gould SF: Anatomy. In Gabbe SG, et al [eds]: Obstetrics: Normal and Problem Pregnancies, 2nd ed. New York: Churchill Livingstone, 1991, p 23.)

fundus, and the lower, fibrous portion is the cervix. The uterus normally is about 9 cm long and 6 cm wide. The uterus generally is flexed anteriorly, although a posterior position is not abnormal. It is supported by the cardinal (Mackenrodt's or lateral cervical) and uterosacral ligaments (Fig. 14–7). The bilateral round ligaments are structures homologous with the spermatic cord (see Fig. 14–1). They originate in the cornua anterior to the fallopian tube, pass through the ipsilateral inguinal canal, and insert in the labium majus. The uterus draws its blood supply from two major and three minor sources on each side. The major sources are the uterine artery and vein, which arise from the internal iliac vessels, and the ovarian artery and vein, which form an anastomotic arcade with the uterine vessels lateral to the uterus (see Fig. 14–7). The minor sources of vascular supply are the artery of the round ligament (Sampson's artery), arising from the inferior epigastric artery; branches of the middle rectal, traveling through the uterosacral ligament; and anastomoses from vaginal vessels whose source is the internal pudendal vessels. Lymphatics follow the blood vessels. The cervix drains to the deep pelvic nodes (obturator, external iliac, and internal iliac); the fundus drains to these and to the aortic nodes directly. Innervation is provided by autonomic nerves. Parasympathetics arise from S-2 through S-4. Sympathetic nerves arise from T-10 through T-12. Pain fibers parallel the sympathetic fibers, also arising from T-10 through T-12. Sympathetic, parasympathetic, and afferent fibers form a plexus lateral to the uterus (Frankenhäuser's plexus) and enter the uterus through the cardinal ligaments.

Ovary and Fallopian Tube

The ovary and the fallopian tube lie medial to the broad ligament, to which they are connected by the mesovarium and the mesosalpinx, respectively (Fig. 14–8). The ovary is situated posterior to the tube and is ovoid in shape. Its longest dimension is up to 4 cm in women of reproductive age, but it is smaller during other stages of life. Each ovary is connected to the fundus of the uterus by a fibrous band called the utero-ovarian ligament (Fig. 14–9). The fallopian tube may be 10 to 12 cm long, with a diameter of up to 1 cm at the proximal end. The fimbriated end of the tube is situated just anterior to the ovary. The tube courses medially, narrowing all the while. The lateral half of the tube is known as the ampulla, and the medial half as the isthmus. The canal of the fallopian tube passes through the cornu of the uterus, emptying into the myometrium. This portion is known as the interstitial portion of the tube.

The ovaries and fallopian tubes derive their blood supply from the ovarian arteries and the uterine arteries. These vessels form an anastomotic arcade inferior to the ovary and the tube. Knowledge of the course of the paired ovarian arteries is vital to surgeons who operate for gynecologic

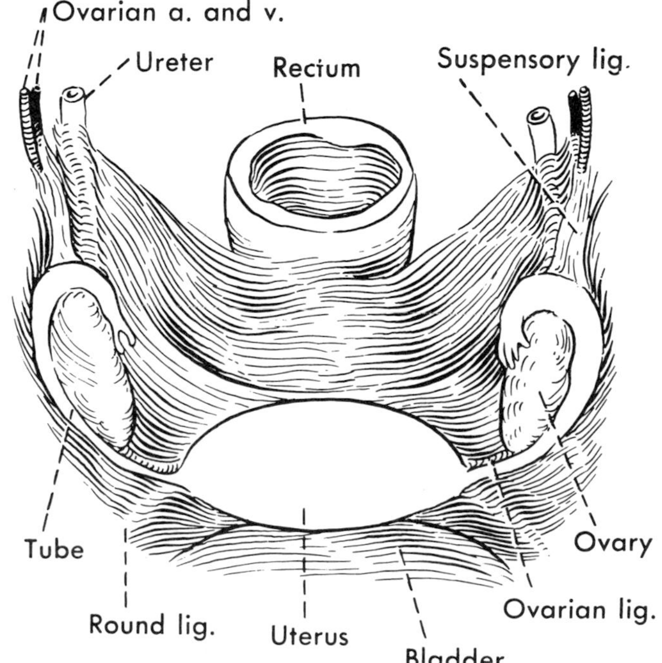

FIGURE 14–8. The mesovarium and mesosalpinx. (From Hollinshead WH: Anatomy for Surgeons, vol 2, The Thorax, Abdomen and Pelvis, 2nd ed. Philadelphia: Harper & Row, 1971, p 789.)

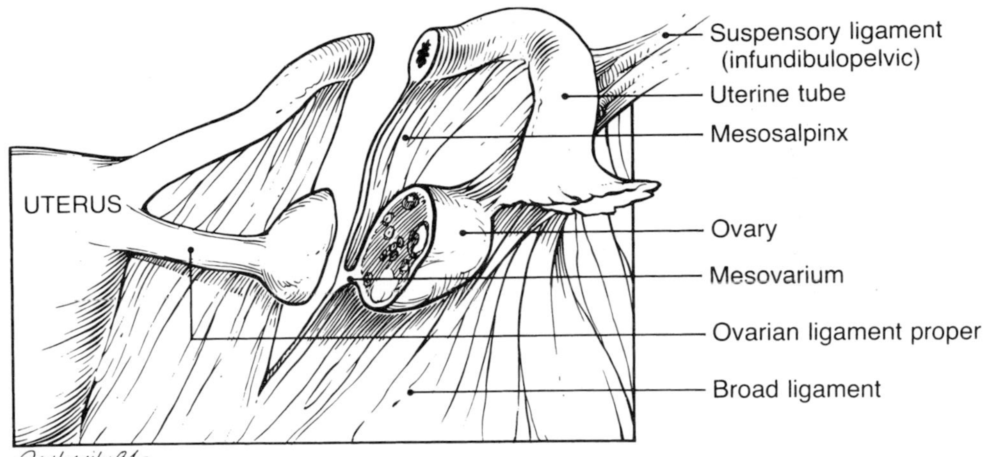

FIGURE 14–9. The adnexal structures, from a posterior view. (From Gould SF: Anatomy. In Gabbe SG, et al [eds]: Obstetrics: Normal and Problem Pregnancies, 2nd ed. New York: Churchill Livingstone, 1991, p 19.)

cancer or other diseases of the abdominal and pelvic retroperitoneum. Ovarian lymphatic vessels drain both to pelvic nodes and to aortic nodes, following both arterial trunks that supply the ovaries. Innervation derives from the lower thoracic roots and reaches the ovary via abdominal plexus.

Bladder and Rectum

The bladder lies anterior to the uterus in the midline and is attached to the cervix and upper vagina by loose connective tissue forming the vesicocervical and vesicovaginal septa. This septum forms a plane that is easily dissected surgically, but it contains numerous small blood vessels originating from the bladder and vagina. It is worth mentioning that the nerves to the bladder pass from the presacral plexus anteriorly through the base of the uterosacral and cardinal ligaments, so they are inevitably subject to injury during radical dissection in the deep pelvis.

The rectum lies posterior to the uterus but, in contrast to the bladder, does not directly abut it. Rather, its peritoneal reflection forms a deep pocket known as the cul-de-sac of Douglas (uterorectal pouch), so that the midline attachment of the rectum at the peritoneal reflection normally is only to the vagina. The septum between the rectum and vagina consists of loose connective tissue that is avascular and easily susceptible to operative lysis. Like the nerves of the bladder, the nerves of the rectum are frequently injured during radical dissection, and prolonged constipation is a side effect of operations such as radical hysterectomy.

DEEP PELVIC STRUCTURES

The peritoneum is enveloped by a muscular wall, except anterior to the vertebral column. This muscular wall serves, for the most part, to move the trunk (although this is not the role of the diaphragm) and to contain the abdominal contents in the appropriate shape. The muscles enveloping the peritoneum lie close to it, with no significant intervening structures, *except in the pelvis.* There, the muscles of the pelvic floor and sidewall lie at some distance from the peritoneum.

The pelvic floor is formed by the levator ani muscle group (Fig. 14–10). This group contains (proceeding anteromedially to posterolaterally) the puborectal, pubococcygeal, and iliococcygeal muscles. The levator ani forms a plate several centimeters caudal to the most caudal peritoneal surfaces. The bladder and urethra anteriorly, the rectum posteriorly, and the uterus and vagina between them occupy the space in the midline between the peritoneum and the levator ani (Fig. 14–11). The vagina pierces this muscle about halfway down its length. Lateral to the bladder and rectum are the paravesical and pararectal spaces (Fig. 14–12). These "spaces" actually contain loose connective tissue. The pararectal space is continuous with the obturator fossa laterally; a plexus of veins is located at its base. Lateral to the cervix and upper vagina is the cardinal ligament, which is a condensation of connective tissue. The uterine artery runs through the cardinal ligament anteriorly, and the bladder innervation runs through it posteriorly. Each cardinal ligament is continuous with a more medial band of connective tissue posterior to the uterus and enveloped on three sides by peritoneum. These bands are called the uterosacral ligaments; anatomy texts regard the uterosacral and cardinal ligaments as one structure called the posterior cervical ligament. The uterosacral ligament is anchored posteriorly near the sigmoid mesentery. Posterior to the rectum lie the rectal stalks, which carry the middle rectal arteries.

VAGINA AND VULVA

Vulva and Groin

The vulva is a term used to describe the external female genitalia (Fig. 14–13). The vestibule is the junction between the vulva and the vagina. It is demarcated by the hymen, which is usually seen as a membranous ring in virgins, but whose remnants are present in circumferential

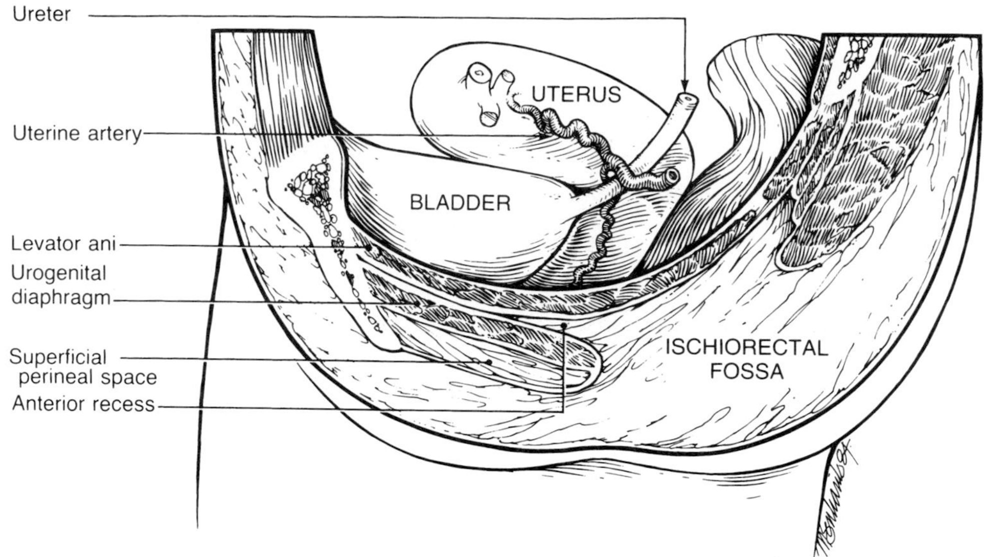

FIGURE 14–10. The levator ani forms the pelvic floor, while the urogenital diaphragm provides additional support for the urethra and perineum. (From Gould SF: Anatomy. In Gabbe SG, et al [eds]: Obstetrics: Normal and Problem Pregnancies, 2nd ed. New York: Churchill Livingstone, 1991, p 14.)

papular tags in sexually active women. Deep and lateral to the vestibule on either side are the bulbocavernous muscles and the vestibular bulbs, which are masses of erectile tissue. Bartholin's glands lie at the posterior aspect of the vestibular bulbs and open into the vestibule. The urethral orifice is situated at the anterior aspect of the vestibule. The labia minora are delicate folds covered by non–hair-bearing skin that lie lateral to the vestibule. The labia majora are thicker folds of hair-bearing skin and subcutaneous tissue that lie lateral to the labia minora. The lateral aspects of the labia majora are demarcated by labiocrural folds.

The paired internal pudendal arteries, which arise from the anterior division of the internal iliac artery, constitute the major blood supply to the vulva (Fig. 14–14). Each has three branches. The clitoral artery runs anteriorly through the urogenital diaphragm, supplying the clitoris, the surrounding tissues of the anterior vulva, and the bulbocavernous muscle. The perineal artery perforates the urogenital diaphragm lateral to the posterior fourchette and supplies the perineum, the labia majora, and the labia minora. The third branch of the internal pudendal artery is the inferior rectal artery. Venous return parallels the arteries.

Most innervation is supplied by the internal pudendal nerve, which is derived mostly from the third and fourth sacral nerve roots. It follows the internal pudendal artery and its branches. Some sensory innervation to the vulvar skin is supplied by other nerves. The ilioinguinal nerve supplies the mons veneris. The posterior femoral nerve innervates the posterolateral vulva. The genitofemoral nerve participates in the innervation of the labia majora.

Lymphatic drainage is directed anteriorly toward the mons veneris, where it turns laterally to terminate in the superficial inguinal lymph nodes (Fig. 14–15). These nodes

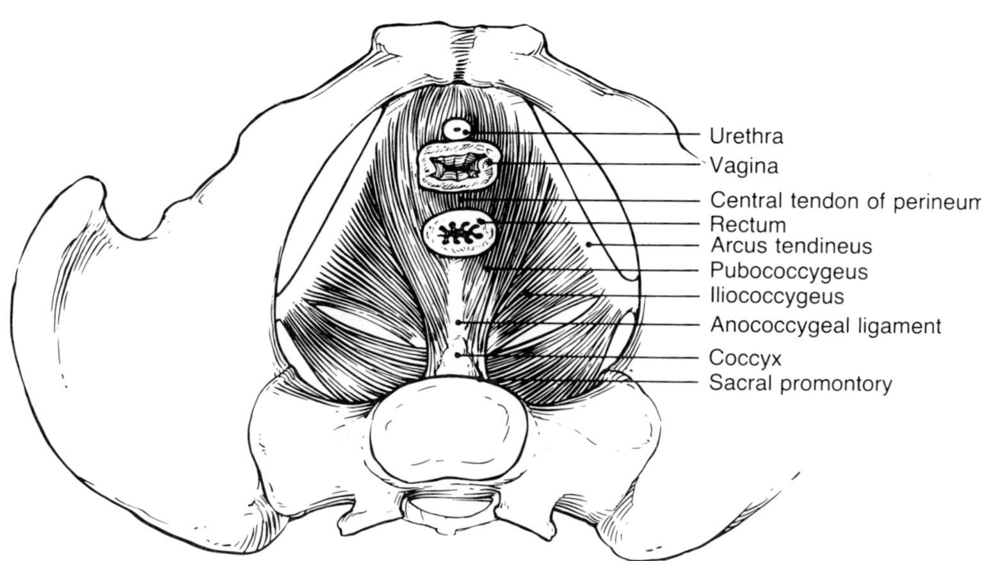

FIGURE 14–11. The component structures of the pelvic floor. (From Gould SF: Anatomy. In Gabbe SG, et al [eds]: Obstetrics: Normal and Problem Pregnancies, 2nd ed. New York: Churchill Livingstone, 1991, p 7.)

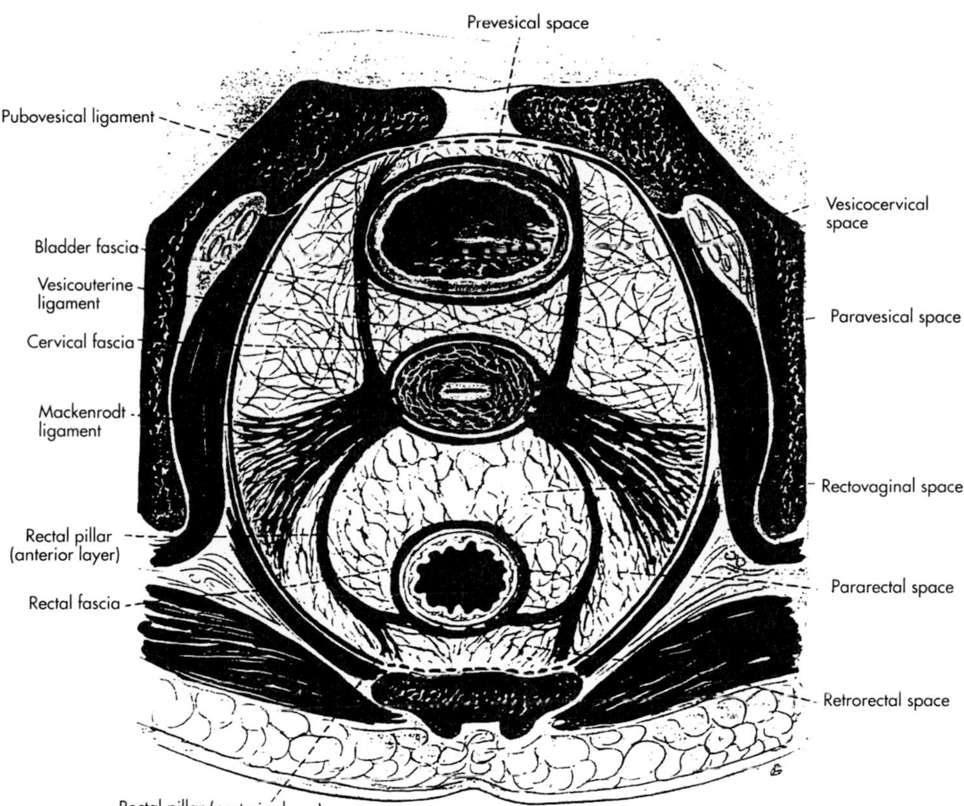

FIGURE 14–12. The paravesical and pararectal spaces, and the other potential spaces of the deep pelvis. (From Von Peham H, Amreich JA: Gynaekologische Operationslehre. Basel, S. Karger, 1930 and Reiffenstuhl G: Practical pelvic anatomy for the gynecologic surgeon. In Nichols DH [ed]: Gynecologic and Obstetric Surgery. St. Louis: Mosby, 1993, p 29.)

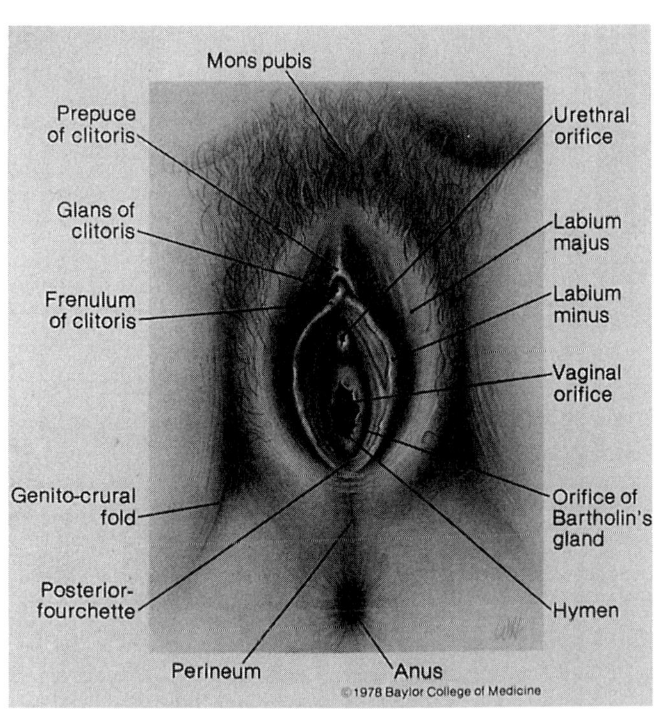

FIGURE 14–13. The cutaneous structures of the external genitalia. (From Kaufman RH, et al: Benign Diseases of the Vulva and Vagina, 3rd ed. Chicago: Year Book Medical Publishers, 1989, p 2.)

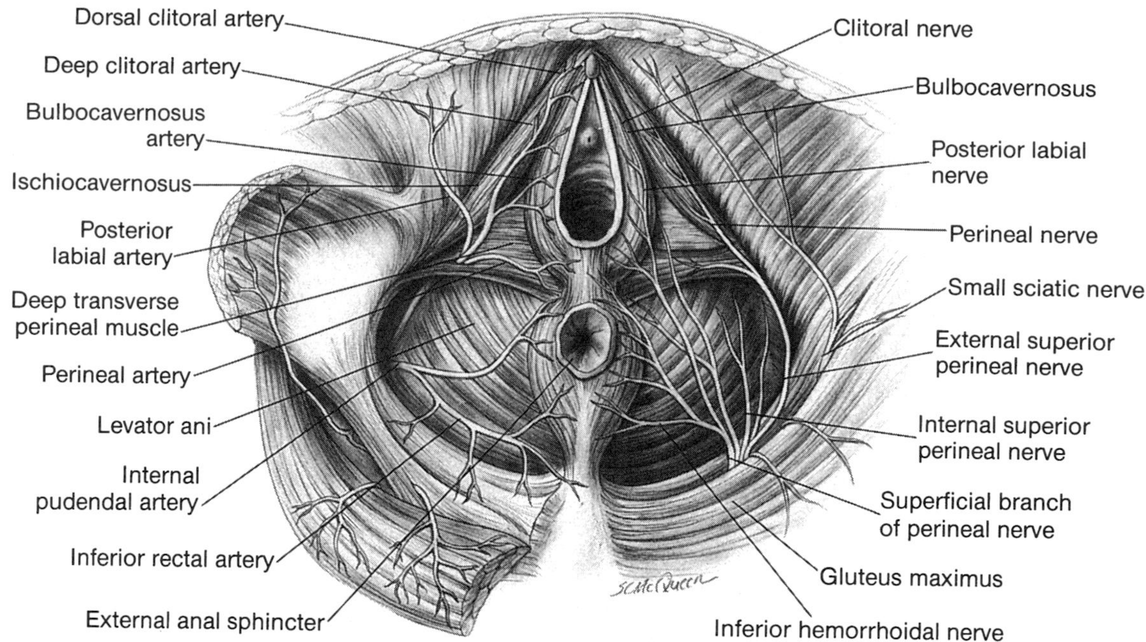

FIGURE 14–14. Blood supply and innervation of the vulva. (From Droegemueller W: Anatomy. In Herbst AL, et al [eds]: Comprehensive Gynecology, 2nd ed. St. Louis: Mosby–Year Book, 1992, p 66, and Mattingly RF, Thompson JD: Te Linde's Operative Gynecology, 6th ed. Philadelphia: JB Lippincott, 1985.)

lie in Scarpa's fascia, between the fascia of Camper superficially and the deep fasciae consisting of the external oblique fascia, the fascia lata, and the cribriform plate (the attenuated fascia lata overlying the femoral triangle). From there, the lymphatic drainage proceeds to the deep femoral nodes (also known as deep inguinal nodes), which lie in a bundle of fat occupying the space in the femoral triangle between the cribriform plate and the femoral vessels. The surgical anatomy of the femoral triangle is of importance in the treatment of vulvar carcinoma (Fig. 14–16). The triangle is bounded by the inguinal ligament cephalad, the sartorius muscle laterally, and the long adductor muscle

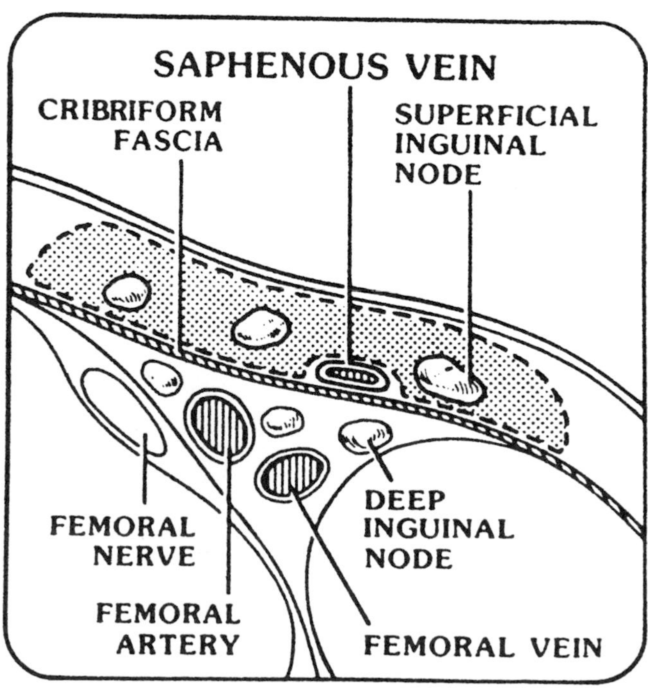

FIGURE 14–15. The cribriform plate separates the superficial from the deep groin nodes. (From Rowley KC, et al: Prognostic factors in early vulvar cancer. Gynecol Oncol 31:45, 1988.)

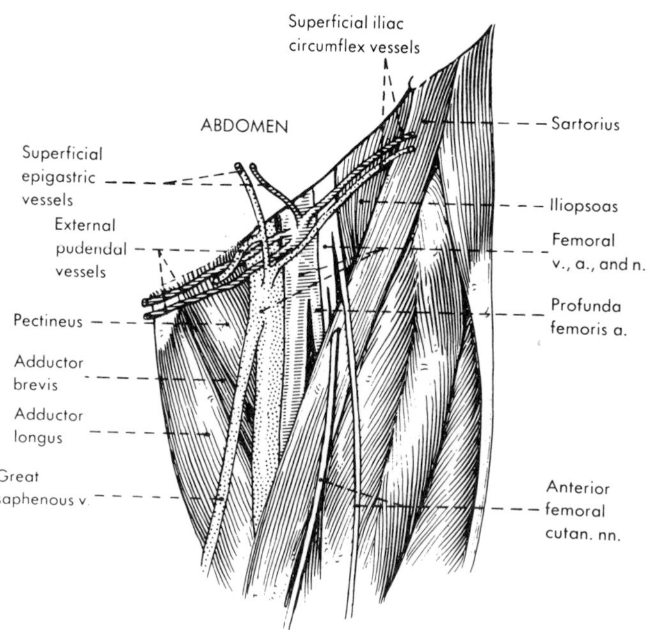

FIGURE 14–16. The femoral triangle. (From Hollinshead WH: Anatomy for Surgeons, vol 3, The Back and Limbs, 3rd ed. Philadelphia: Harper & Row, 1982, p 687.)

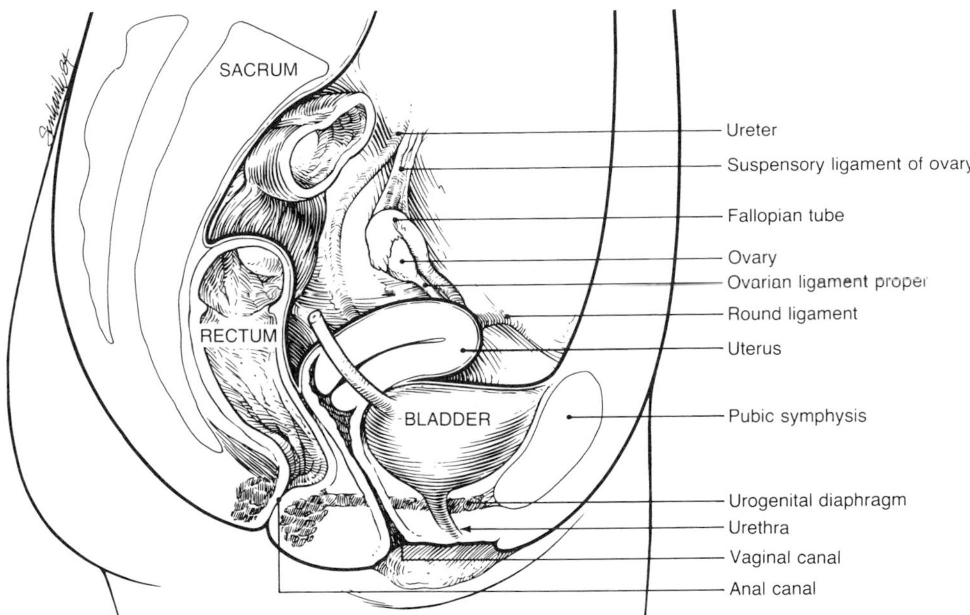

FIGURE 14–17. Anatomic relationships of the vagina. (From Gould SF: Anatomy. In Gabbe SG, et al [eds]: Obstetrics: Normal and Problem Pregnancies, 2nd ed. New York: Churchill Livingstone, 1991, p 18.)

medially. The pectineal muscle forms the posterior floor of the triangle medially, as does the iliopsoas muscle laterally. The femoral artery runs through the triangle in a superoinferior direction, flanked by the femoral vein medially and the femoral nerve laterally. The superficial epigastric artery and the superficial iliac circumflex artery ramify from the anterior aspect of the femoral artery at the superior edge of the triangle, at the inferior margin of the inguinal ligament. Corresponding veins are usually present. Theoretically, there should be a lymph node immediately anterior to these vessels, which is termed Cloquet's node. It represents the most proximal of the deep femoral nodes and is said to be a sentinel node for cephalad extension of tumor. In fact, there is rarely a single distinct lymph node that can be so identified, but this portion of the nodal bundle is often sent as a specimen separate from the other femoral nodes.

Two to 5 cm distal to this, the superficial external pudendal artery branches from the anteromedial aspect of the artery. This is an important anatomic landmark, as the saphenous vein joins the femoral vein just medial to the origin of the superficial external pudendal artery.

Vagina

The vagina is a tubular muscular structure lined with a squamous epithelium that does not have a keratinized superficial layer. Ordinarily, no glands or other skin appendages are present. The anatomic relationships are distally, the vulva; anteriorly, the urethra and bladder (the terminal ureters are immediately anterior to the vagina in its upper third); posteriorly, the rectum and the cul-de-sac of Douglas; laterally, the cardinal ligaments in the upper two thirds; and proximally, the cervix (Fig. 14–17). The vagina is attached to the cervix higher posteriorly than anteriorly. The vagina passes through the levator ani muscles halfway to two thirds of the way toward the introitus, with the urogenital diaphragm enveloping it distal to the levator sling. Most vaginal tumors arise in the upper third, on the posterior wall.

The lower third of the vagina shares the blood vessels, lymphatic drainage, and innervation of the vulva; the upper third shares that of the cervix. The middle third receives contributions from both sources. Lymphatic drainage of the lower third of the vagina is the same as that of the vulva; the upper third drains to the pelvic nodes.

References

1. Droegemueller W: Anatomy. In Herbst AL, Mishell DR Jr, Stenchever MA, Droegemueller W (eds): Comprehensive Gynecology, 2nd ed. St. Louis: Mosby Year Book, 1992, pp 43–77.
2. Gould SF: Anatomy. In Gabbe SG, Niebyl JR, Simpson JL (eds): Obstetrics: Normal and Problem Pregnancies, 2nd ed. New York: Churchill Livingstone, 1991, pp 3–37.
3. Hollinshead WH: Anatomy for Surgeons, vol 2, The Thorax, Abdomen and Pelvis, 2nd ed. Philadelphia: Harper & Row, 1971.
4. Hollinshead WH: Anatomy for Surgeons, vol 3, The Back and Limbs, 3rd ed. Philadelphia: Harper & Row, 1982.
5. Kaufman RH, Friedrich EG Jr, Gardner HL: Benign Diseases of the Vulva and Vagina, 3rd ed. Chicago: Year Book Medical Publishers, 1989.
6. Plentl AA, Friedman EA: Lymphatic System of the Female Genitalia. Philadelphia: WB Saunders, 1971.
7. Reiffenstuhl G: Practical pelvic anatomy for the gynecologic surgeon. In Nichols DH (ed): Gynecologic and Obstetric Surgery. St. Louis: Mosby, 1993, pp 26–71.
8. Rowley KC, Gallion HH, Donaldson ES, et al: Prognostic factors in early vulvar cancer. Gynecol Oncol 31:43–49, 1988.

Cervical Malignancies

Allan J. Jacobs, M.D. • Manjeet Chadha, M.D.

EPIDEMIOLOGY

The American Cancer Society estimates that there will be approximately 15,800 new cases of invasive carcinoma of the cervix diagnosed in the United States in 1995.[1] This will result in approximately 4800 deaths annually. In addition, more than 50,000 new cases of carcinoma in situ will be diagnosed. Risk factors for the disease include geographic location; for example, cervical carcinoma is quite common in Latin America. It is least common in women of Jewish and European descent. The sexual activity, parity, and socioeconomic class of the patient affect the incidence. The disease is more common in women with a history of multiple sexual partners and those who first had intercourse at an early age.[2–4] Prenatal exposure to diethylstilbestrol (DES) may be related to the development of cervical neoplasia.[5] Cigarette smokers are at higher risk for cervical neoplasia,[6] as are women infected with the human immunodeficiency virus (HIV).[7] The human papillomavirus (HPV) has been associated as an etiologic cofactor in genital carcinogenesis.[8] Well over 50% of lesions of high-grade intraepithelial neoplasia[9, 10] and of invasive carcinoma[11–13] contain DNA sequences of certain HPV types, especially types 16 and 18.

LIFE HISTORY

The majority of cervical neoplasias are of squamous cell histology, and the most common site of origin is the portio of the cervix. Squamous cell carcinoma most frequently originates in pre-existing lesions of high-grade cervical intraepithelial neoplasia (CIN). Adenocarcinoma may originate there or from endocervical glands. Adenocarcinoma in situ has been described,[14] but its relationship to the genesis of adenocarcinoma is not well understood.

Invasive cervical carcinoma may metastasize via four pathways. Direct extension is the most common mode of spread. This usually occurs laterally into the cardinal ligaments (which are also known as the parametria). These lesions frequently extend cephalad to the corpus or caudad to the vagina. In advanced cases, the tumor may extend anterior to the bladder, and posterior into the posterior fornix, and then to the cul-de-sac of Douglas and the rectum.

Lymphatic metastasis is the other major route of spread. Involvement of the deep pelvic (obturator, internal iliac, and external iliac) lymph nodes is found in about 15% of stage IB,[15] 30% of stage IIB, and almost 50% of stage IIIB squamous lesions.[16, 17] The tumor may undergo retrograde metastases to the inguinal nodes. More commonly, the tumor travels cephalad to the common iliac, aortic, and mediastinal nodes. Surgical staging studies demonstrate that carcinoma involves aortic nodes in about 25% of women with stage II and stage III squamous lesions.[18] Eventually, supraclavicular nodes are involved. If routine scalene node biopsy samples are taken in all patients with positive aortic nodes, about 25% will show cancer.[19, 20]

Hematogenous dissemination is seen mostly in advanced, recurrent, and poorly differentiated lesions.[21] Anastomoses between pelvic and paravertebral veins allow primary hematogenous metastases to occur in the spine as well as in the lung.

Finally, transperitoneal dissemination may be seen when the tumor has eroded through the entire corpus or into the cul-de-sac of Douglas. Up to 11% of women who undergo laparotomy for cervical carcinoma demonstrate positive peritoneal washings.[22–24] This finding is associated with a dismal prognosis. Women with positive peritoneal cytology findings are apt to experience intraperitoneal recurrence. Ovarian metastases are occasionally encountered in ovaries removed during radical hysterectomy. These metastases presumably arise through peritoneal implantation or transtubal migration of cancer cells. The observation of such spread in adenocarcinoma[25] led the Gynecologic Oncology Group to review its data. It found the incidence of ovarian metastases to be 0.5% (4 of 770) in squamous cell carcinoma and 1.7% (2 of 117) in adenocarcinoma.[26]

Left untreated, most cervical carcinomas grow relatively slowly. Pelvic persistence or recurrence leads to severe pain as a result of infiltration of the lumbar and sacral plexus. Venous compression and lymphatic obstruction may lead to painful and disabling edema of the lower extremities that is not amenable to treatment. Central disease results in painful and malodorous necrosis, as well as vesicovaginal and rectal fistulas. Massive bleeding may sometimes occur. Occasionally there is rectal obstruction, requiring palliative colostomy. Eventually, the ureters become obstructed, and death supervenes. More commonly, death results from distant metastases.

PATHOLOGY

At least 80% of cervical carcinomas demonstrate squamous cell histology; most of the remainder are adenocarci-

TABLE 14–1
Histologic Varieties of Cervical Cancer

Histologic Type	Known Associated Factors
Squamous cell (includes large cell keratinizing, large cell nonkeratinizing, and small cell)	Human papillomavirus (HPV), smoking, immunosuppression
Endocervical type adenocarcinoma	HPV, smoking
Adenoma malignum	Peutz-Jeghers syndrome
Papillary villoglandular adenocarcinoma[203]	—
Clear cell adenocarcinoma	Prenatal DES exposure
Endometrioid adenocarcinoma	—
Serous carcinoma	—
Adenoid cystic carcinoma[204-206]	—
Verrucous carcinoma[207]	HPV
Basal cell carcinoma[208]	—
Adenosquamous carcinoma[47]	HPV
Glassy cell carcinoma[49, 50]	HPV
Mucoepidermoid carcinoma[209]	HPV
Neuroendocrine carcinoma[48, 210]	HPV
Sarcoma (includes endocervical stromal sarcoma, carcinosarcoma, adenosarcoma, and leiomyosarcoma)[209, 211]	—
Embryonal rhabdomyosarcoma[209, 211]	—
Melanoma[212]	—
Lymphoma[209, 211]	—

nomas.[27–31] The remainder are composed of a multitude of histologic types (Table 14–1).

Squamous cell carcinoma arises from the transformation zone of the cervix. This is the annular area of epithelium at the outer margins of the glandular endocervix, which undergoes squamous metaplasia at or after puberty. Squamous cell carcinoma may be keratinizing or nonkeratinizing. It is controversial whether the presence of keratinization or of poor cytologic differentiation worsens the prognosis.[32] Stendahl et al.[33] and Bichel and Jakobsen[34] studied the survival of patients with squamous lesions of all stages who were treated with radiation. They identified risk factors that they have incorporated into a scoring system (Table 14–2). DNA ploidy is also a significant prognostic factor, with a DNA index greater than 1.5 being associated with a worse prognosis.[35]

Squamous cell carcinoma usually arises in a lesion of CIN. This lesion is invisible and symptomless, being detectable only through cytologic screening. It is graded as CIN 1, CIN 2, or CIN 3, depending on the proportion of the cervical epithelium that is involved.[36] The CIN classification is preferable to the older dysplasia–carcinoma in situ classification, as it correlates better with prognosis. CIN 1 lesions usually regress and may be merely observed unless they worsen.[37, 38] Higher-grade CIN should be treated, as it is likely to progress to carcinoma.

Histologically, adenocarcinoma resembles the glandular endocervical epithelium. It may arise de novo, from adenocarcinoma in situ,[14] or from CIN.[39] Adenocarcinoma in situ is a relatively unusual lesion. Its prognosis is unknown, so it should be treated.

An invasive cervical adenocarcinoma of a given stage and size probably has a prognosis similar to that of a comparable squamous lesion. Endocervical carcinomas tend to expand the cervix and spread to the corpus by direct extension. The cephalad and lateral aspects of such tumors are not likely to receive a tumoricidal dose when they are treated using radiation. This may explain why hysterectomy following radiotherapy may confer a survival advantage in stages IB, IIA, and IIB.[40–43] Adenoma malignum (minimal deviation adenocarcinoma) is a variant of adenocarcinoma in which the cells are indistinguishable from normal endocervical cells. It is often seen in patients with Peutz-Jeghers syndrome.[44]

Clear cell carcinoma has a prognosis that, stage for stage, is similar to that of squamous lesions.[45] This unusual tumor is becoming even rarer, as it occurs mostly in young women exposed during early fetal life to DES.[5] That drug has rarely been used in pregnant women since its identification in 1971 as a transplacental carcinogen.[46]

Adenosquamous carcinoma,[47] neuroendocrine carcinoma, mucoepidermoid carcinoma, and glassy cell carcinoma are all HPV-related lesions thought to originate from subepithelial reserve cells. All carry a much worse prognosis than the varieties already discussed, as they are prone to early lymphatic and hematogenous metastasis. These le-

TABLE 14–2
Prognosis Scoring System in Cervical Carcinoma[35]

Parameter	Score*		
	1	*2*	*3*
Structure	Exophytic, papillary solid	Small cords and groups of cells	Marked cellular dissociation
Cell type	Large cell, nonkeratinizing	Large cell, keratinizing	Small cell, nonkeratinizing
Nuclear polymorphism	>75% mature nuclei; few enlarged nuclei	25% to 75% mature nuclei	<25% mature nuclei; numerous irregular nuclei
Mitoses	<1 per high-power field	1–5 per high-power field	>5 per high-power field
Mode of invasion	Well-defined	Cords; less marked	Groups of cells or diffuse growth
Stage of invasion	Minimal stromal invasion	Nodular; into submucosa and connective tissue	Massive; among muscles and vessels
Vascular invasion	None	Possible	Well established
Cellular response (lymphocytes)	Marked (continuous rim)	Moderate (several large patches)	Slight (few small patches or no cells)

*8 to 13: Good prognosis; 14 to 16: moderate prognosis; 17 to 24: poor prognosis.

sions usually recur, even when treated at an early clinical stage. In one series, 11 of 15 stage IB adenosquamous carcinomas recurred after therapy, 9 of them outside the pelvis.[47] The prognosis for neuroendocrine tumors is, if anything, worse; cures are rare or nonexistent, even in early lesions.[48] Recurrence is mostly distant or simultaneously distant and pelvic. Tamimi and colleagues[49] found that, of 24 cases of stage IB glassy cell carcinoma treated by radical hysterectomy, 14 recurred. Twelve of these recurrences were at the vaginal apex, and an additional one was within the pelvis. Lotocki and coworkers[50] improved the long-term survival rate to 87% by administering pelvic radiation after radical hysterectomy.

The other varieties of malignancy listed in Table 14–1 are too unusual to merit discussion here. The accompanying references cite useful articles in the primary literature.

EARLY DETECTION, DIAGNOSIS, AND STAGING

Early Detection

The majority of cases of cervical carcinoma can be prevented by regular cervical cytologic studies (Papanicolaou's smear). This screening technique can also detect many cases at an early stage. Standard American practice is for annual screening of all asymptomatic women who have ever been sexually active and who have never had lower genital tract neoplasia. The American College of Obstetricians and Gynecologists and the American Cancer Society support this practice, with the proviso that after three consecutive negative cytologic examination results, the Pap smear may be performed less frequently at the discretion of the physician.

The Pap smear is obtained by scraping the exocervix with an Ayer spatula and then scraping the endocervix by rotating a stiff brush such as the Cytobrush[51] in the cervical canal. The material on each instrument is transferred to a glass slide by rubbing the instrument against the slide. Fixative is applied immediately; aerosol fixative preparations are available commercially.

Slides should be read using the Bethesda classification (Table 14–3).[52] References in cytology reports to Papanicolaou class should be abandoned, as should vague terms such as koilocytosis and squamous atypia. Opinion is presently in flux regarding the appropriate action when Pap smears are read as atypical squamous cells of undetermined significance (ASCUS) or as low-grade squamous intraepithelial lesion (SIL). The recommendations provided here are those of the American College of Obstetricians and Gynecologists.[53] A reliable patient with a diagnosis of ASCUS can return for repeated examinations in 6 months. A second report of ASCUS warrants colposcopy. Similarly, a cytologic diagnosis of low-grade SIL in a reliable patient warrants repeated examination in 4 to 6 months; a second finding of SIL mandates colposcopy. If the diagnosis is confirmed by colposcopically directed biopsy, ablation or excision may be employed; alternatively, colposcopic observation every 3 to 4 months without active treatment is acceptable, as most low-grade SILs regress spontaneously. The lesion should be treated actively if colposcopic abnormalities persist for a year, however. Colposcopically directed biopsies are mandatory in women with cytologic findings showing high-grade SIL, and treatment should include all documented lesions.

TABLE 14–3
The Bethesda System for Reporting Cervical and Vaginal Cytologic Diagnosis[52]*

Adequacy of the Specimen
Satisfactory for evaluation
Satisfactory for evaluation but limited by (specify reason)
Unsatisfactory for diagnosis (specify reason)

General Categorization
Within normal limits
  Benign cellular changes (see description)
  Epithelial cell abnormality (see description)

Descriptive Diagnosis
Normal
Benign cellular changes
  Infection
    Trichomonas vaginalis
    Fungal organisms (e.g., *Candida*)
    Bacteria morphologically consistent with *Actinomyces* species
    Predominance of coccobacilli consistent with shift in vaginal flora
  Cellular changes associated with herpes simplex virus
  Other (specify)
Reactive changes
  Inflammation (includes typical repair)
  Atrophy with inflammation
  Radiation
  Intrauterine contraceptive device (IUD)
  Other
Epithelial cell abnormalities
  Atypical squamous cells of undetermined significance (ASCUS): qualify
  Low-grade SIL (encompasses HPV and CIN 1)
  High-grade SIL (encompasses CIN 2 and CIN 3)
  Squamous cell carcinoma
Glandular cell abnormalities
  Endometrial cells, cytologically benign, in a postmenopausal woman
  Atypical glandular cells of undetermined significance: qualify
  Endocervical carcinoma
  Endometrial carcinoma
  Extrauterine adenocarcinoma
  Adenocarcinoma, not otherwise specified
Other malignant neoplasms (specify)

SIL, Squamous intraepithelial lesion; HPV, human papillomavirus; CIN, cervical intraepithelial neoplasia.
*Each cytologic report consists of the three elements listed in the table: a statement of the adequacy of the specimen, a general categorization, the descriptive diagnosis.

TABLE 14–4
Indications for Conization

The entire transformation zone is not visible.
Biopsy or cytology demonstrates a neoplastic glandular lesion.
An intraepithelial lesion, or one that is not clearly invasive, is present on endocervical curettage.
Biopsy demonstrates microinvasive carcinoma.
Result of cytologic diagnosis or colposcopic assessment is more severe than the tissue diagnosis.

Colposcopy is performed by staining the cervix with 3% to 5% acetic acid and then examining the cervix using a colposcope. A detailed description of the technique is beyond the scope of this chapter. The entire exocervix is visualized. The colposcopist notes whether the entire transformation zone (TZ) is seen. Endocervical curettage is performed using a Kevorkian curet. Punch biopsy samples are taken of the worst-appearing lesions on the exocervix. If the entire TZ is not seen and no frank invasion is present on cervical biopsy, conization is mandatory. Other findings that mandate conization are listed in Table 14–4. In the absence of these conditions, ablative therapy of CIN is permissible. The colposcopist should be aware that adenocarcinoma in situ, and sometimes adenocarcinoma, is not visible colposcopically. Treatment of CIN is described in more detail below.

Diagnosis

Invasive cervical carcinoma is sometimes detected by cervical cytology in asymptomatic women. More frequently, symptoms call the disease to the attention of the patient. Bleeding following douching or intercourse is the first symptom of an exocervical lesion. As the tumor grows, it may bleed spontaneously or produce a clear discharge. This is the next step in the symptomatology of exocervical lesions and is the first symptom of endocervical cancer. Pelvic pain, back pain, and unilateral edema and pain of the lower extremity are late symptoms. The last is pathognomonic of metastasis to the pelvic sidewall. Weight loss and abdominal distention suggest advanced disease.

Physical examination usually reveals a papillary or ulcerated lesion of the cervix. The cancer may also be endophytic, expanding the cervix without disturbing the epithelium of the cervical portio. An endocervical cancer may not be visible but will be accessible to endocervical curettage or conization. The physical examination should seek metastatic disease in the vagina, the inguinal nodes, and the supraclavicular nodes. Bimanual and rectovaginal examination is performed to determine whether there is anterior spread toward the bladder or posterior spread toward the rectum and cul-de-sac and, most important, whether there is extension into the cardinal ligaments.

Laboratory tests consist of a complete blood count and a general chemistry screen. The platelet count is often elevated in patients with advanced lesions, and many of these patients are also anemic. Squamous cell carcinoma antigen (TA4) may be drawn; this is elevated in many advanced tumors and may be used to monitor the course of treatment.[54]

Staging

Ancillary testing includes imaging and endoscopy. Radiologic testing should determine whether there is hydroureter or lymphadenopathy. Computed tomography (CT) of the pelvis and abdomen using intravenous contrast material achieves both these ends.[55] An intravenous pyelogram may be performed as an alternative to CT with contrast. Barium enema is performed only if indicated by symptoms or general health screening needs. A chest radiograph should be obtained. Cystoscopy should be performed in all patients except those with small lesions confined to the cervix. A bladder biopsy is taken if abnormalities are noted. Lesions larger than 4 cm and those extending beyond the cervix should be staged surgically. Abdominal exploration, washings, and high common and/or aortic lymphadenectomy are performed via laparoscopy or via a flank incision (see below). If enlarged common iliac or aortic nodes are noted on the CT scan, fine-needle aspiration may be performed, and staging lymphadenectomy can be omitted if metastases are found. Similarly, the presence of tumor in supraclavicular nodes or other distant sites obviates the need for staging lymphadenectomy.

A formal stage is assigned using International Federation of Gynecologists and Obstetricians (FIGO) criteria (Table 14–5). It should be noted that FIGO staging is based on clinical evaluation. Results of operative staging (except for conization and superficial biopsy procedures) and CT may not be used to assign a formal stage.

Table 14–5
FIGO Staging System for Cancer of the Cervix

Stage	Definition
I	Cancer is confined to the cervix and corpus
Ia1	Minimal microscopically evident stromal invasion
Ia2	Invasive lesions with depth of invasion up to 5 mm and surface diameter up to 7 mm
Ib	Larger invasive lesions confined to the cervix, whether clinically visible or not
II	Involvement of the upper two thirds of the vagina or involvement of the parametria (cardinal ligaments) but not extending to the pelvic sidewall
IIa	Cancer involving the upper two thirds of the vagina
IIb	Cancer involving the parametria but not extending to the pelvic sidewall
III	Cancer involving the lower third of the vagina or extending to the pelvic sidewall
IIIa	Cancer involving the lower third of the vagina
IIIb	Cancer that extends to the pelvic sidewall or that is coincident with hydronephrosis or a nonfunctioning kidney
IVa	Involvement of bladder or rectal mucosa, which must be demonstrated by biopsy; bullous edema of the bladder is not sufficient to categorize a tumor as stage IVa
IVb	Distant metastasis outside the true pelvis

MODALITIES OF TREATMENT

Surgery

Cone biopsy is an operation used in the treatment of CIN. Some believe that it is sufficient treatment for minimally invasive carcinoma. The operation consists of removal of a cone-shaped section of cervix using a knife, the beam of a carbon dioxide laser, or an electrosurgical loop. The procedure should be performed under colposcopic control to ensure that the entire TZ is removed. The size and shape of the cone depend on the location of both the TZ and the lesion, on the size and shape of the cervix, and on the reproductive desires of the patient. Endocervical curettage should be performed after excision of the cone specimen to confirm that no squamous epithelium remains proximal to the endocervical surgical margin. Laser or loop excision should be used only if the operator is sufficiently skilled to avoid tissue destruction at the tissue margins, so that the specimen can be evaluated histologically for involvement by CIN. The authors perform laser conization using the handpiece held against the dissection plane in the cervix rather than using the laser joystick. First, several circumferential injections into the cervix of 1% lidocaine with epinephrine 1:100,000 are given, for a total of 8 to 10 ml. Conization is then performed using a laser power setting of 50 W. Loop electrosurgical excision procedures (LEEPs) can be performed extremely rapidly. They are well tolerated in an office setting if a cervical block is given using lidocaine with epinephrine, as described above. LEEP is the procedure of choice for a well-trained operator because it is so easily performed.[56] All three methods—cold knife, laser, LEEP—are equally efficacious in curing the patient of CIN.

Intraoperative complications of all types of conization procedures include hemorrhage and uterine perforation. The major postoperative complication is delayed bleeding, which occurs in at least 10% of cases. This typically is seen 5 to 14 days postoperatively, when the eschar sloughs off.[57, 58] Cervical stenosis leading to dysmenorrhea, amenorrhea, and infertility has been widely reported but has not been well quantified. It is easily treated using laser vaporization.[59] Cervical incompetence may lead to recurrent abortion or premature birth, according to most[60–62] but not all[63] authors. The wide disparity in complication rates among various studies makes it difficult to compare cold knife, laser, and LEEP methodologies with regard to safety.

A number of operations used exclusively in the treatment of gynecologic cancer are employed in the treatment of invasive cervical carcinoma. These include three variations of hysterectomy: extrafascial hysterectomy, modified radical hysterectomy, and radical hysterectomy. Piver et al.[64] classified these as, respectively, extended hysterectomy types 1, 2, and 3. The modified radical procedure is often termed a Wertheim hysterectomy,[65] and the radical procedure goes by the eponyms Meigs[66] and Okabayashi.[67] Because these eponyms are often used loosely, they lead to confusion and are best avoided. In addition, three types of exenteration may be used to treat cervical cancer: anterior, posterior, and total exenteration. Finally, staging lymphadenectomy is often employed in the evaluation of advanced cervical carcinoma prior to therapeutic radiation. These procedures and their complications are described in this section; their applications are discussed subsequently.

Hysterectomy

The different types of hysterectomy employed in gynecologic oncology are depicted in Table 14–6. The differences among these procedures are related to the degree of resection of the cardinal ligaments, the uterosacral ligaments, and the vagina. These procedures do not differ with respect to preservation or removal of the ovaries, which may be retained or excised with any of these procedures.

In a standard total abdominal hysterectomy, the lateral plane of dissection enters the cervical stroma just medial to the attachment of the cardinal ligament. Some surgeons also incise the cervix anteriorly. Thus, some peripheral cervical stroma is left behind. The uterosacral ligament is divided at its attachment to the cervix. The vagina is severed at its attachment to the cervix.

The extended extrafascial hysterectomy differs in that the lateral plane of dissection is adjacent to the cervix but does not include cervical stroma. The uterosacral ligament is divided at its attachment to the cervix. A short vaginal cuff of up to 1 cm is taken. This modification of the total abdominal hysterectomy ensures that the entire cervix is removed. This procedure is appropriate for stage Ia1 cervical carcinoma and for cancer of the upper genital tract.

Complications associated with standard and extended extrafascial hysterectomy are similar. The most common postoperative complication of abdominal hysterectomy is infection. Febrile morbidity in reported series varies from 11% to 36%.[68, 69] A large series from 13 collaborating hospitals reported a rate of 31%.[70] The infection rate can be reduced by a brief (<24-hour) course of prophylactic antibiotics; one randomized study reduced febrile morbidity from 20% to 14%, pelvic and wound infections from 21% to 14%, and urinary tract infections from 21% to 9%.[71] Approximately 15% of women undergoing hysterectomy require transfusion.[70, 72] The bladder and ureters are each injured in 0.5% or fewer cases.[73, 74] Bowel injuries and pulmonary emboli are uncommon complications, each occurring in fewer than 1% of cases.[73, 74] Sexual dysfunction and depression have been reported, but their frequency and severity are uncertain. Mortality is 0.1% to 0.3% and generally is due to sepsis or to pulmonary emboli.[73, 74]

A modified radical hysterectomy divides the cardinal ligament about one third to one half of the distance between the cervix and the pelvic sidewall, just medial to the ureter. The ureter is dissected free of its medial and superior attachments but remains adherent to the cardinal ligament laterally. This preserves the blood supply to the ureter,

TABLE 14–6
Varieties of Hysterectomies

Anatomic Feature	Conservative Hysterectomy	Extrafascial Hysterectomy	Modified Radical Hysterectomy	Radical Hysterectomy
Pararectal, paravesical spaces	Not developed	Not developed	Developed	Developed
Cardinal ligament	Dissection plane medial, within cervix	Divided just lateral to cervix	Divided ⅓ to halfway between cervix and sidewall	Divided at pelvic sidewall
Uterosacral ligament	Divided at cervix	Divided at cervix	Divided halfway between cervix and rectum	Divided at rectum
Vagina	Divided at cervix	Minimal cuff; entire cervix removed	2-cm vaginal cuff	⅓ to ½ of vagina removed
Ureters	Identified and traced	Identified and traced	Medial and superior parametrial attachments freed	Totally freed from parametria
Ovaries, lymph nodes	Removal depends on clinical needs	Removal depends on clinical needs	Removal depends on clinical needs	Removal depends on clinical needs

greatly reducing the possibility of ureteral fistula. The uterosacral ligaments are also divided in their midportions, preserving bladder innervation and thus making prolonged catheterization unnecessary. This elegant procedure is rarely performed because it is too extensive for intraepithelial neoplasia and stage IA1 carcinoma but is not sufficiently radical for more extensive lesions. Complications are similar to those for conservative hysterectomy.

Dargent[75] described the treatment of stage IB cervical carcinoma using laparoscopic pelvic lymphadenectomy combined with a vaginal procedure, the Schauta hysterectomy, which achieves the same degree of cardinal ligament, uterosacral ligament, and vaginal ablation as a modified radical hysterectomy. This interesting approach decreases recovery time and, possibly, morbidity. A determination of the applicability of this approach awaits the publication of several investigators' mature survival data for patients with lesions of various histology and size.

Radical hysterectomy involves severing the cardinal ligament at the sidewall and the levator ani. The uterosacral ligaments are also divided near their inferolateral attachment. Many surgeons now conserve 1 cm of the cardinal and uterosacral ligaments to allow more prompt return of voiding. Severing of the cardinal ligament inevitably requires that the ureters be stripped free from all their attachments from their passage into the cardinal ligaments to the ureterovaginal junction. This may render some ureteral segments nonviable because of compromised blood supply. Consequently, radical hysterectomy carries an irreducible ureteral fistula rate of about 2%.[76] The proximal third to half of the vagina is removed during this procedure. Pelvic lymphadenectomy is almost invariably performed with radical hysterectomy.

Radical hysterectomy is associated with certain well-defined acute complications. It can be carried out in obese and elderly women without a significant increase in the acute complication rate, provided the patients are otherwise healthy.[77, 78] At least half of all patients who undergo radical hysterectomy require transfusion.[79] The most frequent acute postoperative complication of radical hysterectomy is urinary tract infection,[76] which occurs in at least 15% of women. In Webb and Symmonds' series,[76] wound infections and deep vein phlebitis each occurred in 5% of cases. Major complications, which occur in 1% to 5% of patients in recent series, include ureteral fistula, bladder fistula, pulmonary embolus, and intestinal fistula or obstruction.[76, 77, 80, 81] Urinary fistulas occur either immediately as a result of unrecognized injury or more than 5 days postoperatively, presumably as a result of devascularization, which is inherent to the operation. Almost all patients have transient urinary dysfunction and require continuous or intermittent catheterization for up to 3 months before they are able to void spontaneously with a postvoiding urinary residual volume under 100 ml. This is said to be due to tonic contraction of the sphincter,[82, 83] inability to initiate detrusor contractions,[84] or both.[85] The cause of this complication is interruption or damage to nerves supplying the bladder; this results from dissection of the bladder base and lateral division of the cardinal and uterosacral ligaments. Since this dissection is an integral part of the procedure, prolonged inability to void is unavoidable; it can be minimized by leaving a cuff of 1 cm when dividing the cardinal and uterosacral ligaments.

Chronic complications may include any complication known to occur after laparotomy. In addition, there are several chronic sequelae specific to this procedure. Many of these involve the urinary tract.

As has been stated, dissection of the entire posterior aspect of the base of the bladder from its posterior attachments, along with lateral dissection of the cardinal and uterosacral ligaments, damages the vesical nerve supply. This damage may persist a long time and often does not completely resolve. Consequently, many patients have permanent voiding dysfunction. This may consist only of loss of bladder sensation. Some women have permanent difficulty initiating voiding. A few must perform the Credé maneuver in order to urinate.

In most patients a functionally unimportant transient

hydroureter develops owing to denervation of the distal ureter. In a few patients, this persists chronically. In occasional patients, clinically significant stenosis of the distal ureter develops due to scarring in the operative bed. This is more prone to develop if radical hysterectomy is followed by pelvic external irradiation.[86, 87]

Interruption of lymphatic drainage from the lower extremity is an inevitable consequence of the extensive lymphadenectomy performed to effect a surgical cure of cervical cancer. Adequate anastomoses usually develop. If they do not, two possible complications may result. Lymphocyst is a frequent complication of radical hysterectomy, occurring after 3% to 20% of these procedures.[88, 89] A lymphocyst is a collection of lymphatic fluid in the pelvic retroperitoneal space, resulting from continued drainage of lymph from severed lymphatics arising in the lower extremity. Lymphocyst is usually harmless. It may result in infection, pain, or ureteral obstruction, the last two resulting from pressure of the fluid. If any of these complications occur, the lymphocyst must be drained and marsupialized. Accurate figures regarding the frequency of lymphocyst are hard to find. Closure of the pelvic peritoneum at the end of the procedure has largely been abandoned over the last 10 years. This allows the lymph to drain into the peritoneal cavity, and the impression of many surgeons is that lymphocyst has become much less common following radical hysterectomy. The second complication that may occur from interruption of lymphatic channels is unilateral or bilateral lower extremity edema. This may be more likely to occur if postoperative radiation is given.

Another common chronic sequela of radical hysterectomy is constipation.[90] This may last for many months. It is a nuisance rather than a serious problem, since it can be managed by laxatives and it eventually resolves. Manometric measurements following radical hysterectomy were abnormal in all patients studied in one series and included altered relaxation of the internal sphincter, increased distention needed to trigger relaxation, and decreased rectal sensation.[90]

Pelvic Exenteration

Exenteration consists of a radical hysterectomy combined with en bloc removal of major adjacent structures. Total pelvic exenteration was described by Brunschwig.[91] In its classic form, it consists of en bloc removal of the uterus, ovaries, fallopian tubes, bladder, rectum, and vagina, together with all soft tissues out to the pelvic sidewall, including the levator ani. As originally described, diversion of waste was accomplished by performance of a ureterosigmoidostomy and end sigmoid colostomy. The Bricker ileal conduit[92] came to be employed as the standard form of urinary diversion, reducing the incidence of chronic pyelonephritis and making bodily wastes less unpleasant for the patient to handle.

Other exenterative procedures include anterior exenteration, in which the rectum is spared, and posterior exenteration, in which the bladder is left behind.

The technique of exenteration has undergone a variety of modifications. The fact that both the terminal ileum and the ureters were irradiated contributed to a high complication rate, so Nelson introduced the transverse colon urinary conduit.[93, 94] The sigmoid colon can also be used for a conduit, with the terminal descending colon brought out as a colostomy; this eliminates the need for an intestinal anastomosis. Total vaginectomy is not necessary when the lesion does not grossly involve the vagina. Under these circumstances, the vagina is amputated at the levator ani and a low rectal anastomosis is performed.[95] This reduces the incidence of pelvic floor complications, the most lethal problem associated with exenteration. In addition, this allows preservation of rectal continence. Continent urinary reservoirs of both the Kock[96] and Indiana[97, 98] types have been employed for urinary diversion. Thus, many women undergoing exenteration no longer need to collect urine or feces in external appliances.

Reconstruction following exenteration must also deal with the vagina and the pelvic floor. If a total vaginectomy is performed, the surgeon must repair the hiatus left distal to the levator ani when the distal vagina, rectum, and urethra are removed. A number of approaches are possible. First, the levators and the urogenital diaphragm can be closed to the greatest possible degree, with any remaining gap allowed to heal by secondary intent. This classic approach leaves the patient without a vagina. Another choice is to create a neovagina using a split-thickness skin graft.[99] Finally, the surgeon may use gracilis myocutaneous flaps either to close the perineum or to create a neovagina.[100]

In addition, the pelvic floor must be repaired to minimize the incidence of pelvic infection and intestinal obstruction. Preferably, this is done using an omental flap.[101] Other closures utilizing the patient's pelvic tissues may be possible.[101] As a last resort, one may create a sling of polygalactin mesh[102]; a foreign body of this size may predispose to infection and obstruction, however.[101] In any event, closed suction drainage of the pelvic floor is highly advisable to prevent fluid collections, which frequently become infected.

A majority of patients who undergo pelvic exenteration experience major morbidity, and in most series, mortality is between 5% and 10%.[92, 103–106] Long operative time, extensive blood loss with concomitant transfusion requirements, and entry of contaminated viscera (vagina, urethra, rectum) are inherent to the operation. Most patients who undergo the procedure have advanced cancer and have had high-dose radiation to the operative field. This compromises healing ability and makes the procedure even more dangerous. Consequently, these women are prone to infection, including wound infections or pyelonephritis. An even more serious infectious complication is pelvic infection, which may be cellulitis or abscess, and may progress to sepsis.[107] Women who have undergone exenteration also are at high risk for development of cardiac complications, adult respiratory distress syndrome, and pulmonary emboli.

Acute enteric complications, however, are the most common disastrous complication of this procedure. The descent of irradiated intestine into an irradiated and denuded pelvic floor predisposes to obstruction and fistulization. The risk is compounded when an intestinal anastomosis is in contact with the pelvic floor, as is likely to be the case following an ileal conduit or a continent reservoir procedure. The rate of major enteric complications may exceed 20%.[108] The incidence of these complications can be minimized by careful pelvic floor reconstruction. Once they occur, they frequently require reoperation, and mortality may exceed 50%.[108]

Enteric obstruction and fistulization may also occur as delayed complications. The most frequent late complications, however, are associated with urinary diversion.[106] These may include stenosis, chronic or recurrent pyelonephritis, prolapsed stoma, incontinent or obstructed reservoir, and calculi in a reservoir. The last is supposedly related to construction of the reservoir using staples. Dehiscence of a ureteral anastomosis used in constructing a urinary diversion constitutes a serious acute complication. It requires reoperation for revision, usually performed after the risk of sepsis and other acute complications subside.

Operative Staging

The primary treatment of stage IIB cervical carcinoma and more extensive lesions is with radiation (see below). The standard external radiation portal includes the deep pelvic and common iliac nodes. The presence of metastases in aortic nodes in more than 25% of these patients[18, 109, 110] raises the question whether routine procedures to detect metastases in these nodes will enhance survival. Fine-needle aspiration of enlarged nodes demonstrable on CT is useful in diagnosis but a negative result is not definitive for two reasons. First, CT demonstrates only enlarged nodes, and metastases often occur in nodes of normal size.[55] Second, it is conceivable that the physical removal of enlarged nodes with metastases could enhance the possibility of cure.[111] Extraperitoneal removal of common iliac and aortic nodes for staging can be done with few complications.[112] A vertical skin incision is made in the anterior axillary line on the side with the greatest volume of tumor. It is carried through the external oblique, internal oblique, and transverse layers. The peritoneum is reflected medially to expose the psoas muscle and the great vessels. Common and aortic lymphadenectomy can usually be performed bilaterally through this incision. Following this, the peritoneum is opened, the pelvis is explored, and washings are taken. Grossly abnormal structures are sampled for biopsy. Complications are unusual and consist of bleeding from the great vessels and wound infection. Even if there is a wound infection, radiation is not delayed with this technique, as the incision is lateral to the radiation field. The complication rate from extraperitoneal lymphadenectomy is lower than that associated with a transperitoneal technique.[113] This is because the transperitoneal technique may produce adherence of intestine to intra-abdominal structures within the anticipated radiation field. Such fixation of intestine predisposes to enteric radiation complications.

Laparoscopic pelvic lymphadenectomy has been performed using extraperitoneal[75] and transperitoneal[114] techniques. When this procedure goes well, pain and length of disability are minimal. It has not been widely demonstrated that endoscopic removal of common iliac and aortic nodes can be accomplished safely and in a reasonable amount of time. If such evidence is forthcoming, this operation likely will supersede the open technique described above.

Radiotherapy

Two main types of radiotherapy are used for treatment of cancer of the cervix: teletherapy (external beam) and brachytherapy (intracavitary or interstitial implants). Typically, treatment is initiated with a course of external irradiation, which distributes a homogeneous dose of radiation to the entire pelvis, including the sidewall. The upper limit of the field is the L4-5 intervertebral space. The lower limit is the midvagina unless the carcinoma involves the vagina. The purpose of external radiation is threefold: to treat all areas at risk at the outset, to shrink the gross tumor so that it can be covered by the effective brachytherapy isodose, and to thus normalize the anatomy to facilitate optimal placement of the applicator.[115, 116] The standard external beam field for cervical cancer encompasses the whole pelvis, which covers both the primary tumor and the lymph nodes that are primarily at risk for metastases. It is recommended that these treatments be given using a four-field technique on a megavoltage machine. In an attempt to minimize treatment-related morbidity, the *normal tissues* in the beam are blocked (Fig. 14–18). A CT-based isodose distribution is illustrated in Figure 14–19. The external therapy dose is usually given as a fractionated course delivering 900 to 1000 cGy/week, for a total pelvic dose of 4000 to 5500 cGy.

Brachytherapy is usually given following the completion of external radiotherapy. It effectively treats the cervix, vagina, and medial parametria. A variety of afterloading cervical applicators are available. Each comprises an intrauterine tandem, which holds up to four intrauterine sources in a line, and two vaginal colpostats, which place one source in each lateral fornix (Fig. 14–20). The most commonly used radioisotope is cesium 137, which delivers gamma rays. The conventional 662 keV dose rate is 40 to 60 cGy/hour to the midparametrium. The high-dose rate applicator is being explored for this disease.[117–119]

The absorbed-dose point system and milligram-hours system[120] are most often used. Neither system adequately expresses the relationship between the dose and the volume being irradiated. Individualized computerized dosimetry is

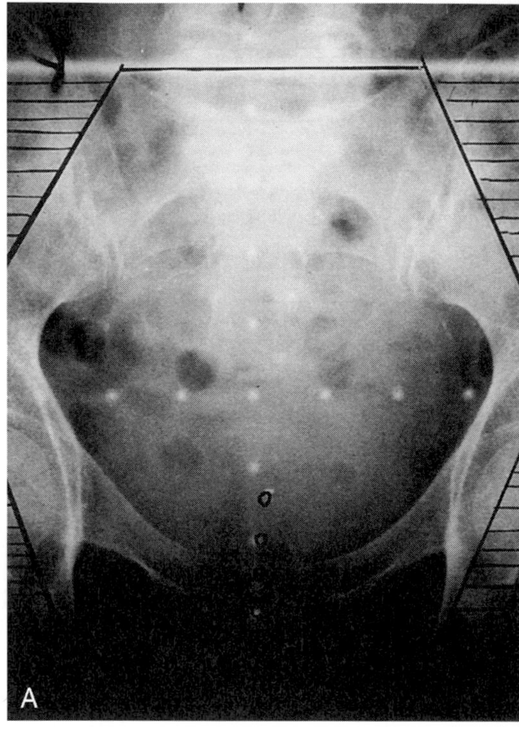

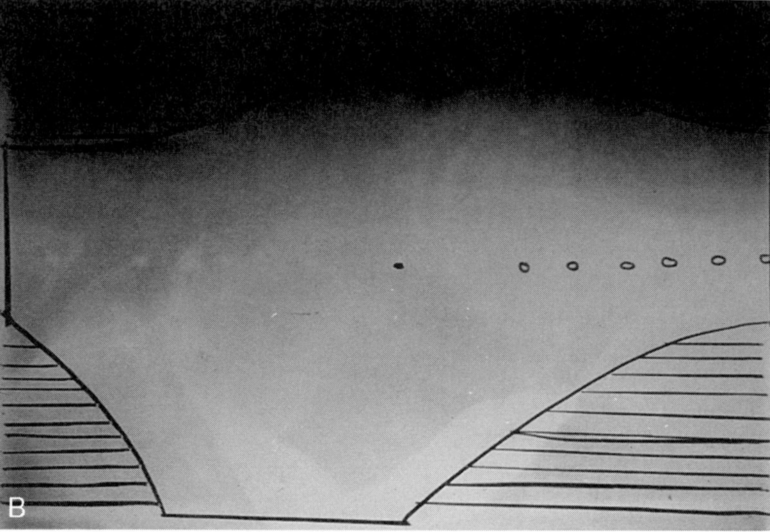

FIGURE 14–18. Treatment localization films for anteroposterior (*A*) and lateral (*B*) external radiation portals. The hatched areas represent areas within the rectangular treatment beam that do not require irradiation. These areas are shielded during treatment using lead blocks.

now widely used to optimize the dosage, so that the cervix, fornices, and parametrium receive the maximum possible dose and the anterior rectum and posterior bladder receive the minimum possible dose.[121] In an attempt to standardize the dosimetry, the International Commission on Radiological Units and Measurements suggested dose and volume specifications for reporting intracavitary therapy in gynecologic procedures.[122]

The organs at risk for radiation morbidity are the ovary, small bowel, rectum, bladder, and vagina, and there may be hematologic complications as well. Radiotherapy ablates the ovarian function in all pre- and perimenopausal women. For the remaining organs, the reported rate of complications ranges from 5% to 15%, being higher in patients with advanced cancer and those receiving higher doses of radiotherapy. The principal site of major chronic complications is the lower colon. Women may develop proctocolitis with hemorrhage, tenesmus, obstruction, or rectovaginal fistula. Enteritis with pain, perforation, or obstruction is common, especially with extended fields. Radiation cystitis is an interstitial cystitis that may be characterized by hemorrhage, diminished bladder capacity, dysuria, constant bladder pain, or all of these. Vaginal atrophy and stenosis often occur following radiotherapy. Therefore, all patients who are not sexually active are advised to use vaginal dilators to maintain patency of the vagina.

Chemotherapy

A number of cytotoxic agents have demonstrable activity against cervical squamous cell carcinoma. Some of these drugs are listed in Table 14–7. The use of combination

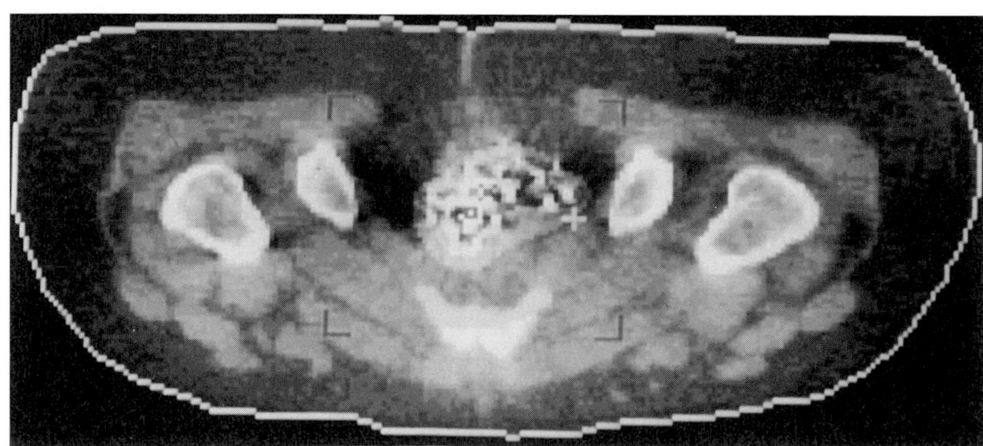

FIGURE 14–19. Transverse image through the cervix obtained through CT. The gray brackets on the film define the area that is to be included in the treatment field.

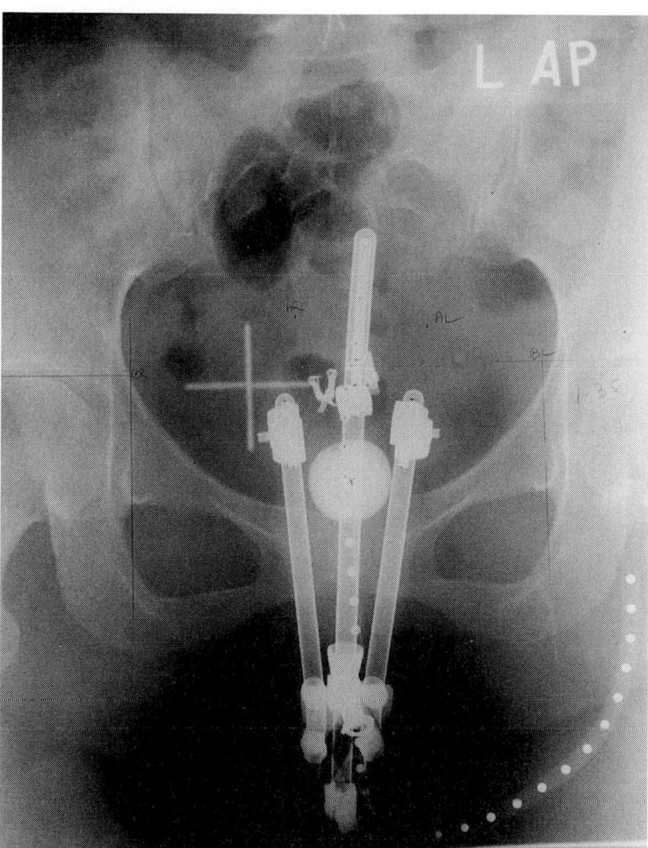

FIGURE 14–20. Supine anteroposterior abdominal film demonstrating correct placement of the central tandem in the uterine cavity and of the two colpostats high in the lateral fornices. The white cross marks the level of the external cervical os to which radiopaque clips are secured. These clips are seen on either side of the tandem, at the level of the cross.

chemotherapy is discussed in the section on metastatic disease. Many of the agents commonly used in combination regimens have little or no efficacy as single agents. In addition, chemotherapy may be given as an adjuvant to radiotherapy. Hydroxyurea is commonly used for this purpose. It has shown efficacy in improving survival in patients with stage IIB and IIIB tumors when combined with radiation,[123] but it is not effective alone.

PRIMARY DISEASE: RESULTS AND COMPLICATIONS OF TREATMENT

Cervical Intraepithelial Neoplasia

CIN is treated as depicted in Table 14–8. This entity should not be treated without a histologic diagnosis obtained by colposcopically directed biopsy. The colposcopic examination determines whether the entire TZ is visible.

CIN 1 need not be treated at the time of diagnosis if the entire TZ is visible, as two thirds of these lesions regress, and fewer than one fifth progress to more severe lesions.[38] Repeated cytologic, and possible colposcopic, tests should be performed every three months until regression or progression occurs. If the lesion persists for a year, treatment is mandatory. Local destruction is an option for patients who do not want to participate in prolonged observation of their low-grade squamous intraepithelial lesions. Destruction can be achieved using cryotherapy,[124–126] carbon dioxide laser ablation,[125–127] or large loop excision of the TZ.[128] In each case, tissue is ablated or excised to a depth of 7 mm, with a margin of 4 to 5 mm beyond the edge of the lesion. Each of these modalities results in cure in over 90% of cases. If the entire TZ is not visible and if cervical cytology, colposcopically directed biopsy, and endocervical curettage all show no lesion worse than CIN 1, observation is permissible, but local destruction is not. Excisional cone biopsy is mandatory for treatment of these patients.

If the entire TZ is visible and if the patient has persistent CIN 1 or 2 after 12 months of observation, the lesion should be treated based on the criteria and using the methods described in the previous paragraph. If a patient is diagnosed with CIN and the entire TZ is not visible, she should not undergo a hysterectomy for any reason without first having a cone biopsy to rule out the presence of an occult invasive carcinoma.

CIN 3 occurring in small lesions may be treated using local destruction. Lesions occupying more than one quadrant, or those in which the entire TZ is not visible on colposcopy, require conization, which cures about 90% of women.[129] Even if surgical margins are involved, more than

TABLE 14–7
Drugs Effective Against 15% or More of Squamous Cell Cervical Carcinomas

Author	Drug	% Response
McGuire et al.[213]	Carboplatin	15
Thigpen et al.[214]	Cisplatin	17
Freeman et al.,[215] Muscato et al.[216]	Chlorambucil	25
Muscato et al.,[216] Wasserman and Carter[217]	Cyclophosphamide	16
Muscato et al.,[216] Piver et al.[218]	Doxorubicin	16
Wong et al.[219]	Epidoxorubicin	48
Wasserman and Carter,[217] Malkasian et al.[220]	Fluorouracil	20
Buxton et al.[221]	Ifosfamide	33
Muscato et al.,[216] Wasserman and Carter[217]	Methotrexate	28
Stehman et al.[222]	Mitolactol	29
Muscato et al.,[216] Wasserman and Carter[217]	Mitomycin C	22

TABLE 14–8
Treatment of Cervical Intraepithelial Neoplasia

Severity of Lesion	Transformation Zone Entirely Seen? Yes	No
CIN 1		
Newly diagnosed	Observe 3 mo*	Observe 3 mo if Pap and colposcopic biopsy both show CIN 1; if Pap is worse, perform cone biopsy
Persistent	Local destruction	Cone biopsy‡
CIN 2	Local destruction	Cone biopsy‡
CIN 3 (limited)	Local destruction†	Cone biopsy‡
CIN 3	Cone biopsy§	Cone biopsy‡

*Local destruction is an acceptable therapeutic alternative.
†Cone biopsy or hysterectomy is an alternative treatment in certain circumstances.
‡Hysterectomy is contraindicated unless carcinoma has been ruled out by cone biopsy.
§Hysterectomy is an alternative treatment in certain circumstances.

half of women will experience no recurrence.[130] Unreliable patients or others who have completed childbearing should consider hysterectomy as an elective procedure for definitive treatment, as invasive cervical carcinoma develops in about 1% of women with CIN 3 following conization.[131] Patients who desire no further children or who have had at least two recurrences of CIN may be treated by vaginal hysterectomy, laparoscopically assisted vaginal hysterectomy, or total abdominal hysterectomy, provided the entire TZ has been evaluated by recent colposcopy or conization.

Cervical Carcinoma

Stage IA1

Microinvasive cervical carcinoma is defined as a lesion that has invaded cervical stroma but whose histologic appearance rules out significant risk of disease beyond the cervix. By definition, such a lesion does not require treatment of a field beyond the uterus in order to effect a cure. Kolstad[132] reports that lesions with invasion less than 1 mm beneath the surface membrane can be treated with conization only. The Society of Gynecologic Oncologists has defined microinvasive cervical carcinoma as a neoplastic lesion that invades the stroma to a depth of up to 3 mm in one or more places and in which no invasion of vascular spaces is present. A number of studies support the conclusion that such lesions demonstrate lymph node invasion in no more than 1% of cases.[131, 133–135]

Establishment of this diagnosis requires a cone biopsy to evaluate the entire lesion. Such lesions are curable with conservative hysterectomy without lymphadenectomy. Cone biopsy may be sufficient treatment for such lesions; there is little documentation to support or refute the belief that conization cures lesions that invade between 1 and 3 mm into the cervical stroma. We advocate hysterectomy for this entity, except in the context of a clinical trial; this has been the treatment reported and advocated in most series and should cure almost all patients. It is reasonable to defer this procedure in a woman who wishes to have children, provided conization has ruled out deeper invasion.

Stages IA2, IB, and IIA (Less Than 4 cm)

Stage IA2 and IB lesions may be treated equally effectively by radical hysterectomy and pelvic lymphadenectomy or by radiation.[136] Most surgical series report 5-year survival rates between 80% and 90%.[136–140] Table 14–9 gives data for survival and pattern of recurrence from three large series of patients treated with radiation for stage IB lesions.[141–143] Stage IIA lesions with minimal vaginal involvement may be treated either surgically or with radiation. Those patients with extensive vaginal involvement are best treated with radiation, using the guidelines specified below.

Surgery is employed more commonly because of the possibility of preserving ovarian function and because chronic complications are unusual. Also, sexual rehabilitation is usually more satisfactory following surgery than following radiation.[144] Specific medical conditions may contraindicate surgery, or a patient may be so obese that the procedure is technically impossible. Old age by itself is not a contraindication.[145] Ovarian conservation should be considered in premenopausal women. Ovarian spread is identified in fewer than 1% of women with stage IB squamous lesions and in 1.7% to 5.5% of those with adenocarcinoma.[26, 146]

If radiation is elected in a medically or technically inoperable patient, or because the expertise for radical hysterectomy is not present in the treating institution, a course of external radiotherapy and preferably two intracavitary applications are given. The midparametrial dose is in the range of 7500 to 8000 cGy, and the pelvic sidewall dose is in the range of 5000 to 5500 cGy.

If examination of the surgical specimen from radical hysterectomy shows involvement of the lymph nodes or the cardinal ligament, 5-year survival is 50% to 70%, provided the surgical margins are free.[147–153] Survival is

TABLE 14–9
Five-Year Survival and Failure Rates in Patients Treated With Radiation for Stage IB Cervical Carcinoma

Author	5-Year Survival (%)	Regional Failure (%)*	Distant Failure (%)*
Coia et al.[141]	74	12	7
Montana et al.[142]	83	3	15
Perez et al.[143]	85	7	14

*Patients with simultaneous regional and distant failure are considered to have failed with distant disease.

correlated with the number of lymph nodes involved and with tumor size, as independent variables (Table 14–10).[147, 148] Most such patients in the United States receive adjuvant pelvic irradiation, sometimes combined with an intracavitary vaginal implant. Such treatment enhances local control, but there is no clear evidence that it increases overall survival.[150–154] Several studies report the use of adjuvant chemotherapy in this situation. Wertheim and colleagues' pilot trial using bleomycin and cisplatin demonstrated 84% at 28 months.[155] Lai and coworkers[156] reported a double-armed trial in which cisplatin (Platinol), vinblastine, and bleomycin (PVB) were given. Three-year survival was 75% in women who received chemotherapy and 47% in those who did not. Ueki et al.[157] found a dramatic increase in survival in patients at high risk for recurrence following radical hysterectomy who were given oral tegafur (a derivative of 5-fluorouracil). Tattersall and colleagues,[158] however, found PVB to be ineffective in 71 patients with lymph node metastases enrolled in a randomized trial.

Stages IB and IIA (Greater Than 4 cm)

These lesions are technically amenable to resection by radical hysterectomy, but survival is higher using radiation. Table 14–11 gives data for survival and pattern of recurrence from three large series of patients treated with radiation for stage IIB lesions.[141, 143, 159]

Survival decreases in patients whose stage IB lesions are greater than 3 to 4 cm in diameter.[160, 161] Patients with these lesions are prone to central, pelvic, and distant recurrence.[116, 162] Our practice is to perform a staging operation prior to treatment with radiation. Operative staging includes examination under anesthesia with cystoscopy and sigmoidoscopy. Any suspicious lesions are sampled for biopsy. Laparoscopy is then performed, with pelvic washings and thorough exploration. Again, biopsy of any suspicious lesions encountered in the pelvic or abdominal peritoneum is performed. Finally, if no intraperitoneal disease is encountered, laparoscopic biopsy of the common iliac and low aortic nodes is done. Standard pelvic irradiation is given to patients with exophytic lesions greater than 4 cm or endophytic lesions of 4 to 6 cm in diameter, provided there is no peritoneal disease or lymphadenopathy in the common iliac nodes or above. If such dissemination is present, treatment is individualized.

Radiation dosimetric guidelines call for a midparametrial dose of approximately 9000 cGy; the pelvic sidewall dose ranges between 6000 and 6500 cGy.

Barrel-shaped stage IB carcinoma describes endophytic lesions of at least 5 to 6 cm without parametrial involvement. They are so named because their expanded diameter gives the uterus a barrel-shaped configuration rather than the usual pear-shaped morphology resulting from the tapered cervix. If such lesions are treated with radiation followed by conservative extrafascial hysterectomy, some investigators have found that pelvic control is better than that which can be obtained using radical hysterectomy or using radiation alone.[163–167] Survival may also be enhanced.[163–167] Perez and Kao,[168] however, using a higher central dose than most other workers, found no difference in local control and survival in patients with large lesions who received adjunctive hysterectomy.

TABLE 14–10
Survival in Women With Stage IB Cervical Carcinoma and Metastases to Pelvic Lymph Nodes Found at Radical Hysterectomy

Number of Nodes With Metastases	Risk Category According to Lesion Size (10-Year Survival, %)		
	<1 cm	*1.1–4 cm*	*>4 cm*
<2	Very low (92)	Low (70)	High (56)
>2	Low (70)	High (56)	Very high (13)

Based on Alvarez RD, et al: Identification of prognostic factors and risk groups in patients found to have nodal metastasis at the time of radical hysterectomy for early-stage carcinoma of the cervix. Gynecol Oncol 35:130–135, 1989.

Stage IIB

Treatment of stage IIB lesions begins with operative staging, as described in the previous section. As with large

TABLE 14–11
Five-Year Survival and Failure Rates in Patients Treated With Radiation for Stage IIB Cervical Carcinoma

Author	5-Year Survival (%)	Regional Failure (%)*	Distant Failure (%)*
Coia et al.[141]	56	27	15
Montana et al.[142]	62	17	18
Perez et al.[143]	68	14	22

*Patients with simultaneous regional and distant failure are considered to have failed with distant disease.

stage IB lesions, pelvic irradiation is given to patients with no dissemination to the peritoneum or to lymph nodes at the level of the common iliac group or higher. Stage IIB squamous lesions are treated using radiation without surgery. Five-year survival rates following standard radiation therapy are approximately 60% to 70%. Concomitant use of hydroxyurea with external irradiation may improve survival.[123] Other adjuvant chemotherapeutic regimens, especially a combination of cisplatin and 5-fluorouracil, have also been used for this purpose.[169] A short course of chemotherapy followed by radical surgery has been proposed to treat stage IIB carcinoma.[170] This is considered investigational at present.

If results of a staging operation show involvement of common iliac or aortic nodes, the external radiation field is extended to include the aortic nodes up to the T-12 vertebra. Series of significant size (>25 patients) show long-term survival of 25% to 40% of patients.[171–173] These series are uncontrolled, but presumably few patients with untreated cancer in the aortic nodes will survive for long. Positive peritoneal cytologic results carry a very poor prognosis, including frequent intraperitoneal recurrences.[24, 174] Appropriate management is uncertain, but whole abdominal irradiation or adjuvant chemotherapy should be considered.

Stages IIIA, IIIB, and IVA

A pretreatment staging operation is performed as described in the previous section. These lesions are treated using irradiation. External radiotherapy and one intracavitary application are given. The dose ranges prescribed are 9000 cGy to the midparametrium and 6500 cGy to the pelvic sidewall. An additional parametrial boost is given if indicated by widespread extension or lymphadenopathy on that side. Conventional radiotherapy alone cures 25% to 45% of patients with stage III lesions.[141, 143, 175, 176] Survival rates are less than 10% in patients with stage IVA lesions.[143] Table 14–12 gives data for survival and pattern of recurrence from three large series of patients treated with radiation for stage III lesions. The high rate of distant recurrence suggests that regional treatment is insufficient to cure the great majority of these patients; the high rate of regional failure offers the hope that better regional treatment techniques may increase rates of survival and cure.

TABLE 14–12
Five-Year Survival and Failure Rates in Patients Treated with Radiation for Stage IIIB Cervical Carcinoma

Author	5-Year Survival (%)	Regional Failure (%)*	Distant Failure (%)*
Coia et al.[141]	33	51	29
Montana et al.[142]	33	40	25
Perez et al.[143]	45	37	32

*Patients with simultaneous regional and distant failure are considered to have failed with distant disease.

The use of chemotherapy along with radiotherapy, as well as altered radiotherapy schedules, is being investigated.[177, 178] Hydroxyurea appears to be a useful adjuvant agent.[123] As with less advanced lesions, the finding of positive peritoneal cytology or aortic nodes worsens the prognosis and calls for more radical treatment. Two randomized trials of neoadjuvant chemotherapy combined with radiotherapy have been reported. Chauvegne et al.[179] found no increase in survival rates when two to four cycles of methotrexate, chlorambucil, vinblastine, and cisplatin were administered to patients with advanced disease prior to radiation. Responders to chemotherapy, however, survived longer than nonresponders. Souhami and colleagues[180] demonstrated poorer survival in a group of patients with stage IIIB disease who received neoadjuvant bleomycin, vincristine, methotrexate, and cisplatin than in controls who received radiation alone. In an interesting pilot study, Rettenmaier and coworkers[181] reported the use of cisplatin by constant intra-arterial infusion simultaneous with radiation in seven women with massive tumors. The catheter was placed in the anterior division of the internal iliac artery. Five of the seven patients achieved remission. Other investigators have given chemotherapy in a neoadjuvant setting to patients with stage IIB tumors or greater. If the tumor shrank enough to render the lesion operable, radical operation was performed. Regimens employed in this manner include PVB;[182, 183] cisplatin, bleomycin, and methotrexate;[184] PVB plus mitomycin;[185] and cisplatin and mitomycin.[186] A majority of patients in all these trials demonstrated an objective response. Responding patients have a lower than expected incidence of lymph node metastases at operation.[182–184] The impact of this approach on survival is unclear.

CENTRAL RECURRENCE OF CERVICAL CARCINOMA

Central recurrence of cervical carcinoma is potentially curable. The appropriate treatment of recurrent cancer in the cervix or at the apex of the vagina depends on how the primary lesion had been treated. Symptoms and signs of possible metastases should be sought. Unilateral lower extremity pain and edema are strongly suggestive of systemic disease, as is inanition. In any case, the patient should undergo a thorough metastatic work-up, including pelvic and abdominal CT, chest radiograph, and bone scan. Enlarged lymph nodes should be subjected to fine-needle aspiration.

If the patient has a tumor of the vaginal cuff recurrent after radical hysterectomy, radiation is the treatment of choice.[187–189] This renders 30% to 40% of patients free of disease.

Patients who have been treated primarily by radiation are unable to tolerate a second therapeutic course of irradiation, however. Vaginal cuff recurrences in such patients are best treated with total pelvic exenteration. It is generally believed that this procedure should be reserved for those with no metastases and whose central recurrence is amenable to operative clearance.[190] Stanhope and Symmonds' observation of 2- and 5-year survival of 46% and 23%, respectively, in women with metastatic nodal disease undergoing exenteration is more optimistic than those of other investigators.[191] Barber and Jones[192] reported 5% 5-year survival in such patients; Creasman and Rutledge[193] also found a high rate of recurrence in this circumstance. Hockel and colleagues[194] proposed ultraradical surgery combined with interstitial radiation implant for central tumor extending to the sidewall. Their results are preliminary and do not address the question of long-term survival.

The choice of exenteration is determined by the possibility of tumor clearance. Posterior exenteration is generally inadvisable in an irradiated patient because of the difficulty of establishing a good surgical plane, the likelihood of anterior extension of the tumor, and the possibility of bladder fistula. Anterior exenteration is seldom used now that it is feasible to perform low anterior rectal resection with anastomosis. The choice of supralevator exenteration versus exenteration with total vaginectomy and proctectomy and the choice of a urinary diverting conduit versus a continent reservoir are complex clinical decisions that must be individualized based on the size and location of the tumor, the general status of the patient, and the experience of the physician. The outcome depends not only on the skill of the surgeon but also on patient selection. DiSaia and Creasman[190] reviewed 13 series totaling 1917 exenterations performed between 1957 and 1989. Five-year survival was 34%, and perioperative mortality was 13%. The more recent series reported an operative mortality between 6% and 10%.[104, 195–197] Five-year survival was 20% to 62%, with a tendency toward greater survival in the more recent series.

PRIMARY OR SECONDARY METASTATIC CERVICAL CARCINOMA

No single agent or combination of drugs demonstrably prolongs life in any category of patients with cervical carcinoma. Nevertheless, patients with symptomatic metastatic tumors often obtain temporary shrinkage of tumors and relief of symptoms with chemotherapy. The combination of bleomycin, ifosfamide, and cisplatin induced an objective tumor regression in 69% of patients, with a complete response rate of 20%.[198] The median duration of response was eight months. Response rates of 50% to 60% have been reported for the combination of cisplatin, bleomycin, methotrexate, and vincristine.[199, 200] Results with the frequently used combination of cisplatin, bleomycin, and vinblastine,[201, 202] and with other combinations, have been more variable. Response rates are consistently higher for lesions that are outside areas previously treated with radiation. All these regimens invariably produce distressing side effects such as nausea, alopecia, anorexia, and fatigue. Many of them are quite toxic. It seems reasonable to utilize chemotherapy for cervical carcinoma only for patients with symptomatic disease or in investigational settings.

POST-TREATMENT CARE AND SURVEILLANCE

Patients are seen every 3 months for 2 years, and then every 6 months, for a history and physical examination, including pelvic examination and cervical or vaginal cytology. Consideration is given to obtaining a chest radiograph and abdominopelvic CT scan every 6 to 12 months for the first 2 to 3 years after treatment.

References

1. Wingo PA, Tong T, Bolden S: Cancer statistics 1995. CA 45:8–30, 1995.
2. Christopherson WM, Parker JE: Relation of cervical cancer to early marriage and childbearing. N Engl J Med 273:235–239, 1965.
3. Keighley E: Carcinoma of the cervix among prostitutes in a women's prison. Br J Vener Dis 44:254–255, 1968.
4. Rotkin ID: Epidemiology of carcinoma of the cervix. III. Sexual characteristics of a cervical cancer population. Am J Public Health 57:815–829, 1967.
5. Herbst AL, Cole P, Colton T, et al: Age-incidence and risk of diethylstilbestrol-related clear cell adenocarcinoma of the vagina and cervix. Am J Obstet Gynecol 128:43–48, 1977.
6. Winklestein W: Smoking and cervical cancer—current status: A review. Am J Epidemiol 131:945–957, 1990.
7. Maiman M, Fruchter R, Serur E, et al: Human immunodeficiency virus infection and cervical neoplasia. Gynecol Oncol 38:377–382, 1990.
8. Boon ME, Susanti I, Tasche MJA, et al: Human papillomavirus (HPV) associated male and female genital carcinomas in a Hindu population: The male as vector and victim. Cancer 64:559–565, 1989.
9. Crum CP, Levine RU: Human papillomavirus infection and cervical neoplasia: New perspectives. Int J Gynecol Pathol 3:376–388, 1984.
10. Reid R, Crum CP, Herschman BR, et al: Genital warts and cervical cancer. III. Subclinical papillomaviral infection and cervical neoplasm are linked by a spectrum of continuous morphologic and biologic change. Cancer 53:943–953, 1984.
11. Prakash SS, Reeves WC, Sisson GR, et al: Herpes simplex virus type 2 and human papillomavirus type 16 in cervicitis, dysplasia and invasive cervical carcinoma. Int J Cancer 35:51–57, 1985.
12. McCance DJ, Campion MJ, Clarkson PJ, et al: Prevalence of human papillomavirus type 16 DNA sequences in cervical intraepithelial neoplasia and invasive carcinoma of the cervix. Br J Obstet Gynaecol 92:1101–1105, 1985.
13. Wilczynski SP, Bergen S, Walker J, et al: Human papillomaviruses and cervical cancer: Analysis of histopathologic features associated with different viral types. Hum Pathol 19:697–704, 1988.
14. Qizilbash AH: In-situ and microinvasive adenocarcinoma of the uterine cervix. A clinical, cytologic and histologic study of 14 cases. Am J Clin Pathol 64:155–170, 1975.
15. Delgado G, Bundy BN, Fowler WC, et al: A prospective surgical pathological study of stage I squamous carcinoma of the cervix: A Gynecologic Oncology Group study. Gynecol Oncol 35:314–320, 1989.
16. Lagasse LD, Ballon SC, Berman ML, et al: Pretreatment lymphangiography and operative evaluation in carcinoma of the cervix. Am J Obstet Gynecol 134:219–224, 1979.
17. Hammond JA, Herson J, Freedman RS, et al: The impact of lymph

node status on survival in cervical carcinoma. Int J Radiat Oncol Biol Phys 7:1713–1718, 1981.
18. Lagasse LD, Creasman WT, Shingleton HM, et al: Results and complications of operative staging in cervical cancer: Experience of the Gynecologic Oncology Group. Gynecol Oncol 9:90–98, 1980.
19. Brandt B III, Lifshitz S: Scalene node biopsy in advanced carcinoma of the cervix uteri. Cancer 47:1920–1921, 1981.
20. Lee RB, Weisbaum GS, Heller PB, et al: Scalene node biopsy in primary and recurrent invasive carcinoma of the cervix. Gynecol Oncol 11:200–206, 1981.
21. Fagundes F, Perez CA, Grigsby PW, et al: Distant metastases after irradiation alone in carcinoma of the uterine cervix. Int J Radiat Oncol Biol Phys 24:197–204, 1992.
22. Imachi M, Tsukamoto N, Matsuyama T, et al: Peritoneal cytology in patients with carcinoma of the uterine cervix. Gynecol Oncol 26:202–207, 1987.
23. Kilgore LC, Orr JW Jr, Hatch KD, et al: Peritoneal cytology in patients with squamous cell carcinoma of the cervix. Gynecol Oncol 19:24–29, 1984.
24. Roberts WS, Bryson SCP, Cavanagh D, et al: Peritoneal cytology and invasive carcinoma of the cervix. Gynecol Oncol 24:331–336, 1986.
25. Mann WJ, Chumas J, Amalfitano T, et al: Ovarian metastases from stage IB adenocarcinoma of the cervix. Cancer 60:1123–1126, 1987.
26. Sutton GP, Bundy BN, Delgado G, et al: Ovarian metastases in stage IB carcinoma of the cervix: A Gynecology Oncology Group study. Am J Obstet Gynecol 166:50–53, 1992.
27. Adcock LL, Potish RA, Julian TM, et al: Carcinoma of the cervix, FIGO stage IB: Treatment failures. Gynecol Oncol 18:218–225, 1984.
28. Dattoli MJ, Gretz HF III, Beller U, et al: Analysis of multiple prognostic factors in patients with stage IB cervical cancer: Age as a major determinant. Int J Radiat Oncol Biol Phys 17:41–47, 1989.
29. Figge DC, Tamimi HK: Patterns of recurrence of carcinoma following radical hysterectomy. Am J Obstet Gynecol 140:213–220, 1981.
30. Hale RJ, Wilcox FL, Buckley CH, et al: Prognostic factors in uterine cervical carcinoma: A clinicopathologic analysis. Int J Gynecol Cancer 1:19–23, 1991.
31. Pejovic M-H, Wolff J-P, Kramar A, et al: Cure rate estimation and long-term prognosis of uterine cervical carcinoma. Cancer 47:203–206, 1981.
32. Robert ME, Fu YS: Squamous cell carcinoma of the uterine cervix—a review with emphasis on prognostic factors and unusual variants. Semin Diagn Pathol 7:173–189, 1990.
33. Stendahl U, Eklund G, Willen H, et al: Invasive squamous cell carcinoma of the uterine cervix. III. A malignancy grading system for indication of prognosis after radiation therapy. Acta Radiol Oncol Scand 20:231–243, 1981.
34. Bichel P, Jakobsen A: Histopathologic grading and prognosis of uterine cervical carcinoma. Am J Clin Oncol 8:247–254, 1985.
35. Jakobsen A, Bichel P, Vaeth M: New prognostic factors in squamous cell carcinoma of the cervix uteri. Am J Clin Oncol 8:39–43, 1985.
36. Richart RM: Natural history of cervical intraepithelial neoplasia. Clin Obstet Gynecol 10:748–784, 1968.
37. Nasiell K, Roger V, Nasiell M, et al: Behavior of mild cervical dysplasia during long-term followup. Obstet Gynecol 67:665–669, 1986.
38. Nasiell K, Nasiell M, Vaclavinkova V: Behavior of moderate cervix dysplasia during long-term follow-up. Obstet Gynecol 61:609–614, 1983.
39. Maier RC, Norris HJ: Coexistence of cervical intraepithelial neoplasia with primary adenocarcinoma of the cervix. Obstet Gynecol 56:361–364, 1980.
40. Berek JS, Castaldo TW, Hacker NF, et al: Adenocarcinoma of the uterine cervix. Cancer 48:2734–2741, 1981.
41. Moberg PJ, Einhorn N, Silfversward C, et al: Adenocarcinoma of the uterine cervix. Cancer 57:407–410, 1986.
42. Moore DH, Fowler WC Jr, Walton LA, et al: Morbidity of lymph node sampling in cancers of the uterine corpus and cervix. Obstet Gynecol 74:180–184, 1989.
43. Rutledge FN, Galakatos AE, Wharton JT, et al: Adenocarcinoma of the uterine cervix. Am J Obstet Gynecol 122:236–245, 1975.
44. McGowan L, Young RH, Scully RE: Peutz-Jeghers syndrome with "adenoma malignum" of the cervix. A report of two cases. Gynecol Oncol 10:125–133, 1980.
45. Herbst AL, Cole P, Norusis MJ, et al: Epidemiologic aspects and factors related to survival in 384 registry cases of clear cell adenocarcinoma of the cervix and vagina. Am J Obstet Gynecol 135:876–883, 1979.
46. Herbst Al, Ulfelder H, Poskanzer DC: Adenocarcinoma of the vagina: Association of maternal stilbestrol therapy with tumor appearance in young women. N Engl J Med 284:878–881, 1971.
47. Gallup DG, Harper RH, Stock RJ: Poor prognosis in patients with adenosquamous cell carcinoma of the cervix. Obstet Gynecol 65:416–422, 1985.
48. Sheets EE, Berman ML, Hrountas CK, et al: Surgically treated, early-stage neuroendocrine small-cell cervical carcinoma. Obstet Gynecol 71:10–14, 1988.
49. Tamimi HK, Ek M, Hesla J, et al: Glassy cell carcinoma of the cervix redefined. Obstet Gynecol 71:837–841, 1988.
50. Lotocki RJ, Krepart GV, Paraskevas M, et al: Glassy cell carcinoma of the cervix: A bimodal treatment strategy. Gynecol Oncol 44:254–259, 1992.
51. Taylor PT, Andersen WA, Barber SR, et al: The screening Papanicolaou smear: Contribution of the endocervical brush. Obstet Gynecol 70:734–738, 1987.
52. Bethesda Workshop: The revised Bethesda system for reporting cervical/vaginal cytologic diagnosis: Report of the 1991 Bethesda Workshop. J Reprod Med 37:383–386, 1992.
53. American College of Obstetricians and Gynecologists: Cervical Cytology: Evaluation and Management of Abnormalities (Technical Bulletin no. 183). Washington, DC: American College of Obstetricians and Gynecologists, 1993.
54. Holloway RW, To A, Moradi M, et al: Monitoring the course of cervical carcinoma with the squamous cell carcinoma serum radioimmunoassay. Obstet Gynecol 74:944–949, 1989.
55. Camilien L, Gordon D, Fruchter RG, et al: Predictive value of computerized tomography in the presurgical evaluation of primary carcinoma of the cervix. Gynecol Oncol 30:209–215, 1988.
56. Wright TC Jr, Gagenon S, Richart RM, et al: Treatment of cervical intraepithelial neoplasia using the loop electrosurgical excision procedure. Obstet Gynecol 79:173–178, 1992.
57. Jones HW III, Buller RE: The treatment of cervical intraepithelial neoplasia by cone biopsy. Am J Obstet Gynecol 137:882–886, 1980.
58. Ohel G: Complications of cone biopsy of the cervix. S Afr Mediese Tydskrif 59:382–384, 1981.
59. Luesley DM, Williams DR, Gee H, et al: Management of postconization cervical stenosis by laser vaporization. Obstet Gynecol 67:126–128, 1986.
60. Jones JN, Sweetnam P, Hibbard BM: The outcome of pregnancy after cone biopsy of the cervix: A case-control study. Br J Obstet Gynaecol 86:913–916, 1979.
61. Moinian M, Andersch B: Does cervix conization increase the risk of complications in subsequent pregnancies? Acta Obstet Gynecol Scand 61:101–103, 1982.
62. Larsson G, Grundsell H, Gullberg B, et al: Outcome of pregnancy after conization. Acta Obstet Gynecol Scand 61:461–466, 1982.
63. Buller RE, Jones HW: Pregnancy following cervical conization. Am J Obstet Gynecol 142:506–512, 1982.
64. Piver MS, Rutledge FN, Smith JP: Five classes of extended hysterectomy for women with cervical cancer. Obstet Gynecol 44:265–272, 1974.
65. Wertheim E: Discussion of the diagnosis and treatment of carcinoma of the uterus. Br Med J 2:689–704, 1905.
66. Meigs JV: Carcinoma of the cervix—the Wertheim operation. Surg Gynecol Obstet 78:195–199, 1944.
67. Okabayashi S: Radical abdominal hysterectomy for cancer of the cervix uteri. Surg Gynecol Obstet 33:335–341, 1921.
68. Cava EF: Hysterectomy in a community hospital. Am J Obstet Gynecol 122:434–438, 1975.
69. White SC, Wartel LJ, Wade ME: Comparison of abdominal and vaginal hysterectomies: A review of 600 operations. Obstet Gynecol 37:530, 1971.
70. Ledger WJ, Child MA: The hospital care of patients undergoing hysterectomy: An analysis of 12,026 patients from the Professional Activity Study. Am J Obstet Gynecol 117:423–433, 1973.
71. Polk BF, Tager IB, Shapiro M: Randomised clinical trial of perioperative cefazolin in preventing infection after hysterectomy. Lancet 1:437–441, 1980.

72. Dicker RC, Greenspan JR, Strauss LT, et al: Complications of abdominal and vaginal hysterectomies among women of reproductive age in the United States. Am J Obstet Gynecol 144:841–848, 1982.
73. Amirikia K, Evans TN: Ten-year review of hysterectomies: Trends, indications, and risks. Am J Obstet Gynecol 134:431–437, 1979.
74. Easterday CL, Grimes DA, Riggs JA: Hysterectomy in the United States. Obstet Gynecol 62:203–212, 1963.
75. Dargent D: A new future for Schauta's operation through presurgical retroperitoneal pelviscopy. Eur J Gynecol Oncol 8:292–296, 1987.
76. Webb MJ, Symmonds RE: Wertheim hysterectomy: A reappraisal. Obstet Gynecol 54:140–145, 1979.
77. Levrant SG, Fruchter TG, Maiman M: Radical hysterectomy for cervical cancer: Morbidity and survival in relation to weight and age. Gynecol Oncol 45:317–322, 1992.
78. Lawton FG, Hacker NF: Surgery for invasive gynecologic cancer in the elderly female population. Obstet Gynecol 76:287–289, 1990.
79. Eisenkop S, Spirtos NM, Montag TW, et al: The clinical significance of blood transfusion at the time of radical hysterectomy. Obstet Gynecol 76:110–113, 1990.
80. Mann WJ Jr, Orr JW, Shingleton HM, et al: Perioperative influences on infectious morbidity in radical hysterectomy. Gynecol Oncol 11:207–212, 1984.
81. Fiorica JV, Roberts WS, Greenberg H, et al: Morbidity and survival patterns in patients after radical hysterectomy and postoperative radiation therapy. Gynecol Oncol 36:343–347, 1990.
82. Forney JP: The effect of radical hysterectomy on bladder physiology. Am J Obstet Gynecol 138:374–382, 1980.
83. Roberts JM, Homesley HD: Observations on bladder function following radical hysterectomy using carbon dioxide cystometry. Surg Gynecol Obstet 147:558–560, 1978.
84. Seski JC, Diokno AC: Bladder dysfunction after radical abdominal hysterectomy. Am J Obstet Gynecol 128:643–650, 1977.
85. Scotti RJ, Bergman A, Bhatia NN, et al: Urodynamic changes in urethrovesical function after radical hysterectomy. Obstet Gynecol 68:111–120, 1986.
86. Buchler DA, Kline JC, Peckham BM, et al: Radiation reactions in cervical therapy. Am J Obstet Gynecol 111:745–750, 1971.
87. Underwood PB, Lutz MH, Smoak DL: Ureteral injury following irradiation for carcinoma of the cervix. Obstet Gynecol 49:663–669, 1977.
88. Mann WJ, Vogel F, Patsner B, et al: Management of lymphocysts after radical gynecologic surgery. Gynecol Oncol 33:248–250, 1989.
89. Petru E, Tamussino K, Lahousen M, et al: Pelvic and paraaortic lymphocysts after radical surgery because of cervical and ovarian cancer. Am J Obstet Gynecol 161:937–941, 1989.
90. Barnes W, Waggoner S, Delgado G, et al: Manometric characterization of rectal dysfunction following radical hysterectomy. Gynecol Oncol 42:116–119, 1991.
91. Brunschwig A: Complete excision of the pelvic viscera for advanced carcinoma. Cancer 1:177–183, 1948.
92. Bricker EM, Butcher HR Jr, Lawler WH, et al: Surgical treatment of advanced and recurrent cancer of the pelvic viscera: An evaluation of 10 years' experience. Ann Surg 152:388–402, 1960.
93. Nelson JH Jr: Transverse colon conduit. In Atlas of Radical Pelvic Surgery, 2nd ed. New York: Appleton-Century-Crofts, 1977, pp 241–259.
94. Schmidt JD, Hawtry CE, Buchsbaum HJ: Transverse colon conduit: A preferred method of urinary diversion for radiation-treated pelvic malignancies. J Urol 113:308–313, 1975.
95. Hatch KD, Gelder MS, Soong S-J, et al: Pelvic exenteration with low rectal anastomosis: Survival, complications, and prognostic factors. Gynecol Oncol 38:462–467, 1990.
96. Kock ND, Nilson AE, Nilsson LO, et al: Urinary diversion via a continent ileal reservoir: Clinical results in 12 patients. J Urol 128:469–475, 1982.
97. Lockhart JL, Bejany DE: Antireflux ureteroileal reimplantation: An alternative for urinary diversion. J Urol 137:867–870, 1987.
98. Penalver MA, Bejany DC, Averette HE, et al: Continent urinary diversion in gynecologic oncology. Gynecol Oncol 34:274–288, 1989.
99. Berek JS, Hacker NF, Lagasse LD: Vaginal reconstruction performed simultaneously with pelvic exenteration. Obstet Gynecol 63:318–323, 1984.
100. McGraw JB, Massey FM, Shanklin KD, et al: Vaginal reconstruction with gracilis myocutaneous flaps. Plast Reconstr Surg 58:176–183, 1976.
101. Webb MJ, Symmonds RE: Management of the pelvic floor after pelvic exenteration. Obstet Gynecol 50:166–171, 1976.
102. Rodier J-F, Janser J-C, Dosier D, et al: Prevention of radiation enteritis by an absorbable polygalactic acid mesh sling. Cancer 68:2545–2549, 1991.
103. Galante M, Hill EC: Pelvic exenteration: A critical analysis of a ten-year experience with the use of the team approach. Am J Obstet Gynecol 110:180–189, 1971.
104. Lawhead RA Jr, Clark DGC, Smith DH, et al: Pelvic exenteration for recurrent or persistent gynecologic malignancies. A 10-year review of the Memorial Sloan-Kettering Cancer Center experience (1972–1981). Gynecol Oncol 33:279–282, 1989.
105. Rutledge FN, Smith JP, Wharton JT, et al: Pelvic exenteration: An analysis of 296 patients. Am J Obstet Gynecol 129:881–892, 1977.
106. Symmonds RE, Pratt JH, Webb MJ: Exenterative operations: Experience of 198 patients. Am J Obstet Gynecol 121:907–918, 1975.
107. Morgan LS, Daly JW, Monif GRG: Infectious morbidity associated with pelvic exenteration. Gynecol Oncol 10:318–328, 1980.
108. Lichtinger M, Averette H, Girtanner R, et al: Small bowel complications after supravesicular urinary diversion in pelvic exenteration. Gynecol Oncol 24:137–142, 1986.
109. Averette HE, Ford JH Jr, Dudan RC, et al: Staging of cervical cancer. Clin Obstet Gynecol 18:215–232, 1975.
110. Nelson JH, Boyce J, Macasaet MA, et al: Incidence, significance and follow-up of para-aortic lymph node metastases in late invasive carcinoma of the cervix. Am J Obstet Gynecol 128:336–340, 1977.
111. Downey GO, Potish RA, Adcock LL, et al: Pretreatment surgical staging in cervical carcinoma: Therapeutic efficacy of pelvic lymph node resection. Am J Obstet Gynecol 160:1055–1061, 1989.
112. Berman ML, Lagasse LD, Watring WG, et al: The operative evaluation of patients with cervical carcinoma by an extraperitoneal approach. Obstet Gynecol 50:658–664, 1977.
113. Weiser EB, Bundy BN, Hoskins WJ, et al: Extraperitoneal versus transperitoneal selective paraaortic lymphadenectomy in the pretreatment surgical staging of advanced cervical carcinoma (a Gynecological Oncology Group study). Gynecol Oncol 33:283–289, 1989.
114. Childers JM, Hatch K, Surwit EA: The role of laparoscopic lymphadenectomy in the management of cervical carcinoma. Gynecol Oncol 47:38–43, 1992.
115. Fletcher GH: Cancer of the uterine cervix: Janeway lecture. AJR Am J Roentgenol 111:225–242, 1971.
116. Perez CA: Uterine cervix. In Perez CA, Brady LW (eds): Principles and Practice of Radiation Oncology, 2nd ed. Philadelphia: JB Lippincott, 1992, pp 1143–1202.
117. Fu K, Phillips TL: High-dose-rate versus low-dose-rate intracavitary brachytherapy for carcinoma of the cervix. Int J Radiat Oncol Biol Phys 19:791–796, 1990.
118. Hall EJ, Brenner DJ: The dose-rate effect revisited: Radiobiological considerations of importance in radiotherapy. Int J Radiat Oncol Biol Phys 21:1403–1414, 1991.
119. Joslin CAF, O'Connell D, Howard N: The treatment of uterine carcinoma using the cathetron. III. Clinical considerations and preliminary reports on treatment. Br J Radiol 40:895–904, 1967.
120. Potish RA, Deibel FC Jr, Khan PM: The relationship between milligram-hours and dose to point A in carcinoma of the cervix. Radiology 145:479–483, 1982.
121. Rosenstein LM: Simple computer program for optimization of source loading in cervical intracavitary applicators. Br J Radiol 50:119–122, 1977.
122. International Commission on Radiological Units and Measurements: Dose and Volume Specification for Reporting Intracavitary Therapy in Gynecology (ICRU Report 38). Bethesda, MD: ICRU, 1985.
123. Hreschyshyn MM, Aron BS, Boronow RC, et al: Hydroxyurea or placebo combined with radiation to treat stages IIIB and IV cervical cancer confined to the pelvis. Int J Radiat Oncol Biol Phys 5:317–322, 1979.
124. Bryson SCP, Lenehan P, Lickrish GM: The treatment of grade 3 cervical intraepithelial neoplasia with cryotherapy: An 11 year experience. Am J Obstet Gynecol 151:201–206, 1985.
125. Paraskevaidis E, Jandial L, Mann EMF, et al: Patterns of treatment failure following laser for cervical intraepithelial neoplasia: Implications for follow up protocol. Obstet Gynecol 78:80–83, 1991.

126. Townsend DE, Richart RM: Cryotherapy and carbon dioxide laser management of cervical intraepithelial neoplasia: A controlled comparison. Obstet Gynecol 61:75–78, 1983.
127. Baggish MS: Management of cervical intraepithelial neoplasia by carbon dioxide laser. Obstet Gynecol 60:378–384, 1982.
128. Bigrigg MA, Codling BW, Pearson P, et al: Colposcope diagnosis and treatment of cervical dysplasia at a single clinic visit. Lancet 336:229–231, 1991.
129. Ahlgren M, Ingemarsson J, Lindberg LG, et al: Conization as treatment of carcinoma in situ of the uterine cervix. Obstet Gynecol 46:135–140, 1975.
130. Holdt DG, Jacobs AJ, Scott JC Jr, et al: Diagnostic significance and sequelae of cone biopsy. Am J Obstet Gynecol 143:312–318, 1982.
131. Kolstad P, Klem V: Long-term followup of 1121 cases of carcinoma in situ. Obstet Gynecol 48:125–129, 1976.
132. Kolstad P: Follow-up study of 232 patients with stage IA1 and 411 patients with stage IA2 squamous cell carcinoma of the cervix (microinvasive carcinoma). Gynecol Oncol 33:265–272, 1989.
133. Maimon MA, Fruchter RG, Di Maio TM, et al: Superficially invasive squamous cell carcinoma of the cervix. Obstet Gynecol 72:399–403, 1988.
134. Seski JC, Abell MR, Morley GW: Microinvasive squamous carcinoma of the cervix: Definition, histologic analysis, late results of treatment. Obstet Gynecol 50:410–414, 1977.
135. Simon NL, Gore H, Shingleton HM: Study of superficially invasive carcinoma of the cervix. Obstet Gynecol 68:19–24, 1986.
136. Morley GW, Seski JC: Radical pelvic surgery versus radiation therapy for stage I carcinoma of the cervix (exclusive of microinvasion). Am J Obstet Gynecol 126:785–798, 1976.
137. Artman LE, Hoskins WJ, Bibro MC, et al: Radical hysterectomy and pelvic lymphadenectomy for stage IB carcinoma of the cervix: 21 years' experience. Gynecol Oncol 28:8–13, 1987.
138. Bianchi UA, Sartori E, Pecorelli S, et al: Treatment of primary invasive cervical cancer. Eur J Gynecol Oncol 9:47–53, 1988.
139. Lee YN, Wang KL, Lin MH, et al: Radical hysterectomy with pelvic lymph node dissection for treatment of cervical cancer: A clinical review of 954 cases. Gynecol Oncol 32:135–142, 1989.
140. Powell JL, Burrell MO, Franklin EW: Radical hysterectomy and pelvic lymphadenectomy. South Med J 77:596–600, 1984.
141. Coia L, Won M, Lanciano R, et al: The patterns of care outcome study for cancer of the uterine cervix: Results of the second National Practice Survey. Cancer 66:2451–2456, 1990.
142. Montana GS, Fowler WC, Varia MA, et al: Analysis of results of radiation therapy for stage IB carcinoma of the cervix. Cancer 60:2195–2200, 1987.
143. Perez CA, Camel HM, Kuske RR, et al: Radiation alone in the treatment of carcinoma of the uterine cervix: A 20-year experience. Gynecol Oncol 23:127–140, 1986.
144. Seibel MM, Freeman MG, Graves WL: Carcinoma of the cervix and sexual function. Obstet Gynecol 55:484–487, 1979.
145. Kinney WK, Egorshin EV, Podratz KC: Wertheim hysterectomy in the geriatric population. Gynecol Oncol 31:227–232, 1988.
146. Toki N, Tsukamoto N, Kaku T, et al: Microscopic ovarian metastasis of the uterine cervical cancer. Gynecol Oncol 41:46–51, 1991.
147. Alvarez RD, Soong S-J, Kinney WK, et al: Identification of prognostic factors and risk groups in patients found to have nodal metastasis at the time of radical hysterectomy for early-stage carcinoma of the cervix. Gynecol Oncol 35:130–135, 1989.
148. Creasman WT, Soper JT, Clarke-Pearson D: Radical hysterectomy as therapy for early carcinoma of the cervix. Am J Obstet Gynecol 155:964–969, 1986.
149. Fuller AF Jr, Elliott N, Kosloff C, et al: Determinants of increased risk for recurrence in patients undergoing radical hysterectomy for stage IB and IA carcinoma of the cervix. Gynecol Oncol 33:34–39, 1989.
150. Hogan WM, Littman P, Griner L, et al: Results of radiation therapy given after radical hysterectomy. Cancer 49:1278–1285, 1982.
151. Kinney WK, Alvarez RD, Reid GC, et al: Value of adjuvant whole-pelvis irradiation after Wertheim hysterectomy for early-stage squamous carcinoma of the cervix with pelvic nodal metastases: A matched-control study. Gynecol Oncol 34:258–262, 1989.
152. Martimbeau PW, Kjorstad KE, Iversen T: Stage IB carcinoma of the cervix, the Norwegian Radium Hospital. II. Results when pelvic nodes are involved. Obstet Gynecol 60:215–218, 1982.
153. Remy JC, di Maio T, Fruchter RG, et al: Adjunctive radiation after radical hysterectomy in stage IB squamous cell carcinoma of the cervix. Gynecol Oncol 38:161–165, 1990.
154. Larson DM, Stringer CA, Copeland LJ, et al: Stage IB cervical carcinoma treated with radical hysterectomy and pelvic lymphadenectomy: Role of adjuvant radiotherapy. Obstet Gynecol 69:378–381, 1987.
155. Wertheim MS, Hakes TB, Daghestani AN, et al: A pilot study of adjuvant therapy in patients with cervical cancer at high risk of recurrence after radical hysterectomy and pelvic lymphadenectomy. J Clin Oncol 3:912–916, 1985.
156. Lai C-H, Lin T-S, Soong Y-K, et al: Adjuvant chemotherapy after radical hysterectomy for cervical carcinoma. Gynecol Oncol 35:193–198, 1989.
157. Ueki M, Okamura S, Maeda T: Individualization of patients for adjuvant chemotherapy after surgical treatment of cervical cancer. Br J Obstet Gynaecol 94:985–990.
158. Tattersall MHN, Ramirez C, Coppelson M: A randomized trial of adjuvant chemotherapy after radical hysterectomy in stage Ib–IIa cervical cancer patients with pelvic node metastases. Gynecol Oncol 46:176–181, 1992.
159. Montana GS, Fowler WC, Varia MA, et al: Analysis of results of radiation therapy for stage IIB carcinoma of the cervix. Cancer 55:956–962, 1985.
160. Hopkins MP, Morley GW: Stage IB squamous cell cancer of the cervix: Clinicopathologic features related to survival. Am J Obstet Gynecol 164:1520–1529, 1991.
161. van Nagell JR, Donaldson ES, Parker JC, et al: The prognostic significance of cell type and lesion size in patients with cervical cancer treated with radical hysterectomy. Gynecol Oncol 5:142–151, 1977.
162. Lu T, Macasaet MA, Nelson JH Jr: The barrel shaped cervix. Am J Obstet Gynecol 124:596–600, 1976.
163. Einhorn N, Patek E, Sjoberg B: Outcome of different treatment modifications in cervix carcinoma, stage IB and IIA. Observations in a well-defined Swedish population. Cancer 55:949–955, 1985.
164. Gallion HN, van Nagell JR, Donaldson ES, et al: Combined radiation therapy and extrafascial hysterectomy in the treatment of stage IB barrel-shaped cervical cancer. Cancer 56:262–265, 1985.
165. Maruyama Y, van Nagell JR, Yoneda J, et al: Dose-response and failure pattern for bulky or barrel-shaped stage IB cervical cancer treated by combined photon irradiation and extrafascial hysterectomy. Cancer 63:70–76, 1989.
166. Nelson AJ, Fletcher GH, Wharton JT: Indications for adjunctive conservative extrafascial hysterectomy in selected cases of carcinoma of the uterine cervix. AJR 123:91–99, 1975.
167. O'Quinn AG, Fletcher GH, Wharton JT: Guidelines for conservative hysterectomy after irradiation. Gynecol Oncol 9:68–79, 1980.
168. Perez CA, Kao MS: Radiation therapy alone or combined with surgery in the treatment of barrel-shaped carcinoma of the uterine cervix. Int J Radiat Oncol Biol Phys 11:1903–1909, 1985.
169. Kuske RR, Perez CA, Grigsby PW, et al: Phase I/II study of definitive radiotherapy and chemotherapy (cisplatin and 5-fluorouracil) for advanced or recurrent gynecologic malignancies. Am J Clin Oncol 12:467–473, 1989.
170. Sardi JE, di Paola GR, Giaroli A, et al: Results of a phase II trial with neoadjuvant chemotherapy in carcinoma of the cervix uteri. Gynecol Oncol 31:256–261, 1988.
171. Berman ML, Keys H, Creasman W, et al: Survival and patterns of recurrence in cervical cancer metastatic to periaortic lymph nodes. Gynecol Oncol 19:8–16, 1984.
172. Nori D, Valentine E, Hilaris B: The role of paraaortic node irradiation in the treatment of cancer of the cervix. Int J Radiat Oncol Biol Phys 11:1469–1473, 1985.
173. Podczaski E, Stryker J, Kaminski P, et al: Extended-field radiation therapy for carcinoma of the cervix. Cancer 66:251–258, 1991.
174. Ito K, Noda K: Peritoneal cytology in patients with uterine cervical carcinoma. Gynecol Oncol 47:76–79, 1992.
175. Hiilesmaa VK, Vesterinen E, Nieminen U, et al: Carcinoma of the uterine cervix. Stage III: A report of 311 cases. Gynecol Oncol 12:99–106, 1981.
176. Montana GS, Fowler WC, Varia MA, et al: Carcinoma of the cervix. Stage III: Results of radiation therapy. Cancer 57:148–154, 1986.
177. Spanos W Jr, Guse C, Perez CA, et al: Phase II study of multiple

daily fractionations in the palliation of advanced pelvic malignancies: Preliminary report of RTOG 8502. Int J Radiat Oncol Biol Phys 17:659–661, 1989.

178. Varghese C, Rangad F, Jose CC, et al: Hyperfractionation in advanced carcinoma of the uterine cervix: A preliminary report. Int J Radiat Oncol Biol Phys 23:393–396, 1992.
179. Chauvergne J, Rohart J, Heron J, et al: Essai randomise dechimiotherapie initiale dans 151 carcinomes du col uterin localement etendus (T2b-N1, T3b, M0). Bull Cancer (Paris) 77:1007–1024, 1990.
180. Souhami L, Gil RA, Allan SE, et al: A randomized trial of chemotherapy followed by pelvic radiation therapy in stage IIIB carcinoma of the cervix. J Clin Oncol 9:970–977, 1991.
181. Rettenmaier MA, Moran MF, Ramsinghani NF, et al: Treatment of advanced and recurrent squamous carcinoma of the uterine cervix with constant intraarterial infusion of cisplatin. Cancer 61:1301–1303, 1988.
182. Giaroli A, Sananes C, Sardi JE, et al: Lymph node metastases in carcinoma of the cervix uteri: Response to neoadjuvant chemotherapy and its impact on survival. Gynecol Oncol 39:34–39, 1990.
183. Kim DS, Moon H, Hwang YY, et al: Preoperative adjuvant chemotherapy in the treatment of cervical cancer stage Ib, IIa, and IIb with bulky tumor. Gynecol Oncol 29:321–332, 1988.
184. Panici PB, Scambia G, Baiocchi G, et al: Neoadjuvant chemotherapy and radical surgery in locally advanced cervical cancer: Prognostic factors for response and survival. Cancer 67:372–379, 1991.
185. Dottino PR, Plaxe SC, Beddoe AM, et al: Induction chemotherapy followed by radical surgery in cervical cancer. Gynecol Oncol 40:7–11, 1991.
186. Deppe G, Malviya VK, Han I, et al: A preliminary report of combination chemotherapy with cisplatin and mitomycin-C followed by radical hysterectomy or radiation therapy in patients with locally advanced cervical cancer. Gynecol Oncol 42:178–181, 1991.
187. Jobsen J, Leer W, Cleton FJ, et al: Treatment of locoregional recurrence of carcinoma of the cervix by radiotherapy after primary surgery. Gynecol Oncol 33:368–371, 1993.
188. Larson DM, Copeland LJ, Stringer CA, et al: Recurrent cervical cancer after radical hysterectomy. Gynecol Oncol 30:381–387, 1988.
189. Potter ME, Alvarez RD, Gay FL, et al: Optimal therapy for pelvic recurrence after radical hysterectomy for early-stage cervical cancer. Gynecol Oncol 37:74–77, 1990.
190. DiSaia PJ, Creasman WT: Invasive cervical cancer. In Clinical Gynecologic Oncology, 4th ed. St. Louis: Mosby, 1993, p 63.
191. Stanhope CR, Symmonds RE: Palliative exenteration—what, when, why? Am J Obstet Gynecol 152:12–16, 1985.
192. Barber HRK, Jones W: Lymphadenectomy in pelvic exenteration for recurrent cervix cancer. JAMA 215:1945–1949, 1971.
193. Creasman WT, Rutledge FN: Is positive pelvic lymphadenopathy a contraindication to radical surgery in recurrent cervical carcinoma? Gynecol Oncol 2:482–485, 1974.
194. Hockel M, Knapstein PG, Kutzner J, et al: A novel combined operative and radiotherapeutic approach for recurrent gynecologic malignant lesions infiltrating the pelvic wall. Surg Gynecol Obstet 173:297–302, 1991.
195. Averette HE, Lichtinger M, Sevin B-U, et al: Pelvic exenteration: A 15 year experience in a general metropolitan hospital. Am J Obstet Gynecol 150:179–184, 1984.
196. Shingleton HM, Soong S-J, Gelder MS, et al: Clinical and histologic factors predicting recurrence and survival after pelvic exenteration for cancer of the cervix. Obstet Gynecol 73:1027–1034, 1989.
197. Soper JT, Berchuk A, Creasman WT, et al: Pelvic exenteration: Factors associated with major surgical morbidity. Gynecol Oncol 35:93–98, 1989.
198. Buxton EJ, Meanwell CA, Hilton C, et al: Combination bleomycin, ifosfamide, and cisplatin chemotherapy in cervical cancer. J Natl Cancer Inst 81:359–361, 1989.
199. Rosenthal CJ, Khulpateea N, Boyce J, et al: Effective chemotherapy for advanced carcinoma of the cervix with bleomycin, cisplatin, vincristine, and methotrexate. Cancer 52:2025–2030, 1983.
200. Rustin GJS, Newlands ES, Southcott BM, et al: Cisplatin, vincristine, methotrexate and bleomycin (POMB) as initial or palliative chemotherapy for carcinoma of the cervix. Br J Obstet Gynaecol 94:1205–1211, 1987.
201. Friedlander M, Kaye SB, Sullivan A, et al: Cervical carcinoma: A drug-responsive tumor—experience with combined cisplatin, vinblastine, and bleomycin therapy. Gynecol Oncol 16:275–281, 1983.
202. Soeters R, Bloch B, Levin W, et al: Combined chemotherapy and radiotherapy in patients with advanced squamous carcinoma of the cervix (cis-platinum-bleomycin-vinblastine). Gynecol Oncol 33:44–45, 1989.
203. Young RH, Scully RE: Villoglandular papillary adenocarcinoma of the uterine cervix: A clinicopathologic analysis of 13 cases. Cancer 63:1773–1779, 1989.
204. Ferry JA, Scully RE: "Adenoid cystic" carcinoma and adenoid basal carcinoma of the uterine cervix: A study of 28 cases. Am J Surg Pathol 12:134–144, 1988.
205. King LA, Talledo OE, Gallup DG, et al: Adenoid cystic carcinoma of the cervix in women under age 40. Gynecol Oncol 32:26–30, 1989.
206. Prempreee T, Villasanta U, Tang C-K: Management of adenoid cystic carcinoma of the uterine cervix (cylindroma): Report of six cases and reappraisal of all cases reported in the medical literature. Cancer 46:1631–1635, 1980.
207. Degefu S, O'Quinn AG, Lacey CG, et al: Verrucous carcinoma of the cervix: A report of two cases and literature review. Gynecol Oncol 25:37–47, 1986.
208. Daroca PJ Jr, Dhurandhar HN: Basaloid carcinoma of the uterine cervix. Am J Surg Pathol 4:235–239, 1980.
209. Fu YS, Reagan JW: Pathology of the Uterine Cervix, Vagina and Vulva. Philadelphia: WB Saunders, 1989.
210. Stoler MH, Mills SE, Gersell DJ, et al: Small-cell neuroendocrine carcinoma of the cervix: A human papillomavirus type 18-associated cancer. Am J Surg Pathol 15:28–32, 1991.
211. Clement PB: Miscellaneous primary tumors and metastatic tumors of the uterine cervix. Semin Diagn Pathol 7:228–248, 1990.
212. Jones HW, Droegemueller W, Makowski EL: A primary melanocarcinoma of the cervix. Obstet Gynecol 111:959–963, 1971.
213. McGuire WP III, Arseneau J, Blessing JA, et al: A randomized comparative trial of carboplatin and iproplatin in advanced squamous carcinoma of the uterine cervix: A Gynecologic Oncology Group study. J Clin Oncol 7:1462–1468, 1989.
214. Thigpen JT, Shingleton H, Homesley H, et al: Cis-platinum in treatment of advanced or recurrent squamous cell carcinoma of the cervix: A phase II study of the Gynecologic Oncology Group. Cancer 48:899–903, 1981.
215. Freeman RS, Herson J, Wharton JT, et al: Single agent chemotherapy for recurrent carcinoma of the cervix. Cancer Clin Trials 3:345–350, 1980.
216. Muscato MS, Perry MC, Yarbro JW: Chemotherapy of cervical cancer. Semin Oncol 9:373–387, 1982.
217. Wasserman TH, Carter SK: The integration of chemotherapy in combined modality treatment of solid tumors. VIII. Cervical cancer. Cancer Treat Rev 4:25–46, 1977.
218. Piver MH, Barlow JJ, Xynos FP: Adriamycin alone or in combination in 100 patients with carcinoma of the cervix or vagina. Am J Obstet Gynecol 131:311–313, 1978.
219. Wong L-C, Choy DTK, Ngan HYS, et al: 4-Epidoxorubicin in recurrent cervical cancer. Cancer 63:1279–1282, 1989.
220. Malkasian GD, Decker DG, Jorgensen ED: Chemotherapy of carcinoma of the cervix. Gynecol Oncol 5:109–120, 1977.
221. Buxton EJ, Blackledge GR, Mould JJ, et al: The role of ifosfamide in cervical cancer. Semin Oncol 16(suppl 3):60–67, 1989.
222. Stehman FB, Blessing JA, McGehee R, et al: A phase II evaluation of mitolactol in patients with advanced squamous cell carcinoma of the cervix: A Gynecologic Oncology Group study. J Clin Oncol 7:1892–1895, 1989.

Uterine Cancers

Allan J. Jacobs, M.D. • Rudy A. Segna, M.D.

EPIDEMIOLOGY

Incidence

According to the American Cancer Society,[1] there are an estimated 31,000 new cases of uterine cancer each year. Approximately 5700 deaths are attributable to these neoplasms. Uterine cancer is the most common gynecologic malignancy, but it is relatively amenable to cure.

Risk Factors

Genetic-Familial

The familial Lynch syndrome II is characterized by hereditary adenocarcinoma of various sites, especially colorectal, but including endometrial carcinoma.[2] This syndrome is inherited as an autosomal dominant trait with varying degrees of penetrance and expressivity. Cytogenetic studies are currently ongoing to identify the potential chromosomal abnormality that may lead to endometrial cancer.[3] No studies to date have identified a genetic association for uterine sarcomas.

Environmental

The most important environmental risk factor associated with the development of endometrial carcinoma is the continuous estrogen stimulation of the endometrium without periodic progesterone to induce maturation. This may occur as a result of the administration of estrogen to postmenopausal women without a concomitant progestin regimen.[4] (Such treatment is now generallyconsidered to be contraindicated in women without a uterus; progestins should be given as part of hormone replacement therapy in such women.) The use of exogenous progestational agents diminishes the risk of endometrial cancer by resulting in the maturation and cyclic sloughing of the endometrium and preventing the development of hyperplasia in response to the exogenous estrogens. Polycystic ovarian syndrome is another syndrome associated with continuous estrogen exposure without modulation by progesterone. By far the most common cause of continuous estrogen stimulation is obesity in postmenopausal women. Obesity is associated with increased aromatization of androstenedione to estrone in the peripheral adipose tissue.[5] This leads to the stimulation of the endometrial lining, with subsequent hyperplasia and cancer. Tamoxifen use, especially the long-term administration in breast cancer patients, can have an estrogenic impact on the endometrium despite being an antiestrogen. An increased risk of endometrial cancer has been identified in these patients.[6]

Other

Diabetic women have also been shown to be at increased risk, even when other confounding variables such as age and weight are controlled.[7] The explanation for this relationship is still elusive. Nulliparity, late menopause, and hypertension have been associated with an increased incidence of endometrial cancer.[7] Prior pelvic radiotherapy has also been associated with an increased risk of uterine cancers, including virulent, poorly differentiated carcinomas and sarcomas.[8] Uterine sarcomas tend to be more common in black women.[9]

LIFE HISTORY

Understanding the patterns of spread of endometrial cancer allows one to appreciate the reasoning behind surgical staging and the type of adjuvant therapy offered. Uterine cancers, like other gynecologic malignancies, may spread by direct extension, lymphatics, hematogenous metastases, or transperitoneally. Direct extension into the myometrium and distally to the cervix is the most common avenue of metastasis.[10] The presence of a lymphatic network in the outer portion of the myometrium explains why the incidence of nodal metastasis increases with greater tumor penetration through the myometrium.[11] Lymphatic dissemination generally leads first to pelvic and then to periaortic node involvement.[11] Occasionally, aortic nodes may be primarily involved due to metastasis via the lymphatics that parallel the ovarian vessels.[11] Inguinofemoral nodal metastasis via the round ligaments rarely occurs. Hematogenous spread, especially in sarcomas and poorly differentiated carcinomas, accounts for distant metastases. The lung is the most common site, followed by bone and liver. Transperitoneal spread via the fallopian tubes and transserosal penetration can result in positive cytology, ovarian metastases, and peritoneal carcinomatosis.[12]

Peritoneal dissemination and consequent intestinal obstruction is a frequent cause of death. Mortality may also arise from pulmonary or hepatic failure, from bilateral ureteral obstruction as a result of pelvic disease, or from disseminated malignancy with malnutrition and infection.

Patterns of recurrence are influenced by the histology, the stage at diagnosis, and the form of treatment. This accounts for differences among series (Table 14–13). Close

TABLE 14–13
Patterns of Recurrence of Endometrial Carcinoma

Site*	Percent of Total	
	Aalders et al.[13]	*Podczaski et al.*[19]
Vagina	22	2
Vault	11	
Distal to vault	11	
Pelvis†	28	14
Distant	50	31
Lung	17	
Upper abdomen	13	
Bone	5	
Other	8	
>1 distant site	7	
Total	100	47
Number of patients	379	300

*Most distant site observed at initial diagnosis of recurrence.
†Includes the uterus.

to half of all recurrences are seen within a year of treatment; three fourths are diagnosed within 3 years of treatment.[13, 14] Isolated vaginal recurrences are not uncommon following treatment of early disease.[13, 15–19] If treatment is unsuccessful, pain, fistulas, and hemorrhagic complications may ensue. Pelvic sidewall recurrence can result in edema of the lower extremities, pain from involvement of the lumbar and sacral plexus, or bowel obstruction. Endometrial carcinoma commonly recurs outside the pelvis, whether the initial disease is early or late stage.[13, 19, 20] If adjuvant radiotherapy is administered, the *relative* chance of a recurrence occurring in the upper abdomen or the lungs is even higher.[19] Angel et al.[21] emphasize that vaginal occurrences of stage I disease are often associated with occult upper abdominal disease. This may account for the low salvage rate seen in these patients.[18]

PATHOLOGY

Approximately 97% of uterine malignancies are epithelial lesions, and 3% are mesenchymal. Histologic type, grade of differentiation, depth of myometrial invasion, and hormone receptor status are important pathologic prognostic indicators in carcinoma. The grade of endometrial carcinoma is based on its architecture. Well-differentiated tumors are defined as those with no more than 5% solid elements exclusive of areas with squamous morphology. Moderately differentiated lesions contain 6% to 50% solid elements. Carcinomas that are more than 50% solid are poorly differentiated. Nuclear grading may be used to raise the FIGO grade one level.

Favorable histologic factors in carcinomas include good differentiation, the presence of benign squamous elements (adenoacanthomas),[22] and the concomitant presence of endometrial hyperplasia. Tumors with favorable histology are usually associated with unopposed estrogen stimulation.[23]

Unfavorable histologic types include moderately to poorly differentiated adenocarcinomas, papillary serous carcinomas, and clear cell carcinomas.[24] These lesions tend to occur in women without the classic risk factors. They often demonstrate peritoneal and lymphatic spread at the time of diagnosis.[24] Papillary serous and clear cell varieties constitute fewer than 20% of endometrial cancers. Five-year survival rates for each of these histologic types is 35%.[25, 26]

Uterine sarcomas, in general, have a poorer prognosis than the adenocarcinomas.[27] These tumors may arise from the myometrium or from the endometrial glands and stroma.

Leiomyosarcomas account for one quarter of all uterine sarcomas.[28] They usually arise de novo from the uterine smooth muscle rather than from pre-existing benign leiomyomas.[29] The number of mitoses per 10 high-power fields (HPF) and the presence of cytologic atypia are the major criteria used to determine the virulence of the tumor.[30] Tumors with 10 or more mitoses per 10 HPF are considered malignant. Those with 5 to 9 mitoses per 10 HPF are considered malignant only if nuclear atypia is present. Without atypia, such tumors are considered borderline. Tumors with cellular atypia but with fewer than 5 mitoses per 10 HPF are benign and are known as cellular leiomyomas.

Seventy percent of uterine sarcomas arise from the endometrium.[27] They are categorized according to two parameters. First, these tumors may be homologous or heterologous. Homologous tumors contain only endometrial stromal elements, and heterologous tumors contain elements not normally found in the uterus (e.g., rhabdomyosarcoma or chondrosarcoma). Second, sarcomas may be pure or mixed. Pure lesions contain only sarcomatous elements, whereas mixed tumors contain malignant endometrial glands as well.

Pure, homologous endometrial stromal sarcomas constitute 15% of uterine sarcomas[27] and are further classified on the basis of mitotic count into low-grade (also known as endolymphatic stromal myosis) and high-grade lesions.[31] Low-grade stromal sarcomas demonstrate fewer than 10 mitoses per 10 HPF, whereas high-grade lesions have more than 10. Low-grade lesions tend to recur locally, and high-grade lesions metastasize via lymphatics and blood.[32] The long-term survival and treatment of each of these entities are quite different.[33] Low-grade lesions are associated with long disease-free intervals and survival. High-grade lesions recur earlier and more frequently. The mainstay of therapy for each type of lesion is surgical extirpation. Low-grade lesions are sensitive to progestins, which are utilized in cases of recurrent or metastatic disease. High-grade lesions do not respond to progestins.

Mixed mesodermal tumors comprise malignant stromal and glandular elements of the endometrium. Some authors reserve this term for heterologous mixed tumors and refer to homologous mixed tumors as carcinosarcomas. These tumors are usually discovered in postmenopausal women and are highly virulent. The 5-year survival rate for patients with mixed mesodermal tumors is 22%.[27] About half of patients with stage I disease are cured.

DIAGNOSIS, SCREENING, EARLY DETECTION, AND STAGING

Approximately 90% of women with uterine cancer present with abnormal uterine bleeding. Pain, increasing abdominal girth, increasing uterine size, weight loss, and ascites are less common presentations. The diagnosis of endometrial cancer is made by histologic sampling of the endometrium. This can be done either by office endometrial biopsy or by dilatation and curettage in the operating room. An office endometrial biopsy should be performed in any of the following circumstances:

1. In women with abnormal uterine bleeding after the age of 35.
2. In women with uterine bleeding more than 6 months after the previous menstrual period (i.e., postmenopausal bleeding).
3. Annually in women receiving tamoxifen.
4. Annually in patients with conditions in which unopposed estrogen stimulation is present (e.g., chronic anovulation, morbid obesity).

A dilatation and fractional endocervical and endometrial curettage should be performed in the following circumstances:

1. If office biopsy is not possible (e.g., because of cervical stenosis, inability of the patient to tolerate the procedure).
2. If further bleeding occurs after outpatient endometrial biopsy.
3. In patients with a tissue diagnosis of atypical hyperplasia on an office biopsy, in order to rule out carcinoma.

Once the tissue diagnosis of endometrial carcinoma is made, almost all patients undergo surgery for therapy and staging of this disease. The preoperative evaluation is directed at diagnosing metastases and establishing medical fitness for the proposed operation. Complete blood count, serum electrolytes and chemistries, chest radiograph, and electrocardiogram are the minimal tests required. A barium enema may be obtained if the patient has any significant bowel symptoms. A computed tomography (CT) scan with contrast, although not required, may provide additional information, such as liver or lymph node involvement, and may detect other intrapelvic and abdominal masses. If a CT scan is not obtained, it is advisable to obtain an intravenous urogram to rule out urinary tract anomalies. In lesions that appear localized, we often perform magnetic resonance imaging (MRI) or transvaginal ultrasonography to estimate the depth of myometrial invasion.[34–37]

The overall inaccuracy of clinical staging may be as high as 50%.[38] Therefore, uterine cancer is now a surgically staged disease (Table 14–14). Prospective studies using surgical staging have identified prognostic factors such as myometrial invasion, histology, grade, peritoneal cytology, lymphatic and vascular space involvement, and hormonal receptor status, all of which may predict length of survival (see below). Surgical staging consists of a total abdominal hysterectomy, bilateral salpingo-oophorectomy, selected pelvic and periaortic lymph node sampling, and peritoneal cytology. The technique is discussed below.

MODALITIES OF TREATMENT

Surgery

The hallmark of treatment of uterine malignancy is the extended extrafascial hysterectomy, which is described on page 396. Bilateral salpingectomy and oophorectomy are almost invariably performed during hysterectomy for uterine lesions. Pelvic washings are routinely taken shortly after the abdomen is entered. This is done by irrigating the pelvis with normal saline, aspirating the fluid, and then

TABLE 14–14
FIGO Staging of Endometrial Carcinoma (1988)*

Stage	Definition
Stage I	Tumor limited to the uterine corpus
IA G1,2,3	Tumor limited to endometrium
IB G1,2,3	Invasion up to half of myometrium†
IC G1,2,3	Invasion greater than half of myometrium†
Stage II	Tumor limited to the uterine corpus and cervix
IIA G1,2,3	Involvement of only endocervical glands
IIB G1,2,3	Invasion of cervical stroma
Stage III	Tumor limited to pelvis and abdominal lymph nodes
IIIA G1,2,3	Positive peritoneal cytology or tumor involves adnexae or uterine serosa
IIIB G1,2,3	Tumor metastatic to vagina
IIIC G1,2,3	Tumor with metastases to bladder or periaortic nodes
Stage IV	Tumor with bladder or rectal involvement, or distant metastases
IVA G1,2,3	Tumor involves mucosa of bladder or rectum
IVB G1,2,3	Distant metastases, including intra-abdominal spread or metastases to inguinofemoral nodes
Grade‡	**Definition**
G1	5% or less of a nonsquamous or nonmorular solid growth pattern
G2	6% to 50% of a nonsquamous or nonmorular solid growth pattern
G3	More than 50% of a nonsquamous or nonmorular solid growth pattern

*Patients with corpus cancer treated primarily by radiation therapy should be graded according to the FIGO clinical staging adopted in 1971.[64] The fact of clinical staging should be noted.

†Optimally, width of the myometrium and width of the tumor invasion should be recorded.

‡Notable nuclear atypia that is inappropriate for the architectural grade raises the grade of a grade 1 or grade 2 tumor by one. In serous, clear cell, and squamous carcinomas, nuclear grading takes precedence. Adenosquamous carcinomas are graded according to the nuclear grade of the glandular component.

sending it for analysis by cytology or cell block or both. The uterus is opened immediately following removal, and a frozen section is taken to determine the grade and myometrial invasion. Additionally, an aliquot of tissue is submitted for progesterone receptors and her-2-*neu* staining.

In order to achieve thorough surgical staging (when indicated), pelvic and aortic lymphadenectomies are performed in conjunction with hysterectomy. The broad ligament incisions in the peritoneum are extended cephalad into the paracolic gutters bilaterally. Medial reflection of the tissues superficial to the psoas muscle identifies the ureter and the great vessels. The precaval nodes are removed on the right, and the periaortic nodes (which lie posterolateral to the aorta) are removed on the left. The superior limit of dissection is the origin of the inferior mesenteric artery, but some surgeons carry the dissection to the level of the renal veins. Adjacent structures subject to damage include the ureters, the lumbar arteries, the vena cava, and tributaries of the great vessels (including the inferior mesenteric and ovarian arteries and the renal veins).[10] This extended staging, when added to an extrafascial hysterectomy, results in little added morbidity.[39–41]

It is possible to perform a hysterectomy with salpingo-oophorectomy by dividing the abdominal pedicles laparoscopically and then dissecting the uterosacral ligament, cardinal ligament, and vaginal cuff vaginally.[42] This so-called laparoscopically assisted vaginal hysterectomy has not been accepted as standard procedure because its safety has not been established, but it seems to be applicable to the treatment of endometrial carcinoma,[43] especially since laparoscopic pelvic and aortic lymphadenectomy has also been reported as feasible.[44, 45] Vaginal hysterectomy may be employed in morbidly obese patients or in women with poor health who are not candidates for abdominal surgery.[46, 47]

Radiotherapy

When external radiation is given to pelvic or extended fields, techniques are the same as those described for cervical carcinoma (see page 399). Whole abdominal irradiation is given as described for ovarian carcinoma (see page 434). Postoperative intracavitary irradiation is given using vaginal cylinders. A single conventional dose rate implant may be employed, delivering 40 Gy to an isodose plane 0.5 cm below the vaginal surface over 2 to 3 days. Alternatively, three high-dose implants are given, each administering 7 Gy in a few minutes to an isodose plane 0.5 cm beneath the vaginal surface.

Chemotherapy

The development of knowledge in this area has been hindered by the fact that most chemotherapy trials have been small and uncontrolled. Different workers employing similar regimens frequently differ in their conclusions regarding efficacy.

Kelley and Baker[48] described the efficacy of progestins in the treatment of metastatic endometrial carcinoma, demonstrating objective responses in 6 of 21 patients. Subsequent reports of extensive series demonstrated a response rate closer to 10%.[49, 50] Responses are almost exclusively confined to well-differentiated tumors that contain progesterone receptors. Several randomized trials failed to confirm the efficacy of progestins as adjuvant therapy in early cancer.[51–54] A few studies of tamoxifen show an objective response rate of 0 to 53%, with a pooled response of about 20%.[55]

Doxorubicin, 5-fluorouracil, cisplatin, and carboplatin are the only single cytotoxic agents whose efficacy against metastatic endometrial carcinoma is consistently demonstrable in clinical trials.[55] Cyclophosphamide and ifosfamide may also be effective.[55] The combination of cisplatin, doxorubicin, and cyclophosphamide appears to induce objective responses in about half of patients with metastatic tumor.[55–57] The combination of cisplatin, doxorubicin, and etoposide provided a 75% response rate (55% complete response) in one trial.[58] Another recent trial showed 60% activity of methotrexate, vinblastine, doxorubicin, and cisplatin.[59]

TREATMENT OF PRIMARY ENDOMETRIAL CARCINOMA

In contrast to the situation with the other common forms of gynecologic cancer, there are few well-controlled studies of the treatment of endometrial cancer. Consequently, therapy must be based on observational studies of the natural history of this tumor with various types of treatment. Many studies attempt to subdivide these tumors according to extent and histologic grade. The remainder assess other variables and attempt to correlate them with known predictors of prognosis, such as extent and grade. These studies are almost all retrospective, and there generally is no standardization of treatment or control for the effects of different modes of therapy. The intellectual exercise involved in conducting and interpreting these studies has three goals. The first is to define a category of low-risk endometrial adenocarcinoma lesions that are so highly curable by surgery alone that postoperative adjuvant treatment is not warranted. The second goal is to define, by exclusion, the complementary category of high-risk tumors that are likely to recur and that can potentially benefit from adjuvant nonoperative therapy. The third goal is to define the sites at which endometrial carcinoma recurs and to quantify the likelihood of recurrence at each of these sites in order to define rational programs of adjuvant therapy for use in clinical trials.

In fact, the process of classifying prognostic subsets of endometrial carcinoma is incomplete. Consequently, there is a third risk category, intermediate risk, for which adjuvant treatment is of uncertain benefit.

TABLE 14–15
Putative Predictors of Prognosis in Stage I Endometrial Carcinoma

Age[62, 67, 72, 75,]
CA 125 level[97, 98]
Cytologic grade[67–69]
DNA ploidy[14, 74, 91–94]
Endometrial hyperplasia, concomitant[82, 83]
Epidemiologic risk factors[23, 76, 100–102]
Estrogen receptors[74, 88, 89] (negative[90])
Histologic grade[61–64, 66, 68, 69, 72–77]
Length of endometrial cavity[63, 76]
Lymph node metastases[64]
Lymphatic vascular space involvement[69, 72, 74, 75, 78–80]
Mitotic index[69, 95]
Myometrial invasion—extent[18, 61–64, 68, 69, 72–77]
Oncogene amplification (c-*neu*)[99]
Peritoneal cytology[77, 85] (negative[75])
Progesterone receptors[74, 77, 88–90]
S-phase index[74, 93, 96]
Tumor size[62, 81]

TABLE 14–16
Effect of Histologic Grade on Clinical Outcome in Stage I Endometrial Carcinoma

Author	No. of Patients	5-Year Survival (%)		
		Grade 1	*Grade 2*	*Grade 3*
Burke et al.[73]	520	98	95	56
DiSaia and Creasman[64]	222	95	87	69
Lotocki et al.[61]	699	96	90	61
Lurain et al.[62]	264	93	86	64
Mittal et al.[69]	181	94	94	73
Ng and Reagan[66]	183	92	80	63
Philipsen and Norgard[18]	1084	97	91	71

Stage I Carcinoma

Assignment of Risk Status

The vast majority of endometrial carcinomas are confined to the fundus, by both clinical[60] and surgicopathologic[10] criteria. Such lesions constitute stage I lesions both in the older clinical and in the current surgical staging systems. Pettersson[60] reported 11,035 of 13,979 lesions (79%) to be clinically confined to the fundus, and an additional 2014 confined to the fundus and cervix, leaving only 1330 (10%) with apparent clinical involvement of extrauterine structures at the time of diagnosis. Surgicopathologic staging was not adopted until 1988, so *almost all the studies cited in this chapter are based on clinical staging.*

It has long been recognized that criteria other than extent of tumor are useful in predicting survival in patients with these tumors. Some of these factors are listed in Table 14–15. Systematic studies of large numbers of patients made it clear that uterine size and endometrial cavity length were not correlated with survival.[61–63] This has led to the elimination of endometrial cavity length as a factor in the formal staging system for endometrial tumors.

In contrast, both histologic grade[18, 62, 64–66] and cytologic grade[67–69] have been strongly associated with survival in almost every study that has examined these variables. Histologic grading has less variability among different observers than cytologic grading.[70] Consequently, it has been studied more frequently than cytologic grading. The results of several studies of the effect of grade on survival are contained in Table 14–16. The International Federation of Gynecologists and Obstetricians (FIGO) staging system for endometrial carcinoma defines histologic grading in a quantitative manner and stipulates that a grade be assigned to each lesion, along with a stage based on the extent of disease.[71] The FIGO system stipulates, however, that cytologic criteria may influence assignment of a grade (see Table 14–14).

After grade, depth of myometrial invasion by the tumor is the variable that is most intensively studied.[18, 61–64, 68, 69, 72–77] Every large study has found an influence of myometrial invasion on prognosis; results of selected series are summarized in Table 14–17. Myometrial invasion and grade appear to affect prognosis independently and additively (Table 14–18).[61, 76]

These studies were responsible for the major changes leading to the current FIGO staging system for endometrial carcinoma adopted in 1988. The clinical staging system was replaced by one based on surgicopathologic criteria. This reflected the knowledge gained by numerous staging studies performed over the previous 20 years (including the ones cited above). The new surgical staging criteria also acknowledged the fact that the standard initial approach to

TABLE 14–17
Effect of Myometrial Invasion on Clinical Outcome in Stage I Endometrial Carcinoma

Author	No. of Patients	5-Year Survival (%)		
		No Invasion	*Inner Half*	*Outer Half*
DiSaia and Creasman[64]*	222	92	87	64
Lurain et al.[62]	264	90	93	70
Morrow et al.[65]*	759	97	87†	68‡
Ng and Reagan[66]	183	88	72	27

*Recurrence, rather than survival, was the end point.
†Inner third.
‡Outer third.

TABLE 14–18
Combined Effect of Myometrial Invasion and Histologic Grade on Survival in Endometrial Cancer[61]

Myometrial Invasion	5-Year Survival (%) Grade 1	Grade 2	Grade 3
None	98	98	80
Inner half	93	87	61
Outer half	91	71	26

endometrial carcinoma had become operative, in contrast to the frequent practice during the 1960s and 1970s of administering preoperative radiotherapy.

Histologic invasion of myometrial lymphatic vessels appears to be an indicator of poor prognosis independent of other histologic factors (Table 14–19).[69, 72–75, 78–80] Other histologic variables that appear to predict tumor behavior are the size of the tumor[62, 81] and the presence of concomitant endometrial hyperplasia in the tumor specimen.[82, 83] The latter finding is associated with better prognosis. Several series show the presence of positive peritoneal cytology to be an important predictor of virulence,[15, 77, 84, 85] but others do not.[75, 86, 87] Kadar and coworkers[75] found that the presence of positive peritoneal washings was often associated with other histologic indicators of poor outcome, but it did not predict recurrence in the absence of other ominous histologic features.

Numerous authors have attempted to correlate various biologic markers with outcome. Patients are generally considered to be at higher risk if their tumors do not contain progesterone receptors[74, 77, 88–90] or estrogen receptors[74, 88, 89] (although some authors[90] have not found that estrogen receptors constitute a prognostic variable). Flow cytometric studies have found that DNA ploidy,[14, 74, 91–94] increased mitotic index,[69, 95] and S-phase index[74, 93, 96] all portend an unfavorable prognosis. Elevated carbohydrate antigen CA 125 levels[97, 98] and amplification of the c-*neu* oncogene[99] are also reported to be ominous indicators.

Younger patients[62, 67, 72, 75, 77] and those with epidemiologic risk factors associated with continuous estrogen stimulation[23, 76, 100–102] enjoy lower recurrence rates and increased survival compared with other women with endometrial carcinoma.

Every recurrence of an operatively staged and treated stage I endometrial carcinoma represents a situation in which an apparently localized tumor was actually metastatic. Recurrence arises from metastatic deposits that are either too small or too inaccessible to be identified by staging procedures. Indeed, staging studies have demonstrated that histologic variables associated with poor outcome are related to an increased incidence of metastasis to lymph nodes.[10, 64] This fact, documented in Table 14–20, has had an important impact on the operative management of this disease.

The information supplied above serves as the basis for treatment recommendations for early endometrial carcinoma (Fig. 14–21 and Table 14–21).

Low Risk

We have previously defined low-risk disease as that for which hysterectomy and bilateral salpingo-oophorectomy, combined with washings, constitute satisfactory treatment and operative evaluation, and for which lymphadenectomy and other extended staging procedures are unnecessary. However, there is not unanimous agreement regarding which tumors belong in this category. The authors consider grades 1 and 2 tumors confined to the endometrium, and grade 1 tumors whose myometrial invasion is confined to

TABLE 14–19
Effect of Lymphatic Vascular Invasion on Recurrence of Endometrial Carcinoma

Classification	Lymphatic Vascular Invasion	Recurrence (%)
Grade		
1	Present	1/1 (100)
	Absent	0/62 (0)
2	Present	3/7 (43)
	Absent	2/22 (9)
3	Present	3/8 (38)
	Absent	0/11 (0)
Myometrial involvement		
<⅓	Present	2/4 (50)
	Absent	2/75 (3)
⅓ to ⅔	Present	4/5 (80)
	Absent	0/17 (0)
>⅔	Present	1/7 (14)
	Absent	0/3 (0)

TABLE 14–20
Association of Various Histologic Factors With Lymph Node Involvement at Diagnosis of Endometrial Cancer

Histologic Factor	Percentage of Involvement: Pelvic Nodes	Aortic Nodes	No. of Patients
Histologic grade			
1	3	2	180
2	9	5	288
3	18	11	153
Myometrial invasion			
None	1	1	87
<⅓	5	3	279
⅓ to ⅔	6	1	116
>⅔	25	17	139
Vessel involvement			
Absent	7	9	528
Present	27	19	93
Peritoneal cytology			
Negative	7	4	537
Positive	25	19	75

Modified from Creasman WT, et al: Surgical pathologic spread patterns of endometrial cancer: A Gynecologic Oncology Group study. Cancer 60:2035–2041, 1987.

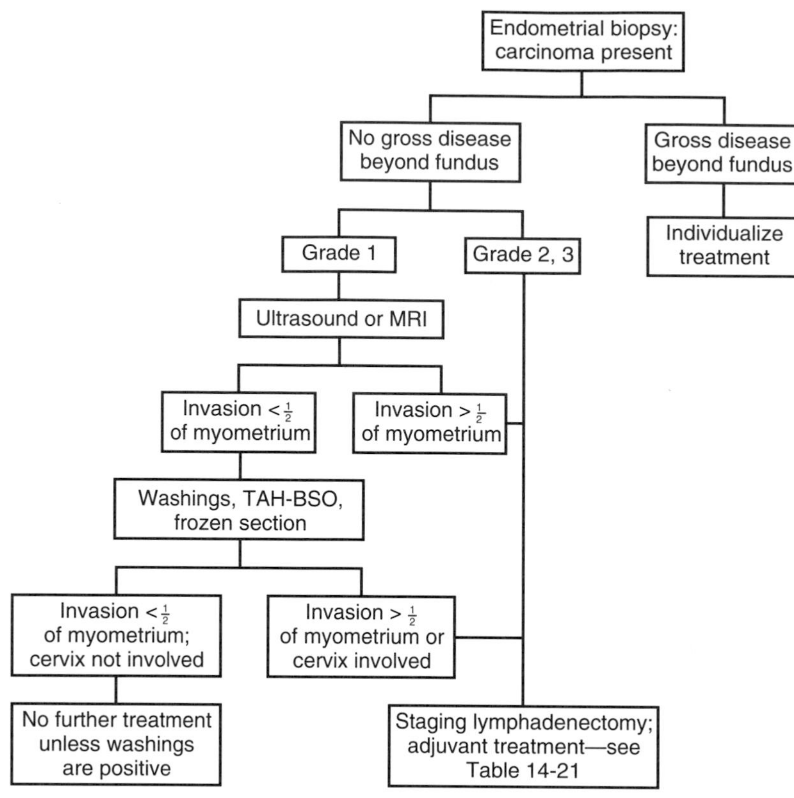

FIGURE 14–21. Initial evaluation and treatment of endometrial carcinoma. TAH-BSO, Total abdominal hysterectomy with bilateral salpingo-oophorectomy.

the inner half, treatable by operation alone. A Gynecologic Oncology Group staging study[65] found no recurrence among 72 patients with no myometrial involvement by grade 1 or 2 tumors, compared with recurrence in one of five patients with grade 3 carcinoma confined to the myometrium. Hording and Hansen[16] found a 96% disease-free survival rate in patients with grade 1 and 2 tumors confined to the inner third of the myometrium.

Therefore, patients with grade 1 or 2 lesions and no evidence of invasion on preoperative imaging may undergo total abdominal hysterectomy with bilateral salpingo-oophorectomy using an extrafascial technique. Pelvic washings are sent for analysis by cytology or cell block or both as soon as the pelvis is exposed. Following removal, the uterus is opened, and the tumor is examined by gross inspection and by frozen section. The intraoperative frozen section correctly predicts the depth of invasion in 95% of patients and provides a more accurate assessment of stage than endometrial biopsy and curettage.[103–105] It is less likely to be accurate in predicting uterine depth when the tumor involves the cornua or isthmus.[106] Patients meeting the criteria of low-risk disease receive no further operative or postoperative therapy. More than half of all patients with endometrial carcinoma belong to the low-risk category.[107] Patients with deep myometrial penetration, occult cervical involvement, or differentiation worse than grade 1 on final report are treated as intermediate-risk patients.

Some patients may be unable to undergo abdominal surgery because of obesity or medical problems. In this case, a vaginal hysterectomy should be performed, with removal of the tubes and ovaries if possible. Most obese patients have low-risk disease, and the actuarial 5-year

TABLE 14–21
Postoperative Adjuvant Treatment Recommendations for Endometrial Carcinoma, Based on Status of Myometrium, Peritoneal Washings, and Retroperitoneal Nodes

Node and Myometrium Status	Negative Washings	Positive Washings
Stage IAG1, 2; IBG1	No adjuvant treatment (no node sampling)	No adjuvant treatment or intraperitoneal ^{32}P colloid
Other stage I; stage IIA		
Nodes negative	Vaginal implant	Whole abdominal radiation or ^{32}P colloid *and* vaginal implant
Pelvic nodes positive	External pelvic radiation; consider vaginal implant	Whole abdominal radiation; consider vaginal implant
Aortic nodes positive	External radiation to pelvic and aortic nodes; consider vaginal implant	Whole abdominal radiation; consider vaginal implant

survival rate following vaginal hysterectomy in inoperable stage I patients is over 90%.[46, 47] Radiotherapy can be employed in patients whose anatomy or medical condition precludes even vaginal hysterectomy. Although survival is inferior to that obtained with hysterectomy, most studies document long-term actuarial survival in stage I carcinoma to be up to 75%.[108–110]

Intermediate Risk

It is known that patients with stage I endometrial carcinoma of certain histologic subtypes have a worse prognosis (see above). It is not clear how these patients are best treated. Widespread American practice is to administer pelvic irradiation following surgery. This technique has, over the last 20 years, replaced the general use of preoperative radiation. Boronow[111] points out that most recurrences from endometrial carcinoma—even from early lesions—are observed beyond the pelvis and suggests that extended field radiation techniques and chemotherapy are more rational techniques in women likely to experience extrapelvic recurrence.

Two randomized trials have been reported that studied the treatment of endometrial carcinoma using pelvic radiation. Weigensberg[112] managed clinical stage I patients using either preoperative external radiation or preoperative intracavitary implants. The group treated by implant demonstrated fewer complications, longer disease-free survival, and longer survival than did the group that received external irradiation. Aalders and colleagues[113] randomized clinical stage I patients to receive either vaginal intracavitary irradiation alone or vaginal implant plus external beam therapy. The group treated with external radiation experienced a lower rate of vaginal and pelvic recurrence but a higher rate of distant recurrence. External irradiation had no effect on survival.

There have been many retrospective studies documenting the effects of multifarious radiation regimens on recurrence and survival. These studies, taken collectively, do not suggest a rational and empirically supported adjuvant radiation regimen that improves disease-free survival. Retrospective data do suggest, however, that adjuvant irradiation, whether intracavitary or external, reduces the incidence of vaginal metastases[17, 65] and possibly the incidence of pelvic recurrence.[65] Since most of these studies did not utilize surgical staging, we have little idea of the impact of adjuvant treatment on the natural history of well-staged FIGO stage I endometrial carcinoma.

If adjuvant therapy is intended only to eliminate vaginal recurrence, intracavitary treatment is the treatment of choice. This seems to be an appropriate goal in stage I patients of intermediate risk, as there is no good reason at present to believe that we can accomplish any more ambitious therapeutic goals with an acceptable rate of treatment complications.

Patients with metastatic disease beyond the uterus, to lymph nodes or the peritoneal cavity, are at overwhelming risk to experience recurrences in the pelvis and beyond. It seems intuitively clear that an attempt should be made to prevent these recurrences through the use of adjuvant treatment, although there are no data describing a series of patients with metastases who did not receive adjuvant treatment. Treatment details for this group of patients are discussed in the following sections as they do not fall into the stage I intermediate-risk category.

Patients with clinically early disease who are not classified as low risk should have pelvic washings, total abdominal hysterectomy, and bilateral salpingo-oophorectomy. In addition, they should undergo extensive bilateral sampling of pelvic and aortic nodes as described above. This can be performed with minimal morbidity, even if followed by extensive irradiation.[114] If no extrauterine disease is present, intracavitary irradiation is administered using dosimetric guidelines detailed previously in the section on radiotherapy.

Stage II Carcinoma

In the absence of gross exocervical involvement, hysterectomy and bilateral salpingo-oophorectomy are performed as for stage I disease. This is true even if results of endocervical curettage are positive for carcinoma. When the uterus is opened immediately following hysterectomy, it is apparent whether there is gross disease in the cervix or close to it in the lower uterine segment of the cervix. If cervical tumor is present, staging lymphadenectomy is performed. Vaginal cuff irradiation is given postoperatively if lymph nodes do not contain carcinoma.

Endometrial carcinoma with gross involvement of the cervix should not be treated in this manner. Such disease may follow metastatic avenues of cervical cancer as well as those of endometrial disease. Treatment must take this into account. Two alternative treatment strategies are appropriate.

First, radical hysterectomy with pelvic and aortic lymphadenectomy may be employed. Such radical surgery is not reasonable for cancer that is grossly confined to the corpus, as it does not enhance survival.[115] When employed in cancer clinically involving the cervix, the 5-year survival rate is 60% to 75%.[116, 117] Preoperative irradiation followed by extrafascial hysterectomy is a more common treatment program. The radiation consists of external therapy alone or followed by an intracavitary implant. Most large series employing this treatment strategy show survival comparable to that obtained with radical hysterectomy.[118–122] Most authors found that patients who received combined treatment fared better than those receiving radiation alone,[119, 120, 122] although Ahmed and coworkers[118] dispute this. As is the case for cervical carcinoma of stage IIB or higher, it seems reasonable to perform surgical staging consisting of aortic lymphadenectomy, abdominal exploration, and peritoneal washings prior to beginning radiotherapy. Occult aortic node metastases and intraperitoneal disease occur frequently, although the precise incidence has not been well documented. Virtually all recurrences occur outside the pelvis.[121] Although most recurrence is distant, there have been no trials of adjuvant chemotherapy reported for gross stage II lesions.

Occult Stage III Carcinoma

Surgical staging has identified a large class of patients with occult stage III carcinoma by virtue of positive peritoneal cytology or lymphadenopathy.

Peritoneal and Adnexal Disease

It is not clear how best to treat patients with positive peritoneal cytologic findings in the absence of other extrauterine disease. Positive peritoneal cytologic findings are more common when other risk factors are present.[12] Whether it is an independent predictor of recurrence is subject to dispute.[15, 62, 75, 85–87, 123–128] Studies in which site and frequency of recurrence were documented suggest that intraperitoneal recurrence is increased in women who demonstrate positive peritoneal cytology.[124, 125] This suggests that this finding is of clinical significance. Soper et al.,[129] in a retrospective study, found a marked improvement in survival when intraperitoneal 32-P chromic phosphate colloid was administered intraperitoneally. The ease of administration and low morbidity of this modality seem to make it the most attractive therapeutic option. Piver and colleagues[130, 131] suggest, on the basis of an uncontrolled trial, that adjuvant treatment consisting of a year of oral progestins may be beneficial. Their lack of therapeutic effectiveness in other clinical circumstances with no postoperative residual disease[53, 54] casts doubt on the efficacy of progestins in this circumstance, however.

Spread to the adnexa and other peritoneal sites has not been studied as closely. MacKillop and Pringle[132] reported 5-year survival of 82% in women with isolated adnexal metastases treated with surgery and postoperative radiation. Greer and Hamburger[133] suggest that the overwhelming majority of patients with small or occult peritoneal metastases will survive at least 5 years if they are given whole abdominal radiation following surgery; Grigsby and associates[134] report similar results. In addition to using it for women with documented peritoneal metastases, it seems rational to consider whole abdominal irradiation as a possible treatment option for women with positive peritoneal cytologic findings who also have other risk factors for recurrence.

Tumor Involving Retroperitoneal Lymph Nodes

The increased use of surgical staging has revealed a group of women who have lymph node metastases that are not clinically apparent. As with peritoneal metastases, it is not entirely clear how best to treat these women, and any recommendations must be based on a few uncontrolled studies. Physicians have been reluctant to rely on surgery alone to treat these women. Pelvic external radiation following lymphadenectomy appears to cure a majority of those with pelvic node metastases.[65, 135] Postoperative radiation to the pelvis and the aortic nodes is associated with 5-year survival of almost half of women with documented carcinoma in aortic nodes.[65, 135, 136]

Gross Extrauterine Extension

Treatment of patients with clinically apparent extrauterine extension presents a difficult challenge to clinicians. Most of these women should undergo operation and irradiation. The specific procedure, the radiation fields and dosimetry, and the sequencing of the two modalities should be tailored to the specific findings and overall condition of the patient. These women should be treated by a team of physicians experienced in the management of this disease. MacKillop and Pringle[132] presented their results and reviewed eight other series, finding that 37% of women with stage III carcinoma enjoy 5-year survival. Chemotherapy should also be considered.

Metastatic Carcinoma

Metastases of endometrial carcinoma that are sufficiently extensive to permit preoperative diagnosis may occur in many sites (Table 14–22).[137] Treatment must be individualized and includes systemic treatment as well as surgery and radiation. The 5-year survival rate in stage IV carcinoma is about 10%. Even in widely metastatic disease, isolated complete responses to chemotherapy accompanied by long-term remission have been reported.[138]

Recurrent Carcinoma

Isolated recurrences are treated to achieve cure. Resection is performed, if possible, and is followed by radiation

TABLE 14–22
Distribution by Site of Extrapelvic Metastases in Patients With Clinical Stage IV Endometrial Carcinoma

Site	No.	%
Lung	30	36
Bladder mucosa	11	13
Inguinal lymph nodes	5	6
Supraclavicular lymph nodes	5	6
Ascites	4	5
Rectal mucosa	3	4
Bone	2	2
Liver	2	2
Brain	1	1
Axillary lymph nodes	1	1
Multiple sites	19	24
Total	83	100

Modified from Aalders JG, et al: Stage IV endometrial carcinoma: A clinical and histopathological study of 83 patients. Gynecol Oncol 17:75–84, 1984.

if the patient has not already received maximum doses to the region. New operative techniques such as ultrasonic aspiration[139] have facilitated cytoreduction. Hormones or cytotoxic chemotherapy is employed in patients whose disease is not amenable to local curative or palliative therapy.

Serous and Clear Cell Carcinoma

Serous carcinoma of the endometrium is recognized to have a worse prognosis than adenocarcinoma whose architecture is endometrioid. Constituting about 10% of all adenocarcinomas, it tends to occur at a more advanced age in patients who lack traditional risk factors.[140] Serous carcinoma has a great predilection to invade the myometrium and lymphatic spaces.[140] It is prone to recur in the upper abdomen,[141, 142] as do the serous ovarian tumors that this lesion resembles. Survival may be as high as 50% in stages I and II,[143, 144] but survival is unusual if the disease extends beyond the uterus at the time of diagnosis. Although sensitive to chemotherapy[145] and radiation,[146] endometrial serous carcinoma responds less well to these modalities than does ovarian serous carcinoma.[147]

Clear cell carcinoma likewise represents a variant of adenocarcinoma with a poor prognosis.[67] It constitutes about 5% of endometrial adenocarcinomas. The natural history and survival data are comparable to those of serous carcinoma.

Management is based on the natural history of this disease. The initial staging operation is more extensive than described above, being similar to that recommended for ovarian carcinoma (see the subchapter on ovarian cancer). Postoperatively, the patient may be given adjuvant chemotherapy[145, 148] or whole abdominal irradiation, although the efficacy of adjuvant therapy is not well established.

Sarcoma

Uterine sarcomas limited to the uterus are treated by total abdominal hysterectomy and bilateral salpingo-oophorectomy. Thorough abdominal exploration is performed; surgical staging with washings and lymphadenectomy are performed as for endometrial cancer. The exception is low-grade endometrial stromal sarcoma (also known as endolymphatic stromal myosis), which tends to recur locally rather than to metastasize to distant sites. Modified radical hysterectomy or radical hysterectomy with pelvic lymphadenectomy is performed for this lesion.

There is no proven role for adjuvant chemotherapy. Postoperative pelvic irradiation has little effect except in mixed endometrial sarcomas (carcinosarcoma and mixed müllerian sarcoma). In these lesions, survival is not improved, but pelvic control is enhanced.[149] Fifty Gy of pelvic irradiation is administered.

Metastatic disease is resected if feasible. Widespread endometrial mixed or pure tumors may be treated using cisplatin[150] or ifosfamide.[151] Although doxorubicin is not active as a single agent, two small studies show high activity for the combination of cisplatin and doxorubicin.[152, 153]

Recurrent or metastatic low-grade endometrial stromal sarcoma is often responsive to progestins for prolonged periods.[154]

Recurrent or metastatic leiomyosarcoma may be treated with doxorubicin,[155] whose activity is greater than that of any other agent.

POST-TREATMENT CARE AND SURVEILLANCE

About half of all recurrences can be detected in asymptomatic individuals.[19] History, physical examination, and vaginal cytology are performed every 3 months for 2 years and then every 6 months indefinitely. Chest radiograph is performed every 6 months. Abdominopelvic CT every 6 to 12 months is optional.

References

1. American Cancer Society: Cancer statistics, 1993. CA 43:1–6, 1993.
2. Lynch HT, Krush AJ, Larsen AL, et al: Endometrial carcinoma: Multiple primary malignancies, constitutional factors, and heredity. Am J Med Sci 252:381–390, 1966.
3. Horgas G, Grubisic G, Spaventi S: Trisomy and tetrasomy of the long arm of chromosome 1 in a direct preparation of human endometrial adenocarcinoma. Cancer Genet Cytogenet 35:269–272, 1988.
4. Ziehl H, Finkle WD: Increased risk of endometrial carcinoma among users of conjugated estrogens. N Engl J Med 293:1167–1170, 1975.
5. La Vecchia C, De Carli A, Fasoli M, et al: Nutrition and diet in the etiology of endometrial cancer. Cancer 57:1248–1253, 1986.
6. Segna RA, Dottino PR, Deligdisch L, et al: Tamoxifen and endometrial cancer. Mt Sinai J Med 59:416–418, 1992.
7. MacMahon B: Risk factors for endometrial cancer. Gynecol Oncol 2:122–129, 1974.
8. Meredith RF, Eisert DR, Kaka Z, et al: An excess of uterine sarcomas after pelvic irradiation. Cancer 58:2003–2007, 1986.
9. Harlow B, Weiss NS, Lofton S, et al: The epidemiology of sarcomas of the uterus. J Natl Cancer Inst 76:399–402, 1986.
10. Creasman WT, Morrow CP, Bundy BN, et al: Surgical pathologic spread patterns of endometrial cancer: A Gynecologic Oncology Group study. Cancer 60:2035–2041, 1987.
11. Plentl AA, Friedman EA: Lymphatic System of the Female Genitalia. Philadelphia: WB Saunders, 1971.
12. McLellan R, Dillon NB, Currie JL, et al: Peritoneal cytology in endometrial cancer: A review. Obstet Gynecol Surv 44:711–719, 1989.
13. Aalders JG, Abeler V, Kolstadt P: Recurrent adenocarcinoma of the endometrium: A clinical and histopathological study of 379 patients. Gynecol Oncol 17:85–103, 1984.
14. Podratz KC, Wilson TO, Gaffey TA, et al: Deoxyribonucleic acid analysis facilitates the pretreatment identification of high-risk endometrial cancer patients. Am J Obstet Gynecol 168:1206–1215, 1993.
15. Grimshaw RN, Tupper WC, Fraser RC, et al: Prognostic value of peritoneal cytology in endometrial carcinoma. Gynecol Oncol 36:97–100, 1990.
16. Hording U, Hansen U: Stage I endometrial carcinoma: A review of 140 patients primarily treated by surgery only. Gynecol Oncol 22:51–58, 1985.
17. Jones HW III: Treatment of adenocarcinoma of the endometrium. Obstet Gynecol Surv 30:147–169, 1975.
18. Philipsen T, Norgard M: Adenocarcinoma of the endometrium. Stage I: Treatment, survival and recurrence. Acta Obstet Gynecol Scand 63:51–55, 1984.

19. Podczaski E, Kaminski P, Gurski K, et al: Detection and patterns of treatment failure in 300 consecutive cases of "early" endometrial cancer after primary surgery. Gynecol Oncol 47:323–327, 1992.
20. Tiitinen A, Forss M, Aho I, et al: Endometrial adenocarcinoma: Clinical outcome in 881 patients and analysis of 146 patients whose deaths were due to endometrial cancer. Gynecol Oncol 25:11–19, 1986.
21. Angel C, DuBeshter B, Dawson AE, et al: Recurrent stage I endometrial adenocarcinoma in the nonirradiated patient: Preliminary results of surgical "staging." Gynecol Oncol 48:221–226, 1993.
22. Zaino RJ, Kurman RJ, Herbold D, et al: The significance of squamous differentiation in endometrial carcinoma. Cancer 68:2293–2302, 1991.
23. Bokhman JV: Two pathogenetic types of endometrial carcinoma. Gynecol Oncol 15:10–17, 1983.
24. Lee KR, Beilinson JL: Recurrence in noninvasive endometrial carcinoma. Am J Surg Pathol 15:965–973, 1991.
25. Christopherson WM, Alberhasky RC, Connelly PJ: Carcinoma of the endometrium. II. Papillary adenocarcinoma: A clinical pathological study. Am J Clin Pathol 77:534–540, 1982.
26. Christopherson WM, Alberhasky RC, Connelly PJ: Carcinoma of the endometrium. I. A clinicopathologic study of clear cell carcinoma and secretory carcinoma. Cancer 49:1511–1523, 1982.
27. Salazar OM, Bonfiglio TA, Patten SE, et al: Uterine sarcomas: Natural history, treatment and prognosis. Cancer 42:1152–1160, 1978.
28. Kempson RL, Hendrickson MR: Pure mesenchymal neoplasms of the uterine corpus: Selected problems. Semin Diagn Pathol 5:172–198, 1988.
29. Schwartz LB, Diamond MP, Schwartz PE: Leiomyosarcomas: Clinical presentation. Am J Obstet Gynecol 168:180–183, 1993.
30. Kempson RL, Hendrickson MR: Pure mesenchymal neoplasms of the uterine corpus. In Fox H (ed): Haines and Taylor's Obstetrical and Gynaecologic Pathology, 3rd ed. Edinburgh: Churchill Livingstone, 1987.
31. Norris HJ, Taylor HB: Mesenchymal tumors of the uterus. I. A clinical and pathologic study of 53 endometrial stromal tumors. Cancer 19:755–766, 1966.
32. Chang KL, Crabtree GS, Lim-Tan SK, et al: Primary uterine endometrial stromal neoplasm. Am J Surg Pathol 14:415–438, 1990.
33. Berchuck A, Rubin SC, Hoskins WJ, et al: Treatment of endometrial stromal tumors. Gynecol Oncol 36:60–65, 1990.
34. Belloni C, Vigano R, del Maschio A, et al: Magnetic resonance imaging in endometrial carcinoma staging. Gynecol Oncol 37:172–177, 1990.
35. Sahakian V, Syrop C, Turner D: Endometrial carcinoma: Transvaginal ultrasonography prediction of depth of myometrial invasion. Gynecol Oncol 43:217–219, 1991.
36. Shipley CF, Smith ST, Dennis EJ III, et al: Evaluation of pretreatment transvaginal ultrasonography in the management of patients with endometrial carcinoma. Am J Obstet Gynecol 167:406–412, 1992.
37. Yazigi R, Cohen J, Munoz AK, et al: Magnetic resonance imaging determination of myometrial invasion in endometrial carcinoma. Gynecol Oncol 34:94–97, 1989.
38. Cowles TA, Magrina JF, Masterson BJ, et al: Comparison of clinical and surgical staging in patients with endometrial carcinoma. Obstet Gynecol 66:413–416, 1985.
39. Larson DM, Johnson K, Olson KA: Pelvic and para-aortic lymphadenectomy for surgical staging of endometrial cancer: Morbidity and mortality. Obstet Gynecol 79:998–1001, 1992.
40. Lewandowski G, Torrisi J, Potkul RK, et al: Hysterectomy with extended surgical staging and radiotherapy versus hysterectomy alone and radiotherapy in stage I endometrial cancer: A comparison of complication rates. Gynecol Oncol 36:401–404, 1990.
41. Orr JW Jr, Holloway RW, Orr PF, et al: Surgical staging of uterine cancer: An analysis of perioperative morbidity. Gynecol Oncol 42:209–216, 1991.
42. Padial JG, Sotolongo J, Casey MJ, et al: Laparoscopy-assisted vaginal hysterectomy: Report of seventy-five consecutive cases. J Gynecol Surg 8:81–85, 1992.
43. Photopolous GJ, Stovall TG, Summitt RL Jr: Laparoscopic-assisted vaginal hysterectomy, bilateral salpingo-oophorectomy, and pelvic lymph node sampling for endometrial cancer. J Gynecol Surg 8:91–94, 1992.
44. Nezhat CR, Nezhat FR, Burrell MO, et al: Laparoscopic radical hysterectomy and laparoscopically assisted vaginal radical hysterectomy with pelvic and paraaortic node dissection. J Gynecol Surg 9:105–120, 1993.
45. Photopulos GJ, Stovall TG, Summitt RL Jr: Laparoscopically-assisted vaginal hysterectomy, bilateral salpingo-oophorectomy, and pelvic lymph node sampling for endometrial cancer. J Gynecol Surg 8:91–94, 1992.
46. Bloss JD, Berman ML, Bloss LP, et al: Use of vaginal hysterectomy for the management of stage I endometrial cancer in the medically compromised patient. Gynecol Oncol 40:74–77, 1991.
47. Peters WA III, Anderson WA, Thornton WN, et al: The selective use of vaginal hysterectomy in the management of adenocarcinoma of the endometrium. Am J Obstet Gynecol 146:285–291, 1983.
48. Kelley RM, Baker WH: Progestational agents in the treatment of carcinoma of the endometrium. N Engl J Med 264:216–222, 1961.
49. Podratz KC, O'Brien PC, Malkasian GD, et al: Effects of progestational agents in treatment of endometrial cancer. Obstet Gynecol 66:106–110, 1985.
50. Thigpen T, Blessing J, DiSaia PJ, et al: Treatment of advanced or recurrent endometrial carcinoma with medroxyprogesterone acetate: A Gynecologic Oncology Group study. Gynecol Oncol 20:250, 1985.
51. DePalo G, Merson M, Del Vecchio M, et al: A controlled clinical study of adjuvant medroxyprogesterone acetate (MPA) therapy in pathologic stage I endometrial carcinoma with myometrial invasion. Proc Am Soc Clin Oncol 4:121, 1985.
52. Lewis GC, Slack NH, Mortel R, et al: Adjuvant progestogen therapy in primary definitive treatment of endometrial cancer. Gynecol Oncol 2:368–376, 1974.
53. MacDonald RR, Thorogood J, Mason MK: A randomized trial of progestogens in the primary treatment of endometrial carcinoma. Br J Obstet Gynaecol 95:166–174, 1988.
54. Vergote I, Kjorstad K, Abeler V, et al: A randomized trial of adjuvant progestagen in early endometrial cancer. Cancer 64:1011–1016, 1989.
55. Moore TD, Phillips PH, Nerenstone SR, et al: Systemic treatment of advanced and recurrent endometrial carcinoma: Current status and future directions. J Clin Oncol 9:1071–1088, 1991.
56. Burke TW, Stringer CA, Morris M, et al: Prospective treatment of advanced or recurrent endometrial carcinoma with cisplatin, doxorubicin and cyclophosphamide. Gynecol Oncol 40:264–267, 1991.
57. Dunton CJ, Pfeifer SM, Braitman LE, et al: Treatment of advanced and recurrent endometrial cancer with cisplatin, doxorubicin and cyclophosphamide. Gynecol Oncol 41:113–116, 1991.
58. Piver MS, Fanning J, Baker TR: Phase II trial of cisplatin, adriamycin, and etoposide for metastatic endometrial adenocarcinoma. Am J Clin Oncol 14:200–202, 1991.
59. Long HJ, Langdon RM, Wieand HS: Phase II trial of methotrexate, vinblastine, doxorubicin, and cisplatin (MVAC) in women with advanced endometrial carcinoma. Proc Am Soc Clin Oncol 10:184, 1991.
60. Pettersson F (ed): Annual Report on the Results of Treatment in Gynecological Cancer, vol 20. Stockholm: International Federation of Gynecology and Obstetrics, 1991.
61. Lotocki RJ, Copeland LJ, DePetrillo AD, et al: Stage I endometrial adenocarcinoma: Treatment results in 835 patients. Am J Obstet Gynecol 146:141–145, 1983.
62. Lurain JR, Rice BL, Rademaker AW, et al: Prognostic factors associated with recurrence in clinical stage I adenocarcinoma of the endometrium. Obstet Gynecol 78:63–69, 1991.
63. Malkasian GD: Carcinoma of the endometrium: Effect of stage and grade on survival. Cancer 41:996–1001, 1978.
64. DiSaia PJ, Creasman WP: Clinical Gynecologic Oncology. St Louis: CV Mosby, 1981, pp 437–440.
65. Morrow CP, Bundy BN, Kumar RJ, et al: Relationship between surgical-pathologic risk factors and outcome in clinical stages I and II carcinoma of the endometrium. A Gynecologic Oncology Group study. Gynecol Oncol 40:55–65, 1991.
66. Ng ABP, Reagan JW: Incidence and prognosis of endometrial carcinoma by histologic grade and extent. Obstet Gynecol 35:437–443, 1970.
67. Christopherson WM, Connelly PJ, Alberhasky RC: Carcinoma of the endometrium. V. An analysis of prognosticators in patients with favorable subtypes and stage I disease. Cancer 51:1705–1709, 1983.

68. Connelly PJ, Alberhasky RC, Christopherson WM: Carcinoma of the endometrium. III. Analysis of 865 cases of adenocarcinoma and adenoacanthoma. Obstet Gynecol 59:569–575, 1982.
69. Mittal K, Schwartz PE, Barwick KW: Architectural (FIGO) grading, nuclear grading, and other prognostic indicators in stage I endometrial carcinoma with identification of high-risk and low-risk groups. Cancer 61:538–545, 1988.
70. Nielsen AL, Thomsen HK, Nyholm HCJ: Evaluation of the reproducibility of the revised 1988 International Federation of Gynecology and Obstetrics grading system of endometrial cancers with special emphasis on nuclear grading. Cancer 68:2303–2309, 1991.
71. Announcements: FIGO stages: 1988 revision. Gynecol Oncol 35:125–127, 1989.
72. Ambros RA, Kurman RJ: Combined assessment of vascular and myometrial invasion as a model to predict prognosis in stage I endometrioid adenocarcinoma of the uterine corpus. Cancer 69:1424–1431, 1992.
73. Burke TW, Heller PB, Woodward JE, et al: Treatment failure in endometrial carcinoma. Obstet Gynecol 75:96–101, 1990.
74. Geisinger KR, Homesley HD, Morgan TM, et al: Endometrial adenocarcinoma: A multiparameter clinicopathologic analysis including the DNA profile and the sex steroid hormone receptors. Cancer 58:1518–1525, 1986.
75. Kadar N, Malfetano JH, Homesley HD: Determinants of survival of surgically staged patients with endometrial carcinoma histologically confined to the uterus: Implications for therapy. Obstet Gynecol 80:655–659, 1992.
76. Malkasian GD, Annegers JF, Fountain KS: Carcinoma of the endometrium: Stage I. Am J Obstet Gynecol 136:872–888, 1980.
77. Sutton GP, Geisler HE, Stehman FB, et al: Features associated with survival and disease-free survival in early endometrial cancer. Am J Obstet Gynecol 160:1385–1393, 1989.
78. Gal D, Recio FO, Zamurovic D: Lymphovascular space involvement—a prognostic indicator in endometrial adenocarcinoma. Gynecol Oncol 42:142–145, 1991.
79. Hanson MB, van Nagell JR, Powell DE, et al: The prognostic significance of lymph-vascular space invasion in stage I endometrial cancer. Cancer 55:1753–1757, 1985.
80. Sivridis E, Buckley CH, Fox H: The prognostic significance of lymphatic space invasion in endometrial carcinoma. Br J Obstet Gynaecol 94:991–994, 1987.
81. Schink JC, Lurain JR, Wallemark CB, et al: Tumor size in endometrial cancer: A prognostic factor for lymph node metastases. Obstet Gynecol 70:216–219, 1987.
82. Deligdisch L, Cohen CJ: Histologic correlates and virulence implications of endometrial carcinoma associated with adenomatous hyperplasia. Cancer 56:1452–1455, 1985.
83. Deligdisch L, Holinka CF: Endometrial carcinoma: Two diseases? Cancer Detect Prev 10:237–246, 1987.
84. Creasman WT, Rutledge F: The prognostic value of peritoneal cytology in gynecologic malignant disease. Am J Obstet Gynecol 110:773–781, 1971.
85. Kadar N, Homesley HD, Malfetano JH: Positive peritoneal cytology is an adverse factor in endometrial carcinoma only if there is other evidence of extrauterine disease. Gynecol Oncol 46:145–149, 1992.
86. Konski A, Poulter C, Keys H, et al: Absence of prognostic significance, peritoneal dissemination and treatment advantage in endometrial cancer patients with positive peritoneal cytology. Int J Radiat Oncol Biol Phys 14:49–55, 1988.
87. Yazigi R, Piver MS, Blumenson L: Malignant peritoneal cytology as prognostic indicator in stage I endometrial cancer. Obstet Gynecol 62:359–362, 1983.
88. Borazjani G, Twiggs LB, Leung BS, et al: Prognostic significance of steroid receptors measured in primary metastatic and recurrent endometrial carcinoma. Am J Obstet Gynecol 161:1253–1257, 1989.
89. Palmer DC, Muir IM, Alexander AI, et al: The prognostic importance of steroid receptors in endometrial carcinoma. Obstet Gynecol 72:388–393, 1988.
90. Utaaker E, Iversen O, Skaarland E: The distribution and prognostic implications of steroid receptors in endometrial carcinomas. Gynecol Oncol 28:89–100, 1987.
91. Britton LC, Wilson TO, Gaffey TA, et al: Flow cytometric DNA analysis of stage I endometrial carcinoma. Gynecol Oncol 34:317–322, 1989.
92. Iversen OE: Flow cytometric deoxyribonucleic acid index: A prognostic factor in endometrial carcinoma. Am J Obstet Gynecol 155:770–776, 1986.
93. Rosenberg P, Wingren S, Simonsen E, et al: Flow cytometric measurements of DNA index and S-phase on paraffin-embedded early stage endometrial cancer: An important prognostic indicator. Gynecol Oncol 35:50–54, 1989.
94. van der Putten HWHM, Baak JPA, Koenders TJM, et al: Prognostic value of quantitative pathologic features and DNA content in individual patients with stage I endometrial adenocarcinoma. Cancer 63:1378–1387, 1989.
95. Pirog EC, Czerwinski W: Diagnostic and prognostic significance of the mitotic index in endometrial carcinoma. Gynecol Oncol 46:337–340, 1992.
96. Yabushita H, Masuda T, Sawaguchi K, et al: Growth potential of endometrial cancers assessed by a Ki-67 Ag/DNA dual-color flow-cytometric assay. Gynecol Oncol 44:263–267, 1992.
97. Fanning J, Piver MS: Serial CA 125 levels during chemotherapy for metastatic or recurrent endometrial cancer. Obstet Gynecol 77:278–280, 1991.
98. Patsner B, Mann WJ, Cohen H, et al: Predictive value of serum CA 125 levels in clinically localized and advanced endometrial carcinoma. Am J Obstet Gynecol 158:399–402, 1988.
99. Boronow RC: Should whole pelvic radiation therapy become past history? A case for the routine use of extended field therapy and multimodality therapy. Gynecol Oncol 43:71–76, 1991.
100. Chu J, Schweid AI, Weiss NS: Survival among women with endometrial cancer: A comparison of estrogen users and nonusers. Am J Obstet Gynecol 143:569–573, 1982.
101. Schwartzbaum JA, Hulka BS, Fowler WC Jr, et al: The influence of exogenous estrogen use on survival after diagnosis of endometrial cancer. Am J Epidemiol 126:851–860, 1987.
102. Smith DC, Prentice RL, Bauermeister DE: Endometrial carcinoma: Histopathology, survival, and exogenous estrogens. Gynecol Obstet Invest 12:169–179, 1981.
103. Malviya VK, Deppe G, Malone JM Jr, et al: Reliability of frozen section examination in identifying poor prognostic indicators in stage I endometrial adenocarcinoma. Gynecol Oncol 34:299–304, 1989.
104. Noumoff JS, Menzin A, Mikuta J, et al: The ability to evaluate prognostic variables on frozen section in hysterectomies performed for endometrial carcinoma. Gynecol Oncol 42:202–208, 1991.
105. Oakley G, Nahhas WA: Endometrial adenocarcinoma: Therapeutic impact of preoperative histopathologic examination of endometrial tissue. Eur J Gynaecol Oncol 10:255–260, 1989.
106. Fanning J, Tsukada Y, Piver MS: Intraoperative frozen section diagnosis of myometrial invasion in endometrial adenocarcinoma. Gynecol Oncol 37:47–50, 1990.
107. Sant Cassia LJ, Weppelmann B, Shingleton H, et al: Management of early endometrial carcinoma. Gynecol Oncol 35:362–366, 1989.
108. Anderson WA, Peters WA III, Fechner RE, et al: Radiotherapeutic alternatives to standard management of adenocarcinoma of the endometrium. Gynecol Oncol 16:383–392, 1983.
109. Lehoczky O, Bosze P, Ungar L, et al: Stage I endometrial carcinoma: Treatment of nonoperable patients with intracavitary radiation therapy alone. Gynecol Oncol 43:211–216, 1991.
110. Pourquier H, Gely S, DuBois JB, et al: Endometrial cancer: A comparative analysis of the therapeutic results and causes of failure after treatment by radiation combined with surgery or radiation therapy alone. Eur J Gynaecol Oncol 9:297–303, 1988.
111. Boronow RC: Should whole pelvic radiation become past history? A case for the routine use of extended field therapy and multimodality therapy. Gynecol Oncol 43:71–76, 1991.
112. Weigensberg IJ: Preoperative radiation therapy in stage I endometrial adenocarcinoma. II. Final report of a clinical trial. Cancer 53:242–247, 1984.
113. Aalders J, Abeler V, Kolstad P, et al: Postoperative external irradiation and prognostic parameters in stage I endometrial carcinoma: Clinical and histopathologic study of 540 patients. Obstet Gynecol 56:419–427, 1980.
114. Homesley HD, Kadar N, Barrett RJ, et al: Selective pelvic and periaortic lymphadenectomy does not increase morbidity in surgical staging of endometrial carcinoma. Am J Obstet Gynecol 167:1225–1230, 1992.

115. Iversen T, Holter J: Radical surgery in stage I carcinoma of the corpus uteri. Br J Obstet Gynaecol 88:1135–1139, 1981.
116. Homesley HD, Boronow RC, Lewis JL Jr: Stage II endometrial adenocarcinoma. Memorial Hospital for Cancer, 1949–1965. Obstet Gynecol 49:604–609, 1977.
117. Wallin TE, Malkasian GD Jr, Gaffey TA, et al: Stage II cancer of the endometrium: A pathologic and clinical study. Gynecol Oncol 18:1–17, 1984.
118. Ahmed K, Kim YH, Deppe G, et al: Radiation therapy in stage II carcinoma of the endometrium. Cancer 63:854–858, 1989.
119. Berman ML, Afridi MA, Kanbour AI, et al: Risk factors and prognosis in stage II endometrial cancer. Gynecol Oncol 14:49–61, 1982.
120. Larson DM, Copeland LJ, Gallager HS, et al: Stage II endometrial carcinoma: Results and complications of a combined radiotherapeutic-surgical approach. Cancer 61:1528–1534, 1988.
121. Rubin SC, Hoskins WJ, Saigo PJ, et al: Management of endometrial carcinoma with cervical involvement. Gynecol Oncol 45:294–298, 1992.
122. Surwit EA, Fowler WC Jr, Rogoff EE, et al: Stage II carcinoma of the endometrium. Int J Radiat Oncol Biol Phys 5:323–326, 1979.
123. Brewington KC, Hughes RR, Coleman S: Peritoneal cytology as a prognostic indicator in endometrial carcinoma. J Reprod Med 34:824–826, 1989.
124. Creasman WT, DiSaia PJ, Blessing J, et al: Prognostic significance of peritoneal cytology in patients with endometrial carcinoma and preliminary data concerning therapy with intraperitoneal radiopharmaceuticals. Am J Obstet Gynecol 141:921–929, 1981.
125. Harouny VR, Sutton GP, Clark SA, et al: The importance of peritoneal cytology in endometrial carcinoma. Obstet Gynecol 72:394–398, 1988.
126. Kennedy AW, Peterson GL, Becker SN, et al: Experience with pelvic washings in stage I and stage II endometrial carcinoma. Gynecol Oncol 28:50–60, 1987.
127. Mazurka JL, Krepart GV, Lotocki RJ: Prognostic significance of positive peritoneal cytology in endometrial carcinoma. Am J Obstet Gynecol 158:303–306, 1988.
128. Turner DA, Gershenson DM, Atkinson N, et al: The prognostic significance of peritoneal cytology for stage I endometrial cancer. Obstet Gynecol 74:775–780, 1989.
129. Soper JT, Creasman WT, Clarke-Pearson DL, et al: Intraperitoneal chromic phosphate P 32 suspension therapy of malignant peritoneal cytology in endometrial carcinoma. Am J Obstet Gynecol 153:191–196, 1983.
130. Piver MS, Lele SB, Gamarra M: Malignant peritoneal cytology in stage I endometrial adenocarcinoma: The effect of progesterone therapy. Eur J Gynaecol Oncol 9:187–190, 1988.
131. Piver MS, Recio FO, Baker TR, et al: A prospective trial of progesterone therapy for malignant peritoneal cytology in patients with endometrial carcinoma. Gynecol Oncol 47:373–376, 1992.
132. MacKillop WJ, Pringle JF: Stage III endometrial carcinoma: A review of 90 cases. Cancer 56:2519–2523, 1985.
133. Greer BE, Hamburger AD: Treatment of intraperitoneal metastatic adenocarcinoma of the endometrium by the whole-abdomen moving-strip technique and pelvic boost irradiation. Gynecol Oncol 16:365–373, 1983.
134. Grigsby PW, Perez CA, Kuske RR, et al: Results of therapy, analysis of failures, and prognostic factors for clinical and pathologic stage III adenocarcinoma of the endometrium. Gynecol Oncol 27:44–57, 1987.
135. Potish RA, Twiggs LB, Adcock LL: Paraaortic lymph node radiotherapy in cancer of the uterine corpus. Obstet Gynecol 65:251–256, 1985.
136. Feuer GA, Calanog A: Endometrial carcinoma: Treatment of positive paraaortic nodes. Gynecol Oncol 27:104–109, 1987.
137. Aalders JG, Abeler V, Kolstad P: Stage IV endometrial carcinoma: A clinical and histopathological study of 83 patients. Gynecol Oncol 17:75–84, 1984.
138. Cohen CJ, Bruckner HW, Deppe G, et al: Multidrug treatment of advanced and recurrent endometrial carcinoma: A Gynecologic Oncology Group study. Obstet Gynecol 63:719–726, 1984.
139. Rose PG, Piver MS: Primary resection of vaginal metastases with the Cavitron ultrasonic surgical aspirator in stage III endometrial carcinoma. Gynecol Oncol 39:264–265, 1990.
140. Hendrickson M, Ross J, Eifel P, et al: Uterine papillary serous carcinoma: A highly malignant form of endometrial adenocarcinoma. Am J Surg Pathol 6:93–108, 1982.
141. Jeffrey JF, Krepart GV, Lotocki RJ: Papillary serous adenocarcinoma of the endometrium. Obstet Gynecol 67:670–674, 1986.
142. Ramirez-Gonzalea CE, Adamsons K, Mangual-Vazquez TY, et al: Papillary adenocarcinoma in the endometrium. Obstet Gynecol 70:212–214, 1987.
143. Chambers JT, Merino M, Kohorn EI, et al: Uterine papillary serous carcinoma. Obstet Gynecol 69:109–113, 1987.
144. Ward BG, Wright RG, Free K: Papillary carcinomas of the endometrium. Gynecol Oncol 39:347–351, 1990.
145. FitzGerald D, Rosenthal S: Uterine papillary serous carcinoma: Complete response to combination chemotherapy. Cancer 56:1023–1024, 1985.
146. Gallion HH, van Nagell JR, Powell DF, et al: Stage I papillary carcinoma of the endometrium. Cancer 63:2224–2228, 1989.
147. Levenback C, Burke TW, Silva E, et al: Uterine papillary serous carcinoma (UPSC) treated with cisplatin, doxorubicin, and cyclophosphamide. Gynecol Oncol 46:317–321, 1992.
148. Rosenberg P, Boeryd B, Simonsen E: A new aggressive treatment approach to high-grade endometrial cancer of possible benefit to patients with stage I uterine papillary cancer. Gynecol Oncol 48:32–37, 1993.
149. Hannigan E, Curtin JP, Silverberg SG, et al: Corpus: Mesenchymal tumors. In Hoskins WJ, Perez CA, Young RC (eds): Principles and Practice of Gynecologic Oncology. Philadelphia: JB Lippincott, 1992, pp 695–714.
150. Gershenson DM, Kavanagh JJ, Copeland LJ, et al: Cisplatin therapy for disseminated mixed mesodermal sarcoma of the uterus. J Clin Oncol 5:618–621, 1987.
151. Sutton GP, Blessing JA, Rosenschein N, et al: Phase II trial of ifosfamide and mesna in mixed mesodermal tumors of the uterus (a Gynecologic Oncology Group study). Am J Obstet Gynecol 161:309–312, 1989.
152. Peters WA III, Rivkin SE, Smith MR, et al: Cisplatin and adriamycin combination chemotherapy for uterine stromal sarcomas and mixed mesodermal tumors. Gynecol Oncol 34:323–327, 1989.
153. Seltzer V, Kaplan V, Vogl S, et al: Doxorubicin and cisplatin in the treatment of advanced mixed mesodermal uterine sarcoma. Cancer Treat Reports 68:1389–1390, 1984.
154. Thatcher SS, Woodruff JD: Uterine stromatosis: A report of 33 cases. Obstet Gynecol 59:428–434, 1982.
155. Omura GA, Major FJ, Blessing JA, et al: A randomized study of adriamycin with or without dimethyl triaminoimidazole carboxamide in advanced uterine sarcoma. Cancer 52:626–632, 1983.

Cancers of the Ovary and Fallopian Tube

Allan J. Jacobs, M.D. • T. Scott Jennings, M.D.

Carcinomas of the ovary and fallopian tube are considered together because of similarities in their natural history, therapy, and response to treatment. Malignancies of the ovary are far more common than those of the fallopian tube.

EPIDEMIOLOGY

Incidence

The American Cancer Society predicts 26,600 new cases of ovarian cancer in 1995, roughly 4% of all cancers in females.[1] The overall incidence rate fluctuated only slightly from 1973 to 1987, between 12.8 and 14.7 per 100,000 population. It has been estimated that 1 in 70 American females will have ovarian carcinoma. This incidence is strongly age-related, with a peak incidence in the eighth decade of life, and approximately half of all cases are diagnosed in women 65 years and older.

Forms of ovarian cancer other than carcinoma constitute no more than 20% of the total. Germ cell tumors characteristically occur in children and young adults,[2] except that dysgerminomas may occur up to age 50.[3] Ovarian stromal tumors may occur in prepubertal girls[4] but are more common in perimenopausal women.[5, 6]

Ovarian cancer is the fifth most common cause of cancer death in American women (fourth most common in the age group 55 to 74 years), with approximately 12,500 deaths attributed to it in 1989.[7] This number is greater than the number of women who die from cervical and endometrial cancer combined. Five-year relative survival rates of women diagnosed from 1981 to 1987 demonstrated an overall survival rate of 36.9%, increased slightly from 34.6% 10 years earlier.[8] The improvement in survival rates for ovarian cancer are most remarkable for patients under the age of 65 years with stage III and IV disease: 31.9% in 1974 to 1976, and 46.3% in 1981 to 1987.[9] More than 65% of all deaths occurred in women 65 years and older, reflecting the discordant mortality risks of elderly women.

Risk Factors

Some of the environmental factors associated with ovarian carcinoma are summarized in Table 14–23.

Demographic

Ovarian carcinoma is more common in nulliparous women[10] and in those with early menarche and late menopause.[11]

Genetic-Familial

Fewer than 10% of women with ovarian carcinoma have a first-degree relative with the disease.[12] Although the large majority of cases are sporadic and presumably related to environmental factors, about 5% of women with epithelial lesions have a predisposing familial syndrome. Three such syndromes have been identified, all of which are transmitted as autosomal dominant traits. These are hereditary site-specific ovarian cancer,[13] the hereditary breast-ovarian cancer syndrome,[14] and Lynch syndrome II,[15] which is associated with adenocarcinomas of multiple sites, including breast, ovarian, endometrial, and gastrointestinal tumors. Individuals with familial ovarian carcinoma of all three types have a younger mean age of onset than women with sporadic ovarian cancer.[16]

Dietary

Obesity[17] and consumption of animal fats[18–20] may be associated with increased risk of epithelial ovarian carcinoma.

Ovulatory Cycle

A common cause of ovarian surface disruption, possibly leading to increased carcinoma, is ovulation. The increased incidence of ovarian tumors in women with more apparent ovulatory cycles (such as women with few or no pregnancies as well as ethnic populations noted to have higher frequencies of multiple births) has implicated "incessant

TABLE 14–23
Relationship Between Environmental Factors and Risk of Ovarian Carcinoma

Author	Factor	Odds Ratio
Demopoulos et al.[10]	Nulliparity	2.3
Parazzini[11]	Late menopause	1.5
Farrow et al.[17]	Obesity (Quetelet index in upper 20%)	1.7
LaVeccia et al.[19]	Animal fat consumption	2.1
Cramer and Welch[25]	Use of talc	1.9
Hankinson et al.[22]	Oral contraceptives	0.6
Whittimore et al.[24]	Fertility drugs (in nulliparous women)	27.0

ovulation" as an etiologic factor in epithelial ovarian tumors.[21] Suppression of ovulation by the use of oral steroid contraceptives has also been firmly related to a decrease in the incidence of ovarian carcinoma.[22]

Hormonal

Hormonal exposure, particularly to gonadotropins, may contribute to ovarian mesothelial proliferation and carcinoma. Administration of gonadotropins for ovarian stimulation of infertile women, for instance, is thought to increase the risk of ovarian cancer.[23, 24] More important to the development of ovarian epithelial carcinoma may be the elevated gonadotropin levels that occur in menopause.[25] With the depletion or destruction of the ovarian follicles in humans, pituitary production of the gonadotropins remains elevated for long periods. Patients with exposure to a number of agents toxic to the ovarian follicles, including mumps virus[26] and polycyclic aromatic hydrocarbons,[27] demonstrate menopausal levels of gonadotropins and a higher incidence of ovarian cancer. Although the development of cancers in these patients can be theorized to be due to the direct carcinogenic effect of the various agents themselves, the indirect effect of longer exposure to gonadotropins in these patients with premature ovarian failure may also be of importance. A long latency period between exposure to gonadotropins and the development of cancer has been theorized, commensurate with the 10- to 15-year delay in the increased incidence of epithelial ovarian cancer after the perimenopausal gonadotropin surge.

Talc

Genital exposure to talc has also been implicated as a potential causative agent in ovarian carcinomas by both direct stimulation of mesothelial proliferation as a foreign body and the carcinogenic effect of the asbestos contamination commonly found in cosmetic powders prior to 1976.[28] The long-term use of talc on diaphragms and sanitary napkins constitutes a significant exposure risk for ovarian cancer but accounts for disease in only a minority of patients.

Other Ovarian Tumors

Little is known about the etiology of tubal carcinoma or of ovarian cancers other than epithelial carcinoma. Germ cell tumors may occur as part of the Li-Fraumeni syndrome[29] and are often found in women with gonadal dysgenesis.[30]

NATURAL HISTORY

Histogenesis

The majority of epithelial ovarian neoplasms are derived from the surface coelomic mesothelium and the immediate underlying stroma.[31, 32] Most of these tumors are believed to originate in mesothelial inclusion cysts in the outer portion of the ovarian cortex rather than on the capsule per se.[25] Such cysts form during healing of the stigma following ovulation. After neoplastic transformation, the tumors proliferate in the inclusion cysts and come to extend to the ovarian surface. Tumors that are identical to ovarian carcinoma histologically, in natural history, and in response to therapy may originate in nonovarian peritoneum.[33, 34]

Patterns of Spread

Ovarian and tubal carcinoma may metastasize by four routes. These are, in declining order of importance, peritoneal seeding, lymphatic embolization, direct extension, and hematogenous metastasis.

Peritoneal Seeding

In 80% of cases of ovarian carcinoma with metastasis, peritoneal dissemination is present. Tumor cells exfoliate into the peritoneal cavity after disruption of the epithelial capsule. These cells implant throughout the abdomen and develop into the numerous macroscopic masses and nodules that are characteristic of advanced ovarian cancer. Intraperitoneal dissemination occurs quite early in the natural history of epithelial ovarian carcinoma, as evidenced by the presence of occult tumor cells in the peritoneal washings of approximately one third of patients with apparent stage I ovarian tumors.[35] Careful operative staging detects metastases in at least a third of patients with ovarian cancer who do not have gross metastases on inspection of the pelvis.[35-37] The tumor cells follow the normal circulatory patterns of peritoneal fluid, from the pelvis to the colonic gutters and preferentially to the undersurface of the right hemidiaphragm. Omental deposits are common, possibly because of the "scavenging" activity of this organ. Involvement of the omentum is a frequent finding also because it contains the bulk of peritoneal mesothelial cells, making it statistically likely to contain peritoneal implants; in addition, it often drapes into the pelvis, where it is in close proximity with the primary tumor. Tumor deposits are common in gravity-dependent sites such as the cul-de-sac of Douglas.

Although it is generally assumed that peritoneal seeding is derived from metastasis, Parmley and Woodruff[38] suggest that it may be due, at least in part, to simultaneous origin of tumor in multiple peritoneal sites.

Lymphatic Embolization

Lymphatic metastasis is seen in at least 15% to 20% of patients with no other extraovarian involvement.[35, 39] Lymphatic embolization to aortic nodes occurs by way of the lymphovascular channels paralleling the ovarian vessels in the infundibulopelvic ligaments. Tumor also may permeate the lymphatic channels of the broad ligament to involve the pelvic lymph nodes. Metastases to the pleura, the most common extra-abdominal site,[40] may be due to lymphatic passages through the diaphragm.

Direct Extension

Local extension occurs as tumor on the outside of the ovary adheres to pelvic structures. The incidence of this is not well documented but is common.

Hematogenous Metastasis

Hematogenous dissemination is seldom seen in primary disease. In one study,[40] 30 of 255 patients presented with stage IV disease, the majority on the basis of pleural metastases. The most common site of parenchymal metastasis is the liver, followed by the lung. Improvements in therapy have allowed considerable prolongation of life, so many patients who do not present with hematogenous metastases now live long enough to develop them terminally in the liver, lungs, brain, and other structures.

Natural Course

If untreated, ovarian malignancies continue to metastasize and proliferate within the peritoneal cavity. Death ensues, usually within a year of diagnosis, from intestinal obstruction with inanition. The terminal course is quite prolonged. It is accompanied by great discomfort due to vomiting from the obstruction and pain from distention by tumor and ascites.

Germ cell tumors follow the same metastatic pathways, except that they may be more likely than epithelial tumors to metastasize to lymph nodes.

Fallopian tube carcinoma follows the same metastatic pathways as ovarian cancer. It is more likely to be associated with lymphatic and distant metastases than is ovarian carcinoma.[41–43]

PATHOLOGY

Ovarian Cancer

The ovary is composed of an outer cortex and an inner medulla. The outer cortex contains the coelomic surface epithelium, the germ cells (oocytes), the specialized hormone-producing stroma (follicular and thecal cells), and unspecialized supporting stromal cells. The surface mesothelium is a single layer that is embryologically distinct from the ovarian follicles. The ovarian medulla is composed of stroma with supporting vascular and lymphatic structures. It is the remnant of that part of the primordial gonad that becomes the testis in males. Almost all ovarian tumors develop from the components of the cortex: epithelial tumors from the mesothelium, germ cell tumors from the primordial germ cells, and sex cord tumors from the granulosa and theca cells.

There are numerous histologic types of ovarian cancer. They are classified according to the World Health Organization histologic typing of ovarian tumors.[32, 44] This classification is based on the discrimination of morphologic characteristics found with light microscopy. Malignancies may arise from any of the constituent cells of the ovary: the ovarian peritoneum (mesothelium), germ cells, specialized stroma, or nonspecialized stroma. In addition, the ovary may harbor metastatic disease. The various cell types exhibit widely variant epidemiology, natural history, and treatment susceptibility. A summary of these histologic types is found in Table 14–24.

The ovarian mesothelium, often known by the misnomer germinal epithelium, gives rise to 80% to 90% of ovarian malignancies.[45] Tumors derived from mesothelium display a number of cell types that are similar to the various epithelia of the female genitourinary tract. These cell types include serous, mucinous, endometrioid, and clear cells, which respectively resemble tubal mucosa, endometrium, endocervix, and the cells found in vaginal adenocarcinoma. There is little difference in clinical behavior among these types, except that clear cell tumors may have a worse prognosis than the other types.[46] Epithelial carcinomas frequently occur bilaterally. Their course and response to treatment are dependent on their stage rather than on their histologic type.[45–47] The influence of grade is controversial, with some studies reporting an influence[45, 47] and others not.[46, 48] It seems to be an important factor in the prognosis of early disease.[49] The proliferation of the ovarian mesothelium, and possibly the interactions of this mesothelium with the hormonally active underlying stromal cells, has

TABLE 14–24
Common Histologic Types of Ovarian Cancer

Type	Derivation (Resemblance)
Epithelial	Capsule
Serous	(Oviduct)
Endometrioid	(Endometrium)
Mucinous	(Cervix, colon)
Clear cell	(Vaginal adenosis)
Brenner	(Transitional cell)
Undifferentiated	—
Mixed	—
Germ cell	Germ cells
Dysgerminoma	(Oocyte)
Embryonal cell	(Primitive embryo)
Teratoma	(Fetus)
Endodermal sinus	(Yolk sac)
Choriocarcinoma	(Chorion)
Mixed	—
Specialized stroma	Hormonally functional cells
Granulosa cell	(Granulosa cells)
Sertoli-Leydig cell	(Sertoli and Leydig cells)
Gynandroblastoma	—
Lipoid cell	—
Unspecialized stroma (includes sarcomas, lymphomas, etc.)	—
Metastatic (especially from endometrium, breast, colon, stomach)	—

been implicated in the pathogenesis of epithelial ovarian tumors. The factors that might contribute to this proliferation were discussed above.

Epithelial ovarian tumors can be classified as benign, low malignant potential (LMP), or frankly malignant. Benign tumors are characterized by bland cells without proliferation. Tumors of LMP demonstrate proliferation without stromal invasion. The tumor cells are well differentiated, closely resembling a müllerian epithelial structure. Frank carcinoma shows invasion as well as proliferation. Malignant tumors are subdivided according to a histologic grade based on architectural appearance, which may deviate considerably from that of the müllerian structure they resemble.

Serous tumors constitute 20% of all benign ovarian tumors and 50% of malignant epithelial carcinomas.[47] These tumors are commonly cystic and unilocular when benign, but multicystic and bilateral when malignant. Although the capsule may be smooth, gross subcapsular papillary projections into cystic structures are usually obvious in carcinomas. The cells are cuboidal and regular, resembling fallopian tube epithelium. Cilia are often present in benign serous tumors and those of LMP. Between one third and two thirds of invasive serous carcinomas are bilateral, and many of these tumors attain sizes in excess of 15 cm. Psammoma bodies are calcified granules that are rarely seen in benign tumors but are present in up to 33% of malignant tumors.

Mucinous tumors constitute 20% of benign epithelial tumors and 6% to 10% of epithelial carcinomas. These tumors are frequently large and sometimes weigh more than 50 kg. Both benign and invasive mucinous tumors commonly range between 15 and 30 cm. Only 5% of benign tumors are bilateral, whereas 25% of malignant mucinous carcinomas are bilateral. The histologic appearance of benign and malignant mucinous tumors is characterized by epithelial, mucin-producing cells.[50] Mucinous carcinomas are more likely than the majority of other ovarian carcinomas to be well differentiated and to be confined to the ovary at the time of presentation.[47] Mucinous tumors often exhibit histologic heterogeneity and may require extensive sampling to demonstrate foci of carcinoma in a lesion that is predominantly benign or of low malignant potential.[51] Pseudomyxoma peritonei may present as a rare complication of any ovarian mucinous tumor. This is a massive accumulation of gelatinous mucin in loculated pockets of the peritoneal cavity. This entity is occasionally seen in concert with appendiceal mucoceles, making the ascertainment of the primary lesion difficult. Surgical treatment is often necessary for recurrences; trials of intraperitoneal sclerotic agents have been less successful. Five-year survival rates of 45% have been reported.

Endometrioid and clear cell ovarian tumors are considered related but distinct histologic subtypes. Both may been seen in malignancies arising from endometriotic implants, but most tumors of these types apparently arise de novo.[52] Endometrioid tumors have a histologic appearance resembling that of endometrial tissue. The rare endometrioid tumor of LMP histologically resembles adenomatous hyperplasia. Endometrioid ovarian carcinoma can exhibit a variety of appearances similar to those of uterine endometrial carcinoma, including the possibility of squamous elements. Endometrioid ovarian carcinomas are the second most common type of epithelial carcinomas, accounting for about 20% of all primary ovarian cancers.[53] Concomitant endometrioid ovarian and endometrial carcinomas are common. They generally carry a favorable prognosis, as both carcinomas usually present at an early stage.[54] Both benign clear cell tumors and clear cell carcinomas of LMP, although rare, have been described. Clear cell carcinomas constitute 5% to 11% of all primary ovarian cancers; 40% are bilateral.[55] Some series have reported clear cell carcinoma of the ovary to have a more aggressive clinical behavior than that of other epithelial malignancies.[56]

Brenner tumors are presumably derived from the coelomic mesothelium of the ovary, despite their urothelial-like transitional cell appearance.[57] The majority of these tumors are solid and less than 8 cm. They are often found incidentally during an operation for other indications. Most are benign, but malignant Brenner tumors occur rarely.

Germ cell tumors are derived from germ cells and resemble primitive germ cells or structures of the conceptus. Tumors resembling primitive germ cells are termed dysgerminomas. They are the only germ cell cancers with a propensity to occur bilaterally; bilateral occurrence is seen in 5% to 10% of cases.[58] Those containing embryonic or fetal structures are teratomas. Most teratomas are benign mature cystic teratomas. Those containing immature embryonic structures are malignant. Tumors containing yolk sac derivatives are known as endodermal sinus tumors. Choriocarcinoma refers to tumors with trophoblastic morphology. Embryonal carcinoma contains large, primitive cells that secrete alpha-fetoprotein. Many germ cell tumors are of mixed histology, consisting predominantly of dysgerminoma, with other elements admixed. The prognosis of mixed germ cell tumors reflects that of the histologically worst element rather than that of the predominant element. All germ cell tumors except for mature teratomas are malignant.

In contrast to epithelial tumors, the clinical behavior of germ cell tumors is heavily dependent on histologic type. Well-differentiated malignant teratomas confined to the ovary are usually cured by unilateral salpingo-oophorectomy.[59] If confined to one ovary, dysgerminomas are usually cured by oophorectomy if less than 10 cm in diameter.[3, 60] Dysgerminomas are usually curable by low doses of radiation[61, 62] but are the only radiosensitive germ cell tumors. Other types of germ cell tumors usually recur without postoperative adjuvant treatment, even when diagnosed at an early stage,[63] but adjuvant chemotherapy usually effects a cure.[64] Germ cell tumors account for 10% to 20% of primary ovarian neoplasms.

Ovarian malignancies arising from specialized stroma constitute about 5% of ovarian neoplasms. They may resemble ovarian stromal elements, testicular elements, or a mixture of both. Granulosa cell tumors have pale, grooved, "coffee bean" nuclei. The cells are arranged in one of a number of characteristic patterns, often forming follicular structures called Call-Exner bodies. They occur at a mean age of 50 years. Their prognosis is related to size. Tumors less than 5 cm in diameter are almost always cured by surgery, but those greater than 15 cm recur almost half the time.[65, 66] Sertoli-Leydig tumors are more prone to metastasize,[67] but their rarity has precluded the development of standard treatment strategies.

Tubal Carcinoma

Virtually all tubal malignancy is papillary serous carcinoma.

DIAGNOSIS, SCREENING, AND STAGING

Diagnosis of Early Ovarian Cancer

The cornerstone of the management of the adnexal mass is that *benign and malignant ovarian masses can not be distinguished clinically.* Therefore, histopathologic evaluation is imperative for the accurate management of an adnexal mass, regardless of the patient's age. This requirement for histologic evaluation has not been obviated by new operative modalities such as laparoscopy. Some small simple cysts (see below) may be observed with frequent physical and ultrasound examination. Most adnexal masses, however, must be removed and subjected to histologic examination to determine whether they are malignant or benign.

Ovarian malignancies are seldom detected at an early stage; by the time of diagnosis, about 80% of ovarian carcinomas have metastasized. The most common presentation of early ovarian carcinoma is palpation of an asymptomatic mass on pelvic examination by a physician. Sometimes a large indolent tumor may grow quite large and present as abdominal distention. Similarly, a large ovarian mass may cause symptoms such as constipation or urinary frequency due to pressure on neighboring structures. The first symptoms of ovarian carcinoma may be vague lower abdominal discomfort. Rarely, torsion of an enlarged malignant ovary is seen. Although epithelial carcinomas seldom present as lesions grossly confined to the ovary, germ cell and specialized stromal tumors usually do so.[66, 68] They are most likely to present with abdominal pain, abnormal vaginal bleeding, or abdominal distention.

Screening of Asymptomatic Women

The desire to diagnose ovarian carcinoma at an early stage has led to attempts to develop technology to detect asymptomatic lesions. A radioimmunoassay for the oncofetal CA 125 has been so employed. Its use has been disappointing because of its low specificity and sensitivity. Serum CA 125 levels are frequently elevated in pregnancy,[69] leiomyomas,[70] and endometriosis,[71] as well as in many other benign[72] and malignant conditions.[70] This limits the usefulness of this assay in the diagnosis of a pelvic mass, let alone in screening asymptomatic women. Conversely, although elevated in most women with metastatic ovarian and tubal carcinoma,[73, 74] serum CA 125 levels are normal in half of women with stage I lesions.[70] These are precisely the lesions that one wishes to detect with a screening test, as it is problematic whether detection of asymptomatic advanced lesions will significantly improve their prognosis.

Pelvic ultrasound examinations have also been employed in an attempt to detect early lesions. Campbell and associates[75] reported the use of abdominal ultrasonography to screen 5479 asymptomatic low-risk postmenopausal women; van Nagell's group screened 1300 women with vaginal ultrasonography.[76] Each of these groups demonstrated adnexal masses in 3% to 4%. Only about 3% of these masses proved to be malignant, most of which were of low grade and stage. These studies report prevalence data rather than incidence data; it is not yet clear how many lesions will be detected during follow-up screening of large numbers of women with negative first screens. It is also unclear whether regular screening will pick up most anaplastic lesions prior to metastasis. Routine ultrasound screening cannot be recommended at present, as it is of unproven efficacy. It seems reasonable that women over 40 years of age with a first-degree relative with ovarian carcinoma should undergo ultrasound screening two to four times annually. Although most of these women will not be at risk for familial ovarian carcinoma, their risk is somewhat higher than that of the general population.

Management of the Adnexal Mass

Physicians must aggressively pursue the diagnosis and treatment of adnexal masses in order to reduce the mortality of ovarian cancer. The differential diagnosis of the adnexal mass is extensive. Etiology can be divided into ovarian, extraovarian, and nongynecologic causes. Adnexal masses may originate from the ovary, the fallopian tube, the uterus or its supporting structures, embryologic remnants of the müllerian or wolffian ducts, the large bowel, the appendix, the kidney or urologic system, and the retroperitoneum. Ovarian masses may be due to benign or malignant neoplasia, inflammation, abscess, endometriosis, ectopic pregnancy, and functional causes.

The age of a patient is strongly correlated with the etiology of ovarian masses. Table 14–25 reports the pathologic diagnoses in one series of women undergoing exploration for pelvic masses. Women over 50 years had ovarian cancer 56% of the time, compared with a 10% rate of

TABLE 14–25
Pathologic Diagnoses in 100 Women Undergoing Surgical Exploration for a Pelvic Mass[220]

Diagnosis	No. (%) of Patients With Diagnosis by Age in Years			
	<31	*31–49*	*>49*	*Total*
Cancer	4 (10)	4 (8)	9 (56)	17
Benign cystic teratoma	13 (33)	3 (7)	1 (6)	17
Endometriosis	5 (13)	12 (27)	0	17
Cystadenoma	4 (10)	8 (18)	4 (25)	16
Tubo-ovarian abscess, hydrosalpinx	5 (13)	9 (20)	0	14
Uterine leiomyoma	2 (5)	6 (13)	2 (13)	10
Functional cyst	3 (8)	0	0	3
Paratubal cyst	2 (5)	1 (2)	0	3
Other	1 (3)	2 (4)	0	3
Total	39	45	16	100

malignancy in women under 30.[77] The common etiologies of adnexal cyst, classified according to menstrual status, are provided in Table 14–26.

Ultrasound examination has been useful in determining the etiology of adnexal masses. The distribution of solid and cystic areas, and their morphology, has proved useful in narrowing the differential diagnosis. Complex cysts, masses with cystic and solid areas, and cystic masses with thickened or irregular capsules are more likely to be malignant.[78] Even simple ovarian cysts may contain cancer, however, especially in postmenopausal women.[77, 79] Furthermore, it is not known how many benign serous and mucinous cystadenomas will undergo malignant transformation if not removed. The blood flow characteristics of the mass may provide further clues regarding the likelihood that a mass is benign or malignant.[80, 81] There is overlap between blood flow findings in benign and malignant ovarian lesions, however.[82] At present, ultrasonography, either alone or in combination with other noninvasive studies, should not be considered sufficiently reliable to differentiate categorically between benign and malignant ovarian masses.

Surgical assessment is the only reliable method of diagnosing an adnexal mass. In the past, laparotomy was universally required for accurate diagnosis and removal; contemporary laparoscopic techniques offer the ability to remove an ovarian mass for histologic assessment. No ovarian masses should be aspirated.[83] Simple cysts less 8 cm in diameter in women under 40 years, and less than 3 cm in older women, may be followed with serial sonography, as they are unlikely to contain cancer. If the cyst grows or changes in appearance, it should be excised. Larger lesions should be removed. If they have a characteristic ultrasound appearance of a benign lesion (e.g., dermoid cyst, endometriosis), laparoscopic cystectomy is permissible in premenopausal patients. Other lesions should be regarded as suspicious for malignancy. It is controversial whether rupture of an ovarian mass may disseminate the disease. Therefore, these lesions should not be removed by laparoscopic cystectomy, which is likely to rupture a cyst. Rather, they should be removed either by oophorectomy (open or laparoscopic) or by open cystectomy, with precautions taken to prevent spilled cyst fluid from coming into contact with the wound or abdomen. This may be achieved by elevating the ovary out of the incision and by surrounding it with sponges during dissection of the cyst. Complex lesions that are suspicious for carcinoma should be approached through a vertical laparotomy incision to allow adequate staging and cytoreduction in the event that they contain cancer. All ovarian masses removed surgically should be reviewed by a pathologist immediately. The operation should not be terminated until a frozen section has established the diagnosis.

Late Symptoms of Ovarian Cancer

Women with metastatic ovarian carcinoma often present with indigestion, anorexia, and constipation. Early satiety—

TABLE 14–26
Common Differential Diagnoses of the Adnexal Mass by Menstrual Status

Premenarchal	Reproductive Years	Postmenopausal
Mesenteric cyst	Ectopic pregnancy	Epithelial ovarian cancer
Benign teratoma	Functional ovarian cyst	Benign ovarian mass
Functional ovarian cyst	Endometriosis	Metastatic ovarian cancer
Germ cell tumor	Benign teratoma	Uterine mass
Other gynecologic tumors	Uterine leiomyoma	Ovarian stromal tumor
	Epithelial ovarian cancer	Colon cancer
	Tubo-ovarian abscess	Diverticulitis
	Benign ovarian epithelial tumor	Tubal carcinoma

the feeling of fullness after eating a small amount—is extremely common. Abdominal distention due to masses or ascites is frequently seen; women with virulent lesions may progress in a few weeks from normalcy to respiratory compromise from massive ascites. The tumor stroma may produce estrogens, leading to metrorrhagia or postmenopausal bleeding as a presenting symptom.[84] Later symptoms include dyspnea and tachypnea from pleural effusions and nausea and vomiting from intestinal tethering or obstruction. There may be marked weight loss despite massive ascites.

Tubal Carcinoma

The most common symptom of tubal carcinoma is vaginal bleeding or discharge, and the next most common symptom is colicky pelvic pain.[41, 42, 85] These occur early in the course of the disease due to blockage of the tube, with resulting distention medially and distal egress of material produced by the tumor. Thus, most tubal carcinomas are diagnosed as stage I or II disease. Hydrops tubae profluens, a profuse watery vaginal discharge, is not seen often,[41, 42, 85] but it is virtually pathognomonic of tubal cancer when present. The diagnosis is sometimes first suspected because of the presence of adenocarcinoma cells on a Papanicolaou smear in an asymptomatic patient.[42]

Physical Findings

The only finding in early ovarian cancer is the presence of an adnexal mass. The ovaries are usually palpated more easily on bimanual rectovaginal examination than on vaginal examination, since the ovaries frequently lie posterior to the uterus. Rectovaginal examination is carried out with the examiner placing the index finger of one hand in the vagina and the middle finger in the rectum. The other hand is placed on the abdomen. The examiner attempts to palpate the uterus and ovaries by squeezing the hands together gently.

The rectal finger can be used to palpate for cul-de-sac masses. It is also useful in assessing whether an adnexal mass is adherent to the sigmoid at the peritoneal reflection; this may have an impact on the operation performed.

Later tumors may give rise to ascites, with the classic findings of abdominal distention, shifting dullness, and fluid wave. Pleural effusions result in decreased breath sounds in the lung bases, accompanied by dullness to percussion. Inguinal and cervical lymph nodes may be palpable in women with advanced disease.

Laboratory and Radiologic Findings

Several tumor markers are widely used to follow the course of ovarian cancer and should be drawn, as appropriate. CA 125 is elevated in 84% of advanced carcinoma[73] as well as in most tubal carcinomas.[74] Unfortunately, it is not very specific. Placental alkaline phosphatase is elevated in up to half of patients with ovarian carcinoma, usually advanced.[86] Alpha-fetoprotein (AFP) and human chorionic gonadotropin (hCG) are sensitive and specific markers for endodermal sinus tumor[87] and choriocarcinoma,[88] respectively. Lactate dehydrogenase (LDH) is less specific but may be used as a marker to follow the course of treatment of germ cell tumors, including dysgerminomas.[89] All three should be drawn immediately upon the diagnosis of any germ cell tumor, including dysgerminoma. Small foci of other elements are often present in dysgerminomas and mandate postoperative chemotherapy. The finding of AFP or hCG in the serum of a woman with apparent dysgerminoma indicates that a mixed tumor actually exists. This implies a need for postoperative chemotherapy even if other elements cannot be found histologically.

If the primary site of a pelvic malignancy is unclear, cervical cytology, endocervical curettage, or endometrial biopsy may be obtained. The frequent association of granulosa cell tumors,[90, 91] endometrioid tumors,[92, 93] and clear cell carcinomas[92, 93] with endometrial carcinoma indicates that endometrial biopsy and possibly hysteroscopy should be performed in women with these ovarian tumors if uterine conservation is contemplated.

Other laboratory studies are of little use, except to indicate whether the patient will be able to tolerate the anticipated treatment.

Certain radiologic studies are important in the evaluation of a woman who may have ovarian or tubal carcinoma. Pelvic ultrasonography, possibly including Doppler flow studies, helps characterize a mass with no obvious metastases. Computed tomography with intravenous contrast may reveal large metastases in the omentum and other peritoneal structures as well as enlarged retroperitoneal lymph nodes. This study also detects ureteral displacement or obstruction; if it is necessary to examine the urinary tract in greater detail, intravenous urography may be obtained. Barium enema or colonoscopy should be obtained to rule out a colonic primary lesion, especially when a pelvic mass is fixed or is on the left side. Mammography is also useful if it was not performed during the previous year.

Staging

Ascribing a Primary Site

Tubal carcinoma is differentiated from ovarian carcinoma by Hu's criteria.[94] In order to diagnose tubal carcinoma, the main tumor must be in the tube and arise from endosalpinx. The histology must resemble tubal carcinoma. The ovaries must either be uninvolved or contain less tumor than the tube. Recognition of serous carcinoma of endometrium as a clinical entity[95] suggests that the absence of endometrial tumor should be added as an additional criterion for the diagnosis of primary tubal carcinoma.

Extraovarian peritoneal serous papillary carcinoma is less common than ovarian carcinoma.[33, 34] It is histologically identical to ovarian carcinoma, but the ovaries show

TABLE 14–27
FIGO Staging System for Ovarian Carcinoma

Stage I: Growth Limited to the Ovaries

- Stage Ia: Growth limited to one ovary; no ascites present containing malignant cells; no tumor on the external surface; capsule intact
- Stage Ib: Growth limited to both ovaries; no ascites present containing malignant cells; no tumor on the external surfaces; capsules intact
- Stage Ic*: Tumor classified as either stage Ia or Ib but with tumor on the surface of one or both ovaries, with ruptured capsule(s), with ascites containing malignant cells present, or with positive peritoneal washings

Stage II: Growth Involving One or Both Ovaries, With Pelvic Extension

- Stage IIa: Extension and/or metastases to the uterus and/or tubes
- Stage IIb: Extension to other pelvic tissues
- Stage IIc*: Tumor classified as either stage IIA or IIB but with tumor on the surface of one or both ovaries, with capsules(s) ruptured, with ascites containing malignant cells present, or with positive peritoneal washings

Stage III: Tumor Involving One or Both Ovaries With Peritoneal Implants Outside the Pelvis and/or Positive Retroperitoneal or Inguinal Nodes

Superficial liver metastasis equals stage III; tumor is limited to the true pelvis but with histologically proven malignant extension to small bowel or omentum

- Stage IIIa: Tumor grossly limited to the true pelvis with negative nodes but with histologically confirmed microscopic seeding of abdominal peritoneal surfaces
- Stage IIIb: Tumor of one or both ovaries with histologically confirmed implants of abdominal peritoneal surfaces, none exceeding 2 cm in diameter; nodes are negative
- Stage IIIc: Abdominal implants greater than 2 cm in diameter and/or positive retroperitoneal or inguinal nodes

Stage IV: Growth Involving One or Both Ovaries, With Distant Metastases

If pleural effusion is present, there must be positive cytologic findings to allot a case to stage IV; parenchymal liver metastasis equals stage IV

*Indicate at the time of operation whether capsular rupture is spontaneous or caused by the surgeon. Also, specify whether the source of malignant cells was peritoneal washings or ascites.

little or no involvement. This cancer may occur even after removal of normal ovaries.[34] It is particularly common in women with one of the familial ovarian cancer syndromes.

Staging of Ovarian and Tubal Cancer

The International Federation of Obstetricians and Gynecologists (FIGO) staging system for ovarian carcinoma, adopted in 1985, is depicted in Table 14–27. This system is a surgicopathologic one, requiring an adequate staging procedure. FIGO has recently adopted a staging system for tubal carcinoma (Table 14–28), which is based on the ovarian schema and is also surgicopathologic.

OVARIAN CARCINOMA: TREATMENT AND RESULTS

The treatment of ovarian carcinoma has evolved from an exercise in palliation to an aggressive and rewarding effort toward long-term remission and even cure.[96] Critical to this evolution has been the utilization of maximal surgical debulking and combination chemotherapy based on platinum coordination compounds. For the purposes of this chapter, a number of definitions are useful:

Adjuvant treatment: the use of therapeutic modalities after surgical excision of gross disease, to obtain or to consolidate remission.

Primary treatment: also called first-line therapy, the first prescribed combination of cytotoxic agents, generally a combination that provides the highest likelihood of cure.

Secondary treatment: the palliative treatment used after failure of primary therapy.

Salvage treatment: the use of new treatment modalities for ovarian cancer in a carefully designed research protocol.

The physician who undertakes the challenge of caring for patients with carcinoma of the ovary should be prepared to manage a chronic disease with a difficult course and often unsuccessful outcome. Ovarian cancer incorporates a wide spectrum of disease, ranging from early tumors curable by surgical extirpation to aggressive, widely disseminated lesions that are beyond the reaches of surgical, chemotherapeutic, and radiotherapeutic attempts at cure. Familiarity with the most recent oncologic advances is critical to optimize each patient's opportunity for survival.

The management of primary ovarian carcinoma may be divided into three phases. Almost all oncologists recommend primary surgery. This is usually followed by adjuvant nonoperative treatment, which usually consists of chemotherapy. Finally, after a predefined course of chemotherapy, disease status is systematically re-evaluated.

Initial Operation

The goal of the initial operation is twofold: to determine the extent of the disease and to remove as much gross disease as possible. It is usually possible to perform a useful cytoreduction, as metastases of ovarian carcinoma have the unique attribute of adhering to peritoneal surfaces without invading deeply. This allows the development of surgical planes where this would not be possible with other tumors.

TABLE 14–28
FIGO Staging System for Fallopian Tube Carcinoma

Stage I:	**Growth Limited to the Fallopian Tubes**
	Stage IA: Growth limited to one tube with extension into submucosa or muscularis but not penetrating serosal surface; no ascites intact
	Stage IB: Growth limited to both tubes with extension into submucosa or muscularis but not penetrating serosal surface; no ascites intact
	Stage IC: Tumor classified as either stage IA or IB but with extension through or onto tubal serosa or with ascites containing malignant cells present or with positive peritoneal washings
Stage II:	**Growth Involving One or Both Fallopian Tubes, With Pelvic Extension**
	Stage IIA: Extension and/or metastases to the uterus and/or ovaries
	Stage IIB: Extension to other pelvic tissues
	Stage IIC: Tumor classified as either stage IIA or IIB but with ascites containing malignant cells or with positive peritoneal washings
Stage III:	**Tumor Involving One or Both Fallopian Tubes, With Peritoneal Implants Outside the Pelvis and/or Positive Retroperitoneal or Inguinal Nodes**
	Superficial liver metastasis equals stage III, tumor is limited to the true pelvis, but with histologically proven malignant extension to small bowel or omentum
	Stage IIIA: Tumor grossly limited to the true pelvis with negative nodes but with histologically confirmed microscopic seeding of abdominal peritoneal surfaces
	Stage IIIB: Tumor of one or both ovaries with histologically confirmed implants of abdominal peritoneal surfaces, none exceeding 2 cm in diameter; lymph nodes are negative
	Stage IIIC: Abdominal implants greater than 2 cm in diameter and/or positive retroperitoneal or inguinal nodes
Stage IV:	**Growth Involving One or Both Fallopian Tubes, With Distant Metastases**
	If pleural effusion is present, there must be positive cytologic findings to allot a case to stage IV; parenchymal liver metastasis equals stage IV

Prior to the operation, the patient is given a bowel preparation adequate for colonic surgery since bowel entry during resection of ovarian carcinoma is common. Most gynecologic oncologists do not obtain preoperative ureteral stenting, in contrast to the frequent practice by general surgeons who intend to perform a procedure involving extensive dissection of the pelvic retroperitoneal spaces. Whether or not the ureters are stented, operations for ovarian carcinoma should be performed only by surgeons who are experienced in dissection of the pelvis, including the retroperitoneal space, and who are familiar with pelvic surgical anatomy.

The operation is performed via laparotomy through a vertical incision initially extending from the pubis to the umbilicus. It is impossible to evaluate the upper abdomen and aortic nodes, let alone to perform an adequate cytoreductive procedure, through a transverse incision in the lower abdomen; indeed, the vertical incision must often be extended well above the umbilicus. The patient must be draped to allow cephalad extension of the incision to the xiphoid, if this proves necessary. If ascites is encountered when the abdomen is opened, an aliquot is sent for cytology. From this point, the conduct of the operation depends on the extent of the disease.

Operative Management of Disease Confined to the Genitalia

It is almost always possible to remove all gross tumor in ovarian carcinoma confined to the pelvis. It is also important that the tumor be adequately staged to facilitate planning of adjuvant therapy. The procedure required for such staging is summarized in Table 14–29. When operating for a pelvic mass, the surgeon collects washings from the pelvis, right diaphragmatic surface, and both paracolic gutters if no ascites is present. This is done by irrigating the appropriate regions with 0.9% sodium chloride and then aspirating. The abdomen is explored and the bowel run. If tumor is present outside the ovary, biopsy samples are taken for frozen section. It is important to know the histology of the tumor. Furthermore, the diagnosis may be a benign disease, such as tuberculosis. If the tumor is derived from germ cells (see Table 14–24), the anesthesiologist is asked to draw blood for serum AFP, hCG, and LDH. If the tumor exhibits borderline histology, a lesser operation may be warranted than for a frankly malignant tumor (see below).

Comprehensive staging is then performed. Total abdominal hysterectomy with bilateral salpingo-oophorectomy is mandatory, *except* in two situations: (1) a borderline tumor confined to one ovary in a patient of any age, and (2) a

TABLE 14–29
Intitial Staging Operation for Patients With Localized Ovarian and Tubal Carcinoma

Vertical incision
Aspiration of ascites or washings from pelvis, both paracolic gutters, and right hemidiaphragm
Thorough abdominal exploration, including visualization of entire intestine
Total abdominal hysterectomy, bilateral salpingo-oophorectomy (perform only unilateral salpingo-oophorectomy without hysterectomy in premenopausal women with lesions grossly limited to the ovary whose histology is low malignant potential or grade 1 epithelial carcinoma or any germ cell or stromal malignancy)
Random biopsy samples from both paracolic gutters, bladder serosa, sigmoid serosa, cul-de-sac of Douglas, both pelvic sidewalls' peritoneum, right hemidiaphragm (two from each site)
Infracolic omentectomy
Lymph node sampling (external iliac, internal iliac, obturator, common iliac, and low abdominal aortic nodes) at least ipsilateral; consider bilateral dissection

stage IAG1 or IAG2 tumor in a woman who desires fertility. Under these circumstances, unilateral salpingo-oophorectomy is the treatment of choice. It is advisable to open the anterior broad ligament on both sides to identify the ureters and great vessels at the outset of hysterectomy or oophorectomy. This maneuver is mandatory if the tumor is adherent to the pelvic sidewall, as damage to the ureter may otherwise occur. If the tumor is in close association with a ureter, the ureter is reflected laterally off the peritoneum and tumor to allow removal.

In addition to washings and ablation of the primary tumor, the infracolic portion of the greater omentum is removed. Biopsy samples are taken of para-aortic, common iliac, external iliac, internal iliac, and obturator nodes on each side. It seems reasonable to remove only ipsilateral nodes for a lesion grossly confined to one ovary, but many protocols of collaborative clinical research require that a bilateral procedure be performed in every case. In addition, small random peritoneal biopsy specimens are taken at the right diaphragm, both paracolic gutters, the bladder serosa, the sigmoid serosa, the cul-de-sac of Douglas, and both pelvic sidewalls. Histopathologic examination of these samples is sufficient to establish the stage and direct further treatment (see Table 14–29).

Operative Management of Extragenital Disease

A large body of literature supports the contention that maximal cytoreduction at the initial operation is associated with prolonged disease-free survival and optimal survival rates.[97–104] A smaller literature questions this assertion.[105] Since the success of treatment is based on a complex interplay among the disease biology, the initial operation, and the postoperative adjuvant therapy, it is difficult to quantitate the role of cytoreduction. Patients with stage IIIC disease reduced surgically to optimal diameter (<2 cm) do not fare as well as those treated with disease found at stage IIIA or IIIB,[106, 107] although they survive longer than women who did not attain optimal cytoreduction at the initial operation.[107] Most gynecologic oncologists recommend optimal cytoreduction at the initial operation.

Total abdominal hysterectomy and bilateral hysterectomy are performed. The retroperitoneal space of the pelvic sidewall is opened at the outset to allow involved sidewall peritoneum to be reflected medially off the ureters and resected with the specimen.

The extent of further tumor resection depends on the possibility of "optimal" cytoreduction. An extensive literature supports the concept that survival is improved when tumor volume is reduced to the point where the largest tumor diameter is less than 2 cm.[99, 101, 104] Below this size, further reduction is said to enhance both median and long-term survival. Some recent literature has called this concept into question,[105] but most authorities advocate extensive operation when this can effect cytoreduction. The operative plan must be individualized and cannot be finalized until laparotomy reveals the exact distribution of tumor. The surgeon must therefore be prepared to execute a wide variety of procedures. It may be necessary to resect bowel, portions of the urinary tract, or even spleen[108] and diaphragm.[109] The degree of operative aggressiveness must be influenced not only by the technical possibility of achieving optimal cytoreduction but also by the medical condition of the patient and her ability to withstand a proposed procedure. Overall, it should be possible to reduce the maximum diameter of the largest residual nodule to 2 cm or less in at least 75% of women presenting with metastatic ovarian carcinoma.[110, 111] The presence of large quantities of tumor at the hepatic portal, the root of the mesentery, or the aortic nodes suggests that cytoreduction is likely to be unfeasible. Clearly, the best results are obtained when operations for ovarian cancer are performed by individuals with appropriate training and wide experience. At least two studies showed that, in both academic[112] and community[113] settings, gynecologic oncologists achieved optimal cytoreduction a higher proportion of the time than did general surgeons or general obstetricians and gynecologists. This translated into longer survival in patients staged by gynecologic oncologists.[112]

When there are tumor nodules in the cul-de-sac, the dissection should include the peritoneum of the cul-de-sac in the specimen. The tumor generally is adherent rather than invasive, and the peritoneum can be peeled anteriorly off the deeper structures.

Tumor on the bladder peritoneum can usually be dissected off by establishing a tissue plane between the tumor and the bladder muscularis. When this is not possible, the tumor may be ablated using an ultrasonic surgery device. Elimination of tumor from the dome of the bladder sometimes requires removal of a segment of bladder. The bladder is then closed primarily after ascertaining the position of the ureters and urethra.

Similarly, tumor on the rectosigmoid is managed by conservative dissection, ablation, or segmental resection of bowel.[110] Primary anastomosis is generally possible if a bowel preparation is done preoperatively, as the tumor rarely invades into the pelvis distal to the level of the peritoneal reflection of the rectum. Use of a circular stapler facilitates such low anterior anastomosis.[110]

The omentum is commonly involved in extraovarian disease. The infracolic omentum should be resected. When gross disease is present in the gastrocolic ligament, total omentectomy is performed. Even when tumor is adherent to the transverse colon, it is usually possible to separate tumor from colon; when this is not possible, partial colectomy should be considered. An omentum infiltrated with tumor may adhere to the spleen, with tumor involving that structure; in this case, splenectomy may be beneficial.[108] When gross disease is present on the small intestine, segmental resection and anastomosis should be considered.

Resection of grossly involved pelvic and low aortic lymph nodes generally is feasible.

The ultrasonic surgical aspirator[114] and the argon beam coagulator[115] allow ablation of tumor from parietal and visceral peritoneal structures with minimal blood loss. In most cases, these tools allow ablation of diaphragmatic tumor.[109] They permit cytoreduction of lesions too extensive or too delicately situated to permit removal by standard techniques. In many instances, ablation of tumor may spare the patient bowel or bladder resection. Although such ablation is tedious, these instruments are relatively easy to operate. Surgeons who operate for ovarian carcinoma should master the use of at least one of these devices.

Major morbidity is comparable to that encountered in other major abdominal oncologic procedures.[110, 116] The problems encountered are those common to extensive laparotomies in general (e.g., hemorrhage, pneumonia, wound infection and dehiscence, pulmonary embolus) and those specific to the operative manipulations involved (e.g., anastomotic dehiscence). One complication that is characteristic in ovarian cytoreduction is the delayed development of pulmonary edema. After an extensive cytoreduction procedure, reaccumulation of ascites and sequestration of fluid in the intestine (third spacing) may necessitate the administration of massive amounts of fluids. There may be a positive fluid balance of 20–25 L. When intestinal function begins to recover on the third to seventh postoperative day, the sequestered fluid is mobilized rapidly. Pulmonary edema may suddenly ensue in a patient who, to all intents and purposes, is recovering clinically.

Surgical mortality for all patients with advanced ovarian carcinoma undergoing primary cytoreductive surgery is 2% to 5%.[110, 116]

Germ Cell and Stromal Malignancies

Germ cell and stromal tumors usually have no gross involvement beyond a single involved ovary. When this is the case and the patient is premenopausal, unilateral salpingo-oophorectomy and careful surgical staging are performed. Hysterectomy and removal of the contralateral ovary are unnecessary.[68] Total abdominal hysterectomy with bilateral salpingo-oophorectomy is usually performed in postmenopausal women, although it is not clear that the more extensive procedure enhances the prognosis. When extraovarian disease is encountered, the maximum possible cytoreduction should be performed.[68] The same principles apply to initial operation for ovarian stromal tumors.

Tubal Carcinoma

Initial operative management of tubal carcinoma is the same as that for ovarian carcinoma of comparable extent.

Adjuvant Postoperative Therapy

Following the initial operation, most patients with ovarian carcinoma, and all patients with tubal carcinoma, should be treated using adjuvant therapy. This generally involves the use of chemotherapy, although in some circumstances there is a role for whole abdominal radiation or for the intraperitoneal use of radionuclide. The most important advance in adjuvant therapy of ovarian epithelial cancer has been the development of chemotherapeutic regimens based on platinum coordination compounds. Patients treated with combinations containing platinum survive longer than patients treated with other chemotherapeutic regimens.[46, 117] Adjuvant chemotherapy regimens for advanced ovarian carcinoma based on organoplatinum compounds offer overall response rates of 60% to 80%,[46, 117–119] with complete response rates as high as 50%. Despite such high clinical response rates, most patients still relapse and later succumb. The later failure of platinum is due to the development of drug resistance of an uncertain mechanism. Most American oncologists combine platinum drugs with another cytotoxic agent in an effort to improve the likelihood of response and cure.

The following recommendations are based on studies of well-staged patients and are based on the premise that surgical staging has been carried out as described above. Oncologists called on to treat patients with apparent early disease that has been inadequately staged face a major problem. Under these circumstances, they may elect to treat according to the apparent stage, treat more aggressively than the apparent stage warrants, or re-explore the patient using laparotomy or laparoscopy to obtain more staging information.

Tumors of Low Malignant Potential

Carcinoma of LMP (also known as borderline tumor) is a concept derived from the "semimalignancy" of Taylor.[120] Although these tumors are intermediate in aggressiveness, between benign tumors (with no cancer-related deaths) and invasive carcinomas, they are definitely malignant, with the potential for extraovarian metastases. The clinical behavior of carcinomas of LMP is characterized by indolent growth, with a 5-year survival rate approaching 100%. Survival at 10 years decreases to 75%, as late recurrence is not unusual, and may take place at 10 to 15 years after diagnosis. Although nuclear atypism and mitotic activity are common, these properties are not related to prognosis.[121] Approximately 75% of carcinomas of LMP are serous and 21% mucinous, as reported in a recent study of 171 patients.[122] In this same study, 21% were found to have extraperitoneal lymphatic metastases and 38% were FIGO stage III by other metastases after full surgical staging. Accurate surgical staging and maximal cytoreduction may be curative; adjuvant chemotherapy or radiotherapy is controversial.[123] Table 14–30 summarizes survival data collected from 16 series reviewed by Massad and colleagues.[124] The subjectivity of the histologic criteria for diagnosis and the relative efficacy of different treatment programs may account for differences among the various series.

TABLE 14–30
Mortality in Patients With Epithelial Tumors of Low Malignant Potential

Stage	Patients	Deaths	Percent	Percent Variation Among Series
I	749	14	1.9	0–10.7
II	85	5	5.9	0–20.0
III, IV	167	35	21.0	0–66.7
All stages	1001	54	5.4	0–30.7

Based on Massad LS Jr, et al: Epithelial tumors of low malignant potential. Obstet Gynecol 78:1027–1032, 1991.

LMP Tumors, Stages I and II

As is the case with frankly malignant tumors, LMP tumors require careful surgical staging, which "upstages" about 25% of these tumors.[122, 125] The majority of these lesions are, however, confined to the pelvis.[126] Young women with tumor grossly limited to one ovary may be treated by unilateral oophorectomy or even by ovarian cystectomy.[127, 128] Even in the unusual circumstance of tumor recurrence, it is likely to recur locally and to be cured by further surgical effort. Serous tumors are more likely to recur than mucinous tumors. Women with well-staged stage I and II tumors require no adjuvant therapy, as virtually all are cured by operation alone.[124, 129]

LMP Tumors, Stage III

Patients with stage III LMP tumors do worse than those with less advanced lesions.[124] The 5-year survival rate is greater than 75%.[130, 131] The rarity of advanced LMP tumors and their long interval to clinical recurrence (up to 20 years after initial treatment) make it difficult to assess the utility of primary therapy. Macroscopic disease frequently responds to combination chemotherapy.[132] It seems reasonable to treat patients with residual macroscopic metastases in a manner comparable to those with frankly malignant stage III carcinomas (see below). Patients with no residual disease may be managed conservatively or given adjuvant treatment, at the discretion of the physician. Pseudomyxoma peritonei is treated using a combination of cisplatin, cyclophosphamide, and doxorubicin,[133] but this therapy is frequently unsuccessful, and most patients with this syndrome die of it.[134]

Frankly Invasive Carcinoma

Different series vary considerably regarding the thoroughness of staging, aggressiveness of cytoreduction, documentation of findings, and treatment regimen. Preliminary data are more frequently reported than mature data. Five-year survival is not tantamount to cure; late recurrences are not uncommon.[135–137] Table 14–31 summarizes the 5-year survival expected in well-staged women treated in a standard manner.

Carcinoma: Stages IA and IB, Grades 1 and 2

These tumors require no adjuvant treatment, as there is 90% survival with operation alone.[67]

Carcinoma: Stages IA and IB (Grade 3), Stage IC (Any Grade), and Stage II With No Gross Residual Disease

Classically, these tumors were treated using 12 courses of melphalan,[138] until it became apparent that as many as 10% of women so treated would develop a universally fatal acute myelocytic leukemia.[139] A large collaborative trial demonstrated that intraperitoneal administration of 15 mCi of phosphorus 32 colloid in this category of patient results in long-term survival equivalent to that obtained with treatment using melphalan (81% at 5 years).[140] The Princess Margaret[141] and Stanford[142] groups suggest that whole abdominal radiation (WAR) is highly efficacious as adjuvant therapy in these women. This treatment involves daily treatment of the entire abdomen and pelvis to 25 to 30 Gy (limiting the renal dose to 22.5 Gy) at the rate of 1.5 to 1.6 Gy daily. The pelvic dose is then boosted to 50 Gy using 1.8 to 2.0 Gy fractions. A randomized trial of these patients showed WAR to result in inferior survival compared with melphalan.[143] Many centers use a course of platinum-based combination chemotherapy.[144–146] The efficacy of such treatment has not been compared with that of other modalities in phase III trials.

Carcinoma: Stage II, With Gross Residual Disease Less Than 2 cm; Stage III, No Gross Residual Disease or Disease Less Than 2 cm

Although the Princess Margaret[141] and Stanford[142] groups suggest that many of these patients do well with WAR, standard therapy for these lesions consists of platinum-based combination chemotherapy. A study from Memorial Sloan Kettering Cancer Center in New York suggests that

TABLE 14–31
Approximate Five-Year Survival After Diagnosis of Ovarian Carcinoma

Stage	5-Year Survival (%)
I	80–90
II	60–80
III	
No residual tumor	40–50
Optimal residual tumor	20–35
Suboptimal residual tumor	<10
IV	<10

5 cycles of treatment may be no more efficacious than 10 cycles.[147] No investigator has yet performed a study in which a group of patients of sufficient size to minimize the beta error is followed for at least 5 years after treatment to determine at what point abbreviation of the number of treatment cycles decreases median and long-term survival. Most centers now offer six to nine cycles of treatment, assuming that progression of disease or severe drug-related complications do not supervene.

Although numerous courses of treatment do not appear to add significant benefit, it seems clear that the likelihood of a good outcome is directly related to the dose intensity of the therapy (i.e., the amount of drug divided by the number of weeks over which the drug was given).[148, 149] Widely used regimens include cisplatin with cyclophosphamide[149] or doxorubicin[117] or both,[46] and carboplatin with cyclophosphamide.[150] It is controversial whether the addition of doxorubicin to a regimen of cisplatin and cyclophosphamide enhances the clinical outcome.[151–154] The survival curve of patients receiving cisplatin versus carboplatin in combination chemotherapy is almost identical.[150, 155, 156] The latter regimen is more attractive because it is less toxic and can be given in an outpatient setting. Its dose-limiting toxicity is thrombocytopenia, whereas that of the cisplatin-based regimens is granulopenia. This allows doses of cisplatin-based regimens to be maintained and increased using colony-stimulating factors,[157] adding to the attractiveness of such regimens. It has not been proved, however, that use of colony-stimulating factors improves clinical outcome. The emergence of paclitaxel as a highly effective drug against ovarian carcinoma is likely to have a major impact on the treatment of this disease in the next few years.[158]

The effectiveness of treatment is monitored using immunologic assays for serum levels of tumor markers such as CA 125,[73] lipid-associated sialic acid,[159] and DK/70.[160] Rising levels of these antigens suggest progressive disease.

Carcinoma: Stage III, Residual Disease Greater Than 2 cm; Stage IV

These tumors are treated using combination chemotherapy as described in the previous section, and the course of treatment is monitored using serum tumor markers. It is clear that radiation has no role in the therapy of this category of tumor.

Reported long-term survival for all patients with stages III and IV ranges from 8%[106] to at least 25%.[96, 161–163] The large difference probably results from differences in the presenting stages of the patients as well as differences in operative and adjuvant chemotherapy.

Germ Cell Tumors

Cytoreduction of advanced disease should be carried out as for epithelial tumors. Incompletely resected lesions fail chemotherapy nearly three times as often as those that are entirely removed at the time of the initial operation if primary VAC chemotherapy is used,[164] and nearly twice as often if PVB chemotherapy is used[64] (see below).

Well-staged dysgerminomas confined to one ovary and measuring less than ten cm need not be treated with postoperative adjuvant therapy. Larger and more extensive tumors in postmenopausal women should be treated using radiation. It is emphasized that mixed tumors must be ruled out before radiation is given. This is done by taking multiple microscopic sections and by demonstrating negative serum levels of AFP and hCG at the time of operation. A variety of regimens are employed,[61, 62, 165] all of which deliver relatively low doses to the abdomen, with a boost to the pelvis, the abdominal aortic nodes, and sometimes the mediastinal nodes. Since this treatment compromises fertility, premenopausal patients are treated using four to six courses of cisplatin (Platinol), vinblastine, and bleomycin (PVB)[166] or bleomycin, etoposide, and Platinol (BEP).[167] The older combination of vincristine, dactinomycin, and cyclophosphamide (VAC)[169, 170] is not as effective and should be reserved for patients failing cisplatin-based therapy.

Mature teratomas have a characteristic appearance on ultrasound examination. They should be excised, as a malignancy will arise in 1–2% of benign teratomas. The bulk of these cancers are squamous cell carcinomas. Cancer arising in a benign teratoma is almost always fatal.[171]

Survival in patients with malignant teratomas depends as much on grade as on stage of the disease. The majority of patients with grade 1 lesions will enjoy prolonged survival, regardless of stage.[59] It is reasonable to treat well-differentiated stage I teratomas by surgery alone. All other immature teratomas should be treated with chemotherapy using PVB, BEP, or VAC,[172] as they are otherwise likely to recur.[59] The majority of lesions will be cured, although some will be left with benign teratomatous implants following treatment.[173] Malignant teratomas are insensitive to radiation.[174]

Other germ cell tumors (endodermal sinus tumors,[175, 176] mixed tumors,[177] pure choriocarcinomas,[88] and embryonal cell tumors) are quite virulent. Stage I lesions usually recur without treatment, and more advanced disease invariably does so. These lesions are insensitive to radiation.[176] The majority are cured using PVB or BEP chemotherapy.[68, 166, 167]

Ovarian Stromal Malignancies

Stage I lesions need no postoperative therapy, as 90% of patients live 5 years, and 75% survive 10 years, without adjuvant treatment.[178, 179] More advanced tumors are treated with systemic chemotherapy such as PVB,[180, 181] cisplatin and doxorubicin,[182] or cisplatin, doxorubicin, and cyclophosphamide.[183] Gonadotropin-releasing hormone agonists may be effective against these tumors.[184]

Fallopian Tube Carcinoma

All patients with carcinoma of the fallopian tube should receive adjuvant therapy, since even early tumors frequently recur when untreated. Some series report a 5-year survival rate of less than 50% for stage I lesions.[185, 186] Because of the frequent metastasis to lymph nodes[43] and distant sites,[41] most clinicians use chemotherapy. Patients with all stages of disease are given six to eight cycles of a combination regimen containing cisplatin.[187] The clinical course in these patients is comparable to that in women with ovarian carcinoma of a similar stage.[187–190]

EVALUATION OF RESPONSE TO TREATMENT

After surgical cytoreduction and completion of a course of a platinum-based cytotoxic drug regimen, careful scrutiny of a patient's response to treatment is essential. If the tumor resolves, the patient should be spared needless exposure to a prolonged course of potentially toxic drugs. Conversely, persistence or growth of tumor should be detected as soon as possible to allow consideration of alternative therapeutic measures.

The behavior of a cancer during therapy may be classified as complete response, partial response, stabilization, progression, or recurrence. *Complete response* is the eradication of all tumor load by therapy. *Partial response* is regression of disease by a significant percentage of the previously measured volume (usually 50% of the product of two dimensions). *Stabilization* of disease is defined as the presence of a tumor without new metastases whose dimensions do not change sufficiently to characterize it as progressive or responding. *Progression* is the appearance of new tumor masses, effusions, or significantly increased tumor volume during therapy (usually a 50% increase in the product of two dimensions). *Recurrence* is the reappearance of tumor following a complete clinical response.

Three varieties of technique are available to monitor the response of ovarian cancer to treatment: measure of clinically evident disease, serum tumor markers, and surgical end-staging.

Clinical Monitoring

Clinical evidence of disease can be demonstrated as a physically palpable mass in an area where tumor is known to be present, as a two- or three-dimensional lesion on imaging studies, or as the accumulation of a malignant effusion. Worsening symptoms identical to those previously attributed to malignant disease are presumptive evidence of tumor progression but should ordinarily be confirmed by objective studies. Knowledge of the sites and sizes of intraperitoneal tumor masses remaining after surgical debulking is imperative. If a patient has unresectable disease after the initial laparotomy, radiographic or clinical measure of the size of the residual tumor mass may accurately reflect the tumor's response to treatment. The clinician should be cautious in interpreting persistence or accumulation of ascites as progression of disease during the first few courses of chemotherapy, as ascites may persist for a long time despite successful tumor cell kill. The reappearance of symptoms that previously brought the patient to medical attention may also herald tumor recurrence. Complaints such as obstipation, epigastric fullness, and increased abdominal girth should always be regarded with concern in a patient with a history of ovarian cancer. Repeated imaging studies are often useful in such patients to document tumor response more objectively.

Because of the ability of gynecologists to achieve optimal surgical cytoreduction at the initial laparotomy for ovarian malignancies, up to 80% of patients with advanced ovarian carcinoma can be left with residual tumor that is unmeasurable by standard radiographic and clinical methods. If there is no tumor mass that can be followed by physical examination or imaging study, more sensitive assays of tumor response may be used to define tumor response.

Biochemical Monitoring

Unfortunately, epithelial ovarian tumors do not secrete a universally useful biochemical marker into the serum, but a number of markers are clinically useful.

In 1981, Bast and associates[73] described CA 125, a monoclonal antibody that is reactive with neoplastic ovarian tissue.[191] This antibody to a cell membrane glycoprotein is elevated in at least 80% of patients with epithelial ovarian cancer.[73] Changes in serum CA 125 values correlate with tumor response of patients treated for epithelial malignancies. Both the rate of decline and the absolute value of CA 125 during therapy have been correlated with tumor response. One small series showed that all complete responders' serum CA 125 levels fell to less than 35 U/ml within 3 months after beginning cytotoxic treatment.[192] Rustin and coworkers[193] demonstrated that a sevenfold decrease in CA 125 values between the first and second courses of treatment correlated with tumor-free survival at 2 years of 58%, compared with 9% if the CA 125 decline was of a lesser magnitude. Mogensen[194] also showed that serum CA 125 values 1 month after the third course of combination chemotherapy are strongly predictive of survival. Patients with CA 125 levels of 10 U/ml or less had a median survival of 5 years, compared with 22 months when the level was 11 to 100 U/ml, and less than a year with a level greater than 100 U/ml. Buller and associates[195] correlated the regression of CA 125 with response to therapy. The accuracy of serum CA 125 is not so precise as to preclude the need for other methods of following tumor response, however. Mucinous tumors generally do not secrete the carbohydrate marker OC 125, the antigen against which CA 125 reacts.[73] Furthermore, CA 125 levels may fall to normal with small volumes of disease present, so they cannot be used to replace second-look operation as a determinant of complete response.[196]

Other tumor markers have been used to evaluate response and tumor status in ovarian carcinoma. These include urinary gonadotropin fragment,[197] NB/70K,[160] and lipid-associated sialic acid.[159] Placental alkaline phosphatase[198] and carcinoembryonic antigen[199] are two oncofetal proteins expressed by only 20% to 50% of ovarian carcinomas. They have limited use in monitoring mucinous carcinomas that are difficult to follow using more conventional markers. Any of these assays may be useful in following tumors in which they are elevated and in which the CA 125 level is normal. No study has yet described the superiority of using multiple markers as compared with using the single marker CA 125.[200] At our institutions, elevated tumor markers are repeated with each treatment. If no elevated marker is noted, CA 125 values are followed at three month intervals.

AFP is a sensitive marker for endodermal sinus tumors and many embryonal cell tumors.[87] hCG is a sensitive marker for nonmetastatic choriocarcinoma.[88] LDH is a highly nonspecific enzyme marker that is elevated in germ cell tumors.[201]

Labeled Monoclonal Antibody Scintigraphy

A mouse monoclonal antibody tagged with indium 111 is available for radionuclide scanning to determine the persistence of disease.[202] This study can be used only once, as development of antibodies against the mouse immunoglobulin occurs after injection. It seems reasonable to reserve this test for patients with clinical complete response in whom second-look surgery is contemplated, or in patients with negative second-look surgery who subsequently have symptoms that raise the specter of recurrence.

Operative Monitoring: Second Look and Secondary Cytoreduction

The most accurate method for determining tumor response to treatment of advanced ovarian carcinoma is surgical assessment at the completion of primary therapy. First described for colon carcinoma,[203] surgical end-staging after the completion of treatment was first applied to ovarian cancer by the M.D. Anderson Cancer Center group.[204] Commonly referred to as second-look laparotomy, surgical end-staging is utilized to assess the entire coelomic cavity and retroperitoneal spaces for tumor at the completion of chemotherapy. It is performed in patients who have achieved a clinical complete response, based on physical examination, computed tomography, and tumor markers.

After bowel preparation, and under general anesthesia, surgical end-staging may begin with laparoscopic evaluation of peritoneal surfaces. If gross tumor is noted, a biopsy sample is taken and the procedure is terminated. If tumor is noted on laparoscopic visual evaluation, or if laparoscopy is not elected, a midline vertical incision is constructed from above the umbilicus to the hypogastrium. Cytologic washings are obtained as in a primary operation for ovarian cancer, after which a careful and thorough evaluation of the peritoneal contents is performed. Biopsy specimens are liberally obtained from any roughened or suspicious peritoneal surfaces. Particular attention is directed to the sites of previous tumor location, especially the stumps of the infundibulopelvic ligaments and the lateral pelvic walls. Any residual infracolic or supracolic omentum is resected, as well as all adhesions of peritoneal surfaces. Careful retroperitoneal exploration, with sampling of pelvic and para-aortic nodal chains, is completed. The number of specimens may be well over 25 if no grossly suspicious findings are noted. Frozen section evaluation of suspicious findings is requested during the procedure, which is terminated if any biopsy samples contain tumor. Up to half of women with normal radiographic and serologic studies prior to second-look procedures are found to have disease at laparotomy.

If gross residual disease is present, the surgeon must decide whether to perform secondary debulking. Some data suggest that effective secondary cytoreduction may prolong life.[205–207] Certainly, the removal of large and easily resectable masses on the intestines may prevent or delay the development of intestinal obstruction. A comparison of the risks and benefits of secondary debulking at the time of positive end-staging involves skilled clinical judgment, which must be tailored to the needs of the individual patient, and for which informative data are unavailable.

Surgical end-staging is controversial because there is no conclusive evidence that it enhances survival or the quality of life.[208] It seems clear that it should be reserved for patients with advanced disease, because it is almost always negative in women with stage I and II carcinoma.[209] Surgical end-staging offers four possible benefits to the patient. First, as a prognostic indicator with unparalleled accuracy in predicting long-term remission and survival, it contributes to the peace of mind of women whose second look shows a complete response. Second, the operation provides a clear rationale for terminating cytotoxic therapy for those patients with negative second-look assessments. Third, patients with residual disease may begin secondary chemotherapy or radiation for attempted cure or palliation when residual disease is minimal and when such secondary treatment is most likely to be effective. Fourth, there is the potential therapeutic advantage of secondary cytoreduction prior to the development of symptomatic recurrence, even in patients destined for chemotherapeutic failure. Secondary cytoreduction of tumor masses resistant to the previously employed chemotherapeutic regimen is possible in up to 52% of patients at second look.[206]

Thirty percent to 40% of women with stage II carcinoma treated with chemotherapy have a complete response as determined by second look, and an additional 10% to 15% demonstrate microscopic disease.[96, 205, 207] Sixty-six percent to 83% of patients with a surgical complete response enjoy disease-free survival for at least 5 years.[96, 130, 137, 207] Five-year survival is about 50% in women with microscopic residual disease and less than 25% in those with macroscopic disease at second look.[96, 207, 210] Presumably, most of these patients had salvage therapy of some sort.

There are three potential disadvantages of surgical end-staging. First is the potential morbidity of repeated surgical assessment. In a recent review of the morbidity of second-look procedures, 23% of 299 patients were noted to experience some sort of surgical, gastrointestinal, pulmonary, cardiac, or urinary tract morbidity.[211] Few of these complications were major, and there was no mortality. As with any procedure, the risks must be weighed against the benefits, but surgical end-staging does not appear to be an extremely morbid procedure. The second potential disadvantage is that end-staging does not accurately define a group of patients in whom freedom from disease is virtually certain. As stated above, many patients with "negative" findings later relapse clinically.[96, 130, 137, 207] Third, it has been stated that there is no statistically significant overall survival advantage to surgical end-staging.[136, 162, 208] Evidence presented above, however, suggests that at least two groups of patients benefit from laparotomy after restaging. First, women with microscopic disease enjoy 50% survival[96, 207, 210]; it is unlikely that this would be true if they did not have the opportunity to receive salvage therapy. Second, survival is prolonged in women with advanced disease that is amenable to cytoreduction.[205–207]

It is unlikely that randomized trials of second-look surgery in any cohort of patients will be performed. Each clinician and patient must decide whether the possible benefit from the operation is worth the risk and discomfort of the procedure. Miller and colleagues[163] estimated that 8% of patients who otherwise would have died will be cured by second-line therapy following second-look surgery. This figure is based on patients treated between 1979 and 1984—most of whom received whole abdominal irradiation. It is therefore possible that a higher proportion of patients is presently salvaged.

Second-look surgery in germ cell tumors is not indicated when there was no residual disease after the first operation. Re-exploration is probably useful in patients with elevated tumor markers (AFP, hCG, LDH) at the end of chemotherapy. These patients probably have gross residual disease. Secondary cytoreduction, if feasible, may augment the effectiveness of secondary chemotherapy. It is not clear whether chemotherapy is useful in patients with gross residual disease and negative tumor markers (as might be the case with malignant teratomas) treated after operation. The authors recommend second-look surgery in these patients.

Considerations regarding end-staging procedures in patients with fallopian tube carcinoma are the same as those in patients with ovarian lesions of the same primary extent.

PALLIATIVE THERAPY

Operative

Ovarian carcinoma is usually fatal, and intestinal obstruction is the usual terminal event. Patients with recurrent ovarian carcinoma in whom intestinal obstruction develops should be evaluated with respect to their performance status. If survival of several months is possible, the number and location of sites of obstruction should be determined by appropriate imaging studies. If there are no more than a few loci of obstruction, palliative bowel resection or diversion may be warranted. There are generally many sites of obstruction, and it is possible to palliate symptoms with intestinal intubation or gastrostomy tube.

Chemotherapy and Radiation

A detailed discussion of salvage therapy is beyond the scope of this chapter. Intravenous paclitaxel[212] and ifosfamide[213] and oral altretamine[214] have been used in this setting with some success. Intraperitoneal chemotherapy has also been used, with mixed results.[215] Most investigators have found palliative whole abdominal radiation to be ineffective and fraught with complications.[216–218] Morgan and associates[219] reported some success using small fractions given as hyperfractionated doses.

POST-TREATMENT CARE AND SURVEILLANCE

Patients should have physical examination, including pelvic examination, and appropriate tumor markers every 3 months for 2 years, and then every 6 months. Imaging studies are optional and should be employed if the clinician believes that it would be beneficial to the care of the patient to detect asymptomatic recurrence.

References

1. Wingo PA, Tong T, Bolden S: Cancer statistics 1995. CA 45:8–30, 1995.
2. Stanhope CR, Smith JP: Germ cell tumors. Clin Obstet Gynaecol 10:357–365, 1983.
3. Bjorkholm E, Lundell M, Gyftodimos E, et al: Dysgerminoma: The Radiumhummet series 1927–1984. Cancer 65:38–44, 1990.
4. Zaloudek C, Norris HJ: Granulosa tumors of the ovary in children: A clinical and pathologic study of 32 cases. Am J Surg Pathol 6:513–522, 1982.
5. Anikwue C, Dawood MY, Kramer E: Granulosa and theca cell tumors. Obstet Gynecol 51:214–220, 1978.
6. Novak ER, Long JH: Arrhenoblastoma of the ovary. Am J Obstet Gynecol 92:1082–1093, 1965.
7. Yancik R: Ovarian cancer: Age contrasts. Cancer 71(Suppl): 517–523, 1993.
8. Ries LAG, Hankey BF, Miller BA, et al (eds): Cancer Statistics Review 1973–88. NIH 91-2789. Bethesda, MD: National Institutes of Health, National Cancer Institute, 1991.
9. Gloeckler Ries LA: Ovarian cancer: Survival and treatment differences by age. Cancer 71(Suppl):524–529, 1993.
10. Demopoulos RI, Seltaer V, Dubin N, et al: The association of parity and marital status with the development of ovarian carcinoma: Clinical implications. Obstet Gynecol 54:150–155, 1979.
11. Parazzini F, La Vecchia C, Negri E, et al: Menstrual factors and the risk of epithelial ovarian cancer. J Clin Epidemiol 42:443–448, 1989.
12. Amos CJ, Struewing JP: Genetic epidemiology of epithelial ovarian cancer. Cancer 71:566–572, 1993.
13. Lynch HT, Albano WA, Black L, et al: Familial excess of cancer of the ovary and other anatomic sites. JAMA 245:261–264, 1981.

14. Prior P, Waterhouse JAH: Multiple primary cancers of the breast and ovary. Br J Cancer 44:628–636, 1981.
15. Lynch HT, Kimberling WJ, Albano WA, et al: Hereditary nonpolyposis colorectal cancer (Lynch syndromes I and II). Parts I and II. Cancer 56:934–951, 1985.
16. Lynch HL, Watson P, Bewtra C, et al: Hereditary ovarian cancer: Heterogeneity in age at diagnosis. Cancer 67:1460–1466, 1991.
17. Farrow DC, Weiss NS, Lyon JL, et al: Association of obesity and ovarian cancer in a case control study. Am J Epidemiol 129:1300–1305, 1989.
18. Cramer DW, Welch WR, Hutchison GB, et al: Dietary animal fat in relation to ovarian cancer risk. Obstet Gynecol 63:833–838, 1984.
19. La Veccia C, Decarli A, Negri E, et al: Dietary factors and the risk of epithelial ovarian cancer. J Natl Cancer Inst 79:663–669, 1987.
20. Rose DP, Boyar AP, Wynder EL: International comparisons of mortality rates for cancer of the breast, ovary, prostate and colon, and per capita food consumption. Cancer 58:2363–2371, 1986.
21. Fathalla MF: Incessant ovulation—a factor in ovarian neoplasia? Lancet 2:163, 1971.
22. Hankinson SE, Colditz GA, Hunter DJ, et al: A quantitative assessment of oral contraceptive use and risk of ovarian cancer. Obstet Gynecol 80:708–714, 1992.
23. Harris R, Whittimore AS, Intyre J, et al: Characteristics relating to ovarian cancer risk. III. Epithelial tumors of low malignant potential in white women. Am J Epidemiol 136:1204–1211, 1992.
24. Whittimore AS, Harris R, Intyre J, et al: Characteristics relating to ovarian cancer risk. II. Invasive epithelial ovarian carcinomas in white women. Am J Epidemiol 136:1184–1203, 1992.
25. Cramer DW, Welch WR: Determinants of ovarian cancer risk. II. Inferences regarding pathogenesis. J Natl Cancer Inst 71:717–721, 1983.
26. Menczer J, Modan M, Ranon L, et al: Possible role for mumps virus in the etiology of ovarian cancer. Cancer 43:1375–1379, 1979.
27. Mattison DR, Thorgeirsson SS: Smoking and industrial pollution and their effects on menopause and ovarian cancer. Lancet 1:187–188, 1978.
28. Harlow BL, Cramer DW, Bell DA, et al: Perineal exposure to talc and ovarian cancer risk. Obstet Gynecol 80:19–26, 1992.
29. Hartley AL, Birch JM, Kelsey AM, et al: Are germ cell tumors part of the Li-Fraumeni cancer family syndrome? Cancer Genet Cytogenet 42:221–226, 1989.
30. Khodr GS, Cadena GD, Ong TC, et al: Y-autosome translocation, gonadal dysgenesis, and gonadoblastoma. Am J Dis Child 133:277–282, 1979.
31. Serov SF, Scully RE, Sobin LH: International Histologic Classification of Tumors. No. 9, Histologic Typing of Ovarian Tumors. Geneva: World Health Organization, 1973, p 37.
32. Scully RE: Tumors of the ovary and maldeveloped gonads. In Atlas of Tumor Pathology, 2nd series, fascicle 16. Washington, DC: Armed Forces Institute of Pathology, 1979.
33. Altaras MM, Aviram R, Cohen I, et al: Primary peritoneal papillary serous adenocarcinoma: Clinical and management aspects. Gynecol Oncol 40:230–236, 1991.
34. Kemp GM, Hsiu J-G, Andrews MC: Papillary peritoneal carcinomatosis after prophylactic oophorectomy. Gynecol Oncol 47:395–397, 1992.
35. Piver MS, Barlow JJ, Lele SB: Incidence of subclinical metastases in stage I and II ovarian carcinoma. Obstet Gynecol 52:100–104, 1978.
36. De Palo G, Musumeci R, Kenda R, et al: The reassessment of patients with ovarian carcinoma. Eur J Cancer 16:1469–1474, 1980.
37. Soper JT, Johnson P, Johnson V, et al: Comprehensive restaging laparotomy in women with apparent early ovarian carcinoma. Obstet Gynecol 80:949–953, 1992.
38. Parmley TH, Woodruff JD: The ovarian mesothelioma. Am J Obstet Gynecol 120:234–241, 1974.
39. Burghardt E, Girardi F, Lahousen M, et al: Patterns of pelvic and paraaortic lymph node involvement in ovarian cancer. Gynecol Oncol 40:103–106, 1991.
40. Dauplat J, Hacker NF, Nieberg RK, et al: Distant metastases in epithelial ovarian carcinoma. Cancer 60:1561–1566, 1987.
41. McMurray EH, Jacobs AJ, Perez CA, et al: Carcinoma of the fallopian tube: Management and sites of failure. Cancer 58:2070–2075, 1986.
42. Peters WA III, Andersen WA, Hopkins MD, et al: Prognostic factors of carcinoma of the fallopian tube. Obstet Gynecol 71:757–762, 1988.
43. Tamimi HK, Figge DC: Adenocarcinoma of the uterine tube: Potential for lymph node metastases. Am J Obstet Gynecol 141:132–137, 1981.
44. Scully RE: Ovarian tumors. A review. Am J Pathol 87:686–720, 1977.
45. Smith JP, Day TG Jr: Review of ovarian cancer at the University of Texas Systems Cancer Center, M. D. Anderson Hospital and Tumor Institute. Am J Obstet Gynecol 135:984–993, 1979.
46. Omura G, Blessing JA, Ehrlich CE, et al: A randomized trial of cyclophosphamide and doxorubicin with or without cisplatin in advanced ovarian carcinoma. A Gynecologic Oncology Group study. Cancer 57:1725–1730, 1986.
47. Malkasian GD, Melton LJ III, O'Brien PC, et al: Prognostic significance of histologic classification and grading of epithelial malignancies of the ovary. Am J Obstet Gynecol 149:274–284, 1984.
48. Jacobs AJ, Deligdisch L, Deppe G, et al: Histologic correlates of virulence in ovarian adenocarcinoma. I. Effect of differentiation. Am J Obstet Gynecol 143:574–580, 1982.
49. Dembo AJ, Davy M, Stenwig AE, et al: Prognostic factors in patients with stage I epithelial ovarian cancer. Obstet Gynecol 75:263–273, 1990.
50. Chaitin BA, Gershenson DM, Evans HL: Mucinous tumors of the ovary. A clinicopathologic study of 70 cases. Cancer 55:1958–1962, 1985.
51. Gramlich T, Austin RM, Lutz M: Histologic sampling requirements in ovarian carcinoma. Gynecol Oncol 38:249–256, 1990.
52. Heaps JM, Nieberg RK, Berek JS: Malignant neoplasms arising in endometriosis. Obstet Gynecol 75:1023–1028, 1990.
53. Czernobilsky B, Silverman BB, Mikuta JJ: Endometrioid carcinoma of the ovary. A clinicopathologic study of 75 cases. Cancer 26:1141–1152, 1970.
54. Ulbright TM, Roth LM: Metastatic and independent cancers of the endometrium and ovary: A clinicopathologic study of 34 cases. Hum Pathol 16:28–34, 1985.
55. Czernobilsky B, Silverman BB, Enterline HT: Clear cell carcinoma of the ovary. A clinicopathologic analysis of pure and mixed forms, and comparison with endometrioid cancer. Cancer 25:762–772, 1970.
56. Jenison EL, Montag AG, Griffiths CT, et al: Clear cell adenocarcinoma of the ovary: A clinical analysis and comparison with serous carcinoma. Gynecol Oncol 32:65–71, 1989.
57. Czernobilsky B: Common epithelial tumors of the ovary. In Kurman RJ (ed): Blaustein's Pathology of the Female Genital Tract, 3rd ed. New York: Springer-Verlag, 1987, pp 560–606.
58. Gordon A, Lipton D, Woodruff JD: Dysgerminoma: A review of 158 cases from the Emil Novak Ovarian Tumor Registry. Obstet Gynecol 58:497–504, 1981.
59. Norris HJ, Zirkin HJ, Benson WL: Immature malignant teratoma of the ovary: A clinical and pathologic study of 58 cases. Cancer 37:2359–2372, 1976.
60. Krepart G, Smith JP, Rutledge F, et al: The treatment for dysgerminoma of the ovary. Cancer 41:986–990, 1978.
61. De Palo G, Lattuada A, Kenda R, et al: Germ cell tumors of the ovary: The experience of the National Cancer Institute of Milan. I. Dysgerminoma. Int J Radiat Oncol Biol Phys 13:853–860, 1987.
62. Lawson AP, Adler GF: Radiotherapy in the treatment of ovarian dysgerminomas. Int J Radiat Oncol Biol Phys 14:431–434, 1988.
63. Kurman RJ, Norris HJ: Malignant germ cell tumors of the ovary. Hum Pathol 8:551–564, 1977.
64. Williams SD, Blessing JA, Moore DM, et al: Cisplatin, vinblastine and bleomycin in advanced and recurrent ovarian germ cell tumors. Ann Intern Med 111:22–27, 1989.
65. Fox H, Agarwal K, Langley FA: A clinicopathologic study of 92 cases of granulosa cell tumor of the ovary with special reference to the factors influencing prognosis. Cancer 35:231–241, 1975.
66. Stenwig JT, Hazelkamp JT, Beecham JB: Granulosa cell tumors of the ovary: A clinicopathologic study of 118 cases with long-term follow-up. Gynecol Oncol 7:136–152, 1979.
67. Young RH, Scully RE: Ovarian Sertoli-Leydig tumors: A clinicopathological analysis of 207 cases. Am J Surg Pathol 9:543–569, 1985.
68. Schwartz PE, Chambers SK, Chambers JT, et al: Ovarian germ

cell malignancies: The Yale University experience. Gynecol Oncol 45:26–31, 1992.
69. Niloff JM, Knapp RC, Schaetzl E, et al: CA 125 antigen levels in obstetrical and gynecological patients. Obstet Gynecol 64:703–707, 1984.
70. Jacobs I, Bast RC Jr: The CA 125 tumour-associated antigen: A review of the literature. Hum Reprod 4:1–12, 1989.
71. Giudice LC, Jacobs AJ, Pineda J, et al: Serum levels of CA 125 in patients with endometriosis: A preliminary report. Fertil Steril 45:876–878, 1986.
72. Rubial A, Encabo E, Martinez-Miralles E, et al: CA 125 seric levels in non malignant pathologies. Bull Cancer (Paris) 71:145–148, 1984.
73. Bast RC Jr, Klug TL, St John E, et al: A radioimmunoassay using a monoclonal antibody to monitor the course of epithelial ovarian cancer. N Engl J Med 309:883–887, 1983.
74. Niloff JM, Klug TL, Schaetzl E, et al: Elevation of serum CA 125 in carcinoma of the fallopian tube, endometrium and endocervix. Am J Obstet Gynecol 148:1057–1058, 1984.
75. Campbell S, Bhan V, Royston P, et al: Transabdominal ultrasound screening for early ovarian cancer. Br Med J 299:1363–1367, 1989.
76. van Nagell JR Jr, De Priest PD, Puls LE, et al: Ovarian cancer screening in asymptomatic postmenopausal women by transvaginal ultrasonography. Cancer 68:458–462, 1991.
77. Herrman UJ, Locher GW, Goldhirsch A: Sonographic patterns of ovarian tumors: Prediction of malignancy. Obstet Gynecol 69:777–781, 1987.
78. Sassone AM, Timor-Tritsch IE, Artner A, et al: Transvaginal sonographic characterization of ovarian disease: Evaluation of a new scoring system to predict ovarian malignancy. Obstet Gynecol 78:70–76, 1991.
79. Luxman D, Bergman A, Sagi J, et al: The postmenopausal adnexal mass: Correlation between ultrasonic and pathologic findings. Obstet Gynecol 77:726–728, 1991.
80. Kurjak A, Schulman H, Sosic A, et al: Transvaginal ultrasound, color flow, and Doppler waveform of the postmenopausal adnexal mass. Obstet Gynecol 80:917–921, 1992.
81. Weiner Z, Thaler I, Beck D, et al: Differentiating malignant form benign ovarian tumors with transvaginal color flow imaging. Obstet Gynecol 79:159–162, 1992.
82. Hata K, Hata T, Manabe A, et al: A critical evaluation of transvaginal Doppler studies, transvaginal sonography, magnetic resonance imaging, and CA 125 in detecting ovarian cancer. Obstet Gynecol 80:922–926, 1992.
83. Hurwitz A, Yagel S, Zion I, et al: The management of persistent clear pelvic cysts diagnosed by ultrasonography. Obstet Gynecol 72:320–322, 1988.
84. Rome RM, Fortune DW, Quinn MA, et al: Functioning ovarian tumors in postmenopausal women. Obstet Gynecol 57:705–710, 1981.
85. Podratz KC, Podczaski ES, Gaffey TA, et al: Primary carcinoma of the fallopian tube. Am J Obstet Gynecol 154:1319–1326, 1986.
86. Eedekens MW, Nouwen EJ, Pollet DE, et al: Placental alkaline phosphatase and cancer antigen 125 in sera of patients with benign and malignant diseases. Clin Chem 31:687–690, 1985.
87. Norgaard-Pederson B, Albrechtsen R, Teilum G: Serum alpha-foetoprotein as a marker for endodermal sinus tumor (yolk sac tumor) or a vitelline component of teratocarcinoma. Acta Pathol Microbiol Scand [A] 83:573–589, 1975.
88. Jacobs AJ, Newland JR, Green RK: Pure choriocarcinoma of the ovary. Obstet Gynecol Surv 37:603–609, 1982.
89. Sheiko MC, Hart WR: Ovarian germinoma (dysgerminoma) with elevated serum lactic dehydrogenase. Case report and review of literature. Cancer 49:994–998, 1982.
90. Antolic ZN, Kovacic J, Rainer S: Theca and granulosa cell tumors and endometrial adenocarcinoma. Gynecol Oncol 10:273–278, 1980.
91. Evans AT III, Gaffey TA, Malkasian GD Jr, et al: Clinicopathologic review of 118 granulosa and 82 theca cell tumors. Obstet Gynecol 55:231–238, 1980.
92. Piura B, Glezerman M: Synchronous carcinomas of endometrium and ovary. Gynecol Oncol 33:261–264, 1989.
93. Eifel P, Hendrickson M, Ross J, et al: Simultaneous presentation of carcinoma involving the ovary and uterine corpus. Cancer 50:163–170, 1982.
94. Hu CY, Taymor ML, Hertig AT: Primary carcinoma of the fallopian tube. Am J Obstet Gynecol 59:58–67, 1950.
95. Hendrikson MR, Ross J, Eifel P, et al: Uterine papillary serous carcinoma. A highly malignant form of endometrial carcinoma. Am J Surg Pathol 6:93–108, 1982.
96. Cohen CJ, Goldberg JD, Holland JF, et al: Improved therapy with cisplatin regimens for patients with ovarian carcinoma (FIGO stages III and IV) as measured by surgical end-staging operation. Am J Obstet Gynecol 145:955–965, 1983.
97. Fioretti P, Gadducci A, del Bravo B, et al: The potential of primary cytoreductive surgery in patients with FIGO stages III and IV ovarian carcinoma. Eur J Gynecol Oncol 9:175–179, 1990.
98. Delgado G, Oram DH, Petrilli ES: Stage III epithelial cancer: The role of maximal cytoreduction. Gynecol Oncol 18:293–298, 1984.
99. Hacker NF, Berek JS, Lagasse LD, et al: Primary cytoreductive surgery for ovarian cancer. Obstet Gynecol 61:413–420, 1983.
100. Griffiths CT, Fuller AF: Intensive surgical and chemotherapeutic management of advanced ovarian cancer. Surg Clin North Am 58:131–142, 1978.
101. Janicke F, Holscher M, Kuhn W, et al: Radical surgical procedure improves survival time in patients with recurrent ovarian cancer. Cancer 70:2129–2136, 1992.
102. McDermott DF, Jaffe EA, Coleman M: The effect of surgical debulking on the response of patients with ovarian carcinoma to chemotherapy. Am J Clin Oncol 11:520–523, 1988.
103. Piver MS, Lele SB, Marchetti DL, et al: The impact of aggressive debulking surgery and cisplatin-based chemotherapy on progression-free survival in stage III and IV ovarian carcinoma. J Clin Oncol 6:983–989, 1988.
104. Schwartz PE: Surgical management of ovarian cancer. Arch Surg 116:99–106, 1981.
105. Hunter RW, Alexander NDE, Soutter WP: Meta-analysis of surgery in advanced ovarian carcinoma: Is maximum cytoreductive surgery an independent determinant of prognosis? Am J Obstet Gynecol 166:504–511, 1992.
106. Hoskins WJ, Bundy BN, Thigpen JT, et al: The influence of cytoreductive surgery on recurrence-free interval and survival in small-volume stage III epithelial ovarian cancer: A Gynecologic Oncology Group study. Gynecol Oncol 47:159–166, 1992.
107. Wharton JT, Herson J: Surgery for common epithelial tumors of the ovary. Cancer 48:582–589, 1981.
108. Deppe G, Zbella EA, Skogerson D, et al: The rare indication for splenectomy as part of cytoreductive surgery in ovarian cancer. Gynecol Oncol 16:282–287, 1983.
109. Adelson MD: Cytoreduction of diaphragmatic metastases using the Cavitron ultrasonic surgical aspitator. Gynecol Oncol 41:220–222, 1991.
110. Heintz APM, Hacker NF, Berek JS: Cytoreductive surgery in ovarian carcinoma: Feasibility and morbidity. Obstet Gynecol 67:783–788, 1986.
111. Piver MS, Baker T: The potential for optimal (<2 cm) cytoreductive surgery in advanced ovarian carcinoma at a tertiary medical center: A prospective study. Gynecol Oncol 24:1–8, 1986.
112. Meyer AR, Chambers SK, Graves E, et al: Ovarian cancer staging: Does it require a gynecologic oncologist? Gynecol Oncol 47:223–227, 1992.
113. Eisenkop SM, Spirtos NM, Montag TW, et al: The impact of subspecialty training on the management of advanced ovarian cancer. Gynecol Oncol 47:203–209, 1992.
114. Adelson MD, Baggish MS, Seifer DB, et al: Cytoreduction of ovarian cancer with the Cavitron ultrasonic surgical aspirator. Obstet Gynecol 72:140–143, 1988.
115. Brand E, Pearlman N: Electrosurgical debulking of ovarian cancer: A new technique using the argon beam coagulator. Gynecol Oncol 39:115–118, 1990.
116. Chen SS, Bochner R: Assessment of morbidity and mortality in primary cytoreductive surgery for advanced ovarian carcinoma. Gynecol Oncol 20:190–195, 1985.
117. Bruckner HW, Cohen CJ, Goldberg JD, et al: Improved chemotherapy for ovarian cancer with *cis*-diamminedichloroplatinum and Adriamycin. Cancer 47:2288–2294, 1981.
118. Belinson JL, Lee KR, Jarrell MA, et al: Management of epithelial ovarian neoplasms using a platinum-based regimen: A 10-year experience. Gynecol Oncol 37:66–73, 1990.
119. Decker DG, Fleming TR, Malkasion GD Jr, et al: Cyclophosphamide plus *cis*-platinum in combination: Treatment program for stage III or IV ovarian carcinoma. Obstet Gynecol 60:481–487, 1982.

120. Taylor HC: Malignant and semimalignant tumors of the ovary. Surg Gynecol Obstet 48:204–230, 1929.
121. Katzenstein AL, Mazur MT, Morgan TE, et al: Proliferative serous tumors of the ovary. Am J Surg Pathol 2:339–356, 1978.
122. Leake JF, Rader JS, Woodruff JD, et al: Retroperitoneal lymphatic involvement with epithelial ovarian tumors of low malignant potential. Gynecol Oncol 42:124–130, 1991.
123. Fort MG, Pierce VK, Saigo PE, et al: Evidence for the efficacy of adjuvant therapy in epithelial ovarian tumors of low malignant potential. Gynecol Oncol 32:269–272, 1989.
124. Massad LS Jr, Hunter VJ, Szpak CA, et al: Epithelial tumors of low malignant potential. Obstet Gynecol 78:1027–1032, 1991.
125. Yazigi R, Sandstad J, Munoz AK: Primary staging in ovarian tumors of low malignant potential. Gynecol Oncol 31:402–408, 1988.
126. Koern J, Trope CG, Abeler VM: A retrospective study of 370 borderline tumors of the ovary treated at the Norwegian Radium Hospital from 1970 to 1982. Cancer 71:1810–1820, 1993.
127. Rice LW, Berkowitz RS, Mark SD, et al: Epithelial tumors of borderline malignancy. Gynecol Oncol 39:195–198, 1990.
128. Tazelaar HD, Bostwick DG, Ballon SC, et al: Conservative treatment of borderline ovarian tumors. Obstet Gynecol 66:417–422, 1985.
129. Bostwick DG, Tazelaar D, Ballon SC, et al: Ovarian epithelial tumors of borderline malignancy. A clinical and pathologic study of 109 cases. Cancer 58:2052–2065, 1986.
130. Gershenson DM, Copeland LJ, Wharton JT, et al: Prognosis of surgically determined complete responders in advanced ovarian cancer. Cancer 55:1129–1135, 1985.
131. Kliman L, Rome RM, Fortune DW: Low malignant potential tumors of the ovary: A study of 76 cases. Obstet Gynecol 68:338–344, 1986.
132. Gershenson DM, Silva FG: Serous ovarian tumors of low malignant potential with peritoneal implants. Cancer 65:578–585, 1990.
133. Jones CM III, Homesley HD: Successful treatment of pseudomyxoma peritonei of ovarian origin with cis-platinum, doxorubicin and cyclophosphamide. Gynecol Oncol 22:257–259, 1985.
134. Mann WJ Jr, Wagner J, Chumas J, et al: The management of pseudomyxoma peritonei. Cancer 66:1636–1640, 1990.
135. Davidson NGP, Khanna S, Kirwan P, et al: Advanced ovarian cancer: Long-term results following chemotherapy and second-look laparotomy. Gynecol Oncol 39:295–299, 1990.
136. Ho AG, Beller U, Speyer JL, et al: A reassessment of the role of second-look laparotomy in advanced ovarian cancer. J Clin Oncol 5:1316–1321, 1987.
137. Rubin SC, Hoskins WJ, Saigo PE, et al: Prognostic factors for recurrence following negative second-look laparotomy in ovarian cancer patients treated with platinum-based chemotherapy. Gynecol Oncol 42:137–141, 1991.
138. Smith JP, Rutledge F, Wharton JT: Chemotherapy of ovarian cancer: New approaches to treatment. Cancer 30:1565–1571, 1972.
139. Kaldor JM, Day NE, Pettersson F, et al: Leukemia following chemotherapy for ovarian cancer. N Engl J Med 322:1–6, 1990.
140. Young RC, Walton LA, Ellenberg SS, et al: Adjuvant therapy in stage I and stage II epithelial ovarian cancer: Results of two prospective randomized trial. N Engl J Med 322:1021–1027, 1990.
141. Dembo AJ, Bush RS, Beale FA, et al: Ovarian carcinoma: Improved survival following abdominopelvic irradiation in patients with a completed pelvic operation. Am J Obstet Gynecol 134:793–800, 1979.
142. Schray M, Martinez A, Cox R, et al: Radiotherapy in epithelial ovarian cancer: Analysis of prognostic factors based on long-term experience. Obstet Gynecol 62:373–382, 1983.
143. Klassen D, Shelley W, Starreveld A, et al: Early stage ovarian cancer: A randomized clinical trial comparing whole abdominal radiotherapy, melphalan, and intraperitoneal chromic phosphate: A National Cancer Institute of Canada Clinical Trials Group report. J Clin Oncol 6:1254–1263, 1988.
144. Dottino PR, Plaxe SC, Cohen CJ: A phase II trial of adjuvant cisplatin and doxorubicin in stage I epithelial ovarian cancer. Gynecol Oncol 43:203–205, 1991.
145. Piver MS, Malfetano J, Baker T, et al: Five-year survival for stage IC or stage I grade 3 epithelial ovarian cancer treated with cisplatin-based chemotherapy. Gynecol Oncol 46:357–360, 1992.
146. Piver MS, Malfetano II, Hempling RE, et al: Cisplatin-based chemotherapy for stage II ovarian adenocarcinoma: A preliminary report. Gynecol Oncol 39:249–252, 1990.
147. Hakes TB, Chalas E, Hoskins WJ, et al: Randomized prospective trial of 5 versus 10 cycles of cyclophosphamide, doxorubicin and cisplatin in advanced ovarian carcinoma. Gynecol Oncol 45:284–289, 1992.
148. Jacobs AJ, Sommers GM, Homan SM, et al: Therapy of ovarian carcinoma: The relationship of dose level and treatment intensity to survival. Gynecol Oncol 31:233–245, 1988.
149. Levin L, Hryniuk W: Dose intensity analysis of chemotherapy regimens in ovarian carcinoma. J Clin Oncol 5:756–767, 1987.
150. Conte PF, Bruzzone M, Carnino F, et al: Carboplatin, doxorubicin and cyclophosphamide versus cisplatin, doxorubicin and cyclophosphamide: A randomized trial in stage III–IV epithelial ovarian carcinoma. J Clin Oncol 9:658–663, 1991.
151. Fanning J, Bennet TZ, Hilgers RD: Meta-analysis of cisplatin, doxorubicin and cyclophosphamide versus cisplatin and cyclophosphamide chemotherapy of ovarian carcinoma. Obstet Gynecol 80:954–960, 1992.
152. Gruppo Interegionale Cooperativo Oncologico Ginecologia: Randomized comparison of cisplatin with cyclophosphamide/cisplatin with cyclophosphamide/doxorubicin/cisplatin in advanced ovarian cancer. Lancet 2:353–359, 1987.
153. Omura GA, Bundy BN, Berek JS, et al: Randomized trial of cyclophosphamide plus cisplatin with or without doxorubicin in ovarian carcinoma: A Gynecologic Oncology Group study. J Clin Oncol 7:457–465, 1989.
154. Ovarian Cancer Meta-analysis Project: Cyclophosphamide plus cisplatin versus cyclophosphamide, doxorubicin and cisplatin chemotherapy of ovarian carcinoma: A meta-analysis. J Clin Oncol 9:1668–1674, 1991.
155. Alberts DS, Green S, Hannigan EV, et al: Improved therapeutic index of carboplatin plus cyclophosphamide versus cisplatin plus cyclophosphamide: Final report by the Southwest Oncology Group of a phase III randomized trial in stages III and IV ovarian cancer. J Clin Oncol 10:706–717, 1992.
156. Swenerton K, Jeffrey J, Stuart G, et al: Cisplatin-cyclophosphamide versus carboplatin-cyclophosphamide in advanced ovarian cancer: A randomized phase II study of the National Institute of Canada Clinical Trials Group. J Clin Oncol 10:718–726, 1992.
157. de Vries EGE, Biesma B, Willemse PHB, et al: A double blind placebo-controlled study with granulocyte-macrophage colony-stimulating factor during chemotherapy for ovarian carcinoma. Cancer Res 51:116–122, 1991.
158. Einzig AI, Wiernik PH, Sasloff J, et al: Phase II study and long-term follow-up of patients treated with Taxol for advanced ovarian adenocarcinoma. J Clin Oncol 10:1748–1753, 1992.
159. Stratton JA, Rettenmaier MA, Phillips HB, et al: Relationship of serum CA125 and lipid-associated sialic acid tumor-associated antigen levels to the disease status of patients with gynecologic malignancies. Obstet Gynecol 71:20–26, 1988.
160. Knauf S: Monoclonal antibody assays for measuring ovarian tumor antigen in blood. Detection of NB/70K in patients with ovarian cancer and nongynecologic diseases. Cancer 62:922–925, 1988.
161. Krag KJ, Canellos GP, Griffiths CT, et al: Predictive factors for long-term survival in patients with advanced ovarian cancer. Gynecol Oncol 34:88–93, 1989.
162. Lund B, Williamson P: Prognostic factors for outcome of and survival after second-look laparotomy in patients with advanced ovarian carcinoma. Obstet Gynecol 76:617–622, 1990.
163. Miller DS, Spirtos NM, Ballon SC: Critical reassessment of second-look exploratory laparotomy for epithelial ovarian carcinoma. Minimal diagnostic and therapeutic value in patients with persistent cancer. Cancer 69:502–510, 1992.
164. Slamon DJ, Godolphin W, Jones LA, et al: Studies of HER-2/*neu* proto-oncogene in human breast and ovarian cancer. Science 244:707–712, 1989.
165. Thomas GM, Dembo AJ, Hacker NF, et al: Current therapy for dysgerminoma of the ovary. Obstet Gynecol 70:268–275, 1987.
166. Williams SD, Blessing JA, Hatch KD, et al: Chemotherapy of advanced dysgerminoma: Trials of the Gynecologic Oncology Group. J Clin Oncol 9:1950–1955, 1991.
167. Gershenson DM, Morris M, Cangir A, et al: Treatment of malignant germ cell tumors of the ovary with bleomycin, etoposide, and cisplatin. J Clin Oncol 8:715–720, 1990.
168. Bajorin DJ, Geller NL, Weisen SF, et al: Two-day therapy in patients with metastatic germ cell tumors. Cancer 67:28–32, 1991.

169. Gershenson DM, Copeland LJ, Kavanagh JJ, et al: Treatment of nondysgerminomatous germ cell tumors of the ovary with vincristine, dactinomycin and cyclophosphamide. Cancer 56:2756–2761, 1985.
170. Slayton RE, Park RC, Silverberg SG, et al: Vincristine, dactinomycin, and cyclophosphamide in the treatment of malignant germ cell tumors of the ovary. A Gynecologic Oncology Group study. (A final report.) Cancer 56:243–248, 1985.
171. Stamp GWH, McConnell EM: Malignancy arising in cystic ovarian teratomas. A report of 24 cases. Br J Obstet Gynaecol 90:671–675, 1983.
172. Curry SL, Smith JP, Gallagher HS: Malignant teratomas of the ovary: Prognostic factors and treatment. Am J Obstet Gynecol 131:845–849, 1978.
173. DiSaia PJ, Saltz A, Kagan AR, et al: Chemotherapeutic retroconversion of immature teratoma of the ovary. Obstet Gynecol 49:346–350, 1977.
174. Malkasian GD, Webb MJ, Jorgensen ED: Observations on chemotherapy of granulosa cell carcinomas and malignant ovarian teratoma. Obstet Gynecol 44:885–888, 1974.
175. Gershenson DM, Del Junco G, Herson J, et al: Endodermal sinus tumor of the ovary: The M.D. Anderson experience. Obstet Gynecol 61:194–202, 1983.
176. Kurman RJ, Norris HJ: Endodermal sinus tumor of the ovary: A clinical and pathological analysis of 71 cases. Cancer 38:2404–2409, 1976.
177. Kurman RJ, Norris HJ: Malignant mixed germ cell tumors of the ovary: A clinical and pathological analysis of 30 cases. Obstet Gynecol 48:579–589, 1976.
178. Pankratz E, Boyes DA, White GW, et al: Granulosa cell tumors: A clinical review of 61 cases. Obstet Gynecol 52:718–723, 1978.
179. Schwartz PE, Smith JP: Treatment of ovarian stromal tumors. Am J Obstet Gynecol 125:402–411, 1976.
180. Colombo N, Sessa C, Landoni F, et al: Cisplatin, vinblastine, and bleomycin combination chemotherapy in metastatic granulosa cell tumor of the ovary. Obstet Gynecol 67:265–268, 1986.
181. Zambetti M, Escobedo A, Pilotti S, et al: Cis-platinum/vinblastine/bleomycin combination chemotherapy in advanced or recurrent granulosa cell tumors of the ovary. Gynecol Oncol 36:317–320, 1990.
182. Jacobs AJ, Deppe G, Cohen CJ: Combination chemotherapy of ovarian granulosa cell tumor with *cis*-platinum and doxorubicin. Gynecol Oncol 14:294–297, 1982.
183. Gershenson DM, Copeland LJ, Kavanagh JJ, et al: Treatment of metastatic stromal tumors of the ovary with cisplatin, doxorubicin, and cyclophosphamide. Obstet Gynecol 70:765–769, 1987.
184. Martikainen H, Penttinen J, Huhtaniemi I, et al: Gonadotropin-releasing hormone agonist analog therapy effective in ovarian granulosa cell malignancy. Gynecol Oncol 35:406–408, 1989.
185. Eddy GL, Copeland LJ, Gershenson DM, et al: Fallopian tube carcinoma. Obstet Gynecol 64:546–552, 1984.
186. Rose PG, Piver MS, Tsukada Y: Fallopian tube cancer: The Roswell Park esperience. Cancer 66:1661–1667, 1990.
187. Jacobs AJ, McMurray EH, Parham J, et al: Treatment of carcinoma of the fallopian tube using cisplatin, doxorubicin, and cyclophosphamide. Am J Clin Oncol 9:436–439, 1986.
188. Muntz HG, Tarraza HM, Goff BA, et al: Combination chemotherapy in advanced adenocarcinoma of the fallopian tube. Gynecol Oncol 40:268–273, 1991.
189. Morris M, Gershenson DM, Burke TW, et al: Treatment of fallopian tube carcinoma with cisplatin, doxorubicin, and cyclophosphamide. Obstet Gynecol 76:1020–1024, 1990.
190. Peters WA III, Andersen WA, Hopkins MD: Results of chemotherapy in advanced carcinoma of the fallopian tube. Cancer 63:836–838, 1989.
191. Bast RC Jr, Feeney M, Lazarus H, et al: Reactivity of a monoclonal antibody with human ovarian carcinoma. J Clin Invest 68:1331–1337, 1981.
192. Lavin PT, Knapp RC, Malkasian G, et al: CA 125 for the monitoring of ovarian carcinoma during therapy. Obstet Gynecol 69:223–227, 1987.
193. Rustin GJS, Gennings JN, Nelstrop AE, et al: Use of CA-125 to predict survival of patients with ovarian carcinoma. J Clin Oncol 7:1667–1671, 1989.
194. Mogensen O: Prognostic value of CA 125 in advanced ovarian cancer. Gynecol Oncol 44:207–212, 1992.
195. Buller RE, Berman ML, Bloss JD, et al: CA 125 regression: A model for epithelial ovarian cancer response. Am J Obstet Gynecol 165:360–367, 1991.
196. Patsner B, Orr JW Jr, Mann WJ Jr, et al: Does serum CA-125 level prior to second-look laparotomy for invasive ovarian adenocarcinoma predict size of residual disease? Gynecol Oncol 38:373–376, 1990.
197. Nam J-H, Cole LA, Chambers JT, et al: Urinary gonadotropin fragment, a new tumor marker. Gynecol Oncol 36:383–390, 1990.
198. Doellgast GJ, Homesley HD: Placental-type alkaline phosphatase in ovarian cancer fluids and tissues. Obstet Gynecol 63:324–329, 1984.
199. Stall KE, Martin EW: Plasma carcinoembryonic antigen levels in ovarian cancer patients: A chart review and survey of published data. J Reprod Med 26:73–79, 1981.
200. Bast RC Jr, Hunter V, Knapp RC: Pros and cons of gynecologic tumor markers. Cancer 60:1984–1992, 1987.
201. Presley RH, Munta HG, Falkenberry S, et al: Serum lactic dehydrogenase as a tumor marker in dysgerminoma. Gynecol Oncol 44:281–283, 1992.
202. Krag DN: Clinical utility of immunoscintigraphy in managing ovarian cancer. J Nucl Med 34:545–548, 1993.
203. Wangensteen OH, Lewis FJ, Tongen LA: The "second-look" in cancer surgery. Lancet 71:303, 1951.
204. Schwartz PE, Smith JP: Second-look operations in ovarian cancer. Am J Obstet Gynecol 138:1124–1130, 1980.
205. Berek JS, Hacker NF, Lagasse LD, et al: Survival of patients following secondary cytoreductive surgery in ovarian cancer. Obstet Gynecol 61:189–193, 1983.
206. Lippman SM, Alberts DS, Slymen DJ, et al: Second look laparotomy in epithelial ovarian carcinoma: Prognostic factors associated with survival duration. Cancer 61:2571–2577, 1988.
207. Podratz KC, Malkasian GD Jr, Hilton JF, et al: Second-look laparotomy in ovarian cancer: Evaluation of pathologic variables. Am J Obstet Gynecol 152:230–238, 1985.
208. Chambers SK, Chambers JT, Kohorn EI, et al: Evaluation of the role of second-look surgery in ovarian cancer. Obstet Gynecol 72:404–408, 1988.
209. Walton L, Ellenberg SS, Major F, et al: Results of second-look laparotomy in patients with early-stage ovarian carcinoma. Obstet Gynecol 70:770–773, 1987.
210. Copeland LJ, Gershenson DM: Ovarian cancer recurrences in patients with no macroscopic tumor at second-look laparotomy. Obstet Gynecol 68:873–874, 1986.
211. Venesmaa P, Ylikorkala O: Morbidity and mortality associated with primary and repeat operations for ovarian cancer. Obstet Gynecol 79:168–172, 1992.
212. McGuire WP, Rowinski EK, Rosenshein NB, et al: Taxol: A unique antineoplastic agent with significant activity in advanced ovarian epithelial neoplasms. Ann Intern Med 111:273–279, 1989.
213. Sutton GP, Blessing JA, Homesley HD, et al: Phase II trial of ifosfamide and mesna in advanced ovarian carcinoma: A Gynecologic Oncology Group study. J Clin Oncol 7:1672–1676, 1989.
214. Manetta A, MacNeill C, Lyter JA, et al: Hexamethylmelamine as a single second-line agent in ovarian cancer. Gynecol Oncol 36:93–96, 1990.
215. Markman M: Intraperitoneal chemotherapy. Semin Oncol 18:248–254, 1991.
216. Hacker NF, Berek JS, Burnison CM, et al: Whole abdominal radiation as salvage therapy for epithelial ovarian cancer. Obstet Gynecol 65:60–66, 1985.
217. Peters WA III, Blasko JC, Bagley CM Jr, et al: Salvage therapy with whole-abdominal irradiation in patients with advanced ovarian carcinoma of the ovary previously treated by combination chemotherapy. Cancer 58:880–882, 1986.
218. Schray M, Martinez A, Howes AE, et al: Advanced epithelial ovarian cancer: Salvage whole abdominal irradiation for patients with recurrent or persistent disease after combination chemotherapy. J Clin Oncol 6:1433–1439, 1988.
219. Morgan L, Chafe W, Mendenhall W, et al: Hyperfraction of whole-abdomen radiation therapy: Salvage treatment of persistent ovarian carcinoma following chemotherapy. Gynecol Oncol 31:122–134, 1988.
220. Hernandez E, Miyazawa K: The pelvic mass: Patients' ages and pathologic findings. J Reprod Med 33:361–364, 1988.

Gestational Trophoblastic Neoplasm

Allan J. Jacobs, M.D.

EPIDEMIOLOGY

Gestational trophoblastic disease (GTD) is an unusual condition arising from pregnancy. It is subdivided into the syndrome of hydatidiform mole (HM) and its malignant sequelae, which collectively are known as gestational trophoblastic neoplasm (GTN). HM arises in 1 in 1000 pregnancies in the United States.[1] No more than 20% of these evolve into GTN.[2] About one third of cases of GTN do not follow molar pregnancy but follow a term pregnancy or an apparently unremarkable abortion.[3] Complete HM arises from dispermic fertilization, with no chromosomal contribution by the mother.[4] The majority of complete moles have 46,XX genotype, but a few are 46,XY. They are characterized by trophoblastic proliferation, hydropic villi, and absence of fetal tissues. Complete moles are more likely to demonstrate malignant sequelae than the less common partial HM.[5] Fetal tissue is present in the latter condition, which also demonstrates a triploid karyotype.[6]

Incidence of HM is related to age, being somewhat higher before 20 years and markedly higher after 40 years.[7] Women who have had a previous mole have a risk 20 times greater than that of the general population of having another.[8] The chances of giving rise to a third mole after having two are in excess of 20%.[9]

The chances of persistence of HM as malignant GTN following evacuation are enhanced by extremes of age,[10] previous HM,[11] and complete (as opposed to partial) HM.

There are no identifiable environmental factors that influence the probability of development of either HM or its malignant sequelae.

LIFE HISTORY

GTN may arise in one of two ways: HM may persist after evacuation, or GTN may follow an ostensibly normal pregnancy or an abortion. GTN may display one of two histologic patterns: Invasive mole is characterized by the presence in the myometrium of viable trophoblast with chorionic villi. This may go on to metastasize. Choriocarcinoma consists of sheets of malignant trophoblast. Either histologic pattern may be seen in the uterus or in metastases. The histologic appearance of GTN has little relationship to the treatment.

GTN metastasizes primarily by the hematogenous route. If pulmonary metastases are absent, it is unusual to find metastases elsewhere. Isolated pelvic and vaginal metastases may be present. They presumably are due to transtubal and lymphatic spread, respectively. Vaginal metastases are identifiable as blue lesions and *should not be sampled for biopsy,* as they are more extensive than they appear on the surface and tend to bleed profusely. The elevated levels of human chorionic gonadotropin (hCG) secreted by the neoplastic trophoblast may cause marked symmetric enlargement of the ovaries due to hyperstimulation of follicles. These theca-lutein cysts are not to be confused with metastases and need not be sampled for biopsy, as they regress after treatment of the GTD. The tumor spreads from the lung to a variety of sites; spread to the liver and brain carries an especially poor prognosis. The presentation, course, and mode of death in GTN are extremely variable. The vast majority of patients are cured, even if they present with metastases. Patients whose GTN is not treated rarely survive two years.

HYDATIDIFORM MOLE

Diagnosis and Staging

The majority of women with GTD present with bleeding in the first half of pregnancy, inability to detect fetal heart tones at an appropriate gestational age, or discrepancy between duration of pregnancy and uterine size. The uterus is large for gestational age in half of women with complete moles. Those with partial moles tend to have small uteri. In contemporary American obstetrics, any of these findings indicates the need for ultrasound examination. HM displays a characteristic homogeneous echogenic appearance. More unusual presentations include passage of grapelike villi (which is pathognomonic), hyperemesis gravidarum, abnormally elevated serum levels of hCG for gestational age, bilateral ovarian enlargement, or onset of thyrotoxicosis or preeclampsia during the first half of pregnancy.

Women with HM should be evaluated with chest radiograph, complete blood count, platelet count, blood type, renal and hepatic function tests, and serum hCG level. Urinalysis is performed to rule out infection. Consideration should be given to DNA probe assays for chlamydia and gonococcus.

Management is operative and usually consists of evacuation using suction curettage.[12] If the uterus is larger than 14-week size, 2 units of packed cells should be available, as blood loss can be brisk when an HM in a large uterus

TABLE 14–32
Hammond Criteria for Low-Risk and High-Risk Gestational Trophoblastic Neoplasm

Low Risk
- Nonmetastatic
- Metastatic with no risk factors

High Risk
- Metastatic with *any* risk factor
  - More than 4 mo since antecedent pregnancy
  - Serum hCG >40,000 mIU/ml
  - Metastasis to brain
  - Metastasis to liver
  - Previous chemotherapy

is evacuated. The procedure should be performed under general or regional anesthesia. The cervix should be dilated carefully, as insertion of dilators deep into the uterine cavity may cause brisk bleeding. Oxytocin infusion or other uterine stimulants are contraindicated prior to evacuation, as they may result in potentially fatal trophoblastic embolization. An oxytocin infusion is given once evacuation has begun. A 9- or 10-mm suction curet may be used in the standard manner. It is optional to use ultrasonography to assess the completeness of evacuation. Many physicians treat the patient postoperatively using a broad-spectrum antibiotic and an ergot derivative. Treatment for a week with a tetracycline is prudent if a patient is infected with chlamydia or if an assay has not been performed.

Since older patients are more prone to malignant sequelae,[10] hysterectomy can be considered as primary treatment for women over 40 years old who have completed their childbearing. This procedure reduces the risk of GTN in such patients to about 5%.[13] The procedure should be performed abdominally. Indications for ovary removal are the same as for women undergoing hysterectomy for other uterine indications. The surgeon should take care not to mistake ovarian theca-lutein cysts, which present as bilateral massive enlargement, for neoplasia. Ovaries involved with theca-lutein cysts should be left undisturbed unless prophylactic oophorectomy is being performed for advancing age. Hysterotomy is rarely if ever indicated.

Regardless of the primary operative treatment, patients are followed with weekly serum hCG levels using an assay specific for the beta unit. The half-life of hCG is 2 to 3 days, so levels should fall 80% to 90% each week if no metabolically active trophoblast is present. Because metabolically active trophoblast is not necessarily capable of proliferation, the hCG levels are followed as long as they fall. If the level plateaus, or rises for 2 successive weeks, then malignant trophoblast is probably present, and the patient is evaluated for chemotherapy. Otherwise, the level eventually becomes undetectable. Levels of hCG are then drawn monthly for 6 months and bimonthly for another 6 months. The patient is maintained on effective contraception (preferably oral contraceptives) for a year, as pregnancy causes a rise in hCG levels that interferes with monitoring the patient for persistent disease. If theca-lutein cysts were present, ultrasonography is performed monthly to document regression.

GESTATIONAL TROPHOBLASTIC NEOPLASM

If GTD is found outside the context of HM, or if hCG levels plateau or elevate after evacuation of HM, the patient has GTN and requires treatment with chemotherapy. Prior to treatment, a chest radiograph, complete blood count, platelet count, blood type, renal and hepatic function tests, and serum hCG level are obtained. In addition, computed tomography of the abdomen, chest, and brain is performed to exclude metastases. If extracranial metastases are present, it is prudent to perform a lumbar puncture to obtain cerebrospinal fluid for hCG levels. If this level is higher than 2% of the serum level, central nervous system metastases are probably present.[14] The disease is categorized according to the Hammond[15] (Table 14–32) and the World Health Organization[16] (Table 14–33) criteria.

Management of GTN is summarized in Figure 14–22. Almost all patients with low-risk disease will be cured with single-agent chemotherapy using methotrexate,[17–19]

TABLE 14–33
World Health Organization Scoring System for Gestational Trophoblastic Neoplasm

	Score*			
Prognostic Factor	*0*	*1*	*2*	*3*
Age	<35	>39	—	—
Antecedent pregnancy	Hydatidiform	Abortion	Term	—
Interval (mo)	<4	4–6	7–12	>12
Serum hCG (mIU/ml)	<1000	1000–10,000	10,000–100,000	>100,000
ABO type (female X male)	—	O × A	B (female)	—
Largest tumor diameter (cm)	<3	3–5	>5	—
Metastatic site	—	Spleen, kidney	Gastrointestinal, liver	Brain
Number of metastases	—	1–4	4–8	>8
Prior chemotherapy	—	—	1 drug	>1 drug

*Risk assignment is based on total score, derived by adding score for each prognostic factor. 0 to 4: Low risk; 5 to 7: intermediate risk; 8 or more: high risk.

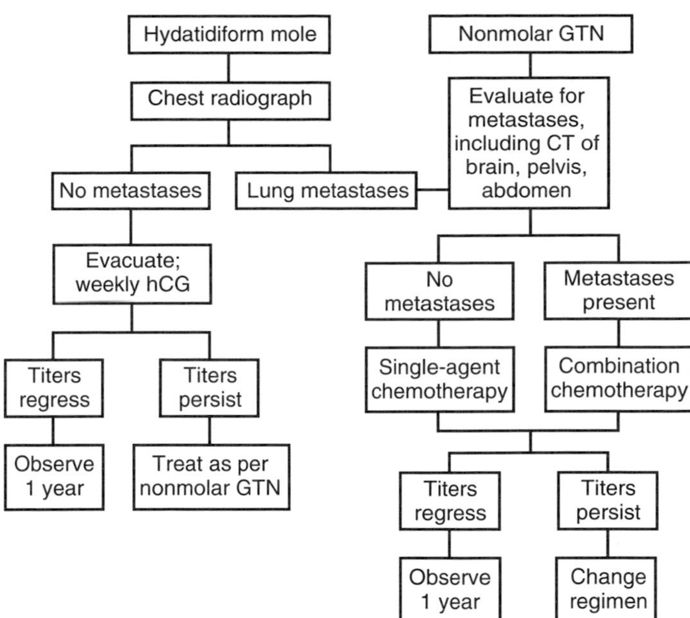

FIGURE 14–22. Algorithm for management of gestational trophoblastic disease. GTN, Gestational trophoblastic neoplasm.

dactinomycin,[20, 21] or etoposide.[22] High-risk patients require combination chemotherapy; if disease is not present in the brain[23] or liver,[24] almost all patients with intermediate-risk disease and about 75% of those with high-risk disease should attain a sustained remission.[25, 26] The vast majority of patients are cured. The reader is referred to other sources for chemotherapy details.[26–28] Brain and liver metastases also require irradiation of the affected site,[22, 23, 29] which is begun simultaneously with chemotherapy. Cure rates are about 50% when disease is present in these sites. Chemotherapy is given for several courses after serum hCG becomes undetectable. Follow-up is the same as for HM.

Operation is required in up to one third of patients with high-risk GTN when chemotherapy alone cannot eradicate the disease. Removal of a uterus with a persistent focus of chemoresistant tumor is the most common such procedure; this ordinarily requires simple total abdominal hysterectomy.[18] Resection of isolated metastases, especially thoracotomy and segmental lung resection for isolated pulmonary lesions, is sometimes required to achieve a cure.[30, 31]

PLACENTAL SITE TROPHOBLASTIC TUMOR

Placental site trophoblastic tumor (PSTT) is a rare variant of GTN. First described by Kurman and associates,[32] it is an infiltrating trophoblastic tumor characterized by lack of chorionic villi, cytotrophoblast, hemorrhage, or necrosis.[33] It may follow HM, spontaneous abortion, induced abortion, or childbirth.[34] The tumor should be suspected following any pregnancy when there is an abnormal pattern of vaginal bleeding (the most common presentation) or amenorrhea. The hCG level is almost invariably less than 500 mIU/ml and may be minimally elevated. PSTT does not respond to chemotherapy. The treatment consists of hysterectomy. Metastatic disease is invariably fatal.

References

1. Grimes DA: Epidemiology of gestational trophoblastic disease. Am J Obstet Gynecol 150:309–318, 1984.
2. Lurain JR, Brewer JI, Torok EE, et al: Natural history of hydatidiform mole after primary evacuation. Am J Obstet Gynecol 145:591–595, 1983.
3. Bagshawe KD: Risk and prognostic factors in trophoblastic neoplasia. Cancer 38:1373–1385, 1976.
4. Yamashita K, Wake N, Araki T, et al: Human lymphocyte antigen expression in hydatidiform mole: Androgenesis following fertilization by a haploid sperm. Am J Obstet Gynecol 135:597–600, 1979.
5. Rice LW, Berkowitz RS, Lage JM, et al: Persistent gestational trophoblastic tumor after partial hydatidiform mole. Gynecol Oncol 36:358–362, 1990.
6. Szulman AE, Surti U: The syndromes of hydatidiform mole. I. Cytogenetic and morphogenetic correlations. Am J Obstet Gynecol 131:665–671, 1978.
7. Hayashi K, Bracken MB, Freeman DH Jr, et al: Hydatidiform mole in the United States (1970–1977): A statistical and theoretical analysis. Am J Epidemiol 115:67–77, 1982.
8. Yen S, MacMahon B: Epidemiologic features of trophoblastic disease. Am J Obstet Gynecol 101:126–132, 1968.
9. Sand PK, Lurain JR, Brewer JI: Repeat gestational trophoblastic disease. Obstet Gynecol 63:140–144, 1984.
10. Bandy LC, Clarke-Pearson DL, Hammond CB: Malignant potential of gestational trophoblastic disease at the extreme ages of reproductive life. Obstet Gynecol 64:395–399, 1984.
11. Federschneider JM, Goldstein DP, Berkowitz RS, et al: Natural history of recurrent molar pregnancy. Obstet Gynecol 55:457–459, 1980.
12. Schlaerth JB, Morrow CP, Montz FJ, et al: Initial management of hydatidiform mole. Am J Obstet Gynecol 158:1299–1306, 1988.
13. Curry SL, Hammond CB, Tyrey L, et al: Hydatidiform mole: Diagnosis, management, and long-term followup of 347 patients. Obstet Gynecol 45:1–8, 1975.
14. Bagshawe KD, Hartland S: Immunodiagnosis and monitoring of gonadotropin-producing metastases in the central nervous system. Cancer 38:112–118, 1976.
15. Hammond CB, Borchert LG, Tyrey L, et al: Treatment of metastatic gestational trophoblastic disease: Good and poor prognosis. Am J Obstet Gynecol 115:451–457, 1973.
16. World Health Organization Scientific Group on Gestational Tropho-

blastic Neoplasms: Technical Report Series No. 692. Geneva: World Health Organization, 1983.
17. Hammond CB, Hertz R, Ross GT, et al: Primary chemotherapy for non-metastatic gestational trophoblastic neoplasms. Am J Obstet Gynecol 98:71–78, 1967.
18. Hammond CB, Weed JC Jr, Currie JL: The role of operation in the current therapy of gestational trophoblastic disease. Am J Obstet Gynecol 136:844–858, 1980.
19. Homesley HD, Blessing JA, Rettenmaier M, et al: Weekly intramuscular methotrexate for nonmetastatic gestational trophoblastic disease. Obstet Gynecol 72:413–418, 1988.
20. Goldstein DP, Winig P, Shirley RL: Actinomycin D as primary agent for gestational trophoblastic disease. Obstet Gynecol 39:341–345, 1975.
21. Petrilli ES, Twiggs LB, Blessing JA, et al: Single-dose actinomycin-D treatment for nonmetastatic gestational trophoblastic disease. A prospective phase II trial of the Gynecologic Oncology Group. Cancer 60:2173–2176, 1987.
22. Wong MA, Choo YC, Ma HK: Primary oral etoposide therapy in gestational trophoblastic disease: An update. Cancer 58:14–17, 1986.
23. Yordan EL Jr, Schlaerth J, Gaddis O, et al: Radiation therapy in the management of gestational choriocarcinoma metastatic to the central nervous system. Obstet Gynecol 69:627–630, 1987.
24. Barnard DE, Woodward KT, Yancey SG, et al: Hepatic metastases of choriocarcinoma: A report of 15 patients. Gynecol Oncol 25:73–83, 1986.
25. Bolis G, Bonazzi C, Landoni F, et al: EMA/CO regimen in high-risk gestational trophoblastic tumor (GTT). Gynecol Oncol 31:439–444, 1988.
26. Newlands ES, Bagshawe KD, Begent RHJ, et al: Developments in chemotherapy for medium- and high-risk patients with gestational trophoblastic tumours (1979–1984). Br J Obstet Gynaecol 93:63–69, 1986.
27. Barter JF, Soong SJ, Hatch KD, et al: Treatment of nonmetastatic gestational trophoblastic disease with oral methotrexate. Am J Obstet Gynecol 157:1166–1168, 1987.
28. DuBeshter B, Berkowitz RS, Goldstein DP, et al: Metastatic gestational trophoblastic disease: Experience at the New England Trophoblastic Disease Center, 1965 to 1985. Obstet Gynecol 68:390–395, 1987.
29. Weed JC, Woodward KT, Hammond CB: Choriocarcinoma metastatic to the brain: Therapy and prognosis. Semin Oncol 9:208–212, 1982.
30. Sink JD, Hammond CB, Young WG: Pulmonary resection in the management of metastases from gestational choriocarcinoma. J Thorac Cardiovasc Surg 81:830–834, 1978.
31. Tomoda Y, Arii Y, Kaseki S, et al: Surgical indications for resection in pulmonary metastases of choriocarcinoma. Cancer 46:2723–2730, 1980.
32. Kurman RJ, Scully RE, Norris HJ: Trophoblastic pseudotumor of the uterus. An exaggerated form of "syncytial endometritis" simulating a malignant tumor. Cancer 38:1214–1226, 1976.
33. Gloor E, Huerlimann H: Trophoblastic pseudotumor of the uterus. Clinicopathologic report with immunohistochemical and ultrastructural studies. Am J Surg Pathol 5:5–13, 1981.
34. Finkler NJ, Berkowitz RS, Driscoll SG, et al: Clinical experience with placental site trophoblastic tumor at the New England Trophoblastic Disease Center. Obstet Gynecol 71:854–858, 1988.
35. Mutch DG, Soper JT, Baker ME: Role of computerized tomography of the chest in staging patients with nonmetastatic gestational trophoblastic neoplasm. Obstet Gynecol 68:348–352, 1986.

Vulvar and Vaginal Malignancies

Allan J. Jacobs, M.D. • Robert Stenson, M.D.

EPIDEMIOLOGY

Incidence

Vulvar carcinoma accounts for approximately 5% of all malignancies of the female genitalia. It is primarily a disease of older women. There does not appear to be a familial component in the pathogenesis of this disease.

The large majority of tumors are squamous lesions. They frequently occur in women who have had other lower genital neoplasms.[1] There appear to be at least two etiologic types of squamous carcinoma—that associated with human papillomavirus (HPV) infection, and that with no such association but with frequent concomitant atypical vulvar dystrophy.[2] Granulomatous vulvar disease and other sexually transmitted diseases have also been associated with vulvar carcinoma.[3] Cigarette smoking may also be a risk factor.[4]

Risk Factors

The identified risk factors include genetic-familial, dietary, social habits (e.g., drugs and alcohol), and environmental and occupational.

LOCAL-REGIONAL ANATOMY AND PATHOLOGY

Patterns of Spread

Vulva

Vulvar cancer may involve the labia minora, labia majora, clitoris, vestibule, posterior fourchette, and perineal skin. Cancers of the Bartholin glands are generally considered to be vulvar malignancies. Vulvar carcinoma can spread by direct extension, lymphatic spread, and hematogenous metastasis.

Local spread may involve the perineum and anus posteriorly, the vagina and distal urethra anteriorly, the labiocrural folds and inner thigh laterally, and the subcutaneous fat and urogenital diaphragm deeply. When a vulvar carcinoma involves medial labial surfaces, satellite lesions may be present on the contralateral labium at the site of contact with the lesion. These "kissing lesions" presumably arise as a result of direct contact with the primary lesion. Carcinoma originating in Bartholin's glands frequently invades the ischiorectal fossa and paravaginal tissues.

The posterior fourchette and perineum share the same lymphatic drainage as the vulva proper. For this reason, cancers arising in those structures are regarded as primary vulvar cancers. Tumors involving the vulva and the perineum simultaneously have the same prognosis as those involving one of these structures, given that the known prognostic factors are the same. The simultaneous presence of tumor on perineum and vulva does not, therefore, affect the staging of the tumor.

In contrast to most other organs, lymphatic drainage from the vulva does not parallel its blood supply. Rather, the lymphatic channels travel anteriorly toward the mons veneris and then turn laterally toward the groin.[5] Lymphatic spread carries vulvar carcinoma first to the superficial inguinal nodes, which lie just anterior to the cribriform plate. The next metastatic station is the deep femoral nodes, which are embedded in a fatty bundle of tissue anterior to the femoral vessels and posterior to the cribriform plate. Tumor can occasionally be found in femoral nodes without concomitant inguinal node involvement.[6] Cloquet's node, the highest femoral node, has been called a sentinel node for further cephalad lymphatic spread of carcinoma. In fact, it is not a reliable indicator, since it is usually not possible to identify a single lymph node as Cloquet's node. Cancer may metastasize cephalad from the femoral chain to the deep pelvic (obturator, internal iliac, and external iliac) lymph nodes regardless of the status of Cloquet's node. From there, the tumor may travel superiorly along the chain of nodes that lies anterior to the great vessels. Caudal spread to the saphenous nodes and the femoral nodes in the distal portion of the femoral triangle is occasionally observed in patients with extensive nodal involvement.

Iversen and Aas[7] studied lymph flow in the vulva by injecting technetium 99 colloid into various sites of the vulva and then following the flow of the isotope by camera scintigraphy and by lymphadenectomy. The clitoris and perineum demonstrated bilateral flow, as did the anterior labia minora. The remainder of the vulva showed only ipsilateral drainage. Iversen[8] also studied the pattern of metastases in women with vulvar carcinoma. Of 39 women with unilateral tumor, he found 14 with unilateral nodes and 3 with bilateral nodes. No patient had contralateral nodes without simultaneous ipsilateral nodes.[8]

Posterior and lateral lesions tend to metastasize to ipsilateral nodes, spreading to contralateral groin nodes only late in their course. Anteromedial lesions are more likely to involve contralateral nodes. Of course, midline lesions or those that involve both sides of the vulva may involve nodes on either or both sides.

It is widely stated in texts without primary citation that clitoral carcinoma metastasizes directly to the deep pelvic nodes. Plentl and Friedman[5] describe lymphatic channels traveling directly from the clitoris to the pelvic nodes. Curry et al.,[9] Ericksson and colleagues,[10] and Piver and Xynos[11] found, in a combined total of 126 carcinomas involving the clitoris, no spread of tumor to pelvic nodes in the absence of groin node metastases.

The incidence of pelvic node spread is much lower than the incidence of groin metastases.[9, 12–14] Also, pelvic nodal metastases almost never occur in the absence of groin involvement. Monaghan and Hammond[15] studied 136 women with vulvar tumors, 55 of whom had metastases to groin nodes. Only three of these women had pelvic node metastases, all of whom also had tumor present in groin nodes. Hacker and associates[16] reviewed 113 women with all stages of disease. Thirty-one had groin adenopathy, six of whom also had positive pelvic nodes. No patient with fewer than three positive groin nodes demonstrated carcinoma in pelvic nodes. Recognition of the predictable sequence of lymphatic spread of vulvar carcinoma has led to the abandonment of treatment of pelvic nodes unless groin nodes are involved.

Ample evidence suggests a strong relationship between tumor size and lymph node metastasis.[15–20] Table 14–34 shows the relationship between the diameter of the lesion and the likelihood of lymph node involvement. The depth of tumor invasion is also correlated with the frequency of groin metastasis (Table 14–35).[21, 22] Increased incidence of positive lymph nodes is also related to worse histologic differentiation of the primary tumor[15, 17] and to vascular space involvement in the primary lesion.[19, 20, 22]

Hematogenous metastases may carry tumor directly to the spine as well as to the lungs. This is because the pelvic veins anastomose with the paravertebral veins. Hematogenous metastases are rarely seen in squamous cell vulvar

TABLE 14–34
Relationship Between Tumor Diameter and Lymph Node Involvement[18, 21, 22]

Tumor Diameter (cm)	Positive Lymph Nodes	
	No.	*%*
Up to 1	7/73	10
1–2	19/137	14
2–4	48/171	28
>4	28/71	40
Total	47/185	25

TABLE 14–35
Relationship Between Depth of Tumor Invasion and Lymph Node Metastases in Vulvar Carcinoma[21, 22]

Tumor Thickness (cm)	Positive Lymph Nodes	
	No.	*%*
Up to 1	1/66	2
1–2	7/75	9
2–3	13/76	17
3–5	41/132	31
>5	19/57	33
Total	62/349	18

carcinoma, except in anaplastic or advanced lesions. Melanomas, adenocarcinomas, and Bartholin's gland tumors, in contrast, frequently display distant metastases arising from hematogenous spread.

Vagina

Primary vaginal cancer constitutes 1% to 2% of female genital tract malignancies.[23] It is one of the rarest gynecologic malignancies, accounting for 0.2% of all cancer in women.[24] In the United States, about 300 deaths a year are caused by vaginal cancer. The mean age at diagnosis is 60.

Risk factors are specific to the histology. Women with squamous cell carcinoma often have a history of infection by HPV,[25] whose DNA may be present in the lesions.[26] Vaginal squamous lesions may also be related to pessary use[27] and to previous pelvic irradiation.[28] Clear cell carcinoma is a rare condition that is usually associated with exposure to diethylstilbestrol (DES) during fetal life, the drug having been ingested by the patient's mother.[29]

Vaginal carcinoma most commonly arises in the proximal third.[5, 30–32] Spread is by local extension, lymphatic involvement, and hematogenous dissemination. By convention, presence of cancer in either the cervix or the vulva classifies the tumor as a primary lesion of those structures rather than of the vagina, no matter how extensive the vaginal involvement or how minimal the involvement of the other structure. The reason for this convention is the rarity of vaginal carcinoma relative to cancer of the cervix or vulva. Direct extension may carry a vaginal carcinoma laterally to the cardinal ligaments, pelvic sidewall, or lower paravaginal tissues. Anteriorly, extension to the bladder, urethra, or pubis is possible. Posterior tumors may invade the rectum or the cul-de-sac of Douglas. In a woman with no cervix, a malignancy of the vaginal cuff may erode into the peritoneal cavity.

Lymphatic metastasis of lesions of the upper third of the vagina tends to follow the same pathways as do cervical lymphatic metastases (see the subchapter on cervical malignancies). Lesions of the lower third tend to spread as do vulvar lesions (see the previous section). There are ample anastomoses among the vaginal lymphatic channels, so any of these tumors may metastasize directly to any lymph nodes, from the deep pelvic nodes proximally to the groin nodes distally.

Hematogenous spread is unimportant compared with the other two routes of metastasis.

Histology

Vulva

Vulvar Intraepithelial Neoplasia (VIN). VIN is the premalignant counterpart to vulvar squamous cell carcinoma.[33] Despite the analogy in nomenclature and histology to the cervix, VIN does not have the same prognostic import as its cervical counterpart. There appear to be two variants of VIN.[34, 35] Those cases associated with HPV infection are detected in women below the age of 50—frequently as young as the third decade of life. They tend to be multifocal. Those not associated with HPV tend to be unifocal and are found in postmenopausal women. Fewer than 10% of untreated VIN lesions progress to invasive cancer,[36, 37] but some studies report that 10% to 20% of patients with apparent VIN that was excised surgically harbor occult invasive carcinoma.[38, 39] Despite adequate treatment, VIN has a marked propensity to recur.

Paget Disease of the Vulva.[40, 41] Paget disease usually presents as a red indurated lesion with a white sheen resembling doughnut frosting. The lesion may be localized or diffuse. It is generally found in elderly white women. Histologically, Paget disease contains characteristic Paget cells, commonly found at the base of the epidermis. These cells may be confused with atypical melanocytes. Paget disease may be definitively distinguished from melanoma by staining for carcinoembryonic antigen, which is present only in Paget cells.[42, 43] Adenocarcinoma is said to underlie 15% to 20% of Paget disease lesions, but it is difficult to find documentation for this figure. When such an adenocarcinoma is present, it is usually easily palpable.[44] DiSaia and Creasman[45] advocate the use of fine-needle aspiration of subcutaneous masses underlying Paget disease in order to establish this diagnosis. Paget disease is notorious for extending histologically well beyond the gross margins.[46]

Squamous Cell Carcinoma. The large majority of cases of vulvar cancer are squamous cell carcinoma (Table 14–36).[5] The majority occur on the labia, but lesions may arise from anywhere on the vulva. The lesion is usually red, although it may be white or pigmented. Carcinomas may be raised or ulcerated. The gross appearance of these lesions is sufficiently protean that they cannot be distinguished from benign lesions by inspection. It has been suggested that those associated with HPV can be distinguished histologically from those that are not (Table 14–37).[2] A keratinizing pattern is said to be characteristic in tumors not associated with HPV, whereas those that contain HPV DNA tend not to keratinize.[2] Both keratinizing and nonkeratinizing vulvar

TABLE 14–36
Incidence of Vulvar Neoplasms by Histologic Type

Histologic Type	%*
Squamous cell	86.2
Melanoma	4.8
Basal cell	1.4
Bartholin's gland	
Squamous cell	0.4
Adenocarcinoma	0.6
Sarcoma	2.2
Adenocarcinoma	0.6
Unidentified, undifferentiated	3.2

From Plentl AA, Friedman EA: Lymphatic System of the Female Genitalia. Philadelphia: WB Saunders, 1971, p. 28.
*Based on 1378 cases from 12 series reported between 1934 and 1964.

TABLE 14–37
Differences Between Vulvar Carcinoma With and Without Presence of HPV Genome

Parameter	HPV-Associated	Non–HPV-Associated
Age (yr)	35–65	55–85
Previous condylomas	Common	Uncommon
Previous STD	Common	Uncommon
Pre-existing lesion	VIN	Inflammation, lichen sclerosus, hyperplasia
Cofactors	Immune status, viral integration	Vulvar atypia, mutated host genes
Histopathology	Basaloid or poorly differentiated	Keratinizing; well differentiated
Cervical neoplasia	High association	Low association
Smoking	High association	Low association
HPV nucleic acids	Frequent	Seldom

Adapted from Crum CP: Carcinoma of the vulva: Epidemiology and pathogenesis. Obstet Gynecol 79:448–454, 1992.
HPV, Human papillomavirus; STD, sexually transmitted disease; VIN, vulvar intraepithelial neoplasia.

tumors tend to grow slowly and to spread by means of direct extension or lymphatic embolization, as described above. There is no known difference in the natural history of lesions containing HPV and those that do not.

Melanoma. Melanomas constitute about 5% of vulvar carcinomas.[5] Conversely, about 7% of all melanomas in women occur on the vulva. Most arise on the clitoris or labia minora. They usually present as pigmented lesions with irregular margins, although they may be amelanotic. They may be raised, flat, or ulcerated. The histologic parameter best correlated with prognosis is depth of invasion.[47, 48] This can be measured by Clark level, which considers the structures into which the tumor has invaded, or by Breslow level, which measures depth of invasion quantitatively. Both of these systems are detailed in Chapter 16. Melanomas follow a different natural course than do squamous tumors, metastasizing by hematogenous spread as well as by lymphatic embolization. Virtually all patients with groin nodes at the time of diagnosis eventually die of the disease. The likelihood of recurrence in a melanoma of a given depth is greater than in squamous tumors.

Basal Cell Carcinoma and Verrucous Carcinoma. Basal cell[49, 50] and verrucous[51] carcinomas are rare lesions. Both may demonstrate local invasion but rarely metastasize.

Bartholin's Gland Carcinoma. Bartholin's gland carcinomas include squamous cell carcinomas, adenocarcinomas, adenoid cystic carcinomas, and transitional cell carcinomas.[52] They tend to infiltrate early into deep tissues, including the ischiorectal fossa and paravaginal tissues.[53–55] Their lymphatic metastasis may bypass the groin nodes for the pelvic nodes.

Other Carcinomas. Unusual vulvar carcinomas whose discussion is beyond the scope of this book include adenocarcinomas, adenosquamous carcinomas, and sarcomas.[56]

Vagina

Over 75% of vaginal malignancies display squamous cell histology. A premalignant entity that is histologically analogous to VIN and cervical intraepithelial neoplasia is termed vaginal intraepithelial neoplasia (VaIN). Its natural history is not well understood.

Clear cell adenocarcinoma develops in about 0.1% of women exposed to DES in utero[57]; it arises in areas of vaginal adenosis that are present in about half of these women. Other rare tumors include verrucous carcinoma, neuroendocrine carcinoma, melanoma, various sarcomas, and (in children) embryonal rhabdomyosarcoma and endodermal sinus tumor.

DIAGNOSIS, SCREENING, EARLY DETECTION, AND STAGING

Vulva

As a result of a decline in social inhibitions to discussing the genitalia and increased frequency of gynecologic examinations, vulvar carcinoma is now diagnosed early in most instances. The most common symptoms that cause the patient to seek care include pruritus, observation of a vulvar mass, or bleeding. Patients with advanced lesions may complain of pain, dysuria, odor, incontinence, or even an inability to sit.

Lesions of vulvar cancer, except for some adenocarcinomas and Bartholin's carcinomas, are obvious on inspection. They are thickened and irregular in outline. As stated above, the appearance of these tumors varies considerably, and cancer cannot reliably be distinguished from benign conditions. Malignant lesions differ in color from normal skin and generally present with thickness and induration. Melanomas may not show induration, however. Adenocarcinomas and Bartholin's gland carcinomas may be situated entirely beneath the skin and present as a subcutaneous mass.

Diagnosis is accomplished by excisional or incisional biopsy. Essentially all abnormal vulvar lesions should be sampled for biopsy. Lesions in young woman that appear to have a pathognomonic appearance (e.g., condyloma acuminatum, chancre, or contact dermatitis) may initially be treated medically or with ablation, as appropriate to the

TABLE 14–38
FIGO Surgical Staging of Primary Vulvar Carcinoma

FIGO Stage	TNM Stage	Definition
I	T1, N0, M0	Tumor confined to vulva and perineum no greater than 2 cm in largest diameter; nodes histologically negative
II	T2, N0, M0	Tumor confined to vulva and perineum greater than 2 cm in largest diameter; nodes histologically negative
III	T1–3, N0, 1, M0	Tumor of any size with extension to urethra, vagina, or anus, and/or groin nodes unilaterally positive by histology
IVA	T1–4, N2, M0	Tumor of any size with extension to urethra, vagina, or anus, and/or fixed to bone; groin nodes bilaterally positive by histology
IVB	T1–4, N0–2, M1	Distant metastases, including pelvic nodes

presumptive condition. Even these should be sampled for biopsy if they do not resolve in several weeks.

The biopsy specimen is taken from the periphery of a lesion in order to avoid a sample consisting exclusively of necrotic tissue. The skin at the site of the biopsy is infiltrated with 1 to 3 ml of 1% lidocaine with 1:100,000 epinephrine using a fine (27-gauge) needle. A 3- or 4-mm Keys punch biopsy instrument is used to core out the specimen, and scissors or a scalpel is used to amputate the base. The sample is submitted in 10% formalin for histopathologic analysis. The base of the wound is cauterized using supersaturated ferric subsulfate solution (Monsel's solution) or silver nitrate sticks. Rarely, sutures are necessary to achieve hemostasis. A presumptive Bartholin's cyst encountered in a women over 40 years of age should be excised rather than drained or marsupialized. Solid vulvar subcutaneous masses should be excised or sampled for biopsy.

Once vulvar carcinoma is diagnosed, the preoperative staging evaluation is simple. When squamous cell carcinoma is present, colposcopy of the cervix and vagina should be performed, as multiple squamous neoplasms of the lower genital tract are common.[58] Chest radiography is also indicated. In melanomas, Bartholin's gland carcinomas, and large squamous lesions, computed tomography of the pelvis should be performed.

Formal staging is surgicopathologic and follows the 1989 recommendations of the International Federation of Gynecologists and Obstetricians (FIGO) (Table 14–38).

Vagina

Annual vaginal speculum examination and cytology should be performed in all patients who have had a hysterectomy or radiation for benign or malignant neoplasia of the lower genital tract. If cytology is abnormal, colposcopy is performed. Colposcopy often does not demonstrate subclinical lesions of VaIN or early cancer, so staining with Lugol's solution should be performed in patients with abnormal vaginal cytology following hysterectomy or radiation. Nonstaining areas are likely to contain neoplasia.

Most vaginal cancer presents with vaginal bleeding. These tumors may also present with abnormal cytology or physical findings on routine examination. The most common site of origin is the upper third of the vagina, on the posterior wall. Vaginal cancer is commonly seen in women who have undergone total hysterectomy.[4] This observation may be because many cancers that actually arise in the vaginas of women with uteri involve the cervix and are classified as cervical lesions.

The staging work-up for vaginal cancer is similar to that for cervical cancer. If the cervix is present, it must be sampled for biopsy.

The FIGO staging system for vaginal cancer is depicted in Table 14–39. Staging is clinical and is based on the physical examination, chest radiograph, intravenous pyelogram, cystoscopy, sigmoidoscopy, and minor operative procedures. Information derived from major operative procedures may not be used to assign a formal stage. Lesions involving the cervix or vulva—no matter how insignificantly—cannot be considered primary vaginal cancer.

TREATMENT MODALITIES

Surgery

Vulvar Laser Ablation with the Carbon Dioxide Laser

Laser ablation is often used to treat intraepithelial lesions of the vulva and vagina. Apparent VIN lesions may harbor occult invasive malignancy.[38, 39] The surgeon must conclusively establish the absence of invasive cancer before ablative treatment of VIN. This may be done by securing multiple biopsy samples of large or diffuse lesions. If there is any doubt about the presence of malignancy, excisional

TABLE 14–39
FIGO Surgical Staging of Primary Vaginal Carcinoma

FIGO Stage	Definition
I	Tumor limited to the vaginal mucosa
II	Tumor has involved the subvaginal tissue but has not extended onto the pelvic wall
III	Carcinoma has extended to the pelvic wall
IVA	Involvement of bladder or rectal mucosa, which must be established by biopsy
IVB	Spread to distant organs

rather than ablative techniques should be employed in order to allow histopathologic analysis.

Laser ablation is best accomplished under general anesthesia. A handpiece or micromanipulator is used, and the laser is operated using a power density of 600 to 800 W/cm^2 on hair-bearing skin and 450 to 600 W/cm^2 on non–hair-bearing skin or vaginal epithelium. The limits of the lesion are identified using application of 5% acetic acid (and, optionally, colposcopy). These are marked with a series of dots using the laser. Vaporization is achieved using a circular motion and is carried down to the junction between the papillary dermis and reticular dermis.[59, 60] Deeper vaporization may result in scarring, and insufficient vaporization compromises the chance of cure. The procedure is usually done as ambulatory surgery. Postoperative care consists of twice-daily sitz baths and application of an ointment containing bacitracin, polymyxin, and neomycin. The patient's activities will be markedly limited for 1 to 2 weeks due to pain, and she may have residual soreness for several additional weeks. Aside from scarring and anesthetic accidents, there are few complications. Infection of the operative bed is unusual.

Laser Thin Section

The laser thin section[61] procedure is also performed as ambulatory surgery under general anesthesia. The lesion is identified and marked as for ablation. A carbon dioxide laser beam of 20 to 25 W set at superpulse is used to amputate the involved vulvar skin in a plane in the superficial reticular dermis. Baggish and colleagues[61] state that the specimen is of sufficient quality that a pathologist can evaluate it for invasion and presence of margins. Postoperative care consists of sitz baths and application of polymyxin-bacitracin-neomycin ointment twice daily. The patient returns to normal activities in 1 to 2 weeks.

Wide Local Excision

Wide local excision of vulvar lesions is best carried out using a scalpel on the skin and electrocautery for the underlying subcutaneous tissue. The distance of the lateral and deep margins from the lesion depends on the nature of the lesion (Table 14–40). An elliptic incision is made, with the ends converging in a point (football shaped) and the long axis in an anteroposterior orientation. The wound is closed in two layers. Both the subcutaneous tissue and the skin may be closed with 3–0 polygalactin or chromic gut suture. The procedure may be done on an ambulatory basis. Complications and disability are minimal.

TABLE 14–40
Optimal Margins in Wide Local Excision of Vulvar Neoplasms*

Neoplasm	Skin Margin	Deep Margin
Vulvar intraepithelial neoplasia	1 cm	Just below dermis
Paget disease	2 cm	Just below dermis
Squamous cell carcinoma (>4 cm)	2 cm†	2 cm†
Melanoma	2 cm	2 cm

*Inappropriate as treatment for multifocal lesions.
†May be as little as 1 cm in thin lesions >2 cm in diameter.

Skinning Vulvectomy with Skin Graft

A skinning vulvectomy with a skin graft is used for large or confluent lesions of VIN. The affected vulvar skin is removed in the avascular plane between the dermis and the subcutaneous fat. Thus, skin appendages are removed, but the contour of the vulva is not disturbed. A 1-cm lateral margin is obtained. A split-thickness skin graft 18/1000 inch (0.45 mm) thick is taken from a donor site on the thigh. It is sewn into place using 4–0 polygalactin suture. With large lesions requiring extensive denudation, the graft may be gridded prior to application. If the graft is not gridded, small perforations are cut into the graft to allow serum to escape. The graft is covered with a foam rubber dressing, and the patient is immobilized in bed for a week. The patient returns to normal activities in about 4 weeks.

Laser Ablation of Vagina

Vaginal epithelium involved with intraepithelial neoplasia may be ablated using a carbon dioxide laser with the same power settings that are appropriate for ablation of the vulva. As is the case with the vulva, invasive carcinoma must be definitively excluded prior to ablative treatment.

Partial Superficial Vaginectomy

A partial superficial vaginectomy may be performed using sharp dissection or laser dissection.[62] In either case, the area to be removed is determined by colposcopy and staining with Lugol's iodine. Following induction of general or regional anesthesia, the operative bed is infiltrated with 1% lidocaine with 1:100,000 epinephrine. An incision is made around the lesion or area that is to be removed using a scalpel, electrocautery, or a sharply focused laser beam. This lesion is carried deep, through the vaginal epithelium. A relatively avascular plane can generally be developed, and the vaginal epithelium is reflected off the subvaginal tissue. Hemostasis is achieved by electrocautery or laser cautery. Re-epithelialization is spontaneous.

Radical Vulvectomy with Inguinofemoral Lymphadenectomy

As will be clear from the section on the treatment of vulvar cancer, a full radical vulvectomy and bilateral groin dissection are seldom required for treatment of the vulva. Modifications of this procedure for ablative treatment of vulvar carcinoma are based on this procedure and use the same dissection planes. Since pelvic lymphadenectomy is no longer indicated in the primary treatment of this disease, it will not be described.

The operation is performed with the patient's legs abducted in Allen stirrups. Either general or regional anesthesia may be used. If a regional anesthetic technique is used, epidural anesthesia is preferable to spinal anesthesia because of the long duration of the operation.

Classic Radical Vulvectomy

The classic operation begins with a curvilinear incision between the anterosuperior iliac spines, about 3 cm cephalad to the inguinal ligament and following Langer's lines in the skin. The skin incision is continued inferomedially and posteriorly from each end of the transverse incision just described by incising on each side along the crease between the thigh and the abdomen and continuing along the labiocrural folds.

After the initial incision is made, inguinofemoral lymphadenectomy is performed. The abdominal incision is developed to the membranous structure separating Camper's fascia from Scarpa's fascia. A dissection plane is established just superficial to Scarpa's fascia, proceeding inferiorly. The subcutaneous tissue at the cephalad aspect of this plane is then incised through Scarpa's fascia to the aponeurosis of the external oblique muscle and the rectus muscles. This plane is developed caudad, toward the inguinal ligaments and the pubic periosteum. As these planes are developed along the anterior thigh, leaving Camper's fascia attached the skin, Scarpa's fascia is mobilized as the most superficial part of the surgical specimen. The lateral border of the specimen is at the lateral margin of the node-bearing tissue of Scarpa's fascia. The cribriform plate is incised at its attachment to the inguinal ligament, and the femoral artery is exposed. The fascia lata is incised at the lateral aspect of the incision, and the specimen is reflected mediolaterally off the sartorius muscle. The dissection proceeds medially, with node-bearing tissue reflected from the femoral artery. The external pudendal artery is ligated as it is encountered. The node-bearing fatty tissue is then mobilized off the femoral vein. The cephalad femoral node (Cloquet's node) may be removed separately and sent as a separate specimen. The saphenous vein is doubly ligated and divided at its entry into the femoral vein. The inferior margin of the inguinofemoral node specimen is defined and dissected on each side. During this dissection, the great saphenous vein is encountered again, at which time it is again doubly ligated and divided. Alternatively, the entire saphenous vein may be spared, leaving behind some of the most distal femoral nodes. The node dissection is now complete. The nodal specimens are attached medially to the vulva. Nodes and vulva will be removed together en bloc.

The vulvectomy is then performed. The labiocrural incisions are extended posteriorly and joined across the perineum to complete the external skin incision. A circumferential vestibular interior incision is constructed in a location that retains the urethral orifice. The perineal incision is developed deep, to the perineal body. The vulva is removed by dissection in a superior direction, with the vestibular incision limiting the extent of the dissection, allowing preservation of the vagina and urethral orifice. The clitoris, the bulbocavernous muscles, and the vestibular bulb are removed, but the urethra, the rectal sphincter, and the perineal body are preserved. The clitoral and perineal arteries are ligated as they are encountered, as is the round ligament.

Removal of the specimen leaves a large hiatus in the groin that must be repaired. The sartorius muscle is detached from its origins on the anterosuperior iliac spine and lateral inguinal ligaments. It is sutured to the proximal adductor longus muscle and the medial inguinal ligament, to cover the femoral vessels. The subcutaneous tissue and skin are approximated if this can be done without much tension on the edges. Suction drains are left between the cutaneous flap and the fascia. If primary skin closure requires tension (as is usually the case), it is preferable to swing tensor fascia lata myocutaneous flaps to fill the defect.[63]

Most patients are mobilized and are eating solid food within 48 hours of the procedure. Parenteral analgesics are required for only 1 to 2 days following the operation.

Complications are frequent following this procedure. At best, when the postoperative course is otherwise uneventful, the classic operation markedly alters the appearance of the vulva, leading to psychologic effects[64] and sexual dysfunction.[65] There is a change in the direction of the urinary stream anteriorly, posteriorly, or laterally, and there may be spraying of urine.[66]

In fact, the postoperative course is rarely uneventful. The mortality rate is less than 5% in all recent series. A list of the more common complications and their incidence in one large series is depicted in Table 14–41. The primary wound breaks down in over half of patients.[67–69] Prevention of this complication is reported elsewhere in this chapter. Small wound disruptions are managed by cleansing, packing, and allowing the wound to heal by secondary intent. If the disruption is large, local measures are used until the wound is clean and there is a good granulation bed. When this occurs, the defect is repaired using a gracilis or tensor fascia lata myocutaneous flap. Prolonged drainage or seromas in the bed of the groin dissection frequently occur and are managed by repeated aspiration. The other common serious complication seen in the immediate postoperative period is deep vein phlebitis, which is managed with anticoagulants in the standard manner. Disruption of the femoral vessels is a disastrous occurrence that arises from severe infection of the groin wound. It can largely be prevented by sartorius muscle transposition.

The most common chronic complication is edema of the lower extremity. The reported incidence is variable but exceeds 50% when carefully sought.[69] Various texts suggest that this can be prevented by the use of prolonged perioperative antibiotics or elastic stockings; there is little evidence

TABLE 14–41
Complications of Radical Vulvectomy and Bilateral Iliofemoral Lymphadenectomy

Type of Complication	No.	%
Early complications		
Wound separation, infection, necrosis	148	85
Urinary tract infection	32	18
Seroma	19	11
Phlebitis	16	9
Necrosis of pubic symphysis	1	<1
Femoral artery hemorrhage	1	<1
Other	17	10
Delayed complications		
Lower extremity edema	120	69
Lymphangitis, cellulitis, phlebitis	22	13
Vaginal stenosis, dyspareunia	22	13
Pelvic relaxation	20	11
Stress urinary incontinence	19	11
Hernia	8	5
Urethral stenosis or prolapse	4	2
Fistula	3	2
Fecal incontinence	1	<1
Rectal prolapse	1	<1
Other	15	9

Modified from Podratz KC, et al: Carcinoma of the vulva: Analysis of treatment and survival. Obstet Gynecol 61:63–74, 1983.

to support these claims. This complication is chronic and can be quite troublesome. Many women who try elastic stockings and leg elevation find these measures as uncomfortable and disruptive as the edema itself. Pelvic relaxation and its consequences,[70] including stress urinary incontinence, total urinary incontinence, and stool incontinence, are frequent postoperative occurrences. They may be corrected operatively several months after the radical vulvectomy. Vaginal stenosis (resulting in dyspareunia) or misdirected urinary stream is corrected after healing has taken place and the postoperative anatomy is stable. Relaxing incisions are made, with appropriate reconstruction.

Three-Incision Technique

In most instances, radical vulvectomy can be performed through three incisions.[71] Bilateral inguinal incisions are used for the inguinofemoral lymphadenectomy. The radical vulvectomy is performed using lateral incisions along the labiocrural folds, which are connected posteriorly across the perineum and anteriorly across the upper mons veneris. The lymph nodes are not removed en bloc with the vulva. Recurrence is rare in the skin bridges intervening between the vulvar and the groin incisions, or in the subcutaneous tissue underneath the skin bridges. Operating time and blood loss are lowered,[72] and the rate of wound breakdown is diminished to 10% to 20%,[68, 71] with no compromise in tumor control in properly selected cases.

Groin Reconstruction Using Cutaneous and Myocutaneous Flaps

Small defects that require tension for closure may be handled using rhomboid flaps swung from adjacent skin and subcutaneous tissue of the buttocks. This may be required to close the perineal wound following a three-incision procedure, especially after extensive dissection of a Bartholin's gland carcinoma. Larger defects, such as those produced by the classic operation with one incision, require a myocutaneous flap. The tensor fascia lata muscle is usually most satisfactory for this purpose, although the gracilis muscle may also be used. Construction of such flaps creates a better cosmetic result, reduces the probability of wound breakdown, and should be considered for routine use. The principal disadvantage is that this adds several hours to the procedure. Furthermore, the flap becomes necrotic up to 25% of the time.

Radical Vaginectomy

Radical vaginectomy consists of removal of the entire vagina and the paravaginal tissues. Reconstruction is by means of skin grafts or myocutaneous flaps. The procedure is used only occasionally for vaginal carcinoma. There are several disadvantages to the procedure. The vagina is quite inaccessible, leading to long operating time and extensive blood loss, which are poorly tolerated by the elderly patients with vaginal cancer. The proximity of the vagina to the urethra, bladder, and rectum precludes the surgeon from achieving good anterior and posterior tumor clearance.

Radiotherapy and Chemotherapy

Radiation treatment of vulvar carcinoma is feasible, but treatment considerations are complex. Discussion of radiation techniques is beyond the scope of this chapter; the applicability of radiation is discussed below. Vaginal carcinoma is usually treated with radiation. Whole pelvic fields are treated with a dose of 1.8 to 2.0 Gy daily; this is followed by brachytherapy in the form of vaginal cylinder or interstitial implant.

Chemotherapy has little role in the treatment of these tumors, except as adjuvant to radiation. This application is also discussed below.

PRIMARY OPERABLE DISEASE OF THE VULVA

Vulvar Intraepithelial Neoplasia

Fewer than 10% of VIN lesions progress to invasive cancer, and progression to malignancy may take many years.[36, 37] Recurrence of these lesions is common, however, no matter how aggressively they are treated. VIN is often found in young women to whom preservation of anatomic appearance and sexual function is extremely important. For these reasons, VIN should be treated as conservatively as possible, keeping in mind that invasive carcinoma is reportedly encountered in 10% to 20% of VIN lesions that are removed surgically.[38, 39] This suggests that every precaution should be taken to exclude invasion if a treatment regimen is planned that involves destruction rather than removal of the lesion. Prior to definitive treatment, the extent of VIN is determined by soaking the entire vulva with gauze saturated with 5% acetic acid for 5 minutes. Areas of skin containing VIN or HPV will blanch. Colposcopy is often helpful in delineating the extent of disease. If such acetowhite areas occur on skin that is grossly normal, they should be sampled for biopsy in order to map the extent of VIN. Thickened areas should be sampled generously. Only when the full extent of the lesion is known is therapy advisable.

Small, discrete lesions can be excised with skin margins of 1 cm and deep margins just below the dermis. Multiple or extensive lesions may be treated primarily by carbon dioxide laser ablation, provided invasive disease has been carefully ruled out in the manner outlined in the previous paragraph. If VIN persists, this procedure may be repeated once or twice. Fifty percent to 75% of patients are reportedly cured by one procedure; the cure rate reaches at least 90% after two or more ablative treatments.[73, 74] Baggish and coworkers[61] report a cure rate in this range using laser thin section. The inherent success of any ablative procedure is limited by the fact that disease may extend deep into the skin appendages in the reticular dermis.[75]

This problem can be overcome using skinning vulvectomy with split-thickness skin graft.[14, 76] Success rates described for this procedure are comparable to those obtained with laser surgery.[77] The added cost and disability of this operation have persuaded most gynecologists to reserve it for disease that persists after several attempts at more conservative management.

Simple vulvectomy, consisting of amputation of the labia, is occasionally indicated in elderly, apareunic women with extensive lesions and multiple medical problems.

Paget Disease of the Vulva

Treatment of Paget disease consists of wide excision with 2-cm lateral margins. The plane of the deep margin should be within the subcutaneous fat to ensure that all skin appendages are removed. This disease is notorious for histologic extension beyond its visible limits. For this reason, treatment, which consists of wide local excision, should be controlled using intraoperative frozen section.[78] Bergen and associates[78] encountered three recurrences in 14 patients treated. Two of the three had positive resection margins when originally treated.

Invasive Squamous Cell Carcinoma

Way[79] and Taussig[80] demonstrated during the 1940s and 1950s that en bloc removal of the vulva, the groin nodes, and all intervening tissues, along with pelvic lymphadenectomy up to the bifurcation of the common iliac, could markedly improve cure rates of squamous cell carcinoma from less than 25% to well over 50% of patients. Exenterative procedures subsequently came to be used for advanced lesions involving the anus, rectum, urethra, and bladder. These achieved a cure rate in at least half of all such patients.[81, 82] Such radical surgery represented the standard of care from 1960 to 1980.[83]

These procedures have high morbidity. In addition, they are somewhat mutilating, leading to psychologic[64] and sexual[65] dysfunction. In the last 20 years, a large volume of clinical investigation has been directed at decreasing the magnitude of operation needed to achieve the present high cure rates. A less extensive operation has proved effective in some categories of early disease. Locally advanced disease has been treated using multimodality therapy in order to avoid exenteration. At present, Way's unmodified technique of radical vulvectomy and bilateral groin dissection is rarely indicated, and exenteration is seldom necessary.

Disease Grossly Limited to the Vulva and Perineum

Lesions with invasion deeper than 1 mm display a significant incidence of lymph node metastases, irrespective of the status of the lymph nodes on physical examination (see Table 14–35).[16, 18, 22, 84] A quarter to a third of women with deeper vulvar carcinoma and palpably suspicious nodes will, in fact, not harbor metastases; a comparable proportion of women with palpably negative nodes will demonstrate metastases on histologic examination.[85, 86] A subset of carcinoma has been defined that consists of lateral lesions in which metastases are rare and are confined to ipsilateral nodes. In these lesions, contralateral nodes are almost never positive. Morris[87] proposed a modification of the Way technique of radical vulvectomy in which only the ipsilateral nodes are removed. Such modification was attempted by Hacker et al,[16] who demonstrated that contralateral lymph node dissection could be safely eliminated in stage I lesions but that further omission of ipsilateral lymphadenectomy resulted in groin recurrence in an unacceptable number of patients. It is also known that pelvic nodes are almost invariably unaffected unless there is tumor in the ipsilateral groin nodes.[9, 21, 88, 89] Consequently, treatment directed at the pelvic lymph nodes is unnecessary unless inguinal nodes are involved. Finally, a large collaborative randomized study conducted by the Gynecologic Oncology Group showed that treating women with positive groin nodes with pelvic irradiation results in higher survival than does pelvic lymphadenectomy.[90] Radiation in this circumstance is no more morbid than is the extended operation. There seems to be little role at the present time for pelvic lymphadenectomy in the treatment of vulvar carcinoma.

Primary operative treatment is now individualized based on the size, location, and status of the groin nodes. An algorithm for the treatment of vulvar carcinoma grossly confined to the vulva and perineum is shown in Figure 14–23.

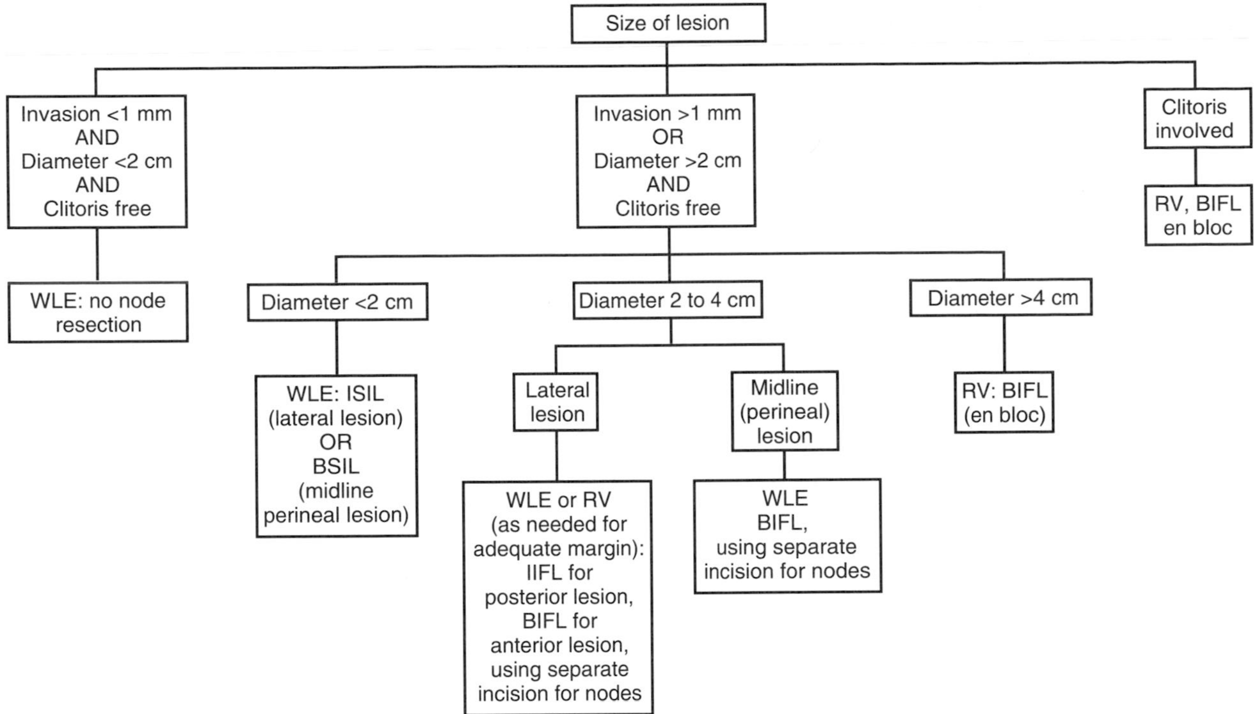

FIGURE 14–23. Treatment of vulvar carcinoma limited to the vulva and perineum.

If ipsilateral inguinofemoral nodes are involved on frozen section, contralateral inguinofemoral lymphadenectomy should be performed. **In all cases, if inguinofemoral groin nodes contain tumor, pelvic radiation should be given.** Radiation should be considered in patients who are medically unfit to undergo an operation.

WLE, Wide local excision; RV, radical vulvectomy; BIFL, bilateral inguinofemoral lymphadenectomy; ISIL, ipsilateral superficial inguinal lymphadenectomy; BSIL, bilateral superficial inguinal lymphadenectomy; IIFL, ipsilateral inguinofemoral lymphadenectomy.

Lesions less than 2 cm in diameter with invasion less than 1 mm below the basement membrane are rarely associated with metastases. These lesions may be excised with skin margins and deep margins of 1 cm, and lymphadenectomy is not warranted.[21, 84, 91]

The surgical treatment of larger carcinomas confined to the vulva and perineum requires two components: adequate resection of the primary lesion and removal of lymph nodes at risk.[71, 92, 93] Wide local excision may be adequate to obtain local control of many of these tumors.[93] Frequent lymph node metastases are present in all categories of lesion discussed below. Omission of lymphadenectomy[71] or even the performance of a superficial lymphadenectomy alone[94] leads to increased incidence of groin recurrence.

Midline and perineal lesions that are greater than 2 cm in diameter or 1 mm in depth (see Tables 14–34 and 14–35), which may occur on either side or bilaterally. They are best treated by radical vulvectomy and bilateral inguinofemoral lymphadenectomy. A posterior lesion may be treated using three incisions,[71] as may most anterior lesions. If an anterior lesion is sufficiently large that the surgeon is concerned about involvement of the skin bridges (i.e., lesions involving or near the clitoris), then the classic en bloc dissection is appropriate. If this is necessary, the defect is best repaired using a tensor fascia lata or other myocutaneous flap to prevent breakdown and to secure a good cosmetic effect.

Small lateral lesions less than 2 cm may be treated using wide local excision and ipsilateral pelvic lymphadenectomy. Lesions larger than 4 cm are treated using radical vulvectomy and ipsilateral groin dissection. All margins of the tumor excision should be 2 cm from the gross border of the lesion. This distance may be compromised somewhat if a 2-cm margin would result in urinary or fecal incontinence. Whether the surgeon removes the skin bridge between the vulva and the groin depends on the location of the lesion. Separate vulvectomy and groin incisions are used if this approach allows for adequate margins. Otherwise, the vulvectomy and groin dissection are performed en bloc. The surgeon must individualize the extent of the operation in women with lateral lesions between 2 and 4 cm in diameter.

When a lesion is sufficiently large to require inguinofemoral lymphadenectomy, the nodes should be submitted for frozen section. If this is positive for tumor, contralateral inguinofemoral lymph node dissection is warranted.

Patients whose medical condition contraindicates general anesthesia may be treated using radiotherapy.[95, 96] External radiation to the vulva and regional nodes is followed by a boost of electrons to the vulva or an interstitial implant of the tumor bed. It has not been demonstrated that this mode of therapy is as effective as and less morbid than the current operative management strategy. Most reported survival rates for patients receiving radiotherapy are inferior to those obtained by operation, but the radiation regimens were usually not administered according to current dosimetric guidelines. Essentially all patients receiving vulvar irradiation experience a temporary, but painful and disabling, moist desquamation of the vulva and perineum.

Alternatively, radical vulvectomy may be combined with irradiation of the groin nodes instead of groin dissection.[97] A recent study published by the Gynecologic Oncology Group[98] randomized women to receive either bilateral inguinofemoral lymphadenectomy or primary groin irradiation following radical vulvectomy. Those receiving radiation had a shorter interval to progression than did the patients who underwent node dissection. The incidence of groin recurrence was 19% in the irradiated patients; no woman experienced groin recurrence following lymphadenectomy.

Regionally Advanced Squamous Cell Carcinoma

As with lesions confined to the vulva and perineum, treatment modification has reduced the intrinsic morbidity of the therapy of vulvar carcinoma affecting the urethra, vagina, anus, and rectum. Pelvic exenteration was at one time the standard of care for these lesions.[81] There may be a role for individualized ultraradical operations involving radical vulvectomy, bilateral iliofemoral lymphadenectomy, and extensive resection of distal urethra or anus with adequate margins, but without urinary or fecal diversion.[67] Such an approach may be relatively satisfactory from the standpoint of tumor cure. The morbidity is even greater than for the standard Way radical vulvectomy, however. Urinary[99] and fecal incontinence are likely even if excretory organs are preserved. Recently, attention has been directed to preoperative irradiation for these locally advanced lesions.[95, 100–102] External irradiation is first employed to shrink the lesion to a sufficient degree that exenteration is unnecessary. This is followed by interstitial implant, wide local excision, vulvectomy, or radical vulvectomy with or without groin dissection, depending on the individual case. Although all reported series are small, local recurrence is only 5%[100] to 25%,[102] and overall survival seems comparable to that in patients treated with exenteration.

Complications of vulvar irradiation include moist desquamation of the vulva and femoral head necrosis. When radiation is combined with operation, the patient is subject to the usual postoperative sequelae.

The success of combined radiotherapy and chemotherapy in squamous cell carcinoma of the anus[103] has led a variety of investigators to attempt this approach in locally advanced vulvar disease. Concurrently with the radiation, the patient is given cytotoxic drugs that are known radiopotentiators. Various centers have employed a wide variety of drugs and radiation doses. Generally, an operation is performed only if there is residual tumor following chemotherapy and radiotherapy. Two trials employing a regimen analogous to that of Nigro and coworkers[103] using mitomycin and 5-fluorouracil[104, 105] demonstrated a complete response rate of 50%. Two recent trials that combined radiation with a cisplatin and 5-fluorouracil regimen demonstrated a combined complete response in 24 of 37 patients.[106, 107] Mature survival data are not yet available. All these trials are small pilot studies from which definitive conclusions cannot be drawn. Moist desquamation and toxic reactions specific to the individual cytotoxic agents are prominent features of all these regimens.

Basal Cell and Verrucous Carcinomas

Basal cell and verrucous lesions are treated using wide local excision,[49, 50, 108, 109] as they are locally invasive but rarely metastasize to lymph nodes.[108, 110, 111] As with their counterparts on other areas of the skin, basal cell lesions may be treated by local irradiation. It is not clear why either a physician or a patient would want to do so, however, since local excision is simpler and less morbid. Verrucous lesions should not be irradiated, as they may undergo anaplastic transformation.[109, 112]

Melanoma

Melanoma lesions are insensitive to radiotherapy and chemotherapy and must be treated by operation. They are solitary, so local resection with 2-cm margins in all directions usually secures local control.[113–115] If inguinal nodes are positive, distant recurrence is almost certain. Nevertheless, avoidance of groin recurrence is highly desirable. Consequently, ipsilateral lymphadenectomy (bilateral for a central lesion, which is common) should be performed for all lesions deeper than Clark (or Breslow) level I.[115] This appears to be successful in reducing the incidence of regional occurrence to a minimum.[116] Almost all patients with level I and II disease will be cured by operation,[116, 117] and more than half of those with level III disease will survive at least 5 years.[115] Level IV and V tumors, or melanomas metastatic to lymph nodes, are usually fatal.[115]

Bartholin's Gland Carcinoma

If localized, Bartholin's gland lesions are managed using wide local excision, which may require extensive lateral and superior dissection. Unilateral or bilateral inguinal lymphadenectomy is performed. Routine postoperative irradiation may improve survival,[53] which is worse than in squamous cell carcinoma.[53, 55]

Outcome of Treatment

Survival in vulvar carcinoma is related to a number of factors. Those relating to the extent of the tumor at the time of diagnosis seem to be the most important (Table 14–42).[118] The more important parameters include the diameter of the lesion, the node status, and the surgical

TABLE 14—42
Analyses of Vulvar Carcinoma Predictors of Survival

Predictor of Survival	Number of Studies: *Examining the Predictor*	*Finding the Predictor Significant*
Age	6	3
Size	7	6
Grade	6	2
FIGO stage (clinical)	7	3
Node status (clinical)	4	2
Node status (surgical)	6	6
Margins	3	1
Lymph vessel involvement	3	3

Adapted from Rutledge FN, et al: Prognostic indicators for invasive carcinoma of the vulva. Gynecol Oncol 42:239–244, 1991.

stage. With the exception of tumors of the clitoris, which frequently are associated with metastases to nodes, the location of the primary vulvar lesion is not related to the probability of metastasis or survival.[8]

If disease is limited to the vulva and perineum, at least 90% of properly treated patients survive for five or more years, which is tantamount to cure.[21, 69, 82, 119] The consensus of recent studies is that five-year survival falls to about 40% if groin nodes contain tumor, and to less than 20% if pelvic nodes are affected. The number of tumor-bearing nodes is also important. Podratz and colleagues[69] report that five-year survival falls to 57% when one node is involved, and to 37% when two nodes are involved. A Gynecologic Oncology Group (GOG) staging study[120] reported 91% survival with no nodes, 75% with one or two nodes, 36% with three or four, 24% with five or six, and no survivors with seven or more nodes. The same study documents a 75% five-year survival with ipsilaterally positive nodes, but less than 30% with contralateral or bilateral involvement.

The diameter of the lesion also affects five-year survival, with lower survival as the tumor exceeds 2 to 3 cm.[69, 120, 121] The GOG study[120] also demonstrated a highly significant influence on survival by histologic grade, vascular invasion, and tumor thickness. The surgical stage correlates closely with five-year survival. This survival was 98% in Stage I, 85% in Stage II, 74% in Stage III, and 31% in Stage IV disease. Its authors defined four risk categories based on tumor diameter and status of nodes which were felt to be more precise predictors of prognosis (Table 14–43).

Recurrence

Most recurrences occur in the vulva and groin (Table 14–44).[12, 69, 123] Treatment of recurrences is highly individualized. Vulvar recurrences may be treated using 45 to 50 Gy of external radiation followed by excision of the tumor bed[12] or an interstitial implant.[124] Most studies indicate that more than half of women with recurrent vulvar carcinoma

TABLE 14–43
Gynecologic Oncology Group Risk Categories for Vulvar Carcinoma[120]

Node Status	Tumor Diameter: *<2 cm*	*2–8 cm*	*>8 cm*
All negative	M	L	I
1 positive	L	I	I
2 positive	I	I	H
>2 positive	H	H	H
Bilaterally positive; any number	H	H	H

M, Minimal: 98% 5-year survival; L, low: 87% 5-year survival; I, intermediate: 75% 5-year survival; H, high: 29% 5-year survival.

confined to the vulvar skin will live 5 years.[69, 123, 125–127] Groin metastases have been treated for attempted cure using radiation[124] or operation,[125] which can be quite radical.[128] Nevertheless, survival following groin metastases is well under 25% at 5 years. Pelvic and distant recurrences are almost never cured. Women with incurable vulvar and groin metastases have a terrible quality of life. They are afflicted by severe pain as a result of involvement of the femoral nerve and the lumbosacral plexus. They generally experience massive edema of the lower extremities. Malodorous friable tumor erodes through the skin. These symptoms may persist many months because of the distance of the groin and vulva from vital structures.

PRIMARY OPERABLE LESIONS OF THE VAGINA

Vaginal Intraepithelial Neoplasia

Laser ablation or wide local surgical excision is the treatment of choice for VaIN. Treatment with 1 ml of 5-fluorouracil cream intravaginally each week for 12 weeks is often effective in extensive or persistent lesions but may result in chronic painful vaginal ulcerations. The medicine is self-administered at night, protecting the vulva using zinc

TABLE 14–44
Site of Recurrence of Vulvar Carcinoma in Five Reports

References	No. Recurrences/Recurrences by Site:* *No. Patients†*	*Vulva*	*Groin*	*Pelvis, Distant*
Krupp[18]	24/153 (16%)	12 (50%)	4 (17%)	8 (33%)
Piura[125]	73/376 (19%)	—	—	—
Podratz[69]	74/224 (33%)	40 (54%)	13 (18%)	21 (27%)
Simonsen[126]	60/244 (25%)	29 (48%)	12 (20%)	19 (42%)
Tilmans[122]	40‡	17 (43%)	12 (30%)	11 (28%)

*Percentages denote patients with recurrence at each site as a percentage of all recurrences.

†Percentages in parentheses denote all patients with recurrence as a percentage of all patients with vulvar carcinoma.

‡The report did not specify the total number of patients treated for vulvar cancer but only the number of recurrences seen at this institution.

oxide ointment. A tampon is inserted after the medicine to prevent it from leaking. Intracavitary radiation using vaginal cylinders is a last resort in elderly women. Operative removal of the lesions may be indicated if more conservative treatment fails. Extensive resection is seldom indicated, although total vaginectomy with reconstruction must occasionally be employed.

Invasive Carcinoma

Most involved patients are elderly, and many have had hysterectomy or irradiation. The vagina is relatively inaccessible, and radical vaginectomy is associated with bleeding and complications. Consequently, radiation is generally employed if the patient has not previously received radiation (Table 14–45).[129] Radical hysterectomy and vaginectomy, or exenteration, together with pelvic or inguinal lymphadenectomy, may be used to treat young women with adenocarcinoma, or women of any age in whom previous radiation precludes another course of radiotherapy. In this case, reconstruction with gracilis myocutaneous flaps or split-thickness skin grafts, or both, may be used to preserve sexual function.

Tumor extending outside the vagina is inoperable and is treated with radiation. If the carcinoma is confined to the pelvis, the intent of therapy is curative.

Other Vaginal Malignancies

Melanoma

Malignant melanoma is the second most common cancer of the vagina, behind squamous cell, accounting for 3% to 5% of all vaginal malignancies.[130] Primary tumors are thought to arise from vaginal melanocytes in otherwise normal women.[131] Any site in the vagina can be involved, but most melanomas occur in the posterior lower third of the vaginal wall.[132] A thorough search for another genital or extragenital primary site is mandatory, as more vaginal melanomas are metastatic rather than primary. Vaginal melanomas are most common between the ages of 40 and 70. Grossly, they show considerable variation in size, color, and growth pattern.[133]

Tumor depth according to the Breslow method[134] (see Chapter 16) should be determined, because this information is the best predictor of survival.[135] In general, this cancer has a poor prognosis, with fewer than 10% of reported patients surviving beyond 5 years.[136]

Wide local excision, with or without hysterectomy, plus inguinal or pelvic lymphadenectomy is the mainstay of therapy. Local control is usually achieved with this therapeutic approach.[135] Pelvic exenteration, which used to be routine treatment, is now rarely indicated. Chemotherapy and radiotherapy are also of limited clinical benefit.[137]

Sarcoma

In adults, leiomyosarcoma is the most common vaginal sarcoma but accounts for only a small percentage of all vaginal lesions. It presents as a firm submucosal mass. Prognosis is based on the histologic grade, which is directly dependent on the frequency of mitoses. Metastatic spread may occur by either lymphatic or hematogenous routes, the latter being more common.

Wide local excision, with or without removal of adjacent organs (e.g., uterus, bladder, or rectum), is the preferred treatment of choice. Adjuvant chemotherapy is of limited value. However, postoperative radiation, particularly when employing modern brachytherapy techniques, may help achieve local control.

Embryonal rhabdomyosarcoma (sarcoma botryoides) is a disease of children and adolescents. It occurs up to age 16, with median occurrence at 2 to 3 years. These tumors grow rapidly, have a grapelike appearance, and are frequently associated with either a vaginal discharge or bleeding. Rhabdomyosarcoma of the vagina is now generally treated with a combined-modality approach. This begins with the most conservative possible local excision, which may involve hysterectomy or other relatively extensive procedures if the uterus is involved or the tumor is extensive. Treatment is consolidated using low-dose irradiation and systemic chemotherapy. The cytotoxic agents of choice

TABLE 14–45
Radiation Treatment of Vaginal Carcinoma

FIGO Stage	External Radiation: *Whole Pelvis*	External Radiation: *Parametrium*	Brachytherapy	Tumor Dose (Total)
VaIN	—	—	IC 65–80 Gy to tumor; 60 Gy to vagina	65–80 Gy
I (superficial)	—	—	IC 65–80 Gy to vagina	65–80 Gy
I (0.5 cm thick)	—	—	IC or IS 65–70 Gy at 0.5 cm depth; 100 Gy at surface	65–70 Gy
II	20 Gy	30 Gy	IC or IS 60–70 Gy TD	70–75 Gy
III, IV	40 Gy	10 Gy	IC 50–60 Gy; IS 20–30 Gy boost to parametrium	80 Gy

From Perez CA: Vaginal cancer. In Perez CA, Brady LW (eds): Principles and Practice of Radiation Oncology, 2nd ed. Philadelphia: JB Lippincott, 1992, pp 1258–1272.

VaIN, Vaginal intraepithelial neoplasia; IC, intracavitary; IS, interstitial (dose calculated at 0.5 cm from plane of implant); TD, total dose.

Note: For distal vaginal lesions, deliver 50 Gy to inguinofemoral nodes at 3 cm.

are vincristine, actinomycin D, and cyclophosphamide (VAC).[138, 139] Survival rates in patients treated with this combined approach are as high as 75% at 5 years.[140, 141] Survivors may retain their future reproductive capabilities if hysterectomy or vaginectomy is not indicated.

Endodermal Sinus Tumor (Yolk Sac Tumor)

Yolk sac tumors of the vagina are rare and occur almost invariably before 2 years of age. They may be pure, or they may contain other germ cell elements. Rhabdomyosarcoma and mesonephric papilloma, a benign müllerian origin lesion, are the main differential diagnostic entities.[24]

The prognosis of these tumors has significantly improved since the introduction of effective adjuvant chemotherapy following local excision.[142] Chemotherapy consists of a combination of either vincristine, dactinomycin, and cyclophosphamide or bleomycin, etoposide, and cisplatin. Serum alpha-fetoprotein serves as a useful marker for monitoring the success of treatment.

References

1. Rose PG, Herterick EE, Boutselis JG, et al: Multiple primary gynecologic neoplasms. Am J Obstet Gynecol 157:261–267, 1987.
2. Crum CP: Carcinoma of the vulva: Epidemiology and pathogenesis. Obstet Gynecol 79:448–454, 1992.
3. Hay DM, Cole FM: Primary invasive carcinoma of the vulva in Jamaica. J Obstet Gynaecol Br Commonw 76:821–830, 1969.
4. Brinton LA, Nasca PC, Mallin K, et al: Case-control study of cancer of the vulva. Obstet Gynecol 75:859–866, 1990.
5. Plentl AA, Friedman EA: Lymphatic System of the Female Genitalia. Philadelphia: WB Saunders, 1971.
6. Chu J, Tamimi HK, Figge DC: Femoral node metastases with negative superficial inguinal nodes in early vulvar cancer. Am J Obstet Gynecol 140:337–338, 1981.
7. Iversen T, Aas M: Lymph drainage from the vulva. Gynecol Oncol 16:179–189, 1983.
8. Iversen T: Squamous cell carcinoma of the vulva: Localization of the primary tumor and lymph node metastases. Acta Obstet Gynecol Scand 60:211–214, 1981.
9. Curry SL, Wharton JT, Rutledge F: Positive lymph nodes in vulvar squamous carcinoma. Gynecol Oncol 9:63–67, 1980.
10. Ericsson E, Eldh J, Peterson L-E: Surgical treatment of carcinoma of the clitoris. Gynecol Oncol 17:291–295, 1984.
11. Piver MS, Xynos FP: Pelvic lymphadenectomy in women with carcinoma of the clitoris. Obstet Gynecol 49:592–595, 1977.
12. Simonsen E: Invasive squamous cell carcinoma of the vulva. Ann Chir Gynaecol 72:331–338, 1984.
13. Krupp PJ, Bohm JW: Lymph gland metastases in invasive squamous cell cancer of the vulva. Am J Obstet Gynecol 130:943–952, 1978.
14. Rutledge F, Sinclair M: Treatment of intraepithelial carcinoma of the vulva by skin excision and graft. Am J Obstet Gynecol 102:806–818, 1968.
15. Monaghan JM, Hammond IG: Pelvic node dissection in the treatment of vulval carcinoma—is it necessary? Br J Obstet Gynaecol 91:270–274, 1984.
16. Hacker NF, Berek JS, Lagasse LD, et al: Individualization of treatment for stage I squamous cell vulvar carcinoma. Obstet Gynecol 63:155–162, 1984.
17. FIGO news: Definitions of the clinical stages in carcinoma of the vulva (correlation of the FIGO, UICC and AJCC nomenclatures). Int J Gynecol Obstet 28:189–190, 1989.
18. Krupp PJ, Lee YL, Bohm JW, et al: Prognostic parameters and clinical staging criteria in epidermoid carcinoma of the vulva. Obstet Gynecol 46:84–88, 1975.
19. Husseinzadeh N, Wesseler T, Schneider T, et al: Prognostic factors and the significance of cytologic grading in invasive squamous cell carcinoma of the vulva: A clinicopathologic study. Gynecol Oncol 36:192–199, 1990.
20. Donaldson ES, Powell DE, Hanson MB, et al: Prognostic parameters in invasive vulvar cancer. Gynecol Oncol 11:184–190, 1981.
21. Hacker NF, Berek JS, Lagasse LD, et al: Management of regional lymph nodes and their prognostic influence in vulvar cancer. Obstet Gynecol 61:408–412, 1983.
22. Sedlis A, Homesley H, Bundy BN, et al: Positive groin lymph nodes in superficial squamous cell vulvar cancer: A Gynecologic Oncology Group study. Am J Obstet Gynecol 156:1159–1164, 1987.
23. Peters WA III, Kumar NB, Morley GW: Carcinoma of the vulva. Cancer 55:892–897, 1985.
24. Young RC, Fuks Z, Hoskins WJ: Cancer of the vagina. In DeVita VT, Hellman S, Rosenberg SA (eds): Cancer: Principles and Practice of Oncology, 3rd ed. Philadelphia: JB Lippincott, 1989, pp 1165–1167.
25. Brinton LA, Nasca PC, Mallin K, et al: Case-control study of cancer of the vagina. Gynecol Oncol 38:49–54, 1990.
26. Okagaki T: Female genital tumors associated with human papillomavirus infection, and the concept of a genital neoplasms-papilloma syndrome (GENPS) (Part 2). Pathol Annu 19:31–62, 1984.
27. Rutledge FN: Cancer of the vagina. Am J Obstet Gynecol 97:635–655, 1967.
28. Way S: Primary carcinoma of the vagina. J Obstet Gynaecol Br Emp 55:739–758, 1948.
29. Herbst AL, Ulfelder H, Poskanzer DC: Adenocarcinoma of the vagina: Association of maternal stilbestrol therapy with tumor appearance in young women. N Engl J Med 284:878–881, 1971.
30. Manetta A, Gutrecht EL, Berman ML, et al: Primary invasive carcinoma of the vagina. Obstet Gynecol 76:639–642, 1990.
31. Benedet JL, Murphy KJ, Fairey RN, et al: Primary invasive carcinoma of the vagina. Obstet Gynecol 62:715–719, 1983.
32. Daw E: Primary carcinoma of the vagina. J Obstet Gynaecol Br Commonw 78:853–856, 1971.
33. Crum CP, Fu YS, Levine RU, et al: Intraepithelial squamous lesions of the vulva: Biologic and histologic criteria for the distinction of condylomas from vulvar intraepithelial neoplasia. Am J Obstet Gynecol 144:77–84, 1982.
34. Bernstein SG, Kovacs BR, Townsend DE, et al: Vulvar carcinoma in situ. Obstet Gynecol 61:304–307, 1983.
35. Husseinzadeh N, Newman NJ, Wesseler TA: Vulvar intraepithelial neoplasia: A clinicopathologic study of carcinoma in situ of the vulva. Gynecol Oncol 33:157–163, 1989.
36. Buscema J, Woodruff JD, Parmley TH, et al: Carcinoma in situ of the vulva. Obstet Gynecol 55:225–230, 1980.
37. Ragnarsson B, Raabe N, Willems J, et al: Carcinoma in situ of the vulva: Long term prognosis. Acta Oncol 26:277–280, 1987.
38. Caglar H, Tamer S, Hreshchyshyn MM: Vulvar intraepithelial neoplasia. Obstet Gynecol 60:346–349, 1981.
39. Chafe W, Richards A, Morgan L, et al: Unrecognized invasive carcinoma in vulvar intraepithelial neoplasia (VIN). Gynecol Oncol 31:154–162, 1988.
40. Creasman WT, Gallagher HS, Rutledge F: Paget's disease of the vulva. Gynecol Oncol 3:133–148, 1975.
41. Curtin JP, Rubin SC, Jones WB, et al: Paget's disease of the vulva. Gynecol Oncol 39:374–377, 1990.
42. Nadji M, Ganji P: The application of immunoperoxidase techniques in the evaluation of vulvar and vaginal disease. In Wilkinson EJ (ed): Contemporary Issues in Surgical Pathology, vol 9. New York: Churchill Livingstone, 1987, pp 239–249.
43. Shah KD, Tabibzadeh SS, Gerber MA: Immunohistochemical distinction of Paget's disease from Bowen's disease and superficial spreading melanoma with the use of monoclonal cytokeratin antibodies. Am J Clin Pathol 88:689–695, 1987.
44. Feuer GA, Shevchuk M, Calanog A: Vulvar Paget's disease: The need to exclude an invasive lesion. Gynecol Oncol 38:81–89, 1990.
45. DiSaia PJ, Creasman WT: Invasive cancer of the vulva. In Clinical Gynecologic Oncology, 4th ed. St. Louis: Mosby, 1993, pp 238–272.
46. Stacy D, Burrell MO, Franklin EW III: Extramammary Paget's disease of the vulva and anus: Use of intraoperative frozen section margins. Am J Obstet Gynecol 155:519–523, 1986.
47. Johnson TL, Kumar NB, White CD: Prognostic features of vulvar melanoma: A clinicopathologic analysis. Int J Gynecol Pathol 5:110–118, 1986.

48. Chung AF, Woodruff JM, Lewis JL Jr: Malignant melanoma of the vulva: A report of 44 cases. Obstet Gynecol 45:638–646, 1975.
49. Breen JL, Neubecker RD, Greenwald E, et al: Basal cell carcinoma of the vulva. Obstet Gynecol 46:122–129, 1974.
50. Deppisch LM: Basal cell carcinoma of the vulva. Mt Sinai J Med 45:406–410, 1978.
51. Isaacs JH: Verrucous carcinoma of the female genital tract. Gynecol Oncol 4:259–269, 1976.
52. Zaino RJ: Carcinoma of the vulva, urethra and Bartholin's gland. In Wilkinson EJ (ed): Pathology of the Vagina and Vulva: Contemporary Issues in Surgical Pathology, vol 9. New York: Churchill Livingstone, 1987, pp 119–137.
53. Copeland LJ, Sneige N, Gershenson DM, et al: Bartholin gland carcinoma. Obstet Gynecol 67:794–801, 1986.
54. Leuchter RS, Hacker NF, Voet RL, et al: Primary carcinoma of the Bartholin gland: A report of 14 cases and review of the literature. Obstet Gynecol 60:361–368, 1982.
55. Wheelock JB, Gopelrud DR, Dunn LJ, et al: Primary carcinoma of the Bartholin gland: A report of ten cases. Obstet Gynecol 63:820–824, 1984.
56. Davos I, Abell MR: Soft tissue sarcomas of the vulva. Gynecol Oncol 4:70–86, 1976.
57. Melnick S, Cole P, Anderson D, et al: Rates and risks of diethylstilbestrol-related clear-cell carcinoma of the vagina and cervix: An update. N Engl J Med 316:514–516, 1987.
58. Spitzer M, Krumholz BA, Seltzer VL: The multicentric nature of disease related to human papillomavirus infection of the lower genital tract. Obstet Gynecol 73:303–307, 1989.
59. Reid R, Elfont EA, Zirkin RM, et al: Superficial laser vulvectomy. II. The anatomic and biophysical principles permitting accurate control over the depth of dermal destruction with the carbon dioxide laser. Am J Obstet Gynecol 152:261–271, 1985.
60. Reid R: Superficial laser vulvectomy. III. A new surgical technique for appendage-conserving ablation of refractory condylomas and vulvar intraepithelial neoplasia. Am J Obstet Gynecol 152:504–509, 1985.
61. Baggish MS, Sze EHM, Adelson MD, et al: Quantitative evaluation of the skin and accessory appendages in vulvar carcinoma in situ. Obstet Gynecol 74:169–174, 1989.
62. Julian TM, O'Connell BJ, Gosewehr JA: Indications, techniques and advantages of partial laser vulvectomy. Obstet Gynecol 80:140–143, 1992.
63. Chafe W, Fowler WC, Walton LA, et al: Radical vulvectomy with use of tensor fascia lata myocutaneous flap. Am J Obstet Gynecol 145:207–213, 1983.
64. Andersen BL, Hacker NF: Psychosexual adjustment after vulvar surgery. Obstet Gynecol 62:457–461, 1983.
65. Weijmar Schultz WCN, van de Wiel HBM, Bouma J, et al: Psychosexual functioning after the treatment of cancer of the vulva. Cancer 66:402–407, 1990.
66. Ilika KL, Duff P: Use of the urinary director appliance for management of voiding problems after radical vulvectomy. Am J Obstet Gynecol 156:72–73, 1987.
67. Cavanagh D, Fiorica JV, Hoffman MS, et al: Invasive carcinoma of the vulva. Changing trends in surgical management. Am J Obstet Gynecol 163:1007–1015, 1990.
68. Lin JY, DuBeshter B, Angel C, et al: Morbidity and recurrence with modification of radical vulvectomy and groin dissection. Gynecol Oncol 47:80–86, 1992.
69. Podratz KC, Symmonds RE, Taylor WF, et al: Carcinoma of the vulva: Analysis of treatment and survival. Obstet Gynecol 61:63–74, 1983.
70. Calame RJ: Pelvic relaxation as a complication of the radical vulvectomy. Obstet Gynecol 55:716–719, 1980.
71. Hacker NF, Leuchter RS, Berek JS, et al: Radical vulvectomy and bilateral inguinal lymphadenectomy through separate groin incisions. Obstet Gynecol 58:574–579, 1981.
72. Helm CW, Hatch K, Austin JM, et al: A matched comparison of single and triple incision techniques for the surgical treatment of carcinoma of the vulva. Gynecol Oncol 46:150–156, 1992.
73. Townsend DE, Levine RU, Richart RM, et al: Management of vulvar intraepithelial neoplasia by carbon dioxide laser. Obstet Gynecol 60:49–52, 1982.
74. Wright VC, Davies E: Laser surgery for vulvar intraepithelial neoplasia: Principles and results. Am J Obstet Gynecol 156:374–378, 1987.
75. Shatz P, Bergeron C, Wilkinson EJ, et al: Vulvar intraepithelial neoplasia and skin appendage involvement. Obstet Gynecol 74:769–774, 1989.
76. DiSaia PJ, Rich WM: Surgical approach to multifocal carcinoma in situ of the vulva. Am J Obstet Gynecol 140:136–145, 1981.
77. Rettenmaier MA, Berman ML, DiSaia PJ: Skinning vulvectomy for the treatment of multifocal vulvar intraepithelial neoplasia. Obstet Gynecol 69:247–250, 1987.
78. Bergen S, DiSaia PJ, Liao SY, et al: Conservative management of extramammary Paget's disease of the vulva. Gynecol Oncol 33:151–156, 1989.
79. Way S: Carcinoma of the vulva. Am J Obstet Gynecol 79:692–697, 1960.
80. Taussig FJ: Cancer of the vulva: An analysis of 155 cases. Am J Obstet Gynecol 40:764–779, 1940.
81. Cavanagh D, Shepard JH: The place of pelvic exenteration in the primary management of advanced carcinoma of the vulva. Gynecol Oncol 13:318–322, 1982.
82. Morley GW: Infiltrative carcinoma of the vulva: Results of surgical treatment. Am J Obstet Gynecol 124:874–888, 1976.
83. Morley GW: Cancer of the vulva: A review. Cancer 48:597–601, 1981.
84. Iversen T, Abeler V, Aalders J: Individualized treatment of stage I carcinoma of the vulva. Obstet Gynecol 57:85–89, 1981.
85. Iversen T: The value of groin palpation in epidermoid carcinoma of the vulva. Gynecol Oncol 12:291–295, 1981.
86. Shanbour KA, Mannel RS, Morris PC, et al: Comparison of clinical versus surgical staging systems in vulvar cancer. Obstet Gynecol 80:827–830, 1992.
87. Morris JM: A formula for selective lymphadenectomy: Its application to cancer of the vulva. Obstet Gynecol 50:152–158, 1977.
88. Benedet JL, Turko M, Fairey RN, et al: Squamous carcinoma of the vulva: Results of treatment, 1938 to 1976. Am J Obstet Gynecol 134:201–206, 1979.
89. Cavanagh D, Roberts WS, Bryson SCP, et al: Changing trends in the surgical treatment of invasive carcinoma of the vulva. Surg Gynecol Obstet 162:164–168, 1986.
90. Homesley HD, Bundy BN, Sedlis A, et al: Radiation therapy versus pelvic node resection for carcinoma of the vulva with positive groin nodes. Obstet Gynecol 68:733–740, 1986.
91. Kelley JL III, Burke TW, Tornos C, et al: Minimally invasive vulvar carcinoma: An indication for conservative therapy. Gynecol Oncol 44:240–244, 1992.
92. Iversen T, Abeler V, Aalders J: Individualized treatment of stage I carcinoma of the vulva. Obstet Gynecol 57:85–89, 1981.
93. Stehman FB, Bundy BN, Dvoretsky PM, et al: Early stage I carcinoma of the vulva treated with ipsilateral superficial inguinal lymphadenectomy and modified radical hemivulvectomy: A prospective study of the Gynecologic Oncology Group. Obstet Gynecol 79:490–497, 1992.
94. Burke TW, Stringer A, Gershenson DM, et al: Radical wide excision and selective inguinal node dissection for squamous cell carcinoma of the vulva. Gynecol Oncol 38:328–332, 1990.
95. Fairey RN, MacKay PA, Benedet JL, et al: Radiation treatment of carcinoma of the vulva, 1950–1980. Am J Obstet Gynecol 151:591–597, 1985.
96. Pao WM, Perez CA, Kuske RR, et al: Radiation therapy and conservation surgery for primary and recurrent carcinoma of the vulva: Report of 40 patients and a review of the literature. Int J Radiat Oncol Biol Phys 14:1123–1132, 1988.
97. Daly JW, Million RR: Radical vulvectomy combined with elective node irradiation for T_xN_0 squamous carcinoma of the vulva. Cancer 34:161–165, 1974.
98. Stehman FB, Bundy BN, Thomas G, et al: Groin dissection versus groin irradiation in carcinoma of the vulva. Int J Radiat Oncol Biol Phys 24:389–396, 1992.
99. Reid GC, DeLancey JO, Hopkins MP, et al: Urinary incontinence following radical vulvectomy. Obstet Gynecol 75:852–857, 1990.
100. Boronow RC: Combined therapy as an alternative to exenteration for locally advanced vulvo-vaginal cancer: Rationale and results. Cancer 49:1085–1091, 1982.
101. Hacker NF, Berek JS, Juillard GJF, et al: Preoperative radiation

therapy for locally advanced vulvar cancer. Cancer 54:2056–2061, 1984.

102. Rotmensch J, Rubin SJ, Sutton HG, et al: Preoperative radiotherapy followed by radical vulvectomy with inguinal lymphadenectomy for advanced vulvar carcinomas. Gynecol Oncol 36:181–184, 1990.
103. Nigro ND, Seydel HG, Considine B, et al: Combined preoperative radiation and chemotherapy for squamous cell carcinoma of the anal canal. Cancer 51:1826–1829, 1983.
104. Evans LS, Kersh CR, Constable WC, et al: Concomitant 5-fluorouracil, mitomycin C, and radiotherapy for advanced gynecologic malignancies. Int J Radiat Oncol Biol Phys 15:901–906, 1988.
105. Thomas G, Dembo A, DePetrillo A, et al: Concurrent radiation and chemotherapy in vulvar cancer. Gynecol Oncol 34:263–267, 1989.
106. Berek JS, Heaps JM, Fu YS, et al: Concurrent cisplatin and 5-fluorouracil chemotherapy and radiation therapy for advanced-stage squamous carcinoma of the vulva. Gynecol Oncol 42:197–201, 1991.
107. Russell AH, Mesic JB, Scudder SA, et al: Synchronous radiation and cytotoxic chemotherapy for locally advanced or recurrent squamous cancer of the vulva. Gynecol Oncol 47:14–20, 1992.
108. Gallousis S: Verrucous carcinoma: Report of three vulvar cases and a review of the literature. Obstet Gynecol 40:502–507, 1972.
109. Japaze H, Dinh TV, Woodruff JD: Verrucous carcinoma of the vulva: Study of 24 cases. Obstet Gynecol 60:462–466, 1982.
110. Hoffman MS, Roberts WS, Ruffolo EH: Basal cell carcinoma of the vulva with inguinal lymph node metastases. Gynecol Oncol 29:113–119, 1988.
111. Sworn MI, Hammond GT, Buchanan R: Metastatic basal cell carcinoma of the vulva: A case report. Br J Obstet Gynaecol 86:332–334, 1979.
112. Demian SDE, Bushkin FL, Echevarria RA: Perineural invasion and anaplastic transformation of verrucous carcinoma. Cancer 32:395–401, 1973.
113. Davidson T, Kissin M, Westbury GV: Vulvo-vaginal melanoma—should radical surgery be abandoned? Br J Obstet Gynaecol 94:473–476, 1987.
114. Rose PG, Piver MS, Tsukada Y, et al: Conservative therapy for melanoma of the vulva. Am J Obstet Gynecol 159:52–55, 1988.
115. Trimble EL, Lewis JL Jr, Williams LL, et al: Management of vulvar melanoma. Gynecol Oncol 45:254–258, 1992.
116. Podratz KC, Gaffey TA, Symmonds RE, et al: Melanoma of the vulva: An update. Gynecol Oncol 16:153–168, 1983.
117. Jaramillo BA, Ganjei P, Averette H, et al: Malignant melanoma of the vulva. Obstet Gynecol 66:398–403, 1985.
118. Rutledge FN, Mitchell MF, Munsell MF, et al: Prognostic indicators for invasive carcinoma of the vulva. Gynecol Oncol 42:239–244, 1991.
119. Hopkins MP, Reid GC, Johnston CM, et al: A comparison of staging systems for squamous cell carcinoma of vulva. Gynecol Oncol 47:34–37, 1992.
120. Homesley HD, Bundy BN, Sedlis A, et al: Assessment of current International Federation of Gynecology and Obstetrics staging of vulvar carcinoma relative to prognostic factors for survival (a Gynecologic Oncology Group study). Am J Obstet Gynecol 164:997–1004, 1991.
121. Krupp P, Bohm JW, Lee FYL, et al: Current status of the treatment of epidermoid carcinoma of the vulva. Cancer 38:587–595, 1976.
122. Tilmans AS, Sutton GP, Look KY, et al: Recurrent squamous carcinoma of the vulva. Am J Obstet Gynecol 167:1383–1389, 1992.
123. Prempree T, Amornmarn R: Radiation treatment of recurrent carcinoma of the vulva. Cancer 54:1943–1949, 1984.
124. Hopkins MP, Reid GC, Morley GW: The surgical management of recurrent squamous cell carcinoma of the vulva. Obstet Gynecol 75:1001–1005, 1990.
125. Piura B, Masotina A, Murdoch J, et al: Recurrent squamous cell carcinoma of the vulva: A study of 73 cases. Gynecol Oncol 48:189–195, 1993.
126. Simonsen E: Treatment of recurrent squamous cell carcinoma of the vulva. Acta Radiol Oncol Scand 23:345–349, 1984.
127. Powell JL, Donovan JT, Reed WP: Hip disarticulation for recurrent vulvar cancer in the groin. Gynecol Oncol 47:110–113, 1992.
128. Perez CA: Vaginal cancer. In Perez CA, Brady LW (eds): Principles and Practice of Radiation Oncology, 2nd ed. Philadelphia: JB Lippincott, 1992, pp 1258–1272.
129. Iversen K, Robins RE: Mucosal malignant melanomas. Am J Surg 139:660–664, 1980.
130. Nigogosyan G, De La Peva S, Pickren JW: Melanoblasts in vaginal mucosa: Origin for primary malignant melanoma. Cancer 17:912–913, 1964.
131. Chung AF, Casey MJ, Flannery JT, et al: Malignant melanoma of the vagina: Report of 19 cases. Obstet Gynecol 55:720–727, 1980.
132. Ragni MV, Tobon H: Primary malignant melanoma of the vagina and vulva. Obstet Gynecol 43:658–664, 1974.
133. Breslow A: Tumor thickness, level of invasion and node dissection in stage I cutaneous melanoma. Ann Surg 182:572–575, 1975.
134. Bonner JA, Perez-Tamayo C, Reid GC, et al: The management of vaginal melanoma. Cancer 62:2066–2072, 1988.
135. Pomante RG: Malignant melanoma primary in the vagina. Gynecol Oncol 3:15–20, 1975.
136. Morrow P, DiSaia PJ: Malignant melanoma of the female genitalia: A clinical review. Obstet Gynecol Surv 31:233–271, 1976.
137. Ortega JA: A therapeutic approach to childhood pelvic rhabdomyosarcoma without pelvic exenteration. J Pediatr 94:205–209, 1979.
138. Piver MS, Rose PG: Long-term follow-up and complication of infants with vulvovaginal rhabdomyosarcoma treated with surgery, radiation therapy and chemotherapy. Obstet Gynecol 71:435–437, 1988.
139. Kilman JM, Clatworthy HM Jr, Newton JA Jr, et al: Reasonable surgery for rhabdomyosarcoma: A study of 67 cases. Ann Surg 178:346, 1973.
140. Hays DM, Shimada H, Raney RB, et al: Sarcomas of the vagina and uterus: The intergroup rhabdomyosarcoma study. J Pediatr Surg 20:718–724, 1985.
141. Young RH, Scully RE: Endodermal sinus tumor of the vagina: A report of nine cases and review of the literature. Gynecol Oncol 18:380–392, 1984.

15

John P. Blandy, D.M. • R.T.D. Oliver, M.D.

Genitourinary Cancer

CANCER OF THE KIDNEY

Embryoma—Wilms' Tumor

Epidemiology

Embryoma is rare: in the United States, 500 new cases occur annually among children in the first 4 years of life, as often in boys as in girls, and in all races. It is seen in adults very rarely.[1, 2]

In 1% of cases there is an inherited autosomal dominant gene[3] on chromosome 11 causing multiple and bilateral tumors with other anomalies (e.g., hypospadias, hemihypertrophy, aniridia)[4] and multicystic dysplastic kidneys with small rests of Wilms' tumor.[5] In 40% of the offspring of those who survive this inherited type, Wilms' tumor develops—ten times more often than in the offspring of those with the usual type.[6]

Local-Regional Anatomy and Pathology

Wilms' tumors are large, easily ruptured on handling, and soft and blotchy on section from hemorrhage. Since Wilms' tumor arises from undifferentiated mesenchyme, it can form any kind of mesodermal cancer, including fibro-, rhabdo-, or leiomyosarcoma. The prognosis depends on how anaplastic these tissues become—that is, it is *favorable,* or *unfavorable* (those with clear cell sarcoma and rhabdomyosarcoma). There is today a 10-fold difference in survival between these two types.[7]

Congenital Mesoblastic Nephroma

This variant of Wilms' tumor is usually noticed soon after birth. There is a lump of spindle cells resembling myoblasts or fibroblasts with scattered primitive glomeruli. It invades only locally, and, if completely excised, the children do well; however, these tumors are by no means benign.[8, 9]

Stage

The staging system in use today is that of the U.S. National Wilms' Tumor Study (Table 15–1).[10]

Diagnosis

Screening and Early Detection

Because other members of the patient's family have an increased risk for development of this tumor, siblings and cousins should undergo abdominal ultrasound scanning. Survivors, and today survival is the rule, should be counseled about the risk to their own offspring and advised to have their children screened.

Clinical Features

Most Wilms' tumors are noticed by the mother when washing the child. Less common symptoms include hematuria, abdominal pain, anorexia, vomiting, and fever. Hypertension occurs in about half these children.

Investigations

Ultrasound scan confirms the mass and may detect tumor in the vena cava. The main task is to distinguish Wilms' tumor from neuroblastoma, the diagnostic features of which are speckled calcification, displacement rather than distortion of the kidney, extension across the midline, and raised urinary vanillylmandelic acid and catecholamines.

Today a computed tomography (CT) scan is obtained, even though this may require a general anesthetic, because it detects metastases in the liver and lungs and tumor in the other kidney, which must be expected in about 5% of

TABLE 15–1
Staging for Wilms' Tumor

Stage I—tumor limited to kidney: complete excision: capsule intact: no spill: no residual tumor beyond margins of resection
Stage II—tumor outside kidney but completely excised: regional extension of tumor: vessel invasion: local spill or previous biopsy: no residual tumor beyond margins of resection
Stage III—residual tumor in abdomen: lymph node involvement: tumor spill: tumor extending beyond resection margins or incompletely removed
Stage IV—metastases in lung, liver, bone, or brain
Stage V—bilateral renal involvement at time of diagnosis

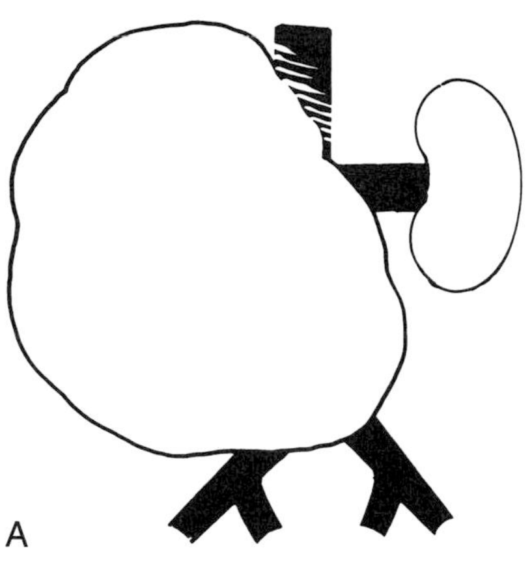

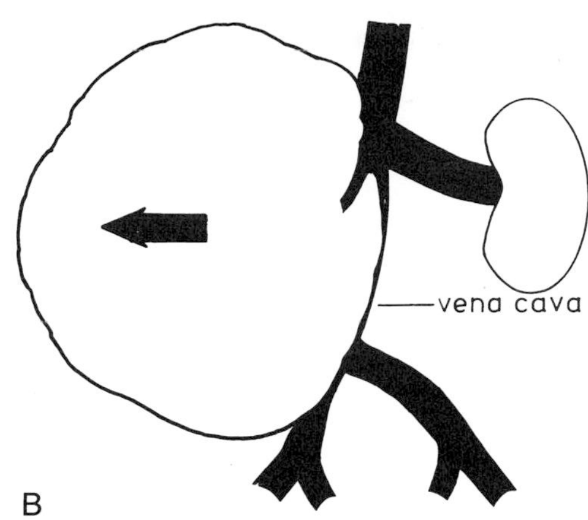

FIGURE 15–1. In a child with a Wilms' tumor, the renal vein that seems to emerge from the right kidney in *A* may be, in fact, the left renal vein as seen in *B*, the true anatomy being obscured by compression and distortion of the cava and the vein emerging from the tumor. (From Blandy JP: Operative Urology, 2nd ed. London, Blackwell Publishers, 1986, p 34.)

cases. Except when partial nephrectomy is contemplated, angiography is no longer needed.

The first line of treatment is radical nephrectomy. Very large tumors should have a preoperative course of chemotherapy—after needle biopsy has confirmed the diagnosis.

Combination Therapy

The triumph in the treatment of Wilms' tumor in recent years has been achieved only by close teamwork. These children should always be referred to a center where many cases are seen and that engages in trials in which every aspect of treatment is under constant audit.[11] The key agents are actinomycin D, vincristine, and doxorubicin.

Today with disease-free survival of stage I cases exceeding 92% and overall survival at 79%, much of the effort of current trials is directed toward reducing toxicity of treatment.[12, 13] Two critical issues remain unresolved. The first is whether radiation is necessary, as there is increasing worry over late toxicity and effects on growth. The second relates to how little doxorubicin can be given in order to minimize cardiac toxicity.

The small number of patients presenting with metastases and the high response even of these cases make it difficult to produce information on new drug activity, and it is these patients more than any others who need to be evaluated in experimental protocols.

Nephrectomy for Wilms' Tumor

Adequate exposure requires a long incision, preferably transverse. The colon and duodenum are reflected off both kidneys so that each side can be examined. The tumor is soft; if it is burst, the prognosis is much worse. If it invades the colon or duodenum, an appropriate length of bowel must be resected en bloc.

There is no therapeutic advantage in removing para-aortic or paracaval lymph nodes, but they should be sampled for staging purposes.

Special care should be taken on the right side to check the inferior vena cava, which may be flattened: it is easy to ligate the left renal vein by mistake (Fig. 15–1).

Bilateral Wilms' Tumors

If tumor is found by CT scan in the opposite kidney and the biopsy result shows favorable histology, preoperative chemotherapy may make partial nephrectomy feasible on one or both sides.[13, 14] Eighty-seven percent of patients with bilateral tumors survived for 2 years, including 19 of the 22 in whom tumor was left behind.[5]

In advanced Wilms' tumors, there is a place for second-look surgery after chemotherapy: inoperable disease may become operable.

These results have focused attention on the possibility of doing a partial nephrectomy under cover of chemotherapy for unilateral tumors in the hope of avoiding the theoretic hazard of late injury to the contralateral kidney.[14]

Results

The 4-year survival rates in a joint study of 1439 patients are shown in Table 15–2.[7]

Wilms' Tumor in Adults

Wilms' tumors are rare in adults and indistinguishable from renal cell cancer until the specimen has been removed; they are unresponsive to chemotherapy.[15, 16]

Once a child has survived 2 years, late metastases are rare but have been reported as long as 15 years later.[17]

TABLE 15–2
Survival Rates for Wilms' Tumor

Stage	Histology	4-Year Survival Rate (%)
I	Favorable	96.5
II	Favorable	92.2
III	Favorable	86.9
IV	Unfavorable	73.0

Adenocarcinoma of the Kidney

Epidemiology

Adenocarcinoma is rare in Africans, uncommon in Indians and Japanese, and most common in North American whites and Scandinavians. It seems to be increasing in the British Isles, especially in Scotland.[18, 19] In the United States, cancer of the kidney accounts for about 9000 deaths per year, 3% of adult cancers.

Renal cancer occurs twice as often in men as in women, mostly in the sixth and seventh decades and very rarely before age 20.[20, 21]

Etiology

In animals, renal cancer may be induced by viruses and radiation.[22] High-incidence strains occur in rodents and primates.[23–25] In humans, it is related to smoking, cadmium, and possibly asbestos.[22]

In some families, an abnormality on the short arm of chromosome 3 causes an increased incidence in one kidney; in others, extra material on chromosome 7 causes bilateral tumors.[22, 26]

In patients who have been on regular hemodialysis for many years, multiple renal cysts develop, and some of these patients go on to have multifocal renal cancer[27] that is very similar to the multiple tumors of von Hippel–Lindau disease (benign hemangioblastoma of the central nervous system, renal cysts, and multiple renal cell carcinomas). Recent results have demonstrated that there is a gene on chromosome 3 that controls this.[28]

Life History

Renal cell carcinomas are identical with the so-called "benign" adenomas of the kidney.[29] By convention, those less than 3 cm in diameter are considered benign, and those greater than 3 cm in diameter malignant—an absurd rule on the basis of observations by Bell,[30] who found that 3 of 62 tumors less than 3 cm in diameter had metastasized.

In a series of 16,294 autopsies, Hellsten et al.[31] found 235 renal tumors that had not been noticed in life, 56 of which had metastasized. Of 82 that were less than 3 cm in diameter, 3 (3.7%) had already metastasized.

Until recently, most tumors were detected only when they were very large, and some of these were observed for up to 35 years without metastasizing.[32, 33] We do not know the doubling time of renal cell cancer and have no idea how long a given tumor has been present, and it is impossible to know if any form of treatment really changes the natural history.

Screening and Prevention

Patients on dialysis, members of families whose members have renal cell cancer, and individuals with central nervous system hemangioblastomas should undergo abdominal ultrasound scanning, which can detect tumors less than 3 cm in diameter, a stage at which they are unlikely to have metastasized.

Local-Regional Anatomy and Pathology

Renal cell cancers are bright yellow, with patches of hemorrhage, cysts, and calcified areas. Microscopically, they are made up of cells from the proximal renal tubule containing glycogen and lipid, which makes them clear in paraffin section. If eosinophilic and spindle cells (resembling sarcoma) are seen, the prognosis is worse.[29] A papillary pattern may mimic a transitional cell carcinoma.

Oncocytoma

Oncocytomas are composed of eosinophilic cells and are possibly a different entity: there is no abnormality on chromosome 3 and they usually have a good prognosis. However, oncocytomas are quite capable of metastasizing and must not be treated as if they were benign.[34, 35]

Grade

There are three grades (1, 2, and 3) according to frequency of mitoses.[36] Cytometry has not improved this subjective assessment, perhaps because it fails to pick out small areas with anaplastic features.[37]

Stage

The International Union Against Cancer (UICC) TNM staging for adenocarcinoma of the kidney is given in Table 15–3.[36]

Prognostic Features

Local extension, size, invasion of veins, and histologic grade determine the prognosis.[38]

Diagnosis

Clinical Features

Hematuria occurs in about 60% of cases,[39] and most of the rest have loin pain or a mass. It is the other syndromes that occur with renal cancer that make it such a challenge clinically. Some of these syndromes are caused by toxins secreted by the renal cell cancer.

1. A pyrogen causes pyrexia, loss of weight, night sweats, and a raised sedimentation rate.[40]

TABLE 15–3
TNM Staging for Adenocarcinoma of the Kidney

T1	Tumor <2.5 cm in diameter, limited to kidney
T2	Tumor >2.5 cm in diameter, limited to kidney
T3	Into major veins, adrenal gland, perinephric tissue but not beyond Gerota's fascia
	T3a Into fat
	T3b Into veins or vena cava below diaphragm
	T3c Into vena cava above diaphragm
N1	Single node <2 cm
N2	Single node >2 cm but <5 cm
N3	Nodes >5 cm
M1	Distant metastases

2. Erythropoietin may cause erythrocytosis without any increase in platelets or splenomegaly.[40]
3. A toxin may suppress the bone marrow, causing anemia.
4. Renin secretion may cause hypertension.
5. Parathormone-like hormone may lead to hypercalcemia, which can be lethal.[41]
6. An hepatotoxin may cause hepatosplenomegaly and disordered liver function.[42]
7. Glucagon may cause diarrhea.[43]
8. A toxic metabolite is thought to cause a form of motor neuron disease.[44]

Proteins from renal carcinoma may form immune complexes, which arrive on the basement membrane and cause glomerulonephritis.[45] Amyloid may be deposited in many tissues, including the contralateral kidney.[45]

Investigations

Intravenous Urography. The urogram, which should be the invariable part of the investigation of hematuria, may show a mass in the parenchyma of the kidney, often with a fleck of calcification.

Ultrasonography. Lack of echoes on ultrasound usually distinguishes a cyst from cancer, but septa between multiple cysts or areas of necrosis or hemorrhage in the tumor may give rise to confusing echoes. Today it is seldom necessary to aspirate the contents of the cyst to settle the question because of the additional information supplied by CT scanning.

Computed Tomography. CT scanning shows not only the Hounsfield number of the contents of the space-occupying lesion but also tumor in the renal vein and vena cava (Fig. 15–2). Lung scanning often shows small metastases missed in routine radiography.

Angiography. Angiography may be helpful when planning a partial nephrectomy for a solitary kidney or when tumor is present on both sides. Preoperative embolization of the renal artery caused discomfort in practice and occasionally caused paradoxical embolism of a cerebral or retinal artery.

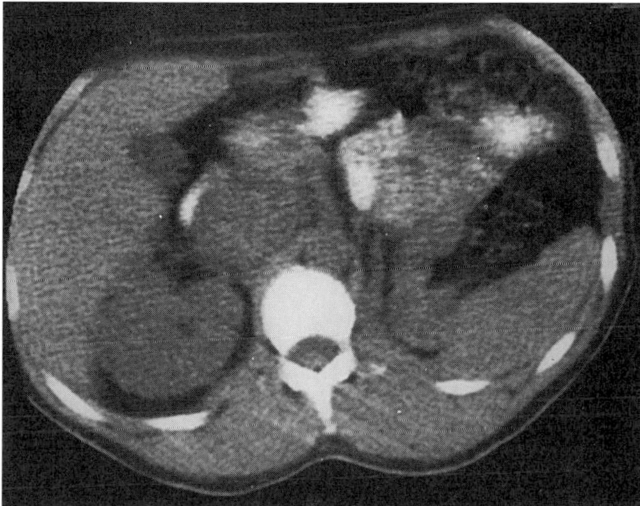

FIGURE 15–2. CT scan of renal cell cancer involving the renal vein. (From Oliver RTD, Blandy JP, Hope-Stone JF: Urological and Genital Cancer. London, Blackwell Publishers, 1989, p 161.)

Magnetic Resonance Imaging (MRI). This imaging study gives very clear images of tumor thrombus in the vena cava and right heart.[46]

Differential Diagnosis

A cortical abscess gives a similar radiologic appearance to cancer, but the history is characteristic. If in doubt, pus can be aspirated from the mass.

A mass around a long-standing calculus is likely to be xanthogranuloma. Even when the kidney is explored, the mass may be mistaken for an inoperable tumor; on frozen section, the macrophages of xanthogranuloma may be mistaken for the clear cells of cancer. Multilocular cystic adenoma is indistinguishable from carcinoma. Angiomyolipoma is recognized by its characteristic CT image. An extra-large column of Bertin should be recognized on the urogram and certainly on the CT scan. Larger sarcomas and hemangiosarcomas of the kidney are recognized only after nephrectomy.

Treatment

The standard treatment for cancer of the kidney is radical nephrectomy, but a partial nephrectomy may be appropriate for small tumors. With a large tumor on the right side, tumor thrombus in the vena cava must be excluded by CT, MRI, or cavography.

Radical Nephrectomy for Cancer

The incision should be big enough to make the subsequent dissection safe. The colon and duodenum are reflected and the renal artery ligated early in the operation, before dividing the renal vein, or there will be needless hemorrhage from collateral vessels (Figs. 15–3 and 15–4).

On the right side, the right renal artery can be found between the aorta and the vena cava. On the left side, the renal artery may be found behind the duodenojejunal flexure, if necessary after dividing the inferior mesenteric vein.

Special care must be taken with lumbar veins. A large one often enters the renal vein at its junction with the cava, and on the left side a large branch may completely encircle the aorta.

Once the renal vessels have been divided, the kidney is removed en bloc with all the tissues inside Gerota's fascia. The ureter is divided at the brim of the pelvis.

Tumor in the Renal Veins. When a small finger of tumor protrudes into the inferior vena cava, it and the opposite renal vein must be isolated with slings. Several pairs of lumbar veins must be divided between ligatures above and below the renal vein to give adequate mobilization. The cava is opened, the thrombus removed, and the vein closed after irrigating it with heparin-saline (Figs. 15–5 to 15–8).

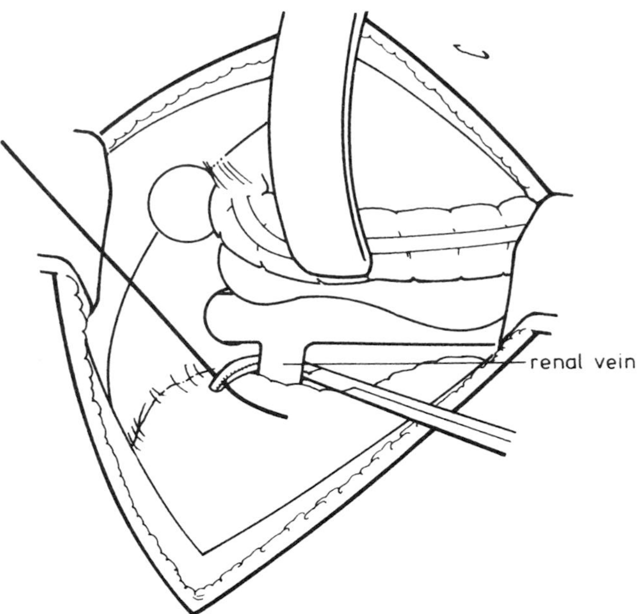

FIGURE 15–3. A stout suture may be passed around the right renal vein but not tied. (From Blandy JP: Operative Urology, 2nd ed. London, Blackwell Publishers, 1986, p 30.)

If the whole thickness of the vena cava is invaded and obstructed, the complete segment may be removed, since in such cases there is always a good collateral circulation.

Tumor thrombus in the left renal vein calls for a wide anterior approach to display the junction of the left renal vein with the cava.

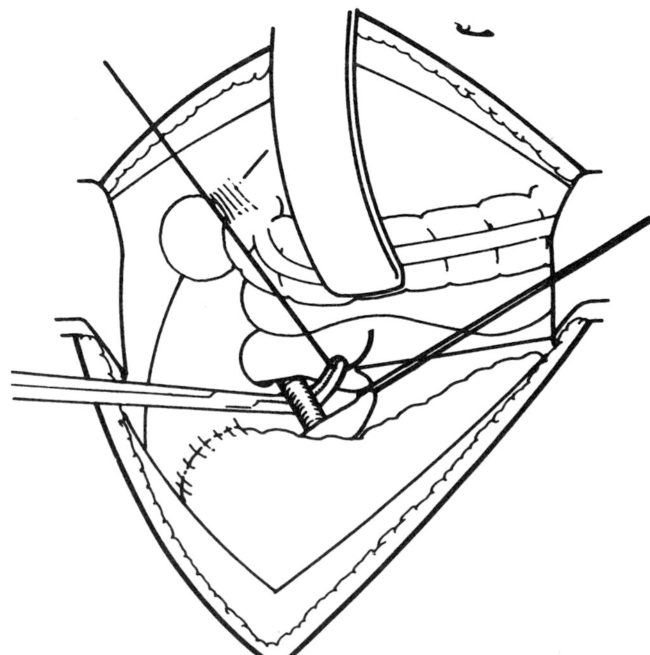

FIGURE 15–4. With retraction of the renal vein, using the previously passed suture, the renal artery may be found and ligated before ligation of the vein. (From Blandy JP: Operative Urology, 2nd ed. London, Blackwell Publishers, 1986, p 30.)

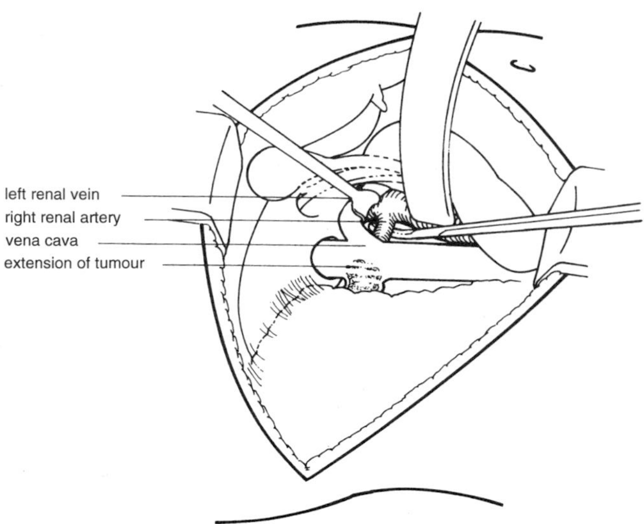

FIGURE 15–5. A tumor of the right kidney extending through the right renal vein into the inferior vena cava. The left renal vein is retracted superiorly to expose the right renal artery between the aorta and the inferior vena cava. (From Blandy JP: Operative Urology, 2nd ed. London, Blackwell Publishers, 1986, p 31.)

Tumor Thrombus Above the Diaphragm. When preliminary investigations show tumor thrombus above the diaphragm, the operation should be planned in collaboration with cardiovascular colleagues. A long midline incision is first made into the abdomen to ensure that the tumor is operable. It is then extended by splitting the sternum, and the inferior vena cava is taped below the right atrium. It may be necessary to cannulate the superior vena cava and aorta and to put the patient on cardiac bypass if the tumor has reached the right atrium. The limiting factor for

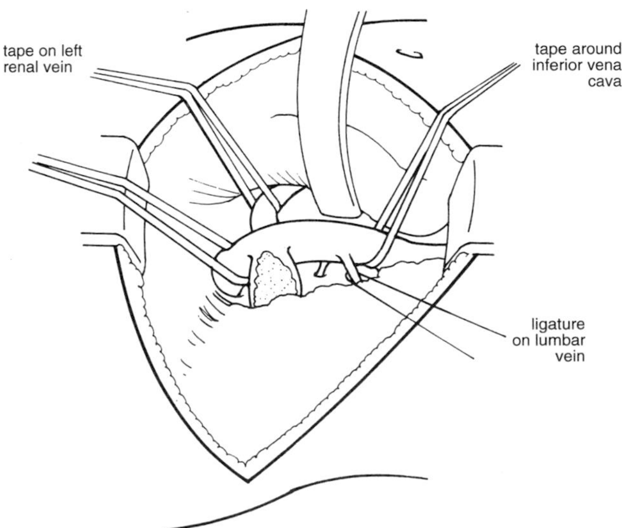

FIGURE 15–6. Vascular tapes are placed around the inferior vena cava above and below the right renal vein. An additional tape is placed on the left renal vein, and ligatures may be looped around the lumbar veins to isolate the cava with its tumor extension. (From Blandy JP: Operative Urology, 2nd ed. London, Blackwell Publishers, 1986, p 31.)

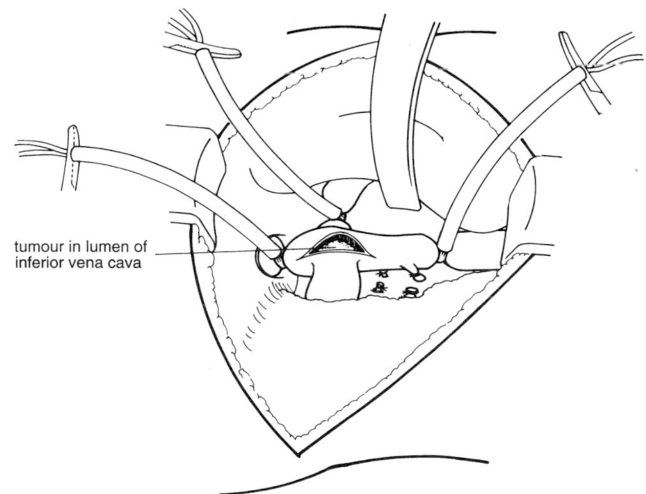

FIGURE 15–7. Tapes are secured and lumbar veins ligated and divided. With the right renal artery ligated previously in continuity, it is safe to open the cava and remove enough caval wall to provide adequate clearance of growth in the lumen. (From Blandy JP: Operative Urology, 2nd ed. London, Blackwell Publishers, 1986, p 32.)

this operation is hepatic ischemia time, to prolong which it may be necessary to lower the body temperature.[47, 48]

One may need to defend such major surgery: despite some operative mortality, those who survive have a 30% chance of surviving for 5 years—more if there is no perinephric spread.[49]

Enthusiasm must be tempered with common sense: at least one bilateral renal cell cancer patient with tumor thrombus extending above the diaphragm survived many years without any operation.[50]

Partial Nephrectomy

Today many more small tumors are being found for which partial nephrectomy is indicated. After the renal artery is occluded, a segment of kidney is removed by a clean guillotine incision together with a good margin of healthy tissue. The flat cut surface of the kidney shows the cut arteries and veins, which are suture ligated with fine catgut (Fig. 15–9). The renal artery is then released and the remaining small vessels secured. No attempt is made

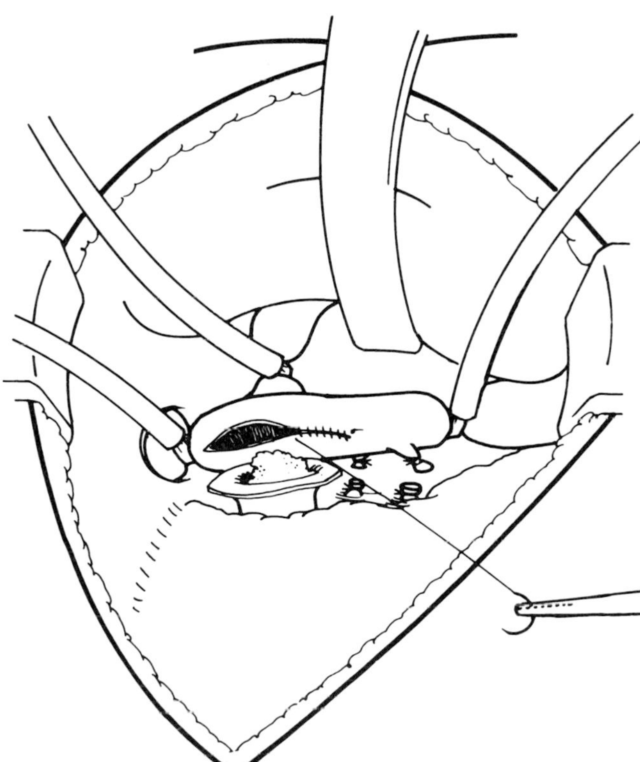

FIGURE 15–8. The caval defect is repaired with running vascular suture. (From Blandy JP: Operative Urology, 2nd ed. London, Blackwell Publishers, 1986, p 32.)

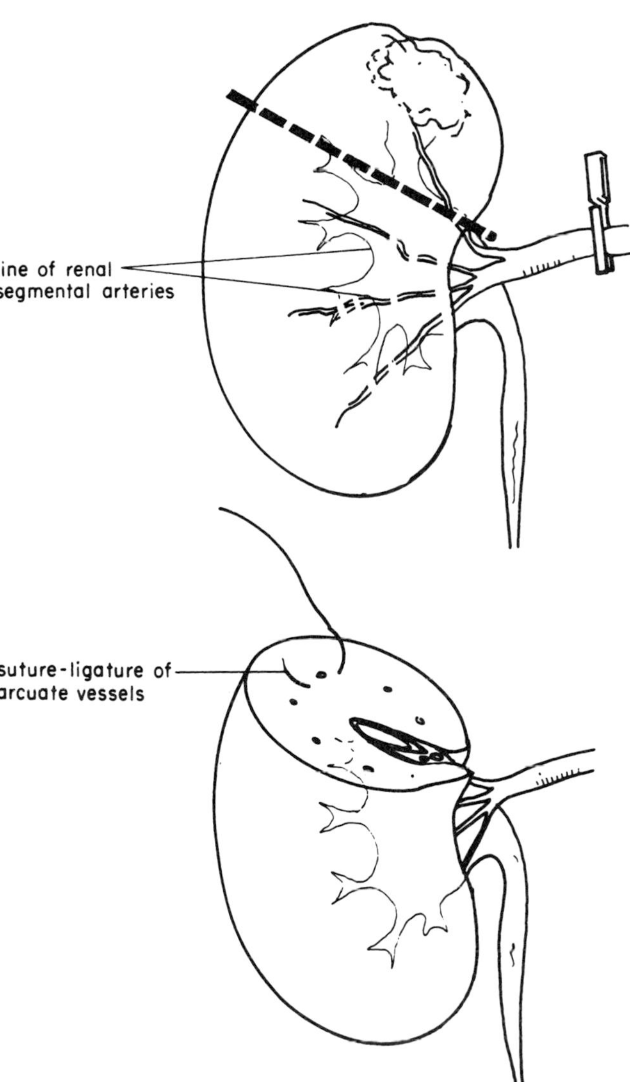

FIGURE 15–9. The technique for partial nephrectomy of a tumor in the superior wall of the kidney. A clip is placed on the renal artery in the segment of kidney to be removed (dotted line above). (From Blandy JP: Operative Urology, 2nd ed. London, Blackwell Publishers, 1986, p 56.)

to cover the raw surface of kidney with capsule, since this increases the chance of hematoma and sepsis.

A tumor in the middle third of the renal cortex may be removed in the same way, taking a broad wedge of tissue, and closing the vessels in each flat surface carefully. As this may take longer, it may be wise to cool the kidney with saline ice slush.

Although much has been made of "bench surgery"—in which the renal artery and vein are cut across, the kidney perfused with transplant solution, and the dissection performed on a "bench" with the help of the dissecting microscope[51]—cases that cannot be dealt with in situ are very rare.[52]

Some have advised "enucleation"—shelling the tumor out of its "capsule." Since tumor has always grown through this capsule, the operation is incomplete and futile. There is no evidence that enucleating these tumors alters the natural history of this unpredictable disease.[53]

Only about 20% of those who live for more than 5 years have metastases by year 10,[54] although metastasis may occur even later. Since spontaneous regression of metastases can occur in up to 12% of late-relapsing (>2 years) cases, and many of these contralateral tumor cases may be quite old, it is important to temper enthusiasm for treating these rare cases.[55]

Regional Lymph Node Dissection

It is impossible to show that para-aortic or paracaval lymph node dissection alters the outlook for this disease despite the passion with which it is advocated.

Adjuvant Radiotherapy

Controlled studies show that radiation worsens the prognosis,[56, 57] perhaps because of immunosuppression.

Hormone Therapy

Medroxyprogesterone acetate is still widely prescribed, even though controlled studies show that it has no benefit.[58]

Immunotherapy

Bacillus Calmette-Guérin (BCG), interferon-α, and interleukin-2 (IL-2) increase host T-cell activity. About 20% of patients get measurable improvement, and 5% get a complete remission. This is double the rate of spontaneous regression.[54, 59]

Blood transfusion does not alter the prognosis, as was once suggested.[60]

Adjuvant Chemotherapy

Single-agent chemotherapy gives only a 9% partial response. As this differs little from the incidence of spontaneous regression, there is little to justify its use, except in the setting of a specific clinical trial, given its toxicity.[61]

Nephrectomy in the Presence of Metastases

Most experienced surgeons have seen metastases resolve after nephrectomy for the primary tumor once or twice in a lifetime, but there is no evidence that this is any more likely to occur following operation than with no treatment. One should think twice before inflicting a painful and perhaps dangerous operation on a patient whose life expectancy is already limited: *primum non nocere.*[62]

Some authors are now reporting complete necrosis of primary tumors after preoperative treatment with IL-2, and a trial is needed to evaluate post-treatment surgical staging in such cases.

Results

The 5-year survival rate for tumors detected when they are very small and removed by radical nephrectomy is greater than 95%; for the usual larger tumors without metastases, it is about 65%.[63]

Carcinoma of the Renal Pelvis and Ureter

Epidemiology

The incidence of urothelial cancers of the kidney and ureter is one-twelfth that of bladder cancer, men are affected twice as often as women, the peak age incidence is around 45, and they occur in about 3% of those with bladder cancer.[64]

Etiology

Analgesic abuse and Balkan nephropathy head the list of etiologic agents that cause cancer of the upper tract, in addition to all those known to cause bladder cancer. An autosomal dominant gene makes certain families susceptible to cancer of the renal pelvis and ureter as well as other organs.[65]

Two types of interstitial nephritis with papillary necrosis are followed, some years later, by multifocal cancer in the urothelium of the renal pelvis and ureter; the more common is caused by analgesics (e.g., phenacetin and phenazone), and the other (probably) by a biologic toxin from mold growing on damp grain in scattered communities in the Balkans.[66–68]

Pathology

The microscopic features and grading system of urothelial cancer in the kidney and ureter are identical to those of cancer in the bladder.[69, 70] Spread is by direct invasion through the renal pelvis and ureter—by lymphatics and veins—and implantation downstream in the ureter and bladder[71] follows sooner or later.

Stage

The UICC TNM staging for cancer of the renal pelvis and ureter is presented in Table 15–4.[72]

TABLE 15–4
Tumor (T) Staging for Cancer of the Renal Pelvis and Ureter

Ta	Papillary, noninvasive tumor
Tis	Carcinoma in situ
T1	Invades subepithelial connective tissue
T2	Invades muscularis
T3	(Pelvis) into peripelvic fat or renal parenchyma; (ureter) into periureteral fat
T4	Adjacent organs, or through kidney into perinephric fat

Diagnosis

Clinical Features

The classic symptom of cancer of the renal pelvis and ureter is hematuria with pain if there is obstruction or infection.

Investigations

The urogram may show a filling defect. In the ureter there is dilatation both above and below the tumor. A retrograde ureterogram adds to the definition. CT and MRI scans help in staging. Ureteroscopy allows the tumor to be sampled for biopsy and destroyed with the laser when very small.

Aneuploid cells in the urine mean that a tumor in the upper tract must be anaplastic; however, finding only "normal" urothelial cells does not rule out a well-differentiated tumor. A ureteral brush provides tissue that gives excellent histologic sections.

Treatment

Radical Nephroureterectomy

Classically, the ureter is removed en bloc with an ellipse of bladder and intramural ureter through a single long midline incision.[73] We[74] find it preferable to use a transverse incision for the kidney and a second Pfannenstiel incision for the lower end of the ureter. In most cases where tumors arise in the upper third of the ureter, Semple's operation can be used.[75] First, a transurethral resection is performed of the ureteral orifice and intramural ureter, well into perivesical fat. Through a transverse incision, the renal pedicle is divided and the kidney freed. The ureter is followed down, and the severed lower end is brought out into the wound. The risk of spilling tumor rules out this method for growths in the lower third of the ureter.

In undifferentiated tumors, the risk of tumor spread makes any surgical removal, however radical, insufficient to prevent recurrence. Adjuvant treatment is needed (see below).

When it is possible to visualize well-differentiated tumors by flexible or rigid ureteroscope up into the renal pelvis, diathermy or laser coagulation can be used. Tumors outside the field of view of the ureteroscope can be treated through a nephroscope, seeding of tumor along the track being avoided by local irradiation.[76]

Results

Treatment of cancer of the renal pelvis and ureter is determined by its grade and stage. For G1 tumors, one can expect a 97% 5-year survival rate,[70] justifying kidney preservation whenever possible. Undifferentiated (G3) tumors are associated with only a 40% survival rate, despite the use of postoperative radiotherapy.[77] This has led to consideration of preoperative radiotherapy.[78] Increasing evidence shows that metastatic G3 renal, pelvic, and ureteric tumors are, like bladder tumors, sensitive to chemotherapy given before resection.[78]

A controlled trial of chemotherapy versus radiation is necessary to show which is effective. Any such trial would require careful cytopathology and grading of the tumors in patients entering the trial.

Squamous and Adenocarcinoma of the Renal Pelvis and Ureter

Ten percent of upper tract tumors are squamous cancers following metaplasia from irritation (e.g., by a stone). They rarely cause hematuria and are diagnosed late with pain from invasion. Similar irritation has occasionally been noted to lead to adenocarcinoma.[79]

Rare Tumors of the Kidney

Multilocular Cystic Adenoma

This benign hamartoma forms a multicystic mass that cannot be distinguished from cancer before operation.[80] When *cystic angioma* is seen with other stigmata of von Hippel–Lindau disease (e.g., angiomatous cysts in the cerebellum, retina, and pancreas), a partial nephrectomy may be performed.[81] Most *angiomyolipomas* are not associated with tuberous sclerosis. The CT scan is characteristic, with a large content of fat. Spontaneous retroperitoneal hemorrhage is a common presentation. Although partial nephrectomy can often be performed, a clear margin is mandatory because malignant elements are present in a quarter of them and metastases have been reported. Very large bilateral tumors have been successfully treated by total nephrectomy with subsequent transplantation in view of the very small risk of metastases.[82, 83]

Hemangioma and *hemangiosarcoma* arise from blood vessels. The benign ones form a more or less solid mass—"Masson's tumor"—anywhere in the urinary tract[83] and are often so small that they are difficult to find. Ureteroscopy may reveal bleeding from one calix, and the tumor may be coagulated with the Nd:YAG laser. Larger lesions tend to have sarcomatous change and require nephrectomy.

Juxtaglomerular Tumor—Reninoma

A variant of hemangioma is derived from the juxtaglomerular cells, which secrete renin, causing hypertension and elevated blood levels of aldosterone and renin. These small tumors are localized by CT scan and are said to be benign.[84]

Sarcoma

Sarcomas may arise from the connective tissues in or around the kidney and must be distinguished from the adult Wilms' tumor by their lack of any renal components. The only effective treatment is wide excision.

CANCER OF THE BLADDER

Epidemiology

The global incidence of bladder cancer has risen steadily, but in the West it may have reached a plateau. Bladder cancer affects white men twice as often as black men, and men four times more than women.[85, 86]

There are many possible causes, of which, worldwide, bilharziasis is the most important. Smoking is suspect, but the incidence differs from lung cancer, perhaps because smokers who get bladder cancer lack liver n-acetyltransferase, which detoxifies tobacco tar carcinogens.

In Taiwan, a toxin in the blackfoot disease endemic area, which causes lower limb ischemia, is associated with bladder cancer.[87]

Industrial bladder cancer was detected in the aniline dye industry[88] and pinpointed to the naphthylamines 60 years later,[89] which were soon found in other occupations (e.g., gas making, rat catching, textiles, and plastics). One feature of industrial carcinogenesis is the long latent interval—up to 40 years—between exposure to the chemicals and the onset of cancer.[90]

Diet may be important. In animals, dietary nitrosamines are converted in the gut to carcinogens. This conversion is inhibited by vitamin C, and the action of the carcinogen is prevented by vitamin A.

Bladder cancer is more common in men with a previous history of condylomata acuminata, and papillomavirus is occasionally found in tumors.[91]

Irritation from many causes (e.g., stricture, calculus, chronic retention, and neuropathy) is associated with bladder cancer.[92]

Local-Regional Anatomy and Pathology

Benign Tumors

Papilloma—It is rare to see a single layer of cells with an intact basement membrane and normal cytology. One variant of this is the *inverted papilloma,* seen by chance on cystoscopy as a smooth, rounded swelling like a sebaceous cyst. *Hemangioma* appears as a knot of veins, usually on one side of the bladder.[93]

Malignant Tumors

Most bladder tumors arise from urothelium, but metaplasia leads to squamous and adenocarcinoma after irritation (e.g., bilharziasis or stone). Adenocarcinoma occurs in exstrophy and remnants of the urachus.

Cystoscopic Appearances

A minority of invasive tumors are pure solid tumors without evidence of any papillary areas. Some authors have suggested that flat carcinoma in situ is always the precursor of these lesions. This condition is usually detected only in field biopsies of apparently normal or, at worst, slightly inflamed areas.

Most carcinomas start as papillary tumors, and then later solid invasive areas develop. In these tumors the original Ta stage is in fact a preinvasive in situ stage and was called Tis.[94] Whichever premalignant type, bladder tumors are often multiple and may be associated with urothelial cancer of the upper tract, particularly those in stage Ta.

Grade

There are three grades, 1, 2, and 3.[95] Flow cytometry gives an objective measure of this[94] and corrects the human observer error in conventional grading.[96]

Stage

The UICC TNM system for bladder cancer (Table 15–5) is based on the depth of invasion of the cancer into the wall of the bladder (Fig. 15–10).[95]

When comparing results of treatment in different centers, it is important to be aware that the "P" (pathologic) stage applies only when the entire bladder is available after total cystectomy. A deep biopsy allows the prefix pT. "T" stage implies that there has been a cystoscopy but no biopsy. Hence, "P" series include more cases with microscopic evidence of invasion undetected in series staged pT or T. Similarly, histologic examination of the lymph nodes removed by radical cystectomy often shows invasion not detected on CT scan.

TABLE 15–5
Tumor (T) Staging for Carcinoma of the Bladder

Stage	Description
Ta	No invasion of lamina propria
Tis	Flat carcinoma in situ
T1	Invasion of lamina propria
T2	Invasion of superficial muscle
T3	a. Invasion of deep muscle
	b. Invasion of fat
	(i) Microscopically
	(ii) Macroscopically
T4	a. Invasion of prostate, uterus, vagina
	b. Invasion of pelvic wall, abdominal wall

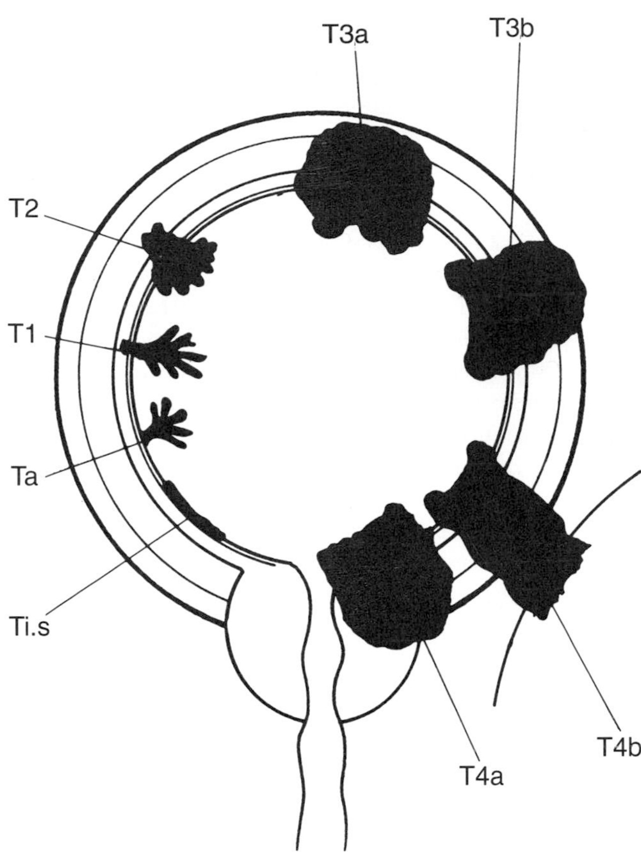

FIGURE 15–10. Depiction of various tumor (T) categories for cancer of the bladder. (From Blandy JP: Operative Urology, 2nd ed. London, Blackwell Publishers, 1986, p 129.)

Carcinoma in Situ (Tis)

The continuous spectrum between normal urothelium, atypia, dysplasia, and carcinoma in situ is susceptible to observer variation.[97, 98] Carcinoma in situ is subdivided into primary when it appears alone and secondary when there is exfoliative tumor elsewhere.

There is an important difference in the prognosis according to whether the basement membrane is penetrated—that is, between Ta and T1[99, 100]—but the traditional distinction between T2 and T3[101] is artificial. It is the access to the lymphatic plexus of the muscle that makes the prognosis so much worse. The imaginary halfway line that distinguishes between T2 and T3 arose from a study in which only 15 cases had muscle invasion, and only 1 of these had metastases.[101]

Once tumor gets outside the bladder, the biologic barrier of peritoneum or Denonvilliers' fascia exists only on the vault and posteriorly.

Tumor Spread

Bladder cancer can spread across the bladder by contact ("kiss cancer"), by direct invasion through the detrusor, and by lymphatic or hematogenous spread. Tumor cells are sometimes implanted onto urethral abrasions or at the vault, carried there on bubbles during transurethral resection.[102]

The local lymph nodes adjoin the internal iliac and obturator arteries. The regional nodes are the paraaortic nodes. Retrograde spread may cause cancer en cuirasse and is occasionally seen late in the disease.

In well-differentiated superficial tumors, hematogenous spread is rare but sometimes occurs, perhaps disseminated by transurethral resection.

With invasion of the prostate, Batson's veins and lymphatics allow metastasis directly to the bone marrow of the femora, pelvis, and lumbar vertebrae and, by allowing access to rectal veins and the portal system, may lead to liver metastases.

Squamous metaplasia, which is premalignant, must be distinguished from the innocent "vaginal metaplasia," a normal finding in the female trigone. Squamous cell cancer seldom has any symptoms, rarely causes hematuria, and so presents late and has a bad prognosis.[103–105]

Adenocarcinoma arising from the urachus or areas of columnar metaplasia is seen in neglected extrophy. Because of the risk of malignant change, the precursors of adenocarcinoma—cystitis glandularis and nephrogenic adenoma—must always be carefully followed.[106] Metaplasia may also give rise to sarcomatoid, microcytic, and trophoblastic variants.

Pheochromocytoma results in paroxysmal hypertension during micturition.[107] The urine vanillylmandelic acid and catecholamine levels are raised. It may be localized with iodine 131 metaiodobenzylguanidine (MIGB).

Presenting as strangury in children, *rhabdomyosarcoma* "botyroides" is best diagnosed by CT scan. Toxic combinations of systemic chemotherapy and radiation in the hands of experienced teams can result in cure in more than 50% of cases.[108]

Leiomyosarcoma may follow cyclophosphamide therapy for Hodgkin's disease.[109]

Diagnosis

Clinical Features

Hematuria is the presenting symptom in more than 80% of patients, often found on routine testing of the urine. About 15% have frequency and dysuria, but the urine is sterile. The remaining patients have a variety of symptoms (e.g., anemia, uremia, distant metastases). Only in advanced cases is induration felt on rectal or suprapubic examination.

Investigations

Urine Cytology. Urine cytology fails to detect differentiated tumors unless whole fronds are found in the urine. False-positive findings occur if mitotic cells from healing urothelium are shed (e.g., after passage of an instrument or a stone). Flow cytometry gives an objective measure of ploidy but will not detect the 80% or so of well-differentiated tumors.

Intravenous Urography. The urogram may reveal filling defects in the bladder. Ureteric obstruction usually means invasion of the muscle.[110]

Ultrasonography. Although in recent years ultrasound scanning has shown some promise in detection of small bladder tumors, it cannot yet detect tumors in the renal pelvis or ureter and does not replace the urogram.[111]

Computed Tomography. The CT scan adds little to the urogram and cystoscopy. It may show large pelvic lymph nodes (Fig. 15–11) and be of value in following response to chemotherapy, but it is not reliable in staging.[112]

Magnetic Resonance Imaging. Some authors have suggested that MRI may be useful in staging and may distinguish edema from cancer.[113] Financial and logistic issues have prevented widespread evaluation of this claim.

Cystoscopy. The flexible cystoscope allows a painless examination in the office, where small tumors can be sampled for biopsy and coagulated with the Nd:YAG laser.[114, 115] If a filling defect is seen on the urogram, cystoscopy is performed under anesthesia, the tumor is resected, and bimanual examination is performed to stage it.

For a small tumor, the resectoscope loop removes it with a divot of underlying muscle.[116] Resection of large papillary tumors is performed in stages: First the stalk is located by removing overhanging tumor. Then the stalk is coagulated and the remainder of the tumor removed in a bloodless field. Finally, the base of the tumor is sampled for staging.

It is pointless to resect a large solid tumor, since it is bound to need some more radical treatment. Deep bites are taken from the edge of the tumor for staging and grading.[116]

Inspection of Diverticula

Diverticula are often found in elderly men, and each one must be thoroughly inspected. Suspicion is raised if there is edema around the mouth of the diverticulum. When this closes the diverticulum completely, it is essential that further studies are carried out (e.g., ultrasound or CT scan) to rule out tumor.

Field Biopsy

Field biopsy samples are taken with cup forceps from the rest of the urothelium because secondary carcinoma in situ may modify the plan of treatment.

Treatment

Superficial Ta, T1 tumors account for more than 80% of bladder tumors, and most can be well managed endoscopically. The exception to this rule is the rare T1, G3 cancer, which has a deadly prognosis and should be treated as if it were already invasive.[117, 118]

Follow-up is done with the flexible cystoscope, although it may be that ultrasound will replace it.

When G1 or G2 tumors recur in large numbers at frequent intervals, intravesical adjuvant therapy is offered after resecting or coagulating the tumors.[119, 120] More recently, a single dose of intravesical mitomycin C (40 mg in 40 ml water) has been shown to halve the number and frequency of subsequent recurrences.[121]

Adjuvant Chemotherapy

Many chemotherapeutic compounds have been used, and all reduce the number and rate of recurrences in about 50% of cases. They differ in their side effects and expense, and where one fails another may succeed.

Of the alkylating agents, thiotepa was the first and cheapest. It is easily absorbed and causes marrow suppression, which is dose-related and avoided by giving 30 mg on alternate days for three doses and checking platelets between each dose.[119] The second, ethoglucid (Epodyl), gives less marrow toxicity, similar results, but more cystitis.[120]

The antibiotics mitomycin C, doxorubicin (Adriamycin), and epirubicin are expensive and give calcification and "white ulcers" at the site of resection, and sometimes severe skin rashes.[121, 122]

Adjuvant Immunotherapy

Morales[123] used BCG to produce an immune response to bladder tumors. Results varied because different strains of

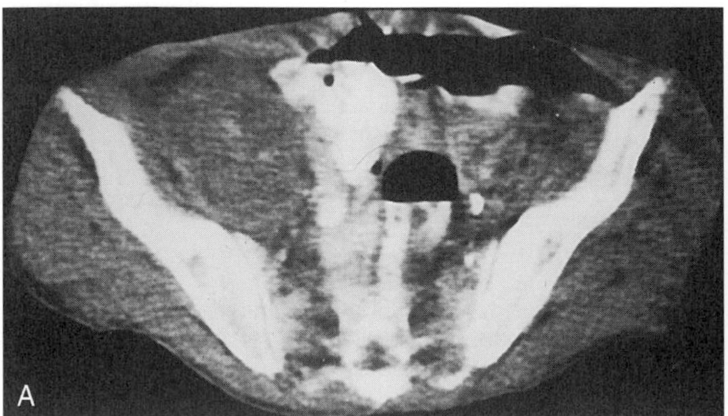

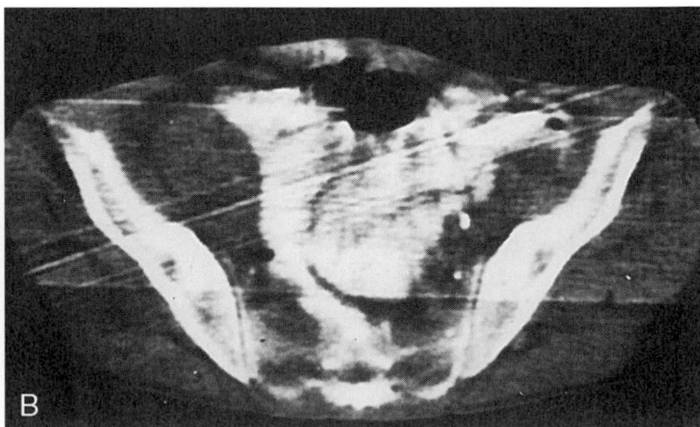

FIGURE 15–11. CT scans demonstrating large pelvic nodes from invasive bladder carcinoma before *(A)* and after *(B)* chemotherapy.

tubercle vaccine had different virulence.[124] The complications are those of local and hematogenous tuberculosis, including severe cystitis, meningitis, and hepatitis, complications that respond to appropriate therapy if diagnosed promptly.[125, 126] Possibly second primary malignancies may be accelerated by BCG.[127]

More patients get a response from BCG than from chemotherapy and it may be more durable. Nonresponders may lack a receptor for BCG resembling the blood group precursor T antigen.[128] In view of the success of BCG, it is disappointing that interferon has given poor results.[129]

Adjuvant Radiotherapy

Colloidal intravesical yttrium was used at one time for superficial tumors,[130] but beam therapy is of value only in the rare G3 superficial tumors.[131]

Adjuvant Phototherapy

To destroy superficial bladder tumors with light after rendering them photosensitive with hematoporphyrin has been the object of research for two decades. So far there is still such a small difference between damage to tumor and to healthy tissue that the method has little practical application.[132]

Failure of Endoscopic and Adjuvant Therapy

When endoscopic treatment, supplemented by adjuvants, fails to control recurrences, total cystectomy is indicated, except for anaplastic tumors, for which radiotherapy is given first.

Treatment of Carcinoma in Situ

Some regard carcinoma in situ as so dangerous that total cystectomy should be the immediate treatment.[133] Complete remissions have been obtained by intravesical chemotherapy, BCG,[134, 135] or systemic cyclophosphamide[136]; these can be tried first as long as follow-up is strict.

Treatment of Tumor Invading Muscle (T2, T3)

Nearly all these tumors are anaplastic (G3) and invade the regional nodes early. The results of radical cystectomy alone were at first so bad that preoperative radiation was added and seemed to improve survival.[137] Later series found equally good results without radiation,[138, 139] and these authors were able to offer the patient a continent diversion.

Other centers continued to use radiation as the first line of treatment, and about 50% of tumors responded. As it was impossible to predict which would respond, all were irradiated, cystectomy being offered to the nonresponders.

Multicenter trials showed no difference in survival between patients treated with radiation followed by cystectomy and those given radical radiotherapy with delayed salvage cystectomy for nonresponders.[140, 141] Half responded, half did not (Fig. 15–12). Overall responders had a 5-year survival rate of nearly 70%: nonresponders only 17%.[142–156]

Routine histologic staging and grading was unable to distinguish between the two groups, nor did flow cytometry. However, there was some suggestion that nonresponders had a higher frequency of metaplastic changes with squamous metaplasia and a higher proportion of the cells secreting beta–human chorionic gonadotropin (βhCG) (Fig. 15–13).[130] It seems possible that these changes may reflect a mutational evolution to escape immune surveillance, because tumors that express βhCG mimic trophoblast in losing expression of human leukocyte antigen (HLA) class I.[148]

Those with radiosensitive tumors can retain their bladders, but radiation bowel injury rules out a continent diversion. Other side effects of radiotherapy as primary treatment include intestinal stricture, persistent bowel or bladder hemorrhage, and contracted bladder, which may require cystectomy. Less than 5% of patients get such serious complications.[149]

Systemic Chemotherapy

Although there are no consistent reports of long-term cure of metastatic bladder cancer by single-agent chemotherapy, there have been a few (< 5%) well-documented instances of durable complete remission, particularly after use of methotrexate.[150] Bladder cancer is one adult solid cancer for which there is evidence from a randomized trial of survival advantage and increased incidence of complete remission of metastatic cases from combination as com-

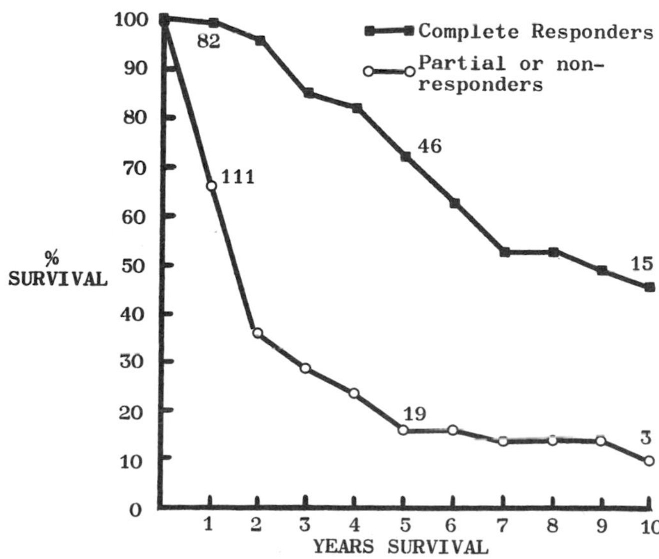

FIGURE 15–12. Effect of response to irradiation on survival of T3 bladder cancer patients.

		BhCG in Tissue Sections +	BhCG in Tissue Sections −
Squamous metaplasia in tissue sections	+	1/23 (4%)	12/37 (32%)
	−	6/6 (100%)	31/34 (91%)

\+ no of complete remissions
++ no treated

FIGURE 15–13. βhCG and squamous metaplasia risk factors in bladder cancer response to chemotherapy.

pared to single-agent chemotherapy.[151] This trial compared single-agent cisplatin with methotrexate, vinblastine Adriamycin, and cisplatin (M-VAC) in combination, demonstrating a 38% versus 12% response rate and a 12.5 months versus 8.2 months median survival.[151] The results in this trial are less impressive than the initial claims of Sternberg et al.,[152] and as yet there is no evidence that this regimen produces any survival advantage when used as an adjuvant for invasive tumors without metastases, though there may be some delay in the onset of metastases.[153–156] Radiation remains the best single agent for primary tumors, as it produces a greater proportion of previously untreated T3 patients in complete remission than M-VAC. The priority for the next decade must be to explore ways of giving chemotherapy and radiation synchronously. A possible approach has been the recent development of a regimen of methotrexate, vincristine, and cisplatin given every 10 days.[157] This has proven to be equally active and less toxic than M-VAC and is currently being studied given concurrently with radiation.

Partial Cystectomy

Partial cystectomy is indicated only for carcinoma arising in a diverticulum or the urachus.

Cancer in a Diverticulum

Through a long midline incision, the superior vesical artery is divided to allow the bladder to be rolled medially. The bladder is opened well away from the diverticulum, and the ureters are catheterized to protect them. Taking a wide cuff, one removes the diverticulum, its surrounding tissue, and the internal and obturator lymph nodes en bloc. It is often necessary to reimplant the ureter.

Carcinoma of the Urachus

The long midline incision encircles the umbilicus, and a wedge of tissue is removed en bloc that includes the urachus and all the tissue between the obliterated hypogastric arteries down to the trigone. A 2-cm rim is left around the ureters and internal meatus, which is closed over a catheter. The bladder regains its normal capacity within 6 weeks; there is no need to add on ileum or colon.

Total Cystectomy

Preliminary Staging Node Dissection

Except for palliation, cystectomy is futile if the lymph nodes contain tumor. Recent developments in laparoscopic surgery make it possible to remove nodes for histologic assessment prior to cystectomy, though as yet there is no evidence of the effect of this procedure on long-term results.[158]

Total Cystectomy Procedure

A long midline incision is made. The bowel is mobilized and packed out of the pelvis. The bladder is separated from the symphysis and retracted medially.

If the lymph nodes have not already been taken laparoscopically, they are removed en bloc with the tumor by opening the connective tissue sheath of the common iliac artery and vein and stripping all the surrounding tissues medially.

All the medial branches of the internal iliac vessels are divided in turn. The ureters are divided and marked with stay sutures. The same is done on the other side (Fig. 15–14).

Except when the tumor is a solitary one, the urethra must be removed en bloc.

For a solitary tumor, the fat is cleaned to define the retropubic veins, and the puboprostatic ligament is incised on either side of them. The veins are divided between suture ligatures. The surgeon pushes the neurovascular bundles laterally (Figs. 15–15 to 15–17).[159] The urethra can then be divided under vision and drawn upward by the catheter.

Between bladder and rectum, the plane within Denonvilliers' fascia is found and opened down behind the prostate and seminal vesicles. The tough fibrous tissue at the apex of the prostate is divided on either side and the specimen lifted out.

If the urethra must be removed,[160] a midline incision is made in the perineum. The corpus spongiosum is separated

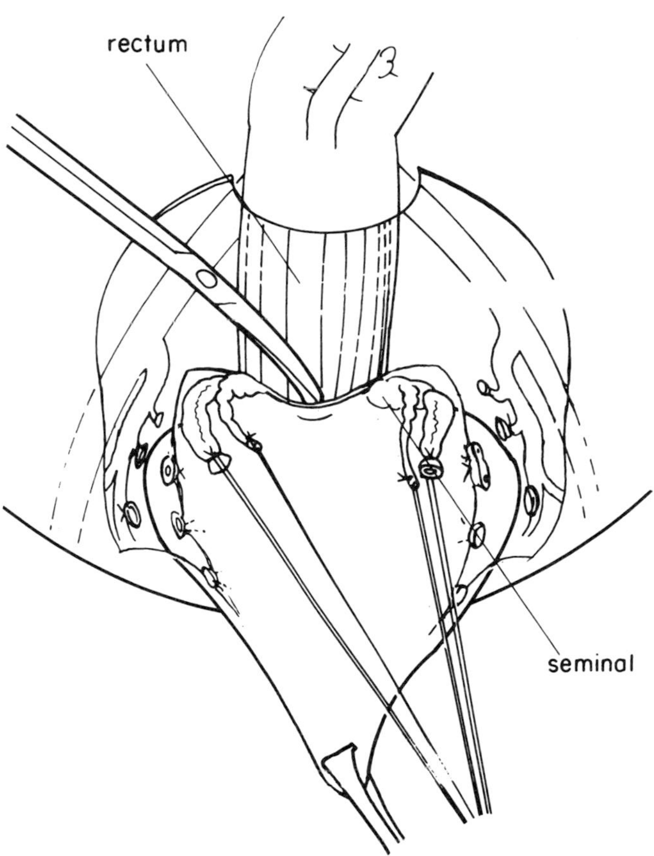

FIGURE 15–14. Traction on both ureters and seminal vesicles facilitating entry into the plane between layers of Denonvilliers' fascia between rectum and bladder. (From Blandy JP: Operative Urology, 2nd ed. London, Blackwell Publishers, 1986, p 138.)

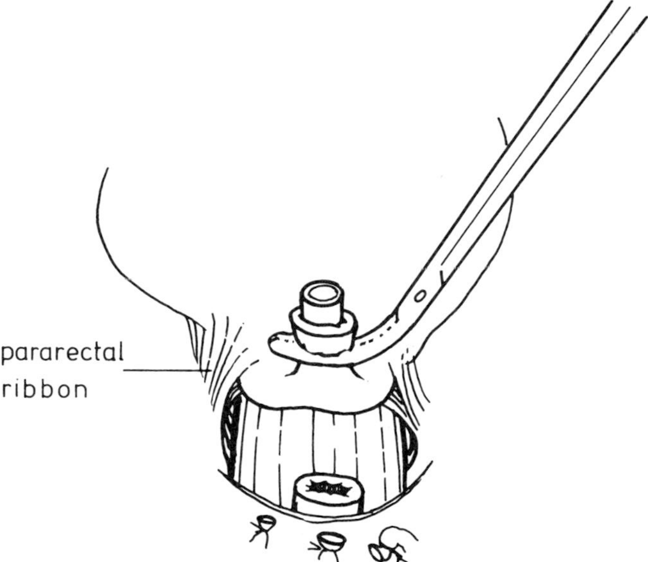

FIGURE 15–16. The pararectal ribbons are divided. (From Blandy JP: Operative Urology, 2nd ed. London, Blackwell Publishers, 1986, p 139.)

from the corpora cavernosa until the penis is turned inside out. The urethra is divided and the penis replaced (Fig. 15–18 to 15–20).

Pulling down the urethra reveals the bulbar arteries and dorsal vessels of the penis. These are divided. The pelvic fascia is incised on either side of the bulb. The rectum is depressed to define the rectoprostatic ligament, which is cut. The specimen is now free and may be drawn up into the pelvis.

The ureters are then anastomosed to an isolated loop of ileum or, if no radiation has been given, to a continent diversion.

Postoperative Care

Good results with total cystectomy require attention to every detail of management.[161] A gastrostomy avoids the discomfort and dangers of a nasogastric tube. Care must be taken with wound closure and to prevent deep vein thrombosis.

Squamous Cell Carcinoma of the Bladder

Squamous cell cancer is seldom diagnosed before it has invaded deeply and, in the West, has a poor prognosis. It

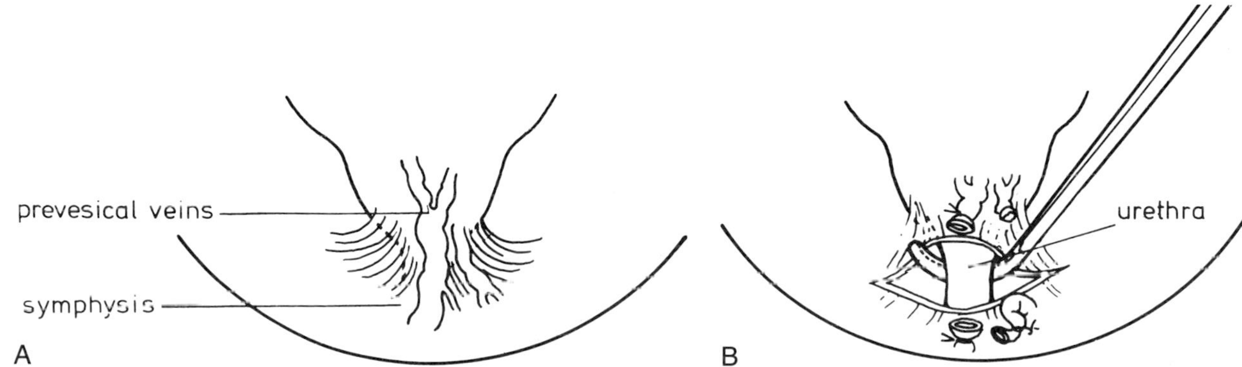

FIGURE 15–15. Separating bladder and prostate from symphysis displays prevesical and preprostatic veins (*A*), which are suture ligated and divided (*B*) in their strands of fibrous tissue. Under the veins lies the superior layer of pelvic fascia, which is divided to allow dissection around the urethra. (From Blandy JP: Operative Urology, 2nd ed. London, Blackwell Publishers, 1986, p 139.)

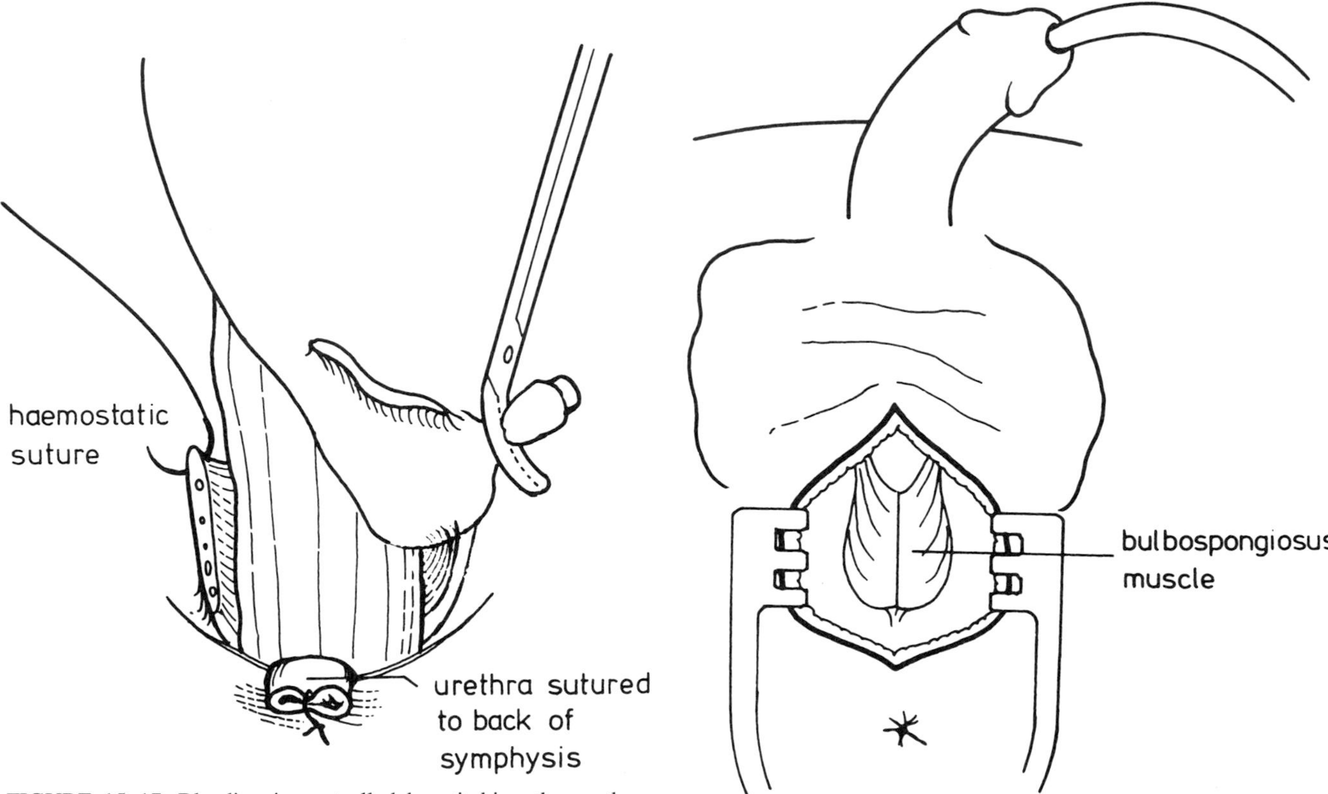

FIGURE 15–17. Bleeding is controlled by stitching the urethra to the back of the symphysis and running a stitch along the pararectal ribbons. (From Blandy JP: Operative Urology, 2nd ed. London, Blackwell Publishers, 1986, p 139.)

FIGURE 15–18. Urethrectomy in the male. A midline perineal incision is made over the bulb. (From Blandy JP: Operative Urology, 2nd ed. London, Blackwell Publishers, 1986, p 140.)

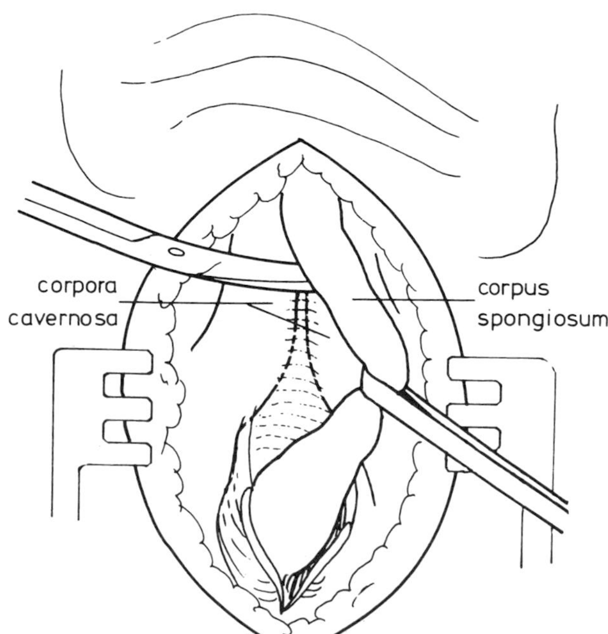

FIGURE 15–19. The corpus spongiosum is separated by sharp dissection from the underside of the united corpora cavernosa. (From Blandy JP: Operative Urology, 2nd ed. London, Blackwell Publishers, 1986, p 140.)

is radioresistant. In Egypt, fibrosis from bilharziasis appears to wall the tumor off, and excellent results are reported with total cystectomy. A low-pressure continent diversion has been devised that avoids reflux.[162]

CANCER OF THE PROSTATE

Epidemiology

Cancer of the prostate is unrelated to industrial pollution, smoking, wealth, or celibacy.[163] It may be less common after circumcision.[164] It occurs three times more in parents or siblings of those who have died of it.[165]

In the United States, about 244,000 new cases are predicted for 1995 with 40,400 deaths.[166] The mortality in white men remains static, at about 21 in 100,000 over the last 50 years, but has risen in black men from 24 to 36 in 100,000.[167]

Remarkable differences are reported in different parts of the world. Mortality for Japanese men in California, although four times higher than for those in Japan, is still only a tenth of that for African-American men in California, who have a ten times higher mortality than those in West Africa. Chinese men in Singapore or Hong Kong have a five times higher mortality than those in Shanghai.[163, 168] Before speculating too much about these data, it is as well to question the validity of some of these reported differences, which may reflect numbers of doctors and postmortem studies.

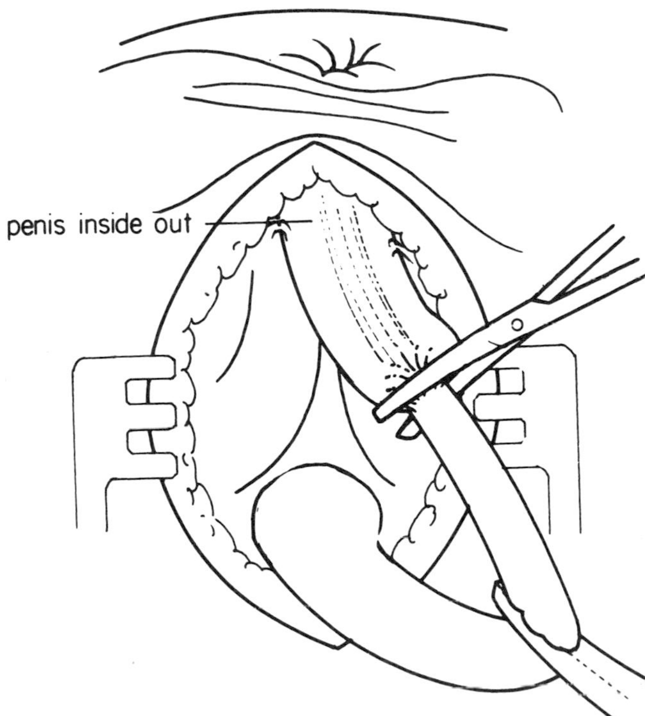

FIGURE 15–20. The urethra is clamped and a Foley catheter cut through. The penis is inverted inside out as the urethra is pulled inside out and divided across at the glans. (From Blandy JP: Operative Urology, 2nd ed. London, Blackwell Publishers, 1986, p 140.)

Local-Regional Anatomy and Pathology

Most adenocarcinomas of the prostate arise from acini; the small number arising from ducts have a worse prognosis.[169] Melanoma, sarcoma, and lymphoma are rarely seen.

Postmortem studies often reveal multifocal cancers too small to be seen or felt.[170] The more and the thinner the histologic sections, the more cancers found. By the age of 80, they are to be found in virtually every prostate,[171] and yet clinical cancer develops in only 3 in 1000 men in the United Kingdom.[172]

The histologic appearances in a single patient are various, making grading difficult. Most systems rely on numbers of mitoses or cytometry.[173–175] Gleason[173] prefers the low-power pattern of the tumor.

Spread is into seminal vesicles, urethra, and trigone, but tumor seldom penetrates the biologic barrier of Denonvilliers' fascia unless breached by biopsy. The "capsule" of the prostate is not a biologic barrier but, rather, the connective tissue that supports the veins[176] and that accompanies vessels and nerves into the substance of the gland. There is also a connective tissue space around each nerve fiber, along which cancer readily spreads.[177] As a result, lymph nodes are invaded in up to 80% of apparently localized cancers.[178, 179]

Bone Invasion

There is a direct connection between the veins and the lymphatics of the prostate and the bone marrow of the femora, pelvis, and lower lumbar vertebrae.[180]

Pathologic Staging

The staging systems vary according to the methods of investigation (Table 15–6), and, as for the bladder, the results based on pathologic staging from the total prostatectomy specimen cannot be compared with those staged by radiology and biopsy.[181–183]

Carcinoma in Situ

Malignant changes in acini without breach of the basement membrane are common near frank carcinoma. This diagnosis is subjective and its significance disputed.[184]

Focal Cancer

Focal cancer initially meant cancers invisible to the naked eye.[170, 172] Later it came to include cancers found by chance after prostatectomy for supposedly benign disease.[185] Today transrectal ultrasound scanning brings a third concept—cancer not felt by rectal examination but shown by ultrasound.

Serial section of radical prostatectomy specimens invariably shows multifocal tumors,[186] and small lesions may skip intervening stages and jump to lymph nodes.[187] Unsuspected lymph node metastasis varies with different observ-

TABLE 15–6
Comparison of Staging Systems for Prostate Cancer

TNM System		Conventional System	
T0	No evidence of prostate cancer		
T1	No palpable lesion	Stage A	Clinically unsuspected disease
T1a	Three or fewer microscopic foci of carcinoma	A1	Focal carcinoma, usually well differentiated
T1b	More than three microscopic foci of carcinoma	A2	Diffuse carcinoma, usually poorly differentiated
T2	Tumor clinically present, limited to the prostate gland	Stage B	Tumor confined to prostate gland
T2a	Tumor 1.5 cm or less in greatest diameter with normal tissue on at least three sides	B1	Small, discrete nodule of one lobe of gland
T2b	Tumor more than 1.5 cm in greatest diameter or in more than one lobe of the prostate	B2	Large or multiple nodules or areas of involvement
T3	Tumor invades prostatic apex, seminal vesicle, bladder neck, or is into or beyond prostatic capsule, but not fixed	Stage C	Tumor localized to the periprostatic area
		C1	Tumor outside prostatic capsule, estimated weight less than 70 g, seminal vesicles uninvolved
T4	Tumor is fixed or invades adjacent structures other than the structures listed in T3 (above)	C2	Tumor outside prostatic capsule, estimated weight more than 70 g, seminal vesicles involved
N	Lymph node metastases	Stage D	Metastatic prostate cancer
N1	Metastasis in a single pelvic node, less than 2 cm in greatest dimension	D1	Pelvic lymph node metastases and/or ureteral obstruction causing hydronephrosis
N2	Metastasis in a single pelvic node, more than 2 cm but less than 5 cm in diameter; or multiple lymph node metastases, none greater than 5 cm in greatest dimension		
N3	Metastasis in a single pelvic lymph node greater than 5 cm in diameter		
M	Distant metastatic disease		
M1	Bone, soft tissue, organ, or distant lymph node metastases	D2	Bone, soft tissue, organ, or distant lymph node metastases

From Glenn JF: AUA Today 4:21–28, 1991.

ers, from 0% to 23% in stage A and from 0% to 50% in stage B.[188]

Other Tumors

Melanin-containing cells are present in up to 4% of prostates and can give rise to melanoma.[189] Leiomyosarcoma may form large tumors in younger men.[190] Lymphoma is occasionally found in the prostate.

Diagnosis

Screening

Today, despite considerable investigation, there is no clear evidence that treatment alters the natural history of cancer in the prostate. As a consequence, to screen for cancer of the prostate, though widely practiced, is illogical.[191] Many symptomless cases are detected by prostate-specific antigen (PSA) examinations done as part of a routine checkup, causing unnecessary anxiety.

Symptoms

The symptoms of cancer are identical with those of benign enlargement of the prostate (frequency, nocturia, urgency, and eventually retention of urine). Ureteric obstruction may cause uremia, blocked lymphatics may give rise to edema, and encirclement of the rectum may lead to large bowel obstruction.[192] In about 10% of cases, distant metastasis brings the patient to the doctor with backache, a pathologic fracture, or paraplegia.

Physical Signs

Few patients have any physical signs. In some, a hard nodule is felt on rectal examination, but about half of the nodules that are felt are caused by some benign condition.[193]

Investigations

Transrectal Ultrasonography. Tissue calcium determines the density of the ultrasonic echo,[194] and cancer may have more, less, or the same amount of calcium. As a result, ultrasound scans detect only a fraction of the multifocal tumors present,[195] and even this observation is subject to considerable observer error.[196]

Computed Tomography. CT scanning does not detect small cancers but may assist in staging (Fig. 15–21).

Magnetic Resonance Imaging. MRI shows invasion of fat and vesicles more clearly.[197]

Tumor Markers. Serum acid phosphatase has been replaced by PSA, but there is a large overlap between benign enlargement and cancer, and it may help to express the PSA as a fraction per volume of prostate as measured by transrectal ultrasonography. PSA is useful in monitoring the response of a patient to treatment. Undifferentiated cells may be unable to make this enzyme, and a normal PSA may be found even though there are widespread metastases.[198, 199]

Most cancers originate in the outer zone of the prostate, while the tissue removed in transurethral resection of prostate (TURP) comes from the inner zone. Thus, cancer is

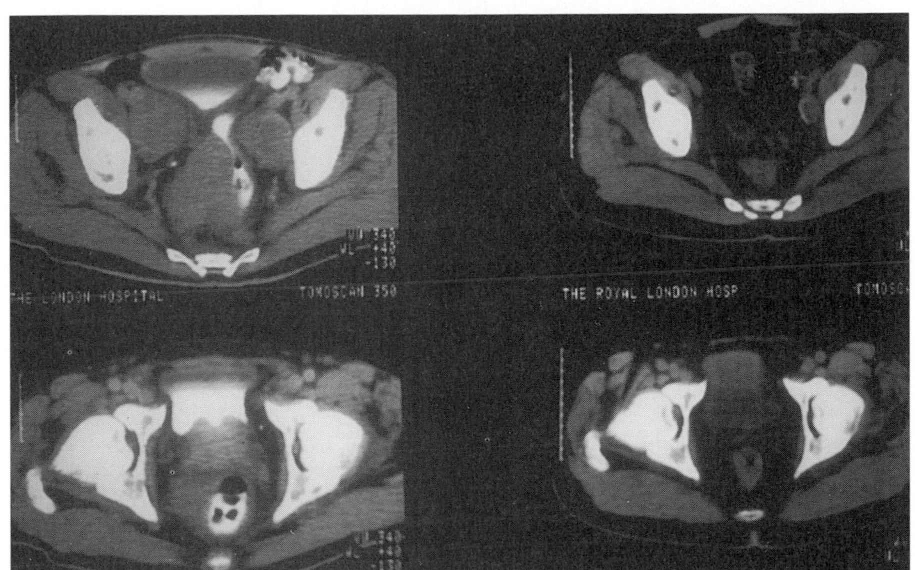

FIGURE 15–21. CT scan of prostate lymph node. (From Oliver RTD, Blandy JP, Hope-Stone F: Urological and Genital Cancer. London, Blackwell Publishers, 1989, pp 68–69.)

often left behind in the periphery, which is better sampled by needle biopsy, preferably under ultrasonic guidance.

Bone Scanning. Technetium Tc 99m MDP is taken up by bone in proportion to the blood flow, so that increased vascularity (e.g., from a metastasis or a fracture) will show a "hot spot" (Fig. 15–22).

Treatment

Cancer Confined to the Prostate (T1-T3, N0, M0)

Many feel deeply that this is a cancer that, when found, is at a stage at which it can be cured. As a consequence, they recommend radical prostatectomy and encourage early diagnosis by screening. Others point out that postmortem studies demonstrate small cancers in the majority of men who are candidates for surgery, which have been present for 10 to 20 years without treatment, and that there is no evidence that any treatment changes life expectancy.[200]

Immediate Versus Deferred Treatment Strategy for Early Cases

With more than 10% of operations for benign hypertrophy revealing occult malignant disease, explaining to a patient that malignancy has been discovered but proposing

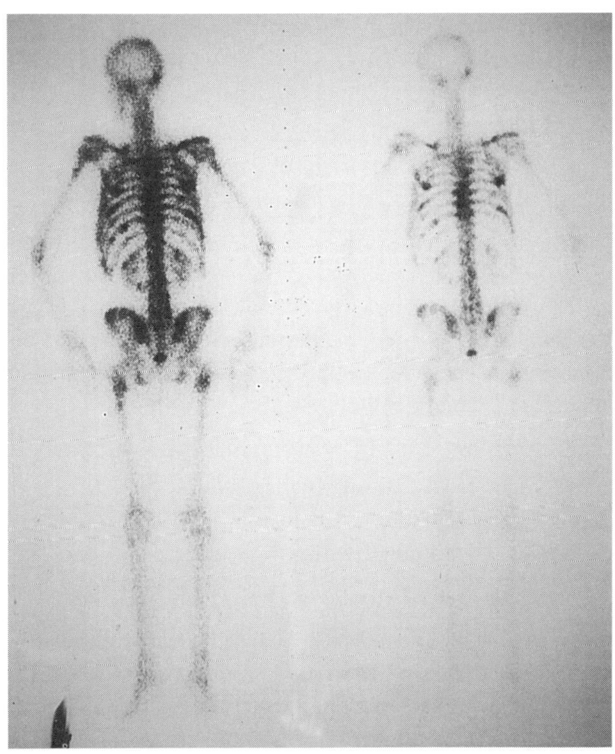

FIGURE 15–22. Bone scan of prostatic cancer metastases. (From Oliver RTD, Blandy JP, Hope-Stone HF: Urological and Genital Cancer. London, Blackwell Publishers, 1989, pp 68–69.)

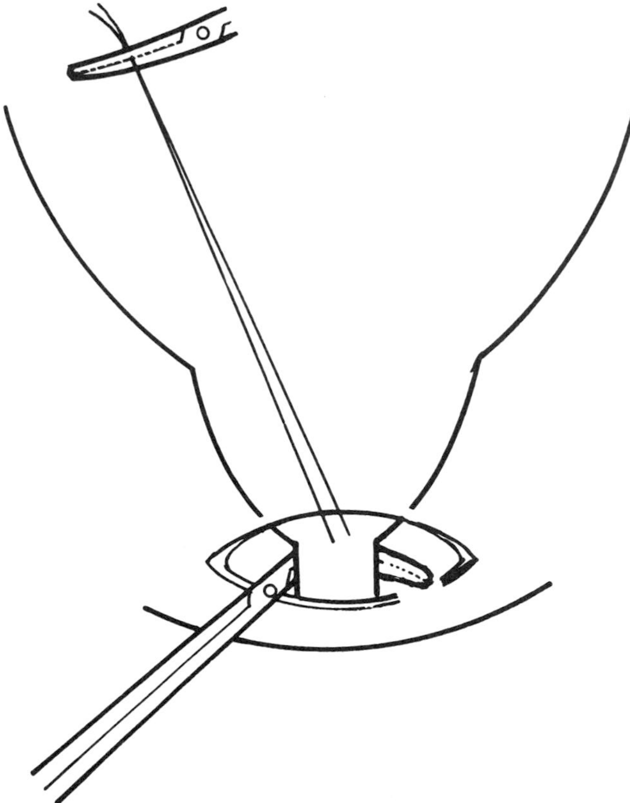

FIGURE 15–23. After the pelvic fascia is incised, the urethra is marked with stay suture and divided just distal to the lower edge of the prostate. (From Blandy JP: Operative Urology, 2nd ed. London, Blackwell Publishers, 1986, p 174.)

that nothing be done about it is one of the most common and most difficult situations a urologist has to handle. However, with the availability of a reliable marker of tumor activity (PSA), the results from doing nothing are demonstrating the safety of such an approach[201, 202] and providing a strong argument against the campaign for universal screening.

Radical Prostatectomy

The long-term results of radical perineal prostatectomy using a technique that did not treat any of the lymph nodes are unrivaled.[203] There is no evidence yet that the newer, nerve-sparing retropubic operation will give similar long-term results, despite its becoming the standard method of treatment in many centers.

Preliminary Laparoscopic Node Dissection

Increasingly, staging node dissection is done by a laparoscopic technique, thus sparing the patient a futile radical operation if the nodes are positive.

Radical Prostatectomy Procedure[204, 205]

Through a long midline incision, the fat is cleaned from the dorsal veins and the pelvic fascia is incised on either side to allow the veins to be suture ligated and divided (Fig. 15–23). The pelvic fascia with the penile neurovascular bundle is displaced laterally on each side. The urethra is drawn up and opened at the apex of the prostate. The rectourethralis muscle is incised, and the penile neurovascular bundles are again displaced laterally. The inferior vesical vessels are divided medial to these bundles.

The bladder neck is opened (Fig. 15–24), and the prostate is lifted up to separate it from the bladder, dividing the pedicle of the seminal vesicles (Figs. 15–25 to 15–28). The bladder neck is then anastomosed to the urethra, making a precise urothelial junction and avoiding the intramural sphincter just distal to the cut edge of the urethra (Fig. 15–29).

Radiotherapy

External Beam Therapy

Parallel opposed beams from a linear accelerator are directed by a CT simulator to include the lymph nodes of the pelvis but to avoid the rectum.[206] Side effects include transient proctitis (responding to hydrocortisone enemas) and impotence (in about 10% of men).

The results of radiotherapy are comparable to those of radical surgery,[206, 207] even though radical prostatectomy provides microscopic staging and cases treated by radiation will inevitably have been understaged.

Interstitial Radiotherapy

Radioactive sources, including iodine 125 seeds, gold Au 198 grains, and iridium wires have been implanted at

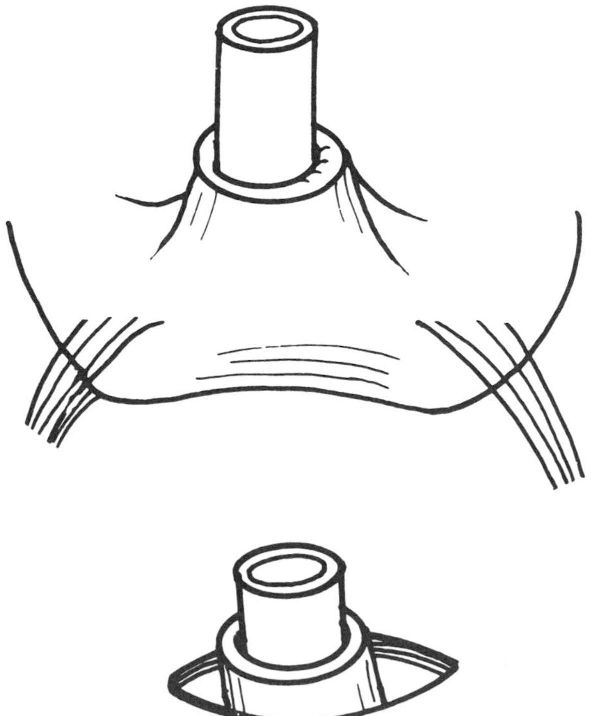

FIGURE 15–24. Dissection behind the prostate: the urethra is cut and lifted upward. (From Blandy JP: Operative Urology, 2nd ed. London, Blackwell Publishers, 1986, p 175.)

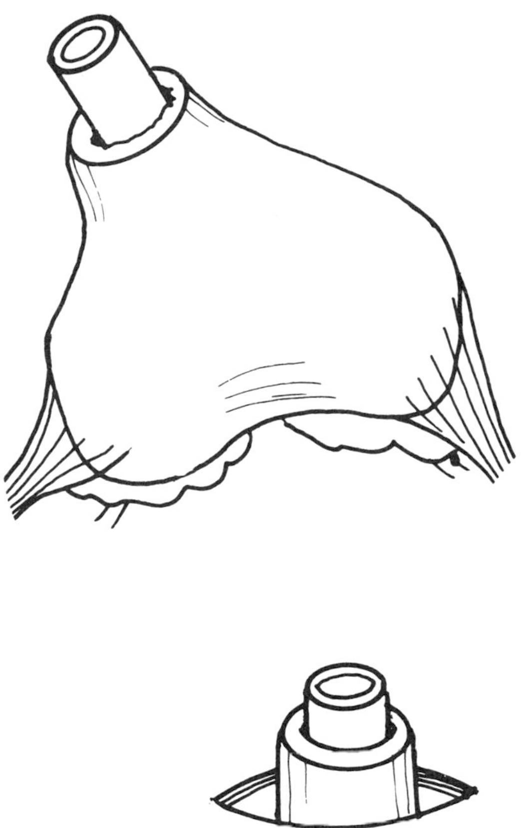

FIGURE 15–25. The prostate is retracted upward, revealing the seminal vesicles and ampullae of the vasa. (From Blandy JP: Operative Urology, 2nd ed. London, Blackwell Publishers, 1986, p 175.)

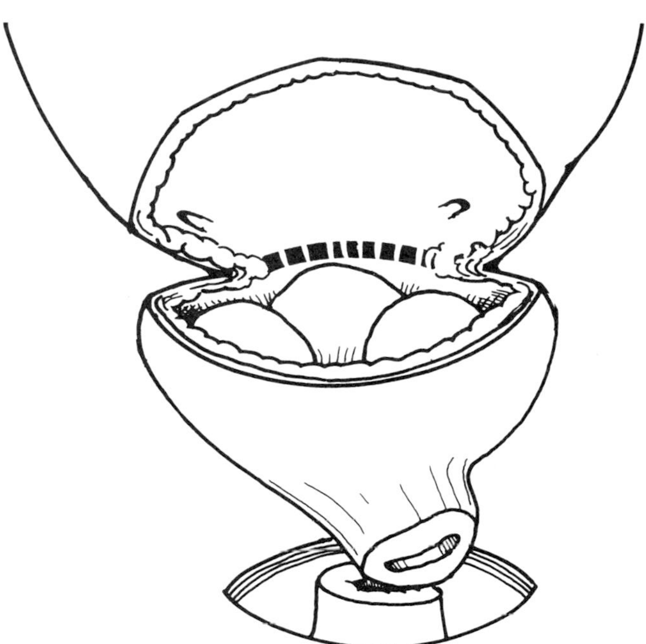

FIGURE 15–27. Incision of the posterior part of the bladder neck well above the prostate, but clear of the ureters. (From Blandy JP: Operative Urology, 2nd ed. London, Blackwell Publishers, 1986, p 175.)

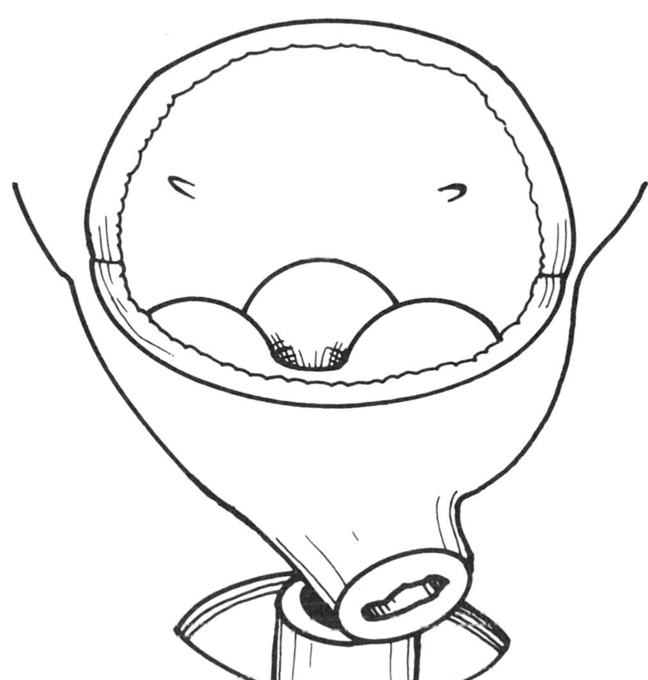

FIGURE 15–26. The bladder neck is cut across just above the prostate. (From Blandy JP: Operative Urology, 2nd ed. London, Blackwell Publishers, 1986, p 175.)

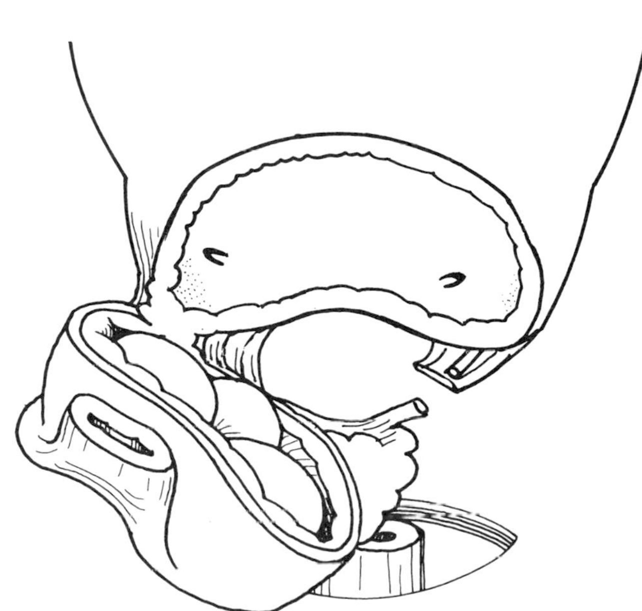

FIGURE 15–28. Division of the vas deferens on the left side. (From Blandy JP: Operative Urology, 2nd ed. London, Blackwell Publishers, 1986, p 175.)

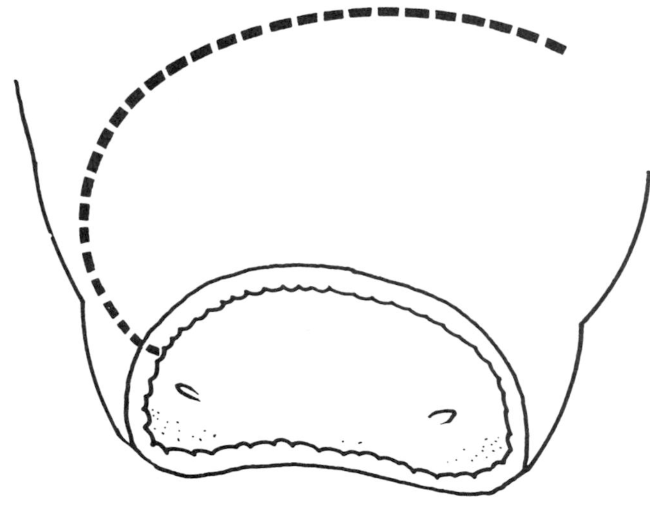

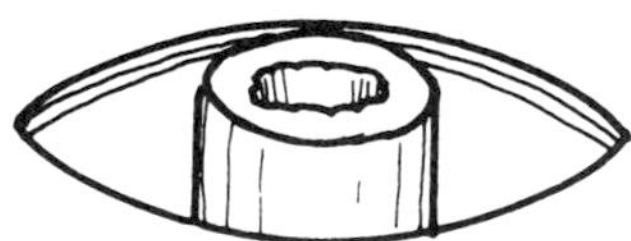

FIGURE 15–29. If the bladder does not come down easily without tension, the gap may be bridged with a tube flap. The dotted line illustrates a flap that may be used to create a tube to reach down to the urethra. (From Blandy JP: Operative Urology, 2nd ed. London, Blackwell Publishers, 1986, p 175.)

open operation, after lymph node dissection, or using an afterloading method with cannulas placed with ultrasound control. The results are similar to those obtained by teletherapy,[208–210] even though irradiated prostates still show cancer cells on biopsy.[209, 210]

Adjuvant Orchiectomy

Adding orchiectomy to radiotherapy or radical surgery may not prolong life but perhaps postpones metastases.[211]

Treatment of Cancer of the Prostate with Metastases

Although it is now more than 50 years since Huggins and Hodges first showed that castration caused metastases to disappear and that diethylstilbestrol would have the same effect,[212] there is still no agreement on the critical question as to whether hormone therapy should be used immediately on diagnosis of the disease or only when symptoms develop.

Unless metastases cause pain or threaten to cause some serious illness (e.g., paraplegia), to delay hormone treatment seems to give equally good results and postpones their side effects.[213] Such patients must be kept under regular review by means of PSA estimations and an occasional bone scan.

Hormone Treatment—The Options

About 80% of prostatic cancers depend on a continuous supply of testosterone. This is nearly all made by Leydig cells of the testes and activated to dihydrotestosterone by the enzyme 5-alpha-reductase within prostate cells. The adrenals secrete inactive precursors, dihydroepiandrosterone and androstenedione, which are converted by the aromatase enzymes into dihydrotestosterone in the prostate cells.

Orchiectomy removes the Leydig cells, is cheap and irreversible, and lowers the level of testosterone in the prostate by 75%.[214] Diethylstilbestrol blocks the action of testosterone even at doses of 1 mg/day. Higher doses have cardiovascular side effects,[215] which have been used to justify the more expensive modern approaches to androgen blockade.

Antiandrogens

Two antiandrogens, cyproterone and flutamide, are currently marketed; others are nearing completion of clinical trials. Cyproterone has been the most extensively studied, and several trials have clearly established that it can produce a transient response in patients who progress after response to orchiectomy and that it equals orchiectomy in previously untreated patients in terms of response and survival.

Flutamide is a pharmacologically purer antiandrogen compared with cyproterone acetate, which has progestrogenic effects. It has the advantage over other approaches to treatment of prostate cancer in that it produces tumor response without impotence, which is invariable with all other endocrine maneuvers. There is no evidence that this drug is equivalent to conventional treatment when used alone in previously untreated patients, and it has been compared with cyproterone in patients who progress after response to orchiectomy.

A third group of drugs, the aromatase inhibitors, have antiandrogenic effects that are occasionally successful in castrated patients who progress after response.[216] The original member of this group of aromatase inhibitor drugs, which inhibit adrenal androgen synthesis, was aminoglutethamide.

Luteinizing Hormone–Releasing Hormone (LH-RH) Agonists

In the last decade, many drugs have been marketed that block release of LH from the pituitary to produce a selective medical hypophysectomy—a functional castration—from lack of LH stimulation of Leydig cells in the testis. They are given as monthly injections in delayed-release formulation. They have been shown to be equal to orchiectomy and do not have the cardiovascular side effects of diethylstilbestrol,[214, 215] but they have no effect on patients failing orchiectomy. Substantially more expensive than orchiectomy and particularly 1 mg/day of stilbestrol, these agents are really justified only when reversal of androgen blockade is considered necessary.

Combined LH-RH Antagonist and Flutamide

Over the last decade, stimulated by laboratory information and many unrandomized phase II studies, there have been several attempts to show that there is an advantage in combining flutamide with an LH-RH antagonist. Although there has been a small benefit in two large randomized trials, the expense is prodigious[217, 218] and the subgroup who benefit are those with earliest extent of spread and least symptoms, the subgroup who also has the most to gain from deferred treatment of any kind.

Symptomatic Control of Painful Bone Metastases

Solitary metastases that cause pain usually respond to local radiotherapy. Pain from generalized bony metastases may be eased by hemibody radiation,[219] phosphorus 32,[220] strontium 89,[221] or diphosphonate.[222]

CANCER OF THE URETHRA

In Males

Etiology

Some benign condylomas caused by papillomavirus can become progressively more malignant until they metastasize.[223] Many urethral tumors are implanted from a primary tumor in the bladder, and some are multifocal—hence the need for urethrectomy in cystectomy for multifocal cancer.[224]

Squamous cell cancer of the urethra is seen with long-standing urethral strictures, especially in Africa,[225] and probably follows squamous metaplasia upstream of a stricture.

Pathology

Benign Tumors

Condylomata acuminata may spread up the urethra, especially in immunosuppressed patients. Benign "polyps" occur near the verumontanum in children. Capillary hemangiomas are an unusual cause of urethral bleeding.[226]

Malignant Tumors

Primary squamous cell cancer may occur in the bulbar urethra without obvious cause. Melanoma is even more rare. Secondary cancer occurs by implantation or infiltration along the wall of the urethra from bladder or prostate.

Tumor Spread

Tumors in the penile urethra spread to the inguinal lymph nodes. Those of the bulb may reach the internal iliac nodes.

Diagnosis

Clinical Features

Any chronic stricture with multiple fistulas should make one suspect cancer. In the West, the symptoms can imitate enlargement of the prostate, but usually the presenting feature is a perineal mass resembling an abscess, the incision of which discloses not pus but cancer.

Investigations

Recurrence after cystectomy can be detected by urethroscopy and biopsy, or with a ureteric brush. Palpable inguinal nodes require fine-needle aspiration biopsy.

Treatment

Condylomata Acuminata

Intraurethral condylomata usually respond to thiotepa, 5-fluorouracil, or mitomycin, but it may be quicker to use diathermy or the Nd:YAG laser. When they are widespread and profuse, it may be necessary to lay open the urethra as in the first stage of a urethroplasty.[227]

Urethral Cancer

Cancer following a chronic stricture does remarkably well with local excision and postoperative radiotherapy: none of our seven cases have metastasized over more than 15 years. In contrast, the outlook for those that arise de novo in the bulbar urethra is appalling.

A preoperative combination of chemotherapy and radiotherapy may shrink the tumor before urethrectomy. The gap in the urethra can be made good by a pedicled tube of scrotal skin.

With positive inguinal nodes, radical node dissection may cure half the patients.[228]

Tumor that recurs after previous resection, or that has invaded the prostate, can be cured only by a radical resection that removes en bloc the bladder, penis, and inguinal and iliac nodes.

In Females

Urethral tumors in women are classified as follows:

Benign
Condyloma acuminatum
Hemangioneurofibroma

Malignant
Squamous cell carcinoma
Adenocarcinoma
Transitional cell carcinoma
Malignant melanoma

Benign Tumors

Most "caruncles" are prolapses of the urethral mucosa complicated by venous thrombosis. Edematous polyps may protrude from the meatus. Condylomata acuminata occur anywhere in the vulva, including the urethra. The rare hemangioneurofibroma forms a characteristic painful red swelling.

Malignant Tumors

Squamous cell cancer of the female urethra may cause frequency and dysuria without obvious cause, and all too often these patients are reassured, dismissed with the spurious diagnosis "urethral syndrome," and treated by dilatation.

The only safe rule is to perform urethroscopy whenever there is any doubt and to sample all urethral swellings for biopsy.[229]

At the cranial end of the female urethra, adenocarcinoma is more common, arising in a paraurethral gland. Primary malignant melanoma of the female urethra causes pain, hematuria, and a brown friable mass.[230] Cancer of the external meatus metastasizes to the inguinal nodes, that of upper third to the internal iliac nodes.

Stage

The UICC system for cancer of the urethra is presented in Table 15–7.[231]

Treatment

Tumors of the lower third of the female urethra are usually cured by interstitial radiotherapy with gold grains, tantalum, iridium, or radium needles; if the tumor recurs, the urethra can be safely excised without loss of continence.

Involved inguinal nodes can be removed en bloc.[232] Localized tumors of the middle third of the urethra can be removed and replaced by a pedicled tube of skin from the labium minus of the vulva with preservation of continence.

Cancers of the upper end of the female urethra spread so early that a course of combination chemotherapy and radiotherapy should precede excision. If the para-aortic lymph nodes are free, cystourethrectomy may be justified for persistent tumor, with up to 36% 3-year survival.[229]

CANCER OF THE PENIS

Etiology

Neonatal circumcision prevents penile cancer,[233] perhaps by removing a common site for its origin, by preventing balanitis, or by removing carcinogens in smegma.[234] When circumcision is performed after the eighth day of life, it protects to a more limited extent.

TABLE 15–7
Tumor (T) Staging for Carcinoma of the Urethra

Tis	Carcinoma in situ
T1	Invasion of subepithelial connective tissue
T2	Invasion of corpus spongiosum, prostate, periurethral muscle
T3	Invasion of corpus cavernosum, beyond prostatic capsule, vagina, or bladder neck
T4	Invasion of other organs

TABLE 15–8
Classification of Penile Tumors

Benign
- Condyloma acuminatum

Precarcinomatous
- Buschke-Löwenstein tumor
  - Erythoplasia of Queyrat
  - Balanitis xerotica obliterans

Malignant
- Squamous cell carcinoma
- Basal cell carcinoma
- Sarcoma fibrosarcoma
- Angiosarcoma—Kaposi's tumor
- Melanoma

Secondary carcinoma, lymphoma, etc.

There is a continuous spectrum from the wart caused by papillomavirus, to the Buschke-Löwenstein "giant" condyloma, to frankly invasive cancer, as seen in Table 15–8.[235] Smoking may be related,[236] as may previous infection with Ducrey's bacillus, *Herpesvirus hominis,*[237] and poor personal hygiene.[238] The wives of men with penile cancer may be more prone to cancer of the cervix.[239] Balanitis xerotica obliterans has been a precursor in up to 20% of cases.[239, 240]

In the West, cancer of the penis is a disease of old men; in India and Russia, it is seen in younger men.[233, 237]

Pathology

Benign Tumors

Condylomata Acuminata (Venereal Warts)

These are transmitted by intercourse. Several strains of virus may be present in the same wart.[235] In immunosuppressed men, they may form a carpet covering the glans and extending up the urethra.

Condylomata acuminata respond to treatment with 10% podophyllin, thiotepa, 5-fluorouracil, mitomycin, diathermy, or the carbon dioxide or Nd:YAG laser.

Precarcinomatous Tumors

Buschke-Löwenstein Tumor

These giant warts contain papillomaviruses[241–243] Local excision was formerly advised, but experience has taught us that they should be treated as malignant from the beginning.

Erythroplasia of Queyrat[244]

This appears as a scaly red patch on the glans in circumcised men, moist and weeping in the uncircumcised. Only by biopsy can it be distinguished from simple balanitis. This will show any stage from carcinoma in situ to invasive carcinoma. The identical carcinoma in situ when found on the shaft of the penis is labeled Bowen's disease and may be a manifestation of occult gastrointestinal cancer.[245]

TABLE 15–9
Tumor (T) Staging for Carcinoma of the Penis

Tx	Cannot be assessed
T0	No evidence of primary tumor
Tis	Carcinoma in situ
Ta	Noninvasive verrucous cancer
T1	Invasion of subepithelial connective tissue
T2	Invasion of corpus spongiosum or cavernosum
T3	Invasion of urethra or prostate
T4	Invasion of other adjacent structures

Erythroplasia of Queyrat responds to topical 5% 5-fluorouracil cream, local irradiation, or coagulation by the carbon dioxide laser, but it must be followed because relapse is common.

Malignant Tumors

Early cancer presents as a shallow fissure or a small "papilloma." Squamous cell carcinoma accounts for 99% of malignancies; basal cell carcinoma occurs in less than 0.5% of cases.[246] Malignant tumors are graded according to the frequency of mitoses.[247] They are usually well differentiated and spread locally for a long time before metastases occur in the inguinal lymph nodes, of which the node on the fossa ovalis is often the first to be involved.[248] Spread along the urethra calls for frozen section at amputation to ensure clear margins.

Clinical Features

It is unusual to see early cancers of the penis. Most present late, with a large, stinking, infected mass behind a phimosis with enlarged inguinal nodes which, at this stage may merely be infected. Enlarged nodes in absence of infection are probably invaded and require aspiration biopsy.[241]

Stage

The UICC system for carcinoma of the penis is presented in Table 15–9.[249] This system has less practical use than that of Jackson (Table 15–10), which is in common use.[250]

Circumcision is the first step in treatment, and it may remove all the tumor. Larger tumors are debulked, and infection is treated. Lymph nodes are reassessed after 3 weeks.

TABLE 15–10
Jackson Staging System for Carcinoma of the Penis

Stage 1	Tumor limited to prepuce or glans
Stage 2	Invasion of the shaft of the penis
Stage 3	Involvement of the scrotum
Stage 4	Invasion of inguinal nodes

Treatment According to Jackson Stage

Stage 1

Local irradiation with gold, tantalum, or iridium 90 gives 100% 5-year survival, but about 25% of patients require partial amputation for residual or recurrent tumor.[241]

In partial amputation, blood loss is prevented with a soft clamp on the base of the penis (Fig. 15–30). A racquet incision is made well clear of the tumor. The corpora cavernosa are amputated 5 mm proximal to the corpus spongiosum, and the margins are checked by frozen section. After suture ligating the penile arteries, the tunicae are closed with catgut, and, to avoid stenosis, the spatulated urethra is sutured to an inverted U-shaped flap of skin (Fig. 15–31).[251]

Stage 2

When the corpora cavernosa are invaded, radiotherapy, although it cures only half the patients by itself, improves the long-term results of amputation, which may be kept in reserve.[251]

Stage 3

Even when the scrotum is invaded, the inguinal lymph nodes may be uninvaded. Amputation is the first step to

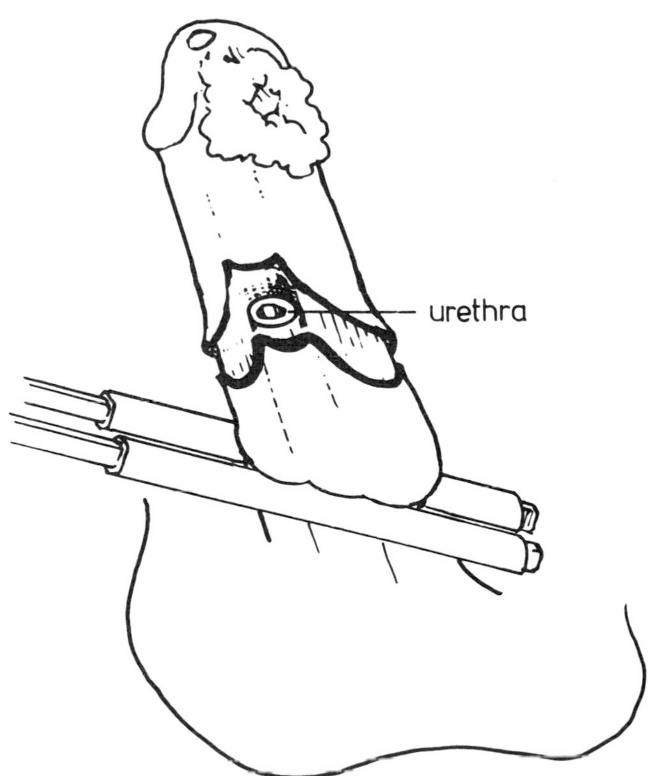

FIGURE 15–30. Partial amputation of the penis. A noncrushing clamp is placed well proximal to the site of the incision to keep the field bloodless. The ventral skin flap is made longer than the dorsal one so that the incision around the penis is elliptic. (From Blandy JP: Operative Urology, 2nd ed. London, Blackwell Publishers, 1986, p 198.)

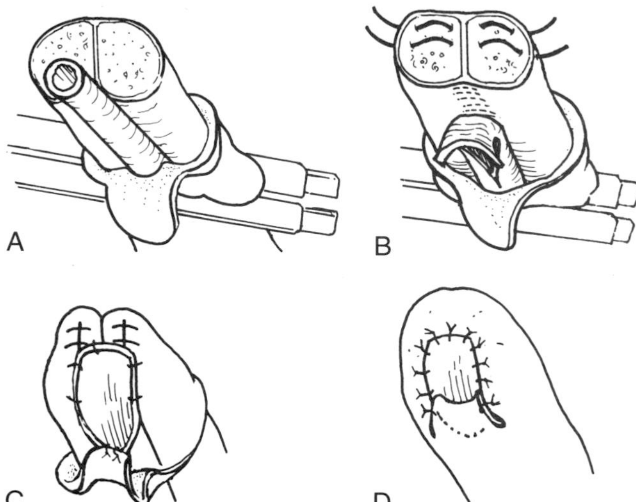

FIGURE 15–31. The skin is retracted and the corpora transected *(A)*. Interrupted sutures are used to close the corpora together *(B)*. The urethra is spatulated and sewn over the united cavernosa *(C)* and the inverted U-shaped flap of skin is used to make an elliptic anastomosis between the skin and the urethra to prevent stricture *(D)*. (From Blandy JP: Operative Urology, 2nd ed. London, Blackwell Publishers, 1986, p 199.)

remove the infected mass.[251] The tumor is enclosed in a glove before preparing the skin. The surgeon cuts around the base of the penis well clear of the tumor. The incision is carried down to make an inverted U-shaped scrotal flap, exposing the entire scrotal contents (Fig. 15–32). It is easier to make a complete excision if the testicles are removed en bloc and all the soft tissues are cleared medially and downward from the external ring, dividing the suspensory ligament and dorsal vessels of the penis (Figs. 15–33 to 15–35).

The surgeon separates the corpus spongiosum from the cavernosa for about 5 cm and cuts it across (Fig. 15–36). The corpora cavernosa are divided near the pubic rami and oversewn with catgut (Fig. 15–37).

After stitching the spatulated urethra to the symphysis, the inverted U-shaped flap of scrotum is anastomosed, forming a long ellipse to prevent stenosis. Closing the wound leaves a perineum resembling a vulva (Fig. 15–38). This resection, which seems so radical, can give 90% long-term survival.[241, 252]

Stage 4

Adjuvant therapy has changed the management of positive inguinal nodes. CT scanning and fine-needle aspiration cytology are used to stage the tumor. If only inguinal nodes are involved, a tumor dose of 4500 cGy is given first, with care to protect the rectum. Any remaining positive nodes call for block dissection.[253]

Block Dissection of the Inguinal Nodes

An oblique inguinal incision is made 2 cm below the inguinal ligament (Fig. 15–39). The contents of the femoral triangle are removed en bloc to strip the femoral artery, vein, and nerve. The femoral vessels are covered by detaching the upper end of the sartorius muscle and swinging it medially to protect them (Figs. 15–40 and 15–41).

When aspiration biopsy shows positive iliac nodes at presentation, a preoperative course of chemotherapy is first given using our current protocol for squamous head, neck, and cervical cancer (i.e., methotrexate, vincristine, cisplatin, and bleomycin), in addition to radiotherapy. After inguinal node dissection has been performed, the iliac fossa is exposed after lifting up a flap of skin and flap. An oblique incision is made 2 cm above the inguinal ligament through the abdominal wall, to enter the retroperitoneal space. A block dissection of the external and internal iliac lymph nodes is performed up to the bifurcation of the aorta.

Sarcoma of the Penis

Sarcomas of the penis usually arise near the frenulum,[254] but hemangiomas may arise anywhere in the erectile tissue and cause priapism. Kaposi's sarcoma of the penile skin is becoming more common owing to the AIDS epidemic.[255] Other sarcomas occur,[256] the most rare of which is melanoma.[257] Surgical excision is not entirely hopeless.

Secondary Cancer of the Penis

Metastases from the prostate or bladder may mimic Peyronie's disease, and, in childhood, deposits of leukemia

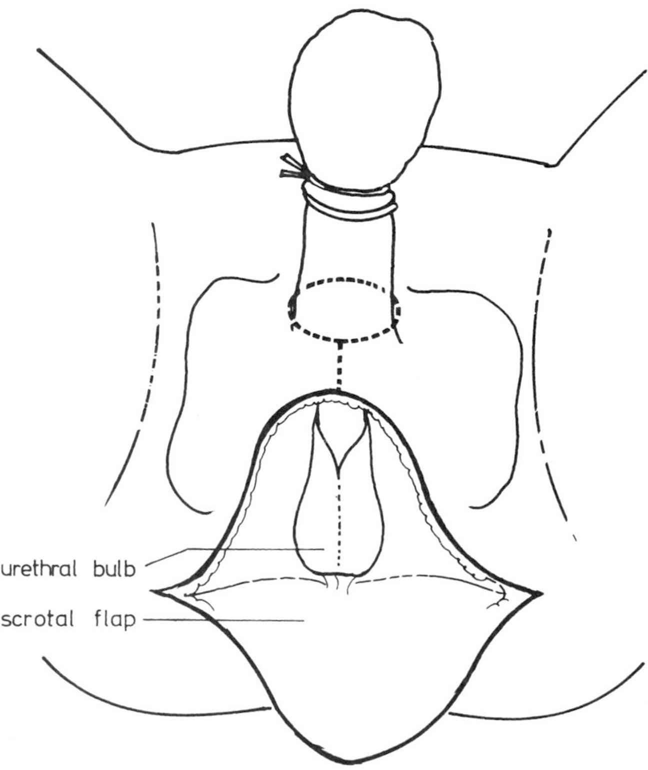

FIGURE 15–32. Radical amputation of the penis is started by raising the inverted U-shaped scrotal flap and exposing the urethra and bulbospongiosus muscles. (From Blandy JP: Operative Urology, 2nd ed. London, Blackwell Publishers, 1986, p 200.)

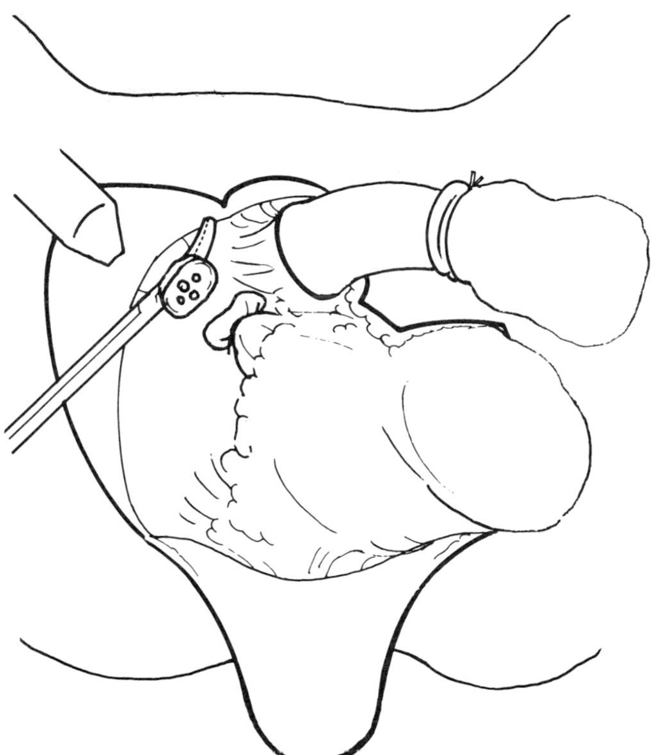

FIGURE 15–33. The spermatic cords are clamped, doubly transfixed, and ligated at the external ring. (From Blandy JP: Operative Urology, 2nd ed. London, Blackwell Publishers, 1986, p 200.)

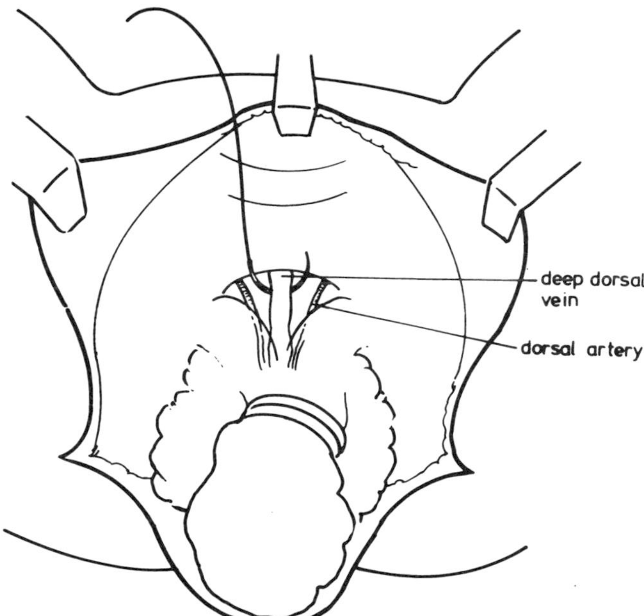

FIGURE 15–35. The deep vein and deep arteries of the penis are suture ligated and divided. (From Blandy JP: Operative Urology, 2nd ed. London, Blackwell Publishers, 1986, p 201.)

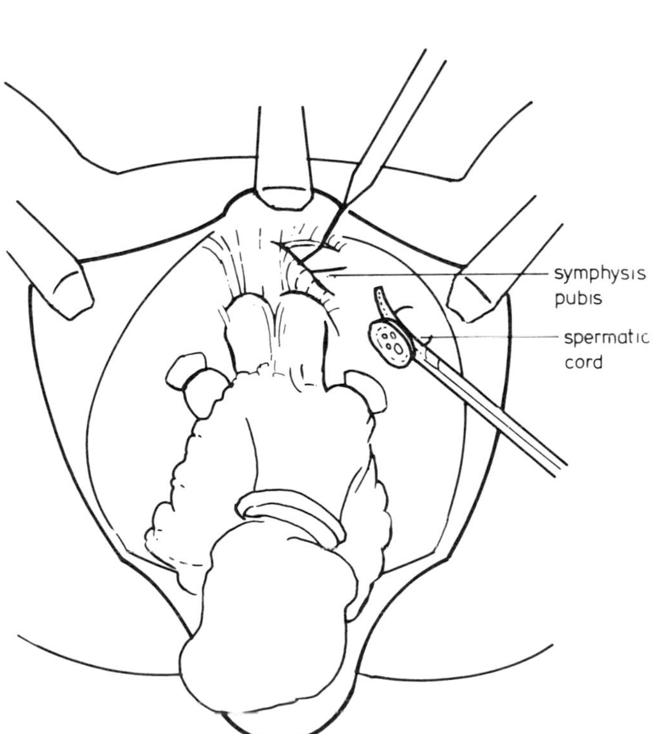

FIGURE 15–34. After the left cord is cut, the suspensory ligament of the penis is divided, clearing tissue away from the front of the symphysis. (From Blandy JP: Operative Urology, 2nd ed. London, Blackwell Publishers, 1986, p 200.)

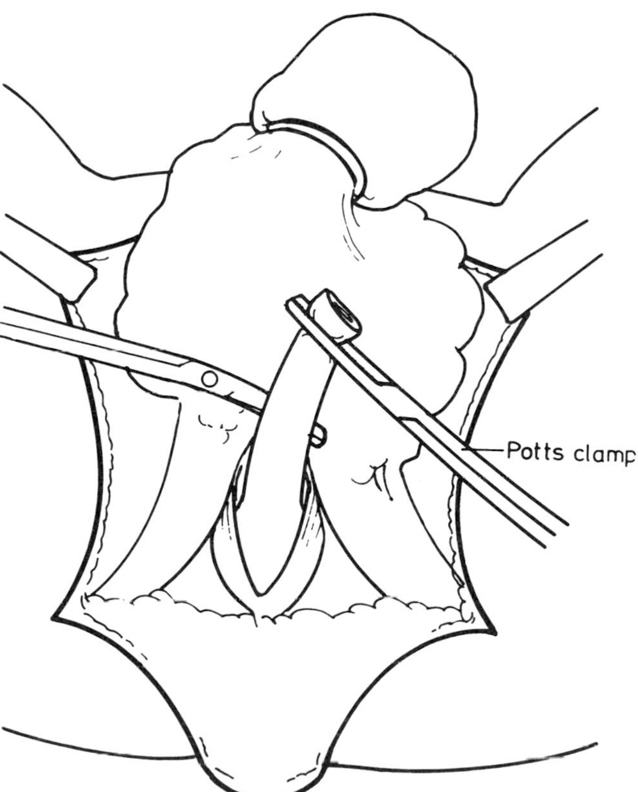

FIGURE 15–36. The corpus spongiosum and urethra are separated from the corpora cavernosa, clamped, and cut across. (From Blandy JP: Operative Urology, 2nd ed. London, Blackwell Publishers, 1986, p 201.)

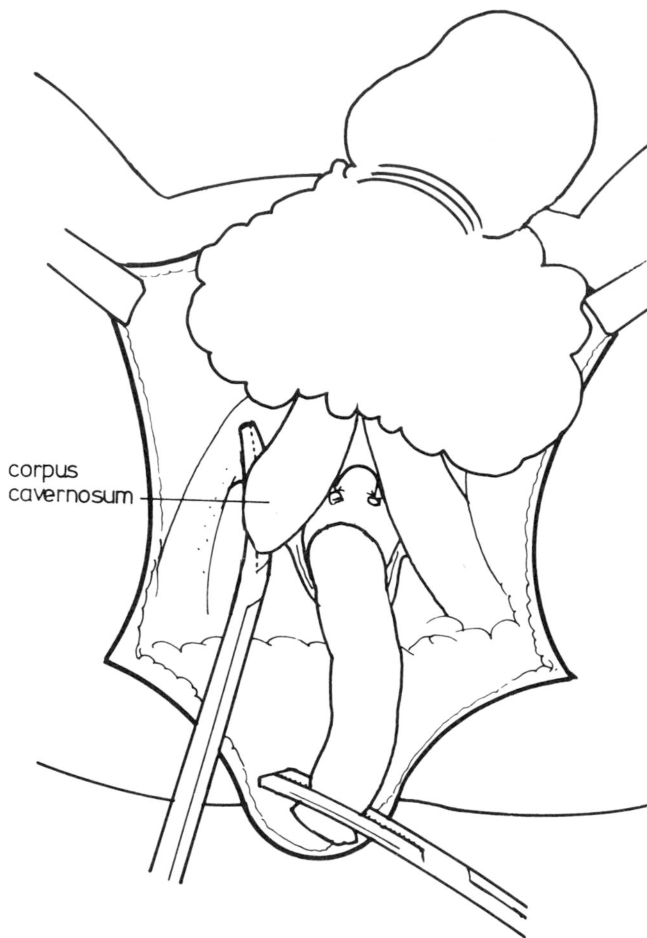

FIGURE 15–37. Each corpus cavernosum is clamped near its attachment to the ischial ramus. (From Blandy JP: Operative Urology, 2nd ed. London, Blackwell Publishers, 1986, p 201.)

are a well-recognized cause of priapism.[258] Surprisingly, metastases from transitional cell cancer respond particularly well to chemotherapy.[259] Occasional patients with prostate and bladder cancer can be cured of primary tumor by radiation and then undergo a urethral recurrence, possibly due to implantation of tumor cells during a traumatic transurethral resection of tumor. Even if resistant to retreatment, an occasional case has been cured by amputation at this stage.

CANCER OF THE ADRENAL GLANDS

Hyperplasia and Tumors

Most cancers of the adrenal form only inactive precursors of hormones, but cortisol from the zona fasciculata causes Cushing's syndrome; androgens from the zona reticularis, virilization; aldosterone from the zona glomerulosa, Conn's syndrome; and catecholamines from the medulla may give rise to paroxysmal hypertension.[260]

Because they are inactive, the majority of adrenal tumors are large and have often metastasized by the time the patient presents. Any nonfunctioning tumor greater than 3.5 cm diameter is probably malignant and behaves like any other retroperitoneal cancer.[261–263]

Adrenocorticotropic hormone (ACTH) from a basophil adenoma of the pituitary or some other cancer (e.g., the lung) may lead to hyperplasia of any of the elements of the adrenal cortex.

In Cushing's syndrome—caused by excess cortisol from zona fasciculata tissue—obesity of the trunk, wasted limbs, moon face, diabetes, buffalo hump, striae, acne, hirsutism, bruising, and hypertension are seen. In Conn's syndrome, the aldosterone from zona glomerulosa cells causes sodium retention, loss of potassium, and polyuria. Clinically, the most important feature is weakness. Hypertension often appears early, but the significance of the associated hypokalemia may be missed because the patient is given diuretics for the hypertension.

Biochemical Diagnosis

To tell whether one of these hormonal syndromes is caused by hyperplasia or a tumor, dexamethasone is given to suppress the action of the pituitary. The hormones from a tumor will remain unchanged, while with hyperplasia they fall.

When Cushing's syndrome is caused by a tumor, the plasma ACTH is elevated and the level of plasma cortisol

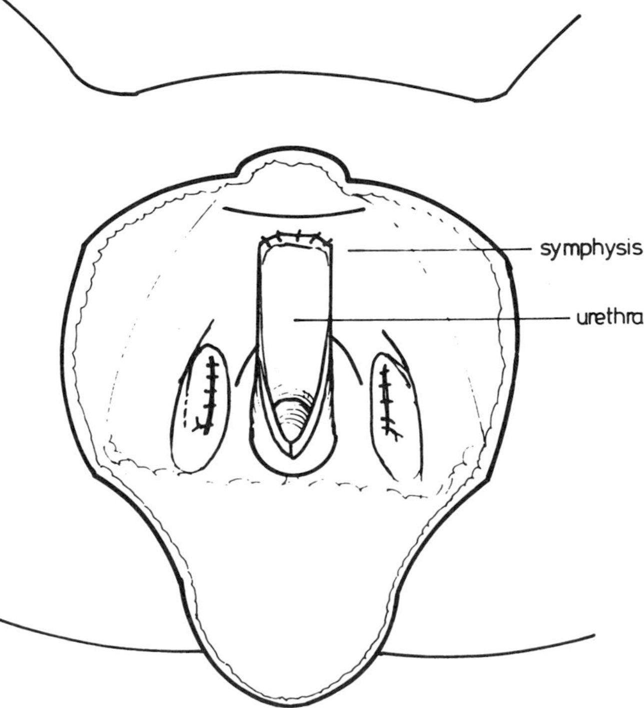

FIGURE 15–38. Both corpora cavernosa are oversewn, and the spatulated urethra is attached to the front of the symphysis. (From Blandy JP: Operative Urology, 2nd ed. London, Blackwell Publishers, 1986, p 201.)

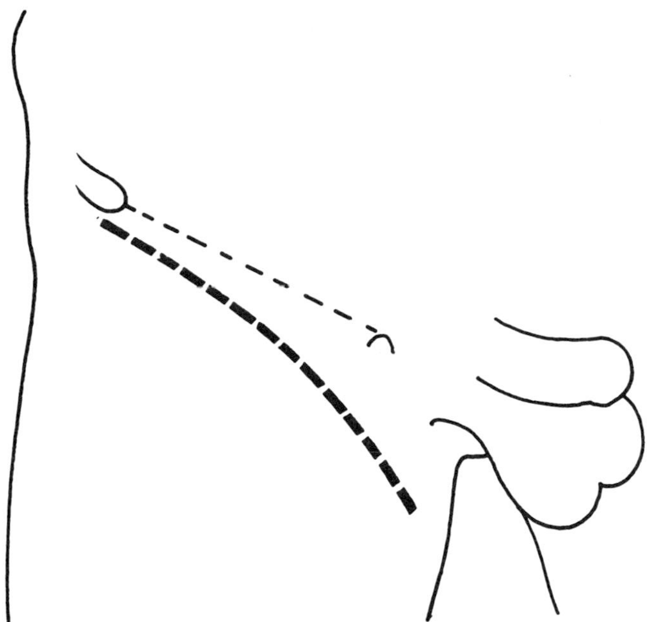

FIGURE 15–39. Incision for inguinal node resection. (From Blandy JP: Operative Urology, 2nd ed. London, Blackwell Publishers, 1986, p 202.)

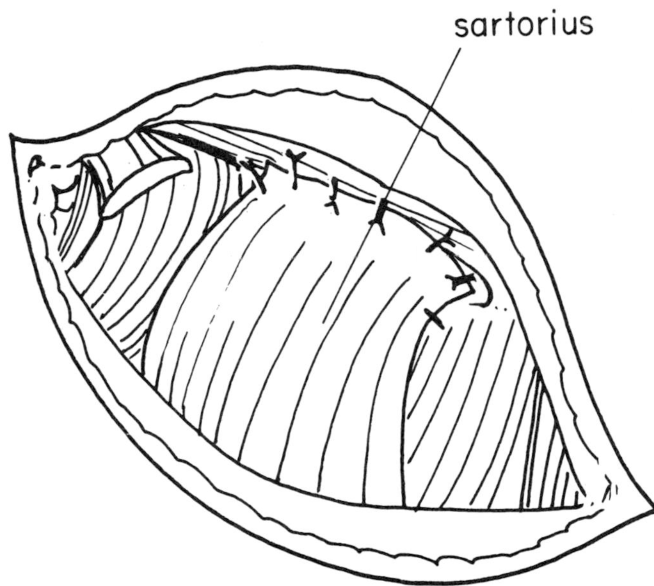

FIGURE 15–41. The detached sartorius muscle sutured to the inguinal ligament to cover and protect the femoral vessels. (From Blandy JP: Operative Urology, 2nd ed. London, Blackwell Publishers, 1986, p 203.)

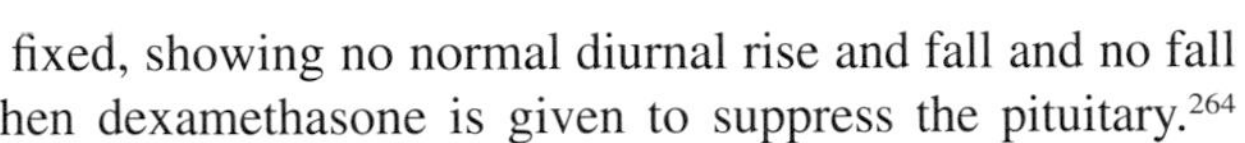

is fixed, showing no normal diurnal rise and fall and no fall when dexamethasone is given to suppress the pituitary.[264]

In virilizing zona reticularis tumors, the raised ketosteroids, testosterone, and other androgens do not rise with ACTH or fall with dexamethasone.[265]

In Conn's syndrome, the elevated plasma aldosterone remains fixed when a saline load is given, and the low plasma renin does not rise when salt is withheld.[266]

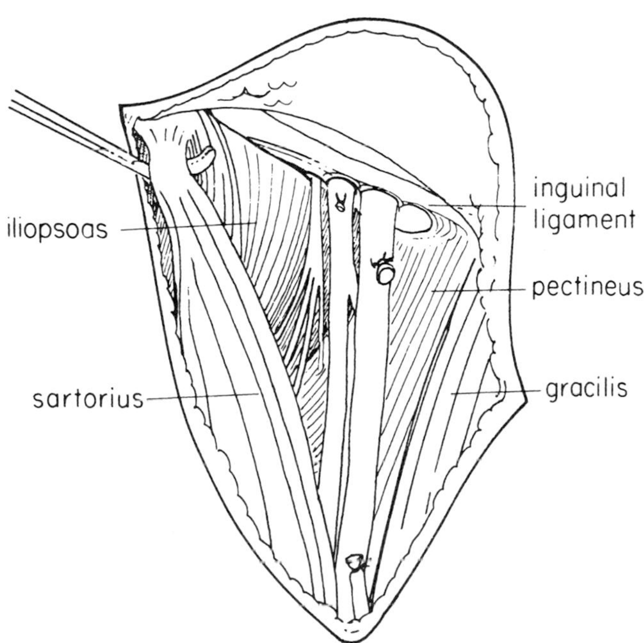

FIGURE 15–40. Structures displayed after inguinal node dissection. (From Blandy JP: Operative Urology, 2nd ed. London, Blackwell Publishers, 1986, p 203.)

Localization

Today these tumors are usually localized with CT scans, which show bilateral adrenal enlargement in cases of hyperplasia. Cortisol-producing tumors of the zona fasciculata are generally small and discrete. Virilizing tumors of the zona reticularis tend to be large and hence often malignant.[263] Aldosterone-secreting zona glomerulosa tumors are small and difficult to find even with CT, and it may be necessary to measure the aldosterone in both adrenal veins to localize the tumor.[264]

Treatment

Surgical excision is the only treatment for malignant cortical tumors, but the results are poor. Claims have been advanced for chemotherapy with 1,1-dichloroethane.[263]

Adrenalectomy

Single small cortical tumors are approached through the bed of the twelfth rib. Traction on the kidney brings down the adrenal. Large tumors may require a thoracoabdominal incision. For hyperplasia, the prone position allows simultaneous exploration of both adrenals through short twelfth rib–tip incisions.

Tumors of the Adrenal Medulla

Pheochromocytoma occurs on its own or as part of a pluriglandular syndrome, either with (1) hyperparathyroidism and carcinoma of the thyroid[267, 268] or (2) renal cell carcinoma and von Hippel–Lindau disease (retinal angiomatosis, cerebellar, and pancreatic cysts).[269] One percent are malignant, 10% are bilateral, and another 10% occur elsewhere than the adrenal (e.g., mediastinum, carotid body, origin of the inferior mesenteric artery, or bladder).[270]

Clinical Features

Paroxysmal hypertension is the classic clinical presentation, with headache, palpitation, and sweating precipitated by smoking, coitus, or other forms of exertion, but in fact sustained hypertension is equally common.[271]

There are seldom any physical signs, and it is dangerous to palpate too firmly to try to feel a tumor, since this may precipitate a paroxysm. Neurofibromas may be present, as well as café au lait patches with a smooth outline.

Biochemical Diagnosis

The biochemical diagnosis is made by finding excess catecholamines in plasma and urine. The simplest test is to measure the urine vanillylmandelic acid, but the other catecholamines—norepinephrine, epinephrine, and metanephrine—can also now be measured.

Localization

CT scan usually discovers the tumor and may be supplemented by scanning with iodine 131 metaiodobenzylguanidine (MIGB) or carbon 11 hydroxyephedrine—analogues of noradrenaline that precisely localize the tumor and any metastases.[272, 273] Angiography shows these tumors very clearly because they have a characteristically profuse blood supply.

Preoperative Preparation

Alpha blockers are given for 2 weeks before operation. The blood volume is measured and restored if found to be low.

Resection of Pheochromocytoma

A transverse abdominal incision is made except for very large tumors, which may require a thoracoabdominal approach.

On the right, the colon and duodenum are mobilized and the liver and gallbladder retracted down to reveal the adrenal. On the left, the splenic flexure and duodenum are mobilized. The adrenal must be handled gently and its vein tied as soon as possible. During the operation, profound hypotension may occur but responds to noradrenaline and hydrocortisone.

All pheochromocytomas should be followed up because it is impossible to predict late metastases.[274]

Neuroblastoma

This is the fourth most common pediatric malignancy and accounts for more than half of all solid cancers in children, usually younger than 2 and rarely older than 5. Most arise near the adrenal medulla, but they may originate anywhere along the course of the sympathetic trunk.

Viruses may have some etiologic influence on these tumors, which may occur in twins.[275] Hematogenous metastases occur early. Spontaneous regression has been reported in the first 6 months of life.

Most neuroblastomas present as a fixed mass, by which time more than a third have metastasized, causing fever and joint pains. The alpha-fetoprotein and carcinoembryonic antigen levels are usually raised, as are the urinary catecholamines. Anemia is common from hemorrhage into the mass or infiltration of the bone marrow.

CT scanning defines the mass, which is distinguished from Wilms' tumor by its scattered calcification and the displacement of the entire kidney.[276]

The only hope of cure is by surgical excision, although a bulky tumor may be shrunk by preoperative radiation. Chemotherapy has been disappointing,[276] although about 25% of patients do become long-term disease-free survivors with modern chemotherapy.[277]

CANCER OF THE TESTIS

Etiology

In the United States, some 2 to 3 new cases of testicular cancer are reported per 100,000 males each year. In England and Wales, the figure is about 4.5, with 157 deaths—less than 1% of cancer in all males, but among men aged 15 to 50, it is 10 times commoner than any other cancer except of the skin,[278] and it is increasing.[279]

Unlike most cancers, which become more common with age, testicular cancer is rare before puberty and peaks at age 25 for nonseminoma and 10 years later for seminoma.[280]

Cancer of the testis is almost unknown in black men, in whom it has a better prognosis.[281] It occurs 10 times more frequently in male first-degree relatives.[282, 283] As yet, there is no clear-cut genetic mechanism: some early studies suggested a linkage to HLA, but this has not been confirmed by a large-scale case control study.[282, 284]

A tenth of all testicular cancer is associated with maldescent of the testis, though occurring in the descended gonad in 10%: the higher the position of the cryptorchid testis, the greater the risk of cancer.[283] Other congenital anomalies are also linked (inguinal hernia, torsion, hypospadias, duplex kidneys, and intersex—dysgenetic gonads being highly prone to cancer).

Inflammation (e.g., mumps) may be a factor.[284]

Trauma is often recalled by men with a cancer of the testis, but it is impossible to know which came first, the lump or the injury.[278]

Hormonal factors may be important: there is an increased risk of maldescent and cancer in the sons of women given diethylstilbestrol in pregnancy, and high natural levels of estrogen have been blamed.[285]

Fertility and Endocrine Factors

Age-incidence curves show that the incidence of germ cell tumors mirrors the level of sexual activity in the male. This supports the view that germ cell tumors are dependent on endocrine factors for their induction. The finding that more than 70% of patients, prior to treatment, have sperm counts in the subfertile range, taken with the high frequency of testicular atrophogenic events, suggests that the effect of increased pituitary gonadotropin (particularly follicle-stimulating hormone) on a diminished number of surviving spermatogonia may be the final common pathway for several risk factors (i.e., infertility, trauma, cryptorchidism, and viral orchitis). A small proportion (0.5% to 5%) of patients with these risk factors have carcinoma in situ as well as testicular atrophy. Study of the cytogenetics of this condition is providing new insight into how these tumors develop.[286]

Pathology

While any tissue in the testicle may become malignant, more than 90% of testicular cancers arise from germ cells.[287] The premalignant stage of this transformation, so-called carcinoma in situ, consists of cells that resemble fetal gonocytes,[288] the primordial germ cell. Because of this, there is an increasing tendency to classify the tumors as malignant gonocytomas. Seminomas, which consist of sheets of cells similar to isolated carcinoma in situ cells, can be considered G1 or well-differentiated gonocytomas, while combined tumors can be considered G2 or intermediate gonocytomas. Pure nonseminomas, given the proof that they are derived from carcinoma in situ, would then be considered undifferentiated or G3 gonocytomas.[289]

Gonocytes can be recognized by having glycogen in their cytoplasm and by staining for placental alkaline phosphatase (PLAP). Some, held up between yolk sac and gonadal ridge, may give rise to *extragonadal germ cell tumors* in the para-aortic region or mediastinum.[290] When they occur in the mediastinum, brain, ovary, or gonads of intersex, they are called *dysgerminomas.*

The currently accepted UICC/World Health Organization (WHO) germ cell tumor classification[291] pays considerably more attention to the multiplicity and variability of fetal elements than to the relationships of tumor subtypes to the premalignant stem cell. It has been routine for solid tumors arising in other tissues, such as bladder and bowel, to use the prefix G1, 2, and 3 to indicate the proportion of cells retaining identity with tissue of origin. Increasingly for these other adult solid cancers, the metaplasia prefix is used to describe minority elements unrelated to original tissue of origin in G2 and G3 bladder tumors.

For germ cell tumors (malignant gonocytomas), designation of the syncytiotrophoblast, cytotrophoblast, yolk sac, and somatic elements such as cartilage neuroglandular and epidermal elements as metaplastic components would bring their pathology into line with that of other solid cancers. It would also fit better into our modern understanding of the role of clonal evolution in cancer development. This is now thought to involve the stepwise accumulation of deletions of genes that suppress mitosis and/or the accumulation of mutations in genes controlling growth factors or their receptors so that the cancer cell is set into a permanent proliferative mode.[292, 293]

Two germ cell tumor subtypes, spermatocytic seminoma[294] and mature teratoma, do not fit this approach to classification. Neither of these is associated with carcinoma in situ in residual tubules. It is possible that they are unrelated to other germ cell tumors, although an alternative explanation is that the carcinoma in situ has been immunologically rejected and only mature elements persist, as occurs in residual masses after chemotherapy.

Epidermoid cyst is rare and probably benign, but it is seldom possible to be certain that the rest of the testis is normal; clinically, it cannot be distinguished from *mature teratoma.*[295]

Classification

A classification has been adopted by the WHO.[291] Cell types can be divided into seminomas and nonseminomas. The latter can be further divided into teratoma, embryonal carcinoma, yolk sac tumor, and choriocarcinoma. Mixtures of these types should be noted. Lymphomas are excluded. Combinations of embryonal carcinoma and teratoma can be designated as teratocarcinoma.

More important than nomenclature is the natural history of these different types of testicular cancer (e.g., pure seminoma metastasizes primarily to lymph nodes late and, in a small proportion of patients, is highly sensitive to radiotherapy and chemotherapy). Choriocarcinoma spreads early—in the majority of patients via the blood stream—and is more resistant to both chemotherapy and radiotherapy, although today a proportion are cured by chemotherapy. Most germ cell tumors fall between these two extremes, and modern cytogenetics suggests that there may be a darwinian type of clonal evolution, with survival of the most malignant clone, to explain the extreme variability seen in these tumors.[292, 293]

Tumor Markers

AFP is the fetal form of albumin[296] and comes from the endoderm of the yolk sac. It is present in many teratomas, in some so-called seminomas, but not in "pure" seminoma or choriocarcinoma. It has a half-life of 6 days. The rise and fall of serum AFP provides a useful marker for the response of metastases to treatment.

The hCG tumor marker is made by syncytiotrophoblast.

TABLE 15–11
TNM Staging for Tumors of the Testis

Primary Tumor (T)
The extent of primary tumor is classified after radical orchiectomy.

pTX	Primary tumor cannot be assessed (If no radical orchiectomy has been performed, TX is used.)
pT0	No evidence of primary tumor (e.g., histologic scar in testis)
pTis	Intratubular tumor: preinvasive cancer
pT1	Tumor limited to the testis, including the rete testis
pT2	Tumor invades beyond the tunica albuginea or into the epididymis
pT3	Tumor invades the spermatic cord
pT4	Tumor invades the scrotum

Regional Lymph Nodes (N)

NX	Regional lymph nodes cannot be assessed
N0	No regional lymph node metastasis
N1	Metastasis in a single lymph node, 2 cm or less in greatest dimension
N2	Metastasis in a single lymph node, more than 2 cm but not more than 5 cm in greatest dimension; or multiple lymph node metastases, none more than 5 cm in greatest dimension
N3	Metastasis in a lymph node more than 5 cm in greatest dimension

Distant Metastasis (M)

MX	Presence of distant metastasis cannot be assessed
M0	No distant metastasis
M1	Distant metastasis

Stage Grouping

Stage 0	pTis	N0	M0
Stage I	Any pT	N0	M0
Stage II	Any pT	N1	M0
	Any pT	N2	M0
	Any pT	N3	M0
Stage III	Any pT	Any N	M1

Its half-life is 36 hours. The beta arm of its molecule can be detected by immunoperoxidase staining in fixed tissue and in plasma. hCG is always raised in choriocarcinoma, often in embryonal carcinoma, and in about 10% of cases of so-called seminoma.[296]

PLAP and lactate dehydrogenase (LDH) are present in the cytoplasm of germ cells and can be useful markers in the treatment of seminoma.[297, 298]

Tumor Spread

Germ cell tumors invade the rete testis, epididymis, tunica albuginea, and scrotum. They readily enter the vessels of the spermatic cord. Local invasion determines the "T" element of the TNM system of classification of the stage of the tumor (Table 15–11).[299]

Lymphatic Spread

The first nodes to be invaded by testicular cancer are adjacent to the origin of the testicular arteries from the aorta.[300] From these para-aortic nodes, secondary spread occurs up to the nodes of the mediastinum and down to those of the pelvis. Invasion of the thoracic duct permits systemic spread.

Hematogenous Spread

Trophoblastic tumors erode veins and spread by the blood stream at an earlier stage and may present without nodal metastases.

Non–Germ Cell Tumors

The other tissues of the testis and epididymis may give rise to benign or malignant neoplasms.

Leydig cell tumors are made up of benign interstitial cells that secrete testosterone and give rise to precocious puberty in boys but, after puberty, may cause feminization and gynecomastia.[301] *Sertoli cell tumors* are even more rare and may cause gynecomastia.[302]

The surrounding tissues may give rise to angioma, fibroma, or neuroma. Benign fibromatous nodules are common in the tunica albuginea, where mesothelioma and fibrosarcoma has occasionally been reported.[303]

A rare benign tumor of müllerian duct origin occurs in the epididymis.[304]

Diagnosis

Clinical Features

The most common symptom is a painless lump, and all lumps in the testis demand exploration. For practical purposes, there are no benign hard lumps in the testicle.[280] Small tumors are easily missed near the epididymis or when surrounded by a thick layer of normal tissue. Today, ultrasound scanning makes it easier to identify these small tumors[305]; however, when in any doubt, the testis must be explored (Fig. 15–42).

Inflammation. Signs of inflammation are present in about 15% of tumors, mimicking epididymo-orchitis or torsion. Ultrasound and color Doppler scans may help, but in the end exploration may be the only safe investigation.

Trauma. About 10% of patients come up with a story of injury. Since the risk of testicular atrophy from a hema-

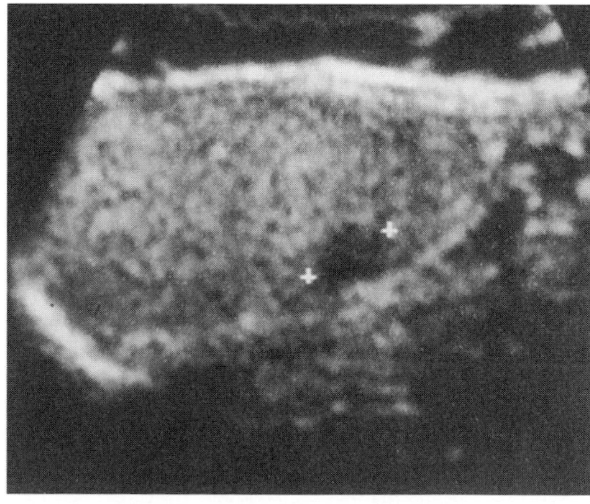

FIGURE 15–42. Ultrasound of the left testicle of a man with pain and site tenderness demonstrates a 0.25-cm echo-poor area, subsequently proven to be early seminoma.

tocele requires every case of trauma to the testis to be explored, a tumor should not be missed, and the patient should always be warned of the chance that exploration may end up as orchiectomy.

Hydrocele. A shallow hydrocele is inevitable with cancer of the testis, but a large one can be a rare method of presentation. Today, every hydrocele calls for confirmation of the diagnosis by ultrasound, and in a young man tumor-marker levels should be obtained as well.[306]

Minor Lesions. One of the most difficult clinical problems is the anxious young man with discomfort in the testicle. Never be reassured to find "only a varicocele." Careful examination of the testicle today requires an ultrasound scan and tumor markers.

The Azzopardi Tumor—The Vanishing Testis. A tumor can eat through the testis and heal up behind. The testis appears to shrink until it is entirely replaced by scar.[307]

Gynecomastia. Gynecomastia can be the first symptom of a testicular tumor, and a "pregnancy test" should form part of the routine examination of every adolescent complaining of this common symptom.

Backache. A young man with persistent backache should always make one think of a testicular tumor, even if the testes appear normal, particularly if the pain is not relieved by extension of the spine. Tumor markers and an abdominal ultrasound are always justified in view of the possibility that the patient has an Azzopardi syndrome tumor.

Investigations

Ultrasound scanning is painless and cheap but can give false-positive findings. A negative exploration is better than missing a testicular tumor when it is curable. Fine-needle biopsy may be performed under ultrasound control, although the risk of dissemination of tumor remains to be quantified.[308]

Tumor Markers. The serum levels of hCG, AFP, PLAP, and LDH should be measured. A pregnancy test is a cheap, readily available qualitative way of detecting a raised hCG level.

Orchiectomy. Scrotal incision should be avoided: it may implant cancer in the scrotal tissues and allow lymphatic spread to the inguinal nodes.[280] Through an inguinal incision, the external oblique is opened and the cord is clamped at the internal ring (Fig. 15–43). When the tumor is very large, it is better to carry the inguinal incision into the neck of the scrotum rather than spill tumor.

Chevassu's Maneuver. When the testis is delivered, there is seldom any doubt about the diagnosis; however, if there is, the wound should be toweled off and the testis sliced along its antimesenteric border. Again, the naked-eye appearance is usually obvious but can be confirmed by frozen section (Fig. 15–44). If the lump proves to be benign, the tunica albuginea is closed with 3–0 catgut. The testicle will survive unharmed and by 6 months cannot be distinguished from the unoperated one.

If cancer is confirmed, the cord is transfixed and divided above the clamp (Fig. 15–45).

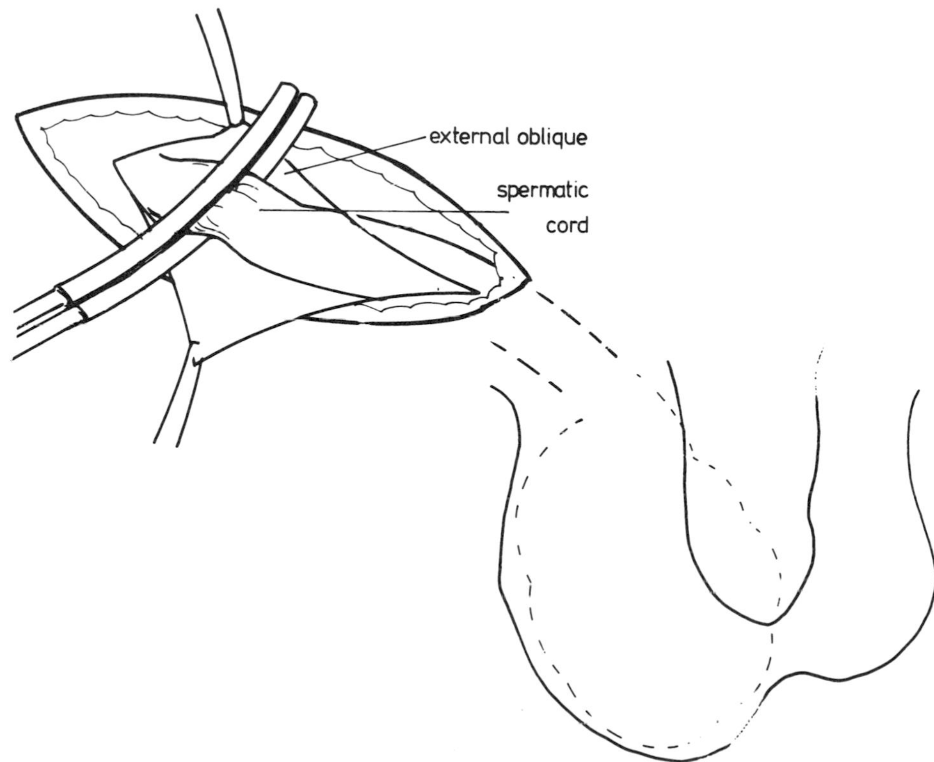

FIGURE 15–43. Orchiectomy for tumor of the testis: the cord is clamped at the internal ring before delivering the testicle from the scrotum. (From Blandy JP: Operative Urology, 2nd ed. London, Blackwell Publishers, 1986, p 249.)

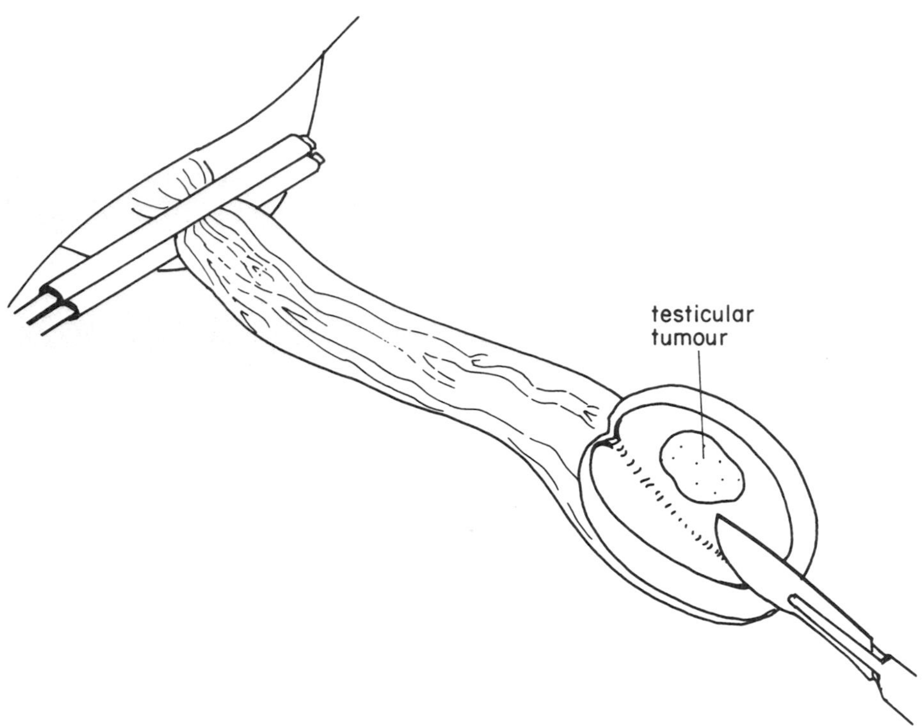

FIGURE 15–44. Chevassu's maneuver. The cord is clamped and delivered through an inguinal incision. After the wound is toweled off, the testis is sliced open. A frozen section may be taken if there is doubt about the diagnosis. (From Blandy JP: Operative Urology, 2nd ed. London, Blackwell Publishers, 1986, p 249.)

Staging the Tumor

CT scanning is performed of the abdomen, mediastinum, and lungs. As this can detect nodes greater than 1 cm in diameter,[303] it has replaced lymphangiography.

An even more invasive but more accurate method of staging is to perform a retroperitoneal node dissection. As well as detecting metastases less than 1 cm diameter in about 20% to 25% of patients, it can establish that 5% to 10% of positive scans are due to postorchiectomy lymphoid hyperplasia and not malignancy.[309] This procedure is not only diagnostic but cures patients with only microscopic metastases and excuses them from unnecessary chemotherapy.[310] By preserving the sympathetic chain, ejaculation is preserved.

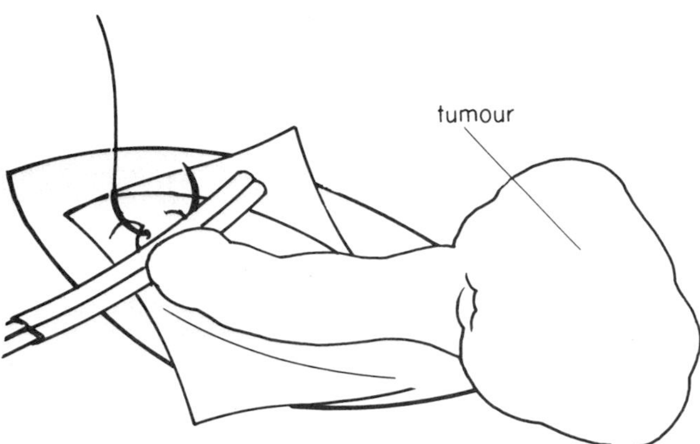

FIGURE 15–45. Orchiectomy for testicular tumor: the cord is doubly transfixed and ligated proximal to the clamp after verifying that the swelling is cancer. (From Blandy JP: Operative Urology, 2nd ed. London, Blackwell Publishers, 1986, p 249.)

Management of Stage I Germ Cell Cancer

When there is no CT evidence of lymph node or distant metastases, and the tumor-marker levels fall after orchiectomy according to their known half-life, subsequent treatment depends on the histology of the tumor. Today there are several equally efficacious approaches.

For seminoma without any other tissue elements present and negative markers, the choice lies between surveillance, a low dose of radiotherapy, and a short course of carboplatin. With surveillance, late retroperitoneal tumor appears in about 25% of patients. Although this (so far) has always been curable, such a high risk justifies some form of treatment because in some patients relapse can take 3 to 4 years to appear and occasionally paraplegia can be the first manifestation of relapse. A low dose of irradiation—3000 cGy to the retroperitoneal tissue—has been the standard for more than 30 years. Recent long-term follow-up studies show a disturbingly large number of second cancers in these men. Early results with one course of carboplatin have been followed by no recurrences and, so far, no second malignancies among 53 patients followed for 2 to 5 years.[311–312]

For stage I nonseminomas there are also three choices:

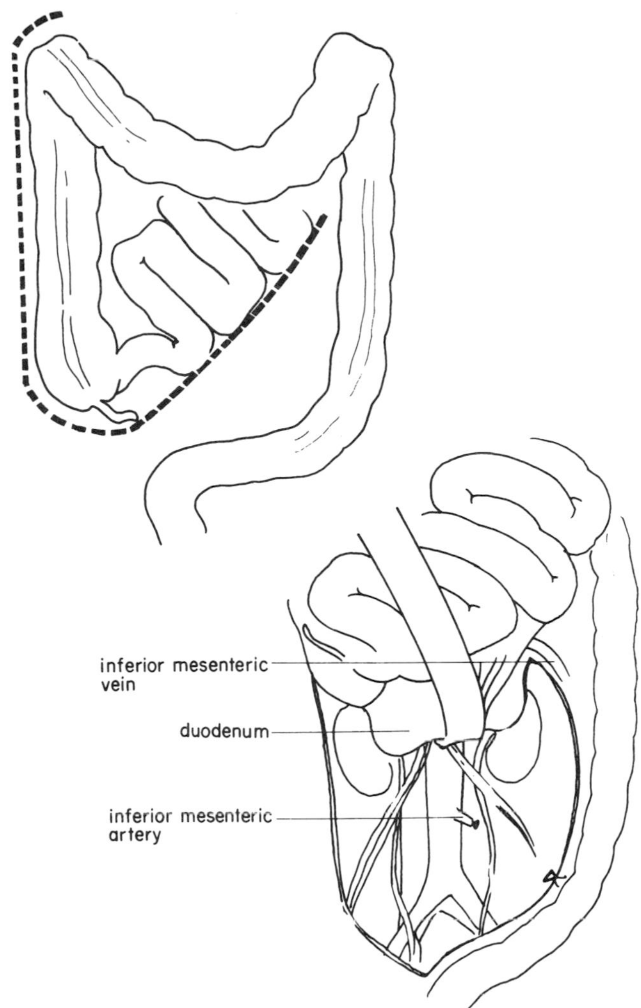

FIGURE 15–46. Radical retroperitoneal node dissection. The entire ascending and transverse colon and all the small intestine are mobilized by incising the mesenteric attachment and, if necessary, the inferior mesenteric artery and vein. (From Blandy JP: Operative Urology, 2nd ed. London, Blackwell Publishers, 1986, p 250.)

surveillance, retroperitoneal lymph node surgery, or adjuvant chemotherapy. As surveillance is associated with a 30% risk of relapse in the first 2 years, there is increasing acceptance of the need for active intervention. This is particularly so in patients with histologic features such as lymphocyte and vascular invasion, presence of undifferentiated cells, and absence of yolk sac elements, which predict relapse in excess of 30%.[312]

Prophylactic Chemotherapy

With increasing confidence that there are no serious late toxic effects of cisplatin-based combination chemotherapy, many centers are now investigating whether prophylactic combination chemotherapy may be preferable to surveillance or node dissection in patients with unfavorable histologic features.[312] With nearly 200 patients treated in four different studies, relapse has occurred so far in less than 5% of patients.[314]

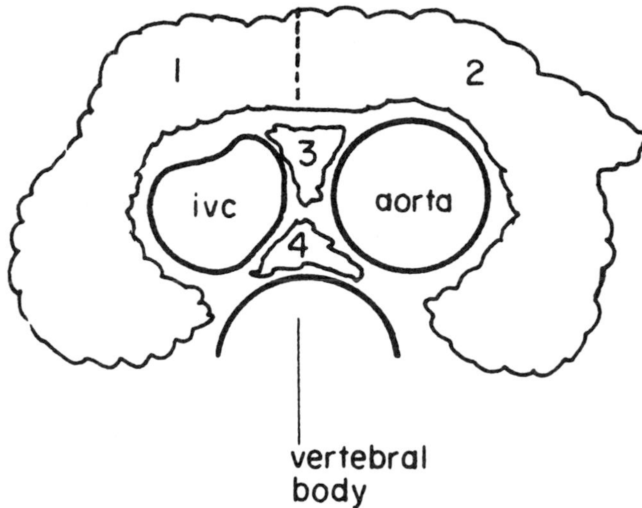

FIGURE 15–47. Line drawing of cross section showing the four wedges of tissue involved in retroperitoneal node dissections. ivc, Inferior vena cava. (From Blandy JP: Operative Urology, 2nd ed. London, Blackwell Publishers, 1986, p 252.)

Retroperitoneal Lymph Node Dissection

This procedure, which combines diagnostic staging with therapeutic removal of micrometastases, has powerful ad-

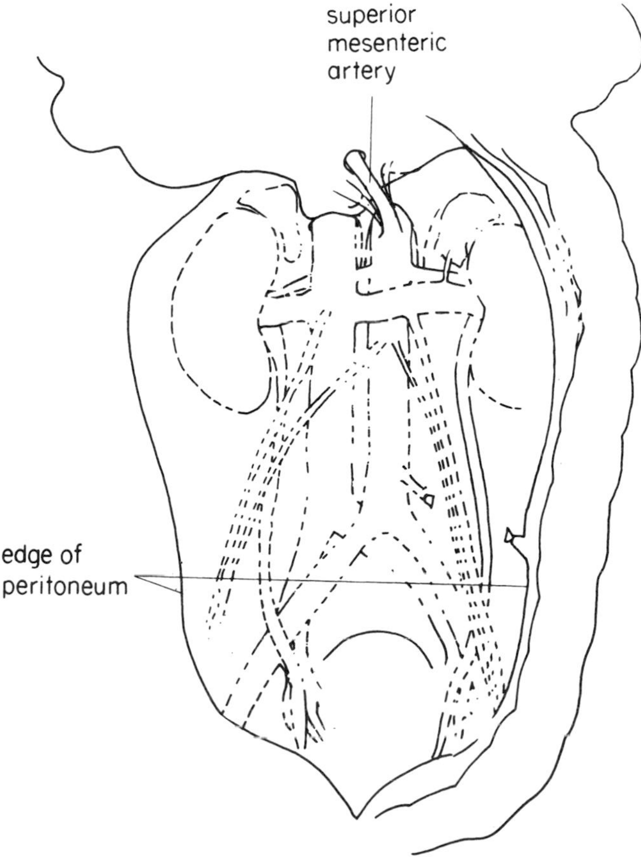

FIGURE 15–48. The structures to be dissected are concealed by lymph nodes and fibrofatty tissue. (From Blandy JP: Operative Urology, 2nd ed. London, Blackwell Publishers, 1986, p 251.)

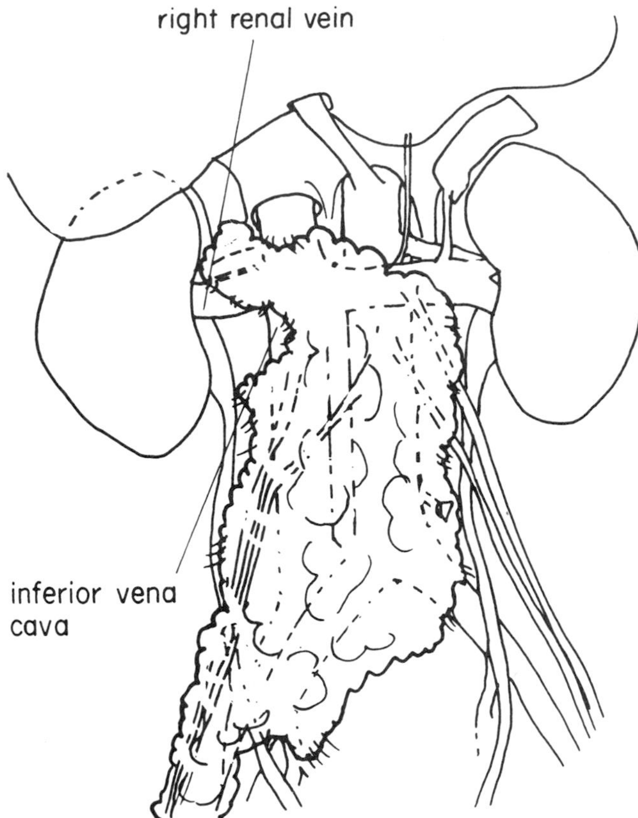

FIGURE 15–49. Fibrofatty and lymphatic tissue is cleared from the right kidney and right side of the inferior vena cava. (From Blandy JP: Operative Urology, 2nd ed. London, Blackwell Publishers, 1986, p 251.)

vocates,[309, 310, 313] especially since new techniques save the sympathetic chain at least on one side and avoid ejaculatory failure. However, 15% to 20% of such surgically staged patients end up needing chemotherapy (i.e., the 10% surgical stage I patients who relapse and at least one third of surgically defined stage II patients).

Through a long midline incision, the ascending colon and small bowel are mobilized, the ligament of Treitz and inferior mesenteric vein are divided, and the bowel is placed on the chest (Fig. 15–46). According to the side of the tumor, a "template" of tissue is removed, which spares the opposite sympathetic chain and presacral nerve.

The para-aortic tissues form four wedges.[291] On the right, the tissue in front of the inferior vena cava is split from the right common iliac artery up to the renal vein. The right testicular vessels (Figs. 15–47 to 15–51) are divided, and the tissue between the vena cava and ureter is removed en bloc down to the internal ring. The lumbar veins are divided to permit the vena cava to be rolled medially (Fig. 15–52).

The tissues along the midline of the aorta are split, taking the inferior mesenteric artery between ligatures, and the anterior wedge of tissue is removed. The aorta is now mobilized by dividing its pairs of lumbar arteries, and when the aorta and vena cava are lifted up, the posterior wedge of tissue between them is dissected off the anterior intervertebral ligament, dividing once more the pairs of lumbar vessels. This allows the left sympathetic chain and presacral nerve to be preserved.

For a left tumor, the template of tissue to be removed includes the left anterior and posterior wedges and spares the wedge on the right with the right sympathetic chain.

TNM Stage N1

When the CT scan shows small nodes, retroperitoneal node dissection is performed in some centers both for cure and to provide exact staging. If only a few nodes are found, chemotherapy can safely be omitted.[314, 315]

Elsewhere where staging is based only on CT scanning, patients are given a full course of combination chemotherapy. For seminoma, radiation is preferred by some.

TNM Stage N2

For nodes greater than 2 cm in diameter, combination chemotherapy is the agreed first-line treatment in most

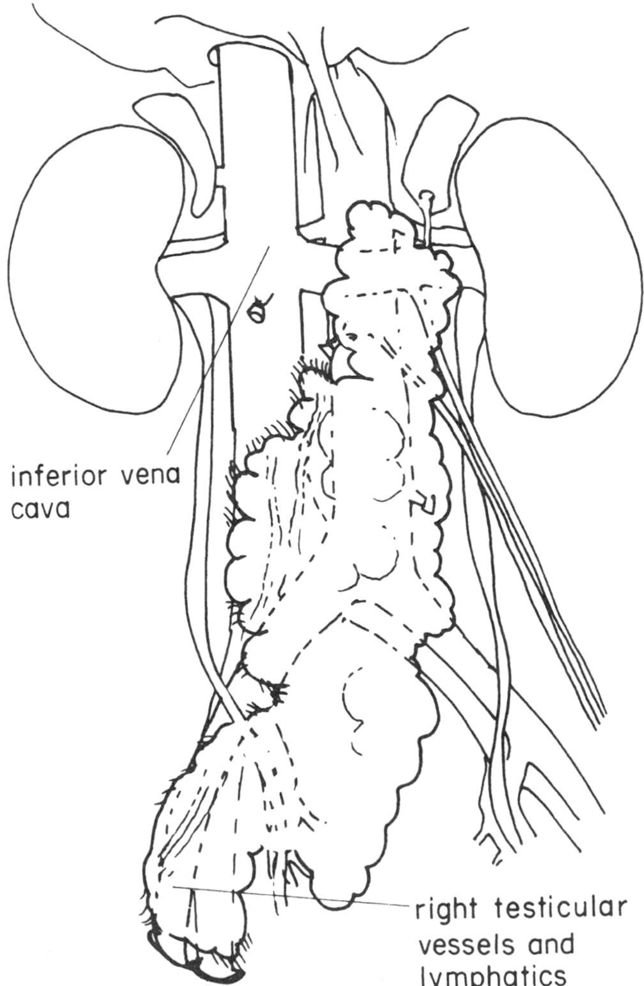

FIGURE 15–50. The cava and renal vein are dissected clean. (From Blandy JP: Operative Urology, 2nd ed. London, Blackwell Publishers, 1986, p 251.)

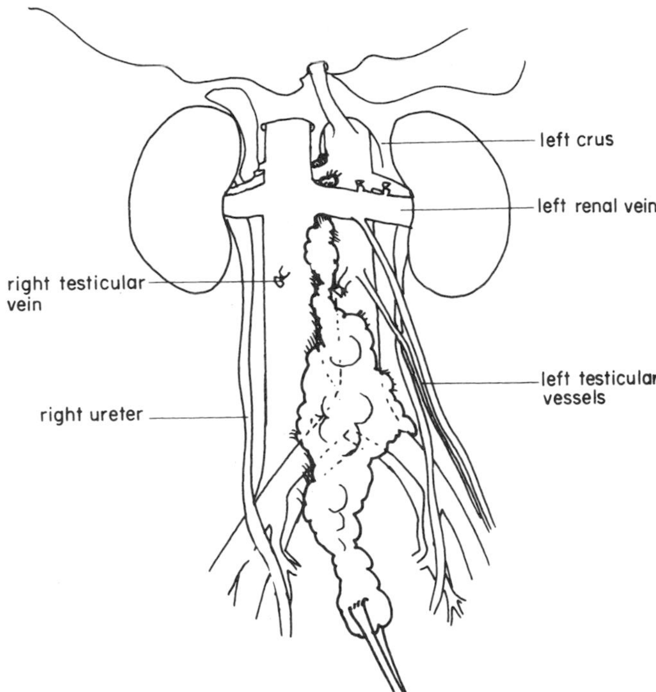

FIGURE 15–51. For right-sided tumors, an attempt is made to preserve the left testicular vessels, but this is not always possible. (From Blandy JP: Operative Urology, 2nd ed. London, Blackwell Publishers, 1986, p 251.)

centers. Many of these patients may need postchemotherapy surgery. These cases require close collaboration between surgeon and physician to build the teamwork and experience to minimize the morbidity of treatment.

TNM Stage N3

Patients with bulky and metastatic tumors are given combination chemotherapy. If the mass found on CT scanning disappears completely, subsequent lymph node dissection virtually never reveals tumor.[316] A mass that persists after two or three cycles of treatment may be fibronecrotic tissue, mature teratoma, or active cancer. It is impossible to tell these apart until the mass has been removed by so-called salvage node dissection (see below).

Unless mature teratoma is removed, it may return within 3 years and be resistant to chemotherapy in up to 30% of cases.[317] Active cancer can sometimes be cured by this dissection, provided excision has a clear margin.[318] If there is any doubt about clear margins, further chemotherapy is usually given. Residual masses in the chest are removed for the same reason.

Technique of Salvage Lymph Node Dissection

The same steps are followed for retroperitoneal lymph node dissection, but the dissection is more difficult and one must be prepared to deal with major operative hazards (e.g., repair or reconstruction of the aorta, cava, and bowel).[316, 318] An attempt is made to preserve one sympathetic chain and presacral nerve, but this is not always possible.[319]

Small masses of tumor behind the crura can be removed through the abdominal approach, but larger ones are more safely dealt with through a thoracotomy.[316]

Residual seminoma is very difficult to remove, although occasionally the attempt is worthwhile, as about 10% have viable cancer or mature teratoma.

Management of N4 and/or M+ Disease

Chemotherapy has completely replaced radiotherapy in this stage of disease for both seminoma and nonseminoma. The Einhorn platinum, vinblastine, bleomycin (PVB) regimen was the first combination regimen to become an international standard.[320] More recent trials have demonstrated that bleomycin, etoposide, and cisplatin (Platinol) (BEP), a combination developed in the United Kingdom,[321] has superior survival, particularly in patients with advanced metastatic disease, as well as less toxicity,[322] and this is now the international standard.

A measure of the exquisite chemosensitivity of germ cell tumors is the fact that although the conventional standard regimen produces 80% to 85% cure, there are at least three different salvage regimens—VePesid, ifosfamide, Platinol (VIP); weekly bleomycin, vincristine (oncovin), and cisplatin (BOP); and high-dose etoposide and carboplatin (EC)—that can produce more than 20% durable cure of

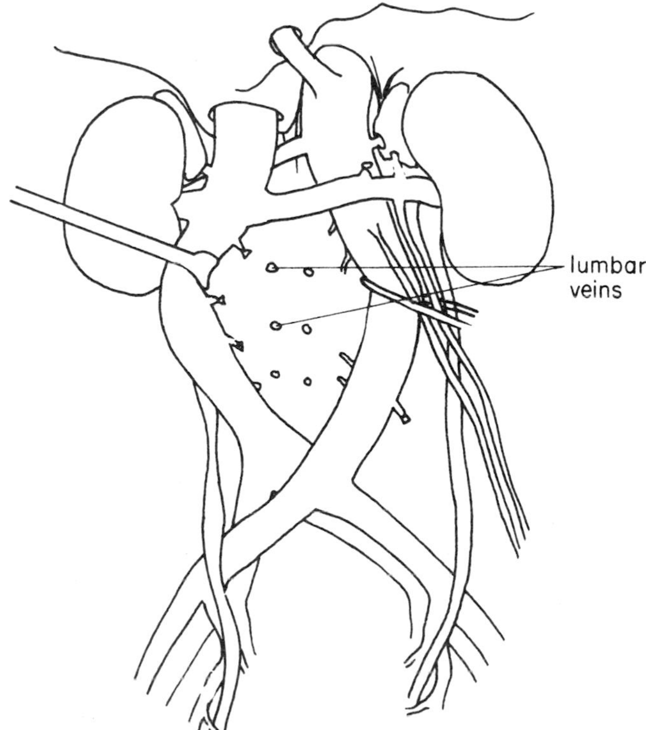

FIGURE 15–52. In order to remove the last part of lymphatic tissue, lumbar veins and often several lumbar arteries are divided. (From Blandy JP: Operative Urology, 2nd ed. London, Blackwell Publishers, 1986, p 252.)

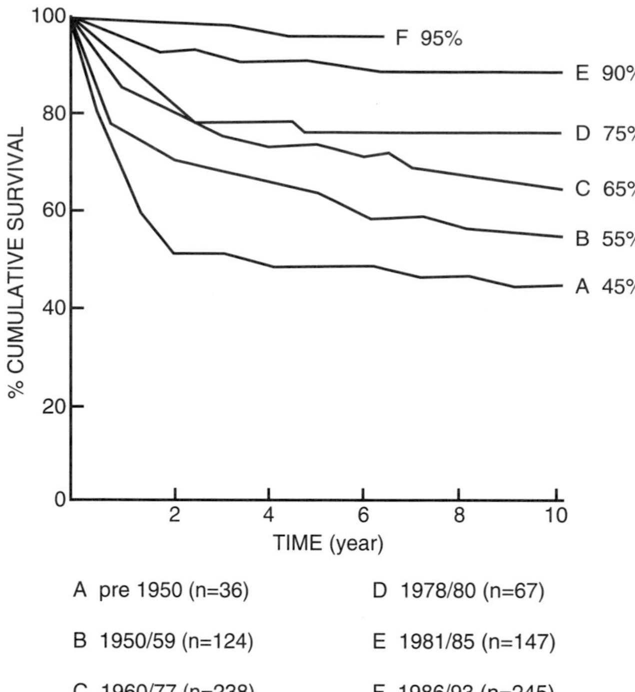

FIGURE 15–53. Changes in survival of germ cell cancer patients treated at the Royal Marsden Hospital.

patients who have failed BEP.[323–325] As yet, none of them have been proven to be better than BEP in previously untreated patients, and, at present, the principal effort is in using clinical prognostic factor analysis to better identify poor-risk patients (Table 15–12).[326]

Even more difficult than identifying poor-risk patients for dose intensification has been risking less treatment for good-risk patients. Two approaches have been applied. The first used a nonnephrotoxic platinum, carboplatin[327]; this has not yet been proven safe.[328] The other approach has been to compare three versus four courses of BEP: one study showed them to be equivalent.[329]

For seminoma, the discovery that single-agent platinum can produce durable complete remission in more than 70% of patients[330, 331] has made it easier to give less treatment because the majority of those failing single-agent treatment can be salvaged by more intensive regimens.[331]

TABLE 15–12
Second U.K. MRC Prognostic Factors Analysis for Metastatic Nonseminoma

Survival by No. of Poor-Risk Features	No. of Patients	3-Year Survival (%)	5-Year Survival (%)
None of the features	528	93	92
Any one of the four	170	78	71
Any two of the four	69	60	48
At least three of the four	28	26	26

From Mead GM, et al: The Second Medical Research Council study of prognostic factors in nonseminomatous germ cell tumours. Medical Research Council Testicular Tumour Working Party. J Clin Oncol 10:85–94, 1992.

Late Toxicity from Chemotherapy

With the overall cure rate of testicular cancer now approaching 95% (Fig. 15–53), increasing attention is being paid to the late effects of treatment. The late risks of second tumor after radiotherapy emerged only after 10 to 15 years. As a consequence, there has been considerable uncertainty about risking chemotherapy in early stages. For the original Einhorn PVB regimen, 10-year follow-up studies are now published, and, apart from a suspicion of extravascular toxicity and hypertension in smokers, there has not been an excess of second nontesticular cancers to date. For BEP, this has not been the case. There have been several anecdotal reports of acute leukemia with a unique chromosomal abnormality, although so far only in patients receiving a high dose.[332] More prolonged follow-up is needed to exclude any later increase in nontesticular solid cancer.

References

1. Mesrobian H-GJ: Wilms tumor: Past, present, future. J Urol 140:231–238, 1988.
2. Breslow NE, Beckwith JB: Epidemiological features of Wilms' tumor: Results of the National Wilms' Tumor Study. J Natl Cancer Inst 68:429–436, 1982.
3. Weissman BE, Saxon PJ, Pasquale SR, et al: Introduction of a normal human chromosome 11 into a Wilms' tumor cell line controls its tumorigenic expression. Science 236:175–180, 1987.
4. Pendergrass TW: Congenital anomalies in children with Wilms' tumor: A new survey. Cancer 37:403–408, 1976.
5. Dimmick JE, Johnson HW, Coleman GU, Carter M: Wilms' tumorlet, nodular renal blastema and multicystic renal dysplasia. J Urol 142:484–485, 1989.
6. Matsunaga E: Genetics of Wilms' tumor. In Vogel F, Motulksy AG (eds): Human Genetics. New York: Springer, 1981, pp 231–246.
7. D'Angio GJ, Breslow N, Beckwith JB, et al: Treatment of Wilms' tumor: Results of the Third National Wilms' Tumor Study. Cancer 64:349–360, 1989.
8. Howell CG, Othersen HB, Kiviat NE, et al: Therapy and outcome in 51 children with mesoblastic nephroma: A report of the National Wilms' Cancer Study. J Pediatr Surg 17:826–831, 1982.
9. Gormley TS, Skoog SJ, Jones RV, Maybee D: Cellular congenital mesoblastic nephroma: What are the options? J Urol 142:479–483, 1989.
10. Farewell VT, D'Angio GJ, Breslow N, Norkool P: Retrospective validation of a new staging system for Wilms' tumor. Cancer Clin Trials 4:167–171, 1981.
11. Pritchard J, Stiller CA, Lennox EL: Overtreatment of children with Wilms' tumour outside paediatric oncology centres. Br Med J 299:835–836, 1989.
12. Tournade MF, Com-Nougue C, Voute PA, et al: Results of the Sixth International Society of Pediatric Oncology Wilms' Tumor Trial and Study: A risk-adapted therapeutic approach in Wilms' tumor. J Clin Oncol 11:1014–1023, 1993.
13. Mclorie GA, McKenna PH, Greenberg M, et al: Reduction in tumor burden allowing partial nephrectomy following preoperative chemotherapy in biopsy proven Wilms' tumor. J Urol 146:509–513, 1991.
14. Montgomery BT, Kelalis PP, Blute ML, et al: Extended follow up of bilateral Wilms' tumor: Results of the National Wilms' Tumor study. J Urol 146:514–518, 1991.
15. Boilletot A, Tournade MF, Delemarre JF, et al: Wilms' tumor in adult patients: SIOP results in 15 patients. In Proceedings of the Third European Conference on Clinical Oncology, Stockholm, 1985, p 179.
16. Williams GB, Colbeck RA, Gowing NFC: Adult Wilms' tumour: Review of 14 patients. Br J Urol 70:230–235, 1992.
17. Rao SP, Miller ST, Wrzolek M, Haller JO, Klotz D: Skeletal muscle

metastasis in a patient with Wilms' tumor and multiple late recurrences. Cancer 71:1343–1347, 1993.
18. Skeet RG: Epidemiology of urogenital tumours. In Chisholm GD, Fair W (eds): Scientific Foundations of Urology, 3rd ed. Oxford: Heinemann, 1990, pp 427–32.
19. Ritchie AWS, Kemp IW, Chisholm GD: Is the incidence of renal carcinoma increasing? Br J Urol 56:571–573, 1984.
20. Wynder EL, Mabuchi K, Whitmore WF: Epidemiology of adenocarcinoma of the kidney. J Natl Cancer Inst 53:1619–1634, 1974.
21. Futrell JW, Filston HC, Reid JD: Rupture of a renal cell carcinoma in a child: Five year tumor-free survival and literature review. Cancer 41:1565–1570, 1978.
22. Delahunt B, Bethwaite PB, Nacel JN: Occupational risk for renal cell carcinoma: A case control study based on the New Zealand Cancer Registry. Br J Urol 75:578–582, 1995.
23. Oliver RTD: Medical management of renal cell carcinoma. In Oliver RTD, Blandy JP, Hope-Stone HF (eds): Urological and genital cancer. Oxford: Blackwell, 1989, pp 180–191.
24. Ratcliffe HL: Familial occurrence of renal carcinoma in rhesus monkey (Macaca mulatta). Am J Pathol 16:619–624, 1940.
25. Reddy ER: Bilateral renal cell carcinoma, unusual occurrence in three members of one family. Br J Radiol 54:8–11, 1981.
26. Meloni AM, Bridge J, Sandberg AA: Reviews on chromosome studies in urological tumors. I. Renal tumors. J Urol 148:253–265, 1992.
27. Brennan JF, Stilmant MM, Babayan RK, Siroky MB: Acquired renal cystic disease: Implications for the urologist. Br J Urol 67:342–348, 1991.
28. Latif F, Tory K, Gnaraa J, et al: Identification of von Hippel–Lindau disease tumour suppression gene. Science 260:1317–1320, 1993.
29. Fuhrman SA, Lasky LC, Limas C: Prognostic significance of morphological parameters in renal cell carcinoma. Am J Surg Pathol 6:655–663, 1982.
30. Bell ET: Renal Disease, 2nd ed. Philadelphia: Lea & Febiger, 1959, p 435.
31. Hellsten S, Berge T, Linell F: Clinically unrecognised renal carcinoma: Aspects of tumour morphology, lymphatic and haematogenous metastatic spread. Br J Urol 55:166–170, 1983.
32. Luungberg B, Duchek M, Hietala S-O, Roos G, Stenling R: Renal cell carcinoma in a solitary kidney: Late nephrectomy after 35 years and analysis of tumor deoxyribonucleic acid content. J Urol 139:350–352, 1988.
33. Woodhouse CRJ: Conservative versus radical surgery for renal transitional cell carcinoma and adenocarcinoma. In Oliver RTD, Blandy JP, Hope-Stone HF (eds): Urological and Genital Cancer. Oxford: Blackwell, pp 171–179, 1989.
34. Zhang G, Monda L, Wasserman FF, Fraley EE: Bilateral renal oncocytoma: Report of 2 cases and literature review. J Urol 133:84–86, 1985.
35. Frydenberg M, Eckstein RP, Saalfield JAAH, Breslin FHD, Alexander JH, Roche J: Renal oncocytomas—an Australian experience. Br J Urol 67:352–357, 1991.
36. Hermanek P, Sobin LH (eds): International Union Against Cancer TNM Classification of Malignant Tumours, 4th ed, 2nd rev. Berlin: Springer, 1992.
37. Grignon DJ, Ayala AG, El-Naggar A, et al: Renal cell carcinoma: A clinicopathologic and DNA flow cytometric analysis of 103 cases. Cancer 64:2133–2140, 1989.
38. Paulson DF: Prognostic factors predicting treatment response. World J Urol 2:99–102, 1984.
39. Best BG: Renal carcinoma: A ten year review 1971–80. Br J Urol 60:100–102, 1987.
40. Samaan NA: Paraneoplastic syndromes associated with renal carcinoma. In Johnson DE, Samuels ML (eds): Clinical Conference on Cancer—Cancer of the Genitourinary Tract. New York: Raven Press, 1979, pp 73–78.
41. Fahn H-J, Lee Y-H, Chen M-T, Huang J-K, Chen K-K, Chang LS: The incidence and prognostic significance of humoral hypercalcemia in renal cell carcinoma. J Urol 145:248–250, 1991.
42. Walsh PN, Kissane JM: Nonmetastatic hypernephroma with reversible hepatic dysfunction. Arch Intern Med 122:214–222, 1968.
43. Gleeson MH, Bloom SR, Polak JM, Henry K, Dowling RN: An endocrine tumour in kidney affecting small bowel structure, motility, and function. Gut 11:1060, 1970.
44. Evans BK, Fagan C, Arnold T, Dropcho EJ, Oh SJ: Paraneoplastic motor neuron disease and renal cell carcinoma: Improvement after nephrectomy. Neurology 40:960–962, 1990.
45. Cronin RE, Kaehny WD, Miller PD, et al: Renal cell carcinoma: Unusual systemic manifestations. Medicine 55:291–311, 1976.
46. Horan JJ, Robertson CN, Choyke PL, et al: The detection of renal carcinoma extension into the renal vein and inferior vena cava: A prospective comparison of vena-cavography and magnetic resonance imaging. J Urol 142:943–947, 1989.
47. Attwood S, Lang DM, Goiti J, Grant J: Venous bypass for surgical resection of renal carcinoma invading the vena cava: A new approach. Br J Urol 61:402–405, 1988.
48. Davits RJAM, Blom JHM, Schroder FH: Surgical management of renal carcinoma with extensive involvement of the vena cava and right atrium. Br J Urol 70:591–593, 1992.
49. Pritchett TR, Lieskovsky G, Skinner DG: Extension of renal cell carcinoma into the vena cava: Clinical review and surgical approach. J Urol 135:460–464, 1986.
50. Schorn A, Marberger M: Long-term survival of untreated bilateral renal cell carcinoma with supradiaphragmatic vena caval thrombus. J Urol 131:108–109, 1984.
51. Marshall FF: The in situ surgical management of renal cell carcinoma and transitional cell carcinoma of the kidney. World J Urol 2:130–135, 1984.
52. Novick AC, Streem S, Montie JE, et al: Conservative surgery for renal cell carcinoma: A single-center experience with 100 patients. J Urol 141:835–839, 1989.
53. Blackley SK, Ladaga L, Woolfitt RA, Schellhammer PF: Ex situ study of the effectiveness of enucleation in patients with renal cell carcinoma. J Urol 140:6–10, 1988.
54. Herrlinger A, Schrott KM, Sigel A, Giedl J: Results of 381 transabdominal radical nephrectomies for renal cell carcinoma with partial and complete en-bloc lymph node dissection. World J Urol 2:114–121, 1984.
55. Freed SZ, Halperin JP, Gordon M: Idiopathic regression of metastases from renal cell carcinoma. J Urol 118:538–542, 1977.
56. Peeling WB, Mantell BS, Shepheard BGF: Post-operative irradiation in the treatment of renal cell carcinoma. Br J Urol 41:23–31, 1969.
57. Finney R: The value of radiotherapy in the treatment of hypernephroma: A clinical trial. Br J Urol 45:258–269, 1973.
58. Pizzocaro G, Piva L, Salvioni R, et al: Adjuvant medroxyprogesterone acetate and steroid hormone receptors in category M_0 renal cell carcinoma. An interim report of a prospective randomized study. J Urol 135:18–21, 1986.
59. Oliver RTD, Nethersell ABW, Bottomley JM: Unexplained spontaneous regression and alpha-interferon as treatment for metastatic renal carcinoma. B J Urol 63:128–131, 1989.
60. Moffat LEF, Sunderland GT, Lamont D: Blood transfusion and survival following nephrectomy for carcinoma of kidney. Br J Urol 60:316–319, 1987.
61. Schornagel JH, Verweij J, ten Bokkel Huinink WW, et al: Phase II study of recombinant Interferon Alpha 2 A and Vinblastine in advanced renal cell carcinoma. J Urol 142:253–256, 1989.
62. Onishi T, Machida T, Masuda F, et al: Nephrectomy in renal carcinoma with distant metastasis. Br J Urol 63:600–604, 1989.
63. Ueda T, Yasumasu T, Uozumi J, Naito S: Comparison of clinical and pathological characteristics in incidentally detected and suspected renal carcinoma. Br J Urol 68:470–472, 1991.
64. Schwartz CB, Bekirov H, Melman A: Urothelial tumors of upper tract following treatment of primary bladder transitional cell carcinoma. Urology 40:509–511, 1992.
65. Lynch HT, Ens JA, Lynch JF: The Lynch syndrome II and urological malignancies. J Urol 143:24–28, 1990.
66. Pommer W, Bronder E, Greiser E, et al: Regular analgesic intake and the risk of end-stage renal failure. Am J Nephrol 9:403–412, 1989.
67. Steffens J, Nagel R: Tumours of the renal pelvis and ureter: Observations in 170 patients. Br J Urol 61:277–283, 1988.
68. Balkan Endemic Nephropathy (BEN), Two International Workshops, Belgrade, Yugoslavia. Kidney Int Suppl 34:S. 1–S. 104, 1991.
69. Mazeman E: Tumours of the upper urinary tract calyces, renal pelvis and ureter. Eur Urol 2:120–126, 1976.
70. Mufti GR, Gove JRW, Badenoch DF, et al: Transitional cell carcinoma of the renal pelvis and ureter. Br J Urol 63:135–140, 1989.
71. Anselmo G, Rissotti A, Felici E, Bassi E, Maccatrozzo L: Multiple

simultaneous bilateral urothelial tumours of the renal pelvis. Br J Urol 60:312–315, 1987.

72. Hermanek P, Sobin LH (eds): International Union Against Cancer TNM Classification of Malignant Tumours, 4th ed, 2nd rev. Berlin: Springer, 1992.
73. Mills C, Vaughan ED: Carcinoma of the ureter: Natural history, management and 5-year survival. J Urol 129:275–277, 1983.
74. Blandy JP: Operative Urology, 2nd ed. Oxford: Blackwell, 1986.
75. Abercrombie GF, Eardley I, Payne SR, Walmsley BH, Vinnicombe J. Modified nephroureterectomy. Long term follow up with particular reference to subsequent bladder tumours. Br J Urol 61:198–201, 1988.
76. Woodhouse CRJ, Kellett MJ, Bloom HJG: Percutaneous renal surgery and local radiotherapy in the management of renal pelvic transitional cell carcinoma. Br J Urol 58:245–249, 1986.
77. Reitelman C, Sawczuk IS, Olsson CA, Puchner PJ, Benson MC: Prognostic variables in patients with transitional cell carcinoma of the renal pelvis and proximal ureter. J Urol 138:1144–1145, 1987.
78. Babaian RJ, Johnson DE: Primary carcinoma of the ureter. J Urol 123:357–359, 1980.
79. Wan J, Ohl DA, Weatherbee L: Primary mucinous adenocarcinoma of renal pelvis in solitary pelvic kidney. Urology 41:292–294, 1993.
80. Thijssen AM, Carpenter B, Jimenez C, Schillinger J: Multilocular cyst (multilocular cystic nephroma) of the kidney: A report of 2 cases with an unusual mode of presentation. J Urol 142:346–348, 1989.
81. Frydenberg M, Malek RS, Zincke H: Conservative renal surgery for renal cell carcinoma in von Hippel Lindau's disease. J Urol 149:461–464, 1993.
82. Webb DW, Osborne JP: New research in tuberous sclerosis. Br Med J 304:1647–1648, 1992.
83. Pirson Y: Renal transplantation in tuberous sclerosis. Br Med J 305:313, 1992.
84. Lam AS, Bedard YC, Buckspan MB, Logan AG, Steinhardt MI: Surgically curable hypertension associated with reninoma. J Urol 128:572–575, 1982.
85. Silverman DT, Hartge P, Morrison AS, Devesa SS: Epidemiology of bladder cancer. Hematol Oncol Clin North Am 6:1–30, 1992.
86. Ross RK, Paganini-Hill A, Henderson BE: Epidemiology of bladder cancer. In Skinner DG, Lieskovsky G (eds): Diagnosis and Management of Genitourinary Cancer. Philadelphia: WB Saunders, 1988, pp 23–31.
87. Chiang HS, Guo HR, Hong CL, Lin SM, Lee EF: The incidence of bladder cancer in the Black Foot Disease endemic area in Taiwan. Br J Urol 71:274–278, 1993.
88. Rehn L: Blasengeschwultse bei fuchsin-arbeitern. Arch Clin Chir 50:588–600, 1895.
89. Hueper WC, Wiley FH, Wolfe HD: Experimental production of bladder tumors in dogs by administration of beta-naphthylamine. J Ind Hyg Toxicol 20:46–84, 1938.
90. Occupational bladder cancer: A guide for clinicians. The BAUS Subcommittee on Industrial Bladder Cancer. Br J Urol 61:183–191, 1988.
91. Sigurgeirsson B, Lindelof B, Eklund G: Condylomata acuminata and risk of cancer: An epidemiological study. Br Med J 303:341–344, 1991.
92. Yaqoob M, McClelland P, Bell GM, Ahmad R, Bakran A: Bladder tumours in paraplegic patients on renal replacement therapy. Lancet 338:1554–1555, 1991.
93. Smith JA: Laser treatment of bladder hemangioma. J Urol 143:282–284, 1990.
94. Masters JRW, Camplejohn RS, Parkinson MC, Woodhouse CRJ: DNA ploidy and the prognosis of Stage pT1 bladder cancer. Br J Urol 64:403–408, 1989.
95. Hermanek P, Sobin LH: International Union Against Cancer TNM Classification of Malignant Tumours, 4th ed, 2nd rev. Berlin: Springer, 1992.
96. Abel PD, Henderson D, Bennett MK, Hall RR, Williams G: Differing interpretations by pathologists of the pT category and grade of transitional cell cancer of the bladder. Br J Urol 62:339–342, 1988.
97. Tannenbaum M, Romas NA, Droller MJ: The pathobiology of early urothelial cancer. In Skinner DG, Lieskovsky G (eds): Diagnosis and Management of Genitourinary Cancer. Philadelphia: WB Saunders, 1988, pp 55–82.
98. Richards B, Parmar MKB, Anderson CK, et al: Interpretation of biopsies of 'normal' urothelium in patients with superficial bladder cancer. Br J Urol 67:369–375, 1991.
99. Abel PD, Hall RR, Williams G: Should pT1 transitional cell cancers of the bladder still be classified as superficial? Br J Urol 62:235–239, 1988.
100. Hendry WF, Rawson NSB, Turney L, Dunlop A, Whitfield HN: Computerisation of urothelial carcinoma records: 16 years experience with the TNM system. Br J Urol 65:583–588, 1990.
101. Jewett HJ, Strong GH: Infiltrating carcinoma of the bladder: Relation of depth of penetration of the bladder wall to incidence of local extension and metastases. J Urol 55:366–372, 1946.
102. Page BH, Levison VB, Curwen MP: The site of recurrences of non-infiltrating bladder tumours. Br J Urol 50:237–242, 1978.
103. Tannenbaum SI, Carson CC, Tatum A, Paulson DF: Squamous carcinoma of the urinary bladder. Urology 22:597–599, 1983.
104. Roehrborn CG, Teigland CM, Spence HM: Progression of leukoplakia of the bladder to squamous cell carcinoma 19 years after complete urinary diversion. J Urol 140:603–604, 1988.
105. Swanson DA, Liles A, Zagars GK: Preoperative irradiation and radical cystectomy for Stages T2 and T3 squamous cell carcinoma of the bladder. J Urol 143:37–40, 1990.
106. Gill HS, Dhillon HK, Woodhouse CRJ: Adenocarcinoma of the urinary bladder. Br J Urol 64:138–142, 1989.
107. Higgins PM, Tresidder GC: Phaeochromocytoma of the urinary bladder. Br Med J 2:274–277, 1966.
108. Broecker BH, Plowman N, Pritchard J, Ransley PG: Pelvic rhabdomyosarcoma in children. Br J Urol 61:427–431, 1988.
109. Thrasher JB, Miller GJ, Wettlaufer JN: Bladder leiomyosarcoma following cyclophosphamide therapy for lupus nephritis. J Urol 143:119–121, 1990.
110. Pereira JH, Towler JM: Ten cases of transitional cell carcinoma of bladder causing ureteric obstruction. Br J Urol 66:628–630, 1990.
111. Spencer J, Lindsell D, Mastorakou I: Ultrasonography compared with intravenous urography in the investigation of adults with haematuria. Br Med J 301:1074–1076, 1990.
112. Voges GE, Tauschke E, Stockle M, Alken P, Hohenfellner R: Computerized tomography: An unreliable method for accurate staging of bladder tumors in patients who are candidates for radical cystectomy. J Urol 142:972–974, 1989.
113. Hendrikx AJM, Barentz JO, v.d. Stappen WAH, Debruyne FMJ, Ruijs SHJ: The value of intravesical echography combined with double-surface coil magnetic resonance imaging in staging bladder cancer. Br J Urol 63:469–475, 1989.
114. Fowler CG, Boorman LS: Outpatient treatment of superficial bladder cancer. Lancet 1:38, 1986.
115. Davies AH, Mastorakou I, Dickinson AJ, et al: Flexible cystoscopy compared with ultrasound in the detection of recurrent bladder tumours. Br J Urol 67:491–492, 1991.
116. Blandy JP, Notley RG: Transurethral Resection, 3rd ed. London: Heinemann, 1993.
117. Jenkins BJ, Nauth-Misir RR, Martin JE, Fowler CG, Hope-Stone HF, Blandy JP: The fate of G3pT1 bladder cancer. Br J Urol 64:608–610, 1989.
118. Birch BRP, Harland SJ: The pT1 G3 bladder tumour. Br J Urol 64:109–116, 1989.
119. England HR, Flynn JT, Paris AMI, Blandy JP: Early multiple-dose adjuvant thiotepa in the control of multiple and rapid T1 tumour neogenesis. Br J Urol 53:588–592, 1981.
120. Mufti GR, Virdi JS, Hall MH: Long-term follow-up of intravesical Epodyl therapy for superficial bladder cancer. Br J Urol 65:32–35, 1990.
121. Tolley DA, Hargreave TB, Smith PH, et al: Effect of intravesical mitomycin C on recurrence of newly diagnosed superficial bladder cancer: Interim report from the Medical Research Council Subgroup on Superficial Bladder Cancer (Urological Cancer Working Party). Br Med J 296:1759–1761, 1988.
122. Bouffioux C, Denis L, Oosterlinck W, et al: Adjuvant chemotherapy of recurrent superficial transitional cell carcinoma: Results of a EORTC randomised trial comparing intravesical instillation of thiotepa, doxorubicin and cisplatin. J Urol 148:297–301, 1992.
123. Morales A: Long term results and complications of intracavitary bacillus Calmette-Guerin therapy for bladder cancer. J Urol 132:457–459, 1984.

124. Morales A, Nickel JC, Wilson JWL: Dose-response of bacillus Calmette-Guerin in the treatment of superficial bladder cancer. J Urol 147:1256–1258, 1992.
125. Deresiewicz RL, Stone RM, Aster JC: Fatal disseminated mycobacterial infection following intravesical bacillus Calmette-Guerin. J Urol 144:1331–1334, 1990.
126. Rawls WH, Lamm DL, Lowe BA, et al: Fatal sepsis following intravesical bacillus Calmette-Guerin administration for bladder cancer. J Urol 144:1328–1330, 1990.
127. Khanna OP, Chou RH, Son DL, et al: Does bacillus Calmette-Guerin immunotherapy accelerate growth and cause metastatic spread of second primary malignancy? Urology 31:459–468, 1988.
128. Dow JA, di Sant'Agnese PA, Cockett ATK: Expression of blood group precursor T antigen as a prognostic marker for human bladder cancer treated by bacillus Calmette-Guerin and interleukin-2. J Urol 142:978–982, 1989.
129. Galvani D, Griffiths SD, Cawley JC: Interferon for treatment: The dust settles. Br Med J 296:1554–1556, 1988.
130. Alcock CJ, Durrant KR, Smith JC, Fellows GJ: Treatment of multiple superficial transitional cell carcinoma of the bladder with intravesical yttrium-90. Br J Urol 58:287–289, 1986.
131. Quilty PM, Duncan W: Treatment of superficial (T1) tumours of the bladder by radical radiotherapy. Br J Urol 58:147–152, 1986.
132. Benson RC, Kinsey JH, Cortese DA, Farrow GM, Utz DC: Treatment of transitional cell carcinoma of the bladder with hematoporphyrin derivative phototherapy. J Urol 1090–1095, 1983.
133. Jakse G, Putz A, Feichtinger J: Cystectomy: The treatment of choice in patients with carcinoma in situ of the bladder? Eur J Surg Oncol 15:211–216, 1989.
134. Harland SJ, Charig CR, Highman W, Parkinson MC, Riddle PR: Outcome in carcinoma-in-situ of bladder treated with intravesical bacille Calmette-Guerin. Br J Urol 70:271–275, 1992.
135. Stricker PD, Grant ABF, Hosken BM, Taylor JS: Topical mitomycin C therapy for carcinoma in situ of the bladder: A follow up. J Urol 1432:34–36, 1990.
136. Jenkins BJ, England HR, Fowler CG, et al: Chemotherapy for carcinoma in situ of the bladder. Br J Urol 61:326–329, 1988.
137. Whitmore WF: Integrated irradiation and cystectomy for bladder cancer. Br J Urol 52:1–9, 1980.
138. Skinner DG, Lieskovsky G: Contemporary cystectomy with pelvic node dissection compared to preoperative radiation therapy plus cystectomy in management of invasive bladder cancer. J Urol 131:1069–1072, 1984.
139. Jacobi GH, Klippel FF, Hohenfellner R: 15 Jahre Erfahrung mit der radikalen Cystecktomie ohne praeoperative Radiotherapie beim Harnblasenkarzinom. Aktuel Urol 14:63–69, 1983.
140. Wallace DM, Bloom HJG: The management of deeply infiltrating (T3) bladder carcinoma: Controlled trial of radical radiotherapy versus pre-operative radiotherapy and radical cystectomy (first report). Br J Urol 48:587–594, 1976.
141. Bloom HJG, Hendry WF, Wallace DM, Skeet RG: Treatment of T3 bladder cancer: Controlled trial of preoperative radiotherapy and radical cystectomy versus radical radiotherapy. Br J Urol 54:136–151, 1982.
142. Blandy JP, England HR, Evans SJW, et al: T3 bladder cancer—the case for salvage cystectomy. Br J Urol 52:506–510, 1980.
143. Blandy JP, Tiptaft RC, Paris AMI, Oliver RTD, Hope-Stone HF: The case for definitive radiotherapy and salvage cystectomy. World J Urol 3:94–97, 1985.
144. Jenkins BJ, Caulfield MJ, Fowler CG, et al: Reappraisal of the role of radical radiotherapy and salvage cystectomy in the treatment of invasive (T2/T3) bladder cancer. Br J Urol 62:343–346, 1988.
145. Shearer RJ, Chilvers CED, Bloom HJG, Bliss JM, Horwich A, Babiker A: Adjuvant chemotherapy in T3 carcinoma of the bladder. A prospective trial: Preliminary report. Br J Urol 62:558–564, 1988.
146. Smaaland R, Akslen LA, Tonder B, Mehus A, Lote K, Albrektsen G: Radical radiation treatment of invasive and locally advanced bladder carcinoma in elderly patients. Br J Urol 67:61–69, 1991.
147. Jenkins BJ, Martin JE, Baithun SI, Zuk RJ, Oliver RTD, Blandy JP: Prediction of response to radiotherapy in invasive bladder cancer. Br J Urol 65:345–348, 1990.
148. Oliver RTD, Nouri AME, Crosby D, et al: Biological significance of beta hCG, HLA and other membrane antigen expression on bladder tumours and their relationship to tumour infiltrating lymphocytes (TIL). J Immunogenet 16:381–390, 1989.
149. Lynch WJ, Jenkins BJ, Fowler CG, Hope-Stone HF, Blandy JP: The quality of life after radical radiotherapy for bladder cancer. Br J Urol 70:519–521, 1992.
150. Oliver RTD: Medical management of bladder cancer with an emphasis on the role of immune modulators and chemotherapy. In Oliver RTD, Hope-Stone HF, Blandy JP (eds): Urological and Genital Cancer. Oxford: Blackwell, 1989, pp 115–124.
151. Loehrer PJ Sr, Einhorn LH, Elson PJ, et al: A randomized comparison of cisplatin alone or in combination with methotrexate, vinblastine, and doxorubicin in patients with metastatic urothelial carcinoma: A cooperative group study. J Clin Oncol 10:1066–1073, 1992.
152. Sternberg CN, Yagoda A, Scher HI, et al: Methotrexate, vinblastine, doxorubicin, and cisplatin for advanced transitional cell carcinoma of the urothelium. Efficacy and patterns of response and relapse. Cancer 64:2448–2458, 1989.
153. Scher H, Herr H, Sternberg C, et al: Neo-adjuvant chemotherapy for invasive bladder cancer: Experience with the M-VAC regimen. Br J Urol 64:250–256, 1989.
154. Stockle M, Meyenburg W, Wellek S, et al: Advanced bladder cancer (Stages pT3b, pT4a, pN1 and pN2) improved survival after radical cystectomy and 3 adjuvant cycles of chemotherapy. Results of a controlled prospective study. J Urol 148:302–307, 1992.
155. Waxman J, Barton C, Biruls R, et al: Bladder cancer: inter-relationships between chemotherapy and radiotherapy. Br J Urol 69:151–155, 1992.
156. Skinner DG, Daniels JR, Russell CA, et al: The role of adjuvant chemotherapy following cystectomy for invasive bladder cancer: A prospective comparative trial. J Urol 145:459–464, 1991.
157. Boshoff C, Oliver RTD: Accelerated cisplatin based combination chemotherapy for bladder cancer: Comparison with 131 patients who received conventional treatment. Proc ASCO 12:242, 1993 (abstract 754).
158. Bowsher WG, Clarke A, Clarke DG, Costello AJ: Laparoscopic pelvic node dissection. Br J Urol 70:276–279, 1992.
159. Tomic R, Sjodin JG: Sexual function in men after radical cystectomy with or without urethrectomy. Scand J Urol Nephrol 26:127–129, 1992.
160. Stockle M, Gokcebay E, Riedmiller H, Hohenfellner R: Urethral tumor recurrences after radical cystoprostatectomy: The case for primary cystoprostatourethrectomy. J Urol 143:41–43, 1990.
161. Frazier HA, Robertson JE, Paulson DF: Complications of radical cystectomy and urinary diversion: A retrospective review of 675 cases in 2 decades. J Urol 148:1401–1405, 1992.
162. Ghoneim MA, Kock NG, Lycke G, el-Din ABS: An appliance-free, sphincter-controlled bladder substitute: The urethral Kock pouch. J Urol 138:1150–1154, 1987.
163. Wynder EL, Mabuchi K, Whitmore WF: Epidemiology of cancer of the prostate. Cancer 28:344–360, 1971.
164. Apt A: Circumcision and prostatic cancer. Acta Med Scand 178:493–504, 1968.
165. Spitz MR, Currier RD, Fueger JJ, Babaian RJ, Newell GR: Familial patterns of prostate cancer: A case control analysis. J Urol 146:1305–1307, 1991.
166. Wingo PA, Tong T, Bolden S: Cancer statistics 1995. CA 45:8–30, 1995.
167. Skeet RG: Epidemiology of urogenital tumours. In Williams DI (ed): Scientific Foundations of Urology. London: Heinemann, 1976, pp 199–211.
168. Lytton B: Demography of prostatic carcinoma. In Fitzpatrick JM, Krane RJ (eds): The Prostate. Edinburgh: Churchill Livingstone, 1989, pp 253–259.
169. Gleason DF: Classification of prostatic carcinoma. Cancer Chemother Rep 50:125–128, 1966.
170. Rich AR: On the frequency of occurrence of occult carcinoma of the prostate. J Urol 33:215–223, 1935.
171. Breslow N, Chan CW, Dhom G, et al: Latent carcinoma of prostate at autopsy in seven areas. Int J Cancer 20:680–688, 1977.
172. Registrar General's Statistical Returns. Office of Population Census and Surveys. Her Majesty's Stationery Office, London, 1987.
173. Gleason DF: Histologic grade, clinical stage and patient age in prostate cancer. NCI Monogr 7:15–18, 1987.
174. Benson MC, Olsson CA: The staging and grading of prostatic cancer. In Fitzpatrick JM, Krane RJ (eds): The Prostate. Edinburgh: Churchill Livingstone, 1989, pp 261–272, 1989.

175. Winkler HZ, Rainwater LM, Myers RP, et al: Stage D1 prostatic adenocarcinoma: Significance of nuclear DNA ploidy patterns studied by flow cytometry. Mayo Clin Proc 63:103–112, 1988.
176. Page BH: The pathological anatomy of digital enucleation for benign prostatic hyperplasia and its application to endoscopic resection. Br J Urol 52:111–126, 1980.
177. Villers A, McNeal JE, Redwine EA, Freiha FS, Stamey TA: The role of perineural space invasion in the local spread of prostatic adenocarcinoma. J Urol 142:763–768, 1989.
178. Arduino LJ, Gluckman MA: Lymph node metastases in early carcinoma of the prostate. J Urol 88:91–93, 1962.
179. Dahl DS, Wilson CS, Middleton RG, Bourne HH: Pelvic lymphadenectomy for staging localised prostatic cancer. J Urol 112:245–246, 1974.
180. Batson O: The function of the vertebral veins and their role in the spread of metastases. Ann Surg 112:138–149, 1940.
181. Wallace DM, Chisholm GD, Hendry WF: TNM classification for urologic tumours. Br J Urol 47:1–12, 1973.
182. Jewett HJ: The present status of radical prostatectomy for Stage A and B prostatic cancer. Urol Clin North Am 2:105–124, 1975.
183. Veterans Administration Co-operative Urological Research Group: Carcinoma of the prostate: Treatment comparisons. J Urol 98:516–522, 1967.
184. Waisman J: Pathology of neoplasms of the prostate gland. In Skinner DG, Lieskovsky G (eds): Diagnosis and Management of Genitourinary Cancer. Philadelphia: WB Saunders, 1988, pp 161–162.
185. Franks LM: Benign nodular hyperplasia of the prostate: Review. Ann R Coll Surg Engl 14:92–106, 1954.
186. Greene DR, Wheeler TM, Egawa S, Weaver RP, Scardino PT: Relationship between clinical stage and histological zone of origin in early prostate cancer: Morphometric analysis. Br J Urol 68:499–509, 1991.
187. Greene DR, Wheeler TM, Egawa S, Dunn JK, Scardino PT: A comparison of the morphological features of cancer arising in the transition zone and in the peripheral zone of the prostate. J Urol 146:1069–1076, 1991.
188. Whitmore WF Jr: Consensus Development Conference on the Management of Clinically Localized Prostate Cancer. Overview: Historical and contemporary. NCI Monogr 7:7–11, 1988.
189. Block NL, Weber D, Schinella R: Blue nevi and other melanotic lesions of the prostate: Report of 3 cases and review of the literature. J Urol 107:85–87, 1972.
190. Shannon RL, Ro JY, Grignon DJ, et al: Sarcomatoid carcinoma of the prostate. A clinicopathologic study of 12 patients. Cancer 69:2676–2682, 1992.
191. Hinman F: Screening for prostatic carcinoma. J Urol 145:126–130, 1991.
192. Barry J, Wild SR: Radiological appearances in prostatic cancer with rectal spread. Br J Urol 67:441–443, 1991.
193. Scott WW, Schirmer HKA: A new oral progestational steroid effective in treating prostatic cancer. Trans Am Assoc Genitourin Surg 58:54–62, 1966.
194. Jones DR, Griffiths GJ, Parkinson MC, et al: Comparative histopathology, microradiography and per-rectal ultrasonography of the prostate using cadaver specimens. Br J Urol 63:508–511, 1989.
195. Palken M, Cobb OE, Simons CE, Warren BH, Aldape HC: Prostate cancer: Comparison of digital rectal examination and transrectal ultrasound for screening. J Urol 145:86–92, 1991.
196. Weaver RP, Noble MJ, Weigel JW: Correlation of ultrasound guided and digitally directed biopsies of palpable prostatic abnormalities. J Urol 145:516–518, 1991.
197. Vapnek JM, Shinohara K, Carroll PR: Staging accuracy of magnetic resonance imaging versus transrectal ultrasound in stages A and B prostatic cancer. J Urol 145:352A, 1991.
198. Babaian RJ, Camps JL, Frangos DN, et al: Monoclonal prostate-specific antigen in untreated prostate cancer. Relationship to clinical stage and grade. Cancer 67:2200–2206, 1991.
199. Oesterling JE: Prostate specific antigen: A critical assessment of the most useful tumor marker for adenocarcinoma of the prostate. J Urol 145:907–923.
200. Adolfsson J: Radical prostatectomy, radiotherapy or deferred treatment for localized prostate cancer. Cancer Surveys 23:141–148, 1995.
201. George NJR: Natural history of localised prostatic cancer managed by conservative therapy alone. Lancet 1:494–497, 1988.
202. Zhang G, Wasserman NF, Sidi AA, Reinberg Y, Reddy PK: Long-term follow up results after expectant management of Stage A1 prostatic cancer. J Urol 146:99–103, 1991.
203. Belt E, Schroeder FH: Total perineal prostatectomy for carcinoma of the prostate. J Urol 107:91–96, 1972.
204. Walsh PC, Mostwin JL: Radical prostatectomy and cystoprostatectomy with preservation of potency. Results using a new nerve-sparing technique. Br J Urol 56:694–697, 1984.
205. Eggleston JC, Walsh PC: Radical prostatectomy with preservation of sexual function: Pathological findings in the first 100 cases. J Urol 134:1146–1148, 1985.
206. Bagshaw MA, Kaplan ID, Cox RC: Prostate cancer. Radiation therapy for localized disease. Cancer 71:939–952, 1993.
207. Lawton CA, Cox JD, Glisch C, Murray KJ, Byhardt RW, Wilson JF: Is long term survival possible with external beam irradiation for stage D1 adenocarcinoma of the prostate? Cancer 69:2761–2766, 1992.
208. Gomella LG, Steinberg SM, Ellison MF, Reeves WW, Flanigan RC, McRoberts JW: Analysis of Iodine-125 interstitial therapy in the treatment of localised carcinoma of the prostate. J Surg Oncol 46:235–240, 1991.
209. Kuban DG, el-Mahdi AM, Schellhammer PF: I-125 interstitial implantation for prostate cancer. What have we learned 10 years later? Cancer 63:2415–2420, 1989.
210. Scardino PT, Wheeler TM: Local control of prostate cancer with radiotherapy: Frequency and prognostic significance of positive results of postirradiation prostate biopsy. NCI Monogr 7:95–103, 1988.
211. Fellows GJ, Clark PB, Beynon LL, et al: Treatment of advanced localised prostatic cancer by orchiectomy, radiotherapy, or combined treatment. A Medical Research Council Study. Urological Cancer Working Party—Subgroup on Prostatic Cancer. Br J Urol 70:304–309, 1992.
212. Huggins C, Hodges CV: Studies on prostatic cancer. I. The effect of castration, of estrogen and of androgen injection on serum phosphatases in metastatic carcinoma of the prostate. Cancer Res 1:293–297, 1941.
213. Geller J: Basis for hormonal management of advanced prostate cancer. Cancer 71:1039–1045, 1993.
214. Waymont B, Lynch TH, Dunn JA, et al: Phase III randomised study of Zoladex versus Stilboestrol in the treatment of advanced prostate cancer. Br J Urol 69:614–620, 1992.
215. Kaisary AV, Tyrrell CJ, Peeling WB, Griffiths K: Comparison of LHRH analogue (Zoladex) with orchiectomy in patients with metastatic prostatic carcinoma. Br J Urol 67:502–508, 1991.
216. McLeod DG: Antiandrogenic drugs. Cancer 71:1046–1049, 1993.
217. Crawford ED, Eisenberger MA, McLeod DG, et al: A controlled trial of leuprolide with and without flutamide in prostatic carcinoma. N Engl J Med 321:419–424, 1989.
218. Janknegt RA, Abbou CC, Bartoletti R, et al: Orchiectomy and nilutamide or placebo as treatment of metastatic prostatic cancer in a multinational double-blind randomized trial. J Urol 149:77–83, 1993.
219. Keen CW: Second-line treatment of advanced prostate cancer: Hemibody radiation. In Alderson AR, Oliver RTD, Hanham IW, Bloom HJG (eds): Urological Oncology: Dilemmas and Developments. Chichester: Wiley, 1991, pp 253–257.
220. Johnson DE, Haynie TP: Phosphorus-32 for intractable pain in carcinoma of prostate. Analysis of androgen priming, parathormone rebound, and combination therapy. Urology 9:137–139, 1977.
221. Laing AH, Ackery DM, Bayly RJ, et al: Strontium-89 chloride for pain palliation in prostatic skeletal malignancy. Br J Radiol 64:816–822, 1991.
222. Elomaa I, Blomqvist C, Grohn P, et al: Long term controlled trial with diphosphonate in patients with osteolytic bone metastases. Lancet 1:146–149, 1983.
223. Kovi J, Tillman RI, Lee SK: Malignant transformation of condyloma acuminatum. Am J Clin Pathol 61:702–710, 1974.
224. Stockle M, Gokcebay E, Riedmiller H, Hohenfellner R (1990) Urethral tumor recurrences after radical cystoprostatectomy: the case for primary cystoprostatourethrectomy. J Urol 143:41–3.
225. Levine RL: Urethral cancer. Cancer 45:1965–72, 1980.
226. Sharma SK, Reddy MJ, Joshi VV, Bapna BC: Capillary haemangioma of male urethra. Br J Urol 53:277, 1981.
227. Kesner KM: Extensive condylomata acuminata of male urethra: Management by ventral urethrotomy. Br J Urol 71:204–207, 1993.
228. Ahlering TE, Lieskovsky G: Surgical treatment of urethral cancer in the male patient. In Skinner DG, Lieskovsky G (eds): Diagnosis

and Management of Genitourinary Cancer. Philadelphia: WB Saunders, 1988, pp 622–633.
229. Skinner EC, Skinner DG: Management of carcinoma of the female urethra. In Skinner DG, Lieskovsky G (eds): Diagnosis and Management of Genitourinary cancer. Philadelphia: WB Saunders, 1988.
230. Dixon FJ, Moore RA: Tumors of the male sex organs. In Atlas of Tumor Pathology VIII. Washington, DC: Armed Forces Institute of Pathology, 1952.
231. Hermanek P, Sobin LH (eds): International Union Against Cancer TNM Classification of Malignant Tumours, 4th ed, 2nd rev. Berlin: Springer, 1992.
232. Woodhouse CR, Flynn JT, Molland EA, Blandy JP: Urethral diverticulum in females. Br J Urol 52:305–310, 1980.
233. Paymaster JC, Gangadharan P: Carcinoma of the penis in India. J Urol 97:110–113, 1967.
234. Editorial: Circumcision and cervical cancer. Br Med J 2:397–398, 1964.
235. O'Brien WM, Jenson AB, Lancaster WD, Maxted WD: Human papillomavirus typing of penile condyloma. J Urol 141:863–865, 1989.
236. Lee PN: Penile cancer and smoking. Br Med J 296:210–211, 1988.
237. Shabad AL: Some aspects of etiology and prevention of penile cancer. J Urol 92:696–702, 1964.
238. Staubitz WJ, Lent MH, Oberkircher OJ: Carcinoma of the penis. Cancer 8:371–378, 1955.
239. Graham S, Priore R, Graham M, Browne R, Burnett W, West D: Genital cancer in wives of penile cancer patients. Cancer 44:1870–1874, 1979.
240. Jamieson NV, Bullock KN, Barker THW: Adenosquamous carcinoma of the penis associated with balanitis xerotica obliterans. Br J Urol 58:730–731, 1986.
241. el-Demiry MIM, Oliver RTD, Hope-Stone HF, Blandy JP: Reappraisal of the role of radiotherapy and surgery in the management of carcinoma of the penis. Br J Urol 56:724–728, 1984.
242. Loewenstein LW: Carcinoma-like condylomata acuminata of the penis. Med Clin North Am 23:789–795, 1939.
243. Alfthan O: Condyloma acuminatum giganticum: Buschke-Loewenstein tumour. Scand J Urol Nephrol 4:71–77, 1970.
244. Graham JH, Helwig EB: Erythroplasia of Queyrat. A clinicopathologic and histochemical study. Cancer 32:1396–1414, 1973.
245. Mikhail GR: Cancers, precancers and pseudocancer on the male genitalia: A review of clinical appearances, histopathology and management. J Dermatol Surg Oncol 6:1027–1035, 1980.
246. Fegen JP, Beebe D, Persky L: Basal cell carcinoma of the penis. J Urol 104:864–866, 1970.
247. Salaverria JC, Hope-Stone HF, Paris AMI, Molland EA, Blandy JP: Conservative treatment of carcinoma of the penis. Br J Urol 51:32–37, 1979.
248. Perinetti E, Crane DB, Catalona WJ: Unreliability of sentinel lymph node biopsy for staging penile carcinoma. J Urol 124:734–735, 1980.
249. Hermanek P, Sobin LH (eds): International Union Against Cancer TNM Classification of Malignant Tumours, 4th ed, 2nd rev. Berlin: Springer, 1992.
250. Jackson SM: The treatment of carcinoma of the penis. Br J Surg 53:33–35, 1966.
251. Blandy JP: Operative Urology, 2nd ed. Oxford: Blackwell, 1986.
252. Johnson DE, Lo RK: Management of regional lymph nodes in penile carcinoma: Five year results following therapeutic groin dissections. Urology 24:308–311, 1984.
253. Blandy JP, Hope-Stone HF, Oliver RTD: Carcinoma of the penis and urethra. In Oliver RTD, Blandy JP, Hope-Stone HF (eds): Urological and Genital Cancer. Oxford: Blackwell, 1989; pp 258–271.
254. Isa SS, Almaraz R, Magovern J: Leiomyosarcoma of the penis. Case report and review of the literature. Cancer 54:939–942, 1984.
255. McNutt NS, Fletcher V, Conant MA: Early lesions of Kaposi's sarcoma in homosexual men. An ultrastructural comparison with other vascular proliferations in skin. Am J Pathol 111:62–77, 1983.
256. Huang DJ, Stanisic TH, Hansen KK: Epithelioid sarcoma of the penis. J Urol 147:1370–1372, 1992.
257. Bracken RB, Diokno AC: Melanoma of the penis and the urethra: 2 Case reports and review of the literature. J Urol 111:198–200, 1974.
258. Powell BL, Craig JB, Muss HB: Secondary malignancies of the penis and epididymis: A case report and review of the literature. J Clin Oncol 3:110–116, 1985.
259. Mathewman PJ, Oliver RTD, Woodhouse CRJ, Tiptaft RC: The role of chemotherapy in the treatment of penile metastases from carcinoma of the bladder. Eur Urol 12:310–312, 1987.
260. Symington T: Functional Pathology of the Human Adrenal Gland. Edinburgh: Churchill Livingstone, 1969.
261. Weiss LM: Comparative histologic study of 43 metastasizing and nonmetastasizing adrenocartical tumors. Am J Surg Pathol 8:163–169, 1984.
262. Venkatesh S, Hickery RC, Sellin RV, Fernandez JF, Samaan NA: Adrenal cortical carcinoma. Cancer 64:765–769, 1989.
263. Chang SY, Lee SS, Ma CP, Lee SK: Non-functioning tumours of the adrenal cortex. Br J Urol 63:462–464, 1989.
264. Donohue JP: Diagnosis and management of adrenal tumors. In Skinner DG, Lieskovsky G (eds): Diagnosis and Management of Genitourinary Cancer. Philadelphia: WB Saunders, 1988, pp 372–389.
265. Hutter AM, Kayhoe DE: Adrenal cortical carcinoma. Clinical features of 138 patients. Am J Med 41:572–580, 1966.
266. Ganguly A, Donohue JP: Primary aldosteronism: Pathophysiology, diagnosis and treatment. J Urol 129:241–247, 1983.
267. Hensle TW, Parkhurst EC: Sipple's syndrome: A urologist's viewpoint. Urology 8:258–262, 1976.
268. Ponder B: Multiple endocrine neoplasia type 2: The search for the gene continues. Br Med J 300:484–485, 1990.
269. Lindau A: Studen ueber Kleinhirncysten: Bau, Pathogenese und Beziehungen zur Angiomatosis Retinae. Acta Pathol Microbiol Scand Suppl 1:1–128, 1926.
270. Neville AM, O'Hare MJ: Aspects of structure, function and pathology. In James VHT (ed): The Adrenal Gland. New York: Raven Press, 1979, pp 52–55.
271. Edwards GA, Smythe GA, Graham PE, Lazarus L: The impact of recent advances in diagnostic technology on the clinical presentation of phaeochromocytoma. Med J Aust 156:153–157, 1992.
272. Ackery DM, Tippett PA, Condon BR, Sutton HE, Wyeth P: New approach to the localisation of phaeochromocytoma: Imaging with iodine-131-meta-iodobenzylguanidine. Br Med J 288:1587–1591, 1984.
273. Shulkin BL, Wieland DM, Schwaiger M, et al: PET scanning with hydroxephedrine: An approach to the localization of pheochromocytoma. J Nucl Med 33:1125–1131, 1992.
274. Nativ O, Grant CS, Sheps SG, et al: Prognostic profile for patients with pheochromocytoma derived from clinical and pathological factors and DNA ploidy pattern. J Surg Oncol 50:258–262, 1992.
275. Mancini AF, Rosito P, Faldella G, et al: Neuroblastoma in a pair of identical twins. Med Pediatr Oncol 10:45–51, 1982.
276. Duckett JW, Koop CE: Neuroblastoma. Urol Clin North Am 4:285–295, 1977.
277. Castleberry RP: Clinical and biologic features in the prognosis and treatment of neuroblastoma. Curr Opin Oncol 4:116–123, 1992.
278. Forman D: Aetiology of Testicular Tumours. In Alderson AR, Oliver RTD, Hanham IWF, Bloom HJG (eds): Urological Oncology: Dilemmas and Developments. Chichester: Wiley, 1991, pp 269–282.
279. Mead GM: Testicular cancer and related neoplasms. Br Med J 304:1426–1429, 1992.
280. Blandy JP: History of the surgery of testicular tumours. In Blandy JP, Hope-Stone HF, Dayan AD (eds): Tumours of the Testicle. London: Heinemann, 1970, pp 1–11.
281. Daniels JL, Stutzman RE, McLeod DG: A comparison of testicular tumors in Black and White patients. J Urol 125:341–342, 1981.
282. Oliver RTD, Stephenson CA, Parkinson MC, et al: Germ cell tumours of the testicle. A model for MHC influence on human malignancy. J Immunogenet 13:85–92, 1986.
283. Brown LM, Pottern LM, Hoover RN, Devesa SS, Aselton P, Flannery JT: Testicular cancer in the United States: Trends in incidence and mortality. Int J Epidemiol 15:164–170, 1986.
284. Chilvers CED, Forman D, Oliver RTD, et al: Social, behavioural and medical factors in the aetiology of testicular cancer—results from the UK study. Br J Cancer 70:513–520, 1994.
285. Bernstein L, Pike MC, Depue RH, Ross RK, Moore JW, Henderson BE: Maternal hormone levels in early gestation of cryptorchid males: A case-control study. Br J Cancer 58:379–381, 1988.
286. Oliver RTD: Clinical relevance of modern understanding of testis cancer epidemiology and aetiology. In Moul JW (ed): Problems in Urology. Philadelphia: JB Lippincott, 1994, pp 12–30.
287. Jacobsen GK: Pathology and cytochemistry of germ cell tumours.

In Oliver RTD, Blandy JP, Hope-Stone HF (eds): Urological and Genital Cancer. Oxford: Blackwell, 1989, pp 322–358.
288. Grigor KM: A new classification of germ cell tumours of the testis. Eur Urol 23:93–103, 1993.
289. Oliver RTD: Grading germ cell tumours as a means to resolve the last twenty five years of Transatlantic conflict over testis tumour classification. Third International Germ Cell Tumour Conference, 1993.
290. Wylie CC, Stott D, Donovan PJ: Primordial germ cell migration. In Browder L (eds): The Cellular Basis of Morphogenesis. New York: Plenum, 1986, pp 433–450.
291. Mostofi FK, Spaander P, Grigor K, Parkingson CM, Skakkebaek NE, Oliver RTD: Consensus on pathological classification of testicular tumours. Prog Clin Biol Res 357:267–276, 1991.
292. Oliver RTD: Clues from natural history and results of treatment supporting the monoclonal origin of germ cell tumours. Cancer Surv 9:333–368, 1990.
293. Oosterhuis JW, Gillis AJM, van Putten WJL, et al: Interphase cytogenetics of carcinoma in situ of the testis. Eur Urol 23:16–22, 1993.
294. Talerman A: Spermatocytic seminoma: Clinicopathological study of 22 cases. Cancer 45:2169–2176, 1980.
295. Shapeero LG, Vordermark JS: Epidermoid cysts of testes and role of sonography. Urology 41:75–79, 1993.
296. Javadpour N: The role of biologic tumor markers in testicular cancer. Cancer 45:1755–1761, 1980.
297. Tucker DF, Oliver RTD, Travers P, et al: Serum marker potential of placental alkaline phosphatase-like activity in testicular germ cell tumours evaluated by H17E2 monoclonal antibody assay. Br J Cancer 51:631–639, 1985.
298. Oliver RTD: Clues from natural history and results of treatment supporting the monoclonal origin of germ cell tumours. Cancer Surveys 9:332–368, 1990.
299. Hermanek P, Sobin LH (eds): International Union Against Cancer TNM Classification of Malignant Tumours, 4th ed, 2nd rev. Berlin: Springer, 1992.
300. Richie JP: Diagnosis and staging of testicular tumors. In Skinner DF, Lieskovsky G (eds): Diagnosis and Management of Genitourinary Cancer. Philadelphia: WB Saunders, 1988, pp 498–507.
301. Davis S, Di Martino NA, Schneider G: Malignant interstitial cell carcinoma of the testis: Report of 2 cases with steroid synthetic profiles, response to therapy and review of the literature. Cancer 47:425–431, 1981.
302. Morin LJ, Loening S: Malignant androblastoma (Sertoli-cell tumor) of the testis. A case report with a review of the literature. J Urol 114:476–480, 1975.
303. Gowing NFC, Morgan AD: Paratesticular tumours of connective tissue and muscle. Br J Urol 36(Suppl):78, 1964.
304. Williams G, Banerjee R: Paratesticular tumours. Br J Urol 41:332–339, 1969.
305. Richie JP, Birnholz J, Garnick MB: Ultrasonography as a diagnostic adjunct for the evaluation of masses in the scrotum. Surg Gynecol Obstet 154:695–698, 1982.
306. Heikkila R, Heilo A, Stenwig AE, Fossa SD: Testicular ultrasonography and 18G biopsy for clinically undetected cancer or carcinoma in situ in patients with germ cell tumours. Br J Urol 71:214–216, 1993.
307. Azzopardi JG, Hoffbrand AV: Retrogression in testicular seminoma with viable metastases. J Clin Pathol 18:135–141, 1965.
308. Vogelzang RL: Real-time scrotal ultrasound with a water bath: Comparison of results using 5 and 8 MHz transducers. J Urol 134:687–690, 1985.
309. Richie JP, Garnick MB, Finberg H: Computerized tomography: How accurate for abdominal staging of testis tumors? J Urol 127:715–717, 1982.
310. McLeod DG, Weiss RB, Stablein DM, et al: Staging relationships and outcome in early stage testicular cancer: A report from the Testicular Cancer Intergroup Study. J Urol 145:1178–1183, 1991.
311. Oliver RTD, Edmonds P, Ong JYH, et al: Pilot studies of 2 & 1 course carboplatin as adjuvant for stage I seminoma: Should it be tested in a randomised trial against radiotherapy? Int J Radiat Oncol Biol Phys 29:3–8, 1994.
312. Oliver RTD, Raja MA, Ong J, Gallagher CJ: Pilot study to evaluate impact of a policy of adjuvant chemotherapy for high risk stage I malignant teratoma on overall relapse rate of stage I cancer patients. J Urol 148:1453–1456, 1992.
313. Donohue JP, Einhorn LH, Perez JM: Improved management of non-seminomatous testis tumours. Cancer 42:2903–2908, 1978.
314. Oliver RTD, Stenning S, Read G, et al: Surveillance as an option in the management of patients with stage 1 germ cell tumours of the testis. In Giuliani L: New Trends in Diagnosis and Treatment of Testis Cancer. Munich, Sympomed, 1992.
315. Donohue JP, Thornhill JA, Foster RS, Rowland RG and Bihrle R: Primary retroperitoneal lymph node dissection in a clinical stage A non-seminomatous germ cell testis cancer. Review of the Indiana University experience 1965–1989. Br J Urol; 71:326–335, 1993.
316. Hendry WF, A'Hern RP, Hetherington JW, Peckham MJ, Dearnaley DP, Horwich A: Para-aortic lymphadenectomy for metastatic non-seminomatous germ cell tumours: Prognostic value and therapeutic benefit. Br J Urol 71:208–213, 1993.
317. Zuk RJ, Jenkins BJ, Martin JE, Oliver RTD and Baithun SI: Findings in lymph nodes of patients with germ cell tumours after chemotherapy and their relation to prognosis. J Clin Path 42:1049–1054, 1989.
318. Williams SN, Jenkins BJ, Baithun SI, Oliver RTD, Blandy JP: Radical retroperitoneal node dissection after chemotherapy for testicular tumours. Br J Urol 63:641–643, 1989.
319. Blandy JP, Jenkins BJ, Badenoch DF, Fowler CG, Oliver RTD: Radical retroperitoneal node dissection after chemotherapy for testicular tumours. EORTC Genitourinary Group Monograph 10: Urological Oncology: Reconstructive surgery, Organ conservation and restoration of function. New York, Wiley-Liss, 1991, pp 399–401.
320. Einhorn LH, and Donohue J: Cis-diaminedichloroplatinum, vinblastine, and bleomycin combination chemotherapy in disseminated testicular cancer. Ann Intern Med; 87:293–298, 1977.
321. Peckham MJ, Barrett A, Liew KH, et al: The treatment of metastatic germ-cell testicular tumours with bleomycin, etoposide and cisplatin (BEP). Br J Cancer 47:613–619, 1983.
322. Williams SD, Birch R, Einhorn LH, Irwin L, Greco FA, Loehrer PJ: Treatment of disseminated germ-cell tumors with cisplatin, bleomycin, and either vinblastine or etoposide. N Engl J Med 316:1435–1440, 1987.
323. Loehrer PJ Sr, Lauer R, Roth BJ, Williams SD, Kalasinski LA, Einhorn LH: Salvage therapy in recurrent germ cell cancer: Ifosfamide and cisplatin plus either vinblastine or etoposide. Ann Intern Med 109:540–546, 1988.
324. Oliver RTD, Ong J, Gallagher CJ: Weekly M-BOP as a second line and VIP plus high dose as third line salvage for germ cell cancer. Proc Am Soc Clin Oncol, 14:249(abstract 671), 1995.
325. Motzer RJ, Bosl GJ: High-dose chemotherapy for resistant germ cell tumors: Recent advances and future directions. J Natl Cancer Inst 84:1703–1709, 1992.
326. Mead GM, Stenning SP, Cullen MH, et al: The Second Medical Research Council study of prognostic factors in nonseminomatous germ cell tumours. Medical Research Council Testicular Tumour Working Party. J Clin Oncol 10:85–94, 1992.
327. Horwich A, Dearnaley DP, Nicholls J, et al: Effectiveness of carboplatin, etoposide, and bleomycin combination chemotherapy in good-prognosis metastatic testicular nonseminomatous germ cell tumors. J Clin Oncol 9:62–69, 1991.
328. Bajorin DF, Motzer RJ, Rodriguez E, Murphy B, Bosl GJ: Acute nonlymphocytic leukaemia in germ cell tumour patients treated with etoposide-containing chemotherapy. J Natl Cancer Inst 85:60–62, 1993.
329. Einhorn LH, Williams SD, Loehrer PJ, et al: Evaluation of optimal duration of chemotherapy in favorable-prognosis disseminated germ cell tumors: A Southeastern Cancer Study Group protocol. J Clin Oncol 7:387–391, 1989.
330. Oliver RTD, Lore S, Ong J: Alternatives to radiotherapy in management of seminoma. Br J Urol 65:61–67, 1990.
331. Horwich A, Dearnaley D, A'Hern R, et al: The activity of single-agent carboplatin in advanced seminoma. Eur J Cancer 28A:1307–1310, 1992.
332. Pedersen-Bjergaard J, Daugaard G, Hansen SW, Philip P, Larsen SO, Rorth M: Increased risk of myelodysplasia and leukaemia after etoposide, cisplatin, and bleomycin for germ-cell tumours. Lancet 338:359–363, 1991.

16

Skin Cancers

Melanoma

Donald L. Morton, M.D. • Richard Essner, M.D.

"What is the Black Spot, Captain?"
"That's a summons, mate."

ROBERT LOUIS STEVENSON, *Treasure Island*

Malignant melanoma now accounts for 3% of all malignancies diagnosed in the United States. It is one of the most rapidly increasing cancers in this country, for reasons that are not fully understood. Most cases of melanoma are limited to a primary cutaneous lesion and can be cured by wide excision. The risk of recurrence or metastatic disease is directly related to the depth of this lesion. Since there is no standard therapy to control metastatic melanoma, prevention and early diagnosis are crucial.

HISTORY

Malignant melanoma—the "black cancer"—has an impressive history that begins thousands of years ago. In Peru, paleopathologists have found Incan mummies exhibiting diffuse metastases to the bones of the skull and extremities as well as rounded melanotic masses in the skin.[1] The occurrence of melanoma in these mummies is startling, considering the infrequency of melanoma in dark-skinned individuals—not to mention the presumably better condition of the ozone layer 2500 years ago. However, this is not an isolated finding; metastatic melanoma lesions have also been reported in fossil evidence from Neanderthal man and in the mummy of an Egyptian pharaoh.

The first descriptions of malignant melanoma belong to the physicians of ancient Greece, most notably Hippocrates (460–375 B.C.) and later Rufus of Ephesus (A.D. 60–120). The next 1650 years brought many other accounts of pigmented malignant cutaneous lesions but no landmarks in melanoma diagnosis or treatment. In 1787, however, British surgeon John Hunter published his report of a 35-year-old man who experienced recurrence of a mass that had been excised 3 years previously from behind the angle of the lower jaw. The recurrent lump enlarged slowly until the patient was struck in the jaw during a drunken brawl, after which the lump rapidly doubled in size. Hunter excised this tumor; according to him, "part of it was white and part spongy, soft and black." Hunter's original specimen is preserved in the Hunterian Museum of the Royal College of Surgeons of England.

Hunter's tumor was identified only as a "cancerous fungous excrescence." The disease itself lacked a more specific label until 1812, when the French physician Rene Theophile Laennec introduced the term *melanosis.*[2] Laennec was the first to describe melanoma as a disease entity (in an unpublished memoir presented in 1806 to the Faculté de Médecine de Paris).

Another nineteenth-century pioneer was William Norris, author of the first case report of melanoma in English literature. Although his 1820 paper describes a case of "fungoid disease," it is nonetheless a remarkable recitation of most of the salient features of malignant melanoma.[3]

The patient, a 59-year-old man, had a tumor in the suprapubic area. Norris described a pigmented halo, the development of satellite tumors, a recurrence after local excision, enlargement of inguinal glands, and progressive dissemination of the disease. He also described melanin in the urine. Norris even noted vertical inheritance of melanoma, concluding that the disease is hereditary (an observation that predated Mendel's experiments by 36 years).

The surgical management of melanoma was pioneered by Oliver Pemberton, whose 1858 report[4] introduced the concept of en bloc regional node dissection—almost a century before it became standard surgical practice. Pemberton described 25 cases of melanoma, advocating wide and deep dissection, carrying the level of excision below the underlying fascia and removing implicated lymph nodes by groin dissection. In 1892, Herbert L. Snow proposed wide excision and routine *elective* lymph node dissection.[5] In his lecture titled "Melanotic Cancerous Disease," Snow focused on "the usually insignificant dimensions of the primary lesion" and "its tendency to rapidly infect the nearest lymph glands." At the turn of the century, Frederic Eve summarized 45 cases of cutaneous melanoma, proposing wide excision and elective regional node dissection as the best surgical approach.[6] In his "Lecture on Melanoma," Eve stated: "The treatment of melanoma of the skin can be given in few words, i.e., free excision or amputation, in accordance with the position and extent of the disease. The removal of the nearest chain of lymphatic glands, whether palpably enlarged or not, should never be omitted; for it may be taken as a matter of certainty that in the great majority of cases they are infected." Eve also deserves credit for considering melanoma as a possible diagnosis in "any case of obscure glandular enlargement."

In 1907, William Sampson Handley described the spread of tumor via the deep and superficial lymphatic channels and the fascial planes.[7] With Eve, he advocated radical (wide) excision of the primary tumor and routine elective lymph node dissection. Handley even recognized the possibility of multiple drainage patterns for certain primary melanomas. Just one year later, J. Hogarth Pringle proposed in continuity or en bloc dissection of the primary melanoma and the regional lymph glands.[8] The recommendations of these early pioneers set the stage for an aggressive surgical approach that characterized the management of melanoma for the next 50 years.

EPIDEMIOLOGY

Incidence

During the past decade, the incidence of melanoma in the United States and Canada has increased faster than that of any other malignancy, except lung cancer in women. In fact, the incidence of melanoma in North America is now increasing 5% to 7% each year.[9] The age-adjusted annual rate in the United States is approximately 10 in 100,000, slightly higher in more temperate climates. According to estimates from the American Cancer Society, in 1995 over 34,000 Americans will be diagnosed with melanoma and 7200 will die of this disese.[9a] If the current rate of increase continues, melanoma will strike 1 of every 75 individuals by the year 2000.

Risk Factors

Although the etiology of melanoma is unknown, a number of factors clearly increase the risk of disease. Foremost among these is skin pigment: melanoma is primarily a disease of individuals with fair complexions. People who tend to burn easily after minimal sun exposure or have a history of severe sunburn are at substantially higher risk, as are those having large numbers of nevi or freckles.[10]

Chronic sun and ultraviolet (UV) light exposure has been implicated as a risk factor for development of melanoma.[11] Adults who migrate to warm climates have a lower risk for development of this disease than individuals born and raised there, which suggests that the duration of sun exposure is important. The overall increase in UV radiation caused by depletion of the ozone layer may be directly responsible for the increasing incidence of cutaneous melanoma.

The correlation between chronic sun exposure and melanoma is strong, but it does not explain why this disease can occur in relatively unexposed skin, such as on the palms, or in completely unexposed sites, such as bowel mucosa. It also does not explain why melanoma is more common in white-collar workers who have occasional sun exposure than in blue-collar workers whose occupations are largely outdoors. The development of melanoma most likely reflects the complex interplay of several known and unknown risk factors.

Familial Melanoma

The mechanism of UV-mediated skin cancers, particularly melanoma, is believed to result from damage to the DNA. UV light produces DNA adducts that lead to genetic mutation of the epithelium and melanocytes.[12] Abnormalities on the short arm of chromosome 1 and on both arms of chromosomes 6 and 7 have been linked to UV-mediated genetic damage.[13–16]

Although a number of earlier studies suggested a heritable form of melanoma, familial melanoma was not documented until Cawley's 1952 report.[17] Subsequent studies by Greene and Fraumeni in 1979[18] used familial and genetic factors to identify a small but distinct population with a higher incidence of melanoma. Familial melanoma has been linked to an abnormality on the short arm of chromosome 1.[14]

Dysplastic Nevus Syndrome

The B-K or dysplastic nevus syndrome,[19] which increases an individual's risk for development of melanoma, is characterized by multiple large and atypical moles that are variable in shape and coloration. These moles commonly appear on the trunk but can occur on any cutaneous site. Diagnosis is confirmed by histopathologic identification of junctional or compound nevi that carry elements of dysplasia. If there is subsequent development of melanoma, the lesion may be adjacent to a dysplastic mole (20% to 50% of cases) or independent of it.[20] The melanoma that develops from dysplastic nevi is usually thin and superficial spreading, which accounts for the favorable prognosis of these patients.

Although dysplastic nevi generally have a familial distribution, the genetic mechanisms of the syndrome and its progression to melanoma are not known. Dysplastic nevus syndrome may be the result of an autosomal dominant single gene with incomplete penetrance,[19] or it may reflect polygenic transmission.[21]

Congenital Nevi

These uncommon melanocytic nevi occur in 1% of newborn infants.[22] They represent hamartomas arising from the neural crest. Congenital nevi are large or small, with irregular borders, increased pigmentation, and hypertrichosis. Large congenital nevi are regarded as precursors of melanoma. The malignant potential of the smaller lesions is not clear, but *all* congenital nevi should be closely monitored. Because the lifetime risk of melanoma in patients with congenital nevi is approximately 20%,[23] these lesions should be excised if possible.

Melanocytes As Precursor Lesions

Melanocytes arise from the neural crest and migrate to the skin, uveal tract, meninges, and ectodermal mucosa. Melanocytes are usually located at the dermal-epidermal interface, and most melanoma lesions arise from the skin. However, melanoma may develop at any of these sites in association with a pre-existing lesion or from apparently normal skin or epithelial surfaces.

PATHOLOGY

Growth

Most cutaneous melanomas can be divided into two distinct biologic growth phases: radial and vertical. During the radial phase, melanoma cells grow in a flat, radial pattern from the primary site. This phase has a low metastatic potential and may persist for many years in superficial spreading, acral lentiginous, or lentigo maligna melanoma. By contrast, this phase is relatively short-lived in nodular melanoma. Eventually *all* melanomas will enter the vertical phase, with initial penetration of the basal lamina. During vertical growth, the lesion's depth, height, and metastatic potential simultaneously increase as it extends down into the dermis and becomes nodular or dome shaped.[24]

Histology

Superficial spreading melanoma (SSM) is the prevalent form of cutaneous melanoma, representing more than 70% of cases. SSM generally arises from a pre-existing nevus and is the most common histologic type in patients with dysplastic nevi. SSM is a typically flat lesion with dark pigment. As this lesion enlarges, its borders become irregular with variable coloration. SSM tends to occur throughout adulthood, particularly in the fifth decade of life.

Lentigo maligna melanoma (LMM) represents only 10% of all melanomas. It arises from lentigo maligna or Hutchinson's freckle, usually appearing on the face of elderly individuals. These large lesions are flat and variable shades of brown. They generally do not invade the basal lamina and have a low metastatic potential. In fact, an LMM lesion may remain clinically static for 5 to 10 years.[25] However, if it enters the vertical growth phase, prognosis depends on the depth of invasion.

Nodular melanoma (NM) is the second most common histologic type, representing 10% to 15% of all cutaneous melanomas.[26] NM may occur at any age and tends to appear more often in men than in women. Typically, the lesion is a dark-brown to black nodule, although some lesions may be amelanotic. NM does not have a radial growth phase; instead, cells rapidly begin vertical growth. For this reason, NM has a worse prognosis than other histologic types.

Acral lentiginous melanoma (ALM) is an unusual entity limited to the palms, soles, or nail beds.[27, 28] ALM typically arises in dark-complected individuals such as Hispanics and Asians, favoring older adults. The lesion has a short radial growth phase and usually presents as a large (~3 cm) ulcerated or fungating mass. Occasionally, lesions are flesh-colored and may be misdiagnosed as benign. Because of its short radial growth phase, ALM is more aggressive and has a greater metastatic potential than LMM or SSM.

Subungual melanoma, a variant of ALM, represents only 2% to 3% of melanomas in whites.[29, 30] Usually diagnosed in older adults, it generally arises under the nail of the big toe or thumb. The most common presenting sign is a brown to black discoloration of the nail bed. Subungual melanoma can easily be misdiagnosed as subungual hematoma, onychomycosis, or ingrown toenail. Biopsy is necessary to establish the diagnosis.

In addition to these major histologic categories of melanoma are several histologic features of prognostic importance. Of particular importance are Breslow thickness and Clark level measurements of vertical growth, as discussed in the next section. In addition, a high mitotic rate,[31] blood vessel or lymphatic invasion,[32] and tumor ulceration and perhaps regression[33] indicate an unfavorable outcome.

TABLE 16–1
Signs and Symptoms of Cutaneous Melanoma

Lesion Characteristic	Percentage of Lesions	
	Depth <0.85 mm	*Depth ≥3.65 mm*
Expansion	55	72
Color change	49	58
Elevation	36	82
Bleeding	13	63
Ulceration	5	50
Tenderness	8	19
Itching	20	46

Adapted from Sober AJ, Day CL Jr, Kopf AW, Fitzpatrick TB: Detection of "thin" primary melanomas. CA Cancer 33:160, 1983.

DIAGNOSIS

In most cases, the diagnosis of melanoma is made early in the natural history of the disease, when cure can be effected by wide excision alone. Melanoma lesions are most often on the lower extremities in women and on the torso in men. Less common are lesions on the head and neck, on the palms of the hands, or on the soles of the feet.

The classic clinical signs and symptoms of melanoma in a pre-existing nevus include darkening or irregular coloration, enlargement, nodularity, ulceration, pruritus, and spontaneous bleeding. However, these changes may not be evident until the lesion is relatively deep and advanced (Table 16–1). About 5% to 10% of lesions lack color and are termed amelanotic. Because a diagnosis of melanoma requires confirmation by histologic examination, any suspicious lesion should be sampled for biopsy by excision. The pathologic features of the lesion affect the approach to treatment.

Staging

One of the earliest and simplest staging systems for melanoma divided patients into three categories according to the presence of clinically observed disease in a primary lesion (stage I), in a regional lymph basin or intransit site (stage II), or at a distant site (stage III).[34] This clinical system, while enviable for its simplicity, failed to consider the prognostic importance of lesion histology. Metastatic potential is determined by characteristics of the primary lesion; any adequate staging system for melanoma *must* include histopathologic features of the primary lesion. In 1953, Allen and Spitz[35] first attempted to predict the biologic behavior of melanoma by histologic characteristics of the primary lesion. Of the many systems developed since then, the microstaging methods of Clark[24] and Breslow[36] are the most useful.

Clark's method categorizes lesions according to their level of invasion through the dermis and subcutaneous fat (Fig. 16–1); the lesion's level of invasion is directly correlated with its metastatic potential. Level I or "in situ" lesions arise in the epidermis and do not penetrate the basal lamina. Level II lesions penetrate the basal lamina and enter the papillary dermis. Level III lesions extend through the papillary dermis to reach the interface of the reticular dermis. Level IV lesions penetrate the reticular dermis. Level V lesions reach into the subcutaneous fat.

Breslow's method is based on lesion thickness rather than invasiveness: the thicker the primary lesion, the higher its metastatic potential. Lesion thickness is defined as the distance from the epidermis to the deepest identifiable layer of contiguous melanoma cells. Breslow's technique has become widely accepted because it is easier and more reproducible than Clark's method.

Because both the Clark level and the Breslow thickness

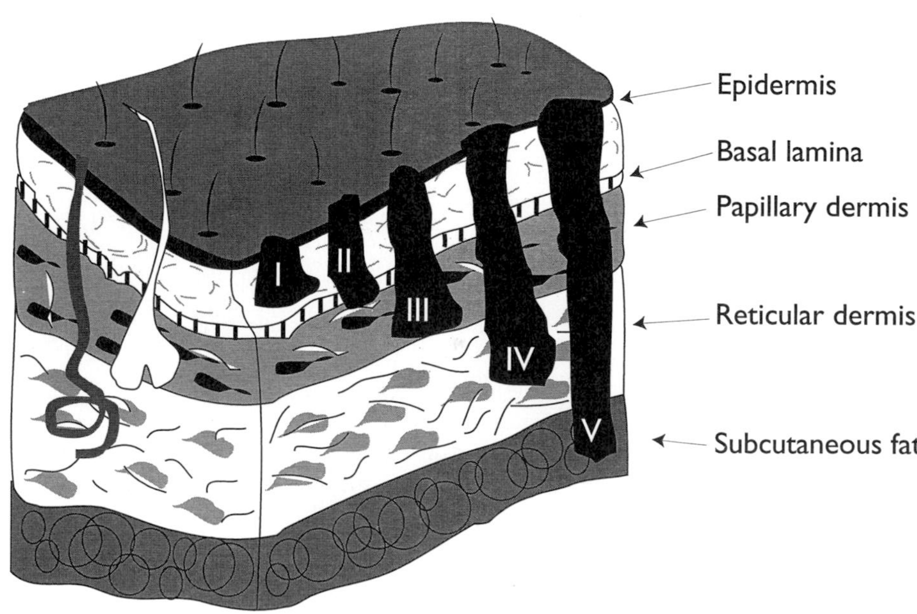

FIGURE 16–1. Clark levels of invasion through the skin.

TABLE 16–2
AJCC/UICC pTNM Staging System*

Stage	Criteria
IA	Primary melanoma ≤0.75 mm thick and/or Clark level II; no nodal or systemic metastases
IB	Primary melanoma 0.76 to 1.50 mm thick and/or Clark level III
IIA	Primary melanoma 1.51 to 4.00 mm thick and/or Clark level IV
IIB	Primary melanoma >4.0 mm thick and/or Clark level V
III	Regional lymph node and/or intransit metastases
IV	Systemic metastases

AJCC, American Joint Committee on Cancer; UICC, International Union Against Cancer.

*When there is a discordance between thickness and level, thickness is used to stage the primary melanoma.

of a primary lesion are important in determining the patient's prognosis, the American Joint Committee on Cancer (AJCC) has adopted a pTNM (primary tumor, nodes, and metastases) staging system that incorporates histopathologic features of both (Table 16–2). The AJCC staging system more accurately defines the malignant potential of the primary lesion than do systems based only on clinical parameters. If Breslow and Clark data are not in agreement, the AJCC system specifies using Breslow thickness for staging. In our experience, however, both staging systems are independently important prognostic indicators. Therefore, when there is a discordance between the two levels of microstaging, we recommend using the system that accords the lesion its *highest* risk.[37]

TREATMENT OF CLINICALLY LOCALIZED MELANOMA

Management of the Primary Lesion

Treatment begins with a biopsy of the primary lesion to provide a specimen for histopathologic verification and microstaging of melanoma. Excisional biopsy yields the most suitable tissue for diagnosis but often is not possible because of the lesion's site or size. For instance, lesions arising on the face, hands, or feet may require incisional biopsy. Punch biopsy is also an acceptable alternative. Shave biopsy is rarely indicated because the lesion cannot be accurately staged if it is not completely resected.

Surgery

The only currently effective therapy for melanoma is surgical excision. Although there is little question of the need for wide excision of the primary lesion, the margins of resection have been actively debated since the turn of the century. In 1907, Handley[7] recommended a 5-cm margin around the primary lesion to prevent local recurrence. More than 50 years later, Peterson's group[38] proposed wide (up to 15 cm) surgical margins for patients at high risk of recurrence. However, others[39–41] claim that the width of surgical excision has no influence on the development of local recurrence or metastatic disease. Elias and associates[42] found no correlation between the initial surgical approach and survival. Olsen[43] reported no difference in recurrence rates for patients having narrow versus wide margins of excision. However, the validity of these studies is impaired by their failure to consider Clark or Breslow histopathology.

Balch and colleagues[44] found the risk of local recurrence to depend on the depth of the primary lesion. Their retrospective study of clinical stage I melanoma found no local recurrences among 36 patients undergoing wide excision of thin (<0.76 mm) primary lesions. They concluded that 2-cm margins of excision are adequate for thin melanomas, while thicker lesions should be excised with margins of 3 to 5 cm.

In 1988, the World Health Organization (WHO) published the results of a randomized trial comparing narrow (1 cm) and wide (3 cm) margins of excision for thin melanomas.[39] The overall survival rate was not significantly different, but the data indicated a higher recurrence rate when narrow margins were used to excise primary lesions greater than 1 mm in depth. Nonrandomized studies also suggest that the rate of local recurrence increases with the depth of the primary lesion.[45, 46]

At the John Wayne Cancer Institute, we recommend 1- to 2-cm margins for excision of primary lesions less than 1 mm deep, and 2- to 3-cm margins for lesions deeper than 1 mm. Narrow margins should be considered only when wide margins would significantly impair cosmetic outcome, as may be the case for lesions on the head, neck, or hands. There is little difference between the cosmetic results of a rotational or an advancement flap when wide versus narrow margins are used. Skin grafts are rarely necessary, except on the hands or feet or distal extremities.

The principles described above apply to all primary lesions, with the following site-specific caveats:

Face: The width of excision margins is determined by three factors: (1) lesion depth, (2) proximity of vital structures, and (3) cosmetic outcome.

Digits: Subungual melanoma is treated by amputating the digit at the distal interphalangeal joint. Larger lesions require more proximal amputation.

Ear: Ear melanomas are surgically removed by wedge excision of the helix, using margins of at least 2 cm; total amputation is rarely necessary. Reconstruction uses primary closure or advancement of the tissue flaps.

Although the defect after wide excision can usually be reconstructed by primary closure, a number of random and axial pattern flaps have been devised to facilitate repair. Rotational flaps (Fig. 16–2) are random flaps that rotate the skin around a fixed point to close the defect. Transposition flaps such as the Limberg or rhomboid flap (Fig. 16–3)

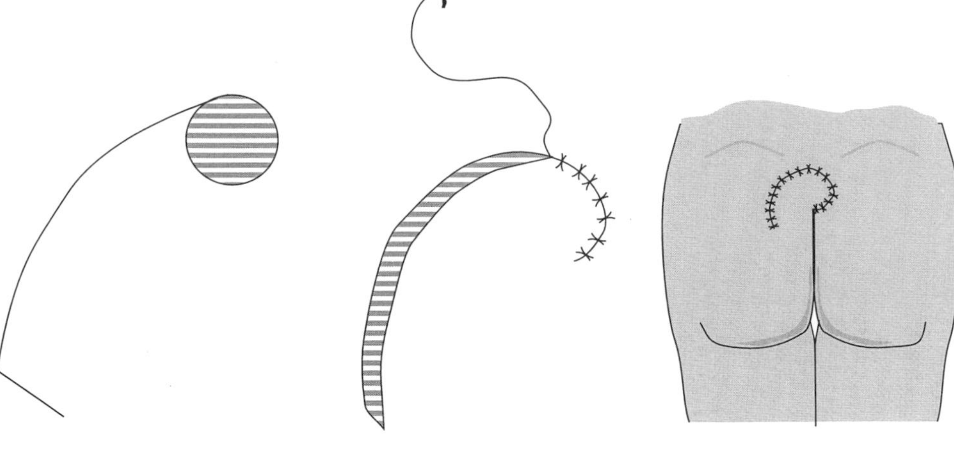

FIGURE 16–2. A rotation flap moves skin in an arc around a fixed point. (Adapted from Fisher J: Basic principles of skin flaps. In Georgiade NG, et al [eds]: Essentials of Plastic, Maxillofacial, and Reconstructive Surgery. Baltimore: Williams & Wilkins, 1987, p 40.)

also rotate skin around a fixed point. Advancement flaps rely on the skin's elasticity, since their primary motion is a straight line. The V-Y advancement flap is particularly useful for repairing amputated digits (Fig. 16–4).

Axial pattern flaps are based on longitudinal cutaneous vessels and random cutaneous perforators. These flaps allow additional skin movement but are limited to sites with an identifiable blood supply, such as the median forehead supplied by supratrochlear vessels, or the dorsal portion of the foot supplied by the dorsalis pedis vessel.

Radiotherapy

Although melanoma is inherently radioresistant, radiotherapy has been reported to have a role in management of the primary lesion. Harwood and Cummings[47] used radiotherapy to treat 28 elderly patients with lentigo maligna melanoma on the face. Local tumor control was achieved in all but two patients; median time to regression was 8 months (range, 1 to 24 months). However, this study was flawed by its failure to consider the depth of the primary lesion.

Radiotherapy has also been used as an adjuvant to surgery when wide excision would produce a functional deficit and/or unacceptable cosmetic result. In a nonrandomized study, Dickson[48] found no survival differences among patients whose primary lesions were managed by local excision (71 patients) versus wide excision (42 patients) versus simple excision plus radiotherapy (121 patients).

Management of the Regional Lymph Nodes

Prophylactic or elective lymph node dissection (ELND) can be undertaken in melanoma patients with clinically uninvolved nodes; however, this procedure remains controversial. ELND is based on the theory that melanoma metastasizes in a predictable and sequential fashion from the

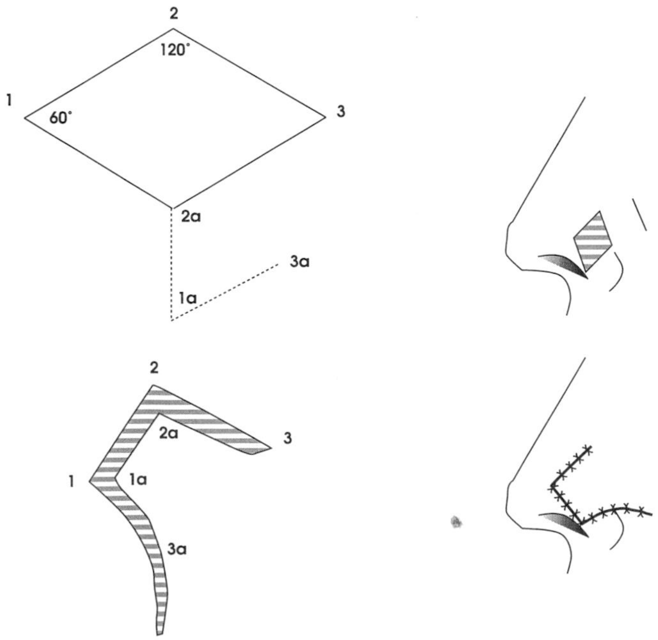

FIGURE 16–3. A Limberg (rhomboid) flap used to close rhomboid defects with angles at 60° and 120° and sides of equal length. (Adapted from Fisher J: Basic principles of skin flaps. In Georgiade NG, et al [eds]: Essentials of Plastic, Maxillofacial, and Reconstructive Surgery. Baltimore: Williams & Wilkins, 1987, p 43.)

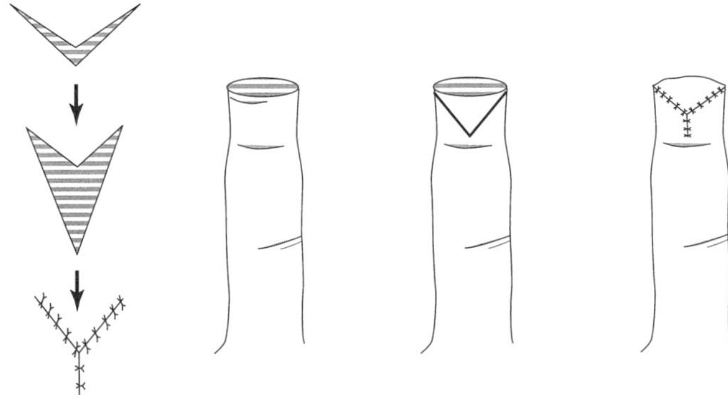

FIGURE 16–4. A V-Y advancement flap used to close the defect left by digital amputation. (Adapted from Fisher J: Basic principles of skin flaps. In Georgiade NG, et al [eds]: Essentials of Plastic, Maxillofacial, and Reconstructive Surgery. Baltimore: Williams & Wilkins, 1987, p 41.)

primary lesion through the lymphatics and then to the regional lymph nodes. Removing clinically uninvolved regional nodes therefore should eliminate a potential source of metastasis early in the natural history of the disease, when the tumor-host relationship favors the host. Multiple nonrandomized studies suggest a survival advantage of up to 25% in those patients undergoing en bloc lymphadenectomy as an elective rather than a therapeutic procedure (Table 16–3).[49–55]

Opponents of ELND advocate a wait-and-watch policy, arguing that the procedure can benefit only the 20% of AJCC stage I or II patients who already have occult regional metastases; the remaining 80% should be cured simply by excision of the primary lesion. Some authors state that clinically uninvolved regional lymph nodes should be left intact and monitored as a marker of systemic metastasis. Others object to ELND because they claim it favors hematogenous spread of disease.

A number of large retrospective analyses have documented a small but significant survival advantage associated with ELND in patients with clinical stage I melanoma of intermediate Clark level or Breslow thickness.[52, 56–58] A large retrospective review from the Sydney Melanoma Unit[58] demonstrated improved survival following ELND in patients with intermediate lesions (0.76 to 4.00 mm) arising on the extremities, torso, or head and neck. ELND was of particularly high potential benefit in males. Similar survival benefits have been observed in studies performed at the University of Alabama,[56] Duke University,[57] and the John Wayne Cancer Institute.[52]

Two important prospective randomized trials, one by Veronesi and the World Health Organization (WHO)[59, 60] and the other by Sim et al. at the Mayo Clinic,[61] have helped clarify the roles of ELND and therapeutic lymph node dissection (TLND) in melanoma. Veronesi's group studied 553 patients: 267 with clinically negative nodes underwent wide excision plus ELND; 286 with clinically negative nodes underwent wide excision and TLND only if regional nodes developed clinical signs of tumor. Overall, there was no statistically significant survival difference between the two groups. The only subgroup of patients to benefit from ELND were those with Clark level IV lesions of intermediate depth (1.0 to 1.99 mm and 3.00 to 3.99 mm). These patients had a 10% better survival (20% at 10 years) than did similar patients treated by TLND, but statistical significance was not achieved because of the small sample size. Another limitation of this study was its predominance of females with extremity lesions, who have a favorable prognosis and therefore are less likely to benefit from ELND. In addition, the trial was initiated before the prognostic importance of histopathologic microstaging was fully understood; thus, patients were not stratified by the primary lesion's Clark level, Breslow thickness, or degree of ulceration.

In the Mayo Clinic trial, 171 patients with AJCC stage I and II melanoma were prospectively randomized into three groups: immediate excision of the regional lymph nodes (54 patients), delayed lymphadenectomy (55 patients), or no lymphadenectomy (62 patients). Patients with primary lesions arising on the head and neck were excluded. There was no difference in survival or metastasis-free survival among the three treatment groups. The 10-year survival rates were 85% for no lymphadenectomy, 87% for immediate lymph node dissection, and 91% for delayed lymphadenectomy. However, most of the primary lesions were thin and therefore had little likelihood of spreading to regional nodes. Moreover, like the WHO study, this trial may have obscured the benefit of ELND by failing to consider important prognostic variables, including the gender of the patient and the anatomic site and histopathologic features of the primary lesion.

Two new randomized trials have been initiated to determine the efficacy of ELND. The Intergroup Melanoma Protocol is comparing the results of four surgical protocols for primary lesions of intermediate thickness (1 to 4 mm) on the torso or extremities. Patients undergo wide excision using either 2- or 4-cm surgical margins, with or without ELND. A similar trial is being conducted by the WHO to determine the role of ELND in patients with primary lesions on the trunk (at least 2 cm from the midline). Wide

TABLE 16–3
Five-Year Survival Rates for Melanoma Patients with Subclinical Versus Clinical Lymph Node Metastases

	Clinical Status of Regional Nodes		
Reference	*Not Palpable or Suspicious (%)*	*Palpable and Suspicious (%)*	Difference (%)
McNeer and Das Gupta[51]	52	19	33
Cohen et al.[54]	55	38	17
Das Gupta[53]	69	20	49
Balch et al.[49]	48	24	24
Callery et al.[55]	48	36	12
Roses et al.[50]	44	20	24
Morton et al.[52]	59	43	16

Adapted from Morton DL, et al: Technical details of intraoperative lymphatic mapping for early stage melanoma. Arch Surg 127:393, 1992.

TABLE 16–4
Estimated Incidence of Regional and Distant Micrometastases in Patients with Clinically Localized Melanoma

Location and Depth (mm) of Primary Lesion	Risk of Occult Regional Metastases Only (%)	Risk of Occult Distant Metastases (± Regional Metastases) (%)
Extremity Lesion in Women		
<0.76	2	1
0.76–1.49	5–7	7–10
1.50–3.99	7–19	10–24
≥4.00	0	48
Extremity Lesion in Men		
<0.76	2	2
0.76–1.49	22–24	22–24
1.50–3.99	24–29	24–34
≥4.00	2	70
Axillary Lesion in Women		
<0.76	8	10
0.76–1.49	14–17	21–29
1.50–3.99	17–21	29–41
≥4.00	0	60
Axillary Lesion in Men		
<0.76	9	14
0.76–1.49	27–28	29–32
1.50–3.99	28–30	32–45
≥4.00	0	79

Adapted from Balch CM, Soong SJ, Milton GW, Shaw HM, McGovern VJ, Maud TM, et al: A comparison of prognostic factors and surgical results in 1786 patients with localized (stage I) melanoma treated in Alabama, USA, and New South Wales, Australia. Ann Surg 196:677, 1982.

excision with 3-cm margins is used alone or in conjunction with ELND.

Identifying Candidates for ELND

Melanoma patients whose disease is limited to the primary site can be cured by wide excision of the lesion and therefore will not benefit from ELND. Melanoma patients with occult distant metastases also will not benefit from ELND.

A number of prognostic factors have been used to determine which patients with clinically negative nodes are likely to harbor occult nodal disease. Tumor site, thickness, level of invasion, ulceration or regression and pattern of growth, plus patient gender should be considered when assessing the aggressive nature of the primary lesion (Tables 16–4 and 16–5).

Lesion Site. Patients with melanoma arising on the extremities have a more favorable prognosis than those with primary lesions arising on the trunk or head and neck[62–64]; however, melanomas on the heels and palms are more aggressive than those on other extremity sites.[27–29] At the John Wayne Cancer Institute, we advocate ELND for intermediate lesions arising on high-risk extremity sites.

Lesion Depth. Tumor thickness can be used as a relative marker for determining the risk of regional or distant metastases. Balch and associates[62] found that thin melanomas (<0.76 mm) are usually associated with localized disease, for which ELND is unlikely to be helpful. However, patients with intermediate-depth primaries (0.76 to 4 mm) have up to a 60% risk of occult regional metastases but less than a 20% risk of distant metastases; therefore, they would theoretically benefit from ELND. By contrast, patients with thick melanomas (>4 mm) have a high risk of regional *and* distant metastases; ELND is less likely to be beneficial in these patients, since many will already have subclinical distant metastases.[44, 49, 56]

Lesion Ulceration and Growth. A lesion's aggressiveness is reflected by the presence and degree of ulceration and regression. Growth pattern is also important; for example, lentigo maligna melanoma (LMM) is relatively static and generally regarded as having little potential for metastasis, while nodular melanoma (NM) spreads at a faster rate and is more likely to affect regional lymph nodes. Urist and colleagues[63] found that 81 of 534 melanoma patients with head and neck lesions had LMM. These patients had significantly better survival rates than patients with superficial spreading melanoma (SSM) or NM. The implication is that ELND is likely to be of greater benefit in patients with SSM or NM rather than LMM. However, the data were not stratified for depth of the primary lesion,

TABLE 16–5
Relationship Between Lesion Microstage, Regional Node Metastasis, and Long-Term Survival

Microstage of Lesion	No. of Patients*	Lymph Node Metastasis (%)	5-Year Survival Rate (%)	10-Year Survival Rate (%)
Breslow Thickness (mm)				
≤0.75	1061	8	98	97
0.76–1.5	1167	20	91	85
1.51–3.99	1166	36	71	64
≥4.00	324	57	46	41
Clark Level				
I/II	1084	9	98	97
III	1600	24	87	82
IV	1403	37	72	64
V	198	53	53	44

*From the John Wayne Cancer Institute melanoma database of 5196 patients (May 1992).

which is probably more important than histologic type, since LMM tends to be a thin, low-risk lesion.

Other Factors. Women have a survival benefit and reduced risk for development of metastases, which may be partly due to the larger proportion of extremity and nonulcerated lesions in females.[49, 65] The patient's age and general medical condition and the presence and type of concurrent illness should also be used to decide for or against ELND.

Identifying Regional Lymphatic Drainage Basins

ELND is undertaken after the regional drainage basin is identified. In some cases, this is obvious: primary lesions arising on the extremities drain to adjacent lymph basins in either the axilla or the groin. However, lesions on the trunk or head and neck often have ambiguous drainage patterns. In 1843, Sappey[66] proposed that lesions arising at least 2 cm superior to the umbilicus drain to the axilla, while lesions at least 2 cm inferior to the umbilicus drain to the groin. However, a recent study demonstrated that up to 59% of lymph node dissections would be misdirected if based on Sappey's approach to truncal primary lesions.[67]

A far more accurate alternative is cutaneous lymphoscintigraphy, introduced in 1977 by the John Wayne group[68] as a method to identify lymphatic drainage patterns from ambiguous sites on the head and neck or on the trunk. A number of different isotopes have been tested, but most produce unacceptable radiation. Technetium Tc-99m–labeled dextran and albumin are now the preferred agents for lymphoscintigraphy.[69] Although lymphoscintigraphy can accurately identify regional lymph basins draining primary lesions, it does not indicate whether or not these basins already contain tumor cells.

Identifying High-Risk Lymph Nodes: Intraoperative Lymphatic Mapping with Selective Lymph Node Dissection

Because the controversy regarding ELND versus TLND for the management of regional lymph nodes has yet to be decided, Morton and associates[70, 71] at the John Wayne Cancer Institute recently introduced a minimally invasive surgical procedure to identify clinical stage I patients with occult regional metastases. Their procedure of intraoperative mapping and selective lymph node dissection (SLND) is based on the premise that tumor cells from a primary cutaneous melanoma pass through subdermal lymphatics to the regional lymphatic basin and then sequentially through the nodes in this basin. Thus, the first sign of regional node metastasis is most likely to be found in the node at the entrance to the basin, the so-called sentinel node. By identifying, removing, and examining this sentinel node, Morton's group is able to determine which patients have regional node metastases and therefore should undergo removal of all nodes in the basin.

Intraoperative mapping is preceded by cutaneous lymphoscintigraphy to identify and confirm the drainage basin and approximate the sentinel node's location by marking the overlying skin. Lymphatic mapping then begins with intradermal injection of 0.5 to 1.0 ml of patent blue-V or isosulfan blue dye at the site of the primary lesion. If the lesion has already been removed, dye is injected on either side of the incision scar. Injections are repeated every 20 minutes during the procedure because the dye rapidly traverses the regional lymphatics and venous drainage paths. A small incision is made in the marked skin that overlies the entrance to the drainage basin, and the flap closest to the primary lesion is dissected free of underlying tissue. Blue-stained lymph from the primary lesion is observed as it enters the lymph basin and drains into the sentinel node. This node is selectively excised ("SLND") for immediate frozen section examination using both routine hematoxylin-eosin and rapid immunohistochemical staining techniques. While the node is being examined, the primary lesion is excised with wide margins, as described above. If the sentinel node contains melanoma cells, a complete regional lymph node dissection is performed in the standard fashion. However, if the sentinel node does not contain micrometastases, the procedure is halted and the patient is spared the costs and potential morbidity of regional en bloc lymphadenectomy.

Morton et al.[70] recently reported their 4-year experience with intraoperative lymphatic mapping and SLND. They were able to identify the sentinel node in 194 (82%) of 237 regional drainage basins. As a control, all patients subsequently underwent en bloc lymphadenectomy, regardless of sentinel node status. Analysis of sentinel and nonsentinel nodes revealed regional metastases in 40 (21%) basins; however, only 2 (0.06%) nonsentinel lymph nodes were the exclusive site of metastasis in any of these basins, a false-negative rate of 1%. Since this initial study, Morton's group has performed intraoperative lymphatic mapping and SLND in more than 200 additional patients. The rate of sentinel node detection increases with practice; at the John Wayne Cancer Institute, it now approaches 100% for surgeons with the most experience. The false-negative rate (tumor cells in nonsentinel nodes only) remains less than 1%. In 1994, the John Wayne group initiated a multicenter trial to determine the efficacy of SLND and its impact on patient survival. Patients with primary melanomas on the head and neck, extremities, and trunk are randomized to wide excision with or without SLND. Only those patients whose sentinel nodes contain tumor cells undergo complete lymph node dissection.

Complications of Regional Lymphadenectomy

Complications associated with intraoperative mapping and SLND are infrequent and of little significance. All patients report the presence of blue dye in their urine during the first 24 hours following the procedure. The rate of wound infection, seroma, or wound necrosis is less than 5%.[70]

Most of the complications from en bloc lymphadenectomy are related to the wound itself: infection, flap necrosis, seroma, and temporary nerve dysfunction.[72, 73] The more severe complications are primarily related to the anatomic site of the lymph basin. In general, axillary lymph node dissection has minimal morbidity; only 1% of patients experience significant arm edema. Cervical node dissections also tend to have low long-term morbidity and infrequently cause functional disorders. By contrast, inguinal node dissection may produce significant edema if the obturator and iliac nodes are removed with nodes in the femoral triangle. Between 2% and 10% of patients undergoing ilioinguinal node dissection experience long-term debilitating edema.[74–76]

TREATMENT OF REGIONAL AND SYSTEMIC METASTASES

Melanoma Metastatic to Lymph Nodes

Surgery

In most cases of cutaneous melanoma, the diagnosis is made while the disease is still confined to the primary site. However, a small proportion of patients present with clinical evidence of regional lymph node disease. Surgical excision is currently the only effective treatment for melanoma metastatic to the regional lymph nodes. When performed for clinically identifiable disease, the procedure is referred to as therapeutic regional lymph node dissection (TLND). Although there is little argument regarding the efficacy of TLND, the 10-year survival rate for patients with clinically palpable lymph nodes is only 15% to 30%.[49–51, 54, 55]

The prognosis of melanoma patients undergoing regional lymph node dissection for proven or suspected metastatic disease depends on patient-related factors, including gender and age,[46, 65] and on lesion-related variables, including Breslow thickness,[77] Clark level,[24] ulceration,[33, 78] and lymphocytic infiltration.[32] It also depends on the extent of lymph node involvement. Coit and Brennan[79] reviewed their experience with 420 patients undergoing superficial or combined superficial and deep groin dissection for melanoma. Poor prognosis was associated with clinical evidence of nodal involvement and with positive superficial *and* deep nodes. The authors failed to find a survival advantage for patients undergoing more extensive lymphadenectomy; they concluded that dissection of the deep pelvic nodes may be of more prognostic than therapeutic value in patients with melanoma. These results differ from those of the John Wayne group, which indicated both a diagnostic and a therapeutic benefit from deep pelvic dissection if superficial groin nodes were not grossly involved.[79a]

A few melanoma patients have lymph node metastases without evidence of a primary cutaneous lesion. TLND is indicated after meticulous inspection for a primary site. At the John Wayne Cancer Institute, patients with an unknown primary lesion represent 14% of all cutaneous melanoma cases, and their prognosis is generally better than that of patients with known primary lesions.[80] In fact, their 5-year survival rate is 46%, equivalent to that of patients with thin primary lesions of the extremities.

Adjuvant Systemic or Limb Perfusion Chemotherapy

Chemotherapy is conceptually a logical adjuvant to surgery in patients with deeply invasive primary lesions or regional lymph node metastases, or both, since the risk of recurrence is as high as 70%. Dacarbazine (DTIC) is currently the only drug considered for adjuvant systemic single-agent chemotherapy.[81–83] However, all trials of DTIC alone or in combination with other chemotherapeutic or immunotherapeutic agents have failed to improve patient survival compared with surgery alone.[84]

The role of isolated limb perfusion as an adjuvant therapy for patients with primary or metastatic melanoma has generated considerable debate. A number of retrospective studies have suggested that hyperthermic, isolated limb perfusion with L-phenylalanine (melphalan) can significantly reduce the rate of recurrence and improve the survival of patients undergoing surgical excision of local or regional lesions.[85, 86] Stehlin and colleagues[87] reported a 5-year survival rate of 43% in melanoma patients undergoing regional lymphadenectomy and perfusion treatment of AJCC stage III disease. With respect to prospective analyses, Ghussen's group[88] demonstrated a significant improvement in disease-free survival when wide excision plus regional node dissection was followed by isolated hyperthermic limb perfusion using L-phenylalanine mustard. However, this prospective study was flawed by an extraordinarily high rate of treatment failures in patients not undergoing limb perfusion. The role of limb perfusion for metastatic melanoma remains unclear.

Adjuvant Radiotherapy

Local-regional failure, particularly in the head and neck region, can significantly increase morbidity and decrease survival. Ang and coworkers[89] reported their series of 83 patients undergoing adjuvant radiotherapy following surgical management (wide excision and cervical lymphadenectomy) of high-risk cutaneous lesions on the head and neck. Local-regional control rates were better than those historically reported for neck dissection alone. However, controlled clinical trials are needed to establish the role of adjuvant radiotherapy for regional metastatic melanoma.

Local Recurrence and Intransit Metastases

Local recurrence is defined as tumor that presents within 5 cm of the primary site after surgical excision of the primary lesion. Although local recurrence may be considered an extension of the primary tumor, it may also be the first manifestation of distant metastases. The overall incidence of local recurrence is approximately 3% but increases threefold when the primary lesion is thick (>4 mm), ulcerated, located on the foot, hand, ear, or scalp, and/or accompanied by nodal metastases.[44, 56, 89a] The potential impact of these risk factors on the patient's overall prognosis is largely responsible for the ongoing controversy regarding adequate surgical margins for excision of primary melanomas.

Intransit metastases are lesions appearing on skin and soft tissue between the primary site and the regional lymph nodes. While local recurrence suggests inadequate treatment of the primary lesion, intransit metastases are the result of tumor emboli established in the lymphatic channels draining the primary lesion. The risk factors for local recurrence also apply to intransit metastases.

There is no standard therapy for locally recurrent or intransit melanoma. In general, the treatment for local recurrence is surgical excision. Patients with a solitary recurrence should undergo re-excision with margins of 2 to 3 cm; this is probably adequate even if the recurrence involves a skin graft. Patients with multiple local recurrences should be considered for re-excision, systemic chemotherapy, or isolated limb perfusion if disease is limited to one extremity. Surgical excision of a recurrent lesion can be curative in about 20% of cases, but most patients eventually have systemic metastases.

The risk of systemic metastases is also high in patients with intransit metastases. Prognosis appears to be related to the number of recurrent lesions and the time interval for their development.[90] Surgical excision can be considered when intransit lesions are few and slow growing, but most patients require systemic chemotherapy, isolated limb perfusion chemotherapy, radiotherapy, or, rarely, amputation.

Another alternative is nonspecific or specific immunotherapy. At the John Wayne Cancer Institute, bacillus Calmette-Guérin (BCG) is administered intralesionally to induce a nonspecific immune response that can control the progression of intransit metastases in up to 60% of patients.[91] Human monoclonal antibodies against ganglioside antigens found on the surface of melanoma cells have been successful in patients whose tumor expresses these antigens.[92, 93] The Institute also uses a melanoma cell vaccine (MCV) that induces an active and specific immune response. MCV is a polyvalent whole-cell preparation of highly immunogenic melanoma cells, which are irradiated prior to administration. As reported recently by Morton and associates,[94] patients receiving MCV for regional skin and soft tissue metastases had a median survival of 44 months and a 5-year survival rate of 38%, significantly better than the 29-month median and 20% 5-year survival statistics for comparable historical controls treated by chemotherapy or non-MCV immunotherapy (Fig. 16–5).

Distant Metastases

Although surgical resection, systemic chemotherapy, radiotherapy, and immunotherapy are used to treat patients

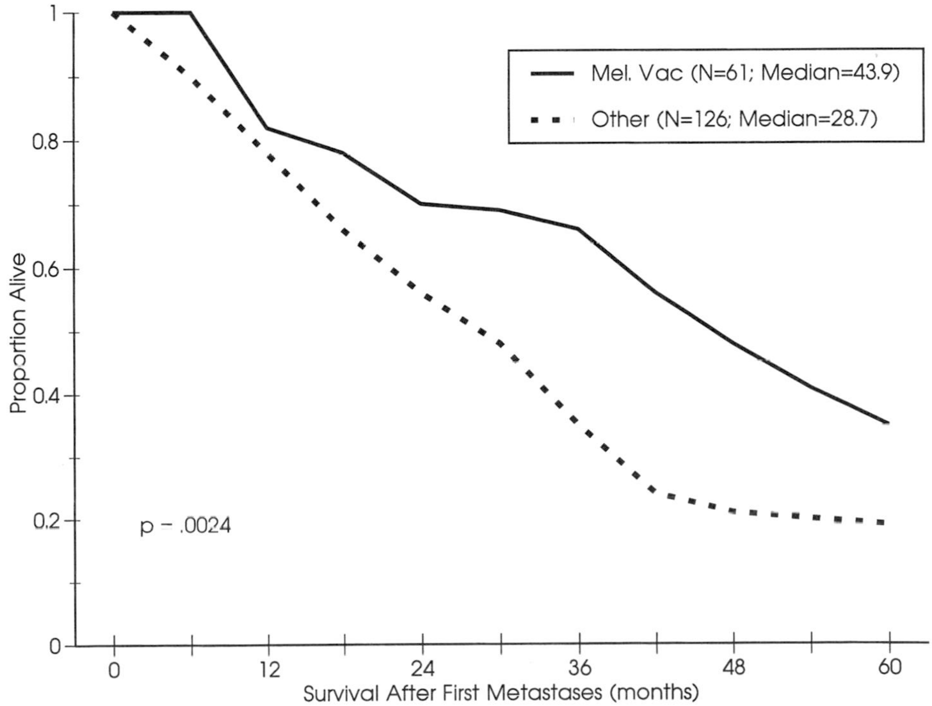

FIGURE 16–5. Survival of AJCC stage IIIA melanoma patients (regional skin and soft tissue metastases) treated with melanoma cell vaccine versus chemotherapy or other immunotherapy. (From Morton DL, et al: Prolongation of survival in metastatic melanoma after active specific immunotherapy with a new polyvalent melanoma vaccine. Ann Surg 216:473, 1992.)

with disseminated melanoma, there is as yet no cure for metastatic disease. Management depends on the anatomic site and rate of progression, both of which are highly variable.

A clinical diagnosis of metastatic melanoma must be confirmed by biopsy, if possible. Before therapy is initiated, the extent of disease should be determined. If a thorough history and physical examination including blood chemistries and chest radiograph reveal no previously unsuspected metastases, further radiologic evaluation is probably not necessary. However, the protean manifestations of metastatic melanoma demand a high index of suspicion with respect to new or persistent symptoms. For example, melanoma metastasizes to the gastrointestinal tract in 8% to 20% of patients with disseminated disease,[95] generally causing chronic bleeding or obstruction. Patients presenting with anemia, intermittent obstruction, and guaiac-positive stools should undergo contrast studies of the gastrointestinal tract. Although brain metastases are clinically apparent in only 12% to 20% of patients with metastatic melanoma,[95] autopsy studies show a 50% rate of cerebral lesions.[96] The most common symptoms of intracranial involvement are headache, mental deficits, and nuchal rigidity; however, seizure can occur. These patients require magnetic resonance imaging of the brain.

The survival of patients with distant metastases depends on the number of involved organs and tissues; median survival is approximately 7 months for patients with only one metastatic site, 4 months for those with two sites, and only 2 months for those with more than two sites. Patients with metastases to the skin, subcutaneous tissue, distant lymph nodes, gastrointestinal tract, lung, or bone have a better prognosis (median survival, 8 to 11 months) than those with metastases to the liver or brain (median survival, 2 to 4 months).

Surgery

Surgery can provide excellent palliation for isolated metastases and, in selected patients, may significantly prolong survival. However, the excision of multiple metastases from multiple organ sites generally does not improve survival. Therefore, surgery should be undertaken only after careful evaluation or observation, or both, has ruled out the possibility of other metastatic sites. Isolated brain or lung metastases are amenable to surgical resection. Symptomatic lesions of the skin, subcutaneous tissue, distant lymph nodes, or gastrointestinal tract can be effectively treated by surgery. However, liver metastases are associated with a poor survival and resection is not generally indicated.[94]

Pulmonary Metastases

The lung is one of the most frequent sites of metastatic melanoma. Most pulmonary metastases are multiple and bilateral and are often associated with hilar and mediastinal disease. However, only those patients with solitary or limited lung involvement may benefit from thoracotomy.

At the John Wayne Cancer Institute, selected patients are followed with serial chest radiographs to determine tumor doubling time (TDT).[97] Patients with a TDT longer than 40 days are considered for thoracotomy. In a study of 47 patients undergoing thoracotomy and resection for metastatic melanoma, Institute investigators found that the estimated 5-year survival rate was 35% when all tumor could be surgically removed.[98] Although similar results have been reported elsewhere,[99] others have been unable to duplicate these findings.[100, 101]

Subcutaneous and Lymph Node Metastases

Surgical excision is the most effective therapy for isolated and accessible subcutaneous or lymph node metastases, or both. Slowly progressing sequential metastases also can be excised. All lesions should be resected before they become large and symptomatic. Median survival is approximately 17 months.

Brain Metastases

Surgical resection of the solitary brain lesion may relieve symptoms but rarely produces long-term palliation. These patients generally also require corticosteroid therapy and postoperative radiation, as discussed below. Patients with multiple brain metastases are not surgical candidates and should receive radiotherapy for palliation.

Gastrointestinal Tract Metastases

Indications for surgery are most commonly associated with acute bowel obstruction from intussusception of the small bowel or chronic anemia. Lesions are typically multiple and predominately involve the jejunum or ileum. Surgical treatment generally consists of segmental bowel resection or partial gastrectomy. The operative mortality is acceptable, but long-term survival is uncommon.

Chemotherapy

Systemic chemotherapy does not improve the survival of patients with disseminated melanoma. Although DTIC reportedly produces response rates of 15% to 30% in large series,[102, 103] most responses last only 5 to 6 months and occur in the more favorable sites such as the skin, subcutaneous tissue, or lymph nodes. Combination therapy based on DTIC and cisplatin may increase response rates: a combination of DTIC, cisplatin, and vindesine reportedly produced an objective response in 30% to 40% of patients,[104, 105] while a similar regimen substituting vinblastine for vindesine was associated with a 40% response rate.[106] A four-drug regimen of DTIC, cisplatin, carmustine (BCNU), and tamoxifen, the so-called Dartmouth protocol, reportedly produced objective responses in more than half of patients.[105, 107] Omitting tamoxifen from this regimen reduced the risk of thrombotic events but also decreased the response rate to 10%.[108] Randomized trials are currently in progress to determine if any of these combined regimens is superior to DTIC alone.

Radiotherapy

The most frequent indication for radiotherapy is palliation of symptoms caused by dermal, subcutaneous, lymph node, bone, and brain metastases. In patients with dermal, subcutaneous, or lymph node metastases, the overall complete and durable response rate is about 65%.[109] The response rate decreases as tumor size exceeds 1 cm^3; response rate is only 20% when lesion diameter is greater than 5 cm.[110]

Indications for radiotherapy of bone metastases are relief of pain and treatment of pathologic fractures of long bones. Pain is effectively relieved with 2-week regimens of 20 Gy in 5 fractions or 30 Gy in 10 fractions. Internal fixation of long-bone fractures is followed by postoperative radiation.

Whole brain irradiation in combination with corticosteroids can palliate the symptoms of brain metastases. After the standard approach of 30 Gy in 10 fractions over 2 weeks, 60% to 70% of patients have improved performance and a 1- to 2-month prolongation of survival.[111, 112] Without surgery, however, long-term survival is rare.

Immunotherapy

Because conventional surgery, chemotherapy, and radiotherapy are of limited usefulness in patients with disseminated melanoma, a number of investigators are pursuing therapies intended to augment or stimulate the patient's immune response. An immunotherapeutic approach to melanoma is validated by the observation that specific cellular and humoral responses against melanoma cells can develop in melanoma patients[113, 114]; moreover, development of an immune response to melanoma generally improves the patient's prognosis.[115]

Active Immunotherapy

Injection of BCG, an attenuated bacterium, can produce a powerful nonspecific immune response against human neoplasms.[91, 116] Eilber and associates[117] demonstrated a fourfold increase in antibodies to tumor-associated antigens on melanoma cells of patients immunized with BCG, and they later described a 50% decrease in the incidence of melanoma metastases in BCG-treated versus control groups. Although other investigators have been unable to reproduce these findings,[118–119a] a WHO report[120] confirmed the efficacy of adjuvant therapy in tuberculin-negative patients. Moreover, there is firm evidence that intralesional BCG can control the progression of up to 60% of injected lesions and 14% of *un*injected lesions in the same patient.[91, 121]

Active Specific Immunotherapy: Melanoma Vaccines

Because of the inconsistent results produced by nonspecific immunostimulation using BCG, a number of investigators have switched to immunotherapy with tumor-associated antigens (TAAs). The immunogenic TAAs found on the surface of melanoma cells can stimulate an active specific immune response. These antigens are injected in purified form, in cell lysates, or in whole-cell preparations. Some melanoma vaccines are whole-cell preparations of allogeneic tumors, xenogeneic tumors, or virus-infected allogeneic tumors. Others are preparations of antigens such as p97; melanoma vaccines have also been developed using murine anti-idiotypes.

The results of these melanoma vaccines are highly variable. Mitchell et al.[122] reported that 5 of 22 melanoma patients responded to treatment using a cell lysate vaccine administered with DETOX for nonspecific immune enhancement; responders had increased levels of cytotoxic T lymphocytes (CTLs). Wallack and coworkers[123] developed a vaccinia melanoma oncolysate vaccine intended to amplify the immune response by expressing viral antigens on the surface of melanoma cells. While this vaccine produces a potent CTL response, the most recent data suggest that this response does not translate into a survival advantage.

In a recent phase II clinical trial of their polyvalent, allogeneic melanoma cell vaccine (MCV), Morton and coworkers[94] reported a 23-month median survival for 75 AJCC stage IV melanoma patients receiving MCV immunotherapy for lung, soft tissue, liver, or brain metastases, compared to a 7.5-month median survival for 1275 historical controls treated with other therapies (Fig. 16–6). The prolonged survival of patients treated with MCV correlated with development of humoral and cell-mediated responses.

Interferons

Interferon (IFN), the prototypical biologic response modifier, enhances melanoma cell surface expression of major histocompatibility antigens and TAAs. Both IFN-β and IFN-γ also enhance the expression of human leukocyte antigen (HLA) class I and class II on monocytes. A number of phase II clinical trials have used IFN-α (2a or 2b) to upregulate antigen expression on melanoma cells; response rates of about 15% have been demonstrated using a variety of dosages and routes.[124–126] IFN-γ adjuvant therapy has been tested in melanoma patients with deep primary lesions or lymph node metastases,[127, 128] but data are not conclusive.

Interleukin-2

Interleukin-2 (IL-2), originally described for its stimulation of T lymphocytes, is now known to activate the immune system, enhance both specific and nonspecific antitumor cytotoxicity, and induce cytokine secretion by immune cells. A number of different IL-2 regimens have been proposed for patients with metastatic melanoma.[129–131] A clinical trial from the National Cancer Institute reported a 21% response rate in metastatic melanoma patients treated with high-dose IL-2 plus lymphokine-activated killer (LAK) cells.[130, 132] More recent investigations have substituted tumor-infiltrating lymphocytes (TILs), which, unlike

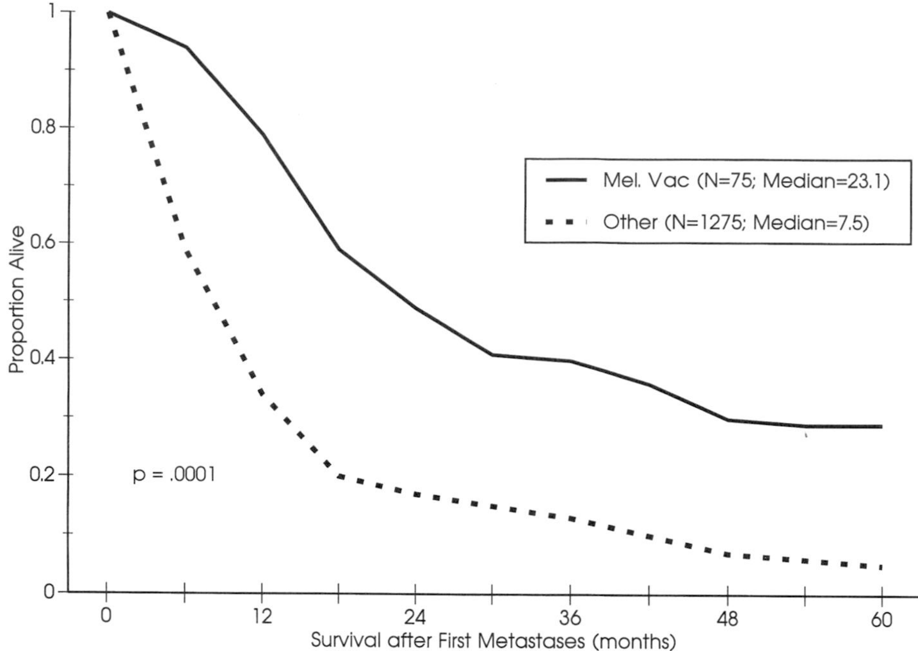

FIGURE 16–6. Survival of AJCC stage IV melanoma patients (distal metastases) treated with melanoma cell vaccine versus chemotherapy or other immunotherapy. (From Morton DL, et al: Prolongation of survival in metastatic melanoma after active specific immunotherapy with a new polyvalent melanoma vaccine. Ann Surg 216:472, 1992.)

LAK cells, can target tumor cells.[132, 133] However, while TILs are less toxic than LAK cells, they grow slowly in culture and are difficult to harvest.

IL-2 has also been combined with IFN-α, IFN-γ, tumor necrosis factor, cyclophosphamide, DTIC, and cisplatin. Although a response rate of 55% was recently reported for the combination of IL-2, IFN-α, and cisplatin, none of these regimens has significantly improved patient survival.

Monoclonal Antibodies (Passive Immunotherapy)

Hybridoma technology and the identification of a number of melanoma TAAs have allowed development of monoclonal antibodies for clinical use. Intralesional injection of human monoclonal antibodies against two melanoma surface gangliosides (GD_2 and GM_2) has been successful in patients whose tumor cells express these particular antigens.[92, 93] Monoclonal antibodies have also been administered with biologic response modifiers such as IL-2, granulocyte-macrophage–colony-stimulating factor, or IFN-α.[134, 135]

Gene Therapies

Recent investigations of gene therapy have focused on the transformation of immune and tumor cells. TILs transformed with the gene for tumor necrosis factor have not proven more effective than nontransformed TILs.[133] Melanoma cells have been transformed in an attempt to enhance their antigen expression.[136, 137] Further genetic manipulations of tumor or immune cells, or both, may eventually lead to better therapies for patients with advanced melanoma.

PROSPECTS FOR THE FUTURE

Since most thin primary melanoma lesions are curable by wide excision alone, early detection remains of paramount importance in the management of melanoma. Outreach programs are necessary to educate the public about the early signs of melanoma (e.g., the American Cancer Society's "ABCDE's of Melanoma") and the importance of using sunscreens to reduce the risk of long-term exposure to UV radiation.

Early detection is also essential for metastatic disease. Use of intraoperative lymphatic mapping and selective lymphadenectomy, as described by Morton and associates,[70] is a minimally invasive technique to identify nodal involvement in patients with no clinical signs of metastatic spread. These patients are excellent candidates for adjuvant therapies.

As yet there is no cure for disseminated melanoma. Vaccine-based immunotherapies are promising; as our understanding of the biology of melanoma improves, more effective and less toxic programs will be devised.

References

1. Urteaga O, Pack GT: On the antiquity of melanoma. Cancer 19:607–610, 1966.
2. Laennec RTH: Sur les melanoses. Bull Fac Med Paris 1:2, 1812.
3. Norris W: Case of fungoid disease. Edinburgh Med Surg J 16:562–565, 1820.
4. Pemberton O: Observations on the History, Pathology and Treatment of Cancerous Diseases. London: J Churchill, 1858.
5. Snow H: Melanotic cancerous disease. Lancet 2:872–874, 1892.
6. Eve F: A lecture on melanoma. The Practitioner 70:165–174, 1903.
7. Handley WS: The pathology of melanotic growths in relation to their operative treatment: Lectures I & II. Lancet 1:927–935, 996–1003, 1907.

8. Pringle JH: A method of operation in cases of melanotic tumours of the skin. Edinburgh Med J 23:496–499, 1908.
9. Graham S, Marshall J, Haughey B, et al: An inquiry into the epidemiology of melanoma. Am J Epidemiol 122:606–619, 1985.
9a Wingo PA, Tong T, Bolden S: Cancer statistics, 1995. CA 45:8–30, 1995.
10. MacKie RM, Freudenberger T, Aitchison TC: Personal risk-factor chart for cutaneous melanoma. Lancet 2:487–490, 1989.
11. Lee JAH: Melanoma and exposure to sunlight. Epidemiol Rev 4:110–136, 1982.
12. Tormanen VT, Pfeifer GP: Mapping of UV photoproducts within *ras* proto-oncogenes in UV-irradiated cells: Correlation with mutations in human skin cancer. Oncogene 7:1729–1736, 1992.
13. Balaban GB, Herlyn M, Clark WH Jr, Nowell PC: Karyotypic evolution in human malignant melanoma. Cancer Genet Cytogenet 19:113–122, 1986.
14. Bale SJ, Dracopoli NC, Tucker MA, et al: Mapping the gene for hereditary cutaneous malignant melanoma-dysplastic nevus to chromosome 1p. N Engl J Med 320:1367–1372, 1989.
15. Becher R, Gibas Z, Sandberg AA: Chromosome 6 in malignant melanoma. Cancer Genet Cytogenet 9:173–175, 1983.
16. Becher R, Gibas Z, Karakousis C, Sandberg AA: Non-random chromosome changes in malignant melanoma. Cancer 43:5010–5016, 1983.
17. Cawley EF: Genetic aspects of malignant melanoma. Arch Dermatol 65:440–450, 1952.
18. Greene MH, Fraumeni JF Jr: The hereditary variant of malignant melanoma. In Clark WH Jr, Goldman LI, Mastrangelo MJ (eds): Malignant Melanoma. New York: Grune & Stratton, 1979, p 139.
19. Clark WH Jr, Reimer RR, Greene M, et al: Origin of familial malignant melanomas from heritable melanocytic lesions. The 'B-K mole syndrome.' Arch Dermatol 114:732–738, 1978.
20. Ackerman AB: What nevus is dysplastic, a syndrome, and the commonest precursor of malignant melanoma? A riddle, and an answer. Histopathology 13:241–256, 1988.
21. Wallace DC, Beardmore GL, Exton LA: Familial malignant melanoma. Ann Surg 177:15–20, 1973.
22. Rhodes AR, Melski JW: Small congenital nevocellular nevi and the risk of cutaneous melanoma. J Pediatr 100:219–224, 1982.
23. Consensus Conference: Precursors to malignant melanoma. JAMA 251:1864–1866, 1984.
24. Clark WH Jr, From L, Bernardino EA, Mihm MC Jr: The histogenesis and biologic behavior of primary human malignant melanomas of the skin. Cancer Res 29:705–727, 1969.
25. McGovern VJ, Shaw HM, Milton GW, Farago GA: Is malignant melanoma arising in a Hutchinson's melanotic freckle a separate disease entity? Histopathology 4:235–242, 1980.
26. Clark WH Jr, Ainsworth AM, Bernardino EA, et al: The developmental biology of primary human malignant melanomas. Semin Oncol 2:83–103, 1975.
27. Coleman WP III, Loria PR, Reed RJ, Krementz ET: Acral lentiginous melanoma. Arch Dermatol 116:773–776, 1980.
28. Paladugu RR, Winberg CD, Yonemoto RH: Acral lentiginous melanoma. A clinicopathologic study of 36 patients. Cancer 52:161–168, 1983.
29. Feibleman CE, Stoll H, Maize JC: Melanomas of the palm, sole and nailbed: A clinicopathologic study. Cancer 46:2492–2504, 1980.
30. Patterson RH, Helwig EB: Subungual malignant melanoma. A clinicopathologic study. Cancer 46:2074, 1980.
31. Elder DE, Guerry D, Van Horn M, et al: The role of lymph node dissection for clinical stage I malignant melanoma of intermediate thickness (1.51–3.99 mm). Cancer 56:413–418, 1985.
32. Ronan SG, Han MC, Das Gupta TK: Histologic prognostic indicators in cutaneous malignant melanoma. Semin Oncol 15:558–565, 1988.
33. Day CL Jr, Sober AJ, Kopf AW, et al: A prognostic model for clinical stage I melanoma of the upper extremity. The importance of anatomic subsites in predicting recurrent disease. Ann Surg 193:436–440, 1981.
34. Goldsmith HS: Melanoma: An overview. CA 29:194–215, 1979.
35. Allen AC, Spitz S: Malignant melanoma. A clinicopathological analysis of criteria for diagnosis and prognosis. Cancer 6:1–45, 1953.
36. Breslow A: Prognostic factors in the treatment of cutaneous melanoma. J Cutan Pathol 6:208–212, 1979.
37. Morton DL, Davtyan DG, Wanek LA, et al: Multivariate analysis of the relationship between survival and the microstage of primary melanoma by Clark level and Breslow thickness. Cancer 71:3737–3743, 1993.
38. Peterson NC, Bodenham DC, Lloyd OC: Malignant melanoma of the skin: A study of the origin, development, etiology, spread, treatment and prognosis. Br J Plast Surg 15:49, 97, 1962.
39. Veronesi U, Cascinelli N, Adamus J, et al: Thin stage I primary cutaneous malignant melanoma. Comparison of excision with margins of 1 or 3 cm. N Engl J Med 318:1159–1162, 1988.
40. Goldman LI, Byrd R: Narrowing resection margins for patients with low-risk melanoma. Am J Surg 155:242–244, 1988.
41. Rogers GS: Narrow versus wide margins in malignant melanoma. J Dermatol Surg Oncol 15:33–34, 1989.
42. Elias EG, Didolkar MS, Goel IP, et al: A clinicopathologic study of prognostic factors in cutaneous melanoma. Surg Gynecol Obstet 144:327–334, 1977.
43. Olsen G: The malignant melanoma of the skin: New theories based on a study of 500 cases. Acta Chir Scand Suppl 365:1–22, 1966.
44. Balch CM, Murad TM, Soong S-J, et al: Tumor thickness as a guide to surgical management of clinical stage I melanoma patients. Cancer 43:883–888, 1979.
45. Bagley FH, Cady B, Lee A, Legg MA: Changes in clinical presentation and management of malignant melanoma. Cancer 47:2126–2134, 1981.
46. Schmoeckel C, Bockelbrink A, Bockelbrink H, et al: Is wide excision necessary in malignant melanoma? J Invest Dermatol 76:424, 1981 (abstract).
47. Harwood AR, Cummings BJ: Radiotherapy for malignant melanoma: A reappraisal. Cancer Treat Rep 8:271–282, 1981.
48. Dickson RJ: Malignant melanoma: A combined surgical and radiotherapeutic approach. Am J Roentgenol 79:1063–1070, 1958.
49. Balch CM, Soong S-J, Murad TM, et al: A multifactorial analysis of melanoma. III. Prognostic factors in melanoma patients with lymph node metastases (stage II). Ann Surg 193:377–388, 1981.
50. Roses DF, Provet JA, Harris MN, et al: Prognosis of patients with pathologic stage II cutaneous melanoma. Ann Surg 201:103–107, 1985.
51. McNeer G, Das Gupta TK: Prognosis in malignant melanoma. Surgery 56:512–518, 1964.
52. Morton DL, Wanek LA, Nizze JA, et al: Improved long-term survival after lymphadenectomy of melanoma metastatic to regional nodes: Analysis of prognostic factors in 1134 patients from the John Wayne Cancer Institute. Ann Surg 214:491–499, 1991.
53. Das Gupta TK: Results of treatment of 269 patients with primary cutaneous melanoma: A five-year prospective study. Ann Surg 186:201–209, 1977.
54. Cohen MH, Ketcham AS, Felix EL, et al: Prognostic factors in patients undergoing lymphadenectomy for malignant melanoma. Ann Surg 186:635–642, 1977.
55. Callery C, Cochran AJ, Roe DJ, et al: Factors prognostic in patients with malignant melanoma spread to the regional lymph nodes. Ann Surg 196:69–75, 1982.
56. Balch CM, Soong S-J, Milton GW, et al: A comparison of prognostic factors and surgical results in 1,786 patients with localized (stage I) melanoma treated in Alabama, USA and New South Wales, Australia. Ann Surg 196:677–684, 1982.
57. Reintgen DS, Cox EB, McCarty KS Jr, et al: Efficacy of elective lymph node dissection in patients with intermediate thickness primary melanoma. Ann Surg 198:379–385, 1983.
58. McCarthy WH, Shaw HM, Milton GW: Efficacy of elective lymph node dissection in 2,347 patients with clinical stage I malignant melanoma. Surg Gynecol Obstet 161:575–580, 1985.
59. Veronesi U, Adamus J, Bandiera DC, et al: Stage I melanoma of the limbs. Immediate versus delayed node dissection. Tumori 66:373–396, 1980.
60. Veronesi U, Adamus J, Bandiera DC, et al: Inefficacy of immediate node dissection in stage I melanoma of the limbs. N Engl J Med 297:627–630, 1977.
61. Sim FH, Taylor WF, Pritchard DJ, Soule EH: Lymphadenectomy in the management of stage I malignant melanoma: A prospective randomized study. Mayo Clin Proc 61:697–705, 1986.
62. Balch CM, Milton GW, Cascinelli N, Sim FH: Elective lymph node dissection: Pros and cons. In Balch CM, Houghton AN, Milton GW,

et al (eds): Cutaneous Melanoma, 2nd ed. Philadelphia: JB Lippincott, 1992, pp 345–366.
63. Urist MM, Balch CM, Soong S-J, et al: Head and neck melanoma in 534 clinical stage I patients. A prognostic factors analysis and results of surgical treatment. Ann Surg 200:769–775, 1984.
64. Essner R, Wanek LA, Morton DL: Ominous prognosis of malignant melanoma originating on the scalp. Presented at the Pacific Coast Surgical Association 1993 Meeting.
65. Balch CM, Soong S-J, Shaw HM, et al: An analysis of prognostic factors in 8500 patients with cutaneous melanoma. In Balch CM, Houghton AN, Milton GW, et al (eds): Cutaneous Melanoma, 2nd ed. Philadelphia: JB Lippincott, 1992, pp 165–187.
66. Sappey MPC: Injection preparation et conservation des vaisseau lymphatiques. These pour le doctorate en medecine, No 241. Paris: Rignoux Imprimeur de la Faculté de Médecine, 1843.
67. Norman J, Cruse CW, Espinosa C, et al: Redefinition of cutaneous lymphatic drainage with the use of lymphoscintigraphy for malignant melanoma. Am J Surg 162:432–437, 1991.
68. Robinson DS, Sample WF, Fee HJ, et al: Regional lymphatic drainage in primary malignant melanoma of the trunk determined by colloidal gold scanning. Surg Forum 28:147–148, 1977.
69. Wanebo HJ, Harpole D, Teates CD: Radionuclide lymphoscintigraphy with technetium antimony sulfide colloid to identify lymphatic drainage of cutaneous melanoma of ambiguous sites in the head and neck and trunk. Cancer 55:1403–1413, 1985.
70. Morton DL, Wen D-R, Wong JH, et al: Technical details of intraoperative lymphatic mapping for early stage melanoma. Arch Surg 127:392–399, 1992.
71. Morton DL, Wen D-R, Foshag LJ, et al: Intraoperative lymphatic mapping and selective cervical lymphadenectomy for early-stage melanomas of the head and neck. J Clin Oncol 11:1751–1756, 1993.
72. Urist MM, Maddox WA, Kennedy RE, Balch CM: Patient risk factors and surgical morbidity after regional lymphadenectomy in 204 melanoma patients. Cancer 51:2152–2156, 1983.
73. Baas PC, Koops HS, Hoekstra HJ, et al: Groin dissection in the treatment of lower-extremity melanoma. Short-term and long-term morbidity. Arch Surg 127:281–286, 1992.
74. Beitsch P, Balch CM: Operative morbidity and risk factor assessment in melanoma patients undergoing inguinal lymph node dissection. Am J Surg 164:462–466, 1992.
75. Karakousis CP, Heiser MA, Moore RH: Lymphedema after groin dissection. Am J Surg 145:205–208, 1983.
76. Shaw JHF, Rumball EM: Complications and local recurrence following lymphadenectomy. Br J Surg 77:760–764, 1990.
77. Balch CM, Murad TM, Soong S-J, et al: A multifactorial analysis of melanoma. Prognostic histopathological features comparing Clark's and Breslow's staging methods. Ann Surg 188:732–742, 1978.
78. Balch CM, Wilkerson JA, Murad TM, et al: The prognostic significance of ulceration of cutaneous melanoma. Cancer 45:3012–3017, 1980.
79. Coit DG, Brennan MF: Extent of lymph node dissection in melanoma of the trunk or lower extremity. Arch Surg 124:162–166, 1989.
79a. Finck SJ, Giuliano AE, Mann BD, Morton DL: Results of ilioinguinal dissection for stage II melanoma. Ann Surg 196:180–186, 1982.
80. Wong JH, Cagle LA, Morton DL: Surgical treatment of lymph nodes with metastatic melanoma from an unknown primary site. Arch Surg 122:1380–1383, 1987.
81. Hill GJ II, Krementz ET, Hill HZ: Dimethyl triazeno imidazole carboxamide and combination therapy for melanoma. IV. Late results after complete response to chemotherapy. Cancer 53:1299–1305, 1984.
82. Kaiser LR, Burk MW, Morton DL: Adjuvant therapy for malignant melanoma. Surg Clin North Am 61:1249–1257, 1981.
83. Houghton AN, Legha S, Bajorin DF: Chemotherapy for metastatic melanoma. In Balch CM, Houghton AN, Milton GW, et al (eds): Cutaneous Melanoma, 2nd ed. Philadelphia: JB Lippincott, 1992, pp 498–508.
84. Veronesi U, Adamus J, Aubert C, et al: A randomized trial of adjuvant chemotherapy and immunotherapy in cutaneous melanoma. N Engl J Med 307:913–916, 1982.
85. Krementz ET, Creech O Jr, Ryan RF, Reemtsma K: An appraisal of cancer chemotherapy by regional perfusion. Ann Surg 156:417–428, 1962.
86. Krementz ET, Ryan RF: Chemotherapy of melanoma of the extremities by perfusion. Fourteen years clinical experience. Ann Surg 175:900–917, 1972.
87. Stehlin JS, Giovanella BC, de Ipolyi PD, et al: Hyperthermic perfusion of extremities for melanoma and soft tissue sarcomas. In Rossi-Fanelli A, Cavaliere R, Mondoni B, Moricca G (eds): Selective Heat Sensitivity of Cancer Cells. Berlin: Springer-Verlag, 1977, pp 171–185.
88. Ghussen F, Kruger I, Smalley RU, Groth W: Hyperthermic perfusion with chemotherapy and melanoma of the extremities. World J Surg 13:598–602, 1989.
89. Ang KK, Byers RM, Peters LJ, et al: Regional radiotherapy as adjuvant treatment for head and neck malignant melanoma. Arch Otolaryngol Head Neck Surg 116:169–172, 1990.
89a. Roses DF, Harris MN, Rigel D, et al: Local and intransit metastases following definitive excision for primary cutaneous malignant melanoma. Ann Surg 198:65–69, 1983.
90. Wong JH, Cagle LA, Kopald KH, Swisher SG: Natural history and selective management of intransit melanoma. J Surg Oncol 44:146–150, 1990.
91. Morton DL, Bertelsen CA: Intralesional immunotherapy: An important tool for local treatment of melanoma. Primary Care Cancer, September 7–11, 1985.
92. Irie RF, Morton DL: Regression of cutaneous metastatic melanoma by intralesional injection with human monoclonal antibody to ganglioside GD_2. Proc Natl Acad Sci USA 83:8694–8698, 1986.
93. Irie RF, Matsuki T, Morton DL: Human monoclonal antibody to ganglioside GM_2 for melanoma treatment. Lancet 1:786–787, 1989.
94. Morton DL, Foshag LJ, Hoon DSB, et al: Prolongation of survival in metastatic melanoma after active specific immunotherapy with a new polyvalent melanoma vaccine. Ann Surg 216:463–482, 1992.
95. Das Gupta T, Brasfield R: Metastatic melanoma. A clinicopathological study. Cancer 17:1323–1339, 1964.
96. Patel JK, Didolkar MS, Pickren JW, Moore RH: Metastatic pattern of malignant melanoma. A study of 216 autopsy cases. Am J Surg 135:807–810, 1978.
97. Morton DL, Joseph WL, Ketcham AS, et al: Surgical resection and adjunctive immunotherapy for selected patients with multiple pulmonary metastases. Ann Surg 178:360–366, 1973.
98. Wong JH, Euhus DM, Morton DL: Surgical resection for metastatic melanoma to the lung. Arch Surg 123:1091–1095, 1988.
99. Cahan WG: Excision of melanoma metastases to the lung: Problems in diagnosis and management. Ann Surg 178:703–709, 1973.
100. Marincola FM, Mark JBD: Selection factors resulting in improved survival after surgical resection of tumors metastatic to the lungs. Arch Surg 125:1387–1393, 1990.
101. Mathisen DJ, Flye MN, Peabody J: The role of thoracotomy in the management of pulmonary metastases from malignant melanoma. Ann Thorac Surg 27:295–299, 1975.
102. Luce JK: Chemotherapy of malignant melanoma. Cancer 30:1604–1615, 1972.
103. Wagner DE, Ramirez G, Weiss AJ, Hill G Jr: Combination phase I–II study of imidazole carboxamide (NCS45388). Oncology 26:310–316, 1972.
104. Gundersen S: Dacarbazine, vindesine, and cisplatin combination chemotherapy in advanced malignant melanoma: A phase II study. Cancer Treat Rep 71:997–999, 1987.
105. Czarnetzki BM, Macher E, Behrendt H, Lejeune F: Current status of melanoma chemotherapy and immunotherapy. Recent Results Cancer Res 80:264–268, 1982.
106. Legha SS, Ring S, Papadopoulous N, et al: A prospective evaluation of a triple drug regimen containing cisplatin, vinblastine, and dacarbazine (CVD) for metastatic melanoma. Cancer 64:2024–2029, 1989.
107. McClay EF, Mastrangelo MJ, Bellet RE, Berd D: Combination chemotherapy and hormonal therapy in the treatment of malignant melanoma. Cancer Treat Rep 71:465–469, 1987.
108. McClay EF, Mastrangelo MJ, Sprandio JD, et al: The importance of tamoxifen to a cisplatin-containing regimen in the treatment of metastatic melanoma. Cancer 63:1292–1295, 1989.
109. Bentzen SM, Overgaard J, Thames HD, et al: Clinical radiobiology of malignant melanoma. Radiother Oncol 16:169–182, 1989.
110. Sause WT, Cooper JS, Rush S, et al: A randomized trial evaluating fraction size in external beam radiation therapy in treatment of melanoma. Int J Radiat Oncol Biol Phys 20:429–432, 1991.

111. Patchell RA, Tibbs PA, Walsh JW, et al: A randomized trial of surgery in the treatment of single metastases to the brain. N Engl J Med 322:494–500, 1990.
112. Ziegler JC, Cooper JS: Brain metastases from malignant melanoma. Conventional v. high-dose per fraction radiotherapy. Int J Radiat Oncol Biol Phys 12:1839–1842, 1986.
113. Bumgland TF, Reisfeld RA: Unique glycoprotein-proteoglycan complex defined by monoclonal antibody on human monoclonal cells. Proc Natl Acad Sci USA 79:1245–1249, 1987.
114. Seigler HF, Wallack MK, Vervaet CE, et al: Melanoma patient antibody response to melanoma tumor-associated antigen defined by murine monoclonal antibodies. J Biol Response Mod 8:37–52, 1989.
115. Briele HA, Beattie CW, Ronan SG, et al: Late recurrence of cutaneous melanoma. Arch Surg 118:800–803, 1983.
116. Nathanson L: Use of BCG in the treatment of human neoplasms. A review. Semin Oncol 1:337–349, 1974.
117. Eilber FR, Morton DL, Holmes EC, et al: Adjuvant immunotherapy with BCG in treatment of regional lymph node metastasis from malignant melanoma. N Engl J Med 294:237–240, 1976.
118. Quirt IC, DeBoer G, Kersey PA, et al: Randomized controlled trial of adjuvant chemoimmunotherapy with DTIC and BCG after complete excision of primary melanoma with a poor prognosis or melanoma metastases. Can Med Assoc J 128:929–933, 1983.
119. Spitler LE, Sagebeil R: A randomized trial of levamisole versus placebo as adjuvant therapy in malignant melanoma. N Engl J Med 303:1143–1147, 1980.
119a. Czarnetzki BM, Macher E, Suciu S, et al: Long-term adjuvant immunotherapy in stage I high risk malignant melanoma, comparing two BCG preparations versus non-treatment in a randomised multicentre study (EORTC Protocol 18781). Eur J Cancer 29A:1237–1242, 1993.
120. Balch CM, Smalley RV, Bartolucci AA, et al: A randomized prospective clinical trial of adjuvant *C. parvum* immunotherapy in 260 patients with clinically localized melanoma (Stage I): Prognostic factors analysis and preliminary results of immunotherapy. Cancer 49:1079–1084, 1982.
121. Bast RC, Zhar B, Bursos T, et al: BCG and cancer. N Engl J Med 290:1413–1419, 1974.
122. Mitchell MS, Karn-Mitchell J, Kempf RA, et al: Active specific immunotherapy for melanoma: Phase I trial of allogeneic lysate and a novel immunostimulant. Cancer Res 48:5883–5893, 1988.
123. Wallack MK, Bash JA, Leftheriotis E, et al: Positive relationship of clinical and serologic responses to vaccinia melanoma oncolysate. Arch Surg 122:1460–1463, 1987.
124. Creagan ET, Ahmann DL, Frytak S, et al: Phase II trials of recombinant leukocyte alpha-interferon in disseminated malignant melanoma. Results in 96 patients. Cancer Treat Rep 70:619–624, 1986.
125. Keilholz U, Scheibenbogen C, Tilgen W, et al: Interferon-alpha and interleukin-2 in the treatment of metastatic melanoma. Comparison of phase II trials. Cancer 72:607–614, 1993.
126. Robinson WA, Mughal TI, Thomas MR, et al: Treatment of metastatic malignant melanoma with recombinant interferon alpha-2. Immunobiology 172:275–282, 1986.
127. Creagan ET, Ahmann DL, Long HJ, et al: Phase II study of recombinant interferon-gamma in patients with disseminated malignant melanoma. Cancer Treat Rep 71:843–844, 1987.
128. Ernstoff MS, Trautman T, Davis CA, et al: A randomized phase I/II study of cutaneous versus intermittent intravenous interferon-gamma in patients with metastatic melanoma. J Clin Oncol 5:1804–1810, 1987.
129. Lotze MT, Chang AE, Seipp CA, et al: High-dose recombinant interleukin 2 in the treatment of patients with disseminated cancer. Responses, treatment-related morbidity, and histologic findings. JAMA 256:3117–3124, 1986.
130. Rosenberg SA, Lotze MT, Yang JC, et al: Experience with the use of high-dose interleukin-2 in the treatment of 652 cancer patients. Ann Surg 210:474–484, 1989.
131. Mitchell MS, Kempf RA, Harel W, et al: Effectiveness and tolerability of low-dose cyclophosphamide and low-dose intravenous interleukin-2 in disseminated melanoma. J Clin Oncol 6:409–424, 1988.
132. Rosenberg SA, Packard BS, Aebersold PM, et al: Use of tumor-infiltrating lymphocytes and interleukin-2 in the immunotherapy of patients with metastatic melanoma. A preliminary report. N Engl J Med 319:1676–1680, 1988.
133. Rosenberg SA, Aebersold P, Cornetta K, et al: Gene transfer into humans—immunotherapy of patients with advanced melanoma, using tumor-infiltrating lymphocytes modified by retroviral gene transduction. N Engl J Med 323:570–578, 1990.
134. Kushner BH, Cheung N-K: GM-CSF enhances 3F8 monoclonal antibody-dependent cellular cytotoxicity against human melanoma and neuroblastoma. Blood 73:1936–1941, 1989.
135. Munn DH, Cheung N-K: Interleukin-2 enhancement of monoclonal antibody–mediated cellular cytotoxicity against human melanoma. Cancer Res 47:6600–6605, 1987.
136. Uchiyama A, Hoon DSB, Morisaki T, et al: Transfection of interleukin-2 gene into human melanoma cells augments cellular immune response. Cancer Res 53:949–952, 1993.
137. Ogasawara M, Rosenberg SA: Enhanced expression of HLA molecules and stimulation of autologous human tumor infiltrating lymphocytes following transduction of melanoma cells with gamma-interferon genes. Cancer Res 53:3561–3568, 1993.

Basal and Squamous Cancers of the Skin

Donald L. Morton, M.D. • Richard Essner, M.D.

EPIDEMIOLOGY

Incidence

Although melanoma is the most lethal of skin cancers, basal cell carcinoma (BCC) and squamous cell carcinoma (SCC) are much more frequent, with an estimated 800,000 new cases annually.[1, 2] BCC and SCC are primarily diseases of individuals with fair complexions and light eyes and hair color.[3, 4] Men are more likely to have these lesions, probably due to occupational sun exposure and ultraviolet (UV) light. The incidence in blacks and Asians is much lower than that in whites.[5]

BCC is the most common malignancy of the skin. This tumor does not metastasize, and its cure rate approaches 100% with early treatment. Deaths from BCC usually are the result of failure to seek or to provide treatment in a timely manner. Although BCC tumors grow slowly, they may have periods of rapid growth. Destructive forms of this tumor can invade cartilage, bone, and soft tissue and may result in death.

SCC is the second most common skin malignancy, arising as a primary tumor or as the result of actinic keratoses or leukoplasia. SCC can occur on any area of the skin or mucous membranes but is most often found on the face or the dorsum of the hands. Its clinical course depends on its primary site, etiology, and histologic differentiation. Although high-risk primary lesions can be associated with lymph node metastasis, the overall incidence of metastases from SCC is only 0.3% to 4.0%.[5a, 5b] The cure rate is very high when SCC lesions are treated early in their development.

Risk Factors

Among the many different etiologic agents of skin cancer are ionizing radiation, chemical carcinogens, scars, chronic wounds, discoid lupus, and particular genotypes. The most important factor is ionizing radiation from UV light, which causes actinic damage.[1, 6] Particular genetic mutations have been demonstrated after sunlight exposure; these mutations have been suggested to produce skin cancer.

In the past, skin tumors occurred in individuals with occupational x-ray exposure, particularly dentists. Skin cancer may develop in patients who have received radiotherapy for benign disease.[7, 8] These tumors tend to occur in multiple sites and ulcerate more often than do skin cancers induced by other factors. They may be associated with chronic radiation dermatitis secondary to treatment for diseases such as acne, hirsutism, psoriasis, hemangiomas, and benign ulcers. The latency period is typically many years and may be related to the nonlethal radiation doses. These lesions are typically BCC on the face and SCC on other sites. BCC and SCC are fairly uncommon sequelae of radiotherapy for malignant disease, since the higher radiation fractions may produce irreversible skin cell damage and death.

Chronic arsenic exposure can lead to the development of SCC and BCC.[5, 8, 9] Long-term exposure to contaminated drinking water, pesticides, and medications may induce these tumors. Scrotal SCC develops in chimney sweeps after chronic exposure to the products of combustion from shale, coal, or petroleum.[9]

Chronic skin damage or irritation is another etiologic agent of skin cancer. Patients with fistulous tracts, stasis ulcers, amputation stumps, burn wounds, Marjolin's ulcer, or chronic skin infections are at high risk for development of skin cancer. Patients with xeroderma pigmentosum lack the ability to repair DNA damaged from UV light exposure.[6] Those patients with basal cell nevus syndrome develop BCC on multiple skin sites.

Skin cancer is being increasingly discovered in those patients who are immunosuppressed following transplantation or chemotherapy.[1, 8, 10] In renal transplant patients, the risk for development of skin cancer is 35-fold higher than in the population at large.[11, 12] Patients who receive methotrexate therapy for psoriasis or who suffer from lymphocytic lymphoma or leukemia are at higher risk for development of SCC.[13]

PATHOLOGY AND DIAGNOSIS

There are several variants of BCC: noduloulcerative, superficial, pigmented, and morphealike. Typically, BCC is a small, waxy nodule that enlarges slowly over a number of years. A central depression leads to ulceration. A few telangiectatic vessels develop on the surface of the nodule. The pigmented type of BCC is similar to the noduloulcerative variant, with the addition of brown or black coloration. Superficial BCC is characterized by slowly enlarging, red scaly areas on the back or chest. Morphealike BCC is a white, scarred plaque with ill-defined borders. This lesion is more aggressive than other forms of BCC.

SCC usually appears as a rapidly growing nodule with raised borders and central ulceration; however, some SCC lesions may have a verrucoselike appearance without ulceration. Actinic keratoses are considered the biologic equivalent to carcinoma in situ and occur after long-term sun exposure.

Suspicious skin lesions can easily be diagnosed by incision or excisional biopsy.

STAGING

Because the incidence of metastasis is so low, a classification system that considers nodal or distant disease is not generally used to stage BCC and SCC. In 1932, Broders[14] introduced a classification system for SCC determined by the degree of differentiation of the tumor. In grade I lesions, more than 75% of cells are differentiated; in grade II, 50%; in grade III, greater than 25%; and in grade IV, less than 25%. The degree of atypia and the depth of lesion penetration into the underlying tissue are also important for staging these lesions. There is no suitable staging system for BCC.

TREATMENT

Early sun-induced skin cancers such as actinic keratoses are potentially preventable by avoiding excessive sunlight and using sunscreens and clothing to prevent sun exposure in fair-complected patients.[15] Curettage or surgical excision is curative. Cryosurgery with liquid nitrogen is another effective and reliable method to treat actinic keratoses.[16] Topical therapy with 5-fluorouracil (5-FU) produces an inflammatory response 3 to 5 days after treatment and can be repeated for unresponsive lesions.[17, 18] Systemic toxicity is rare following use of 5-FU in this manner. This agent probably acts by blocking DNA synthesis through inhibition of thymidylate synthetase rather than through a direct caustic effect.[17, 18] Radiotherapy is not generally indicated for treatment of actinic keratoses.

Conventional treatment of BCC and SCC depends on adequate removal or destruction of the primary lesion using surgical excision, curettage, or radiotherapy, or a combination. These treatment modalities are usually curative. Although the treatment of certain tumors may be more difficult due to functional or cosmetic limitations, delayed or incomplete intervention may result in loss of vital structures and death. In general, recurrence is due to inadequate treatment of the primary lesion.[19]

Surgical treatment of BCC and SCC is usually accomplished by excisional biopsy of the primary lesion. Generally, the margin of excision should equal the greatest radius of the tumor.[20, 21] Since most primary lesions can be resected under local anesthesia, it is important to mark the borders of resection before injecting local anesthetic. Careful palpation is often necessary to delineate the borders of the lesion. Whenever possible, the lines of excision should follow the natural skin lines. The excision should include the full thickness of the skin down into the subcutaneous fat. If the tumor status of excision margins is unclear, frozen section should be performed. Most wounds can be closed by primary repair. The larger wounds can be reconstructed by random or axial-based flaps (see Figs. 16–2 and 16–3). Large primary tumors may be managed by initial incisional biopsy followed by wide excision and planned reconstruction.

If the permanent section reveals extension of the tumor to the margins of excision, a second procedure should be performed to eliminate the residual tumor. Approximately 30% of lesions recur if the histologic margins are positive.[19, 20] Patients whose tumors have a morpheaform histology or are incompletely excised, or both, have a higher risk of recurrence; they require treatment and should not be observed.

Curettage and electrodesiccation can be used to treat either BCC or SCC, although it is more commonly used for BCC. The technique depends on the difference in texture between normal and malignant tissue. After infiltration of local anesthesia, the tumor is curetted and examined by pathologic sectioning and the diagnosis is confirmed. The base and sides of the wound are then electrodesiccated, and the entire procedure is repeated until suitable margins are obtained. Curettage plus desiccation is excellent for excising large BCC lesions but should not be used for morpheaform BCC, BCC and SCC that penetrate bone or soft tissue, or SCC that is poorly differentiated. The recurrence rate varies from 3% to 6% with this technique.[21, 22] Most recurrences are in the scar, and excision of the scar is necessary for treatment.

Radiotherapy for BCC and SCC produces cure rates similar to those of other modalities but requires the patient to return for multiple treatments. On the other hand, it is painless and does not require anesthesia. Recurrence rates as low as 5% to 10% have been reported by a number of groups treating either SCC or BCC.[23–25] Underestimation of tumor size is probably the main reason for treatment failures. Radiation is best used in sites that are not desirable for surgery, such as the face, eyelids, tip of the nose, or ear.[25] Lesions on the trunk or extremities also respond to radiation, but the cosmetic result may be better after surgery. Morpheaform BCC and radiation-induced skin cancer are best treated by other modalities.

Other approaches to the management of BCC and SCC include cryosurgery, chemosurgery, topical chemotherapy, and immunotherapy. Cryosurgical technique destroys cancer cells by freezing the tumor mass. Liquid nitrogen is introduced either topically or via a probe, and the tumor is frozen and thawed through two cycles. This technique is most effective for small (<15 mm) lesions on flat surfaces away from the borders of the eyelids and lips. It should not be used for poorly differentiated SCC or infiltrative BCC. Cure rates of approximately 95% have been demonstrated,[26, 27] and serious complications are rare with this technique.

In the 1930s, Frederic Mohs developed the technique of chemosurgery for the treatment of skin cancers.[28, 29] This technique, now referred to as cutaneous micrographic surgery (CMS), entails excision of the bulk of the lesion and careful mapping of the excised tissues by permanent (fixed tissue) or frozen (fresh tissue) section. Mapping is repeated until the margins show no histopathologic evidence of tumor cells. The fixed tissue technique is rarely used because it must be performed over successive visits, whereas the fresh tissue method can be performed in one procedure. Cure rates from either method approach 97%.[28–31] In Mohs' experience, recurrence rates were less than 1%.[28, 29] Large tumors in difficult anatomic sites are particularly well treated by this technique. Many authors prefer CMS for treatment of recurrent or infiltrative BCC.[30–32] CMS is equally effective for treatment of SCC. Recurrence rates as low as 3% have been reported following use of CMS to treat recurrence, poorly differentiated SCC, or other high-risk SCC.[29, 33, 34] The main disadvantages of this technique are its expense, technical difficulty, and inaccuracy for tumors that are not limited to a single mass.

A variety of chemotherapeutic agents have been employed for the treatment of skin cancer. Topical 5-FU has shown the most promising results in the treatment of superficial SCC and BCC, with cure rates better than 80%.[35–37] Topical 5-FU is not generally recommended for treatment of recurrent or infiltrative tumors. Systemic toxicity is rare from this treatment modality.

Immunotherapy is used for those patients who have multiple skin cancers that would be difficult to treat by other modalities. Patients who have xeroderma pigmentosum, nevoid basal cell syndrome, or long-term exposure to toxic chemicals or radiation may have a large number of tumors. Immunotherapy has centered on the use of a number of immunogens that produce a delayed-type hypersensitivity reaction. Dinitrochlorobenzene, purified protein derivative, bacillus Calmette-Guérin, and other nonspecific immune-enhancing agents have been used. Pilot studies have shown excellent responses to intralesional injection of interferon-α for treatment of nodular and superficial BCC.[38, 39]

CONCLUSION

BCC and SCC are the most common forms of skin cancer, with about 800,000 new cases annually. A number of etiologic agents have been identified, but most skin cancers can be prevented by avoiding excessive sunlight and tanning. The treatment of these lesions can be accomplished in most cases by surgical excision, although a number of different modalities can provide similar cure rates. Initial treatment must be successful to avoid the risk of recurrence and the danger of potential disfigurement, metastasis, or death.

References

1. Kwa RE, Campana K, Moy RL: Biology of cutaneous squamous cell carcinoma. J Am Acad Dermatol 26:1–26, 1992.
2. Wingo PA, Tong T, Bolden S: Cancer statistics, 1995. CA 45:8–30, 1995.
3. Kopf AW: Computer analysis of 3531 basal-cell carcinomas of the skin. J Dermatol 6:267–281, 1979.
4. Chuang TY, Popescu NA, Su WP, Chute CG: Squamous cell carcinoma. A population-based incidence study in Rochester, Minn. Arch Dermatol 126:185–188, 1990.
5. Miller SJ: Biology of basal cell carcinoma (part I). J Am Acad Dermatol 24:1–13, 1991.
5a. Asarch RG: A review of the lymphatic drainage of the head and neck: Use in evaluation of potential metastases. J Dermatol Surg Oncol 8:869–872, 1982.
5b. Dinehart SM, Pollack SV: Metastases from squamous cell carcinoma of the skin and lip. An analysis of twenty-seven cases. J Am Acad Dermatol 21:241–248, 1989.
6. Reed WB, Landing B, Sugarman G, et al: Xeroderma pigmentosum. Clinical and laboratory investigation of its basic defect. JAMA 207:2073–2079, 1969.
7. Levine HL, Ratz JL, Bailin P: Squamous cell carcinoma of the head and neck. Selective management according to site and stage—skin. Otolaryngol Clin North Am 18:499–503, 1985.
8. Miller SJ: Biology of basal cell carcinoma (part II). J Am Acad Dermatol 24:161–175, 1991.
9. Hanke CW: Squamous cell carcinoma. In Roenigk RK, Roenigk HH Jr (eds): Dermatologic Surgery—Principles and Practice. New York: Marcel Dekker, 1989, p 665.
10. Maize JC: Skin cancer in immunosuppressed patients. JAMA 237:1857–1858, 1977 (editorial).
11. Barr BB, Benton EC, McLaren K, et al: Human papilloma virus infection and skin cancer in renal allograft recipients. Lancet 1:124–129, 1989.
12. Liddington M, Richardson AJ, Higgins RM, et al: Skin cancer in renal transplant recipients. Br J Surg 76:1002–1005, 1989.
13. Marshall V: Premalignant and malignant skin tumours in immunosuppressed patients. Transplantation 17:272–275, 1974.
14. Broders AC: Practical points on the microscopic grading of carcinoma. NY J Med 32:667–1932.
15. Marks VJ: Actinic keratosis. A premalignant skin lesion. Otolaryngol Clin North Am 26:23–35, 1993.
16. Marks R: The role of treatment of actinic keratoses in the prevention of morbidity and mortality due to squamous cell carcinoma. Arch Dermatol 127:1031–1033, 1991.
17. Abadir DM: Combination of topical 5-fluorouracil with cryotherapy for treatment of actinic keratoses. J Dermatol Surg Oncol 9:403–404, 1983.
18. Bercovitch L: Topical chemotherapy of actinic keratoses of the upper extremity with tretinoin and 5-fluorouracil: A double-blind controlled study. Br J Dermatol 116:549–552, 1987.
19. Pascal RR, Hobby LW, Lattes R, Crikelair GF: Prognosis of "incompletely excised" versus "completely excised" basal cell carcinoma. Plast Reconstr Surg 41:328–332, 1968.
20. Epstein E: How accurate is the visual assessment of basal cell carcinoma margin? Br J Dermatol 89:37–43, 1973.
21. Kopf A, Bart R, Schrager D, et al: Curettage-electrodesiccation treatment of basal cell carcinomas. Arch Dermatol 113:439–443, 1977.
22. Spiller W, Spiller R: Treatment of basal cell epithelioma by curettage and electrodesiccation. J Am Acad Dermatol 11:808–814, 1984.
23. Fishbach A, Sause W, Plenk H: Radiation therapy for skin cancer. West J Med 133:379–382, 1980.
24. Fitzpatrick P, Thompson G, Easterbrook W, et al: Basal and squamous cell carcinoma of the eyelids and their treatment by radiotherapy. Int J Radiat Oncol Biol Phys 10:449–454, 1984.
25. Goldschmidt H: Radiotherapy of skin cancer. Modern indications and techniques. Cutis 17:253–261, 1976.
26. Biro L, Price E, Brand A: Cryosurgery for basal cell carcinomas of the eyelids and nose. Five-year experience. J Am Acad Dermatol 6:1042–1047, 1982.
27. Graham G: Statistical data on malignant tumors in cryosurgery: 1982. J Dermatol Surg Oncol 9:238–239, 1983.
28. Mohs FE: Chemosurgery: A microscopically controlled method of cancer excision. Arch Surg 42:279–295, 1941.
29. Mohs FE: Chemosurgery: Microscopically controlled surgery for skin cancer—past, present and future. J Dermatol Surg Oncol 4:41–54, 1978.
30. Robins P: Chemosurgery. My 15 years of experience. J Dermatol Surg Oncol 7:779–789, 1981.
31. Roenigk R, Ratz J, Bailin P, Wheeland R: Trends in the presentation and treatment of basal cell carcinomas. J Dermatol Surg Oncol 3:860–865, 1986.
32. Menn H, Robins P, Kopf AW, et al: The recurrent basal cell epithelioma. A study of 100 cases of recurrent re-treated basal cell epitheliomas. Arch Dermatol 103:628–635, 1971.
33. Rowe DE, Carroll RJ, Day CL Jr: Prognostic factors for local recurrence, metastasis, and survival rates in squamous cell carcinoma of the skin, ear, and lip. Indications for treatment modality selection. J Am Acad Dermatol 26:976–990, 1992.
34. Swarson NA: Mohs' surgery: Technique, indications, application, and the future. Arch Dermatol 119:761–773, 1983.
35. Klein E, Case RW, Burgess GH: Chemotherapy of skin cancer. Cancer 23:228–231, 1973.
36. Stoll HL Jr, Klein E, Case RW: Tumors of the skin. VII. Effects of varying concentrations of locally administered 5-fluorouracil on basal cell carcinomas. J Invest Dermatol 49:219–224, 1967.
37. Sturm HM: Bowen's disease and 5-fluorouracil. J Am Acad Dermatol 1:513–522, 1979.
38. Greenway HT, Cornell RC, Tanner DJ, et al: Treatment of basal cell carcinoma with intralesional interferon. J Am Acad Dermatol 15:437–443, 1986.
39. McDonald RR, Georgouras K: Treatment of basal cell carcinoma with intralesional interferon alpha: A case report and literature review. Australas J Dermatol 33:81–86, 1992.

Rache M. Simmons, M.D. • Eva Rubin, M.D.
Julianna Pisch, M.D.

17

Breast Cancer

INCIDENCE AND MORTALITY

Worldwide, breast cancer is the leading cause of cancer death in women.[1] It is estimated that by the year 2000, 1 million women a year will receive a diagnosis of breast cancer.[2] In the United States, breast cancer accounts for nearly one third of female cancers (excluding nonmelanoma skin cancer and carcinoma in situ) and is responsible for 18% of cancer deaths, exceeded only by lung cancer with 24%.[3] Current projections indicate that 12.5% of women in the United States will be diagnosed with breast cancer and that 3.5% will die of the disease.[4] The age-adjusted breast cancer death rate in the United States is 22.4 in 100,000 women and ranks sixteenth in the world. The highest breast cancer death rates are in the British Isles and Denmark, the lowest are in the Far East. The Republic of Korea has a breast cancer death rate of only 2.6 in 100,000, and Japan's rate is only 6 in 100,000.

Age-adjusted breast cancer mortality has remained fairly steady in the United States since at least 1930.[5] Incidence, on the other hand, has risen sharply. On the basis of data from the Surveillance, Epidemiology, and End Results (SEER) program of the National Cancer Institute, the incidence of breast cancer rose slowly through the 1970s, with one major upswing occurring in 1974 thought to be related to increased public awareness resulting from the diagnosis of breast cancer in the wives of the president and vice president of the United States and from the initiation of screening by the Breast Cancer Detection Demonstration Projects.[6]

Incidence continued to rise slowly through 1981 and then took a sharp jump between 1982 and 1986.[7] The most recent data indicate a continued rise in 1987, with declining rates in the next 2 years, the last for which accurate figures are available at the time of this publication.[8]

The media attention to breast cancer in recent years and the well-intended promotion of breast cancer screening by organizations such as the American Cancer Society have resulted in both increased public awareness and anxiety. The widely publicized figure of a 1 in 8 lifetime risk for American women,[8] compared with 1 in 10 two years ago and 1 in 20 thirty years ago, has to some extent resulted in exaggeration of perceived risk by many women.[9] It has been suggested that such misperceptions may be minimized by defining risk in three ways: (1) lifetime risk by 5-year intervals, (2) risk for development of breast cancer by age X if one has attained age Y without breast cancer, and (3) risk of dying from breast cancer.[10]

The reasons for the overall rising incidence as well as the more recent sharp rise remain speculative. A study from the Seattle–Puget Sound SEER registry showed a 31% increase in incidence between 1974 and 1978 and 1986 and 1987.[8] Analysis of these data suggest that for women age 45 to 64, most of the increased incidence was attributable to early detection by mammography, since the increase was almost entirely in early-stage disease and smaller-sized tumors. However, for women under age 45 and over age 64, increases in incidence were even more substantial than in the 45- to 64-year-old age group. Since there is relatively less participation in mammographic screening by these age groups, this was thought to represent a true rise in incidence.

Epidemiologic factors may have influenced the increase in incidence. Trends in childbearing, particularly increased rates of nulliparity, which is a risk for development of breast cancer, may be responsible for some of the rise in incidence in young women.[11] The incidence of breast cancer significantly increases with age. The rising age of the population and the decreased force of mortality from competing causes of death also tend to increase breast cancer incidence in the older population.[12] Until recently, participation in screening by postmenopausal women has been at a relatively low rate ($\leq$15%)[13] and has not appreciably affected overall mortality.

In general, the nonparallelism of the mortality rate (flat) and incidence curves (rising) for breast cancer can be viewed positively as an indication that current strategies for earlier diagnosis and treatment are somewhat effective.

The impact of screening is likely to become more apparent in the next decade.

Although overall breast cancer mortality has remained stable since case registries were first established in the 1930s, there are differences in some subsets of the population. During the 50-year period between 1930 and 1980, mortality rates for women over age 50 remained level while mortality for women age 30 to 50 was initially level and then declined.[14] The decreasing mortality in younger women has occurred without significant change in the stage distribution of cancers in this age group.[15] This would imply that the effect is not due to screening or other methods of early detection but rather to improved treatment, notably chemotherapy.[16]

Breast cancer is more common in higher socioeconomic groups, women who remain unmarried, women living in urban areas, Jewish women, and women born in northern Europe and the northern United States.[17] The extent to which such associations may be due to improved access to health care in these populations is uncertain.

There are differences in breast cancer incidence and mortality according to race. Mortality rates of black women have steadily increased since 1975 and are currently higher than for white women.[18] A study of Atlanta SEER registry data from 1979 to 1980 showed a 26% increase in incidence of breast cancer in white women and a 45% increase in black women. The authors could attribute only 45% of the increase in whites and 15% to 25% in blacks to mammographic screening.[19] The explanations for the rising mortality in black women are likely more complex and may in part be due to improved reporting of deaths in this population and relatively late stage of disease at diagnosis.[20]

Within specific ethnic groups, there is a difference in the occurrence of breast cancer according to age. White women in their fifties and sixties have a higher incidence of breast cancer than black women of that age, while black women in their thirties and forties have a higher incidence than white women of those age groups.[21] It has been speculated that the increased incidence of breast cancer at a young age in blacks is due to a higher prevalence of hereditary breast cancer in blacks.[22]

RISK FACTORS

There are few diseases for which as many risk factors are known as breast cancer. Yet, despite the wealth of information and research in this area, there is no known acceptable primary preventive measure. The strongest risk factors for breast cancer are sex and age. Breast cancer is 200 times more common in women than in men[23] and 400 times more common in women age 50 than in women age 20.[24] It is estimated that three fourths of women in whom breast cancer develops have no identifiable risk factor other than age.[25]

Aside from sex and age, the strongest risk factors for breast cancer are a personal history of having had the disease and certain types of family history. Women who have had breast cancer have a risk of contralateral cancer that approaches 0.7% per year (14% at 20 years).[26]

Relative risk of a second breast cancer is inversely related to age at diagnosis and is directly related to stage of the original breast cancer.[27] The risk of a second primary breast cancer is higher among women with a family history of breast cancer.[28]

To understand the risk associated with family history, one must make a distinction between truly hereditary breast cancer and other types of familial breast cancer in which the risk may be environmental rather than genetic. The risk associated with hereditary breast cancer is substantial. Recently, a gene has been identified, mutations of which are strongly implicated in the development of breast cancer. Women with genetically acquired alterations of this gene, called BRCA1, have an 85% chance for development of breast or ovarian cancer, or both, with 50% of cases occurring before the age of 50 and a significantly increased risk of bilaterality.[29] While research in this area appears promising and will provide a valuable genetic marker for breast cancer, it appears that only 2% to 4% of breast cancers are due to familial inheritance of alterations of this gene. The extent to which somatically acquired mutations occur, the cause of them, and the extent to which they are implicated in sporadically occurring breast cancers are as yet unknown.

The risk with other mechanisms of family history varies from only mildly elevated to moderately increased. Since breast cancer is relatively common in elderly women, a woman whose mother had breast cancer in her late postmenopausal years has little added risk compared with that of a woman without a family history. This fact is often misunderstood, resulting in inordinately high perceptions of risk by some women and by their physicians. On the other hand, a woman with a family history of premenopausal breast cancer, particularly if bilateral and occurring in multiple first- and second-degree relatives, has a risk of breast cancer that is three to five times higher than that of other women.

A number of pathologic factors have been positively correlated with breast cancer risk. Women with proliferative breast disease found at breast biopsy have mild to moderate elevations of risk while women with atypical hyperplasia in their biopsy specimens have a significantly increased risk of breast cancer compared with women without proliferative change. Family history in a first-degree relative elevates risk even further for women with proliferative disease and atypia on biopsy.

Reproductive factors (menarche before age 12, menopause after age 55, nulliparity, and first pregnancy after age 30) are well-recognized risk factors associated with only mild elevations in risk (relative risk <2). The common thread in all of these may be their association with an increased number of ovulatory cycles, resulting in increased exposure to estrogen during critical periods of breast development.

Pregnancy, particularly if occurring early in life, has a modest protective effect that may be mediated by differentiation of mammary ductal epithelium, rendering the ductal cells relatively insensitive to carcinogenic influences. Lactation appears to have a weakly protective effect. Whether it has an effect independent of its association with parity and early first birth is unclear.[30] Recent studies have shown an association between the number of months of breastfeeding and reduced risk of breast cancer in premenopausal women. This may be related to the cessation of ovulation and decreased estrogen production associated with breastfeeding.[31]

Early bilateral oophorectomy also exerts a protective effect against breast cancer, supporting the hypothesis that ovarian hormone production is an important etiologic factor. The lifetime reduction in risk associated with bilateral oophorectomy before age 40 is estimated to be approximately 50%.[32]

The increased relative risks associated with exogenous hormone use, in the form of either oral contraceptives or postmenopausal estrogen replacement therapy, appear to be quite small and are not consistently demonstrated in all studies. The risk associated with oral contraceptive use does not appear to be affected by dose, brand, or type of hormone in most studies.[33] However, subgroup analyses suggest an elevated risk for some oral contraceptive users, such as those with greater number of years of use and those with other known breast cancer risk factors, such as family history and nulliparity.

Similarly, studies of hormone replacement therapy and breast cancer risk have yielded inconclusive results. The most current studies indicate either no elevation in risk or at most only a mild elevation (relative risk 1.5 to 2). Some studies do indicate an increase in risk associated with higher doses or increased number of years of use. Combined estrogen-progestin replacement, which does decrease endometrial cancer incidence, does not clearly decrease breast cancer incidence and may increase it.

Dietary factors, in particular high-fat diets, have long been considered major culprits resulting in elevated breast cancer risk. This opinion is supported by animal data,[34] significant correlations between per capita fat intake and breast cancer incidence and mortality,[35] studies of migrant populations,[36] and temporal increases and decreases in breast cancer incidence related to higher (or lower) rates of fat intake.[37] A recently published study using data from the Nurses' Health Study[38] did not find a correlation between breast cancer risk and the amount of fat in the diet. Critics of this study have maintained that the study did not truly compare high- and low-fat diets, since the American "low-fat" diet is still relatively high in fat. In addition, the effect of high fat intake may be most pronounced early in life, which may not have been reflected by fat intake measured later in life. Nonetheless, the study did find a significant correlation between colon cancer and high-fat diets, suggesting that the discrimination between high- and low-fat diets was accurate or that dietary fat at the levels measured in the study affects carcinogenesis in the colon but not in the breast.

Alcohol consumption is associated with modest elevations in breast cancer risk in many, but not all, studies. The variability of risk with type and amount of alcohol consumed has not been consistent in the studies showing elevated risk. A meta-analysis of these studies favors an association between alcohol consumption and increased breast cancer risk, but it is not clear whether alcohol itself is an etiologic agent or whether the risk is associated with some other confounding factor that is present in women who drink alcohol.

Body build is associated with breast cancer risk. Many studies show an association between tallness and increased breast cancer risk. Obesity is associated with increased risk in postmenopausal women, while thinness is associated with a higher risk of premenopausal breast cancer. Exercise has been shown to be associated with a decreased risk of breast cancer in some studies, but it is not clear that this effect is independent of its influence on body weight.

Other lifestyle factors and environmental exposures have been studied in relation to breast cancer risk. These include caffeine consumption, cigarette smoking, use of hair dyes, certain drugs, stress, and depression. None of these appears to have a significant influence on risk. Other factors currently being investigated include electromagnetic fields and pesticides, particularly DDT, metabolites of which are concentrated in breast milk.

From the above discussion, it is apparent that few of the known major risk factors for breast cancer are amenable to primary preventive measures. Since there are no known means of primary prevention short of extreme methods such as bilateral prophylactic mastectomy, the only proven effective measure for reduction of breast cancer mortality is early detection, through the use of screening mammography, routine monthly breast self-examination, and annual examination by a physician.

SCREENING

Screening for breast cancer includes three separate components. These are mammography, breast self-examination, and physical examination by a physician or trained nurse practitioner.

The first randomized controlled trial of breast cancer screening was begun 30 years ago under the auspices of the Health Insurance Plan (HIP) of New York. This trial showed a 20% reduction in breast cancer mortality through 18 years of follow-up for the women allocated to the screening arm. Screening in the HIP trial involved annual physical examination and mammography for 5 years. Compliance was relatively poor compared with that in later trials, the mammography used was antiquated by today's standards, and comparatively few cancers diagnosed were so-called "minimal" breast cancers (invasive cancer <1 cm in size or in situ ductal cancer). Nonetheless, the trial was important in demonstrating that breast cancer death rates could be reduced by screening with mammography and physical examination.

Two randomized controlled trials performed in Sweden in the early 1970s, the Swedish W-E (two-county) trial[39] and the Malmo trial,[40] demonstrated that similar reductions in breast cancer mortality were achievable with use of mammography alone. Compliance was better than in the HIP trial, mammography was more sophisticated, and only a single-view mammogram was performed at 2- to 3-year intervals. At 12 years of follow-up, the Swedish two-county trial showed a 30% reduction in mortality among the women invited to undergo screening.

Several other randomized controlled trials, as well as case-control studies,[41–45] have been performed. The trials are not equivalent in many ways, differing in study design, type and quality of mammography, compliance rates, screening intervals, and length of follow-up. There has been a tendency to regard all the trials as equivalent, leading to projections regarding the efficacy of current mammography that cannot be justified based on the available data. The data from the randomized controlled trials are too disparate to be suitable for a meta-analysis. Regrettably, there is no available trial that indicates what is achievable with state-of-the-art mammography of the 1990s performed at yearly intervals. Still, it is possible to conclude that significant mortality reductions can be expected from mammographic screening of women from age 50 to 65.

The available mammographic screening data are less compelling for women under age 50. While breast cancer is a major cause of mortality in this age group, the prevalence of the disease is considerably lower than in older women. The results of the National Breast Screening Study (NBSS), often referred to as "the Canadian trial," have been interpreted as demonstrating that screening mammography is ineffective in younger women. This trial accrued women in the early 1980s to be screened with annual mammography and physical examination. Quality control of mammography, particularly in the early years of patient accrual, was considerably less than ideal. In addition, for reasons still poorly explained, a disproportionate number of women with advanced-stage breast cancer were allocated to the screening arm of the trial. This fact, along with significant contamination of the control arm resulting from a 26% rate of mammography among the women allocated to the control group, makes interpretation of the early mortality data hazardous.

Insufficient numbers of women were screened in the NBSS trial to make up for the selection bias and contamination that occurred. The impact of screening is delayed in younger women because breast cancer deaths—other than those resulting from advanced-stage disease on which screening has no impact—take longer to occur and accumulate; therefore, it is possible that benefit, even if it occurred under the suboptimal conditions of the NBSS trial, will not be demonstrable for several more years.[46]

Mammographic Examination

Until recently, most breast cancers were self-detected (presence of a palpable mass). Currently, more than 50% of breast cancers are mammographically detected.

The increased proportion of mammographically detected cancers has resulted in lowering of stage for the majority of breast cancers detected. There has also been a small decrease in advanced-stage disease, suggesting that most mammographically detected cancers would ultimately result in mortality once they reached clinically detectable size. This raises the hope that, despite the rising incidence, mortality rates will significantly decrease in the next decade.

Although both self-examination and physical examination are capable of detecting breast cancers, for the most part, neither of these detects breast cancer at an early curable stage. The threshold for physical detection of breast cancer by skilled examiners appears to be about 6 mm (Fig. 17–1). Even the majority of those up to 1.5 cm in size are not detectable by palpation. Once breast cancers exceed this size, most are detectable by both palpation and mammography.

X-ray mammography is currently the only proven method that reliably detects breast cancer while it is still curable. A distinction must be made between screening mammography, the performance of mammography in a woman without significant signs or symptoms of breast cancer, and diagnostic mammography, a tailored study performed to evaluate a significant sign or symptom. In the first instance, the object of the examination is simply to identify whether a potentially significant abnormality is present; in the second, the object is to characterize an abnormality as well as possible in order to determine whether intervention is indicated.

In the screening setting, most examinations can be expected to be normal. Screening of women over age 40 in the United States should yield approximately 6 to 8 breast cancers in 1000 women screened (prevalence screen). If screening of these same women were to continue, the rate of detection would approach that of newly emerging cancers—that is, 1 to 2 in 1000 women (incidence screen).

The detection rate of breast cancer by mammography is highly correlated with the mammographic density of the breast. Assuming optimal technique and positioning, nearly all cancers arising in breasts of predominantly adipose tissue should be detectable. The detection rate of cancer in a breast consisting predominantly of fibrous or glandular tissue may be as low as 50% or 60%. Cancers that manifest

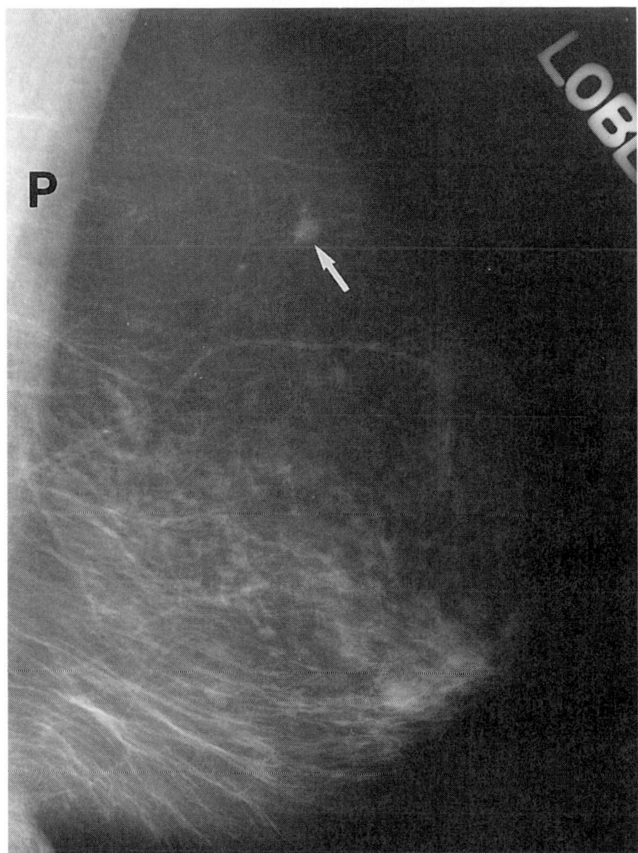

FIGURE 17–1. Mediolateral oblique view of left breast of 74-year-old woman. The 5-mm invasive duct cancer, manifest as a tiny spiculated mass in the upper breast (arrow), is easily detected against the gray background of this fatty replaced breast. P, Pectoral muscle.

as microcalcifications are still detectable in such breasts (Fig. 17–2), but cancers developing as nondescript soft tissue densities fail to be appreciated until they either distort the surrounding parenchyma or are large enough or superficial enough to produce an abnormality in contour or a secondary sign such as skin thickening or retraction (Fig. 17–3*A* to 3*D*). The corollary to this is that breast cancers are more easily detected in the breasts of elderly women whose breasts are largely fatty and more difficult to detect in the breasts of young women whose breasts are largely glandular.

The current move to eliminate, or at least severely curtail, mammographic screening of women under age 50 is somewhat misguided. Rather than denying women age 40 to 50 the only reliable means of detecting early breast cancer, especially if they happen to have predominantly fatty breast tissue, it would appear more sensible to find means to supplement the x-ray mammogram in women of any age with dense breast tissue.

Breast cancer may present on mammography as an area of asymmetric density or architectural distortion, a focal mass or masses, localized or diffuse calcification, or some combination of these. Although the mammogram is rarely pathognomonic, in the presence of certain findings (e.g., a spiculated mass in the absence of a history of trauma or biopsy, clustered pleomorphic calcifications in ductal or segmental distribution, or both), the likelihood of malignancy is exceedingly high. Unfortunately, many occult cancers, especially at the smallest detectable sizes, present as nondescript areas of soft tissue density or asymmetric nodularity, which require further imaging work-up or intervention for clarification.

One of the major criticisms of screening mammography is the large number of unnecessary benign biopsies performed owing to the inherent high false-positive rate of the method. The routine use of breast ultrasound for evaluation of mass lesions detected on mammography has significantly decreased the number of biopsies performed for simple cystic disease of the breast. The present move to increase utilization of methods such as fine-needle aspiration cytology and core biopsy for clinically occult breast lesions should also lead to a decrease in the number of benign breast biopsies performed for mammographically detected abnormalities.

These data do not suggest that self-examination and physical examination of the breasts should be abandoned. The false-negative rates for mammography cover a broad range, from a low of 5% to a high of 69%.

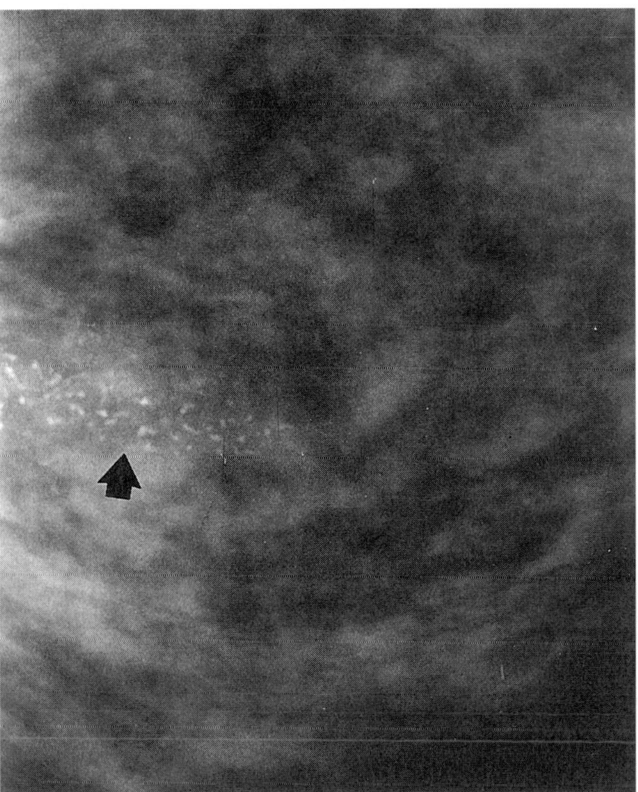

FIGURE 17–2. Detail of left lower breast near chest wall from oblique view of screening mammogram of 34-year-old woman. Pleomorphic linearly distributed calcifications (arrow) typical for comedocarcinoma are readily appreciable despite the background of dense fibroglandular tissue.

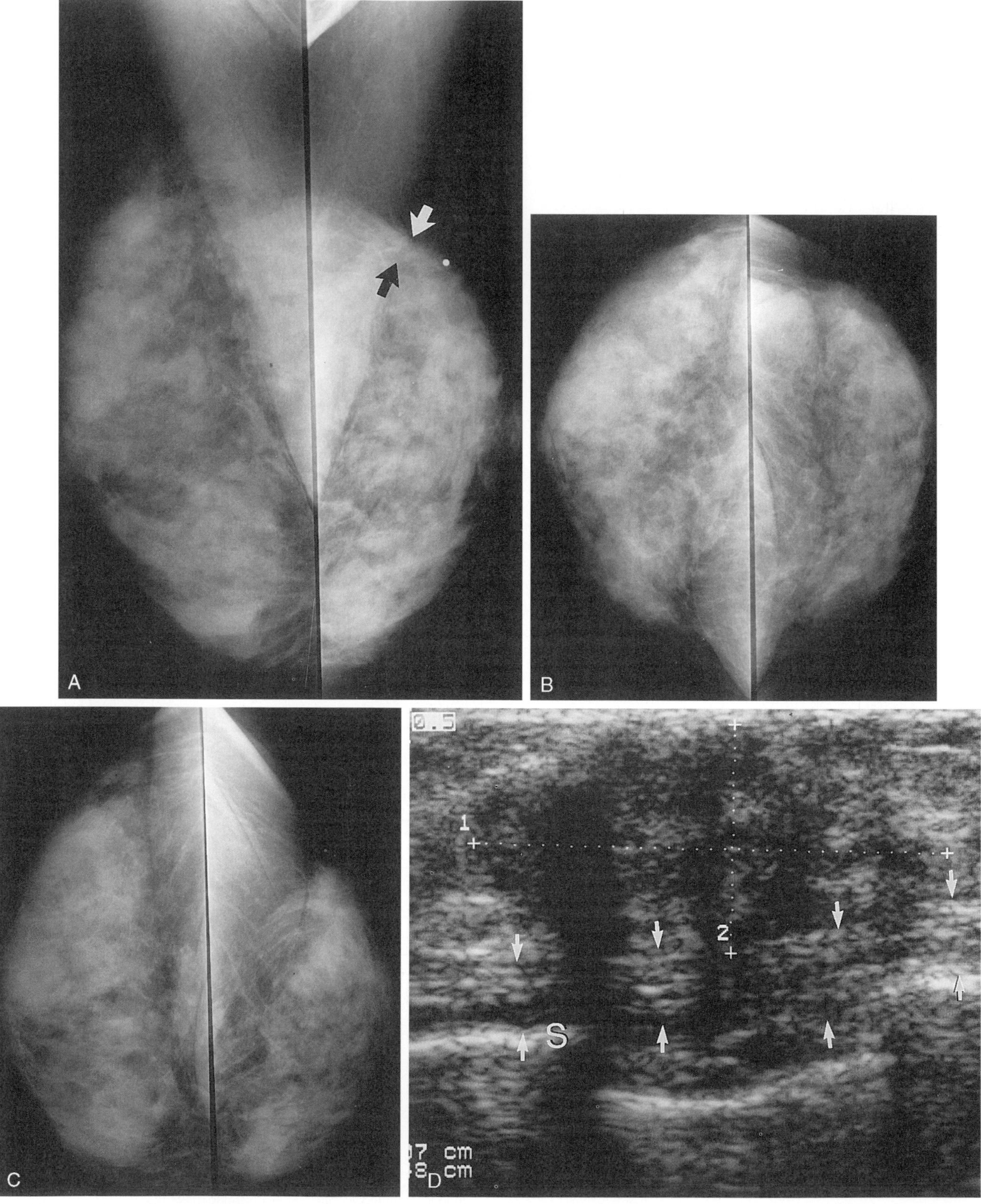

FIGURE 17–3. *A,* Bilateral oblique views of 51-year-old woman with mammographically dense breasts and a palpable mass in the left upper outer quadrant. A radiopaque marker has been placed over the area of the mass. Parenchymal distortion (arrows) is visible, but the margins of the mass are obscured by the surrounding dense tissue. *B,* Craniocaudal views of same patient. Again, there is apparent distortion, but the margins of involvement are not distinct. *C,* Laterally extended craniocaudal views of same patient. These supplemental views may be necessary to visualize the most lateral portions of breast tissue not visible on standard projections in 10% to 15% of women. The distortion in the left breast is seen to involve a fairly large area, but accurate measurement of a mass is not possible. *D,* Ultrasound image of mass shows maximum dimension of about 3 cm. The mass has irregular margins and inhomogeneous echotexture and demonstrates areas of attenuation of the ultrasound beam (S, shadowing). The posterior margin of the mass abuts the pectoral muscle (arrows) but does not appear to involve it. Histology showed a 3-cm invasive duct cancer extending to within 0.1 cm of the muscle.

Self-Examination

Some studies have shown that women who routinely perform self-examination detect their cancers at a more favorable stage than those who do not. It is probably desirable to encourage self-examination and annual physical examination of the breasts by a physician for those women whose mammograms are most likely to result in a false-negative result—that is, any woman with dense breast tissue. Whether there is significant benefit to be derived by physical examination of the breasts in women whose breasts are fatty-replaced and who are having annual mammography of high quality can be questioned. The current American Cancer Society guidelines recommend that women begin breast self-examination at the age of 20 and have annual physical examinations of their breasts by a physician beginning at age 30.

Breast self-examination should begin with inspection of the breasts in front of a mirror, first with the arms at the sides, then with the arms raised, and finally with the hands on the hips and pushing onto the hips. Women should be instructed to look for swellings, dimpling, discoloration, and changes in the appearance of the nipple.

The palpation portion of breast examination should be performed upright as well as supine with a pillow under the shoulder of the breast to be examined. Because it is advantageous for the skin of the breast to be moist during palpation, it is often suggested that the upright examination be performed in the shower with soapy fingers and that lotion or oil be applied to the breast for the supine examination.

Palpation should be performed with the pads of the middle three fingers applied to the breast, the right hand being used to examine the left breast, and the left hand for the right. Palpation can be performed with three methods: (1) a circular motion in an elliptic pattern; (2) a vertical up-and-down motion in a rectangular pattern; and (3) a wedge motion in a radial pattern. Women are counseled to feel for lumps, hard areas, and thickenings.

Breast self-examination should be performed monthly. Premenopausal women should choose the time following their menstrual period. Postmenopausal women should choose a particular day of the month and consistently examine their breasts on that day each month.

Women who practice breast self-examination must learn to appreciate the differences in texture between the normal adipose and fibroglandular elements of their breasts. Any persistent abnormality should be brought to the attention of a physician, even if a recent mammogram has shown no suspicious finding.

Physical Examination

The physical examination begins with the patient in the sitting position. The physician looks for any asymmetry of the breasts (Fig. 17–4), skin retraction or discoloration (Figs. 17–5 and 17–6), and nipple crusting (Fig. 17–7), irritation, discharge, or retraction (Fig. 17–8). Edema of the breast skin, sometimes called peau d'orange, as it resembles the skin of an orange, can be secondary to lymphatic obstruction with extensive axillary nodal involvement or inflammatory carcinoma (Fig. 17–9). Retraction of the skin may indicate carcinoma involving Cooper's ligaments of the breast. Erythema of the breast can be indicative of mastitis or inflammatory carcinoma. Erosion or scaling of the nipple can be due to Paget disease. Nipple discharge should be evaluated for an intraductal papilloma or papillary carcinoma. Nipple retraction can be representative of an underlying cancer.

With the patient's arms raised above her head and with her hands on her hips pushing down, any skin dimpling or retraction is accentuated. The axillae should be examined with the ipsilateral arm relaxed to allow thorough examination of the axillary fossa. If lymph nodes are palpated, it

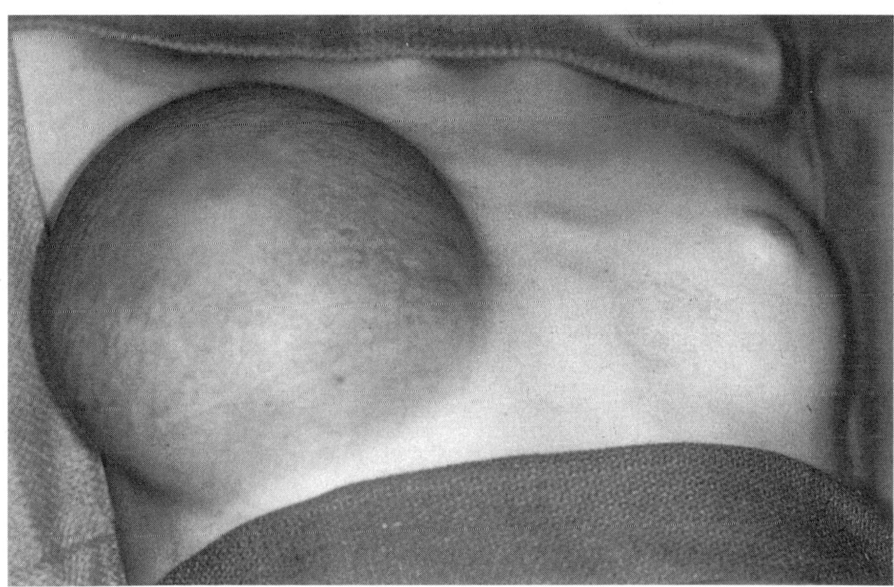

FIGURE 17–4. Marked breast asymmetry in a patient with a rapidly enlarging mass.

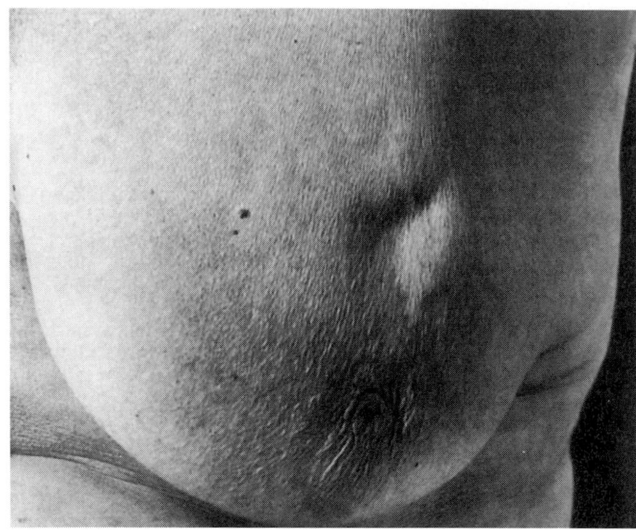

FIGURE 17–5. Broad shallow dimple in the skin over a carcinoma of the upper outer sector of the breast. (From Haagensen CD: Diseases of the Breast. Philadelphia: WB Saunders, 1986, p 531.)

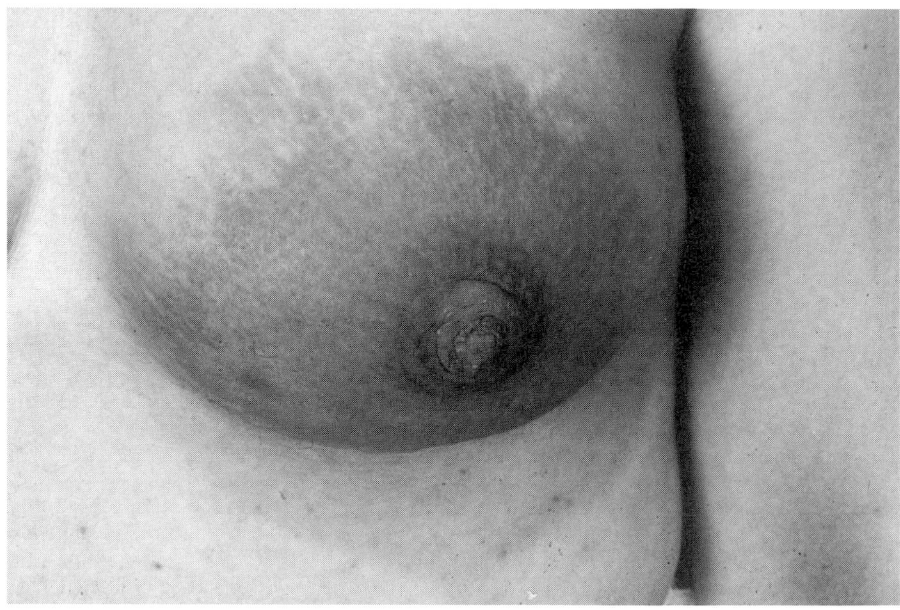

FIGURE 17–6. Skin erythema of a patient with inflammatory breast carcinoma.

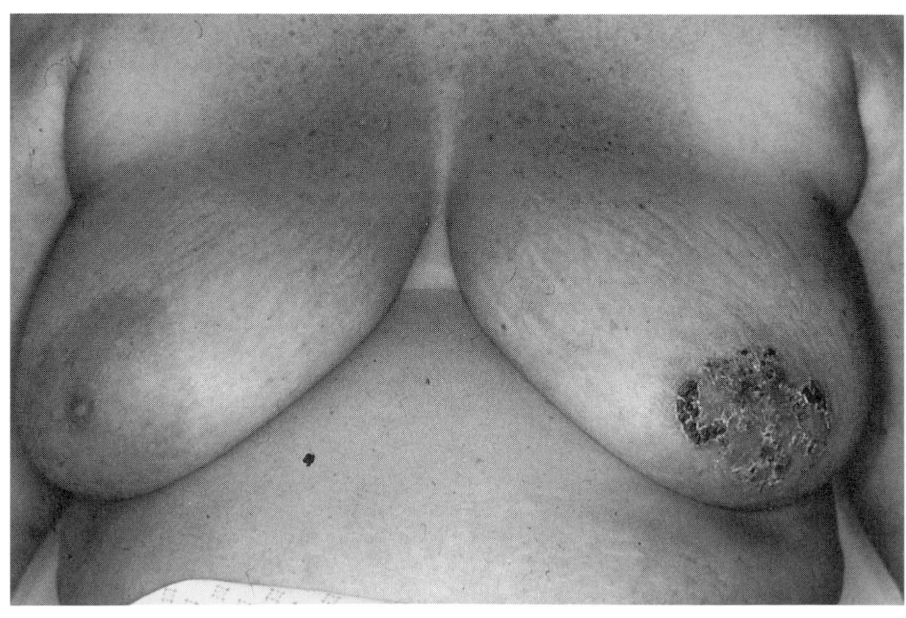

FIGURE 17–7. Paget disease of the left breast.

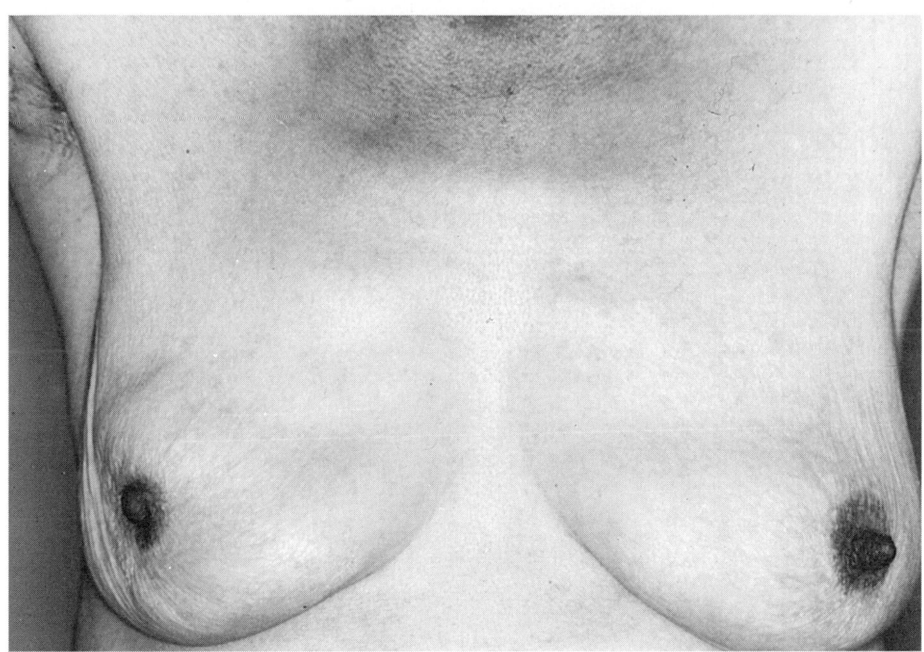

FIGURE 17–8. Right breast nipple retraction in patient with invasive breast cancer.

should be noted whether they are single, multiple, matted, mobile, fixed, soft, or firm. The supraclavicular fossa is also examined for palpable lymph nodes.[47]

Palpation of the breast can be performed in the upright position but is much more sensitive and accurate in the supine position.[48] With the patient in a supine position and her arms above her head, the entire breast should be examined by the physician. A popular method is to start at the nipple and continue in enlarging concentric circles until the entire breast, including the tail of Spence, has been examined. If a mass is discovered, it is important to note the size, firmness, mobility from underlying and overlying structures, and regularity of borders.

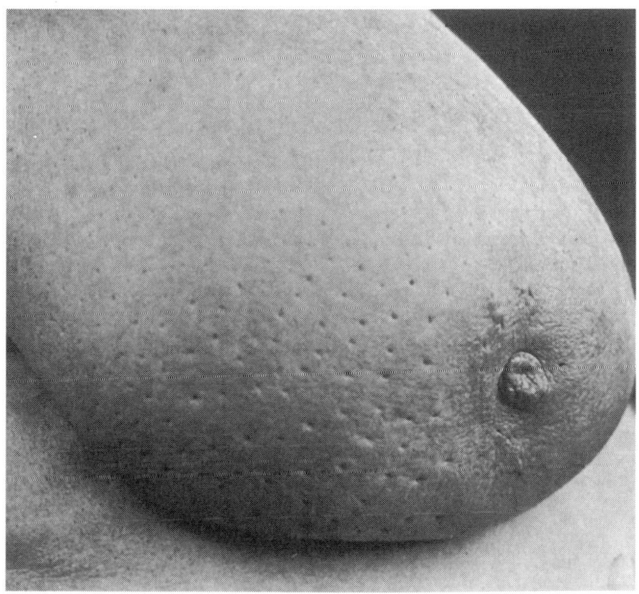

FIGURE 17–9. Extensive edema of the skin of the breast due to carcinoma. (From Haagensen CD: Diseases of the Breast. Philadelphia: WB Saunders, 1986, p 521.)

EVALUATION OF A PALPABLE BREAST MASS

It is important in the evaluation of a breast lump to obtain a clinical history in regard to the duration of the mass, cyclic variation in size in relation to the patient's menstrual cycle, history of previous similar masses, and presence of tenderness. The patient's age and risk factors for development of breast cancer, especially family history of breast cancer and personal history of breast cancer, carcinoma in situ, or atypical hyperplasia, are important in the evaluation. Typically, breast masses in young women represent benign lesions, often fibroadenomas and cysts, while masses in postmenopausal women are cancer until proven otherwise.

If a cyst is suspected clinically in a young menstruating woman, the patient should be re-examined immediately after her next menstrual cycle. If the mass is observed to resolve during this time, one can feel confident that the mass represented a benign cyst. If the mass does not resolve after 2 months or enlarges, a breast ultrasound or needle aspiration should be performed.

A safe, simple, inexpensive method for potential diagnosis and treatment is cyst aspiration. Cyst fluid may be clear, yellow, brown, or green. Bloody discharge is worrisome for malignancy. If with aspiration of fluid the mass does not completely resolve, the fluid is bloody, or the cyst recurs multiple times, a surgical biopsy is indicated. Cystic fluid cytology is typically not very helpful and is not generally recommended unless the fluid is grossly bloody.[47]

If a mass is found to be solid by aspiration, some advocate fine-needle aspiration. The accuracy with this technique for diagnosis is quite variable. The false-negative rate is 1% to 35% and the false-positive rate is 1% to 18%.[49] These results are due in part to variability in the specimen obtained and to the expertise of the cytologist.

A mammogram is recommended for any noncystic mass in the breast. In young women with dense breasts and in women who are pregnant, an ultrasound is recommended.[49] It is important to remember that a cancerous mass may not be seen on a mammogram, and a normal mammogram does not preclude a biopsy in a clinically suspicious mass.

In a young woman with a benign-appearing mass by examination and ultrasound, the therapeutic options include surgical excision or core biopsy; in selected cases, close observation may be considered.[47]

BREAST DEVELOPMENT AND ANATOMY

An understanding of the anatomy and physiology of the breast is essential in the management of benign, preneoplastic, and neoplastic disorders.

Embryology and Normal Breast Development

In human fetal development, the ectodermal primitive milk streak develops from the axilla to the groin on the embryonic trunk by the fifth gestational week. In 2% to 6% of adult women, incomplete regression of the primitive milk streak leads to accessory breast tissues or accessory nipples, or both.[47] While the vast majority of breast cancers develop in mammary tissue on the chest wall, it is important to recognize that breast cancer can develop from mammary tissue anywhere along the milk streak.

At 7 to 8 weeks of gestation, a thickening occurs in the mammary tissue, followed by invagination into the chest wall mesenchyme. Between 12 and 16 weeks, mesenchymal cells differentiate into the smooth muscle of the nipple and areola. At 16 weeks, epithelial buds develop and then branch to form strips of epithelium that represent the future secretory alveoli. It is believed that, phylogenetically, breast parenchyma develops from sweat gland tissue. The special apocrine glands (Montgomery's glands) around the nipple are a less differentiated form of sweat glands.[47]

In the neonate, the stimulated mammary tissue secretes colostral milk (sometimes called witch's milk), which can be expressed from the nipple of most neonates of both sexes for the first 4 to 7 days of life. This secretion declines over a 3- to 4-week period owing to involution of the breast after withdrawal of placental hormones.[47]

Normal Breast Development During Puberty

Puberty in girls born in industrialized nations begins at the age of 10 to 12 years, with the sex hormones inducing the growth and maturation of the breasts and genital organs. The physiologic effect of estrogens on the maturing breast is to stimulate longitudinal growth of ductal epithelium. Terminal ductules also form buds that develop into breast lobules. Simultaneously, periductal connective tissues increase in volume and elasticity, with enhanced vascularity and fat deposition. The evolution of breast development from childhood to maturity has been divided into five phases by Tanner (Table 17–1).

Abnormal Breast Development

The most frequently observed abnormality seen in both sexes is an accessory nipple (polythelia), which may occur at any point along the milk streak from the axilla to the groin. Rarely, accessory true mammary glands develop (polymastia). These are most often located in the axilla. During pregnancy and lactation, an accessory breast may swell, and occasionally, if there is an associated nipple, it may function.[47]

Other developmental abnormalities include hypoplasia, which is the underdevelopment of the breast; amastia, the congenital absence of a breast; and amazia, the lack of breast tissue but the presence of a nipple. Amazia is most often iatrogenic as a consequence of excision of the breast bud, resulting in marked deformity during and after puberty. The prepubertal use of radiotherapy in the region of the developing breast may also result in amazia.[47]

Unilateral hypoplasia of breast, thorax, and pectoral muscles is called Poland's syndrome. There are often associated abnormalities of the hand, such as synbrachydactyly, a hypoplasia of the middle phalanges, and central skin webbing.[50]

Anatomy of the Breast

The adult breast lies between the second and sixth ribs in the vertical axis and between the sternal edge and the midaxillary line in the horizontal axis (Fig. 17–10).[47] Breast tissue also projects into the axilla as the tail of Spence. Fifteen to twenty segmental ducts converge at the nipple in a radial arrangement. The breast parenchyma is divided into 15 to 20 lobes corresponding to the arborization of each segmental duct. The segmental ducts drain each lobe

TABLE 17–1
Phases of Breast Development

Phase I (age: puberty): Preadolescent elevation of the nipple with no palpable glandular tissue or areolar pigmentation.

Phase II (age: 11.1 ± 1.1 yr): Presence of glandular tissue in the subareolar region. The nipple and breast project as a single mound from the chest wall.

Phase III (age: 12.2 ± 1.09 yr): Increase in the amount of readily palpable glandular tissue with enlargement of the breast and increased diameter and pigmentation of the areola. The contour of the breast and nipple remains in a single plane.

Phase IV (age: 13.1 ± 1.15 yr): Enlargement of the areola and increased areola pigmentation. The nipple and areola form a secondary mound above the level of the breast.

Phase V (age: 15.3 ± 1.7 yr): Final adolescent development of a smooth contour with no projection of the areola and nipple.

From Harris JR, et al: Breast Diseases. Philadelphia: JB Lippincott, 1991, p 2.

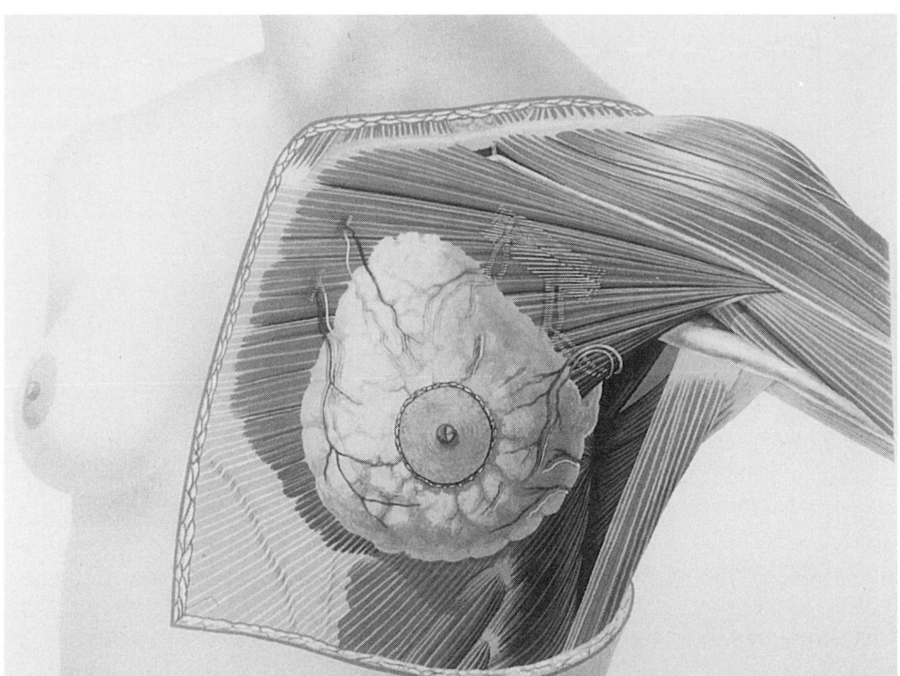

FIGURE 17–10. Normal anatomy of the breast and pectoralis major muscle. (Adapted from Harris JR, et al: Breast Diseases. Philadelphia: JB Lippincott, 1991, p 3.)

into the collecting ducts. Between five and ten collecting ducts open at the nipple. Expanded areas of the ducts just before they enter the nipple are called lactiferous sinuses.[47]

Within the parenchyma and subcutaneous tissues of the breast are fat, connective tissue, blood vessels, nerves, and lymphatics. Morgagni's tubercles, located near the periphery of the areola, are elevations formed by the openings of the ducts of Montgomery's glands. Enveloping the breast is the superficial pectoral fascia, which is continuous with the superficial abdominal fascia of Camper, and the deep pectoral fascia, covering the pectoralis major and serratus anterior muscles. Between these are fibrous bands, Cooper's ligaments, which connect the superficial and deep fascial layers.[47]

Blood Supply

The breast is supplied with blood primarily from the internal mammary and lateral thoracic arteries. The anterior perforating branches of the internal mammary artery supply mainly the medial and central parts of the breast. The lateral thoracic artery supplies mainly the upper quadrant of the breast. Other minor contributions to the blood supply are the pectoral branch of the thoracoacromial artery; the lateral branches of the third, fourth, and fifth intercostal arteries; and the subscapular and thoracodorsal arteries (Fig. 17–11).[47]

Lymphatic Drainage

The subepithelial lymphatic drainage of the breast is part of the subepithelial lymphatic system of the body surface. Lymph flows in a unidirectional fashion from the superficial to the deep plexus.

Flow from the breast lymphatic vessels moves centrifugally toward the axillary and internal mammary lymph nodes.[51] The majority of lymphatic drainage of the breast flows to the axilla. It has been documented that about 3% of the lymph flows to the internal mammary nodes and 97% flows to the axillary nodes. All quadrants of the breast drain some lymph to the internal mammary chain. This has been observed following dye injections of the breast.[52]

There are several groups of axillary lymph nodes. They consist of the subclavicular nodes, the axillary vein lymph nodes, the interpectoral (Rotter's) nodes, the scapular group, and the central nodes.

A method of measuring metastatic progression is to divide the axillary lymph nodes into arbitrary levels, I to III.[53] Lymph nodes lying lateral to the lateral border of the pectoralis minor muscle are designated level I, those behind the pectoralis minor muscle level II, and those located medial to the medial border of the pectoralis minor muscle level III (Fig. 17–12). The internal mammary nodes lie in the intercostal spaces in the parasternal region close to the internal mammary vessels.

Muscular and Neural Anatomy

The muscles of interest in the region of the breast and axilla are the pectoralis major and minor, serratus anterior, and latissimus dorsi muscles, as well as the aponeuroses of the external oblique and rectus abdominis muscles.

The pectoralis minor muscle arises from the outer aspect of the third, fourth, and fifth ribs and is inserted into the medial border of the upper surface of the coracoid process of the scapula. The muscle is innervated by the medial pectoral nerve. This nerve passes either through the muscle itself (in 62% of cases) or around the lateral border as a single branch (in 38% of cases).[55] The nomenclature of the pectoral nerves (i.e., medial and lateral) refers to their

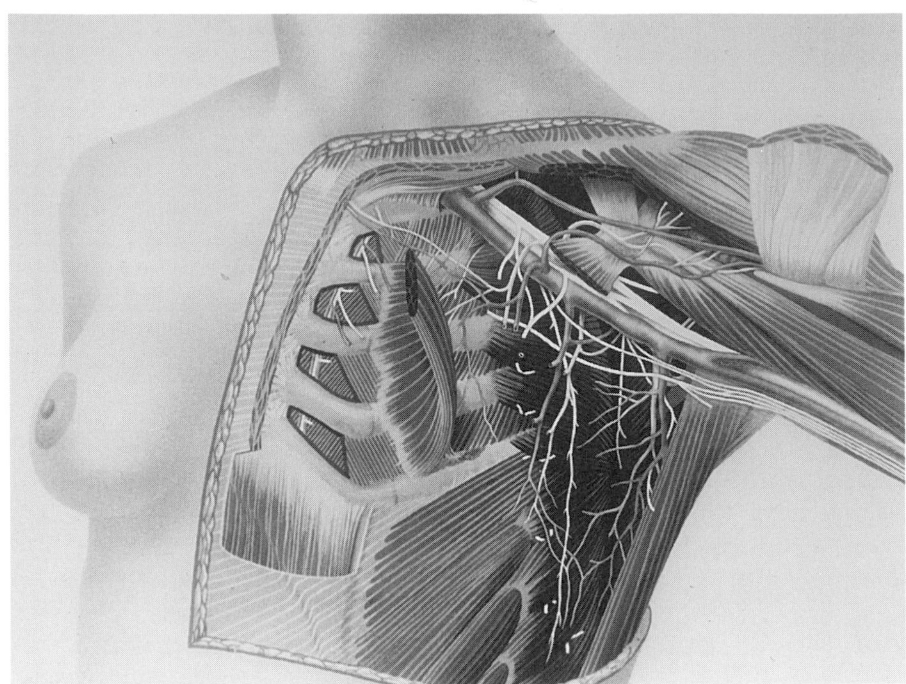

FIGURE 17–11. Chest wall muscles and vascular anatomy. (Adapted from Harris JR, et al: Breast Diseases. Philadelphia: JB Lippincott, 1991, p 6.)

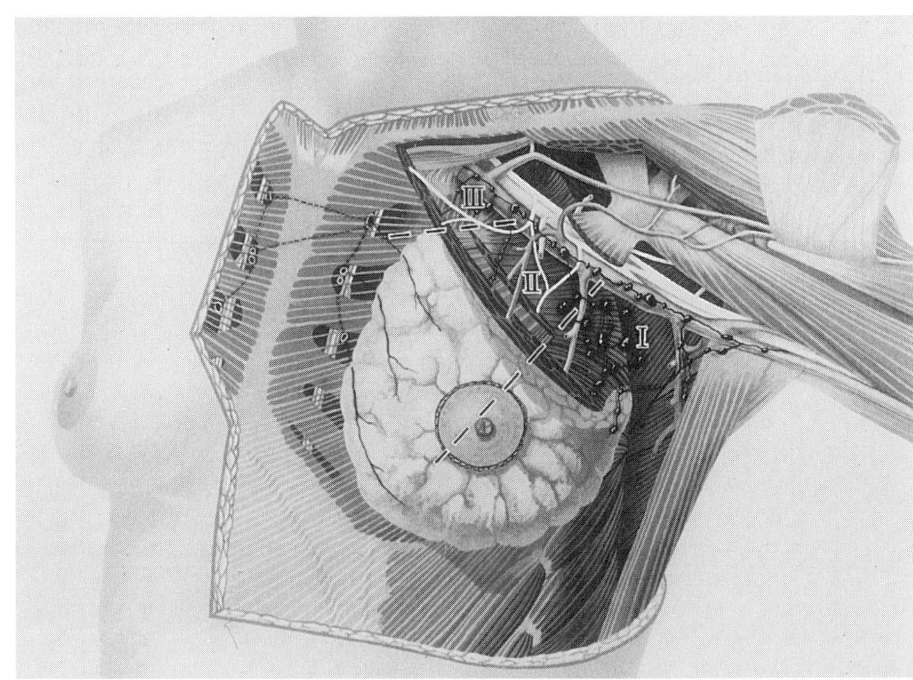

FIGURE 17–12. The lymphatic drainage of the breast showing lymph node groups and levels. (Adapted from Harris JR, et al: Breast Diseases. Philadelphia: JB Lippincott, 1991, p 8.)

brachial plexus origin rather than to their anatomic positions. The arrangement of these nerves is of particular importance in performing the modified radical mastectomy.

The serratus anterior muscle arises by a series of digitations with the external oblique from the upper eight ribs laterally. The muscle inserts into the vertebral border of the scapula and is important to stabilize the scapula. It is supplied by the long thoracic nerve of Bell, which lies superficial to the fascia overlying the anterior serratus muscle. Preservation of this nerve is essential to avoid "winging" of the scapula.[47]

The latissimus dorsi muscle has its origin from the spinous processes and supraspinous ligaments of the seventh thoracic vertebra downward, including all the lumbar and sacral vertebrae. The muscle inserts onto the humerus and is supplied by the thoracodorsal nerve. The nerve courses from behind the axillary vein, passing anterior to the scapular vessels to enter the medial surface of the muscle. Damage of this nerve does not result in any significant cosmetic or functional defect; nevertheless, it should be preserved when possible.[47]

An important landmark in the apex of the axilla is Halsted's ligament. This is formed by two layers of the clavipectoral fascia fusing together to form a well-developed band, which stretches from the coracoid process to the first costochondral junction. At this point, the axillary vessels enter the thorax, passing over the first rib and beneath the clavicle.[47]

PATHOLOGY

Benign Breast Pathology

The benign breast conditions, often grouped together in the catch-all term "fibrocystic disease," can be observed in one half of normal women during their reproductive years. An understanding of the spectrum of benign breast changes is necessary to optimize appropriate treatment and counseling of patients. Various studies have suggested some benign breast changes to be associated with an increased risk for development of breast cancer.[56–59]

The confusion and controversy regarding the relationship between benign breast changes and increased risk derive from the imprecise terminology used to describe benign breast changes (Table 17–2) and the indecisiveness regarding what lesions should be included under the term benign breast changes. Pathologic entities commonly grouped as such include cystic duct dilation, blunt duct adenosis, apocrine metaplasia, fibroadenoma, sclerosing adenosis, radial scar, ductal ectasia, epithelial hyperplasia, and atypical ductal and lobular hyperplasia. To discuss the relative risk for development of breast cancer associated with benign lesions, they are best divided into nonproliferative and proliferative disease.

TABLE 17–2
Terminology Commonly Used for Benign Breast Conditions

Fibrocystic disease	Mastopathy
Schimmelbusch's disease	Papillomatosis
Mastitis	Blue-dome cysts
Cystic mastitis	Adenofibromatosis
Cystic disease	Mazoplasia
Fibroadenomatosis	Adenosis
Mammary dysplasia	Epitheliosis
Chronic cystic mastitis	Nodular hyperplasia

From Simmons R, et al: Pathologic considerations in the high-risk breast patient. Clin Plas Surg 15:656, 1988.

Nonproliferative Disease

Cystic Duct Dilation

Cystic duct dilation is a common clinically and mammographically observed benign breast change. Palpable cysts usually present as soft, pliant nodules, although they can feel quite firm. Cysts may occur as a solitary nodule or in complex clusters. In premenopausal women, cysts often fluctuate in size with the menstrual cycle, typically reaching a maximum in the late luteal phase (postovulation, premenstrual) and diminishing with the onset of menstruation. Clinically evident cysts often resolve with menopause. Macrocysts, or large cysts, may be visible grossly on examination of excised breast tissue. Microscopically, cysts are lined either with apocrine metaplastic cells or a flattened epithelium.

There is no evidence that cystic duct dilation represents a significantly increased risk for development of breast cancer.[58, 60, 61] In a study of 7100 patients with cysts diagnosed by surgical biopsy and followed 30 years, none were observed to have breast cancer.[62] Dupont and Page[63] followed 10,366 patients with breast cysts for 17 years, observing a relative risk of 0.86 in this group compared with that in the general population (risk of 1.0). Cystic duct dilation is found with equal or lesser frequency in cancerous breasts than in benign breast specimens.[64, 65]

Blunt Duct Adenosis

Blunt duct adenosis is usually an incidental finding on breast biopsy performed for another reason. This lesion consists of ducts that end abruptly and do not terminate in lobules. These ducts are lined by normal ductal epithelium.[65]

Blunt duct adenosis has not been shown to represent an increased risk for the development of breast cancer.[64, 66]

Apocrine Metaplasia

Apocrine metaplasia describes a change in the epithelial lining of dilated ducts and cysts. Histologically, apocrine metaplasia consists of tall, large cylindric cells with bright, eosinophilic cytoplasm.

Apocrine metaplasia is not considered to be associated with an increased relative risk for development of breast cancer[58, 64, 65] and has even been considered by some to represent a decreased relative risk.[66]

Fibroadenoma

A fibroadenoma presents as a firm, well-circumscribed mass that is freely mobile within the breast. Fibroadenomas can enlarge rapidly or remain stable in size for years. These are the most common breast tumors in women younger than 25 years of age. They consist of fibrous masses with glandular epithelium compressed into cords by connective tissue, often with a pseudocapsule.

There is doubt among some authorities that fibroadenoma is associated with an increased risk for development of breast cancer.[58, 66]

Sclerosing Adenosis

Sclerosing adenosis can be observed clinically to mimic cancer both on physical examination, as a firm, fixed, poorly circumscribed mass, and on mammogram, as an irregular or stellate lesion, microcalcifications, or both.[67] However, these lesions are most often discovered incidentally on pathologic examination of the breast tissue at biopsy or mastectomy for another reason.[64, 65] The distorted histologic pattern can give the impression of invasion of the surrounding stroma and can be mistaken for invasive breast cancer by less experienced pathologists.

Sclerosing adenosis is not considered to represent an increased risk for the development of breast cancer by some investigators.[58, 60, 61, 65, 66]

Radial Scar

Radial scars usually present mammographically as a stellate mass that mimics a malignancy. They appear histologically as fibroelastic centers with radiating dilated ducts.

Radial scars probably do not represent an increased risk for development of breast cancer.[68]

Ductal Ectasia

Ductal ectasia can present as a palpable tumor or as breast pain and tenderness. Nipple discharge may also be noted. Histologically, ductal ectasia consists of a dilated duct with inspissated material. Leakage into the surrounding tissue may cause an intense inflammatory reaction. The presence of plasma cells in the periductal inflammatory infiltrate results in the condition called plasma cell mastitis.

Ductal ectasia does not represent an increased relative risk for development of breast cancer.[65]

Proliferative Disease

The distinction between nonproliferative disease and proliferative disease is significant with respect to associated breast cancer risk. Proliferative disease should be further subdivided according to the presence or absence of atypia.

Epithelial Hyperplasia

Proliferative disease is almost always an incidental finding in a biopsy specimen. Epithelial proliferation is the multiplication of the ductal epithelial cells within existing ductal and lobular structures.

Women with epithelial hyperplasias are at an increased relative risk for development of breast cancer. Epithelial hyperplasia is found more frequently in cancerous breasts.[69] Conversely, when women with epithelial hyperplasia are followed, their incidence of breast cancer is higher than in women without epithelial hyperplasia.[60, 61] Women with proliferative disease without atypia have a 1.9- to 2.4-fold increased relative risk over women without proliferative disease.[58, 59, 63, 70]

Atypical Epithelial Hyperplasia

Atypical ductal and lobular hyperplasia are described as lesions resembling ductal carcinoma in situ and lobular carcinoma in situ, yet not having all the components necessary to designate them as true in situ carcinomas. If there is any question as to the diagnosis of atypical changes versus in situ carcinoma, the slides should be reviewed by a pathologist who specializes in this area. The borderlines between proliferative lesions, atypical hyperplasias, and in situ carcinomas are not discrete, and interobserver variation, even among expert pathologists, is common.

Atypical hyperplasia does represent an increased risk for development of invasive breast cancer. Several studies have shown atypical epithelial hyperplasia to be present more often in cancerous breasts and breasts contralateral to a cancerous breast than in noncancerous breasts.[60, 64, 66, 69, 71] Atypical epithelial hyperplasia represents a four to six times increased risk for development of breast cancer.[59, 63, 64, 70, 72]

Page et al.[73] followed 10,542 patients with biopsies showing atypical hyperplasia for an average of 17 years. The average time interval to the development of invasive breast cancer from the diagnosis of atypical ductal hyperplasia was 8.2 years (range, 1.4 to 24.3 years) and from the diagnosis of atypical lobular epithelial hyperplasia was 11.9 years (range, 4.6 to 21.9 years). In patients with atypical lesions, the risk for development of breast cancer was 4% to 5% at 30 months, 9% at 46 months, and 10% at 55 months.[74]

The relative risk of atypical hyperplasia greater than doubles when associated with a positive family history. This represents a relative risk of 11 times that of women who have no proliferative disease and no family history of breast cancer (Fig. 17–13).[63] Twenty percent of the women with atypia and family history had breast cancer within 15 years versus 8% with atypia but no family history.[63]

Ductal Carcinoma In Situ

Ductal carcinoma in situ (DCIS; intraductal carcinoma) is most often an incidental finding on pathologic examination unless associated with mammographic calcifications. However, when extensive and involving large volumes of breast tissue, DCIS may be palpable. The histologic patterns of DCIS are solid, cribriform, papillary, and comedo. In the comedo type, the ducts often have expressible cores

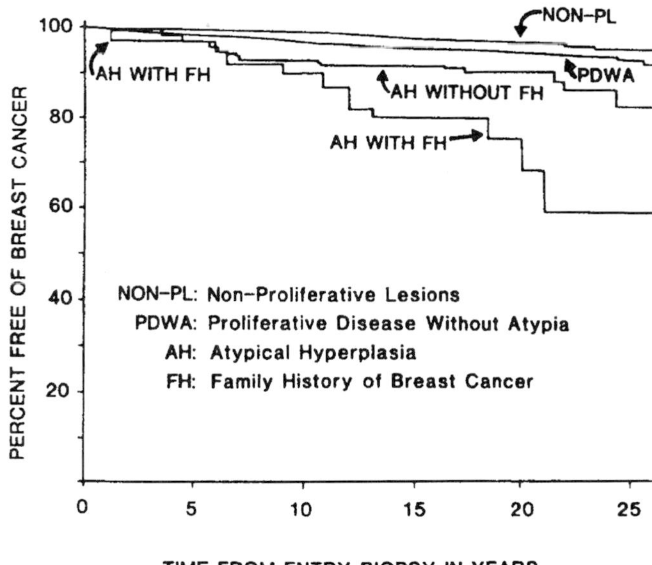

FIGURE 17–13. Proportion of patients free of invasive breast cancer, as a function of time since the entry biopsy. (From Dupont WD, Page DL: Risk factors for breast cancer in women with proliferative disease. N Engl J Med 312:146–151, 1985.)

of soft necrotic material. This central plug of necrotic material resembles a comedo, thus the name "comedo carcinoma" for this form of DCIS (Fig. 17–14).

DCIS is frequently present in breasts containing invasive cancer.[69, 75] It is frequently multifocal.[69, 76, 77] The rate of multicentricity is 33%[76, 77] to 36%.[78] The subsequent invasive breast cancer is usually ipsilateral.[75]

In patients with DCIS treated with biopsy alone, infiltrating breast cancer developed in the same breast in 39%, with an average latency period of 10 years.[79] The average interval from diagnosis of DCIS to the development of clinically detectable invasive breast cancer is 9.7 years in patients treated with biopsy alone.[79, 80]

In a study by Cutuli and colleagues,[81] the local recurrence rate for DCIS was compared with treatment of radical mastectomy and breast conservation. At 55 months, the local recurrence rate of the radical mastectomy group was 3% and the local recurrence rate of the conservative treatment group was 9%. Similar results were found by Lagios et al.,[82] with a 10% 10-year local recurrence in DCIS treated with local excision without irradiation.

In the National Surgical Adjuvant Breast Project (NSABP) B-06 trial, the results of lumpectomy alone versus lumpectomy and radiation for DCIS were evaluated. Of those women treated with lumpectomy alone, 23% recurred within or close to the initial surgical site in a period up to 53 months. Only 7% of those who received radiation as well had a local recurrence.[83]

In patients with DCIS, an axillary node dissection is not justified. In a study by Silverstein and coworkers,[84] only 1 patient with DCIS of 175 who had axillary lymph node dissections was positive. In patients with microinvasion, axillary node dissection may be justified. With microinvasion, there is a positive axillary node dissection in 2% to 20% of patients.[85–88]

Lobular Carcinoma In Situ

Lobular carcinoma in situ (LCIS) is clinically asymptomatic. It is associated with an increased frequency of subsequent invasive carcinoma, either ductal or lobular invasive.

LCIS is a proliferation of the epithelial cells in the terminal lobular unit, until this proliferation fills the acini (Fig. 17–15). This pathologic entity was described in a classic article by Foote and Stewart in 1940.[89]

LCIS is often seen in mastectomy specimens associated with invasive cancer.[71, 90, 91] It is frequently multifocal,

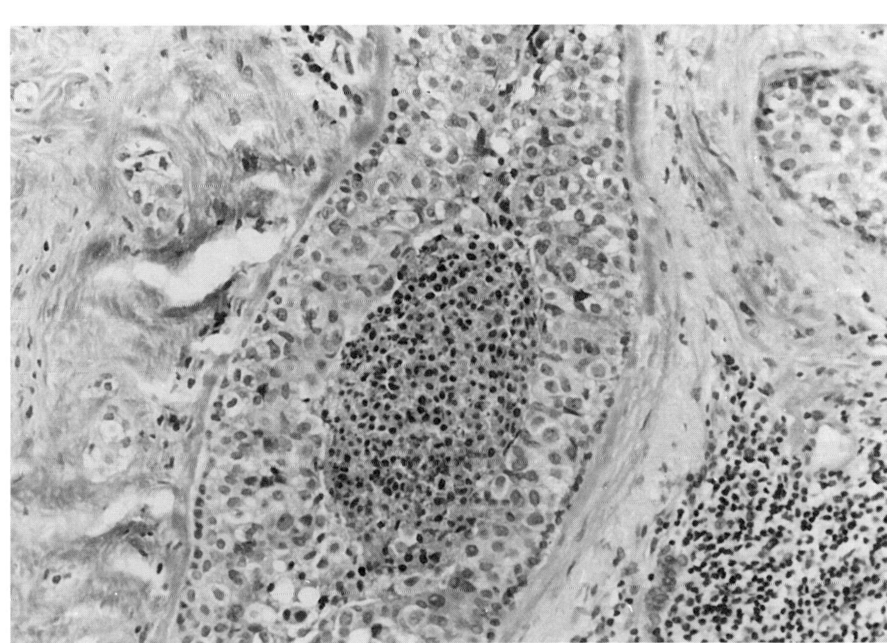
FIGURE 17–14. Ductal carcinoma in situ/comedocarcinoma: Mammary duct containing pleomorphic neoplastic cells, with central necrosis. (Courtesy of Dr. Syed Hoda, Department of Pathology, New York Hospital–Cornell Medical Center.)

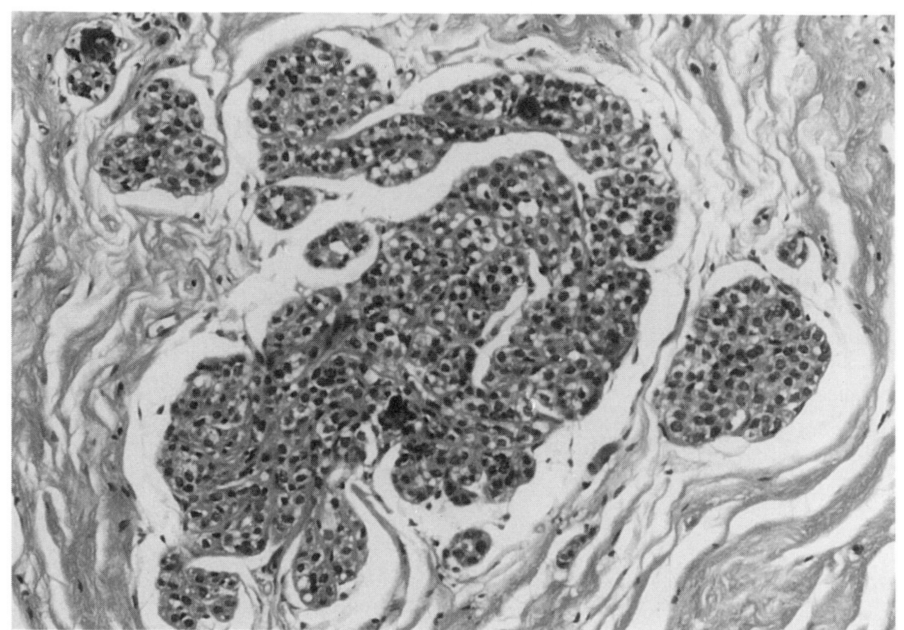

FIGURE 17–15. Lobular carcinoma in situ: Normal lobular epithelium replaced by neoplastic uniformly rounded cells that fill and distend the acinar glands. (Courtesy of Dr. Syed Hoda, Department of Pathology, New York Hospital–Cornell Medical Center.)

multicentric, and bilateral.[65, 90, 92] Multicentricity has been noted in 42.9%[77] to 90% of specimens studied. In patients treated for LCIS with mastectomy, 4% to 6% of the breast specimens contain invasive cancer.[91] The probability of development of invasive cancer is equal for the contralateral and the ipsilateral breast.[91, 93, 94] In women with LCIS treated with local excision, the incidence of development of subsequent invasive cancers is nine times the relative risk.[95] In approximately 25% to 33% of these women, a subsequent carcinoma develops.[91]

With LCIS treated with local excision, the incidence of ipsilateral invasive breast cancer at 5 years was 8%, at 10 years 15%, at 15 years 27%, and at 20 years 35%.[98] Similar results were found by Walt et al.,[96] with a 14.8% incidence rate in a follow-up period of 96 months.

The contralateral incidence at 10 years was 10%, at 15 years 15%, and at 20 years 25%.[97] Of the recurrences, only half appeared in the first decade after initial surgical treatment.[98]

The ipsilateral interval to development of invasive breast cancer ranged from 2 to 31 years, with 32% occurring after 20 years. The contralateral interval ranged from 3 to 30 years, with 44% occurring at more than 20 years. In 38% of the patients in whom invasive breast cancer eventually developed, there was no evidence of disease until more than 20 years.[99] The incidence of future invasive breast cancer after the diagnosis of LCIS did not vary with the age of the patient at the time of the initial LCIS diagnosis.[100]

Malignant Breast Pathology

Infiltrating Ductal Carcinoma

Infiltrating ductal carcinoma, not otherwise specified (IFDC,NOS), is the most common of the invasive breast cancers, representing 65% to 80% of breast tumors.[101] This is typically a solid tumor that presents as a hard mass on examination. In cutting the tumor, the consistency is often gritty. There is often DCIS present with IFDC,NOS.

The prognosis is the poorest of the invasive breast cancers, excluding inflammatory carcinoma (Fig. 17–16).

Tubular Carcinoma

Tubular carcinoma is a subtype of invasive ductal carcinoma, representing 2% of breast cancers.[47] This is typically well differentiated, with proliferation of tubular ductal structures.[101]

The prognosis is generally good, with axillary metastases rarely found (Fig. 17–17).[101]

Medullary Carcinoma

Less than 5% of invasive breast cancer is of the medullary type.[47] These tumors often grow rapidly in sheets rather than forming glands. On presentation, they are often large, with central hemorrhage or necrosis present.

The prognosis is typically good, with fewer axillary metastases than with IFDC,NOS.[101]

Mucinous Carcinoma

Mucinous carcinoma, sometimes called colloid or gelatinous carcinoma, represents 1% to 3% of invasive breast cancer. The growth of these tumors is usually slow. They are characterized by a gelatinous matrix containing clusters of malignant cells within it.

The prognosis is generally good compared with that in IFDC,NOS (Fig. 17–18).[101]

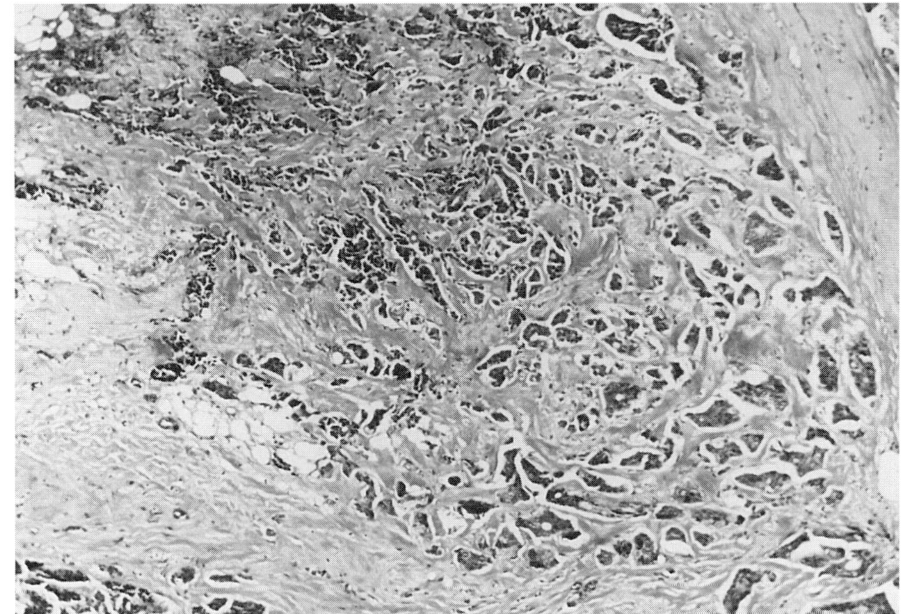

FIGURE 17–16. Infiltrating duct carcinoma: Tumor, with a tendency to form glands, infiltrating mammary stroma. Grading of infiltrative duct carcinoma is an estimate of differentiation and takes into consideration extent of tubule formation, nuclear grading, and mitotic rate. This is an intermediate (grade II) infiltrative carcinoma. (Courtesy of Dr. Syed Hoda, Department of Pathology, New York Hospital–Cornell Medical Center.)

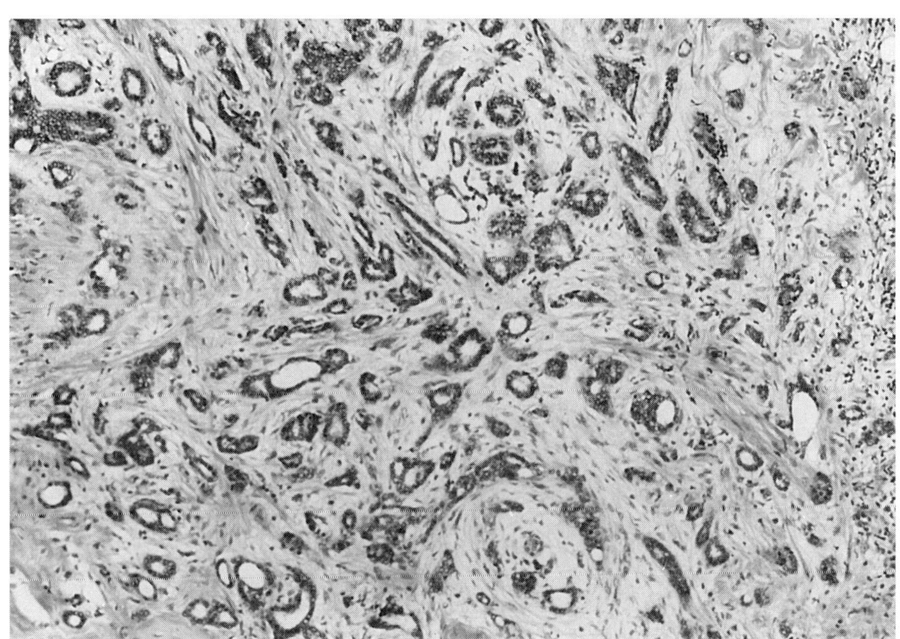

FIGURE 17–17. Tubular carcinoma: Randomly arranged neoplastic glands, with oval to angulated contours, invading collagenous stroma. (Courtesy of Dr. Syed Hoda, Department of Pathology, New York Hospital–Cornell Medical Center.)

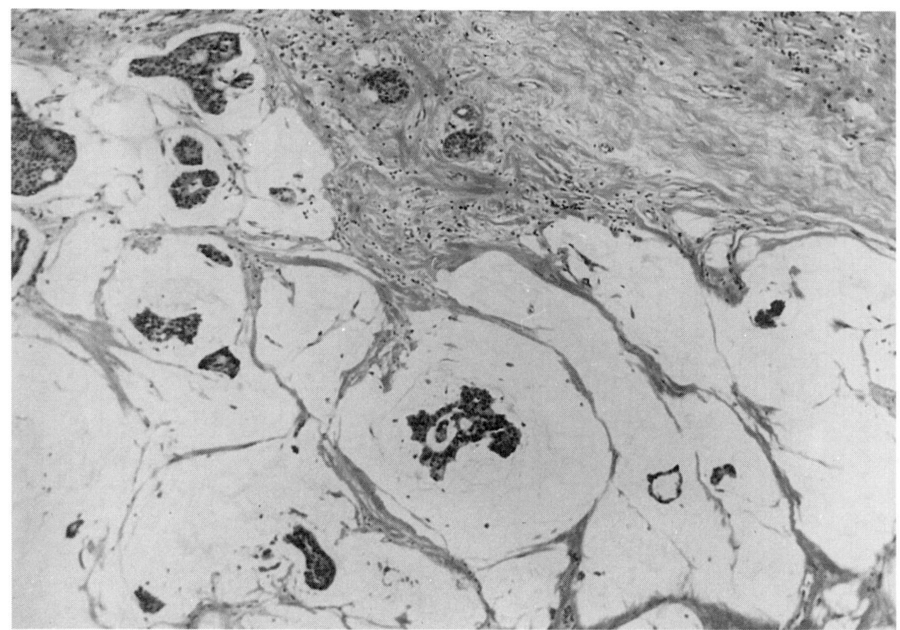

FIGURE 17–18. Mucinous carcinoma: Clusters of neoplastic cells lying in a background of mucinous secretion. (Courtesy of Dr. Syed Hoda, Department of Pathology, New York Hospital–Cornell Medical Center.)

Papillary Carcinoma

Most papillary intracystic cancers are noninvasive. The nonmalignant form of similar appearance is an intraductal papilloma. These tumors present with serous or bloody nipple discharge in 22% to 34% of cases (Fig. 17–19).[101]

Infiltrating Lobular Carcinoma

Infiltrating lobular carcinoma represents 5% to 10% of invasive breast cancer. These tumors may present as a palpable mass that is ill-defined or as a vague thickening, unlike the hard mass of IFDC,NOS.[101] Histologically, they are characterized by small cells in a linear arrangement called "Indian filing."[101] These tumors are prone to multicentricity and bilaterality.[101] The likelihood of axillary involvement and the prognosis are similar to those in IFDS,NOS (Fig. 17–20).[101]

Inflammatory Carcinoma

This is not a histologic type but a clinical entity. The presentation is typically of an erythematous, indurated, edematous, warm breast, often with peau d'orange, resembling an inflammatory reaction (see Fig. 17–6). The diagnosis is confirmed by the presence of involvement of the dermal lymphatics of the breast. The pathology of the underlying cancer is usually IFDC,NDOS. The tumor is generally poorly differentiated. Axillary lymph nodes are positive in 91% of these patients.[47]

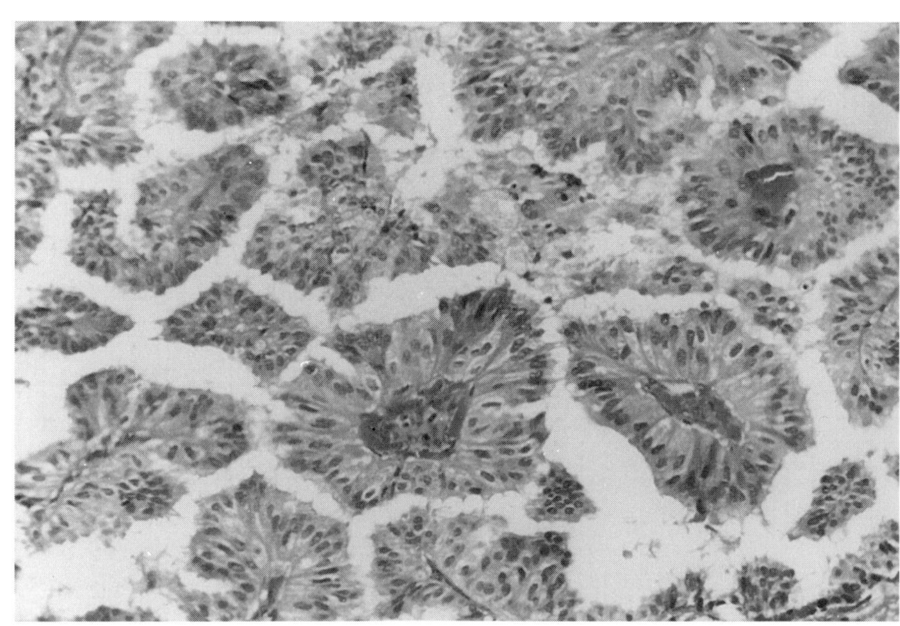

FIGURE 17–19. Papillary carcinoma: Crowded neoplastic columnar cells cover papillary fibrovascular fronds. (Courtesy of Dr. Syed Hoda, Department of Pathology, New York Hospital–Cornell Medical Center.)

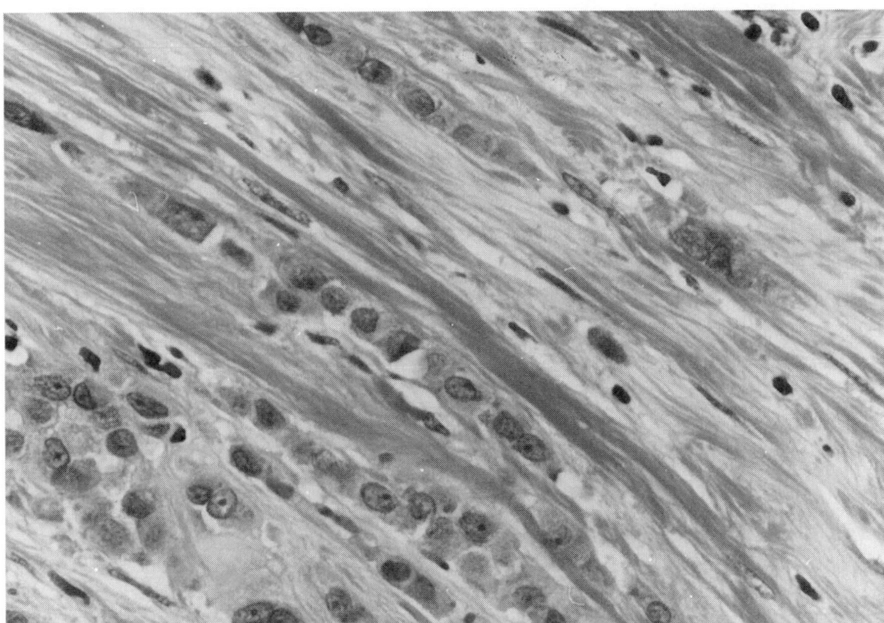

FIGURE 17–20. Infiltrating lobular carcinoma: Classic linear growth pattern of neoplastic cells in infiltrating lobular carcinoma (so-called "Indian filing"). (Courtesy of Dr. Syed Hoda, Department of Pathology, New York Hospital–Cornell Medical Center.)

These patients have an extremely poor prognosis, and the best treatment for inflammatory breast cancer is upfront chemotherapy and radiation followed by mastectomy.[102–104] Surgery should follow radiation in 2 to 4 weeks. In the postsurgical period, chemotherapy is resumed with doxorubicin (Adriamycin).

The feasibility of breast conservation surgery after induction chemotherapy has been investigated.[102, 105, 106] Considerably higher local failure rates (20% vs. 52%) were found in patients treated with breast conservation than in those with mastectomy.[102]

Paget Disease

Paget disease represents 1% to 4% of breast cancer. It typically presents as a crusting, scaling, erosion of the nipple, similar in appearance to eczema (see Fig. 17–7). Owing to its confusion with benign dermatologic changes, the diagnosis is often delayed. The diagnosis is made by a punch or incisional biopsy of the nipple. Histologically, there are large cells with pale cytoplasm and prominent, irregular nuclei (Paget cells) present in the epidermis of the nipple (Fig. 17–21). These nipple changes are associated with underlying carcinoma, typically DCIS or IFDC, NOS.

The standard treatment, especially with evidence of diffuse malignancy, is total mastectomy and axillary dissection. Segmental resection and radiation have been used occasionally. The prognosis of this tumor is the same as that of the underlying tumor and its axillary involvement.[101]

Cystosarcoma Phyllodes

These fleshy tumors resembling fibroadenomas can be benign or malignant. Although historically most phyllodes tumors presented as very large masses, many are now detected at a small size owing to mammography. When malignant, they infrequently metastasize to axillary nodes but, rather, act more consistently with other sarcomas, with metastases to the lung initially.

The recommended treatment is surgical excision with a 2-cm tumor-free margin with malignant tumors or total mastectomy. Even the benign tumors recur if incompletely excised. Because of the type of metastases, axillary dissection is not recommended. If metastatic disease is present, it is treated with adjuvant chemotherapy as with other sarcomatous tumors.[47]

Miscellaneous

Other tumors, such as angiosarcoma, lymphoma, and squamous cell carcinoma, uncommonly present in the breast. These are generally treated as in other parts of the body, with mastectomy and radiation or chemotherapy for sarcomas and squamous cell carcinomas and with biopsy diagnosis and radiation or chemotherapy, or both, for lymphoma.[47]

PROGNOSIS

Clinical Staging

Clinical staging is done by examining and assessing the breast and the axillary, supraclavicular, and cervical lymph nodes. Operative findings, such as the size of the primary tumor and invasion of the chest wall and gross involvement of regional lymph nodes, are included in the clinical staging. Any preoperative metastatic disease work-up is also considered part of the clinical staging.

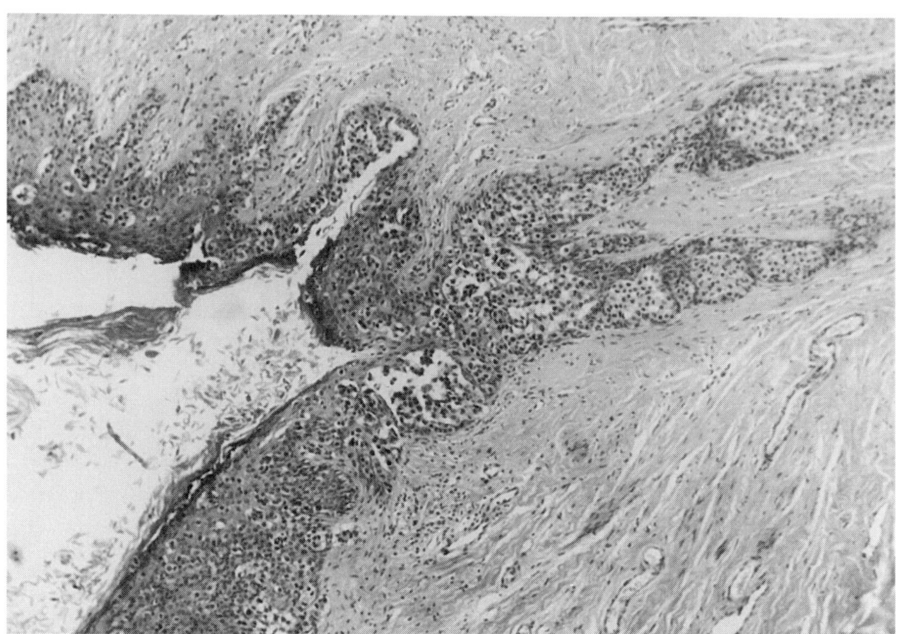

FIGURE 17–21. Paget disease of nipple: Terminal portion of lactiferous ducts at its junction with the nipple epidermis. The duct contains intraductal carcinoma, and there is contiguous Paget disease in the epidermis. (Courtesy of Dr. Syed Hoda, Department of Pathology, New York Hospital–Cornell Medical Center.)

Pathologic Staging

The pathologic staging is determined by evaluation of the pathologic specimen.

TNM Classification

The standard method of classifying breast cancers is with the American Joint Committee on Cancer (AJCC) tumor (T), nodal status (N), and metastasis (M) system. This classification is presented in Table 17–3. Several points of the classification may need further elaboration:

In Situ Tumor: If there is an in situ and an invasive component of a tumor, the invasive component is the measured value for staging.

Multiple Simultaneous Ipsilateral Primary Carcinomas: The largest primary tumor is used to classify the tumor size.

Simultaneous Contralateral Primary Carcinomas: Each tumor is classified separately.

Paget Disease of the Nipple: If there is no associated invasive carcinoma in the specimen, it is classified Tis. If there is an invasive component of the tumor, it is considered as any other tumor.

Prognostic Factors

Axillary Lymph Node Status

The number of positive nodes is predictive of survival when broken down into three or less and four or more.[107] The 5-year freedom from distant relapse is 86% in node-negative patients, 78% in those with one to three involved nodes, and 45% in those with four or more involved nodes.[108]

Tumor Size

The size of the primary tumor is a significant predictor of patient prognosis, generally with the risk of recurrence increasing with increasing tumor size.[109, 110] In tumors ≤1 cm, there is an excellent prognosis, with less than 10% recurrence in 10 years.[109] The size of the primary tumor is directly related to the likelihood of involved positive nodes.[110, 111] Tumor size is a particularly significant predictor of prognosis in node-negative patients.[110, 112] Even in patients with positive lymph nodes, the size of the tumor (≤2 cm or >2 cm) is predictive of survival.[109]

Histologic Type

Several well-differentiated subtypes of breast cancer have a relatively favorable prognosis. These include medullary, tubular, colloid (mucinous), and papillary carcinomas. Inflammatory carcinoma has an extremely poor prognosis.

Hormone Receptor Status

Estrogen receptor (ER) protein of the primary cancer and progesterone receptor (PR) protein levels are measured in fentimoles (fmol) per milligram of cytosol protein. A tumor with a level above 10 fmol is usually considered positive, although there may be some variability in particular laboratories.

Fisher et al.[113] evaluated the predictive power of ER, PR, and histologic grade as to disease-free survival, distant disease-free survival, and overall survival in node-negative patients. In ER-positive, node-negative patients, the disease-free survival and survival were significantly better than in those patients with ER-negative tumors. PR status made no independent prediction of prognosis. The advan-

TABLE 17–3
TNM Classification for Breast Cancer

Primary Tumor (T)	
TX	Primary tumor cannot be assessed
T0	No evidence of primary tumor
Tis	Carcinoma in situ: intraductal carcinoma, lobular carcinoma in situ, or Paget disease of the nipple with no tumor
T1	Tumor 2 cm or less in greatest dimension
	T1a 0.5 cm or less in greatest dimension
	T1b More than 0.5 cm but not more than 1 cm in greatest dimension
	T1c More than 1 cm but not more than 2 cm in greatest dimension
T2	Tumor more than 2 cm but not more than 5 cm in greatest dimension
T3	Tumor more than 5 cm in greatest dimension
T4	Tumor of any size with direct extension to chest wall or skin
	T4a Extension to chest wall
	T4b Edema (including peau d'orange) or ulceration of the skin of the breast or satellite skin nodules confined to the same breast
	T4c Both (T4a and T4b)
	T4d Inflammatory carcinoma
Regional Lymph Nodes (N)	
NX	Regional lymph nodes cannot be assessed (e.g., previously removed)
N0	No regional lymph node metastasis
N1	Metastasis to movable ipsilateral axillary lymph node(s)
N2	Metastasis to ipsilateral axillary lymph node(s) fixed to one another or to other structures
N3	Metastasis to ipsilateral internal mammary lymph node(s)
Distant Metastasis (M)	
MX	Presence of distant metastasis cannot be assessed
M0	No distant metastasis
M1	Distant metastasis (includes metastasis to ipsilateral supraclavicular lymph node(s))

Stage Grouping			
Stage 0	Tis	N0	M0
Stage I	T1	N0	M0
Stage IIA	T0	N1	M0
	T1	N1	M0
	T2	N0	M0
Stage IIB	T2	N1	M0
	T3	N0	M0
Stage IIIA	T0	N2	M0
	T1	N2	M0
	T2	N2	M0
	T3	N1	M0
	T3	N2	M0
Stage IIIB	T4	Any N	M0
	Any T	N3	M0
Stage IV	Any T	Any N	M1

tage of positive ER and PR is only 8% to 10%, however, after 5 years.[106] Also, in patients with positive axillary nodes, the ER and PR status is predictive of survival.[107, 110]

Histologic Grade

Histologic grade is determined by the architectural arrangement of cells, the degree of nuclear differentiation, and the mitotic rate. Generally, a higher nuclear grade is associated with an increased risk of recurrence.[109, 113] The 5-year freedom from distant relapse is 96% and 75% for histologic grades I-II and III, respectively.[108]

S Phase

The S phase is a measurement of cell proliferative rate. In node-positive patients, the S-phase fraction is predictive of survival. As the S phase increases, the survival decreases accordingly.[107, 114] Higher S-phase levels have also been shown to be associated with increased recurrence rates. With S-phase fractions greater than or equal to 10%, there were three times more recurrences than in patients with lower S-phase fractions.

Other Factors

Other tumor characteristics, such as the presence of HER-2/neu and cathepsin D, may be associated with a poor prognosis. These as well as numerous other putative prognostic indicators are currently under investigation.

TREATMENT

There has been a significant shift in the prevailing paradigms of the natural history of breast cancer over the last few decades that has resulted in a revolution in both surgical and nonsurgical approaches to this disease and in opinions regarding the curability of breast cancer and the effectiveness of strategies such as screening mammography. The Halsted paradigm, which hypothesized contiguous, orderly local advance of breast cancer through the breast and thence to adjacent skin and lymph nodes in the axilla and from these distantly but in continuity, has largely been replaced by the Fisher paradigm, which theorizes that breast cancer is a disease that is systemic from very early on in its course if not at its inception. In the Fisher paradigm, axillary nodes are conceived of not as barriers to the further spread of disease but rather as indicators of disease aggressiveness. Thus, removal of lymph nodes provides a prognostic marker of some importance but has little impact on disease progression. The implication of the Halsted paradigm is that more intensive local treatment leads to a higher rate of cure, while the Fisher paradigm suggests that local treatment has relatively little impact on long-term survival.

In reality, none of the paradigms used to explain the evolution and course of breast cancer, from the early Galenic hypothesis that the disease resulted from an excess of black bile to the biologic models of Halsted and Fisher, adequately explain the highly variable nature of this disease. Knowledge derived from modern molecular biology can be used to support some of what seems so fanciful in the early humoral hypotheses of disease origin. Breast cancer cells are known to secrete growth factors that are in turn influenced by hormones such as estrogen. Halsted's ideas regarding the importance of local control were likewise not entirely unfounded. Breast cancer does have a predilection to both arise and recur at the site of the breast itself. Such recurrences, often occurring many years after

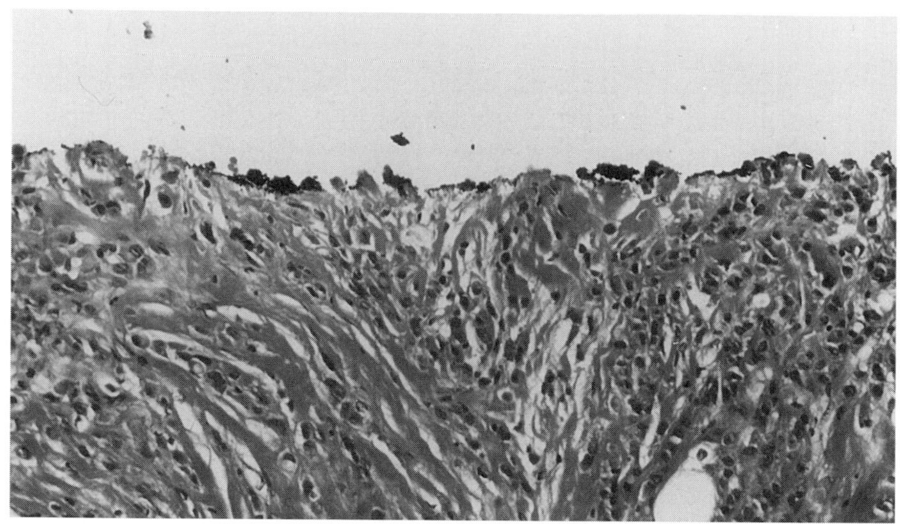

FIGURE 17–22. Mammary carcinoma at inked margin: Positive margin with infiltrative carcinoma of resection. (Courtesy of Dr. Syed Hoda, Department of Pathology, New York Hospital–Cornell Medical Center.)

the original diagnosis, are not adequately explained by a hypothesis that proposes early systemic spread as the origin of all distant metastases.

Surgical Procedures

Surgical Biopsy

In the United States, the ratio of biopsies performed for each cancer detected ranges from 3 to over 10. Unless other diagnostic methods, such as fine-needle aspiration and core biopsy, are used, it is difficult to exceed a true positive biopsy rate of 30% to 40% without missing the smallest occult cancers. True positive rates higher than this suggest one of three possibilities: (1) the threshold rate for recommending biopsy is too high (i.e., only the most definitively diagnosable lesions are being selected for biopsy); (2) overdiagnosis by the pathologist (i.e., borderline lesions are diagnosed more frequently as cancers rather than atypical hyperplasia or other benign hyperplastic conditions); or (3) preselection of cases has been accomplished by means of fine-needle aspiration cytology or core biopsy. Experience in Europe suggests that preselection can raise the true positive yield to 40% to 60%, or approximately one benign biopsy for each cancer detected.

Incisional Biopsy

On very large breast masses, an incisional biopsy should be done for diagnosis only. After the confirmation of cancer, the appropriate definitive surgical procedure can be performed either during the same operation or as another procedure.

Excisional Biopsy

Once the specimen with grossly clean margins is resected, it should be submitted to pathology in its intact, unfixed form. It is often helpful for designing any further surgical procedure to have the specimen oriented relative to the lateral and superior margins with sutures or clips. A frozen section diagnosis may or may not be performed, as appropriate for the given surgical case. On malignancies that are of sufficient size, a portion of the specimen should be submitted for hormone receptor analysis. All specimens should be inked by the pathologist for microscopic margin evaluation. Electrocautery should not be used because the thermal effect may cause tissue distortion and thus difficulty in evaluating the surgical margins (Fig. 17–22).

Needle Localization Biopsy

Surgical excision of a suspicious mammographic abnormality that is not palpable requires special techniques in order to ensure that the appropriate area is removed without sacrifice of large amounts of uninvolved breast tissue. Various methods of preoperative localization have been developed for this purpose. In this country, needle localization methods are the most popular; localization with dyes and inert carbon are somewhat more frequently used in Europe. Two critical steps are involved in localization methods: (1) placement of a marker (e.g., needle, wire, dye, carbon) in or near the lesion to be removed using x-ray mammographic, ultrasound, or stereotactic guidance, and (2) performance of a specimen radiograph of the excised tissue, preferably at the time of surgery. Specimen radiographs should be performed during all breast biopsies requiring localization to ensure that the appropriate tissue has been excised (Figs. 17–23*A* to *D* and 17–24*A* to *D*).

The successful needle localization is a cooperative effort involving the patient, radiologist, surgeon, and pathologist. For needle localizations performed with x-ray mammographic guidance, the needle is inserted using the position that provides the shortest distance to the lesion. Although this can be performed freehand, estimating distance and position from preliminary orthogonal views, most American radiologists prefer to use a localizing grid and an

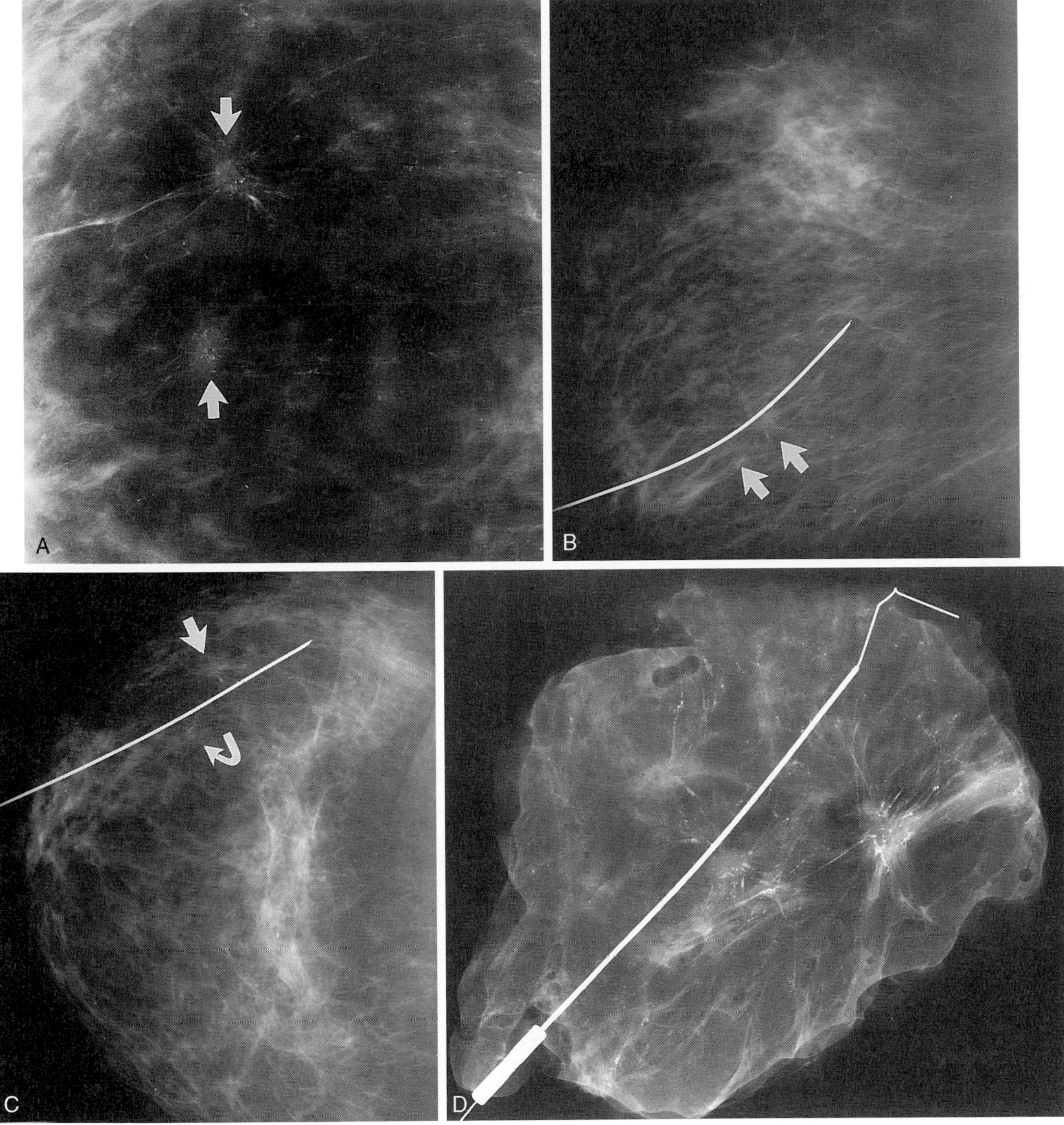

FIGURE 17–23. *A,* Detail of magnified craniocaudal view of right breast of 59-year-old woman on tamoxifen after contralateral mastectomy for invasive breast cancer 2 years previously. At least two tiny spiculated areas (arrows) are visible, each containing microcalcifications. Calcification extends along the spicules, and there is also extensive calcification in surrounding tissue. *B,* Lateral view following freehand introduction of localization needle. The spiculated areas (arrows) are just below the axis of the needle, which courses through the area containing microcalcifications. *C,* Corresponding craniocaudal view shows one of the spiculated areas (straight arrow) just lateral to the axis of the needle and another (curved arrow) just medial to it. There is fine calcification all along the course of the wire. *D,* Specimen radiograph with hook wire and stiffening cannula in position shows at least four spiculated masses and extensive malignant calcification. Histology showed multifocal invasive duct cancer with an extensive intraductal component extending to the margin at several sites.

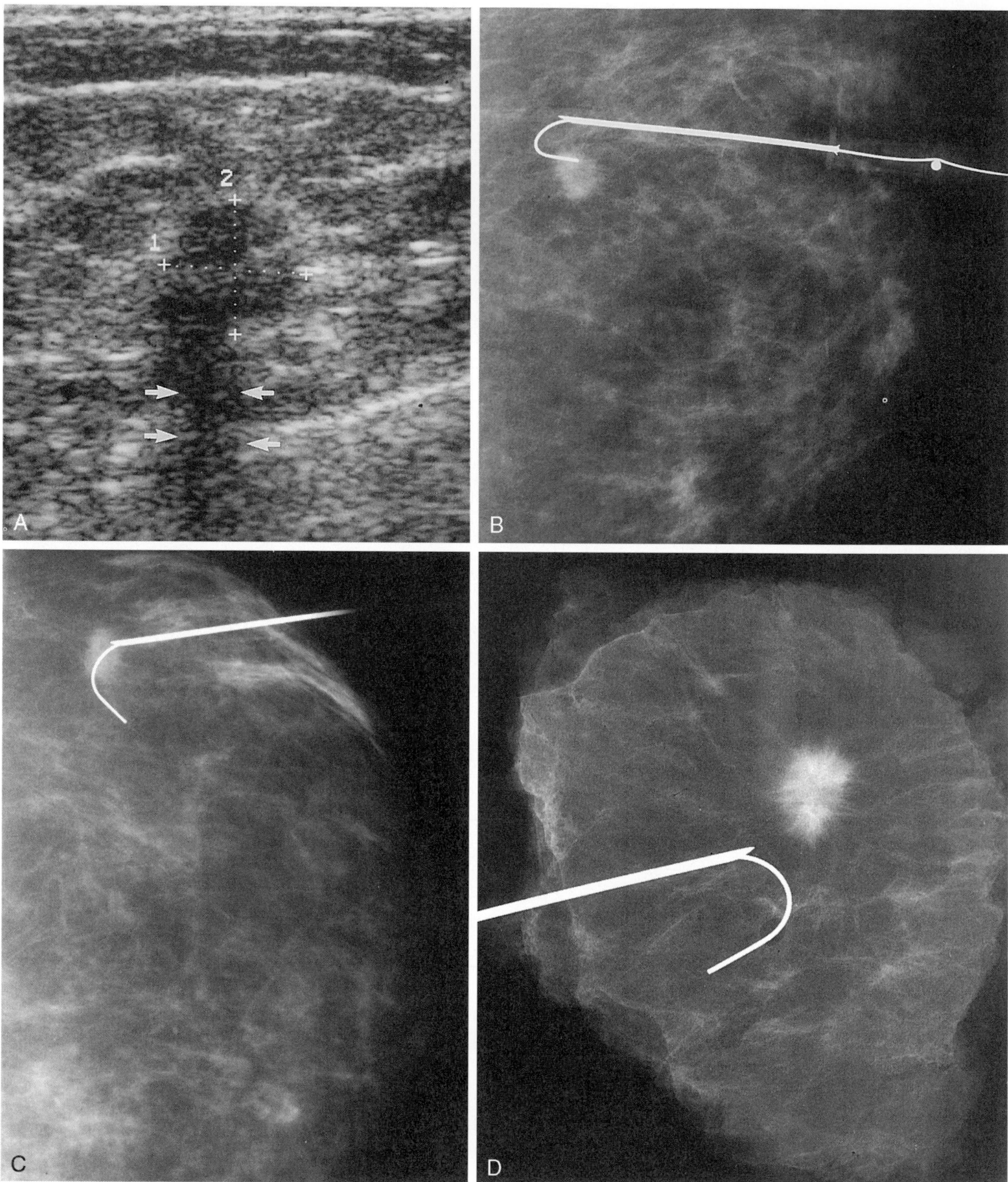

FIGURE 17–24. *A,* Ultrasound of 1-cm solid irregular nodule with distal acoustic shadowing (arrows) shown on mammogram as spiculated mass in fatty breast. *B,* Lateral view following introduction of curved wire under ultrasound guidance for localization of mass shown in *A*. The wire extends around the posterosuperior margin of the mass. *C,* Corresponding craniocaudal view showing appropriately positioned wire. *D,* Specimen radiograph demonstrating the excised noncalcified spiculated mass. Histology showed a 1-cm invasive duct cancer.

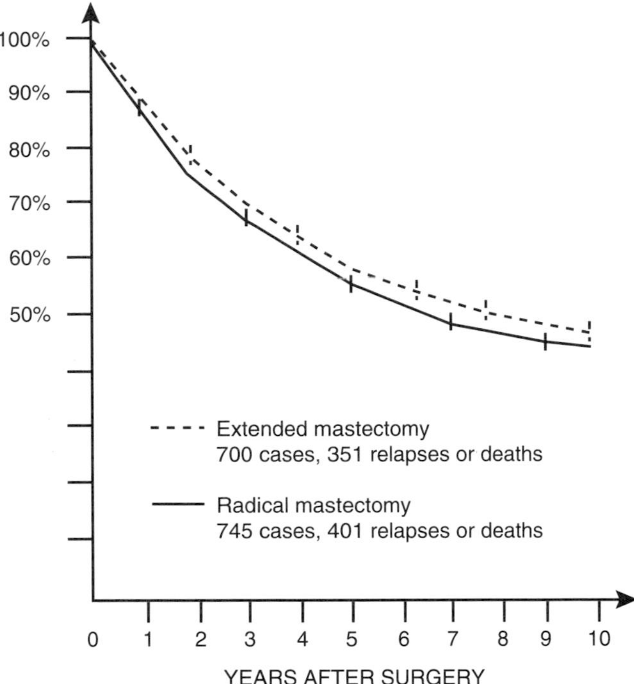

FIGURE 17–25. Ten-year relapse-free survival curves by treatment. (From Lacour J, et al: Radical mastectomy versus radical mastectomy plus internal mammary dissection: Ten year results of an international cooperative trial in breast cancer. Cancer 51:1941–1943, 1983.)

approach that parallels the chest wall. The skin over the chosen needle entry site is prepared, and local anesthesia is often administered. A needle containing a thin wire is then inserted through an opening in the plastic compression plate immobilizing the breast and is advanced fully or until a lesion is encountered. A mammogram in the appropriate projection is then obtained to assess depth of the needle relative to the area being localized. Adjustment is made if necessary, and the wire is extruded from the needle. In most cases, the needle is then withdrawn. A final set of mammograms is obtained to show the position of the lesion relative to the tip of the wire. More than one wire may be placed to bracket a more extensive area of involvement or to localize multiple lesions.

Extended Radical Mastectomy

The extended radical mastectomy involves the removal of the breast, pectoral muscles, axillary contents, and internal mammary lymph nodes on the ipsilateral side. Conceptualized by Halsted in 1889, this operation was popularized in the United States in the 1950s.[115]

The results of an international cooperative trial comparing radical and extended radical mastectomy showed no statistically significant differences between the 10-year relapse-free survival rate, overall survival rate, and local recurrence rate (Figs. 17–25 and 17–26).[116] These results are supported by a randomized trial at the University of Chicago comparing extended radical and standard radical mastectomy. Overall, the 10-year survival rate was not statistically significant.[117]

There is a difference in outcome with lateral versus central and medial tumors. Although there is no evidence of improved survival with lateral tumors, an improvement in survival has been shown with central and inner quadrant tumors treated with extended radical mastectomy. However, survival rate and risk of distant metastasis in central and inner quadrant tumors were equal with internal mammary nodes by either dissection or radiation.[117, 118] With improvement in the quality of radiotherapy, and less enthusiasm for radical surgery, the extended radical mastectomy is seldom used in current surgical practice.

Radical Mastectomy

Popularized by Halsted, the radical mastectomy involves en bloc resection of the breast, pectoral muscles, and axillary contents. Although the modified radical mastectomy has mostly replaced the radical mastectomy in current surgical practice, the radical mastectomy still offers an excellent palliative treatment in advanced cases in which there is pectoral muscle invasion or Rotter's node involvement.

Modified Radical Mastectomy

Modified radical mastectomy, as described by Patey, involves resection of the breast, with the overlying skin to

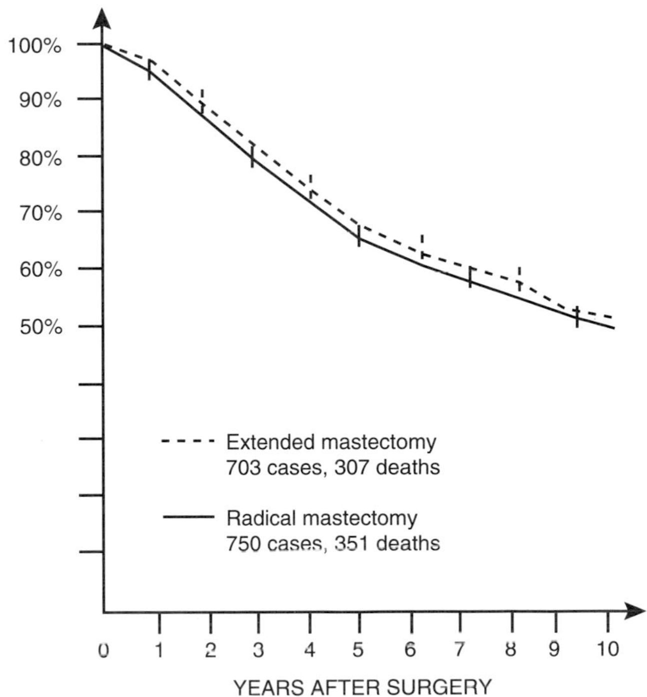

FIGURE 17–26. Ten-year overall survival curves by treatment. (From Lacour J, et al: Radical mastectomy versus radical mastectomy plus internal mammary dissection: Ten year results of an international cooperative trial in breast cancer. Cancer 51:1941–1943, 1983.)

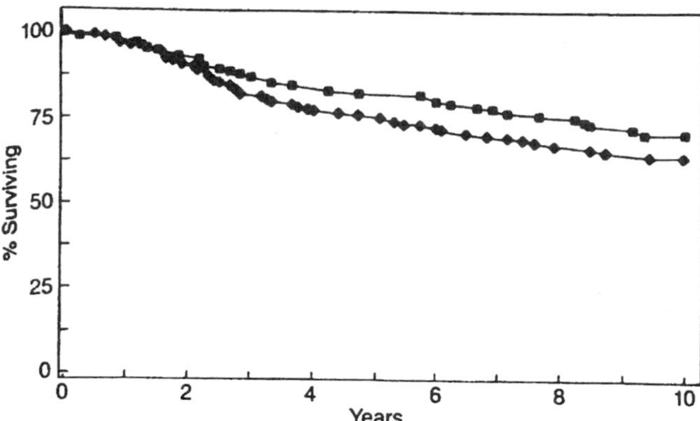

FIGURE 17–27. Overall survival of patients who underwent radical (squares, n = 136) and modified radical (diamonds, n = 175) mastectomy. (From Maddox WA, et al: Does radical mastectomy still have a place in the treatment of primary operable breast cancer? Arch Surg 122:1317–1320, 1987.)

include the previous biopsy incision, pectoralis major fascia, pectoralis minor muscle, and axillary lymph nodes, with preservation of the pectoralis major muscle. Auchincloss[120] supports preservation of the pectoralis minor muscle as well.

Several trials have compared the modified radical mastectomy with the radical mastectomy, finding no advantage to the radical mastectomy in terms of total survival (Fig. 17–27).[121, 122] Overall survival was better, however, in certain groups of patients, such as those with T2 tumors with clinically positive nodes and those with T3 tumors, when radical mastectomy was compared with modified radical mastectomy.[121]

There is a slight increase in local recurrence rates in the patients treated with the modified operation, with a 10-year local recurrence rate of 11% in the modified radical group and 6% in the radical group (Fig. 17–28).[121]

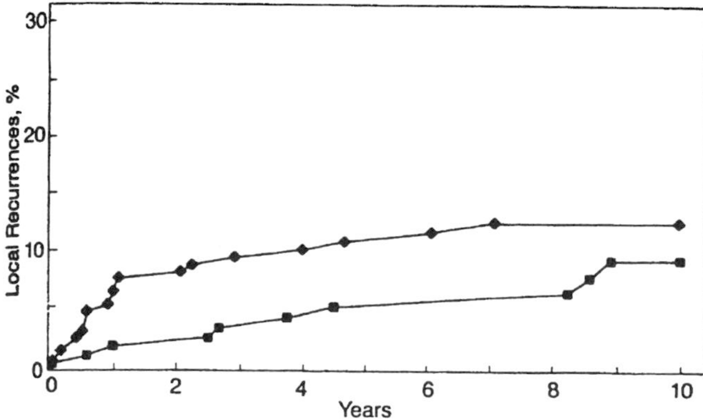

FIGURE 17–28. Overall local recurrence rates in patients who underwent radical (squares, n = 136) and modified radical (diamonds, n = 175) mastectomy. Local recurrence rate was significantly higher after modified radical mastectomy. (From Maddox WA, et al: Does radical mastectomy still have a place in the treatment of primary operable breast cancer? Arch Surg 122:1317–1320, 1987.)

Total Mastectomy

Total mastectomy involves complete resection of the breast and the pectoral fascia without dissection of the axillary lymph nodes.

There is controversy about the role of axillary dissection in affecting disease outcome. It has been proposed that total mastectomy plus radiation is as effective as radical mastectomy. The findings at 10 years comparing radical mastectomy, total mastectomy with regional radiation of the axilla, and total mastectomy with subsequent removal of axillary lymph nodes if they became clinically positive show no difference in disease-free or overall survival in patients with no clinical evidence initially of axillary lymph node involvement.[123]

A survival advantage was observed in a group undergoing radical mastectomy compared with total mastectomy plus radiation to the axilla in another study. Indeed, the local recurrence rate in the axilla was markedly higher in patients treated by total mastectomy and radiation than in the group having radical mastectomy.[124] These results imply that leaving behind axillary lymph nodes containing metastatic disease increases the frequency of distant disease.

Total mastectomy appears to be quite effective in the treatment of DCIS. The increase in breast cancer awareness and the improvement in screening techniques have increased the number of in situ cancers that are diagnosed. The treatment of choice for DCIS remains controversial, although the evidence suggests that for lesions greater than 25 mm in diameter and for multicentric lesions, total mastectomy is the procedure of choice.[125]

In a study following 112 patients with DCIS treated with total mastectomy, only 1 patient had a recurrence.[126] Axillary node involvement is rare with DCIS. Although axillary dissection is unnecessary for prognostic purposes, axillary node sampling is both acceptable and reassuring for the patient.[125]

There are multiple contraindications to mastectomy (Table 17–4).

Partial Mastectomy

The procedures included under the term "partial mastectomy" have been defined as follows:

1. Lumpectomy (local excision, excisional biopsy, par-

TABLE 17–4
Contraindications to Mastectomy

Inflammatory breast cancer
Supraclavicular lymph node metastasis
Chest wall (rib) fixation of the primary tumor
Ipsilateral arm edema
Satellite lesions beyond proposed skin incision
Distant metastatic disease
Concurrent medical contraindications to general anesthesia

From Osborne MP, Borgen PI: Role of mastectomy in breast cancer. Surg Clin North Am 70:1023–1046, 1990.

tial mastectomy): excision of all gross tumor without microscopic control of the surgical margins.
2. Limited resection, wide local excision: excision of tumor with margins microscopically free of tumor.
3. Quadrantectomy: en bloc excision of a quadrant of the breast including the overlying skin and underlying pectoralis major fascia.[127]

Breast conservation surgery and radiation treatment are recommended as appropriate methods of primary therapy for the majority of women with stage I and II breast cancer.

Considering the multicentricity of breast cancer, radiation of the remaining breast is critical. Additional foci of carcinoma within a breast containing a cancer have been documented in several studies. Rosen and associates[128] found microscopic residual carcinoma in 26% of patients with tumors less than 2 cm who had mastectomy and simulated partial mastectomy. This was true in 38% of patients with tumors greater than or equal to 2 cm and 80% of patients with subareolar tumors.

In the NSABP B-06 trial, total mastectomy was compared with lumpectomy and axillary dissection with and without radiotherapy. Lumpectomy followed by irradiation showed similar results in disease-free and overall survival. The results of this study show that local recurrence rates are significantly higher in patients treated by lumpectomy without radiotherapy, with a 90% disease-free survival in those irradiated and 61% in those not receiving radiation. Irradiation improved disease-free survival in both node-negative and node-positive patients (Fig. 17–29). Overall survival is not influenced in the three groups.[129]

An earlier trial from Milan compared the removal of a quarter of the breast (quadrantectomy), axillary dissection, and radiation (QUART) with radical mastectomy for tumors less than 2 cm and no palpable axillary lymph nodes. At 7 years of follow-up, there was no difference in the disease-free or overall survival rates of these two groups (Fig. 17–30).[130]

A wide margin of excision of the tumor is also important. With decreasing margins of excision, the extent of local recurrence is significantly increased.[131] Complete excision with adequately wide margins can be done at the time of the initial diagnostic biopsy or subsequently with a re-excision (Figs. 17–31 and 17–32).

Placement and orientation of the incision are important for convenience of excision and also for cosmesis. The incision is best made directly over the lesion. Circumareolar incisions are ideal for cosmesis but should be used only when complete excision of the lesion will not be compromised and there is no risk of seeding a subcutaneous tunnel with malignant cells. Curvilinear incisions corresponding to Langer's lines are preferred (Fig. 17–33). In closure of the defect, the best cosmetic result has been found with closure of the dead space with degloving of the breast skin and underlying fat from the under-

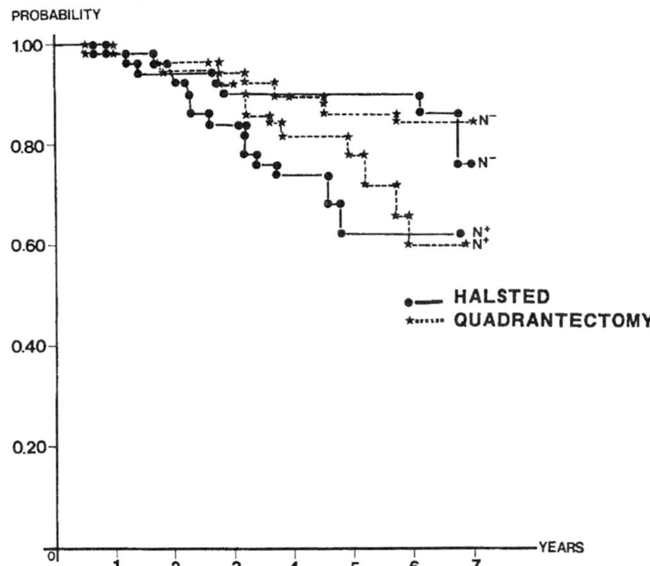

FIGURE 17–30. Actuarial overall survival in patients treated with Halsted mastectomy or quadrantectomy, axillary dissection, and radiotherapy. (From Veronesi U, et al: Comparing radical mastectomy with quadrantectomy, axillary dissection, and radiotherapy in patients with small cancers of the breast. N Engl J Med 305:6–11, 1981.)

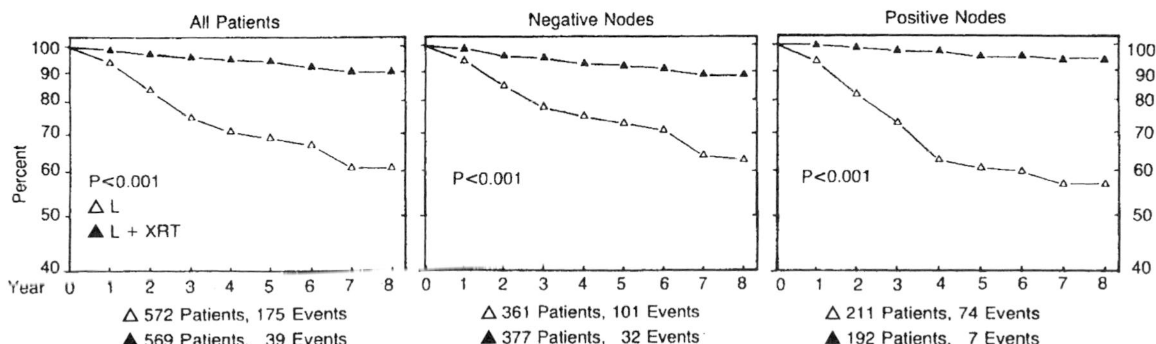

FIGURE 17–29. Life-table analysis showing the percentage of patients who remained free of breast tumor after lumpectomy (L) or after lumpectomy and breast irradiation (L + XRT). (From Fisher B, et al: Eight-year results of a randomized clinical trial comparing total mastectomy and lumpectomy with or without irradiation in the treatment of breast cancer. N Engl J Med 320:822–828, 1989.)

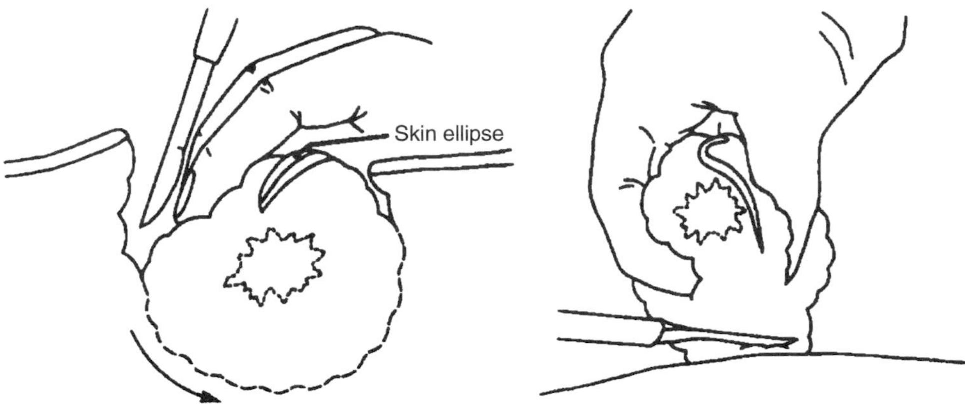

FIGURE 17–31. Palpating fingers guide the surgeon to a complete spherical excision of breast mass. (From Margolese R, et al: The technique of segmental mastectomy [lumpectomy] and axillary dissection: A syllabus from the national surgical adjuvant breast project workshops. Surgery 102:828–834, 1987.)

lying breast parenchyma. The skin is then closed as it falls naturally.

Along with local excision, a level I-II axillary lymph node dissection is performed. This can easily be approached through a transverse or curvilinear incision in the inferior portion of the axillary hairline. The borders of the dissection include laterally the medial border of the latissimus dorsi muscle, medially the medial border of the pectoralis minor muscle, and superiorly the axillary vein. There is preservation of the pectoralis minor muscle, long thoracic nerve, thoracodorsal vessels and nerve, and intercostal brachial nerve (Fig. 17–34).[132]

Segmental resection and radiotherapy are the alternative methods for treatment of DCIS. With local excision alone, the local recurrence rate is 43%; in those treated with local excision and radiotherapy, the local recurrence rate is only 7%. The average time to recurrence was 35 months (range, 4 to 118 months).[133] Similar results are found with a 38% local recurrence rate (mean follow-up, 96.5 months; range, 24 to 198 months) of DCIS treated by local excision alone, with 50% recurring as DCIS and 50% as infiltrating ductal carcinoma.[134]

DCIS patients who are candidates for conservative surgery and radiation include those with tumor size less than 4 to 5 cm; focal microcalcifications; no evidence of multicentric disease; negative resection margins, or, if positive, only focally positive; and a postbiopsy mammogram demonstrating no residual microcalcifications.[135–141] Patients for whom wide excision alone may represent the sole treatment include those with mammographically detected microcalcifications or detection as an incidental finding, negative resection margins, negative postbiopsy mammogram, and histologic subtype of noncomedo or low nuclear grade or both. Currently, multiple randomized trials are under way evaluating conservative surgery with or without radiation for DCIS. The results of these trials will further clarify the role of wide excision alone or in combination with irradiation for treatment of noninvasive ductal carcinomas.

There are some relative and absolute contraindications for breast conservation (Table 17–5). Pregnancy, because

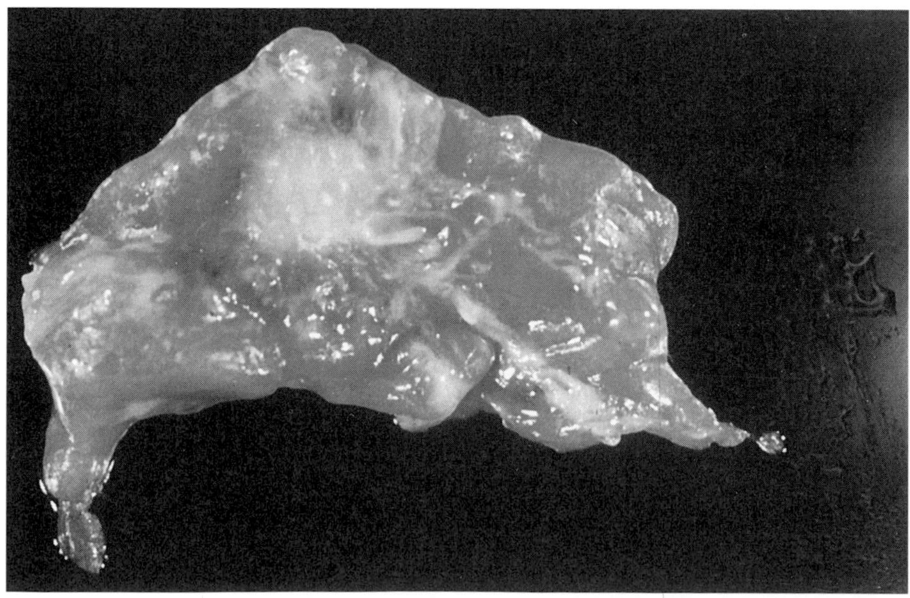

FIGURE 17–32. Surgical specimen containing surgically excised breast cancer. Margins are grossly and histologically free of tumor.

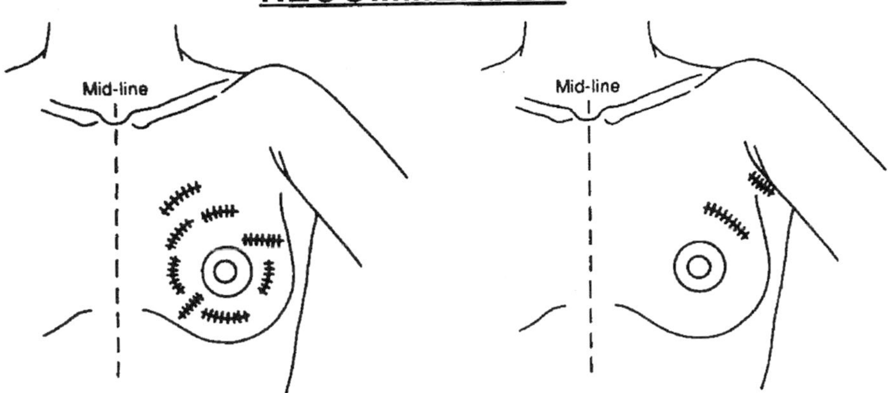

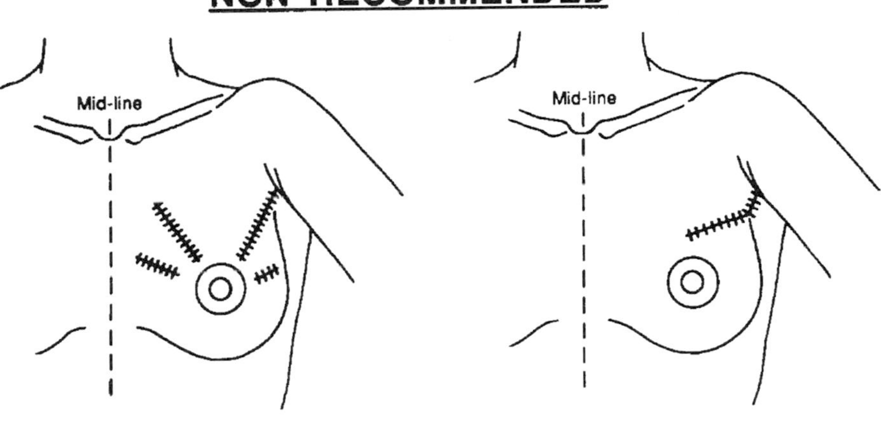

FIGURE 17–33. Tranverse or curvilinear incision is preferred. Radial incisions are acceptable in the inferior breast. Incisions should not be prolonged to encompass the axillary dissection. (Adapted from Margolese R, et al: The technique of segmental mastectomy [lumpectomy] and axillary dissection: A syllabus from the national surgical adjuvant breast project workshops. Surgery 102:828–834, 1987.)

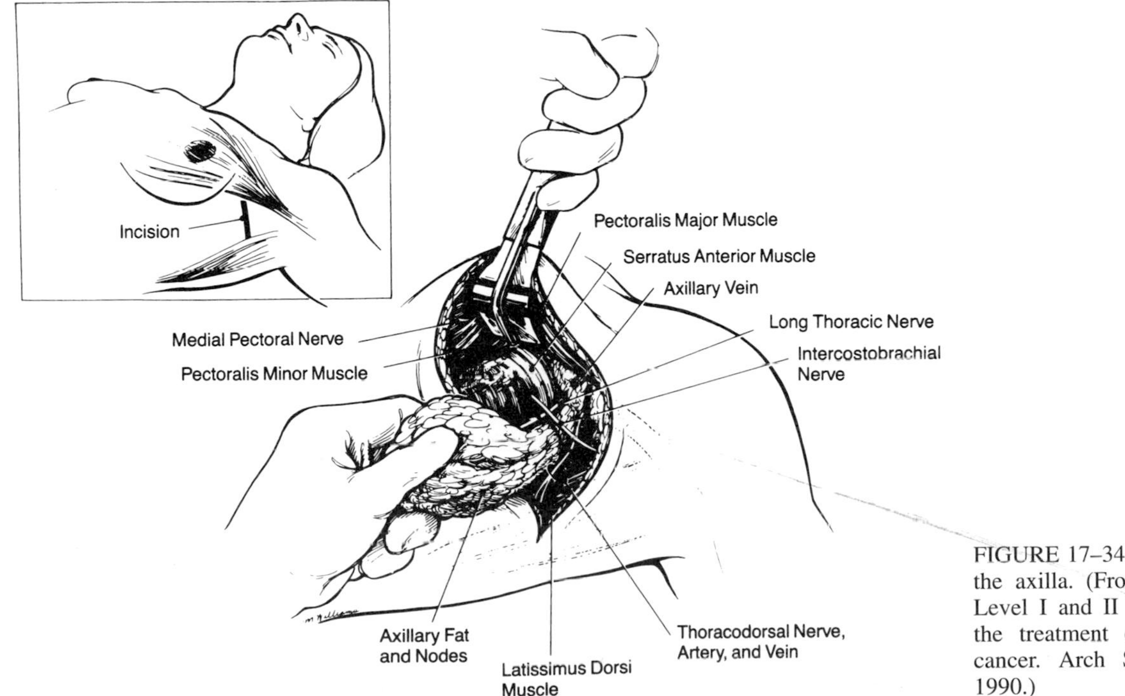

FIGURE 17–34. Surgical approach to the axilla. (From Siegel BM, et al: Level I and II axillary dissection in the treatment of early-stage breast cancer. Arch Surg 125:1144–1147, 1990.)

TABLE 17–5
Indications for Mastectomy

Absolute	Relative
Tumor >5 cm	Tumor 3–5 cm (depends on breast size)
Pregnancy	Central lesion
Prior irradiation	Infiltrating lobular carcinoma
Male patient	Ductal carcinoma in situ
Two ipsilateral tumors in different quadrants	Occult cancer presenting as axillary metastasis
Extensive intraductal carcinoma	Unreliable patient
Diffuse mammographic calcifications	Bulky axillary disease
Inability to obtain tumor-free margins	
High-quality radiotherapy not available	
Inability to comply with radiation protocol	
Failed breast conserving therapy	

From Osborne MP, Borgen PI: Role of mastectomy in breast cancer. Surg Clin North Am 70:1023–1046, 1990.

the radiation scatter has potential teratogenic effects, and prior radiation, such as mantle irradiation for Hodgkin's disease, are absolute contraindications. Extensive intraductal carcinoma, the presence of two noncontiguous ipsilateral tumors, or diffuse mammographic calcifications do not allow acceptable local-regional control with breast preservation.[125]

Adjuvant Therapy

Adjuvant therapy is systemic treatment of breast cancer. Both surgical and radiation treatments are ineffective if metastases are established at the time of initial treatment. The use of adjuvant therapy to improve survival is considered standard for any patient with lymph node involvement. It is more likely to be effective with smaller tumor burdens.

Radiotherapy Technique in Postlumpectomy Patients

Following excision of the primary tumor and dissection of the axilla, radiation is directed to the entire breast to a total dose of 4500 to 5000 cGy in a period of 4.5 to 6 weeks. Often this is followed by a supplemental boost or radiation to the surgical bed. Variations in radiotherapy techniques affect cosmetic outcome and the incidence of early and late complications. Indeed, prolongation of the overall treatment time with less than 8 Gy weekly is associated with higher local recurrence rates.[142, 143] Also, adverse cosmetic results are observed with the use of daily radiation doses in excess of 2.5 Gy or with total doses higher than 50 Gy.

Whether a "boost" should be used, and to what radiation dose, is not yet clearly defined. Preliminary data show no difference for patients with tumors less than 3 cm in size with negative margins whether or not a radiation boost is given. In patients with positive margins of resection or unknown margins, the addition of a boost appears to decrease the incidence of local recurrence. Surgical clips marking the area of excision are helpful for localizing the appropriate area to be boosted.[144–146]

Management of Locally Advanced Breast Cancer

Postoperative irradiation of the chest wall or the chest wall and regional lymphatics following mastectomy is given to minimize the risk of uncontrolled local-regional recurrence that will ultimately impair the quality of life and decrease the duration of survival. Indications for postoperative radiation include N2 or N3 nodal status, T4 tumor, involvement of the pectoralis fascia, and the combination of a tumor greater than 5 cm in size and more than four positive nodes. Indications are less clear in situations in which the tumor is greater than 5 cm in size but there are less than four positive nodes, or when the tumor is less than 5 cm in size but there are more than four involved nodes. However, receptor status, extranodal extension, and histologically positive margins should be included in the evaluation process.

The Oslo trials[147] show increased survival in patients who received postoperative irradiation. In the Helsinki trial,[148] both disease-free survival and overall survival were increased with the addition of radiation to postoperative chemotherapy.

The dose to the chest wall is in the range of 50 to 60 Gy, with electron energies selected to correspond to chest wall thickness measured on multiple computed tomography scan sections. Positive tumor margins and areas of extracapsular extension usually require higher doses to a limited area.

There is as yet no firm recommendation on how to combine external irradiation and chemotherapy. McCormick et al.,[149] in a retrospective review, compared local recurrence rates in three groups of patients in relation to the timing of radiotherapy and chemotherapy. In patients treated conservatively, no differences in local control were noted despite delays in the delivery of primary radiation until after adjuvant chemotherapy was delivered. Stefanik and colleagues[150] also did not show an increase in local-regional recurrence in mastectomy patients during the period of chemotherapy; therefore, they concluded that there was no harm in delaying radiation until completion of chemotherapy. A randomized trial in South Africa did not show benefit from early chemotherapy in stage III breast cancer, indicating that chest wall irradiation may be "sandwiched" between chemotherapy administrations.[151]

Chemotherapeutic Drugs

Of the single drug therapies, doxorubicin is the most effective. Multiple drug combinations seem more effective than single-agent therapy. The most commonly used combinations of chemotherapeutic drugs are cyclophosphamide, methotrexate, and 5-fluorouracil (CMF), or cyclophosphamide, doxorubicin (Adriamycin), and 5-fluorouracil (CAF).

In a study by Bonadonna et al.,[152] patients treated with mastectomy having positive axillary lymph nodes were randomized into those receiving adjuvant chemotherapy with CMF and controls receiving no adjuvant therapy. The treatment failures were found to occur significantly more often in the control group. This was true for all patients regardless of the number of axillary nodes involved but was especially significant when there were four or more nodes involved (Figs. 17–35 to 17–37). There was no difference in the relapse rate in pre- and postmenopausal patients.

Hormonal Manipulation

There is a definite correlation between positive hormonal receptors and response to hormonal manipulative therapy. Fifty percent of hormone receptor–positive patients respond to hormonal therapy, whereas less than 10% of those that are hormone receptor–negative respond.[153]

The adjuvant treatment of breast cancer in patients with

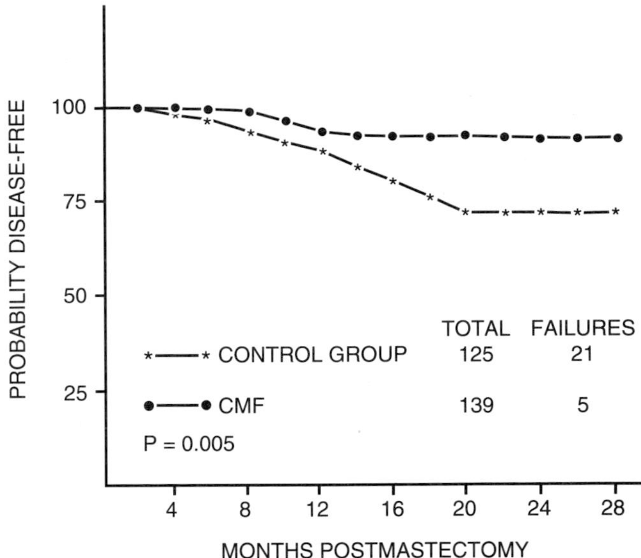

FIGURE 17–36. Treatment-failure time distribution of patients with one to three axillary lymph nodes. (From Bonnadonna G, et al: Combination chemotherapy as an adjuvant treatment in operable breast cancer. N Engl J Med 294:405–410, 1976.)

histologically negative axillary nodes and ER-positive tumor levels (≥ 10 fmol) with tamoxifen compared with placebo controls has been studied. Tamoxifen was found to decrease the rate of treatment failure locally and distantly.[154] There was also a reduction in development of contralateral breast cancers.[155]

The combination of chemotherapy consisting of L-phenylalanine mustard and 5-fluorouracil with tamoxifen has been investigated. In those patients with ER and PR levels

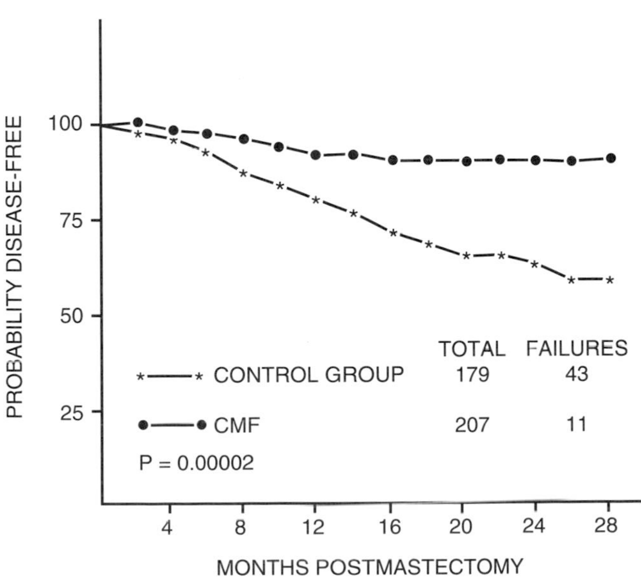

FIGURE 17–35. Treatment-failure time distribution in all evaluable patients. (From Bonnadonna G, et al: Combination chemotherapy as an adjuvant treatment in operable breast cancer. N Engl J Med 294:405–410, 1976.)

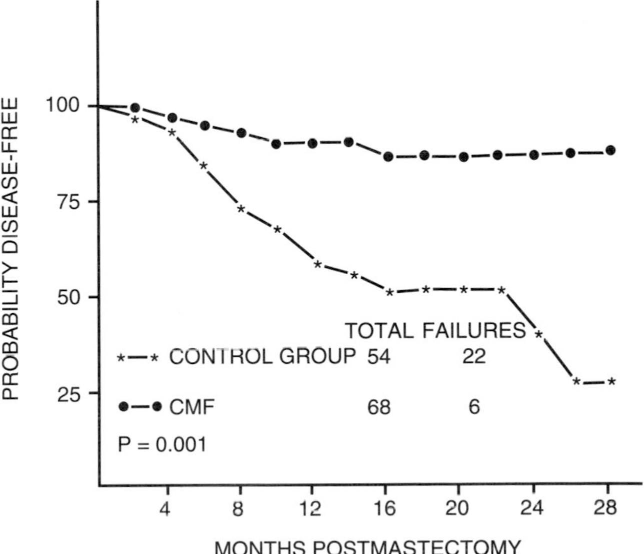

FIGURE 17–37. Treatment-failure time distribution of patients with four or more positive axillary lymph nodes. (From Bonnadonna G, et al: Combination chemotherapy as an adjuvant treatment in operable breast cancer. N Engl J Med 294:405–410, 1976.)

equal to or above 10 fmol, the recurrence of disease was reduced with the addition of tamoxifen. Higher ER levels showed a greater likelihood of disease-free survival. Treatment failure was significantly reduced with the addition of tamoxifen in patients greater than or equal to 50 years old. In patients less than 50 years old, the only significant reduction in failure was in those patients with four or more positive nodes and high ER and PR levels.[156, 157]

Therapeutic Oophorectomy

The benefit of therapeutic oophorectomy in premenopausal patients with four or more positive axillary lymph nodes has been evaluated. In a study by the Ludwig Cancer Study Group, patients were randomized into those receiving CMF and oophorectomy and those receiving CMF alone. The disease-free survival and overall survival were no different in the two groups. This study concluded that adjuvent oophorectomy is of no benefit in premenopausal women, even at high risk of recurrence with four or more axillary nodes positive.[158]

LOCAL RECURRENCE AFTER BREAST CONSERVATION SURGERY

The incidence of local recurrence after partial mastectomy and radiotherapy has been shown in multiple studies to range from 9.3% to 22% at 10 years for stage I and II breast cancer. These local-regional recurrences, although grouped together, probably represent several different processes. There are recurrences at the original site of a primary tumor that usually appear directly beneath the previous incision. Other recurrences, that develop in the quadrant of the primary tumor, probably represent the evolution of multifocal, in situ, or minimally invasive disease that was present at the time of the original surgery. There are recurrences elsewhere in the breast that represent a new primary cancer. There are also those rare primary breast cancers that are induced by radiation of the original tumor.[159]

Fortunately, most local recurrences after breast conservation surgery represent operable disease. Only 5% of these patients have distant disease at the time of local recurrence.[160] The majority of local recurrences (76%) are detected within the first 2 years after the original surgery.[161]

These local-regional recurrences are usually detected by the finding of a palpable mass on physical examination (70% to 96%). They are also usually detectable by mammogram (67% to 85%). Obtaining mammograms as follow-up in these patients is important, since 12% to 42% of mammographically detectable abnormalities do not present with a palpable mass.[161–165] Most of these recurrences (64%) are 2 cm or less at presentation.[161]

Sixty percent of the local recurrences are within the same quadrant as the original tumor, with 28% within 2 cm of the original incision. Another 22% are located in an adjacent quadrant of the breast.[161] The histologic type of the recurrence is usually the same as that of the original tumor.[166]

After local-regional recurrence, salvage mastectomy offers good disease control. In women followed a median period of 5 years after local-regional recurrence treated with salvage mastectomy, the local-regional recurrence rate is 15%. At 5 years, the disease-free survival ranges from 51% to 63% and the survival rate ranges from 48% to 79%. The disease-free survival at 10 years is 50% to 57%.[159, 161, 163, 164, 167–171]

The prognosis at salvage mastectomy is related to several factors, many similar to prognosis at diagnosis of the primary tumor. The size of the recurrence is important, with those measuring less than 2 cm having a better prognosis. The extent of the recurrence within the breast is significant, with those having dermal or diffuse breast involvement having a poorer prognosis. Those patients with involved axillary nodes and increasing number of axillary nodes at both treatment of the original tumor and recurrence had a worse prognosis than those without lymph node involvement. Those recurrent tumors detected on mammogram alone had a better prognosis than those palpable at the time of diagnosis.[159]

SPECIAL TOPICS

Nipple Discharge

Nipple discharge is not an uncommon finding. The most important issue to clarify in evaluating this problem is whether the discharge is pathologic or physiologic.

Physiologic discharge is often a result of breast manipulation, which is then often encouraged by continued manipulation in an anxious patient. Galactorrhea typically produces a milky white discharge. It is often from multiple ducts and usually is bilateral but can be unilateral. Discharge that is serous or bloody and originates from a single duct is suspicious for carcinoma.

The etiology of persistent galactorrhea includes medications, such as oral contraceptives, antihypertensives, and tranquilizers, and endocrine abnormalities, including hypothyroidism and pituitary adenomas. In evaluating galactorrhea, a prolactin level and thyroid panel should be obtained.

The majority of patients with nipple discharge have benign disease. The most common causes of discharge are intraductal papilloma, papillomatosis, duct ectasia, and fibrocystic disease. Carcinoma is found in only 11% of patients.

In the evaluation of nipple discharge, cytology of the discharge fluid is notoriously inaccurate, with high false-negative and false-positive rates. A mammogram is important to review for obvious abnormality as an etiology or need for surgical biopsy. Galactography has not been shown to be helpful in differentiating benign from malignant causes of nipple discharge.

If the discharge is suspicious, the surgical procedure of choice is a major duct excision. This is performed by a circumareolar incision partially around the areola in the quadrant of the suspected duct. A probe may be inserted into the duct to facilitate the dissection. The areola is reflected to allow exposure of the ductal system. The suspicious duct or collection of ducts is dissected for several centimeters into the breast and resected (Fig. 17–38).[47]

Male Breast Cancer

Carcinoma of the male breast is an unusual occurrence; it represents less than 1% of all breast cancer. Because it is unusual, the diagnosis is often delayed, and thus the stage at presentation is often advanced.[65, 172, 173]

The most common presenting symptom in male breast cancer is a painless, firm subareolar breast mass.[65, 174] Other symptoms include retracted nipple, nipple discharge, ulceration, axillary swelling, and breast pain.[65]

The main differential diagnosis is gynecomastia. A history of use of particular drugs, alcohol abuse, bilaterality, a discoid shape to the mass, and tenderness favors gynecomastia. Mammograms may be helpful in that a dense, irregular, or spiculated mass is more consistent with breast cancer, as is true in women.[173]

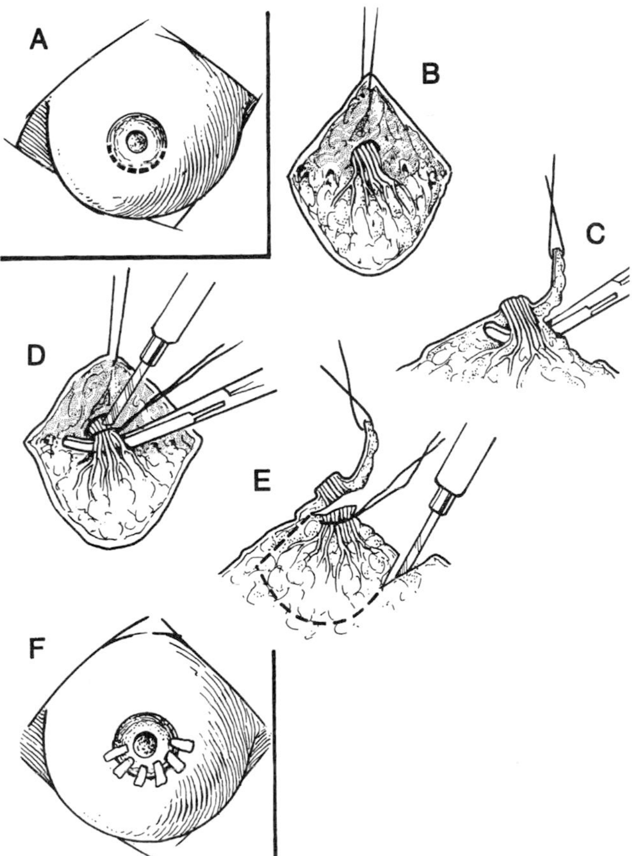

FIGURE 17–38. Excision of the major duct system. Circumareolar incision *(A);* undermining areola *(B);* isolating lactiferous sinuses *(C);* transecting end of major duct system *(D);* removing core of surrounding breast tissue *(E);* incision closed *(F)*. (From Harris JR, et al: Breast Diseases. Philadelphia: JB Lippincott, 1991, p 76.)

The most common pathology is infiltrating ductal carcinoma, as in female breast cancer.[174, 175] Paget disease is also occasionally seen in the male breast and acts similarly clinically and pathologically to the disease in women.[65] The majority of male breast cancers are ER- and PR-positive.[174]

The diagnosis of a suspicious breast mass can be made with fine-needle aspiration or excisional biopsy.[174] The standard of treatment is a radical mastectomy. This is because of the typical later presentation, with the close proximity of the pectoralis major muscle often necessitating sacrifice of the pectoralis muscles.[173] When axillary metastases are present, combination chemotherapy or tamoxifen, or both, after primary surgical treatment is indicated.[174]

Male breast cancer has a reputation for being difficult to cure; however, it is often diagnosed at an advanced stage.[65] The most powerful predictor of outcome is the status of the axillary lymph nodes.[176] The prognosis stage for stage is identical in male and female breast cancer.[174–177]

Gynecomastia

Unilateral or bilateral benign enlargement of the male breast is called gynecomastia. The causes of gynecomastia can be hormonal influences on the male breast tissue, the effect of systemic diseases, or drug use, or it can be idiopathic.

Pubertal and senescent gynecomastia is due to hormonal influences. This is usually bilateral and self-limited. Gynecomastia is also associated with Klinefelter's syndrome.

Systemic diseases associated with gynecomastia include hyperplasia or carcinoma of the adrenal cortex, pituitary adenomas, and hyperthyroidism. Hepatic disease and renal failure have also been found to cause gynecomastia.

A common cause of gynecomastia is drug use, including prescription and nonprescription drugs and illegal drugs such as marijuana and heroin (Table 17–6). The use of estrogens and androgens can cause gynecomastia, including diethylstilbestrol for prostate cancer.

The obvious concern in evaluating a patient for gynecomastia is to rule out male breast cancer. Childhood and adolescent gynecomastia is almost always benign and usually resolves spontaneously. In an older patient, or in any patient in whom a mass persists, levels of serum estrogen, testosterone, prolactin, luteinizing hormone, and follicle-stimulating hormone should be obtained to evaluate for an endocrine abnormality. On physical examination, findings that are usually associated with benign etiology are bilaterality, discoid shape limited to the margins of the areola, free mobility from the underlying pectoralis major muscle, and soft or rubbery consistency. A biopsy should be performed on any mass that is hard, fixed, or persistent, particularly in an older male patient.[47]

TABLE 17–6
Drugs That Can Cause Gynecomastia

Antacid	***Hormone/Hormonelike***
Cimetidine	Clomiphene
Ranitidine	Diethylstilbesterol
Antibiotic	Estramustine
Isoniazid	Estrogen
Metronidazole	Flutamide
	Leuprolide
Antihypertensive	Tamoxifen
Guanabenz	***Narcotic***
Methyldopa	Heroin
Reserpine	Methadone
Antinausea	***Tranquilizer***
Prochlorperazine	Chlorpromazine
Thiethylperazine	Fluphenazine
Antineoplastic	Perphenazine
Busulfan	Thioridazine
Methotrexate	Trifluoperazine
Procarbazine	***Other***
Vincristine	Amphetamines
Cardiac	Anabolic steroids
Calcium channel blockers	Auranofin
Digoxin	Diazepam
Propranolol	D-Penicillamine
Diuretic	Ergotamine tartrate
Amiloride	Ketoconazole
Spironolactone	Marijuana
Thiazide	Neuroleptic drugs
	Phenothiazines
	Sulindac
	Theophylline
	Tricyclics

From Harris JR, et al: Breast Diseases. Philadelphia: JB Lippincott, 1991, p 47.

Pregnancy-Associated Breast Cancer

One in 3000 pregnancies has an associated diagnosis of breast cancer.[178] This represents 2% to 3% of all breast cancers.[179]

There is often a delay in diagnosis because the hypertrophy of the breast during pregnancy makes it difficult to detect a mass.[180] Any mass that persists or enlarges must be considered potentially a malignancy and be treated as such.[181] Inflammatory cancer may be mistaken for mastitis, so all incision and drainage procedures of an abscess cavity occurring during pregnancy should include biopsy of the cavity wall.[182]

The standard of treatment of breast cancer diagnosed during pregnancy is a modified radical mastectomy. Breast conservation is not an option because of radiation effects to the fetus.[179, 180, 182] Unless the patient is within weeks of delivery, operative treatment should not be delayed for completion of the pregnancy.[180] The administration of bromocriptine prior to surgical biopsy decreases the risk of subsequent milk fistulas.[179]

The majority of tumors diagnosed during pregnancy are ER- and PR-negative.[179, 182] Termination of pregnancy is not routinely recommended and has no effect on prognosis.[179, 182, 183] If, however, chemotherapy is indicated, the pregnancy should be terminated.[179, 182, 184]

The prognosis of pregnancy-associated breast cancer is no different at the same stage and age as in women who are not pregnant.[178, 182, 184] Owing to delay in diagnosis, pregnant women are often diagnosed at a later stage than in nonpregnant women. In pregnancy-associated breast cancer, 53% to 89% are axillary lymph node–positive at diagnosis.[179, 184]

There does not appear to be a difference in survival in women who choose to become pregnant subsequent to the diagnosis of breast cancer.[179, 183]

References

1. World Health Organization: World Health Statistics. Annuals, 1987–1991. Geneva: WHO.
2. Miller AB, Bulbrook RO: UICC multi-disciplinary project on breast cancer: The epidemiology, aetiology and prevention of breast cancer. Int J Cancer 37:173–177, 1986.
3. Wingo PA, Tong T, Bolden S: Cancer statistics, 1995. CA 45:8–30, 1995.
4. Harris JR, Lippman ME, Veronesi U, Willett W: Breast cancer (first of three parts). New Engl J Med 327:319–328, 1992.
5. U.S. Department of Health and Human Services: Cancer Statistics Review 1973–1987. NIH Publication 90-2789. Bethesda, MD: National Cancer Institute, 1990.
6. Miller BA, Feuer EJ, Hankey BF: Recent incidence trends for breast cancer in women and the relevance of early detection: An update. CA 43:27–41, 1993.
7. White E, Lee CY, Kristal AR: An evaluation of the increase in breast cancer incidence in relation to mammography use. J Natl Cancer Inst 82:1546–1552, 1990.
8. Liff JM, Sung JFC, Chow WH, Greenbery RS, Flanders WD: Does increased detection account for the rising incidence of breast cancer? Am J Public Health 81:462–465, 1991.
9. Feuer EJ, Wan L-M, Boring CC, Flanders WD, Timmel MJ, Tong T: The lifetime risk of developing breast cancer. J Natl Cancer Inst 85:892–897, 1993.
10. National Center for Health Statistics: Vital Statistics of the United States, 1989. Washington, DC: Public Health Service, 1992.
11. Ries LAG, Hankey BF, Edwards BK: Cancer Statistics Review 1973–1987. NIH Publication 90-2789. Bethesda, MD: Division of Cancer Prevention and Control, National Cancer Institute, 1990.
12. Swanson GM: Breast cancer risk estimation: A translational statistic for communication to the public. J Natl Cancer Inst 85:848–849, 1993.
13. Swanson GM: Breast cancer in the 1990s. JAMA 47:140–148, 1992.
14. Blot WJ, Devesa SS, Fraumen JF Jr: Declining breast cancer mortality among young American women. J Natl Cancer Inst 78:451–454, 1987.
15. Wells BL, Horm JW: Stage at diagnosis in breast cancer: Race and socioeconomic factors. Am J Public Health 82:1383–1385, 1992.
16. Howard J: Using mammography for cancer control: An unrealized potential. CA 37:33–48, 1987.
17. Ephross SA, Morris DL, Hulka BS: Increases in breast cancer incidence and mortality rates between 1975 and 1986 in white and black Americans: A screening effect or an alarming trend? Am J Epidemiol 132:790, 1990.
18. Early Breast Cancer Trialists' Collaborative Group: Systemic treatment of early breast cancer by hormonal, cytotoxic, or immune therapy: 151 randomized trials involving 32,000 recurrences and 25,000 deaths among 77,000 women. Lancet 339:1–15, 71–85, 1992.
19. White E: Projected changes in breast cancer incidence due to the trend toward delayed childbearing. Am J Public Health 77:495–497, 1987.
20. Thomas DB, Jimenez LM, McTiernan A, et al: Breast cancer in men: Risk factors with hormonal implications. Am J Epidemiol 135:734–748, 1992.
21. Gordon NH, Crowe JP, Brumberg DJ, Berger NA: Socioeconomic factors and race in breast cancer recurrence and survival. Am J Epidemiol 135:609–618, 1992.

22. Kelsey JL, Gammon MD: The epidemiology of breast cancer. CA 41:147–165, 1991.
23. Kelsey J, Berkowitz G: Breast cancer epidemiology. Cancer Res 48:5616–5623, 1988.
24. Healey EA, Cook EF, Orav EJ, Schnitt SJ, Connolly JL, Harris JR: Contralateral breast cancer: Clinical characteristics and impact on prognosis. J Clin Oncol 11:1545–1552, 1993.
25. Hall JM, Lee MK, Newman B, et al: Linkage of early-onset breast cancer to chromosome 17q21. Science 250:1684–1689, 1990.
26. Hayes DF, Schnitt SJ: Risk factors, epidemiology, and development of breast cancer. In Hayes DF (ed): Atlas of Breast Cancer. London: Mosby Europe, 1993.
27. de Waard F, Trichopoulos D: A unifying concept of the aetiology of breast cancer. Int J Cancer 41:666–669, 1988.
28. McTiernan A, Thomas D: Evidence for a protective effect of lactation on risk of breast cancer in young women: Results from a case-control study. Am J Epidemiol 124:353–358, 1986.
29. Hankey BF, Curtis RE, Naughton MD, et al: A retrospective cohort analysis of second breast cancer risk for primary breast cancer patients with an assessment of the effect of radiation therapy. J Natl Cancer Inst 70:797–804, 1983.
30. United Kingdom National Case-Control Study Group: Breast feeding and the risk of breast cancer in young women. Br Med J 307:17–20, 1993.
31. Welsch CW: Relationship between dietary fat and experimental mammary tumorigenesis: A review and critique. Cancer Res 52(suppl):2040–2048, 1992.
32. Goodwyn PJ, Boyd NF: Critical appraisal of the evidence that dietary fat intake is related to breast cancer risk in humans. J Natl Cancer Inst 79:473–485, 1987.
33. Armstrong BK: Oestrogen therapy after the menopause—boon or bane? Med J Aust 148:213–214, 1988.
34. Buell P: Changing incidence of breast cancer in Japanese–American women. J Natl Cancer Inst 51:1479–1483, 1973.
35. Rose DP, Boyar AP, Wynder EL: International comparisons of mortality rates for cancer of the breast, ovary, prostate, and colon, and per capita food consumption. Cancer 58:2363–2371, 1986.
36. Willett WC, Hunter DJ, Stampfer MJ, et al: Dietary fat and fiber in relation to risk of breast cancer: An eight-year follow-up. JAMA 268:2037–2044, 1992.
37. Prentice RL, Thomas DB: On the epidemiology of oral contraceptives and disease. Adv Cancer Res 49:285–301, 1987.
38. Romieu I, Berlin JA, Colditz G: Oral contraceptives and breast cancer: Review and meta-analysis. Cancer 66:2253–2263, 1990.
39. Tabar L, Fagerberg G, Duffy SW, Fay NE: Update of the Swedish Two-County Program of mammographic screening for breast cancer. Radiol Clin North Am 30:187–210, 1992.
40. Andersoon I, Aspergren K, Janzon L: Mammographic screening and mortality from breast cancer: The Malmo mammographic screening trial. Br Med J 297:943–948, 1988.
41. Roberts MM, Alexander FE, Anderson TJ: Edinburgh trial of screening for breast cancer: Mortality at seven years. Lancet 335:241–246, 1990.
42. Morrison AS, Brisson J, Khalid N: Breast cancer incidence and mortality in the Breast Cancer Detection Demonstration Project. J Natl Cancer Inst 80:1540–1547, 1988.
43. Verbeek ALM, Hendriks JHCL, Holland R, Mravunac M, Sturmans F: Mammographic screening and breast cancer mortality: Age-specific effects in the Nijmegen project, 1975–1982. Lancet 1:411–416, 1985.
44. Collette HJA, Rombach JJ, Day NE, deWaard F: Evaluation of screening for breast cancer in a non-randomized study (the DOM project) by means of a case-control study. Lancet 1:1224–1226, 1984.
45. Paci E, Ciatto C, Buiatti S, Palli D, del Turco MR: Early indicators of efficacy of breast cancer screening programmes. Results of the Florence district programme. Int J Cancer 46:198–202, 1990.
46. Kopans DB, Feig SA: The Canadian National Breast Screening Study: A critical review. AJR 161:755–760, 1993.
47. Harris JR, Hellman S, Henderson IC, Kinne DW: Breast Diseases. Philadelphia: JB Lippincott, 1991.
48. Sabiston D: Textbook of Surgery. Philadelphia: WB Saunders, 1991.
49. Donegan WL: Evaluation of a palpable breast mass. N Engl J Med 327:937–942, 1992.
50. Beals RK, Crawford S: Congenital absence of the pectoral muscles. Clin Orthop 119:166, 1976.
51. Turner-Warwick RT: The lymphatics of the breast. Br J Surg 46:574, 1959.
52. Hultborn KA, Larsen LG, Raghnult I: The lymph drainage from the breast to the axillary and parasternal lymph nodes: Studied with the aid of colloidal AU^{198}. Acta Radiol 43:52, 1955.
53. Berg JW: The significance of axillary node levels in the study of breast carcinoma. Cancer 8:776, 1955.
55. Moosman DA: Anatomy of the pectoral nerves and their preservation in modified mastectomy. Am J Surg 139:883–886, 1980.
56. Davis HH, Simons M, Davis JB: Cystic disease of the breast: Relationship to carcinoma. Cancer 17:957–978, 1964.
57. Donnelly PK, Baker KW, Carney JA, O'Fallon WM: Benign breast lesions and subsequent breast carcinoma in Rochester, Minnesota. Mayo Clinic Proc 50:650–655, 1975.
58. Hutchinson W, Thomas D, Hamlin W, et al: Risk of breast cancer in women with benign breast disease. J Natl Cancer Inst 65:13–20, 1980.
59. Kodlin D, Winger EE, Morgenstern NL, Chen U: Chronic mastopathy and breast cancer. Cancer 39:26033–2607, 1977.
60. McCarty K Jr, Kesterson G, Wilkinson W, Georgiade N: Histologic study of subcutaneous mastectomy specimens from patients with carcinoma of the contralateral breast. Surg Gynecol Obstet 147:682–688, 1978.
61. Page DL, Zwaag RV, Rogers LW, et al: Relation between component parts of fibrocystic disease complex and breast cancer. J Natl Cancer Inst 61:1055–1063, 1978.
62. Bloodgood JC: Borderline breast tumors. Ann Surg 93:235–249, 1931.
63. Dupont WD, Page DL: Risk factors for breast cancer in women with proliferative disease. N Engl J Med 312:146–151, 1985.
64. Foote FW, Stewart FW: Comparative studies of cancerous versus noncancerous breasts. Ann Surg 121:6–53, 197–249, 1945.
65. Haagensen CD: Diseases of the Breast. Philadelphia: WB Saunders, 1986.
66. Black MM, Barclay THC, Cutler SJ, et al: Association of atypical characteristics of benign breast lesions with subsequent risk of breast cancer. Cancer 29:338–343, 1972.
67. Georgiade N, Serafin D, Georgiade G, McCarty K: Subcutaneous mastectomy: An evolution of concept and technique. Ann Plast Surg 8:8–19, 1982.
68. Andersen JA, Gram JB: Radial scar in the female breast. Cancer 53:2557–2560, 1984.
69. Wellings SR, Jensen HM, Marcum RG: An atlas of subgross pathology of the human breast with special reference to possible precancerous lesions. J Natl Cancer Inst 55:231–273, 1975.
70. Dupont WD, Parl FF, Hartmann WH, et al: Breast cancer risk associated with proliferative breast disease and atypical hyperplasia. Cancer 71:19–26, 1992.
71. Kern WH, Brooks RN: Atypical epithelial hyperplasia associated with breast cancer and fibrocystic disease. Cancer 24:668–675, 1969.
72. Dupont WD, Page DL: Breast cancer risk associated with proliferative disease, age at first birth, and a family history of breast cancer. Am J Epidemiol 125:769, 1987.
73. Page DL, Dupont WD, Rogers LW, Rados MS: Atypical hyperplastic lesions of the female breast. Cancer 55:2698–2708, 1985.
74. Ashikari R, Humos AG, Snyder RE, et al: A clinicopathologic study of atypical lesions of the breast. Cancer 33:310–317, 1974.
75. Page DL, Dupont WD, Rogers LW, Landenberger M: Intraductal carcinoma of the breast: Follow-up after biopsy only. Cancer 49:751–758, 1982.
76. Lagios MD, Westdahl PR, Margolin FR, Rose MR: Duct carcinoma in situ: Relationship of extent of noninvasive disease to the frequency of occult invasion, multicentricity, lymph node metastases, and short-term treatment failures. Cancer 50:1309–1314, 1982.
77. Neilsen M, Jensen J, Andersen J: Precancerous and cancerous breast lesions during lifetime and at autopsy. Cancer 54:612–615, 1984.
78. Ashikari R, Huvos AG, Snyder RE: Prospective study of non-infiltrating carcinoma of the breast. Cancer 39:435–439, 1977.
79. Betsill WL, Rosen PP, Lieberman PH, et al: Intraductal carcinoma: Long-term follow-up after treatment by biopsy alone. JAMA 239:1863–1867, 1978.
80. Rosen PP, Braun DW, Lyngholm B, et al: Lobular carcinoma in

situ of the breast: Preliminary results of treatment by ipsilateral mastectomy and contralateral breast biopsy. Cancer 47:813–819, 1981.
81. Cutuli B, Teissier E, Piat J-M, et al: Radical surgery and conservative treatment of ductal carcinoma in situ of the breast. Eur J Cancer 28:649–654, 1992.
82. Lagios MD, Margolin FR, Westdahl PR, et al: Mammographically detected duct carcinoma in situ. Cancer 63:618–624, 1989.
83. Fisher ER, Sass R, Fisher B, et al: Pathologic findings from the National Surgical Adjuvant Breast Project (protocol 6). I. Intraductal carcinoma (DCIS). Cancer 57:197–208, 1986.
84. Silverstein MJ, Gierson ED, Colburn WJ, et al: Axillary lymphadenectomy for intraductal carcinoma of the breast. Surg Gynecol Obstet 172:211–214, 1994.
85. Schuh ME, Nemoto T, Penetrante RB, et al: Intraductal carcinoma: Analysis of presentation, pathologic findings and outcome of disease. Arch Surg 121:1303–1307, 1986.
86. Rosner D, Warren WL, Penetrante R: Ductal carcinoma in situ with microinvasion. Cancer 67:1498–1503, 1991.
87. Kopald KH, Hiatt JR, Irving C, et al: The pathology of nonpalpable breast cancer. Am Surg 56:782–787, 1990.
88. Patchefsky AS, Schwartz GF, Finkelstein SD, et al: Heterogeneity of intraductal carcinoma of the breast. Cancer 63:731–741, 1989.
89. Foote FW, Stewart FW: Lobular carcinoma in situ: A rare form of mammary cancer. Am J Pathol 17:491–497, 1940.
90. Haagensen CD, Lane N, Bodian C: Coexisting lobular neoplasia and carcinoma of the breast. Cancer 51:1468–1482, 1983.
91. Hutter R: The management of patients with lobular carcinoma in situ of the breast. Cancer 53:798–802, 1984.
92. Rosen PP, Braun DW, Kinne DE: The clinical significance of preinvasive breast carcinoma. Cancer 46:919–9255, 1980.
94. Rosen PP: Lobular carcinoma in situ: Recent clinicopathologic studies at Memorial Hospital. Pathol Res Pract 166:430–455, 1980.
95. Rosen PP, Braun DW, Kinne DE: The clinical significance of preinvasive breast carcinoma. Cancer 46:919–925, 1980.
96. Walt AJ, Simon M, Swanson M: The continuing dilemma of lobular carcinoma in situ. Arch Surg 127:904–907, 1992.
97. McDivitt RW, Hutter RVP, Foote FW, Stewart FW: In situ lobular carcinoma. JAMA 201:96–100, 1967.
98. Hutter RVP, Foote FW Jr: Lobular carcinoma in situ. Long term follow up. Cancer 24:1081–1085, 1969.
99. Rosen PP, Lieberman PH, Braun DW, et al: Lobular carcinoma in situ of the breast: Detailed analysis of 99 patients with average follow-up of 24 years. Am J Surg Pathol 2:225–251, 1978.
100. Andersen JA: Lobular carcinoma in situ of the breast: An approach to rational treatment. Cancer 39:2597–2602, 1977.
101. DeVita VT Jr, Hellman S, Rosenberg SA: Cancer: Principles and Practice, 3rd ed. Philadelphia: JB Lippincott, 1989.
102. Brun B, Otemezguine Y, Feuilhade F, et al: Treatment of inflammatory breast cancer with combination chemotherapy and mastectomy versus breast conservation. Cancer 61:1096–1103, 1988.
103. Fields JN, Kuske RR, Perez Ca, Fineberg BB, Bartlett N: Prognostic factors in inflammatory breast cancer. Univariate and multivariate analysis. Cancer 63:1225–1232, 1989.
104. Thoms WW, McNeese MD, Fletcher GH, Buzdar AU, Singletary E, Oswald MJ: Multimodal treatment for inflammatory breast cancer. Int J Radiat Oncol Biol Phys 17:739–745, 1989.
105. Singletary E, McNeese MD, Hortobagyi GN: Feasibility of breast-conservation surgery after induction chemotherapy for locally advanced breast carcinoma. Cancer 69:2849–2852, 1992.
106. Mourali N, Tabbane F, Muenz LR, et al: Ten-year results utilizing chemotherapy as primary treatment in non-metastatic, rapidly progressing breast cancer. Cancer Invest 11:363–370, 1993.
107. Clark GM, Wenger CR, Beardslee S, et al: How to integrate steroid hormone receptor, flow cytometric, and other prognostic information in regard to primary breast cancer. Cancer Suppl 71:2157–2162, 1993.
108. Epstein AH, Connolly JL, Gelman R, et al: The predictors of distant relapse following conservative surgery and radiotherapy for early breast cancer are similar to those following mastectomy. Int J Radiat Oncol Biol Phys 17:755–760, 1989.
109. Dorr FA: Prognostic factors observed in current clinical trials. Cancer 71:2163–2168, 1992.
110. Crowe JP, Gordon NH, Sheenk RR, et al: Primary tumor size, relevance to breast cancer survival. Arch Surg 127:910–916, 1992.
111. Carter CL, Allen C, Henson DE: Relation of tumor size, lymph node status, and survival in 24,740 breast cancer cases. Cancer 63:181–187, 1989.
112. Donegan WL: Prognostic factors; stage and receptor status in breast cancer. Cancer 70:1755–1764, 1992.
113. Fisher B, Redmond C, Fisher ER, et al: Relative worth of estrogen or progesterone receptor and pathologic characteristics of differentiation as indicators of prognosis in node negative breast cancer patients: Findings from National Surgical Adjuvant Breast and Bowel Project protocol B-06. J Clin Oncol 6:1076–1087, 1988.
114. Stål O, Dufmats M, Hatschek T, et al: S-phase fraction is a prognostic factor in stage I breast carcinoma. J Clin Oncol 11:1717–1722, 1993.
115. Urban JA, Baker HW: Radical mastectomy in continuity with en bloc resection of the internal mammary lymph-node chain. Cancer 5:992–1008, 1952.
116. Lacour J, Monique L, Caceres E, et al: Radical mastectomy versus radical mastectomy plus internal mammary dissection: Ten year results of an international cooperative trial in breast cancer. Cancer 51:1941–1943, 1983.
117. Meier P, Ferguson D, Karrison T: A controlled trial of extended radical versus radical mastectomy. Cancer 63:188–195, 1989.
118. Lacour J, Lê MG, Kramar A, et al: Is it useful to remove internal mammary nodes in operable breast cancer? Eur J Surg Oncol 13:309–314, 1987.
120. Auchincloss H: Significance of location and number of axillary metastases in carcinoma of the breast: A justification for a conservation operation. Ann Surg 158:37–46, 1962.
121. Maddox WA, Carpenter JT, Laws HT, et al: Does radical mastectomy still have a place in the treatment of primary operable breast cancer? Arch Surg 122:1317–1320, 1987.
122. Turner L, Swindell R, Bell WGT, et al: Radical versus modified radical mastectomy for breast cancer.
123. Fisher B, Redmond C, Fisher ER, et al: Ten-year results of a randomized clinical trial comparing radical mastectomy and total mastectomy with or without radiation. N Engl J Med 312:674–681, 1985.
124. Langlands AO, Prescott RJ, Hamilton T: A clinical trial in the management of operable cancer of the breast. Br J Surg 67:170–174, 1980.
125. Osborne MP, Borgen PI: Role of mastectomy in breast cancer. Surg Clin North Am 70:1023–1046, 1990.
126. Ashikari R, Hajdu SI, Robbins GF: Intraductal carcinoma of the breast. Cancer 5:1182–1187, 1971.
127. Harris JR, Hellman S, Kinne DW: Limited surgery and radiotherapy for early breast cancer. N Engl J Med 313:1365–1368, 1985.
128. Rosen PP, Fracchia AA, Urban JA, et al: "Residual" mammary carcinoma following simulated partial mastectomy. Cancer 35:739–747, 1975.
129. Fisher B, Redmond C, Poisson R, et al: Eight-year results of a randomized clinical trial comparing total mastectomy and lumpectomy with or without irradiation in the treatment of breast cancer. N Engl J Med 320:822–828, 1989.
130. Veronesi U, Saccozzi R, DelVecchio M, et al: Comparing radical mastectomy with quadrantectomy, axillary dissection, and radiotherapy in patients with small cancers of the breast. N Engl J Med 305:6–11, 1981.
131. Ghossein NA, Alpert S, Barba J, et al: Breast cancer: The importance of adequate surgical excision prior to radiotherapy in the local control of breast cancer in patients treated conservatively. Arch Surg 127:411–415, 1992.
132. Siegel BM, Mayzel KA, Love SM: Level I and II axillary dissection in the treatment of early-stage breast cancer. Arch Surg 125:1144–1147, 1990.
133. Fisher B, Leeming R, Andersen S, et al: Conservative management of intraductal carcinoma (DCIS) of the breast. J Surg Oncol 47:139–147, 1991.
134. Graham MD, Lakhani S, Gazet JC: Breast conserving surgery in the management of in situ breast carcinoma. Eur J Surg Oncol 17:258–264, 1991.
135. Sollin LJ, Yeh I-T, Kurtz J, et al: Ductal carcinoma in situ (intraductal carcinoma) of the breast treated with breast-conserving surgery and definitive irradiation. Cancer 71:2532–2542, 1993.
136. Swain SM: Ductal carcinoma in situ. Cancer Invest 10:443–454, 1992.

137. Bland KI, Frykberg ER: Selective management of in situ carcinoma of the breast. Breast Dis 3:11–22, 1992.
138. Bradley SJ, Weaver DW, Bouwman DL: Alternatives in the surgical management of in situ breast cancer. A meta-analysis of outcome. Am Surg 56:428–432, 1990.
139. Solin LJ, Fowble BL, Schultz DJ, Yeh I, Kowalyshyn MJ, Goodman RL: Definitive irradiation for intraductal carcinoma of the breast. Int J Radiat Oncol Biol Phys 19:843–850, 1990.
140. Kuske RR, Bean JM, Garcia DM, et al: Breast conservation therapy for intraductal carcinoma of the breast. Int J Radiat Oncol Biol Phys 26:391–396, 1993.
141. McCormick B, Rosen PP, Kinne D, Cox L, Yaholom J: Duct carcinoma in situ of the breast: An analysis of local control after conservation surgery and radiotherapy. Int J Radiat Oncol Biol Phys 21:289–292, 1991.
142. Jacquemier J, Kurtz JM, Amalric R, Brandone H, Ayme Y, Spitalier J-M: An assessment of extensive intraductal component as a risk factor for local recurrence after breast-conserving therapy. Br J Cancer 61:873–976, 1990.
143. Wood WC, Barringer TA, Daly JM, et al: Results of the NCI early breast cancer trial. In Proceedings of the National Institutes of Health Consensus Development Conference on Early Stage Breast Cancer, June 1990, pp 32–33.
144. Bedwinek J: Breast conserving surgery and irradiation: The importance of demarcating the excision cavity with surgical clips. Int J Radiat Oncol Biol Phys 26:675–679, 1993.
145. Regine W, Ayyamgan W, Komarnicky L, Bhandane N, Mansfield C: Computer-CT planning of the electron boost in definitive breast irradiation. Int J Radiat Oncol Biol Phys 20:121–125, 1991.
146. Solin L, Chu T, Larsen R, Fowble B, Galvin T, Goodman R: Determination of depth for electron breast boosts. Int J Radiat Oncol Biol Phys 13:1915–1919, 1987.
147. Host H, Brennhovd IO, Loeeb M: Postoperative radiotherapy in breast conserving and radiation: The delay of primary radiation after adjuvant chemotherapy does not influence local control. Proc ASCO 11:55, 1992 (abstract).
148. Klefstron P, Grohn P, Heinonen E, Holsti L, Holsti P: Adjuvant postoperative radiotherapy, chemotherapy and immunotherapy in Stage III breast cancer. II. 5-Year results and influence of levamisole. Cancer 60:936–942, 1987.
149. McCormick B, Hakes T, Yahalom J, Kinne D, Norton L: Breast conserving surgery and radiation: The delay of primary radiation after adjuvant chemotherapy does not influence local control. Pro ASCO 11:55, 1992 (abstract).
150. Stefanik D, Goldberg R, Byrne P, et al: Local-regional failure in patients treated with adjuvant chemotherapy for breast cancer. J Clin Oncol 3:660–665, 1985.
151. Derman DP, Browde S, Kessel IL, et al: Adjuvant chemotherapy (CMF) for stage III breast cancer: A randomized trial. Int J Radiat Oncol Biol Phys 17:257–261, 1989.
152. Bonadonna G, Brusamolino E, Pinuccia V: Combination chemotherapy as an adjuvant treatment in operable breast cancer. N Engl J Med 294:405–410, 1976.
153. Sheth SP, Allegra JC: What role for concurrent chemohormonal therapy in breast cancer? Oncology 1:19–27, 1987.
154. Fisher B, Costantino J, Redmond C, et al: A randomized clinical trial evaluating tamoxifen in the treatment of patients with node-negative breast cancer who have estrogen-receptor–positive tumors. N Engl J Med 320:479–484, 1989.
155. Stewart HJ: The Scottish trial of adjuvant tamoxifen in node-negative breast cancer. Treatment of early-stage breast cancer. NCI Monogr 11:117–120, 1992.
156. Fisher B, Redmond C, Brown A, et al: Treatment of primary breast cancer with chemotherapy and tamoxifen. N Engl J Med 305:1–6, 1981.
157. Fisher B, Costantino J, Redmond C, et al: Adjuvant chemotherapy with and without tamoxifen in the treatment of primary breast cancer: 5-Year results from the National Surgical Adjuvant Breast and Bowel Project trial. J Clin Oncol 4:459–471, 1986.
158. Ludwig Breast Cancer Study Group: Chemotherapy with or without oophorectomy in high-risk premenopausal patients with operable breast cancer. J Clin Oncol 3:1059–1067, 1985.
159. Osborne MP, Borgen PI, Wong GY, et al: Salvage mastectomy for local-regional recurrence after breast conserving surgery and radiation therapy. Surg Gynecol Obstet 174:189, 1992.
160. Stotter A, McNeese M, Ames F, et al: Predicting the rate and extent of locoregional failure after breast conservation therapy for early breast cancer. Cancer 64:2217, 1989.
161. Cajucom C, Tsangaris T, Nemoto T, et al: Results of salvage mastectomy for local recurrence after breast conserving surgery without radiation therapy. Cancer 71:1774, 1993.
162. Dershaw D, McCormick B, Cox L, et al: Differentiation of benign and malignant local tumor recurrence after lumpectomy. Am J Roentgenol 155:35, 1990.
163. Kurtz J, Amalric R, Brandone H, et al: Local recurrence after breast conserving surgery and radiotherapy. Cancer 63:1912, 1989.
164. Abner A, Recht A, Eberlein T, et al: Prognosis following salvage mastectomy for recurrence in the breast after conservative surgery and radiation therapy for early stage breast cancer. J Clin Oncol 11:44, 1993.
165. Dershaw D, McCormick Osborne M: Detection of local recurrence after conservative therapy for breast carcinoma. Cancer 70:493, 1992.
167. Recht A, Schnitt S, Connolly J, et al: Prognosis following local or regional recurrence after conservative surgery and radiotherapy for early stage breast carcinoma. Int J Radiat Oncol Biol Phys 16:3, 1989.
168. Fowble B, Solin LJ, Schultz DJ, et al: Breast recurrence following conservative surgery and radiation: Patterns of failure, prognosis and pathologic findings from mastectomy specimens with implications for treatment. Int J Radiat Oncol Biol Phys 19:833, 1990.
169. Harris J, Recht A, Amalric R, et al: Time course and prognosis of local recurrence following primary radiation therapy for early breast cancer. J Clin Oncol 2:37, 1984.
170. Haffty B, Goldberg N, Fischer K, et al: Conservative surgery and radiation therapy in breast carcinoma: Local recurrence and prognostic implications. Int J Radiat Oncol Biol Phys 17:727, 1989.
171. Fourquet A, Campana F, Zagrani B, et al: Prognostic factors of breast recurrence in the conservative management of early breast cancer. A 25-year follow-up. Int J Radiat Oncol Biol Phys 17:719, 1989.
172. Ouriel K: Carcinoma of the male breast. NY State J Med 8:291–292, 1988.
173. Kinne DW: Management of male breast cancer. Oncology 5:45–48, 1991.
174. Jaiyesimi IA, Buzdar AU, Sahin AA, Ross MA: Carcinoma of the male breast. Ann Intern Med 117:771–775, 1992.
175. Lefor AT, Numann PJ: Carcinoma of the breast in men. NY State J Med 8:293–296, 1988.
176. Borgen PI, Wong GY, Vlamis V, et al: Current management of male breast cancer: A review of 104 cases. Male breast cancer. 215:451–457, 1992.
177. Guinee VF, Olsson H, Moller T, et al: The prognosis of breast cancer in males. Cancer 71:154–161, 1993.
178. Tobon HH, Horowitz LF: Breast cancer during pregnancy. Breast Dis 6:127–134, 1993.
179. Saunders CM, Baum M: Breast cancer and pregnancy. J R Soc Med 86:162–165, 1993.
180. van der Vange N, van Dongen JA: Breast cancer and pregnancy. Eur J Surg Oncol 17:1–8, 1991.
181. Barnavon Y, Wallack MK: Management of the pregnant patient with carcinoma of the breast. Surg Gynecol Obstet 171:347–352, 1990.
182. Petrek JA: Breast cancer and pregnancy. Breast Dis 809–816, 1991.
183. Nugent P, O'Connell TX: Breast cancer and pregnancy. Arch Surg 120:1221–1224, 1985.
184. Harvey JC, Rosen PP, Ashikari R, et al: The effect of pregnancy on the prognosis of carcinoma of the breast following radical mastectomy. Surg Gynecol Obstet 153:723–725, 1981.

18

Narayan Sundaresan, M.D. • George Krol, M.D.
Mark Reiner, M.D. • Alfred A. Steinberger, M.D.

Tumors of the Sacrum

Tumors of the sacrum comprise a diverse group of neoplasms encompassing a wide range of histopathology.[1–6] The majority of tumors expand predominantly into the presacral space, often being asymptomatic until they attain large size. The last decade has witnessed a dramatic evolution in the concepts of surgical management of these tumors because of earlier diagnosis and improved delineation of anatomy achieved through the use of imaging by computed tomography (CT) and magnetic resonance imaging (MRI).

The operative approach to sacral tumors requires a multidisciplinary team of surgical oncologists, spine surgeons, and plastic surgeons. The involvement of these subspecialties minimizes the chances of intraoperative catastrophies and maximizes the chances of adequate functional and cosmetic results. The postoperative management should include the anticipation of potential complications, since the end results of resection may produce a neurogenic bladder with bowel and sexual dysfunction as well as loss of mobility from extensive muscle and ligamentous resection.

Sacral tumors are classified, on the basis of their biologic behavior, as benign tumors, locally aggressive low-grade malignant tumors, and highly aggressive or high-grade malignant tumors. Aneurysmal bone cysts or osteoblastoma are examples of benign tumors, while chondromas, giant cell tumors, and chondrosarcomas constitute the low-grade malignant tumors. High-grade malignant tumors are osteosarcomas and cancers invading the spine by direct local extension.[6]

Indications for surgery range from open biopsy for diagnosis, to decompressive laminectomy for intraspinal benign lesions, to partial sacrectomy for benign bone and neural tumors. Extensive resections done in conjunction with pelvic posterior exenteration are reserved for locally invasive or recurrent cancers such as those originating in the cervix or rectum.[1, 7–11] Although intralesional curettage by decompressive laminectomy was accepted treatment for many low-grade malignant tumors such as chordomas and giant cell tumors, this surgery is followed by high rates of local recurrence. These tumors are best treated by en bloc resection without violation of tumor pseudocapsule.[12] A variety of surgical techniques are available, including anterior, posterior, or combined anterior-posterior approaches. En bloc sacrectomies are used for the treatment of high-grade malignancies: indications for this procedure have been extended to include cases of recurrent local pelvic cancers.[7–10, 13, 14]

SURGICAL ANATOMY

Five or occasionally six vertebrae are fused in the adult to form the sacrum, a single wedge-shaped bone with its base lying in the superior position. The sacrum forms the back wall of the pelvis and lies between the two innominate bones. Its anterior surface is concave from side to side and from above downward (Fig. 18–1). There are four anterior sacral foramina on each side in parallel rows. Lateral to these foramina are lateral masses marked by the neural grooves. The lateral margin of the sacrum has a notch (sacral notch) opposite the second segment and ends below the fourth foramen in the inferior lateral angle.

The posterior surface of the sacrum is composed of fused neural arches that house the central canal (Fig. 18–2). Bony surface projections include the midline spinal crest and a narrow sacral groove bounded laterally by a row of tubercles, the articular crest. The four posterior sacral foramina are lateral to this structure. The sacral groove and its neighboring processes give origin to the posterior spinous muscles (erector spinae, sacrospinalis, multifidus). The articular crests end below in the sacral cornu, which articulates with the coccyx. The area between the articular crests is deficient below the fourth segment and is termed the hiatus sacralis.

The lateral mass has a rough double hollow on its posterolateral aspect, opposite the first two segments. This provides a broad surface area of attachment for the sacroil-

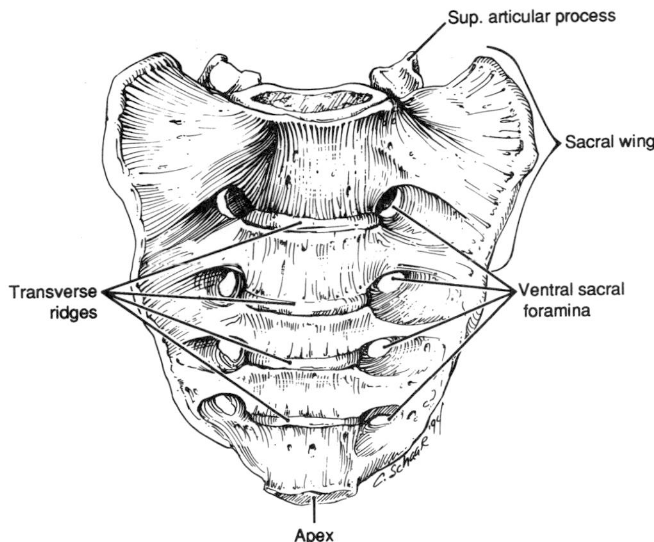

FIGURE 18–1. Anterior surface of the sacrum. Prominent features include neural foramina and transverse ridges.

iac ligaments. The base of the sacrum demonstrates the sacral body centrally flanked on either side by the ala. Behind the body is the upper opening of the sacral canal. A large superior articular process present on each side is separated from the sacral body by a vertebral notch. A mamillary tubercle is below the outer edge on the back of the superior articular facet. The lumbosacral angle of 210° in the erect position is formed between the first sacral and the last lumbar segments, with its angle being rounded off by the intervertebral disc.

Normally, the articular surface of the sacrum extends back onto the posteroinferior spine. The sacrotuberous ligament is attached to the posterior aspects of the inferior spine extending inferiorly to the tranverse fibers and coccyx. The gluteus maximus and multifidus originate along the posterior aspect of the sacrum and from the sacrotuberous ligament (Fig. 18–3). Inferiorly, the attachment of the coccygeus fibers extends down to the coccyx. The back and upper fibers of this sheet are ligamentous and constitute the sacrospinal ligament.

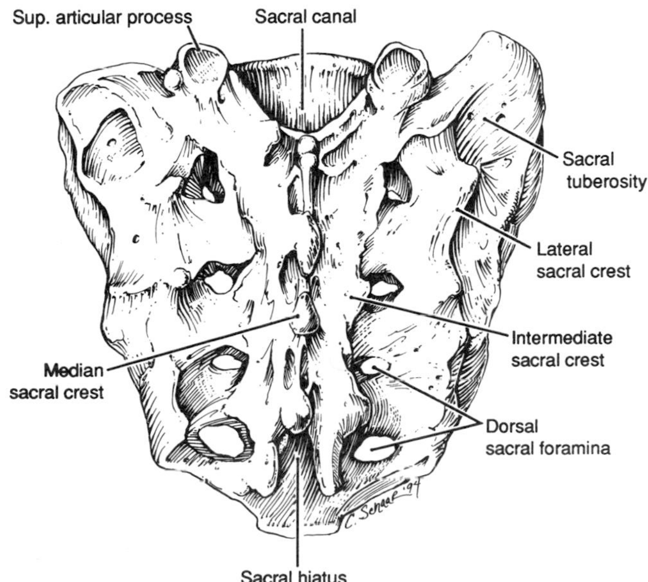

FIGURE 18–2. Sacrum, posterior view. Neural arches and midline crest comprise the posterior wall of the spinal canal. Foramina are situated between intermediate and lateral sacral crests.

The anterior surface of the bodies may show longitudinal markings, which represent a portion of the anterior longitudinal ligaments (Fig. 18–4). The presacral space is a crescent-shaped defect located between the posterior wall of the rectum and the anterior surface of the sacrum and coccyx. This space has an anterior lining comprising the fascia propria of the rectum, and a posterior sheath made up of the fascia pelvis parietalis, or Waldeyer's fascia. The presacral space is limited superiorly by the peritoneal reflection at the S-2 level and inferiorly by the coccygeal ligament and levator ani muscles.

Sacral stability comes predominantly from the lateral sacral ala of the first three sacral vertebrae and the iliac bones. Some mobility and resilience are provided by the sacroiliac joint. This articulation consists of a synovial joint and a strong interosseous sacroiliac ligament, which is located posterior to the joint cavity. Degenerative changes in this joint occur, especially in men over 50 years of age, and can result in early fusion. The ventral and dorsal sacroiliac ligaments function to reinforce the stability of the sacroiliac joint by resisting forward rotation. Both the sacrotuberous and the sacrospinous ligaments provide torsional stability and prevent rotation of the lower sacrum. Gunterberg et al.[15] showed that an osteotomy through the first sacral segment results in approximately 50% loss of strength in the pelvic girdle but still allows the vertical load of the body to be resisted. Our observations confirm these studies, since resections carried through the first sacral segment do not always require stabilization.

INCIDENCE AND CLINICAL PRESENTATION

The first recorded case of a sacral tumor was by Luschka, but the first detailed description was a congenital sacrococcygeal tumor in a 1-year-old child, discussed in 1885 by Middledorpf. As a result, all congenital tumors were initially called Middledorpf tumors.

The true incidence of primary tumors of the sacrum is difficult to ascertain, since the majority of sacral tumors are metastatic or secondary to the direct extension of previously resected pelvic cancers. It is estimated that approximately 25% of rectal cancers locally recur within the pelvis following curative resection. In women, the incidence of intrapelvic recurrences in stage III cancer of the cervix treated by external beam irradiation may range from 50% to 80%; this figure may drop to between 20% and 50% if

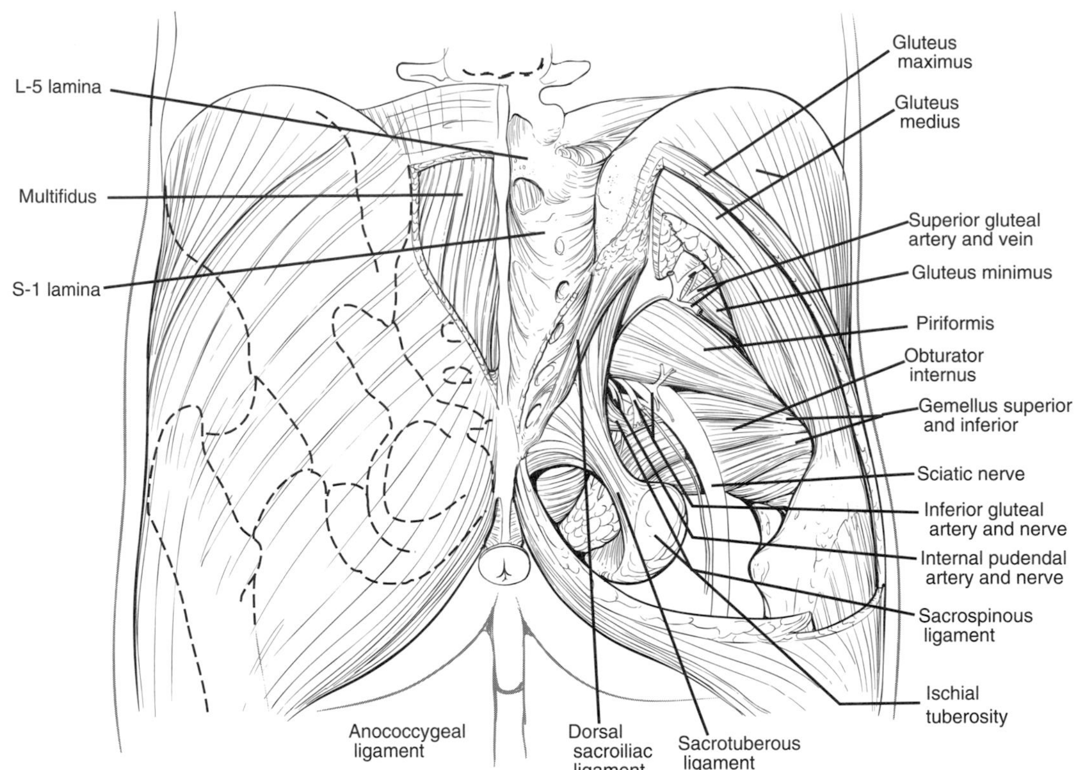

FIGURE 18–3. Diagram of the posterior sacroiliac region. Left: gluteus maximus muscle intact. Exposed in the window are posterior paraspinal muscles. Right: structures lying beneath gluteus major.

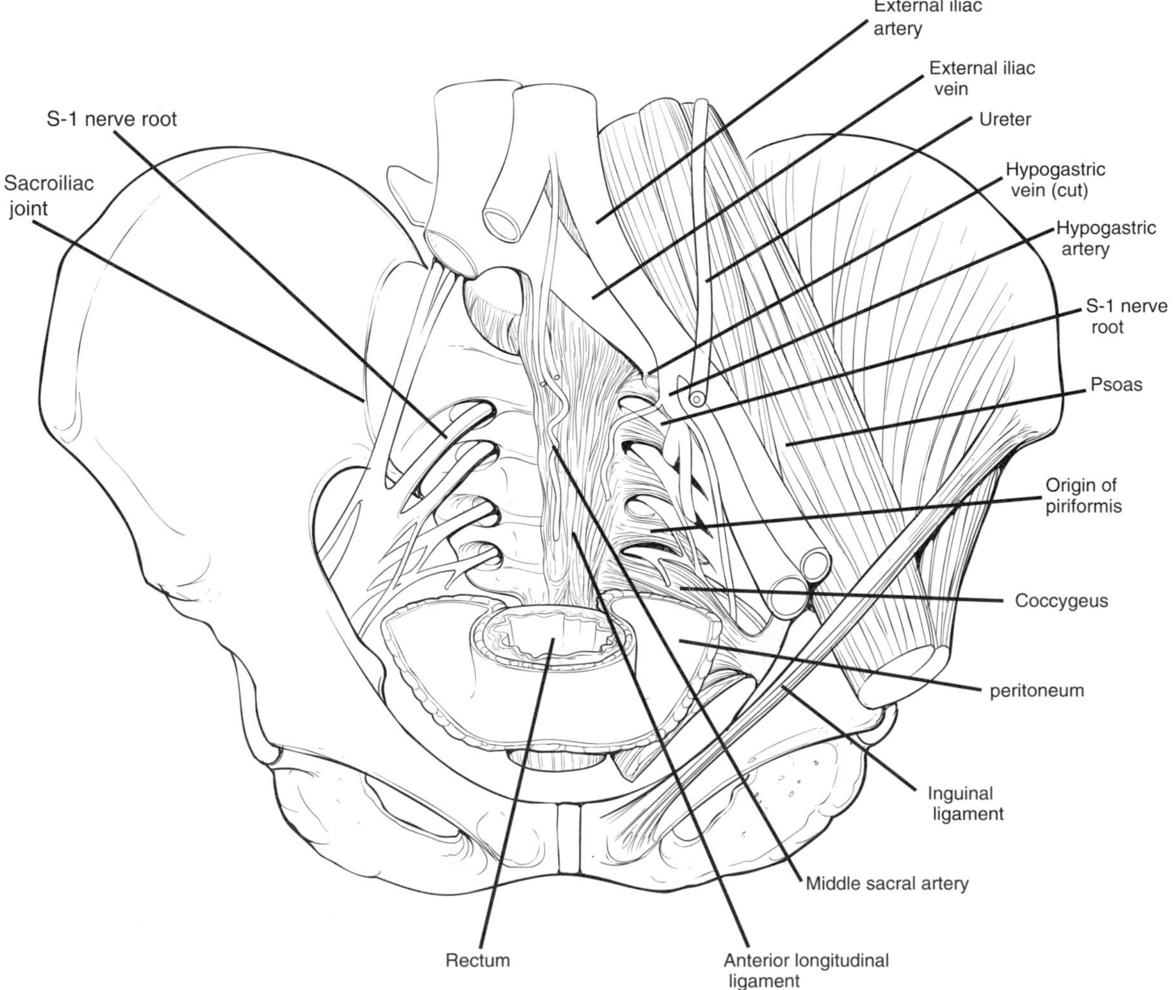

FIGURE 18–4. Relationship of major vascular structures and neural pathways to the anterior sacrum.

additional brachytherapy or intracavitary radiation is used. A small proportion of these patients have local failures within the pelvis that are amenable to pelvic exenteration.

Tumors involving the sacrum can be classified into different categories based on tissue of origin: congenital, neurogenic, osseous, metastatic, and miscellaneous. The largest single institutional series is that of Xu and colleagues[6] from Beijing. This study had 87 patients seen over a 30-year period. Ages ranged from 14 to 66 years, with an average of 41 years. Seventeen patients had benign bone tumors, 62 had low-grade malignant tumors (chordoma or giant cell tumors), and 8 had high-grade malignant tumors. In the practice of most surgical oncologists, the chordoma is the most commonly seen primary sacral tumor. Though it makes up only 1% to 4% of all bone tumors, approximately half of all chordomas originate in the sacrococcygeal region.

The clinical presentation of benign tumors is generally nonspecific. More than three quarters of patients report back pain without localization.[2] Others may have no complaints, with the tumor being diagnosed during a routine physical or gynecologic examination. Such benign tumors may grow to extremely large sizes, often exceeding 10 cm in diameter. Most patients with chordomas, or low-grade malignant tumors, present with back pain and may give a recent history of trauma. Since localized or radicular pain is a feature of these tumors, long delays in diagnosis are relatively common because early symptoms may mimic disc disease. The presence of leg pain or sciatica-like symptoms may frequently lead the clinician to suspect a lumbar disc syndrome. Thus, the majority of patients with sacral pain are usually evaluated by the orthopedist, and in some series approximately 20% have undergone inappropriate lumbar discectomy as initial treatment. In others, the presence of a large presacral mass may lead to rectal dysfunction, including tenesmus, obstipation, or constipation.[16] Rectal bleeding may result from secondary hemorrhoids resulting from straining. In patients with rectal cancer, the presence of recurrent or new onset of pelvic and perineal pain may herald the earliest recurrence of pelvic cancer. In such patients, the recurrence may not always be accompanied by rising tumor markers such as carcinoembryonic antigen (CEA) levels. In most patients, rectal examination should confirm the presence of a large retrorectal mass.

RADIOGRAPHIC EVALUATION

Plain radiographic evaluations are often difficult to interpret owing to overlying gas shadows and curvature of the sacrum. Although the lateral view may not show enough bony detail, the presence of scalloping or reactional bony sclerosis should raise the possibility of a benign long-standing lesion (Figs. 18–5 and 18–6). Similarly, on a spot film of the sacrum, enlargement of the neural foramina may suggest the diagnosis of neurofibroma.

CT and MRI scans are very sensitive in detecting sacral tumors and presacral masses that are not seen on plain radiography. The presence of bone destruction is usually caused by a malignant process (Figs. 18–7 and 18–8). The most common radiologic finding in sacral chordomas is the destruction of several segments of the sacrum associated with a soft tissue tumor mass anterior to it; the incidence of calcifications may vary from 40% to 80%. Frequently, the soft tissue mass is disproportionately larger than the area of bone destruction, and the superior limit of the mass may be above the level of bone involvement.[3, 16, 17] Al-

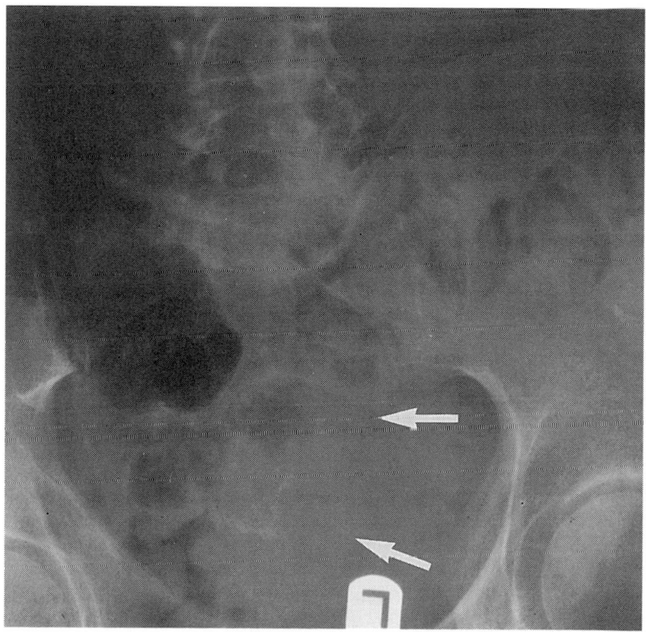

FIGURE 18–5. Anterposterior radiograph of the pelvis. Loss of definition of left lateral border and distal aspect of the sacrum is due to lower sacral chordoma (arrows).

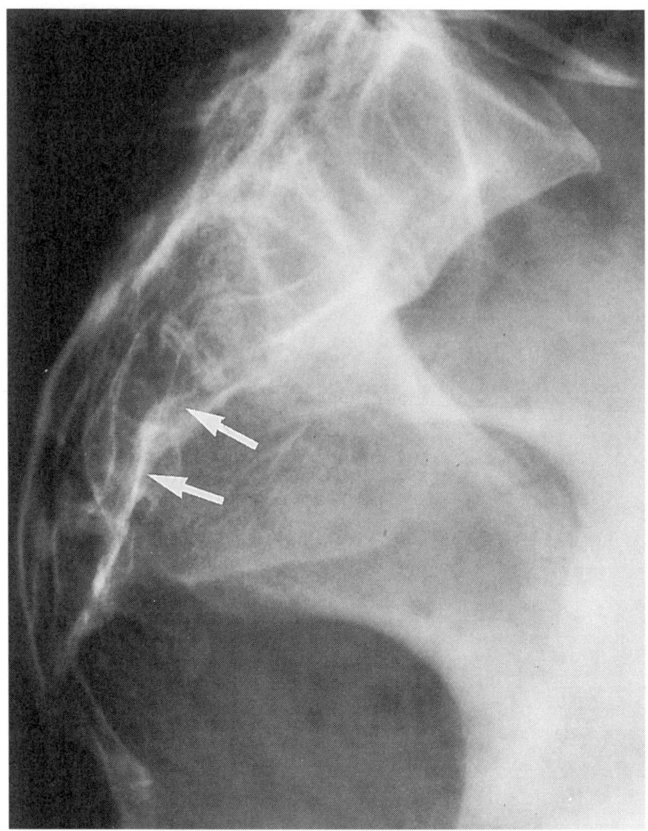

FIGURE 18–6. Sacrum, lateral view. Focal pressure erosion of the anterior cortex (arrows) without bone destruction, characteristic of a long-standing process (neurofibroma).

though previous radiographic methods of tumor imaging included indirect evidence of tumor mass by means of barium enemas and intravenous pyelography, these studies have largely been replaced by CT and MRI.[18] MRI has been shown to be superior to CT because of its multiplanar imaging capacity, which allows assessment of tumor extension into soft tissues, nerves, and adjacent viscera (Fig. 18–9*A* and *B*). Rectal invasion should be sought, although the rectum is rarely involved in benign tumors. The CT scan is superior in demonstrating cortical and trabecular bone detail and demonstrates tumor calcification much more clearly. For a proper radiologic diagnosis, both CT and MRI should be performed. Another major advantage of CT is the ability to obtain CT-guided biopsies using percutaneous techniques. In many cases, this allows a tissue diagnosis to be made.

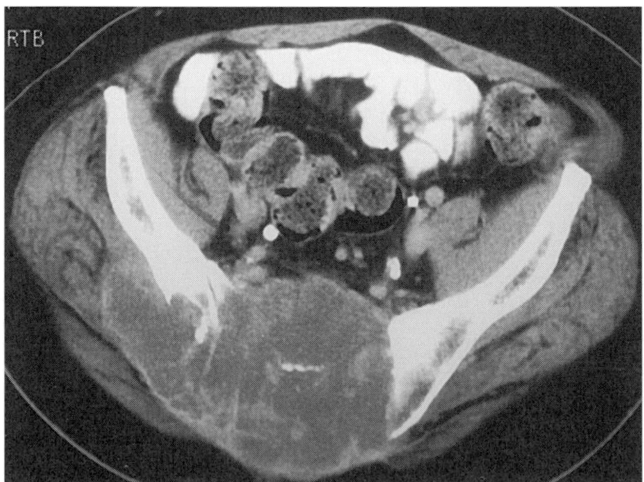

FIGURE 18–7. Advanced sacral chordoma. Axial CT section through the lower pelvis. There is extensive destruction of the entire sacrum and part of the right ilium, associated with large, lobulated, inhomogeneous soft tissue mass.

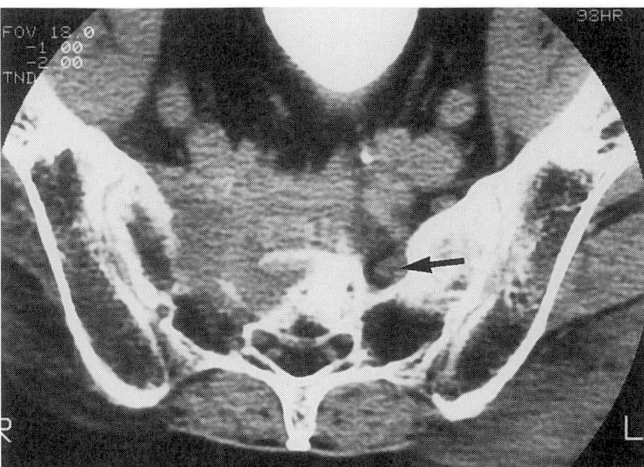

FIGURE 18–8. Direct extension of the rectal carcinoma into the sacrum. There is invasion of the S-3 foramen and obliteration of the corresponding nerve. Normal nerve on the left (arrow).

In selected cases, angiography is recommended to demonstrate tumor neovascularity and to embolize highly vascular lesions presurgically. We routinely evaluate all primary tumors of the sacrum by angiography, since most sacral tumors are extremely hypervascular and surgical morbidity can be reduced by embolization. Angiography has also been used for selective introduction of therapeutic drugs (such as intraarterial infusion of cisplatin in osteosarcoma).

BIOPSY

Biopsy is performed for definitive diagnosis. The biopsy may be an open or Tru-Cut needle biopsy performed from a posterior approach. Sufficient tissue must be obtained for routine histology and immunoperoxidase stains.[19] Frequently, if soft tissue extension is seen, a CT-guided biopsy (Fig. 18–10) is sufficient to make an accurate diagnosis.[20] In general, transrectal biopsies are avoided. The biopsy site should be planned so that the tract can be excised at the subsequent operation.

SURGICAL TREATMENT

All patients referred for resection of malignant sacral tumors should be assessed completely for systemic and

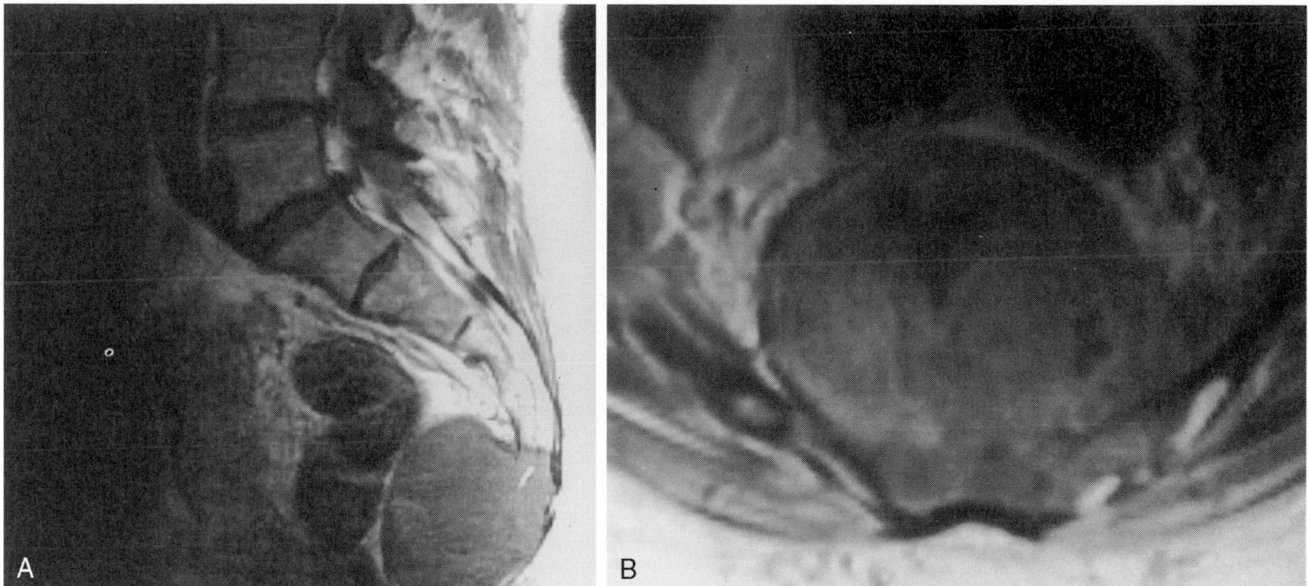

FIGURE 18–9. Chordoma of distal sacrum. There is superb demonstration of the tumor extension on these T1-weighted sagittal *(A)* and axial *(B)* MR images.

local spread. This may require CT evaluation of the abdomen and chest, bone scan, and intravenous pyelography. In nonirradiated patients, some advocate a course of preoperative radiation of 45 Gy over 4½ weeks to the pelvis.[10] Nutritional supplements may be required, and a preoperative bowel regimen is generally used. A low-residue diet is advised for several days prior to admission. The patient is generally hospitalized 24 hours prior to surgery on a liquid diet and appropriate antibiotics, such as neomycin and erythromycin; in addition, mechanical cleansing of the bowel is carried out.

Most procedures involving sacral resections may be complicated by profuse blood loss. Preparation for management of intraoperative blood loss should include the use of a Cell Saver, Level One transfusion device and large-bore intravenous catheters. In the elderly, a Swan-Ganz catheter is inserted for monitoring. Those with symptoms of coronary disease may require preoperative evaluation by stress testing or thallium myocardial scans.

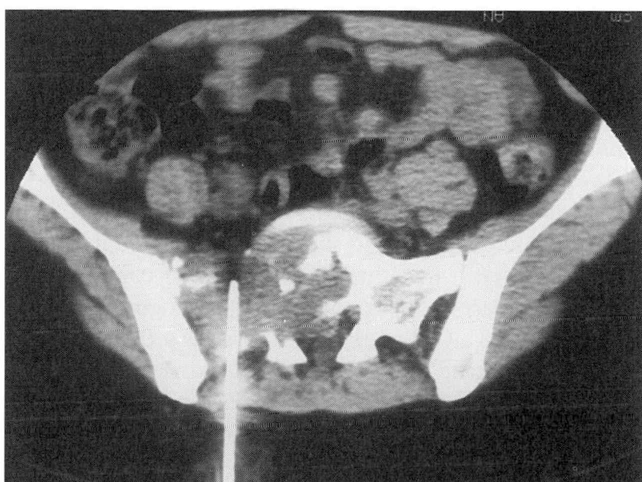

FIGURE 18–10. Biopsy of the sacral lesion, subsequently diagnosed as poorly differentiated spindle cell sarcoma. CT guidance allows for precise placement of the biopsy instrument within the desired portion of the tumor.

Posterior Laminectomy

In the earlier literature, the standard operative procedure was a posterior approach performed in the prone position.[21, 22] This approach is applicable only for small tumors below the S-3 segment or for intraspinal lesions such as dumbbell neurofibromas, in which the intradural component has to be resected as part of a staged operation. The major advantage of this procedure is its familiarity and technical ease, clear identification and preservation of neural tissue, and low morbidity. In addition, the prone position allows proper radiographic placement of screws with fluoroscopic monitoring.

Staged Anterior-Posterior Resection

For larger tumors (Fig. 18–11*A* and *B*) that extend to the second sacral segment, or those with large presacral extensions, several authors have proposed a staged anterior-posterior operation.[1, 7, 9, 10, 23] In the initial operation, the abdomen is opened through a midline laparotomy, which allows determination of resectability of the tumor and detection of intra-abdominal metastases that would preclude curative resection. In addition, the anterior approach allows bilateral ligation of the hypogastric arteries to minimize blood loss during the sacrectomy portion of the procedure.[1, 8, 11] Sung et al.[5] reported on 54 patients undergoing hypo-

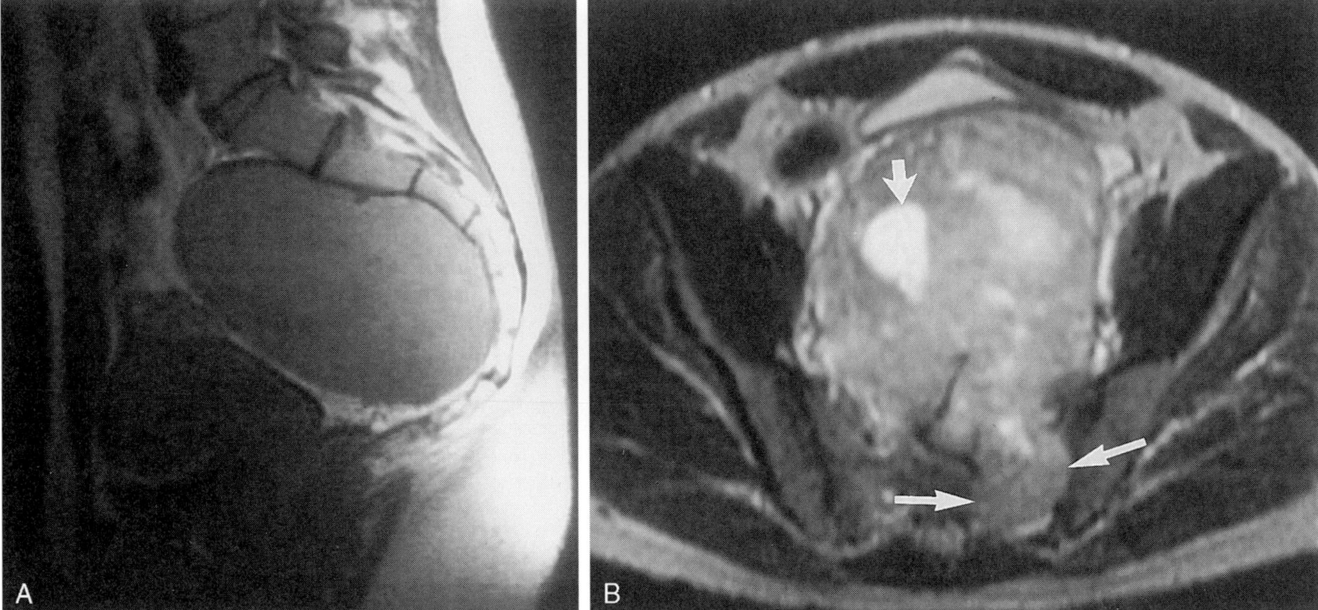

FIGURE 18–11. Giant neurofibroma with large presacral component. *A,* Sagittal T1-weighted MR image. There is preservation of the adjacent cortical bone, and signal intensity of the bone marrow is normal. *B,* Axial T2-weighted image. There is marked enlargement of the foramen, characteristic of neural tumors (horizontal arrows). Oval hyperintensity within the mass (vertical arrow) probably represents an area of cystic degeneration.

gastric artery ligation, with no specific complications related to ischemic injury.

In the staged approach, the patient is generally placed supine with the legs supported by stirrups. To facilitate access, a pad is placed under the distal lumbar spine to elevate the sacrum off the table. An initial laparotomy is performed. After assessment of resectability, the main mass should be mobilized by sharp dissection at least 1 cm beyond the mass. The sidewall of the pelvis is cleared at the level of the endopelvic fascia, including the lymph nodes and internal iliac vessels. When necessary, the fascia and muscle of the lateral pelvic walls are resected to obtain clear margins; this may include the internal obturator, piriformis, and branches of the lumbosacral plexus. The sacrum above the tumor is prepared for subsequent transection. If exposure in the pelvis is difficult, the central pubis is excised and the pelvic bony ring is spread.

The perineal portion of the operation is begun only when the entire specimen is free laterally, anteriorly, and posteriorly at the level of the sacrum. During the perineal portion of the dissection, the aorta may be crossclamped to minimize bleeding. A skin margin of 2.5 to 3 cm is obtained around the tumor, and the tissues attached to the dorsal sacrum are freed up to the level of intended transection.

Reconstruction is required if the bladder is sacrificed. The pelvic defect is often massive, and omentum may be brought over to cover the brim. This can be supplemented by a Dexon or Marlex mesh sutured to the margins of the pelvis to help hold the bowel. The perineal cavity needs to be covered by a myocutaneous flap: the tensor fascia lata, gluteus maximus, or rectus abdominis flap may be used. Suction Silastic drains are inserted to prevent seromas in the pelvis.

Combined Abdominosacral Approach

For the majority of chordomas and benign neurofibromas, we favor the lateral position using a simultaneous combined abdominosacral approach, initially described by Localio et al.[25–26]

The patient is positioned in the right lateral position, although the nature of tumor extension may favor a right-sided approach. The skin is prepared to allow simultaneous access to the front and back of the sacrum; two operating teams are required.

For the left-sided approach, an oblique incision is made parallel to the left inguinal ligament and carried through all layers with cautery (Fig. 18–12). The sigmoid colon is rotated medially and its lateral attachments divided. The left ureter is mobilized and tapes placed around it. Along the retroperitoneal plane, the dissection is carried into the pelvis on the fascia propria of the rectum. The right ureter is identified and swept laterally. The tumor with its pseudocapsule can be seen in the hollow of the sacrum. The plane between Waldeyer's fascia and rectum is developed as far distally as possible. The common iliac and both internal and external hypogastric arteries and veins are identified and mobilized. This is relatively easier to perform in the nonirradiated patient. If vessel loops are placed for vascular control of these vessels, we do not believe it necessary to ligate the hypogastric arteries (Fig. 18–13). Once vascular

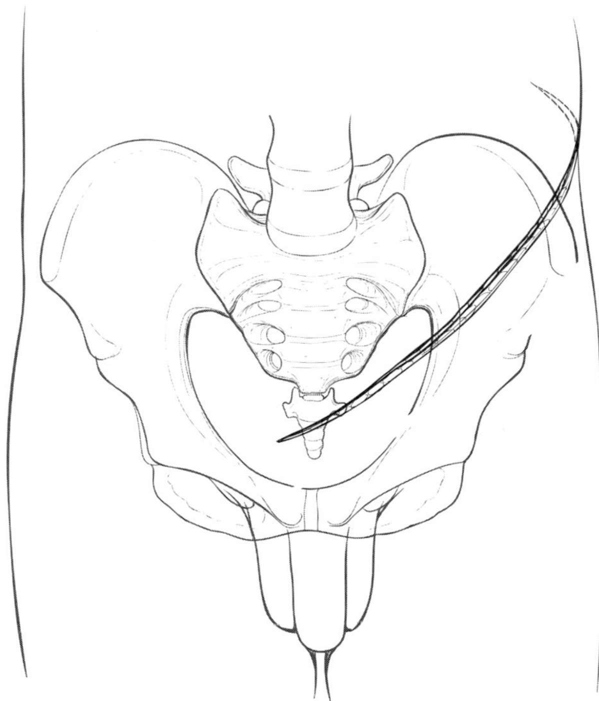

FIGURE 18–12. Left anterior modified incision (Pfannensteil) used in combined anterior-posterior approach.

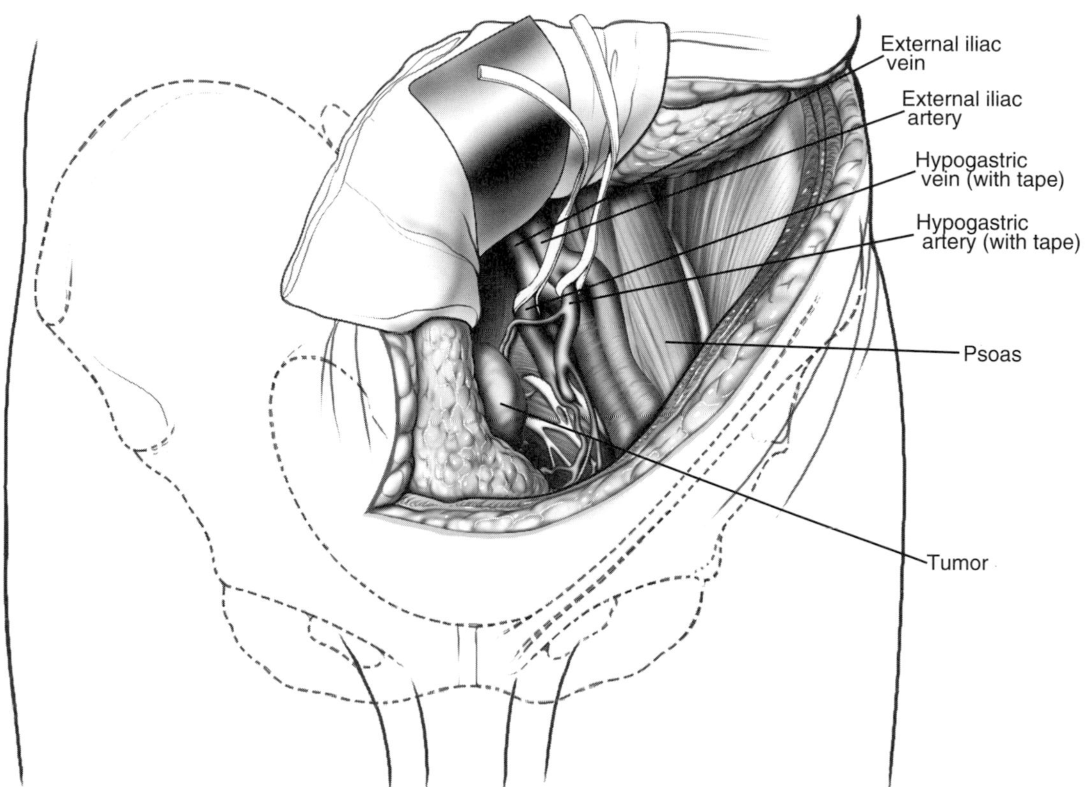

FIGURE 18–13. Following retraction of the abdominal contents medially, the hypogastric vessels are identified and mobilized with vessel loops.

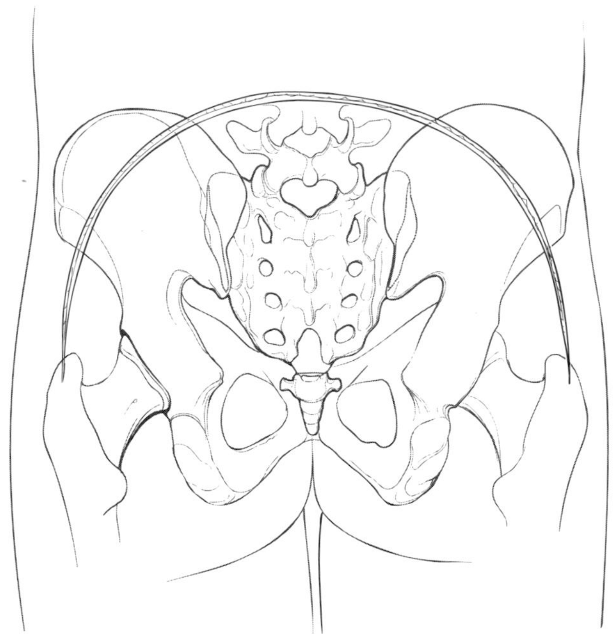

FIGURE 18–14. Posterior incision (omega shaped) used for posterior phase of operation.

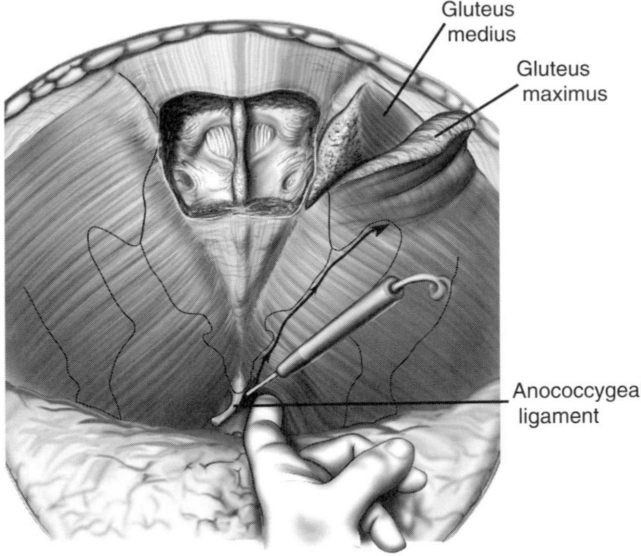

FIGURE 18–16. Separation of the gluteus maximus from the iliac crest and, inferiorly, from the sacrum. Note finger in the presacral space.

control is achieved and the anterior pole of the tumor is freed from the rectum, the posterior phase of the operation is begun.

For the posterior phase, we favor an elliptic incision (omega shaped) with a broad base and limbs carried inferiorly (Fig. 18–14). Midline incisions over the lumbosacral junction are notoriously slow to heal, especially in irradiated patients. A broad flap down to the fascia is developed and reflected inferiorly. An ellipse of skin and subcutaneous fat is left attached to the sacrum to avoid entering the tumor (Fig. 18–15). The gluteus maximus muscle is stripped with cautery off the iliac crests, and this muscle is transected at the lateral border of the sacrum (Fig. 18–16). Inferiorly, the flap should extend to the anal verge, and the anococcygeal ligament is divided. The posterior surface of the rectum is identified at the levators. By developing the plane behind the rectum, an effort is made to meet the abdominal dissection. The inferolateral attachments of the sacrum are divided from below upward. The sacrotuberous and sacrospinous ligaments and portions of the piriformis are divided (Fig. 18–17). During these maneuvers, the lower border of the sciatic foramen is opened; the sciatic nerve should be

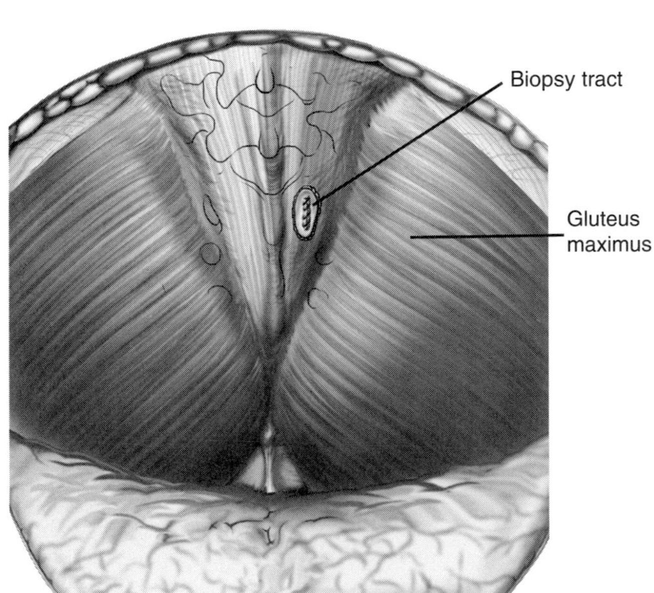

FIGURE 18–15. Skin and subcutaneous flaps reflected to show attachments of gluteus maximus to the sacrum.

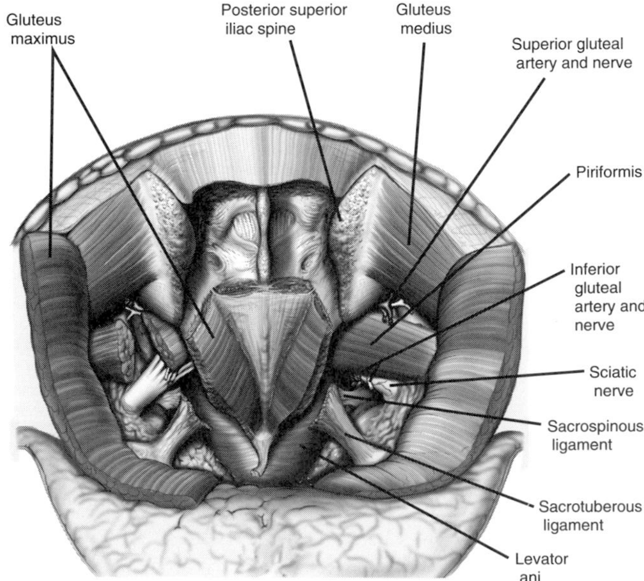

FIGURE 18–17. Detachment of sacrum and tumor by sectioning of the sacrotuberous and sacroiliac ligaments.

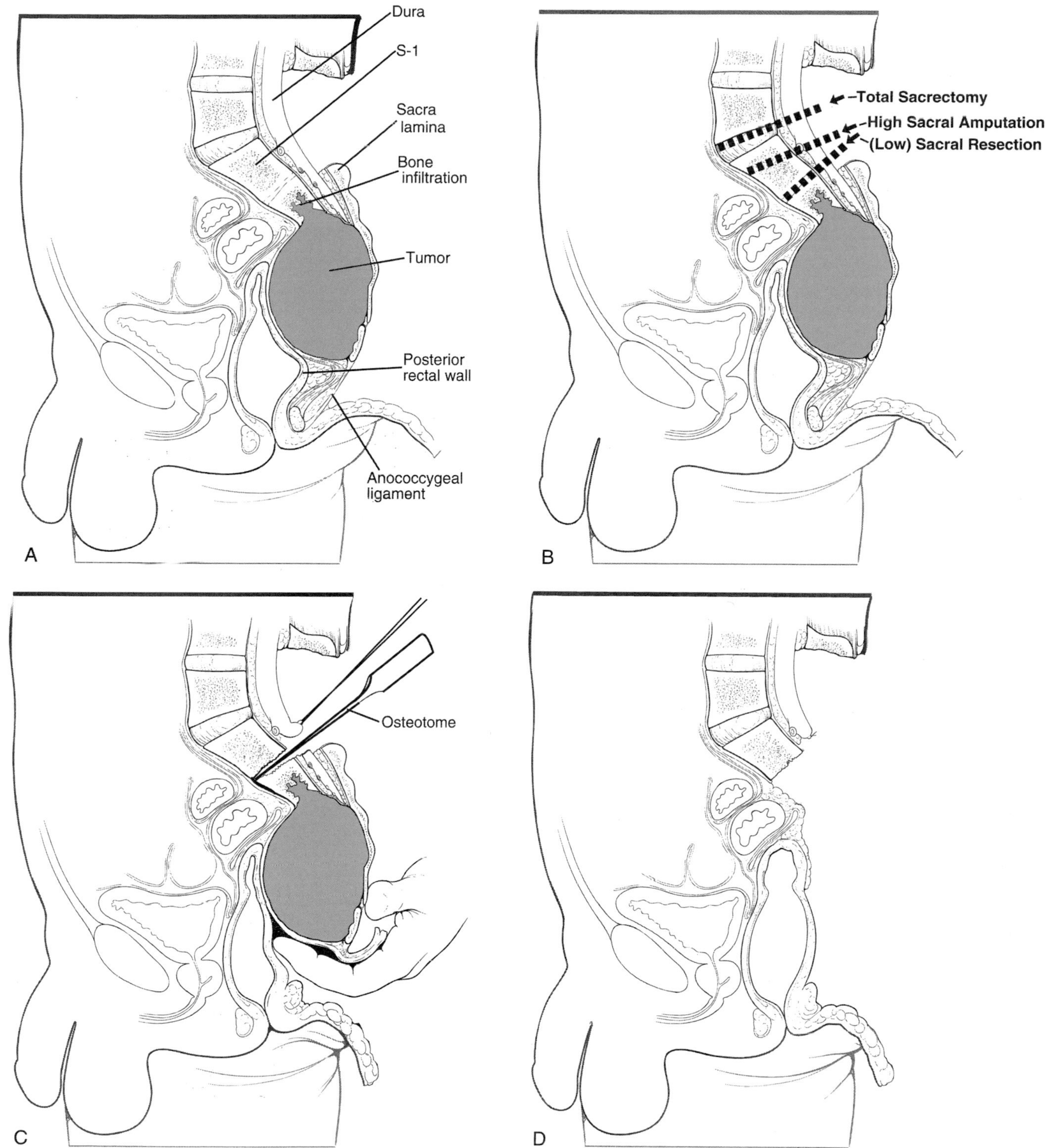

FIGURE 18–18. *A,* Sagittal diagram showing typical chordoma with presacral extension and involvement of the S-2 sacral segment. *B,* Surgical planes frequently used during resection of malignant sacral tumors. *C,* Osteotomy carried out one segment above the soft tissue extension of the tumor. *D,* En bloc completed resection.

carefully protected. Both the sciatic nerve and the inferior gluteal artery are identified at the lower border of the piriformis muscles. The piriformis muscles are resected and the sciatic nerves swept laterally to protect the S-1 and S-2 nerve roots.

After this stage, the exact level of the sacral osteotomy has to be chosen (Fig. 18–18*A* to *D*). We frequently perform a sacral laminectomy at the lumbosacral junction to identify the dural sac and extend the laminectomy laterally to identify and follow the S-1 and S-2 nerve roots to their exit foramina anteriorly. The dura below S-2 is transected and the osteotomy level chosen to include a normal vertebra above the level of tumor involvement (Fig. 18–19*A* to *C*).

During the sacrectomy, iliac vessels are temporarily occluded and the abdominal surgeon guides the positioning of the osteotomy cuts. The specimen is thus removed en bloc, and hemostasis is secured with bipolar cautery and ligatures around larger arterioles.

To close the defect, soft suction drains are placed in the pelvis and led through stab wounds. In healthy nonirradiated patients, we use a Marlex mesh reconstruction of the sacral defect (Fig. 18–20) to prevent postoperative herniation of the rectum into the subcutaneous tissue, which poses some difficulty in bowel evacuation. In all previously irradiated patients, wound healing is a major problem; we thus recommend the use of a myocutaneous or microvascular free flap reconstruction. Although the gluteus muscle is easily available and can be rotated to cover the defect, it has a high failure rate in the irradiated patient. To perform the plastic closure properly, it may be necessary to have the patient completely prone for adequate muscle mobilization.

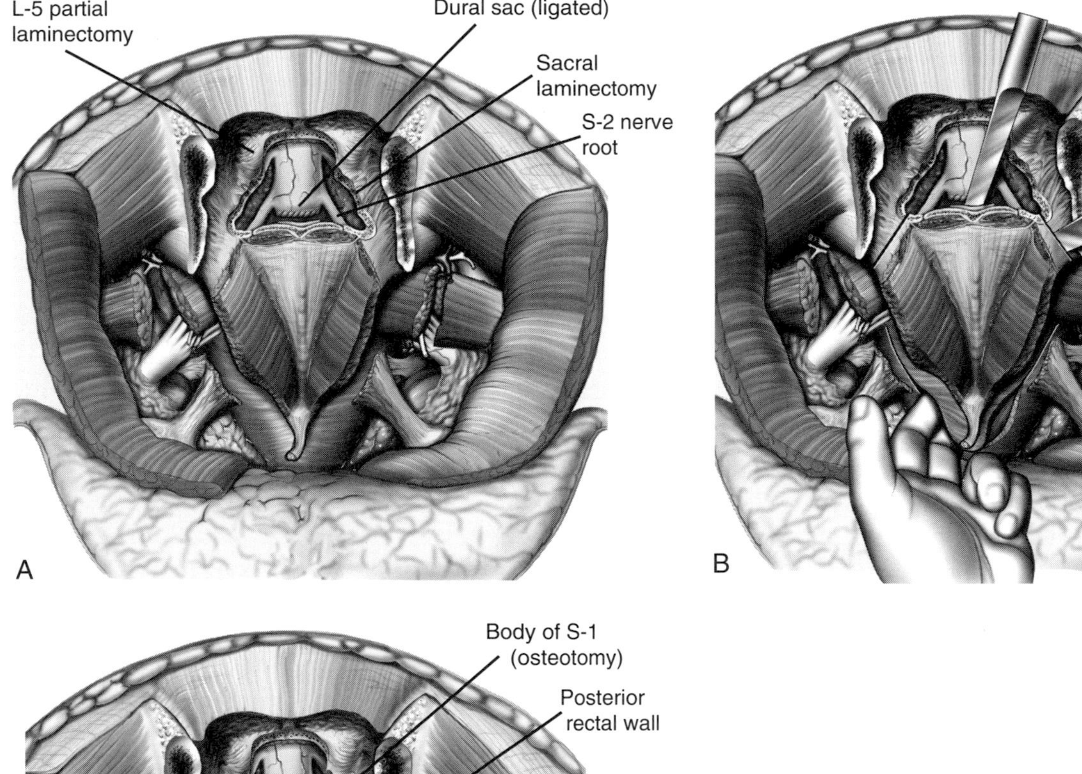

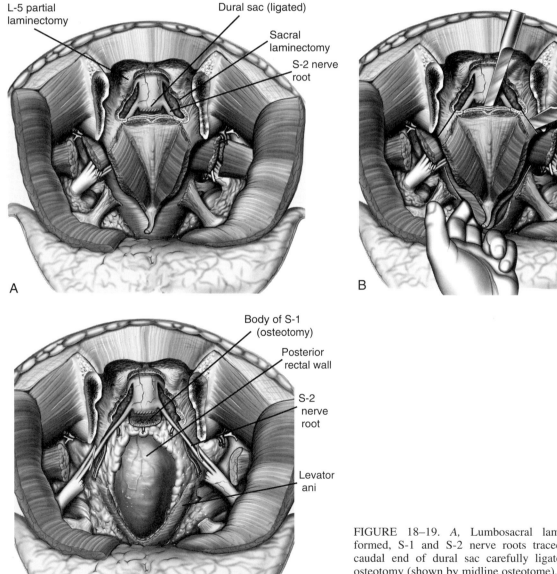

FIGURE 18–19. *A,* Lumbosacral laminectomy performed, S-1 and S-2 nerve roots traced laterally, and caudal end of dural sac carefully ligated. *B,* Prior to osteotomy (shown by midline osteotome), the sacral roots are traced laterally. *C,* Completed sacral resection with bilateral preservation of both S-2 roots.

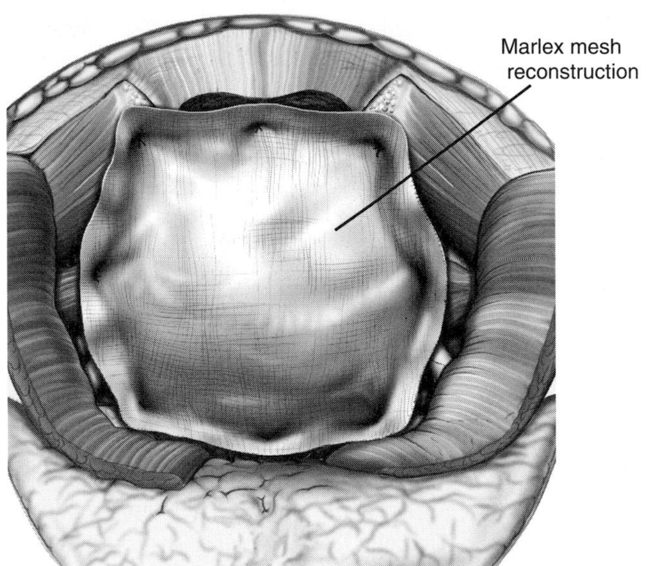

FIGURE 18–20. Following resection, reconstruction of the defect is carried out with Marlex mesh prosthesis.

High Sacral Amputation and Total Sacrectomy

For tumors extending into the first sacral segment, several options are available. If the goal of operation is cure, an en bloc resection must be performed.[12] This is true of chordomas, which involve the first sacral segment and extend superiorly into the soft tissues by lifting the periosteum of the sacrum and presacral fascia. The canal of S-1 runs obliquely forward and in an anteroinferior direction and then exits between the S-1 and S-2 segments. A sacral laminectomy and careful identification of the dura and S-1 nerve roots are mandatory unless the tumor extends to this level. If the tumor extends laterally into the ala, a portion of the posterior iliac crests should be removed because they overlie the first sacral segment. In addition, tumors extending anteriorly involve the piriformis muscle and may extend outside the pelvis by protruding through the greater sciatic notch.

The functional effects of sacral resection include loss of bladder function, since the urinary bladder and urethral sphincters become denervated. If the S-2 nerves are sectioned bilaterally, sexual (erection) and bowel function as well as bladder function will be lost. It is therefore important to preserve the S-2 nerve roots whenever possible by tracing them out to their exit foramina (Fig. 18–21). Lacking any detrusor function, patients will have to depend on the abdominal muscles and manual pressure to void. In general, abdominal pressure maneuvers may result in reflux backward and hydronephrosis. By far the preferred method is the technique of intermittent self-catheterization. Loss of genital function results in loss of sensation of the external genitalia and vagina. Penile erection is possible, but ejaculation will be weak. Loss of anorectal function results in incontinence but can be controlled with a constipating diet and manual digital evacuation. The patient will have no control over flatus or intermittent episodes of incontinence and should be instructed to wear a diaper.

For the anterior operation, the patient is positioned in the lithotomy position with the legs in stirrups, and the anus is closed by a pursestring suture. For the posterior

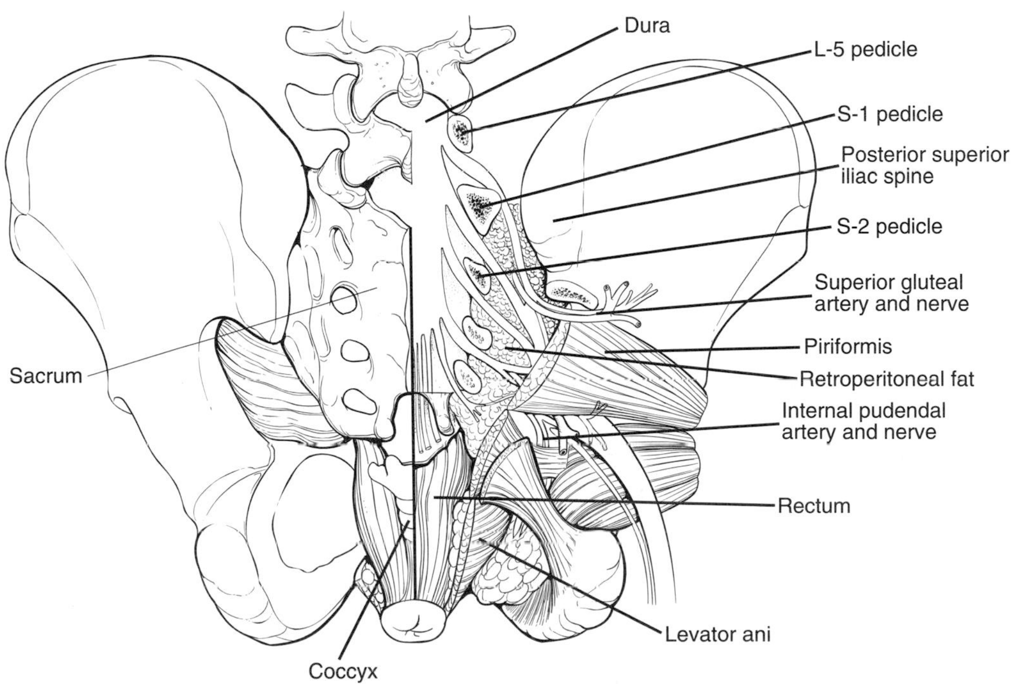

FIGURE 18–21. Roots of lower lumbosacral plexus, carrying innervation to the pelvic organs. If possible, both S-2 roots should be preserved.

phase, the patient is positioned prone on a radiographic table, especially if stabilization is indicated.

The anterior exposure can be performed completely extraperitoneally by using a low semicircular incision. The tendon of the rectus abdominis muscle is severed bilaterally about 1 cm above the pubis. The anterior parietal peritoneum is retracted medially on both sides, and the dissection should meet in the midline over the sacral promontory. If the procedure requires resection of the rectum, the abdomen should be opened and the bowel resection performed at this stage.

The internal iliac vessels are divided separately and the cut ends secured by suture ligatures. The lateral and median sacral arteries and veins are ligated and divided. The periosteum over the sacral promontory is stripped down to the level of the sacral osteotomy, which requires division of the sympathetic nerve trunk. On either side, the lumbosacral nerve trunk (L4-5) passing anterior to the sacral wing and sacroiliac joint is released so that it can be protected during the sacral resection. An osteotomy is made through the sacrum and through the sacroiliac joint. The anterior wound is closed and the patient then turned prone.

The posterior incision is generally an elliptic one or may be midline for benign tumors. Any biopsy scar should be excised. The superior aspect of the incision should include the posterior elements of the L-5 vertebra. After the flap is raised, the gluteus maximus is stripped off the iliac crests and cut lateral to the sacral edges. Both the superior and the inferior gluteal arteries and veins are isolated and ligated, but an effort must be made to preserve the superior gluteal nerve, which innervates the gluteus medius and minimus and the tensor fascia lata. At the lumbosacral level, the sacrospinalis muscles are sectioned transversely, and a partial laminectomy of L-5 is performed. The sacrum is unroofed as far distally as the first posterior sacral foramina. In addition, using Kerrison rongeurs, the S-1 and S-2 nerve roots are traced laterally and the dural sac is ligated.

Once the dural sac has been ligated and transected, the actual amputation of the sacrum can be performed. The osteotomy is outlined by using a finger passed anteriorly to identify the previously marked anterior cuts on the sacrum. The sacral nerves, excluding the first and second, may have to be transected to be included in the specimen. Once the transection of bone has been completed, and all sacral contributions to the sciatic nerve have been severed, the specimen can be removed. Closure of the flaps with drainage is then performed.

Stabilization

After high sacral resections, or total sacrectomy, surgical stabilization is indicated. The most widely applicable technique is the Galveston technique: rods or screws are placed into the ilium under fluoroscopic control and hooked in tandem to pedicle screws inserted in the lumbar spine. Both prebent Luque rods and iliac screws with the Isola system (Fig. 18–22*A* and *B*) are equally effective in maintaining lumbopelvic stability.[27] In addition, stabilization by screw fixation to the sacrum is often required after surgery of lumbosacral tumors.[27–30] To prevent rotational stresses, both iliac bones must be compressed together by the use of compression rods or plates between the iliac wings.[31] After complete sacrectomy for benign tumors, anterior reconstruction using bone grafts between the ilium and the lumbar vertebra is indicated in conjunction with posterior lumbosacral instrumentation.

Postoperative Morbidity and Results

In the past, curative resections were often not possible for chordomas because of their large size and extension to the first sacral segment at the time of initial presentation. In addition, many patients with sacral chordomas are elderly and may have significant comorbid factors that may preclude curative resection. Although radiotherapy has been widely used to attempt local control after subtotal resection, we do not believe that radiation should be used as a substitute for adequate operation. Most locally aggressive tumors, including giant cell tumors, chordomas, and sarcomas, respond poorly to conventional radiation, and the use of radiation has been implicated in the malignant transformation of these relatively indolent tumors. Other treatment modalities include cryosurgery, in which liquid nitrogen is used for palliative treatment of unresectable tumors.[32] Unfortunately, skin necrosis, poor healing, and potential fractures and neural damage are the limiting factors to effective cryosurgery of sacral tumors.

A major potential cause of morbidity is the extensive blood loss from sacral resections. During operation, blood loss may range from 5000 to 10,000 ml for large tumors. The only death in our series resulted from intraoperative hypotension and myocardial infarction in a patient with unsuspected coronary disease. It is therefore mandatory to work with experienced teams that can manage sudden blood loss and replacement, which is often required in these procedures. The mortality rate from sacral resection ranges from 5% to 15% and is dependent on age, comorbid factors, and type of tumor. Irradiated cancer patients have the highest morbidity.

Urinary retention and urosepsis are common, especially in older men. In some patients, prophylactic transurethral resection should be considered. The majority of patients have saddle anesthesia and describe deafferentation pain, which requires appropriate medications. Rehabilitation is begun as soon as possible, since extensive sacral resections often result in considerable loss of muscle mass.

In virtually all patients seromas develop because of the large posterior flaps used. Between 25% and 40% of irradiated patients may have wound dehiscence, requiring additional plastic closure. To avoid this, we recommend that closure be performed by an experienced plastic surgery team.

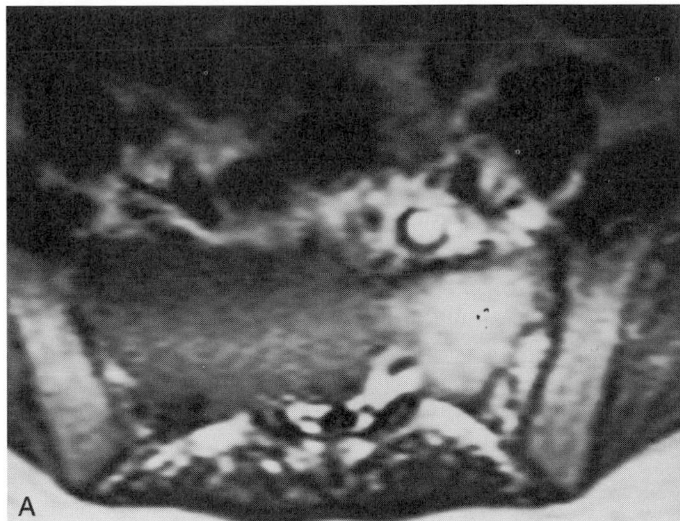

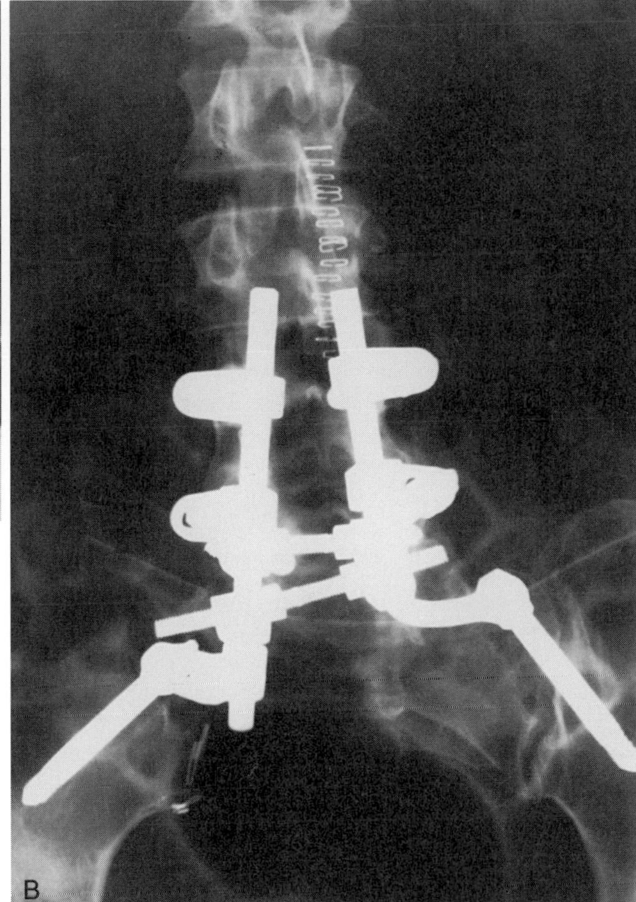

FIGURE 18–22. *A,* Sacral osteosarcoma. Axial T1-weighted MR image shows infiltrative lesion on the right side, extending about 2 cm across the midline. *B,* Postoperative anteroposterior radiograph of the lumbosacral spine. Stabilization using prebent Luque rods affixed to lumbar segments with Isola pedicle screws and to the pelvis with iliac screws (Galveston technique).

Although the morbidity following surgery is considerable, especially in the cancer patient, long-term palliation in a small subset of patients can be achieved. While the overall median survival in recurrent cancer patients ranges from 12 to 16 months, approximately 15% to 25% of patients with localized invasive cancers are effectively palliated for 3 to 5 years.[7, 9, 13, 14] Since the results of failed therapy include intractable pain from sacral plexopathy along with bladder and bowel dysfunction, surgery for both long-term palliation as well as short-term improvement of pain is indicated.

The major experience with radical extended operations has been reported from several different centers.[7, 8, 10, 14] In Wanebo and colleagues' series of 24 patients,[14] half underwent complete pelvic exenteration. There were three postoperative deaths, and five patients were alive in excess of 4 years. Pearlman and associates reported the results of 21 patients with recurrent rectal cancer; all but 3 had prior radiation. Of the 16 patients who had potentially curative surgery, 8 were free of recurrence with follow-up of 6 to 48 months. Excellent local control of tumor and pain relief were obtained in the majority of patients.

In patients with low-grade malignant tumors, both local control and long-term disease-free results are gratifying. We are currently able to control local tumor in more than 80% of patients with chordoma and other low-grade malignant tumors with surgery alone, without the need for radiation. Even in patients with local recurrences following attempted curative resection, surgery remains an important therapeutic option.

References

1. Cody H, Marcove R, Quan S: Malignant retrorectal tumors: 28 Years experience at Memorial Sloan-Kettering Cancer Institute. Dis Colon Rectum 24:501–506, 1981.
2. Feldenzer J, McCauley J, McGillicuddy J: Sacral and presacral tumors: Problems in diagnosis and management. Neurosurgery 25:884–891, 1989.
3. Sundaresan N, Schmidek H, Schiller A, Rosenthal D: Tumors of the Spine: Diagnosis and Clinical Management. Philadelphia: WB Saunders, 1990.
4. Goldman A, Gluckert K, Exner G: Treatment of tumors of the sacrum. Z Orthop 127:404–409, 1989.
5. Sung H, Hsu W, Wang H, et al: Surgical treatment of primary tumors of the sacrum. Clin Orthop 215:91–98, 1987.
6. Xu W, Song X, Yue S, Cai Y, Wu J: Primary sacral tumors and their surgical treatment. A report of 87 cases. Chin Med J 103:879–884, 1990.
7. Pearlman N, Donohue R, Stiegmann G, et al: Pelvic and sacropelvic exenteration for locally advanced or recurrent anorectal cancer. Arch Surg 122:537–541, 1987.
8. Sugarbaker P: Partial sacrectomy for en bloc excision of rectal cancer with posterior fixation. Dis Colon Rectum 25:708–711, 1987.
9. Takagi H, Morimoto T, Hara S, Suzuki R, Horio S: Seven cases of

pelvic extension combined with sacral resection for locally recurrent rectal cancer. J Surg Oncol 32:184–188, 1986.
10. Temple W, Ketcham A: Sacral resection for control of pelvic tumors. Am J Surg 163:370–374, 1992.
11. Touran T, Frost D, O'Connell T: Sacral resection. Operative technique and outcome. Arch Surg 125:911–913, 1990.
12. Stener B, Gunterberg B: High amputation of sacrum for extirpation of tumors: Principles and technique. Spine 3:351–356, 1978.
13. Brunschwig A, Daniel W: Pelvic exenteration operations: With summary of sixty six cases surviving more than 5 years. Ann Surg 151:571–576, 1960.
14. Wanebo H, Whitehill R, Gaker D, et al: Composite pelvic resection. Arch Surg 122:1401–1406, 1987.
15. Gunterberg B, Romanus B, Stener B: Pelvic strength after major amputation of the sacrum. Acta Orthop Scand 47:635–642, 1976.
16. Sundaresan N, Galicich J, Chu F, Huvos A: Spinal chordomas. J Neurosurg 50:312–319, 1979.
17. Sundaresan N, Huvos A, Krol G, Brennan M: Spinal chordoma: Results of surgical treatment. Arch Surg 122:1478–1482, 1987.
18. Wetzel L, Levine E: MR imaging of sacral and presacral lesions. Am J Roentgenol 154:771–775, 1990.
19. Walaas L, Kindblom L: Fine-needle aspiration biopsy in the preoperative diagnosis of chordoma: A study of 17 cases with application of electron microscopic, histochemical, and immunocytochemical examination. Human Pathol 22:22–28, 1991.
20. Krol G, Sundaresan N, Deck M: Computed tomography of axial chordomas. J Comput Assist Tomogr 7:286–298, 1983.
21. Kraske P, Perry E, Hinrichs B: Extirpation Hochsitzender Mastdarmkrebse. Aust NZ J Surg 59:421–424, 1989.
22. MacCarty C, Waugh J, Mayo C, Coventry M: The surgical treatment of presacral tumors: A combined problem. Proc Staff Meet Mayo Clinic 27:73–84, 1952.
23. Karakousis C: Sacral resection with preservation of continence. Surg Gynecol Obstet 163:270–273, 1980.
24. Huth J, Dawson E, Eilber F: Abdominosacral resection for malignant tumors of the sacrum. Am J Surg 148:157–161, 1984.
25. Localio S, Francis K, Rossano P: Abdomino-sacral resection of sacrococcygeal chordomas. Ann Surg 166:394–402, 1967.
26. Localio S, Eng K, Ranson J: Abdominosacral approach for retrorectal tumors. Ann Surg 91:555–560, 1980.
27. Allen B Jr, Ferguson R: The Galveston technique of pelvic fixation with L rod instrumentation of the spine. Spine 9:388–394, 1984.
28. Carlson G, Abitbol J, Anderson D, et al: Screw fixation in the human sacrum: An in vitro study of the biomechanics of fixation. Spine 17:196–203, 1992.
29. McCarthy R, Dunn E, McCullough F: Luque fixation to the sacral ala using the Dunn-McCarthy Modification. Spine 14:281–283, 1989.
30. Mirkovic S, Abitbol J, Steinmann J: Anatomic considerations for sacral screw placement. Spine 16:289–294, 1991.
31. Tomita K, Tsuchiya H: Total sacrectomy and reconstruction for huge sacral tumors. Spine 15:1223–1227, 1990.
32. Vries de J, Oldhoff J, Hadeless H: Cryosurgical treatment of sacrococcygeal chordoma. Report of four cases. Cancer 50:2340–2354, 1986.

Index

Note: Page numbers in *italics* refer to illustrations; page numbers followed by (t) refer to tables.

ISBN 0-7216-5173-9